Clinical Diagnostic Ultrasound

Clinical Diagnostic Ultrasound

Second Edition

EDITED BY

Grant M. Baxter
FRCR
Consultant Radiologist, Department of Radiology
Western Infirmary, Glasgow

Paul L.P. Allan
MB, BS, BSc, FRCP, FRCR, DMRD
Honorary Consultant Radiologist, Department of Radiology
Royal Infirmary, Edinburgh

Patricia Morley
MB, BS, FRCP, FRCR, DMRD
Consultant Radiologist (retired), Department of Radiology
Western Infirmary, Glasgow

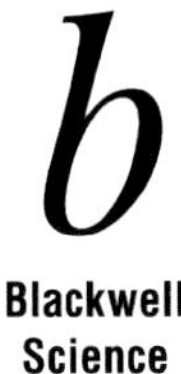

Blackwell
Science

Editorial Offices:
Osney Mead, Oxford OX2 0EL
25 John Street, London WC1N 2BL
23 Ainslie Place, Edinburgh EH3 6AJ
350 Main Street, Malden
MA 02148 5018, USA
54 University Street, Carlton
Victoria 3053, Australia
10, rue Casimir Delavigne
75006 Paris, France

Other Editorial Offices:
Blackwell Wissenschafts-Verlag GmbH
Kurfürstendamm 57
10707 Berlin, Germany

Blackwell Science KK
MG Kodenmacho Building
7–10 Kodenmacho Nihombashi
Chuo-ku, Tokyo 104, Japan

First published 1986
Second edition 1999

Set by Excel Typesetters Co., Hong Kong
Printed and Bound in Great Britain
at the Alden Press, Oxford and
Northampton
Bound by MPG Books Ltd, Bodmin,
Cornwall

A catalogue record for this title
is available from the British Library

ISBN 0-632-03744-X
Library of Congress
Cataloging-in-publication Data

Clinical diagnostic ultrasound / edited by
Grant M. Baxter, Paul L.P. Allan,
Patricia Morley.—2nd ed.
p. cm.
Includes bibliographical references
and index.
ISBN 0-632-03744-X
1. Diagnosis, Ultrasonic. I. Baxter,
Grant M. II. Allan, Paul L.P.
III. Morley, Patricia.
[DNLM: 1. Ultrasonography. WB
289 C641 1998]
RC78.7.U4C574 1998
616.07'543—dc21
DNLM/DLC
for Library of Congress 98-25578
CIP

For further information on
Blackwell Science, visit our website:
www.blackwell-science.com

DISTRIBUTORS
Marston Book Services Ltd
PO Box 269
Abingdon, Oxon OX14 4YN
(*Orders*: Tel: 01235 465500
Fax: 01235 465555)

USA
Blackwell Science, Inc.
Commerce Place
350 Main Street
Malden, MA 02148 5018
(*Orders*: Tel: 800 759 6102
781 388 8250
Fax: 781 388 8255)

Canada
Login Brothers Book Company
324 Saulteaux Crescent
Winnipeg, Manitoba R3J 3T2
(*Orders*: Tel: 204 837-2987)

Australia
Blackwell Science Pty Ltd
54 University Street
Carlton, Victoria 3053
(*Orders*: Tel: 3 9347 0300
Fax: 3 9347 5001)

Contents

List of contributors

P.L.P. Allan
Consultant Radiologist, Department of Radiology, Royal Infirmary, Lauriston Place, Edinburgh EH3 9YW, UK

C.I. Bartram
Consultant Radiologist, Intestinal Imaging Centre, St Mark's Hospital, Northwick Park, Watford Road, Harrow HA1 3UJ, UK

G.M. Baxter
Consultant Radiologist, Department of Radiology, Western Infirmary, Dumbarton Road, Glasgow G11 6NT, UK

N. Bom
Director, Department of Biomedical Engineering, Thorax Centre, Erasmus University Rotterdam, Dr Molewaterplein 50, 3015 GE Rotterdam, The Netherlands

K.M. Carroll
Consultant Radiologist, Department of Radiology, Queen Elizabeth Hospital, Edgbaston, Birmingham B15 2TH, UK

D.O. Cosgrove
Professor, Department of Radiology, Hammersmith Hospital, Du Cane Road, London W12 0HS, UK

A. Deaner
Consultant Cardiologist, Department of Cardiology, King George Hospital, Barley Lane, Goodmayes, Ilford, Essex IG3 8XJ, UK

K.C. Dewbury
Consultant Radiologist, Department of Radiology, Southampton General Hospital, Tremona Road, Southampton SO9 4XY, UK

C. di Mario
Associate Director, Catheterization Laboratories, Columbus Clinic and San Raffaele Hospital, Via Michelangelo Buonaroti 48, 20145 Milan, Italy

T.J. Edwards
Cardiology Registrar, Department of Cardiology, General Hospital, Tremona Road, Southampton SP9 4XY, UK

P. Farrant
Superintendent Research Sonographer, Department of Radiology, King's College Hospital, Denmark Hill, London SE5 9RS, UK

P.J. Fish
Reader, School of Electronic Engineering, University of Wales, Bangor LL57 1UT, UK

J.E.E. Fleming
Honorary Research Associate, Department of Obstetrics and Gynaecology, University of Glasgow, The Queen Mother's Hospital, Yorkhill, Glasgow G3 8SJ, UK

S. Gorman
Physicist, Department of Medical Physics and Bioengineering, University of Wales College of Medicine, Heath Park, Cardiff CF4 4XW, UK

K.P. Hanretty
Consultant, The Queen Mother's Hospital, Yorkhill, Glasgow G3 8SJ, UK

A.S. Hollman
Consultant Paediatric Radiologist, Department of Radiology, Royal Hospital for Sick Children, Yorkhill, Glasgow G3 8SJ, UK

P.R. Hoskins
Principal Physicist, Department of Medical Physics and Medical Engineering, Royal Infirmary and University of Edinburgh, Edinburgh EH3 9YW, UK

A. Houston
Consultant Paediatric Cardiologist, Department of Cardiology, Royal Hospital for Sick Children, Yorkhill, Glasgow G3 8SJ, UK

H.C. Irving
Consultant Radiologist, Department of Radiology, St James's University Hospital, Leeds LS9 7TF, UK

P.R. John
Consultant Paediatric Radiologist, Radiology Department, Birmingham Children's Hospital, Steelhouse Lane, Birmingham B4 6NH, UK

W. Li
Senior Lecturer, Department of Biomedical Engineering, Thorax Centre, Erasmus University Rotterdam and Interuniversity Cardiology Institute of The Netherlands, Rotterdam 3015 GE, The Netherlands

S. Lilley
Ultrasound Manager, Department of Cardiology, Royal Hospital for Sick Children, Yorkhill, Glasgow G3 8SJ, UK

L.M. Macara
Consultant, The Queen Mother's Hospital, Yorkhill, Glasgow G3 8SJ, UK

W.N. McDicken
Professor, Department of Medical Physics and Medical Engineering, University of Edinburgh, Edinburgh EH3 9YW, UK

T. McDonagh
Lecturer, Department of Cardiology, Western Infirmary, Dumbarton Road, Glasgow G11 6NT, UK

J.R. MacKenzie
Consultant Radiologist, Glasgow Royal Maternity Hospital, Rottenrow, Glasgow G4 0NA, UK

N.C. McMillan
Consultant Radiologist, Department of Radiology, Western Infirmary, Dumbarton Road, Glasgow G11 6NT, UK

E.G. McNally
Consultant Musculoskeletal Radiologist, Department of Radiology, Nuffield Orthopaedic Centre, Windmill Road, Oxford OX3 7LD, UK

A.M. Mathers
Consultant Obstetritian, Glasgow Royal Maternity Hospital, Rottenrow, Glasgow G4 0NA, UK

H. Meire
Consultant Radiologist, Department of Radiology, Kings College Hospital, Denmark Hill, London SE5 9RS, UK

C.M. Moran
Research Associate, Department of Medical Physics and Medical Engineering, University of Edinburgh, Edinburgh EH3 9YW, UK

P. Morley
Consultant Radiologist (retired), Department of Radiology, Western Infirmary, Dumbarton Road, Glasgow G11 6NT, UK

S.A. Moussa
Consultant Radiologist, Department of Radiology, Western General Hospital, Crewe Road, Edinburgh EH4 2XU, UK

D.A. Nicholson
Consultant Gastrointestinal Radiologist, Department of Radiology, Hope Hospital, Stott Lane, Salford, Manchester M6 8HD, UK

M. Nicolson
Senior Lecturer, Wellcome Unit for the History of Medicine, University Gardens, University of Glasgow, Glasgow G12 8QQ, UK

N. Pugh
Principal Physicist, Department of Physics and Bioengineering, University of Wales College of Medicine, Heath Park, Cardiff CF4 4XW, UK

S.D. Pye
Principal Physicist, Department of Medical Physics and Medical Engineering, Western General Hospital and University of Edinburgh, Crewe Road, Edinburgh EH4 2XU, UK

J.C. Rodger
Consultant Physician, Department of Medicine, Monklands District General Hospital, Airdrie, Lanarkshire ML6 6NT, UK

R.S.C. Rodger
Department of Renal Medicine, Western Infirmary, Dumbarton Road, Glasgow G11 6NT, UK

C.A. Roobottom
Consultant Cardiovascular Radiologist, Department of Radiology, Derriford Hospital, Derriford Road, Plymouth PL6 8DH, UK

P.S. Sidhu
Consultant Radiologist, Department of Radiology, Kings College Hospital, Denmark Hill, London SE5 9RS, UK

I.A. Simpson
Consultant Cardiologist, Department of Cardiology, General Hospital, Tremona Road, Southampton SO9 4XY, UK

I.H. Spencer
Lecturer, School of Nursing and Midwifery, The Queen's University of Belfast, College Park East, Belfast BT7 1LQ, UK

G.R. Sutherland
Consultant Cardiologist, Department of Cardiology, Western General Hospital, Crewe Road, Edinburgh EH4 2XU, UK

A.F.W. van der Steen
Thorax Centre, Erasmus University Rotterdam and Interuniversity Cardiology Institute of The Netherlands, Rotterdam 3015 GE, The Netherlands

J.M. Wardlaw
Reader, Department of Clinical Neurosciences, Western General Hospital and University of Edinburgh, Crewe Road, Edinburgh EH4 2XU, UK

J. Weir
Professor, Department of Radiology, Aberdeen Royal Infirmary, Foresterhill, Aberdeen AB25 2ZN, UK

P.N.T. Wells
Chief Physicist and Honorary Professor, Department of Medical Physics and Bioengineering, Bristol General Hospital, Bristol BS1 6SY, UK

P. Wilde
Consultant Cardiac Radiologist, Department of Radiology, Bristol Royal Infirmary, Malborough Street, Bristol BS2 8HW, UK

J.P. Woodcock
Professor, Department of Medical Physics and Bioengineering, University of Wales College of Medicine, Heath Park, Cardiff CF4 4XW, UK

Foreword

It is a pleasure and privilege to have been invited to write a foreword to this book with which I was associated as co-editor of the first edition, 13 years ago. In the rapidly developing and expanding field of diagnostic ultrasound such a long interval has rendered much of the original text incomplete, if not obsolete. Therefore, for all practical purposes, the second edition is a completely new textbook and not merely an update of the previous edition.

The original aim of the book has been preserved, namely to provide an up to date comprehensive text covering all aspects of diagnostic ultrasound likely to be encountered in clinical practice. Each chapter has been completely re-written with refreshing additional contributions from many new authors, all widely recognized as experts in their fields. The reader can, therefore, accept that the information given is authoritative and represents the present state of the art.

The usual format of an introductory section on physics and instrumentation has been continued, although it is now more extensive than in the first edition, and will provide a valuable source of reference.

Echocardiology is now much more widely practised by general radiologists, in addition to cardiologists. Therefore this major section of over 100 pages is timely, particularly with regard to the practical application of Doppler flow scanning and the introduction of transoesophageal echocardiography which have become standard procedures. A small but significant contribution on paediatric cardiology has been included.

The vascular section is one of the largest. It has been completely transformed and expanded, and incorporates new work on the carotids and peripheral arterial and venous applications of diagnostic ultrasound. An introduction to intravascular ultrasound is included. The practical and authoritative text contained in this section will be welcomed in view of the rapid development of a vascular ultrasound service in many general radiological departments, replacing standard radiological procedures.

As would be expected, ultrasound of the abdomen and pelvis, including the liver, biliary system, pancreas and urinary tract, is a major part of the book. The text is enhanced by new contributions on transplants, lithotripsy and endoscopic ultrasound.

The section on obstetrics is much larger and more comprehensive than in the first edition and reflects the wide practical experience of the authors. Small parts scanning, including the breast, neck, testes and orbits, has been completely updated. The small section on the musculoskeletal system is a new addition.

I consider that this new book will fill the void that exists for an up to date authoritative, but practical and comprehensive, textbook for radiologists and clinicians with a special interest in diagnostic ultrasound, and should prove to be a valuable reference book for consultants generally and radiologists in training. The editors and contributors are to be congratulated on this excellent publication which undoubtedly is an outstanding addition to the literature.

E. Barnett

Preface

The aim of this book is to serve as a 'bench book' for reference and also to assist in both the education and teaching of ultrasound. Whilst some books concentrate on specific areas of ultrasound in great detail, for example musculoskeletal imaging or gynaecological imaging, this book has been aimed as a general reference book suitable for all those who practise ultrasound in the everyday world and for trainees wishing to obtain more knowledge of the subject. We feel that this book will be of value to radiologists and sonographers as well as being a useful adjunct for those involved in sonographic training.

The book has been split into sections, beginning with a brief discussion of the history of ultrasound and followed by the physical principles and instrumentation involved in image production. Specific, focused clinical areas include echocardiology, vascular scanning, small parts scanning, the abdomen and pelvis, obstetrics and paediatrics, concluding with musculoskeletal imaging. Within each section, we have tried to give an up to the minute account of ultrasound; however, in such a dynamic and changing field, this is never always completely achievable but we have tried to cover the practical knowledge required in day-to-day examinations.

The first edition of this book was published many years ago, edited by two well recognized and highly regarded radiologists with specific interests in ultrasound, namely Dr Patricia Morley and Dr Ellis Barnett. Both have made significant contributions in the ultrasound field, promoting Glasgow as one of the major centres in the development of ultrasound as a clinical tool. It is indeed a great honour to be associated with these two highly regarded individuals and to be asked to edit the second edition of this book. Although both have now retired from clinical practice, the initial idea and individual enthusiasm for a second edition was that of Dr Morley herself, whilst Dr Barnett was also very encouraging in this undertaking.

Clearly, such a diverse book with such a wide range of specific specialist areas could not be covered by one or two individuals and therefore we have contributions from a large number of authors, all of whom are well respected in their fields. It has indeed been an enlightening experience to see firsthand exactly what is involved in publishing such a book, and certainly our admiration for the work of all the contributors and section editors has only increased during this undertaking. We very much appreciate their support in the project and thank them for their time and effort. It has been an extremely fruitful and generally enjoyable period of time. All of us who have been closely involved with the book have made new friends and acquaintances during the period of preparation.

One of our main aims was to produce an eclectic array of contributions covering all aspects of ultrasound for the general and sub-specialist radiologist within one volume. We hope we have gone some way to achieving this. We hope that those involved in clinical practice will appreciate the comprehensive nature of this book, and that it will provide them with practical, critical and useful information which they will be able to use throughout their working practice.

Finally, we all wish to thank our families and friends who have supported us during this project over the past few occasionally stressful years. Specifically we would like to thank our wives Nuala and Helen, together with our children, who are now owed some 'quality time' and an opportunity to regain access to their fathers' computers.

GMB
PLA

Acknowledgements

To publish a new integrated textbook covering all areas of ultrasound, one the most rapidly expanding subspecialities within radiology, requires a large amount of effort, enthusiasm and dedication across the board, and such a project would have been impossible without the help, support and encouragement of many of the individuals involved in writing, illustrating, typesetting, designing, proofreading and printing this book. Regretfully, we cannot thank all individually in print. However, we do wish to thank them collectively for their co-operation and help in producing the finished product.

The editors are aware of the time, effort and dedication involved for the contributors to this book and would like to thank them for this. In addition, specific thanks should be given to Dr P.R. Hoskins who acted as section editor for the physics and instrumentation section. Special thanks are also given to Dr D.M. Cowan who reviewed the echocardiology section, and Dr J.R. MacKenzie who reviewed and guided the contributions in the obstetrics section.

We would also like to acknowledge the forbearance of both our families and colleagues during the preparation of this book, and the patient work of Dr Baxter's secretary Mrs R. MacQueen. Last, but not least, both Drs Baxter and Allan would like to acknowledge the contribution of Dr P. Morley, who was not only one of the main editors of the first edition, but was the initiating, organizing and driving force behind this updated second edition.

GMB
PLA

Chapter 1: Medical ultrasound — germination and growth

J.E.E. Fleming, I.H. Spencer & M. Nicolson

The earliest attempts to use ultrasound for medical diagnosis were in the late 1930s by the neurologist K.T. Dussik who tried to make 'hyperphonograms' of the head [1]. By the early 1950s a few more pioneers were beginning to explore other possibilities. The following 20 years transformed ultrasound into a recognized diagnostic method and the next 20 years into a common feature of modern medicine. The current range of applications described in this book are evidence of the apparent foresight of those early pioneers. At the time, however, it was far from clear where experiments with ultrasound would lead, or whether they were even of value. In the 1950s ultrasound could be likened to a tiny plant just unfolding its cotyledons from the soil, a stage at which it was unclear what it would become, let alone that it would develop into a major feature in the diagnostic 'garden'. It is all too easy from the viewpoint of the late 1990s to look at the well-established plant and describe a simple progression from germination to maturity. It is more difficult to imagine the environment of the 1940s, 1950s or even the early 1960s, when just a handful of machines existed, and then to extrapolate a few decades into the future. Particularly the future of the late 1990s when it is estimated that there are about 250000 machines in the world being used to perform nearly 250 million scans per year [2,3] (Fig. 1.1).

Achieving a clear understanding of the growth of a new technique and its effects requires considerable effort. The rewards to be aimed for are the development of an understanding of the medical, social, professional and commercial consequences of this aspect of technology, a reduction of myth and the recognition of the efforts of individuals, organizations and associations. Also it could lead to a better understanding of the conditions in which such germination and growth is possible. To do this requires sources of material, historical collections and archives. Over the last 10–20 years efforts have been made to establish these. In particular the American Institute for Ultrasound in Medicine (AIUM), the British Medical Ultrasound Society (BMUS) and the German Society of Ultrasound in Medicine (DEGUM) have established collections and archives.

Notably in 1988 Professor Barry Goldberg (Fig. 1.2) organized the first History of Medical Ultrasound Symposium (HMUS) in Washington, DC. As a result an archive was established and is now housed at the AIUM. This contains contributions from at least 70 pioneers from more than 15 countries in the form of written and pictorial material and recordings, both audio and video. Additionally, the work and lives of another 50 were described and acknowledged.

In 1995 the Wellcome Unit for the History of Medicine (WUHM), University of Glasgow, commenced a 3-year study of the developments which took place in Glasgow. This work is based on the resources of the BMUS collection and archives. Additional material is being acquired from a series of interviews being conducted by the WUHM with many of the pioneers, and their associates. Work on this large and increasing resource has been undertaken [4–6] and is planned to continue. A chronological listing of events is being assembled and this was used as the basis for the brief list of major events at the end of this chapter (Appendix 1).

The German collection was established in 1995 with the aim of collecting material from the early period of ultrasound with a special interest in the work which took place in the German-speaking countries of central Europe. More details of these collections are given at the end of this chapter (Appendix 2).

Apart from these collections and archives there are historical accounts, some written from personal experience [7–15]. Then there are the scholarly works such as the theses of Coste [2] and Koch [16]. Complementing these is a survey of the mature ultrasound industry by Blackwell [3] which contains factual and projected data for 1994–2000.

When reading of the efforts of the medical ultrasound pioneers between the late 1930s and the late 1960s the stories seem to be dominated by the development of equipment. This is especially evident in the frequency with which pictures of equipment appear. For example, in the Kodak booklet [17] there are 104 pictures, 73 show pieces of equipment, 25 show images and 23 pioneers. The equipment was usually developed from military or industrial instruments. From the military side came the technology of radar, which had developed rapidly during World War II, and in which the basic system is virtually the same as used in medical ultrasound. From industry came ultrasonic flaw detection developed to meet the particular needs of metal fabrication, from high pressure boilers to aircraft structures; ultrasound fulfilled the need for testing without the use of hazardous and time-consuming radiographic methods (B. Donnelly, 1996, interview in the I.H. Spencer, BMUS Collection and Archive).

But radar and flaw detectors did not have an obvious place in medicine. Who made the leap from these existing technologies to medicine? How did it happen? Someone must have planted the seed, or seeds, so that they could germinate. The existence of, in retrospect, such obviously suitable technology alone was insufficient; an initiator was needed.

Exploring the archives shows that in the majority of cases the initiator was a medical doctor. Making this connection between medicine and engineering was remarkable at a time when ultrasound was so little known, when there were few publications on ultrasound, or 'supersonics' as it was known in industry, and easily searched databases and bibliographies [18] were not available. It seems that the burden of a clinical problem prompted the question, can ultrasound help?

The question having been asked the next crucial element was the availability of a physicist or engineer, initially to discuss and advise and later to actively co-operate. To quote Hertz [9] '. . . at every point in this development [echocardiology] the engineering advance had to be carried to a certain stage before the apparatus could be used in medical research. Then the engineer had to wait until the physician had amassed enough experi-

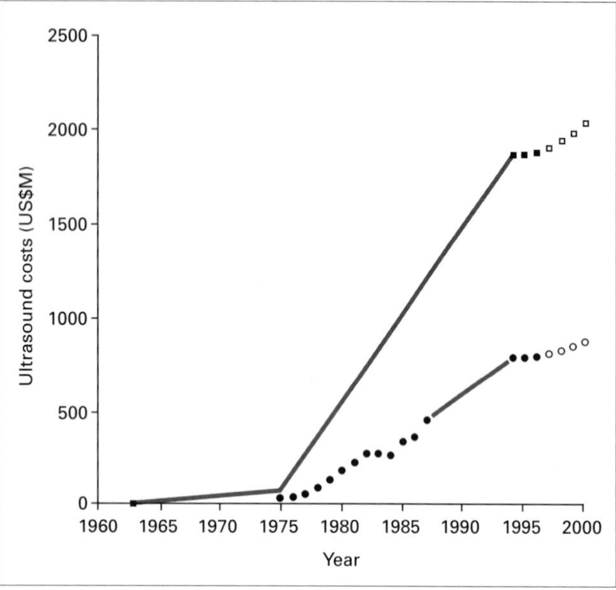

Fig. 1.1 The colossal expansion of the market from 1975 has been called 'the real-time boom'. This chart shows the World (■) and US domestic (●) markets for medical ultrasound in millions of US$. The 1975–87 points are from Coste [2] and for 1994–2000 from Blackwell [3] whose predicted figures are shown as unfilled symbols (World, □; US domestic, ○). The lines represent our interpolations and the 1963 point our estimate of the sales of KH Diasonographs.

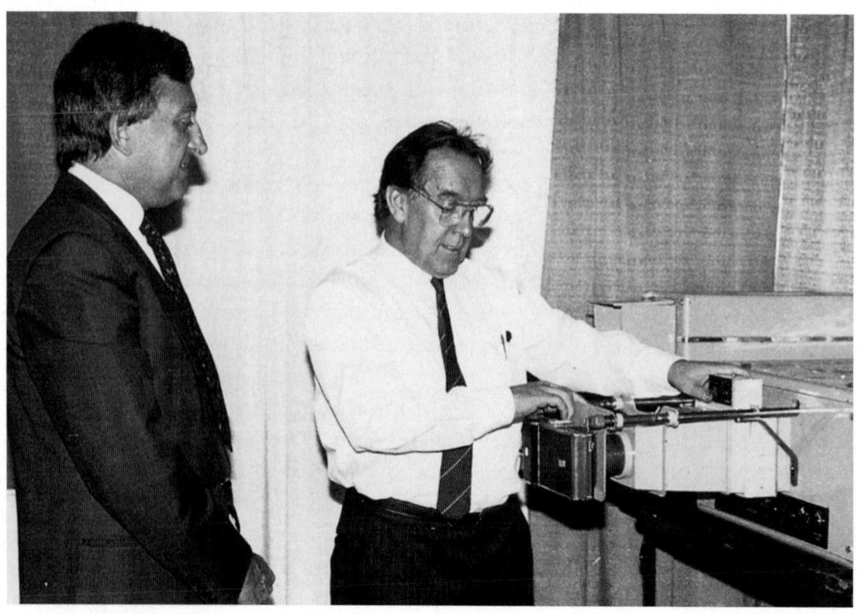

Fig. 1.2 Exhibition at the History of Medical Ultrasound Symposium, Washington, 1988. Professor Barry B. Goldberg (left), Chairman of the Symposium organizing committee with Mr Tom Brown (see text) who is demonstrating the method of recording patient data and an ultrasound image using the Polaroid camera on the machine shown in Fig. 1.6. (Courtesy of the BMUS Historical Collection.)

ence to point out new possible improvements to the engineer'. Today such co-operation would not seem an unusual occurrence, just a normal activity of a department of medical physics. However, it was not always so; in the introduction to Koch's thesis [16] she states that she analysed 'the evolving relationships of one innovator, John Wild, and a medical community which was unaccustomed to dealing with research on machines'. In her conclusions she indicates some of the difficulties and explains the historical importance of the machines by saying of the individuals involved in research on ultrasound '[They] had to reconcile their differences of opinion about how research on ultrasound should be conducted and applied to clinical practice. As a result, the ultrasonic instrument was the crux of the relationship between individuals with very disparate interests, who might otherwise have nothing in common'.

Such relationships would be more likely to be successful if the medical practitioner had an interest in machines and the problems of invention and engineering. This carries with it the acceptance that invention does not work perfectly first time and that modification and adaptation will be needed. Wild is someone with that trait, and Koch described him succinctly and aptly as a 'tinkerer'.

Then there were deterrents to physicists, engineers or technologists moving into biology or medicine. Both may appear fuzzy and slippery subjects compared with the more defined and measurable world of engineering and technology. And the medical research community of the 1950s, at least in America, was not inviting. To quote Koch again [16] '. . . technological knowledge and the activities leading to its development were not valued—or at least were grossly undervalued compared with scientific knowledge . . .'.

Given that clinical medicine and physics had come together advances occurred most readily when the clinical problem related to the heart, the eye or the abdomen of a sick gynaecological patient. These are the regions of the body most amenable to ultrasound imaging. The heart is a well-defined structure of relatively simple form made more apparent by its dynamic nature. The eye being a simple structure, within the resolution of ultrasound, was also suitable and successful although it did present contact problems which required the use of water baths or bags or a steady hand placing the transducer directly onto the closed eyelid.

In retrospect it is clear that it was gynaecological patients, particularly those with large cysts or tumours who provided the most suitable subjects. In these patients the abdomen is almost entirely soft tissue or fluid ultrasonically similar to water. As the spine is positioned posteriorly, and the gas-containing bowel is commonly displaced by the mass, the two principal barriers to ultrasound are avoided. Later when pregnant patients were examined at mid or late term similarly obliging conditions existed. There could of course be fetal bone but being thin, soft and part of an easily recognizable structure this only served to enhance the images. The scale of the structures seen in these two groups of patients were also ideal as they were clearly resolvable even by the low frequency (1.5–2.5 MHz), poor resolution systems of the time. Furthermore, the deformable abdominal surface facilitated contact scanning.

In contrast the most unsuitable region was the head. This, however, in addition to Dussik's work mentioned above, attracted much attention in the early years, reflecting the many associated clinical problems. Unfortunately, in spite of considerable effort clinical value was difficult to establish [12,13]. Then X-ray computed tomography arrived and completely supplanted ultrasound. However, the technology has changed, Doppler and contrast enhancement have brought ultrasound back into the study of the head as evidenced by a recent congress on cerebral haemodynamics [19] in which there were 169 presentations, involving over 400 authors.

The crucial elements—an initiator with a clinical problem, ultrasonically suitable anatomy, co-operation with a physicist or engineer together with sponsorship and support—came together in varying ways in various places and over a number of years to allow 'germination' to occur. These are summarized Table 1.1. Less definable and not shown in the table, but perhaps of equal importance, was the strength of will to engage in the long haul of convincing a very sceptical medical community and of positively promoting this new technology.

As space does not allow inclusion of the stories from all of the centres, the events in Glasgow are taken as an example of ultrasound germination. The initiator was Ian Donald, the distended female abdomen presented the clinical problem, Tom Brown provided engineering insight and Kelvin Hughes (KH) supplied substantial support and facilities.

Ian Donald was born in 1910, a time of great advances in engineering and technology; the Wright brothers were at the height of their powers, Bleriot had recently flown the English Channel and Asdic, or Sonar as it became known, was developing. Ian Donald's sister Dame Allison Munro recalls (interview by I.H. Spencer, 1997 BMUS Collection and Archive) that as a child 'Ian was very good with his hands, boat building and things like that, and this man Hawkhurst, I think he was called, taught him something about electronics. . . . Ian built himself this wireless with a "cat's whisker", it was the first time I ever heard the wireless'. Later as a medical student he developed a device for bladder irrigation. As a registrar he developed a negative pressure ventilator for the newborn, and a spiroscope to

Table 1.1 A selection of initiators of research in ultrasound imaging; their speciality, when and where they began, region of application, initial objective, collaborators (individuals and firms/organizations) and how they came together

Initiator (year work began)	Place of study	Speciality	Part of body	(a) First reason for interest in ultrasound (b) Knowledge of other work	Co-operation Co-worker(s) Firm/organization	How they met and other notes
Dussik, K.T. (1937)	Salzburg, Austria	Neurology	Head	(a) Seeking method of visualizing non-calcified brain tumours (b) Had learnt that ultrasound was used for finding fish and non-destructive testing	Dussik, F. (physics)	Brothers
Denier, A. (1946)	France	Physiotherapy		(a) To produce images of interior body structures (b) –		
Howry, D.H. (1948)	Denver, CO	Radiology	Neck, limbs	(a) Wanted to make a soft tissue 'X-ray' (b) –	Bliss, W.R. (eng) Posakony, G. (eng)	
Wild, J.J. (1949)	Minneapolis, MN	Surgery	Bowel	(a) To detect malignancy in bowel by measurement of bowel wall thickness. 'Wild was trying to demonstrate to other surgeons the difference between obstruction of the bowel and paralysis' (b) From Finn Larsen (Honeywell) designer of radar simulator using ultrasound for US Navy	Neal, D. (eng) Reid, J. (eng) US Navy	
Edler, I. (1953)	Lund, Sweden	Cardiology	Heart	(a) Need for a method of detecting mitral regurgitation. co-operation with Lars Leksell (b) Only learned later of work in USA	Hertz, H. (physics) Siemens	Edler said he sought out Hertz who says they met by chance. The first echocardiogram was recorded October 1953
Donald, I. (1954)	Glasgow, UK	Obstetrics/ gynaecology	Female abdomen	(a) To differentiate between cyst and tumours (b) Donald had heard J.J. Wild talk about ultrasound, Brown said didn't know of Howry's work	Brown, T.G. (eng) MacVicar, J. (obstetrics/ gynaecology) Kelvin Hughes Ltd	As described in text
Leksell, L. (1955)	Lund, Sweden	Neurology	Head	(a) – (b) By co-operation with Edler and Hertz		
Mundt, G.H., Hughes, W.F. (1956)		Physicians	Eye		Smith Kline Precision Inc.	
Kossoff, G. (1959)	Melbourne, Australia	Physics	Obstetrics	(a) Garrett quotes diagnosis of placenta praevia as aim (b) At start did not know of Donald's work in Glasgow	Garrett, W.J. (obstetrics/ gynaecology) Robinson, D.E. (eng.) Comm. Acoustic Labs	
Kratochwil, A. (1964)	Austria	Obstetrics/ gynaecology	Obstetrics/ gynaecology	(a) As alternative to radionuclides for placental localization (b) In head	Kretz, C. (eng) KretzTechnic	

eng, engineering.

aid his studies of neonatal breathing. During World War II, as a member of the medical branch of the Royal Air Force, he became aware of the development of radar. Possibly this awareness was increased to some extent because his sister worked with Robert Watson-Watt the radar pioneer. Later while Reader in Obstetrics at the Hammersmith Hospital, London, Donald heard of the medical possibilities of ultrasound from a lecture by a surgeon, J.J. Wild (Fig. 1.3), who had been experimenting in Minneapolis since 1949 [20]. Initially, Wild had been seeking a means of measuring bowel wall thickness and had contacted Finn Larsen, a physicist, who had designed a radar simulator using 15 MHz pulsed ultrasound. This consisted of a water tank containing a relief map of a land area; this was scanned by an ultrasound transducer which simulated the radar antenna. By the time Donald heard him speak, Wild's interest had moved to using the whole echo pattern to differentiate one tissue from another.

Some time after Wild's lecture Donald was appointed to the Regius Chair of Midwifery at Glasgow University. On his arrival in Glasgow in 1954 Donald had in his own words '. . . a rudimentary knowledge of radar and a continuing childish interest in machines, electronic and otherwise—or what my wife would refer to as my "toys" [7]'; altogether a suitable background for being involved in invention and development. In his clinical practice he was commonly faced with grossly distended female abdomens and the problem of making a differential diagnosis. By chance one of his patients was the wife of a Director of Babcock and Wilcox (now Mitsui Babcock) a major firm in Glasgow's heavy engineering industry. This contact led to a visit to their works on 21 July 1955 with a quantity of cysts and tumours removed during operations that morning. These were 'tested' using the company's ultrasonic flaw detector. As a camera was not available the A-scan traces were sketched by the company artist; Donald related that '. . . these [results] were beyond my wildest dreams and clearly showed the difference between a fibroid and an ovarian cyst'.* The Babcock equipment had been manufactured by KH, also in Glasgow, and through this connection Ian Donald visited Professor Mayneord at the Royal Marsden Hospital, London. Mayneord had been using a KH Mk2 flaw detector (Fig. 1.4) in an attempt to examine the brain through the intact skull, but as was later recognized this presented major difficulties. Thus it is no surprise that Donald formed the view '. . . that they knew a good deal about the subject, enough in fact to be thoroughly discouraged' [7] and that soon after it was agreed that Mayneord's apparatus could be loaned to Donald.

Kelvin Hughes had interests other than ultrasound and were installing an experimental shadowless lamp in Donald's operating theatre in the Western Infirmary in Glasgow (WIG) where one of the KH staff heard that 'The doctor was using a flaw detector on people'. Later he mentioned this to his colleague Tom Brown, a young design engineer, who that evening phoned Professor Donald. He later described this 'as the most fateful telephone call I ever made', but it was the start of a fruitful and exciting period. Brown visited Donald at the WIG and found that

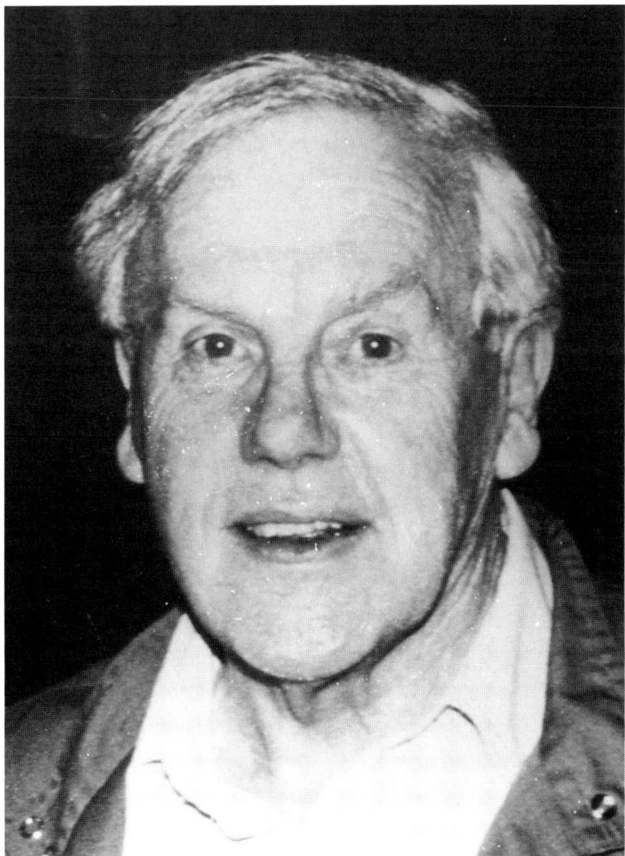

Fig. 1.3 J.J. Wild at the History of Medical Ultrasound Symposium, Washington, 1988. Dr Wild began his ultrasound experiments in 1949.

* As part of the work in the WUHM Ian Donald's first experiments were re-enacted on 19 July 1996. A KH Mk4 flaw detector as used in Babcock and Wilcox in the 1950s was borrowed from Axiom (NDT) Ltd; with only a few minor repairs this still worked after more than 40 years and the difference between 'cysts and tumours' could be distinguished. To avoid ethical problems these were simulated by using animal material: water-filled bladders and samples of muscle tissue (see Fig. 1.19). These were provided by Professor Jack Boyd in whose Department of Veterinary Anatomy, University of Glasgow, the re-enactment was carried out. As many people as possible who had been around at the time of the original experiments were invited [38]. Video recordings were made of the flaw detector traces and of the whole 3 h of activity. Extracts of this were used in a video [39].

the A-scan instrument from Mayneord had, as was common at that time, been designed to use a transducer with separate transmit and receive elements. Unfortunately, it had been inexpertly modified to use a single transducer resulting in paralysis for hundreds of microseconds after the transmit pulse. Donald's solution was to use a large water stand-off device, both clumsy and inconvenient. Brown overcame this by making another phone call, this time to Alec Rankine (interview with I.H. Spencer, 1996, BMUS Collection and Archive). In Brown's words 'Alec never respected formalities' and within days a brand new KH Mark 4 flaw detector (Fig. 1.5) worth £600 in 1956 was on its way from the factory in London to Glasgow.

The echo patterns from cysts, solid masses and normal bowel could be distinguished but Tom Brown realized the limitations of the A-scan as a means of presenting the enormous amount of echo information which was returning from inside the abdomen. He concluded that 'we needed some sort of automatic plotting device' but 'I found it difficult to fire Ian Donald or John MacVicar [Donald's Registrar at the time and later Professor of Obstetrics and Gynaecology in Leicester] with my "dream"; or even make them understand it' (T.G. Brown, 1988, personal communication). Was Donald blinkered by Wild's efforts to use ultrasound to differentiate between tissues? Just at this juncture it was suggested to Donald by physicians at the WIG that he try his apparatus on a woman '. . . supposedly dying with massive ascites due to portal obstruction from a radiologically demonstrated carcinoma of the stomach'. The A-scan showed well-separated echoes and MacVicar observed 'that it seems like a large cyst' [7]. It turned out that the physicians were uncertain of their diagnosis. After transfer to Donald's care, the lady was operated on and made a rapid recovery. This was just what was needed to secure financial support and enabled the KH deputy chairman, Bill Slater, to conjure up £500, later described by Tom Brown as 'a rather elastic sum'. This allowed him to build his 'dream'—the first contact scanner (Fig. 1.6).

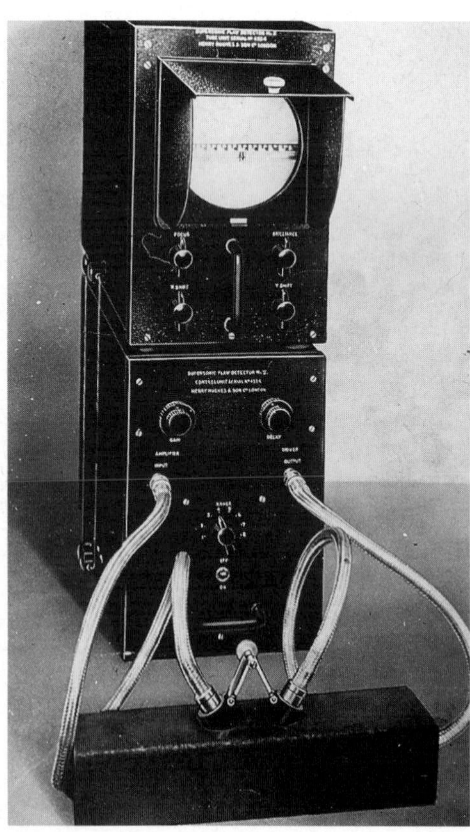

Fig. 1.4 Kelvin Hughes Mk2 flaw detector. This was based on an airborne radar set and was the type of instrument used by Professor Mayneord at the Royal Marsden Hospital, London, and then by Professor Ian Donald in his first experiments. An example of this unit is in the collection of the Science Museum, London.

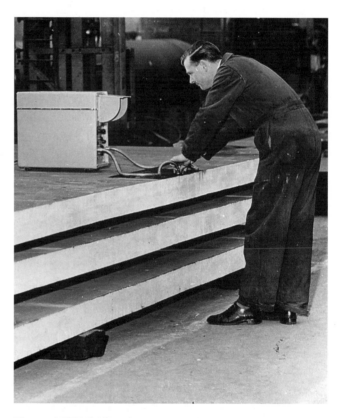

Fig. 1.5 A KH Mk4 flaw detector, *c.* 1956 being using by Mr Jim Davis in the Babcock and Wilcocks factory to test steel plates. Soon after his first meeting with Professor Ian Donald, Tom Brown arranged the loan of an instrument of this type from KH to replace the Mk2 (Fig. 1.4). The Mk4 was used for most of the early A-scan experiments and then became part of the contact B-scan machine in Fig. 1.6.

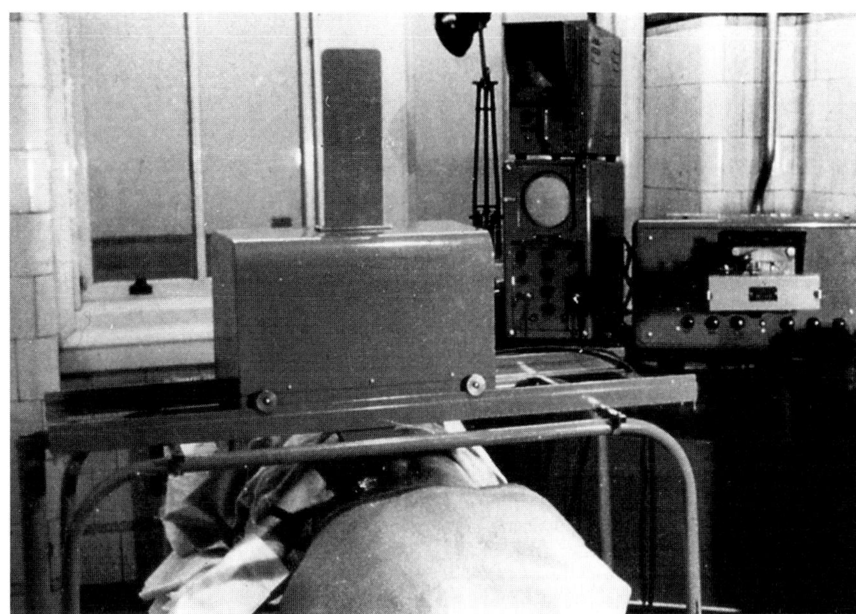

Fig. 1.6 The contact scanner in the Western Infirmary, Glasgow. This manually operated scanner was designed by T.G. Brown, at KH and used by Professor Ian Donald and Dr John MacVicar [22]. See text for more details.

This scanner had a transducer which could be moved freely in one plane while being kept in contact with the patient thus avoiding the use of a water bath, as was thought necessary by other experimenters of the time. To explain this different approach Brown wrote 'I was unaware at the time of Howry's beautiful neck pictures using a water bath. I was aware from my industrial experience, of the reverberation problems. But the most compelling reason was quite unrelated to technical considerations. The patients I was seeing in Donald's gynaecology wards were often elderly, and generally quite unwell, I could not see any technique being well received which involved disturbing these old ladies any more than necessary' (T.G. Brown, 1988, personal communication).

The first recorded image from this scanner was of a massive ovarian cystic carcinoma. At the 1988 Symposium Brown said 'I remember it being made and being rather disappointed by it' [21]. Images from this machine, such as Fig. 1.7, were published in the *Lancet* [22]. This paper was regarded by Ian Donald as his most important. Presumably the *Lancet* was chosen in order to reach a wide audience and promote the concept that pulsed ultrasound could be applied to more than obstetrics and gynaecology.

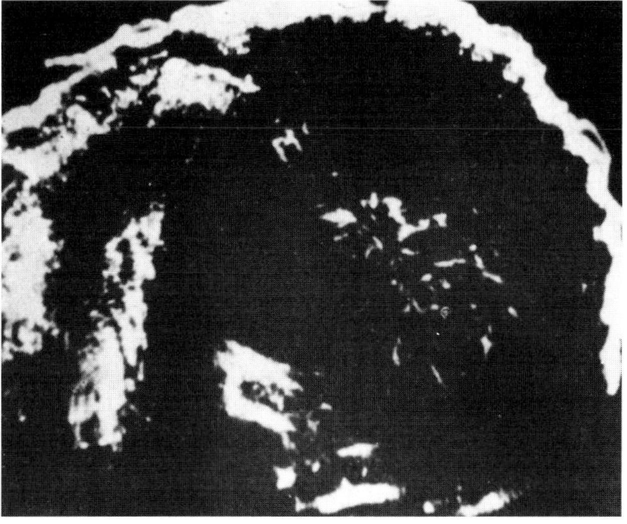

Fig. 1.7 Typical image, *c.* 1957, from contact scanner in Fig. 1.6. This transverse scan was recorded as being of a 'complex ovarian tumour (multilocular pseudomucinous cystadenoma)'. The somewhat irregular hand scanning is seen in the tracing of the almost semicircular abdominal surface.

Brown, however, could see that the prototype was difficult to use and that the pictures were probably influenced by the way in which the operator handled the probe. Howry [23] (Figs 1.8, 1.9) had quite separately expressed similar reservations. However, it was difficult in the prevailing Victorian atmosphere of the 1950s for Brown, an engineer without medical qualification, to take direct control of the scanning. He therefore did so indirectly by designing and building an automatic scanner largely funded by a grant from the National Research and Development Corporation. This monster of a machine (Fig. 1.10) produced thousands of images which are clearly recognizable in publications from Glasgow by the consistent scanning pattern (Fig. 1.11). This sort of devel-

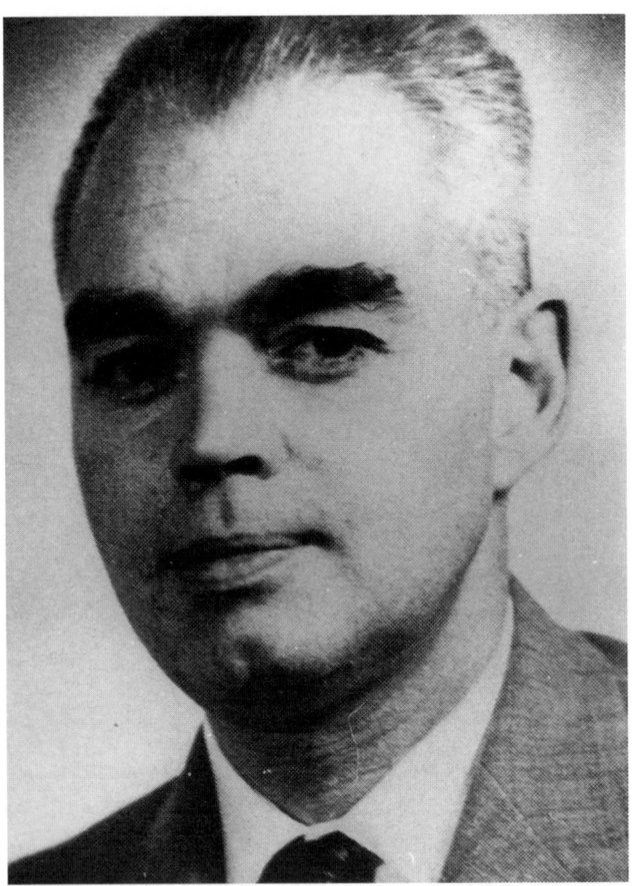

Fig. 1.8 Douglas H. Howry, *c.* 1960. (Courtesy of AIUM Archives.)

opment cost a great deal of money so that the arrival of an obstetrician, Bertil Sunden, with a grant to buy an ultrasound machine must have appeared as a godsend. Following an introduction to A-scan by a neurologist, Lars Leksell, who also worked in Lund, Sweden, Sunden heard of Donald's work in Glasgow. In 1962 a machine was delivered to Sunden (Fig. 1.12). This was based on the original manual contact scanner; experience with the autoscanner having shown that the operator did not unduly affect the images. Sunden's subsequent MD thesis [24] provided independent confirmation of Donald's findings.

Having sold one machine KH, by then known as S. Smith & Sons, saw the prospect of a return on its investment. A development engineer (JEEF) was employed to work on the design of a scanner to go into production. This was in turn based on the Sunden machine and became the first scanner to be built in quantity. Twelve of these 1-ton Diasonographs (Fig. 1.13) were delivered to hospitals in the UK, USA and Iraq. In spite of this success and the large potential market (evident with hindsight) Smith's decided to close the Glasgow factory. Fortunately in 1967, the medical ultrasound interest was purchased by Nuclear Enterprises, Edinburgh, who went on to produce more to the Smith's design. They then took the bold and successful step of redesigning the system, the gantry was improved and the circuits redesigned using semiconductor devices to replace the by then outdated thermionic valves. Over 200 machines of the new design, in various versions—NE4102, NE4200, etc.—were sold before problems arose from the involvement of the parent company, EMI, in the computed tomography market. After complex manoeuvrings three small highly active Scottish companies* have continued in the ultrasound business.

Although there were unique aspects to the Glasgow story, events elsewhere in place and time were broadly similar. Particularly interesting was the earlier development of echocardiography initiated by Inge Edler in a search for a means to detect mitral regurgitation. Cooperation with Hellmuth Hertz and the loan of equipment from Siemens led, in 1953, to the first routine clinical application of diagnostic ultrasound (Fig. 1.14). The details of this development are described both, fully [1] and clearly and concisely [11].

Even as late as 1964 a similar story unfolded in Austria where Alfred Kratochwil was looking for an alternative to radionuclides for placental localization [25]. Hearing of the interest of a neurologist in the use of ultrasound led Kratochwil to borrow an A-scan from Kretztechnic, (Fig. 1.15). The move to two dimensions took place when Kratochwil became aware of the work of Donald *et al.* and persuaded Kretztechnic to build a B-scanner.

Notably different was the work at the Commonwealth Acoustics Laboratory in Australia. At this laboratory an ultrasonics institute was established and George Kossof, a physicist, started work on medical ultrasound (Fig. 1.16). Here to quote his colleague, obstetrician Bill Garrett, 'The difference between the Australian activities and those in North America and continental Europe was, we were physics advised by medicine, whereas almost all the others were medicine advised by physics. And this meant quite a lot in the outcome. For instance when we first started in 1959 we were not aware of Donald's work, . . . [Our] first pictures came out in 1962, clinical pictures, but the important thing was that we had superb images, better than those from people who used modified flaw detectors' [26]. Even though the work was initiated by a physicist it has to be noted that Garrett stated that their prime objective had been placental localization as the

* BCF Technology, 8 Brewster Square, Brucefield Industrial Park, Livingston, W. Lothian EH54 9BJ, UK. Diagnostic Sonar Ltd, Kirkton Campus, Livingston, W. Lothian EH54 7BX, UK. Dynamic Imaging Ltd, 9 Cochrane Square, Brucefield Industrial Park, Livingston, W. Lothian EH54 9DR, UK.

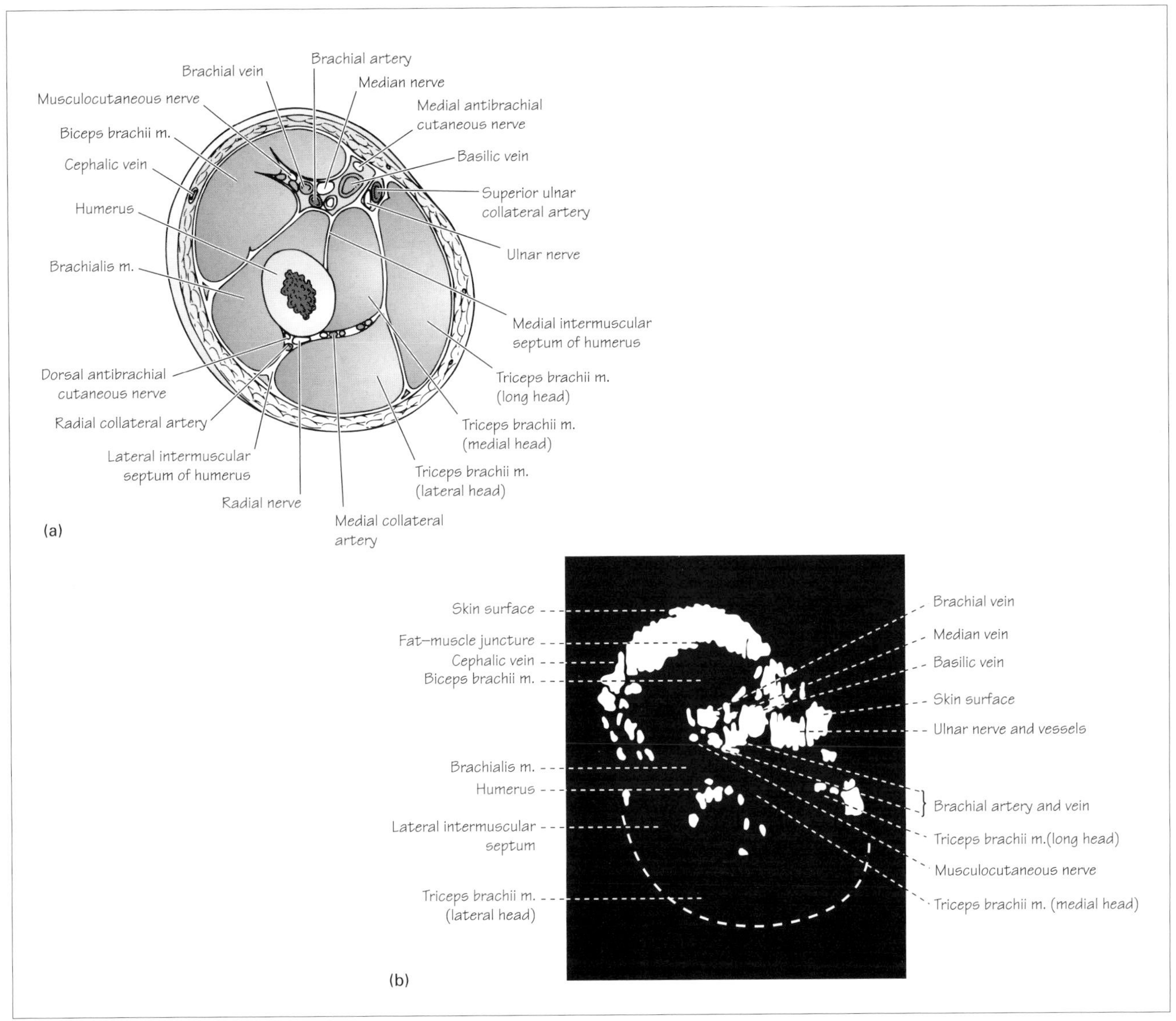

Fig. 1.9 An image from Howry's Somascope [40]. (a) Cross-section and (b) somagram through the mid-third of the right arm. (Courtesy of AIUM Archives.)

available methods of the time 'were very poor'. Their pictures particularly of fetal anatomy were truly remarkable (Fig. 1.17) and a clear demonstration of the importance of grey scale. This led to a rejection of storage tubes, both the bistable type, which showed only black and white, and the variable persistence ones which produced very few grey tones between black and white.

The combined momentum of the work in these various areas, geographical and clinical, was to change ultrasound from an 'eccentricity' as described by Donald [27] to something with possibilities. Then began the long haul to establish ultrasound as a routine diagnostic tool which could be widely applied. Even in Glasgow there was reluctance to accept this new-fangled ultrasound technique. When that reluctance subsided there was more reaction not against ultrasound *per se*, but just reaction towards the new. For example, even Ian Donald dismissed Doppler as not being of any real value. And real-time was seen as a step backwards; perhaps this is understandable because the first real-time scanners exhibited serious shortcomings; limited field of view, poor resolution, poor beam shape and gaps in the image [28]. Also, these scanners had been developed specifically to examine the heart and there was only a gradual realization that they could be of value on many parts of the body. Of course it is now clear that it had great advantages; they were easier to use and demonstrations were far easier hence sales improved (see Fig. 1.1), encouraging further development. The market enlarged, sales increased even more and the real price of machines fell dramatically in spite of greatly increased electronic complexity. Real-time had given an enormous impetus to ultrasound [29].

As can be seen from the brief chronology at the end of this chapter the development of Doppler ran almost in parallel with the development of 2D imaging. Doppler ultrasound had been in industrial use, then in 1957 Satomura [30] demonstrated its use to record heart valve motion. Four years later Kaneko *et al.* [31] were able to show that blood flow could be detected. From these observations tremendous development followed resulting in the simple but useful fetal heart detector to instruments for measuring blood velocity, the development of real-time spectral analysis and the combining of B scan and Doppler in duplex systems. Then an almost unnoticed paper by Namekawa *et al.* [32] working at Aloka laid the foundations for colour Doppler, rapid development and improvement followed leading to 2D images overlaid with colour to indicate blood or tissue velocity. More recently we have seen the development of power Doppler to give a display indicating tissue perfusion.

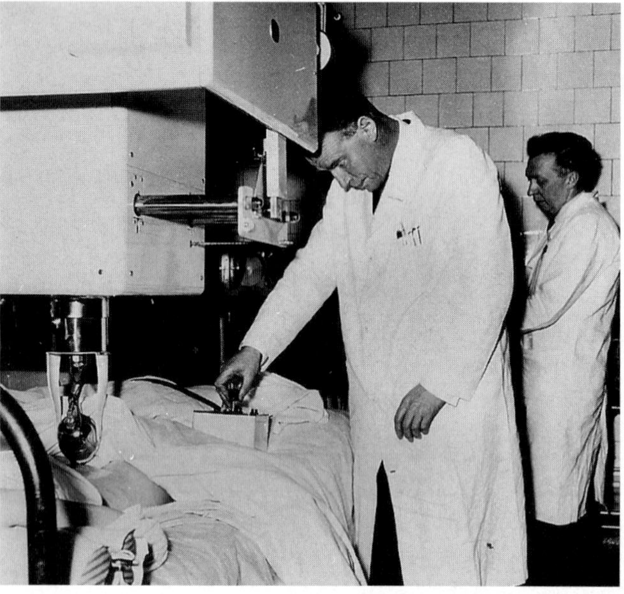

Fig. 1.10 The Kelvin Hughes automatic contact scanner designed by Tom Brown and used by Professor Ian Donald (left) and Dr John MacVicar to produce thousands of scans from 1959 to *c.* 1967. The electronic units on the trolley were previously used with the manually operated scanner (Fig. 1.6).

Three-dimensional ultrasound is now advancing rapidly; this too has a long and complex history. Its earliest manifestations were seen in the work of Howry and more significantly Brown who designed a 3D capability, albeit unused, into the autoscanner used by Ian Donald (T.G. Brown, 1988, personal communication). The problems of displaying 3D images inhibited its use. However, in 1972 at Sonicaid Ltd Brown designed the Multiplanar scanner (Fig. 1.18) the first commercial 3D machine [33]. This did not become a commercial success; one factor was the lack of a clinical problem requiring its capability. Now technology has advanced and some of the limitations forced upon Brown have disappeared. Additionally, clinical practice now has greater demands and expectations so that there is a growing desire to view in 3D. Among the indicators that its time has come was the first congress, in 1997, on 3D in obstetrics and gynaecology [34].

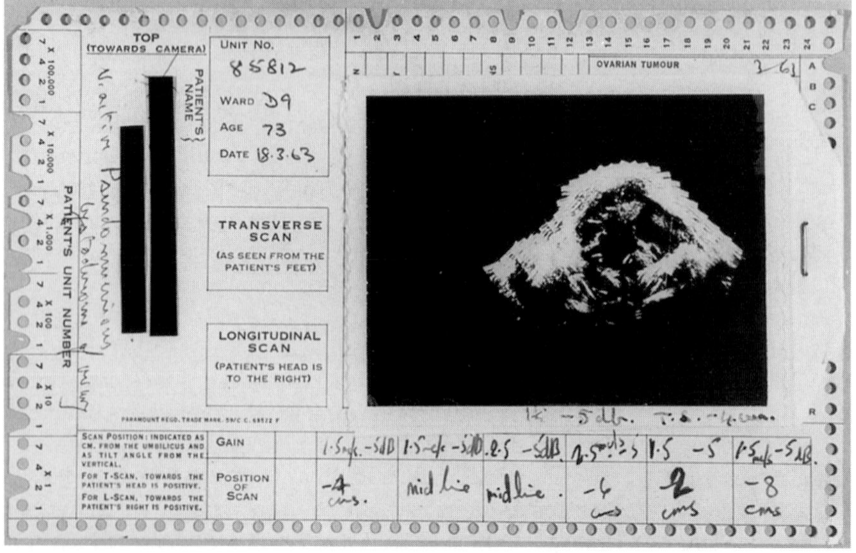

TOP (TOWARDS CAMERA)

PATIENT'S NAME

UNIT NO. 85812

WARD D9

AGE 73

DATE 18.3.63

OVARIAN TUMOUR 3-61

TRANSVERSE SCAN (AS SEEN FROM THE PATIENT'S FEET)

LONGITUDINAL SCAN (PATIENT'S HEAD IS TO THE RIGHT)

PATIENT'S UNIT NUMBER

PARAMOUNT REGD. TRADE MARK. 59/C C. 68522 F

SCAN POSITION: INDICATED AS CM. FROM THE UMBILICUS AND AS TILT ANGLE FROM THE VERTICAL. FOR T-SCAN, TOWARDS THE PATIENT'S HEAD IS POSITIVE. FOR L-SCAN, TOWARDS THE PATIENT'S RIGHT IS POSITIVE.

GAIN		1·5 -5dB	1·5 -5dB	2·5 -5dB	2·5 -5	1·5 -5	1·5 -5dB
POSITION OF SCAN		-4 cms.	mid line	midline	-6 cms	2 cms	-8 cms

Fig. 1.11 Image and record card (partly annotated by JEEF) from autoscanner, March 1963. This transverse scan was interpreted as showing a 'cystadenocarcinoma of ovary' and found to be 'very active multilocular pseudomucinous carcinoma with almost solid portions, microscopically malignant'.

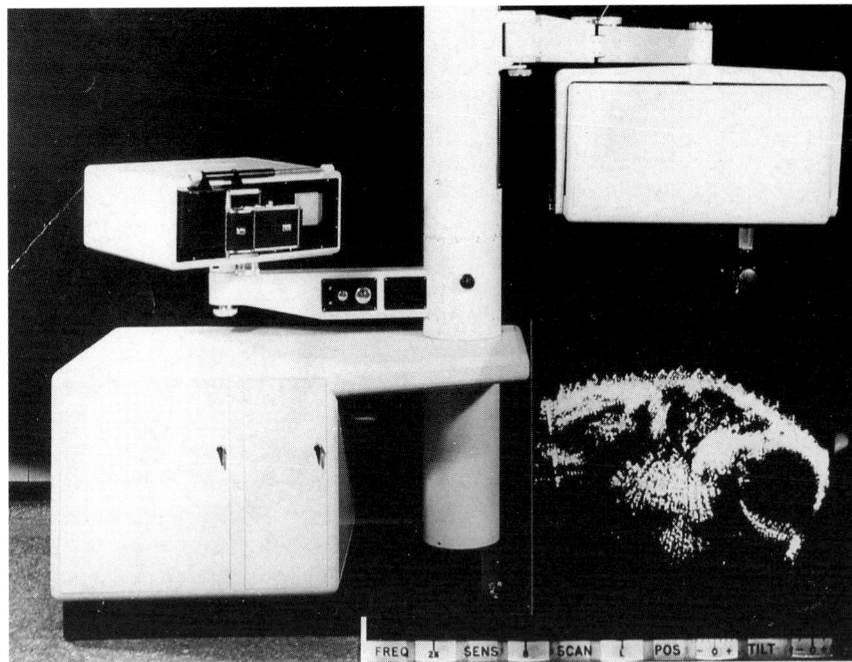

Fig. 1.12 The machine delivered to Dr Bertil Sunden, Lund, Sweden, in 1962. The images seen on the insert, have a characteristically 'spotty' appearance due to the very low pulse repetition rate of $25\,s^{-1}$. This low rate was used to ensure a low acoustic output and thus minimize exposure of the patient and required the operator to scan slowly and therefore more evenly across the patient. (Courtesy of the BMUS Historical Collection.)

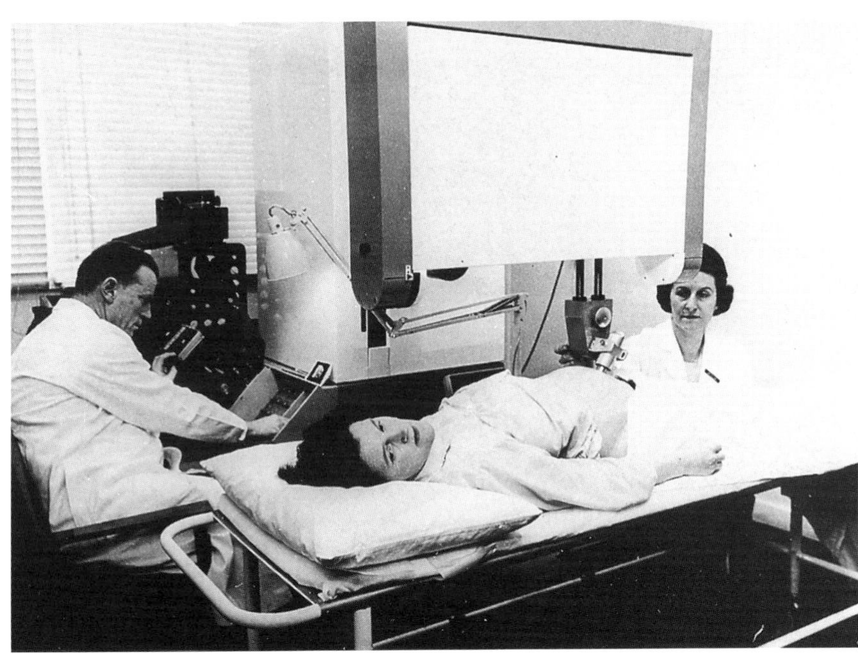

Fig. 1.13 Professor Ian Donald and Mrs Ida Miller posing with the KH diasonograph in the then recently opened Queen Mother's Hospital, Glasgow *c.* 1964. The scanning frame was supported by a substantial and very stable gantry to allow scans in virtually any plane. The electronics used thermionic valves in circuits derived from the Mk7 industrial flaw detector. At this time the Mk7 seen in the background was still used with an electronic caliper unit for fetal cephalometry.

Ultrasound is now so widely used that some radiologists claim it provides 40% of all medical imaging. Its use has spread to almost every medical speciality. This chapter has attempted to give some insight into the complex nature of the factors which allowed medical ultrasound to develop and grow. Perhaps if nothing more it will foster sympathy for today's new ideas—they may have a potential just as great as ultrasound had 50 years ago. An even broader view is possible as portrayed by Ellen Koch [35] when addressing the audience of ultrasound pioneers at the HMUS 'You should consider yourselves as pioneers in a much broader context than the

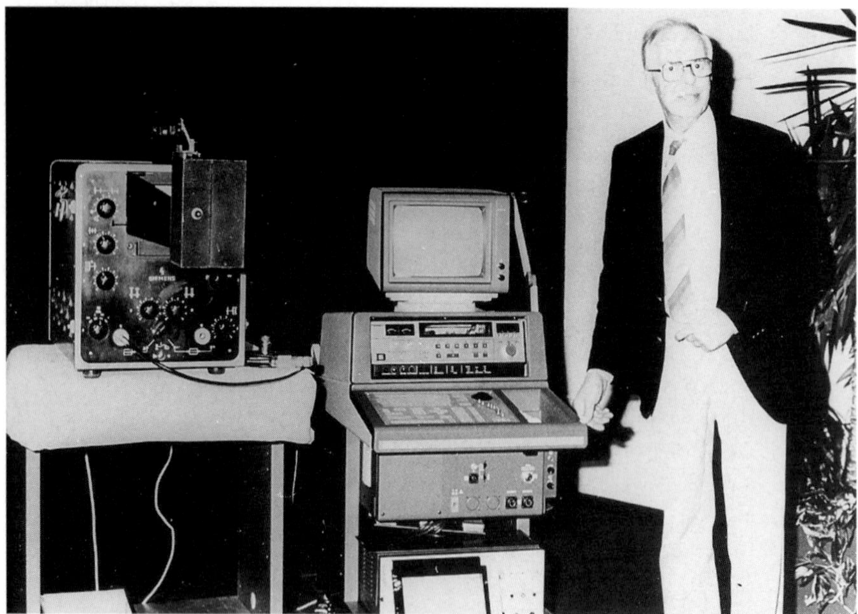

Fig. 1.14 The late Professor Hertz pictured here with, on the left, the Siemens Ultraschall-Impulsgerat which he modified for cardiology. Inge Edler and Hellmuth Hertz used this apparatus to produce the first echocardiograms in 1953. This picture taken in 1982 also shows in the centre a Siemens Sonoline CD echocardiography scanner.

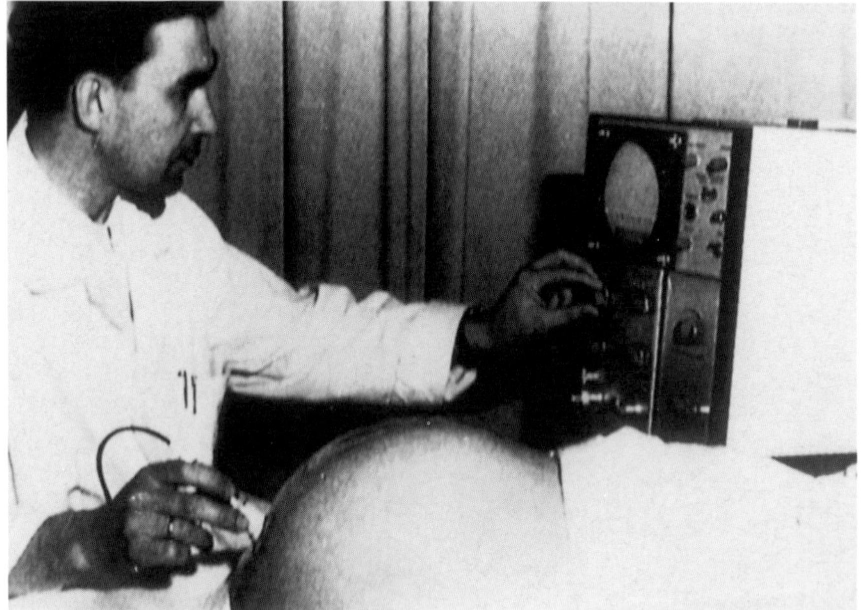

Fig. 1.15 Dr Alfred Kratochwil using a Kretz A-scan instrument in 1965.

research and practice of ultrasonography. As you work together in the next two days framing the history of ultrasound you are in a unique position to put aside the questions of priority or the nitty-gritty detail of technical developments and consider instead how the emerging interest in ultrasonics continued or diverged from existing research traditions in each country. How non-scientific factors played a role in shaping scientific and medical practice, and how the interactions of individual researchers and practitioners served to carve out a fruitful new style of clinical research incorporating the skills of the physicist, the engineer and physician alike'.

Acknowledgements

We would like to acknowledge the support of the Wellcome Trust, the British Medical Ultrasound Society and the Department of Obstetrics and Gynaecology, University of Glasgow.

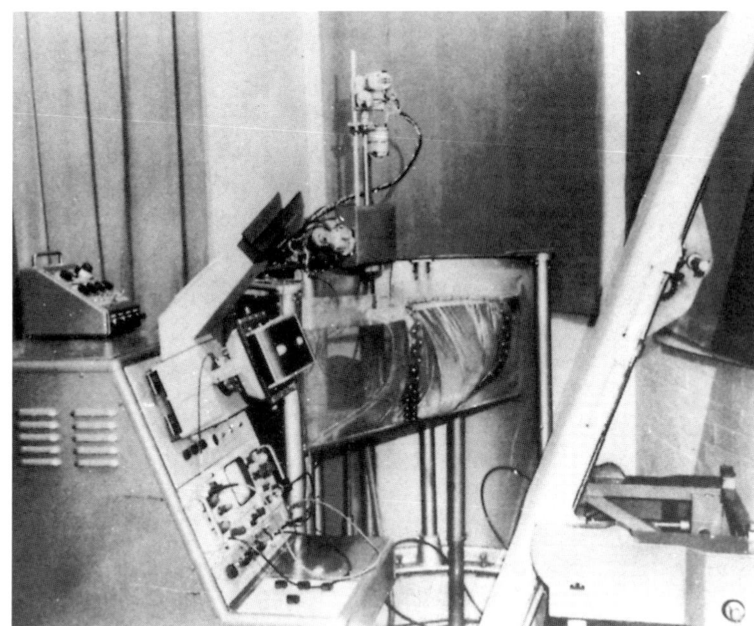

Fig. 1.16 The CAL Echoscope designed by Dr George Kossof [41]. The transducer in the water-filled coupling tank (centre of picture) scanned the patient who was positioned with the abdomen against the membrane while supported by the tilting stretcher on the right.

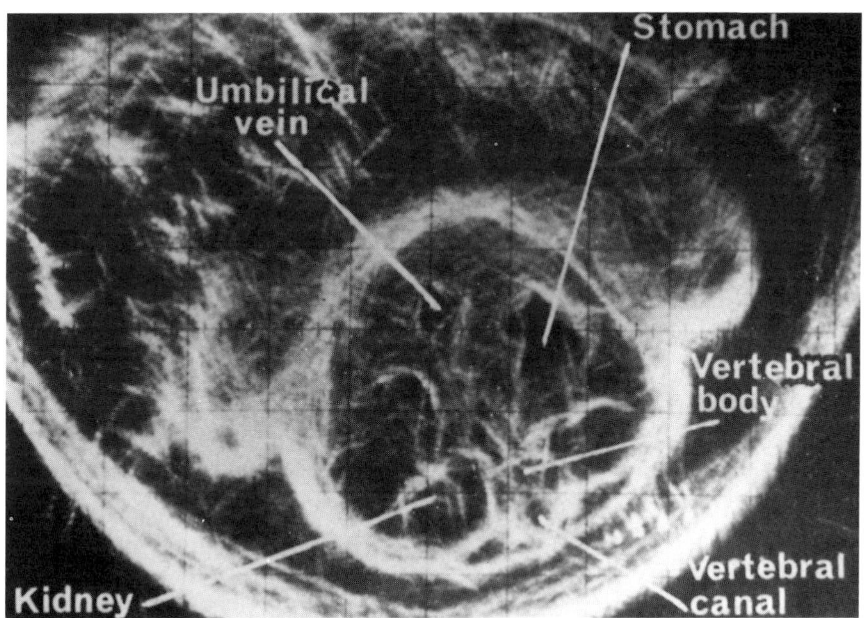

Fig. 1.17 An image from Kossoff and Garrett [42]; transverse scan showing fetal abdomen, vertebral column, kidneys, stomach and umbilical vein. This image is later than the Echoscope in Fig. 1.16 but displays the excellent grey scale and resolution seen in their earliest images.

Appendix 1: Diagnostic ultrasound—historical landmarks

This very brief, rather selective, set of 'landmarks' acknowledges only a few of the multitude of people who over the last hundred or more years have contributed to the development of diagnostic ultrasound.

1842 J.C. Doppler (Austria), paper on the Doppler effect.

1880 J. and P. Curie (France), discovered piezoelectric effect.

1917 P. Langevin (France), built first piezoelectric transducers, found lethal effects on fish.

1929–49 S. Sokolov (USSR), suggested use of ultrasound for imaging flaws in material, subsequent research led to at least two patents.

1937–50 K.T. Dussik (Austria), efforts to use through-transmission in neurology.

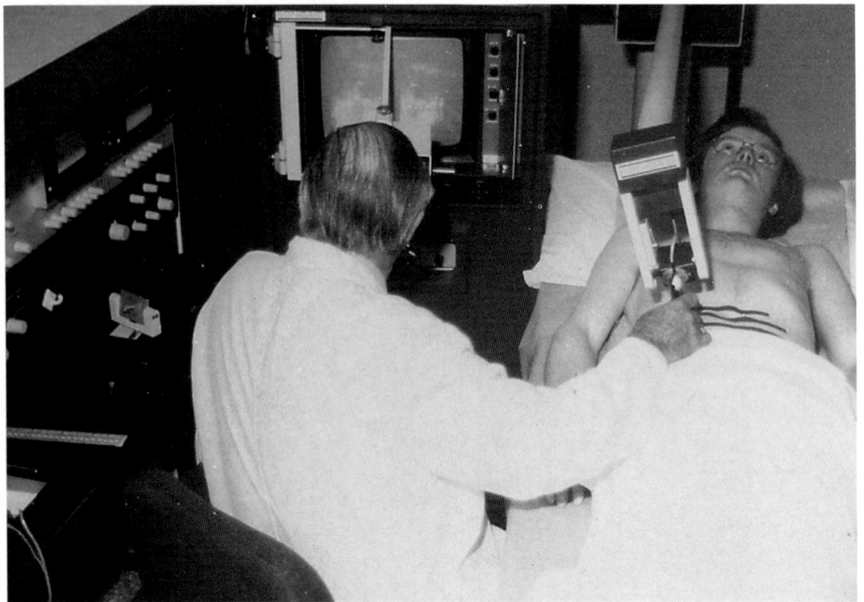

Fig. 1.18 Sonicaid 5000 Series multiplanar scanning system seen here in use by Dr G.B. Young, Edinburgh. The transducer is free to move in three dimensions. The image could be a conventional B-scan, by restraining the transducer to movement in one plane, or a series of parallel transverse scans could be viewed from an oblique viewpoint, these appeared one behind the other as in a perspective drawing. Longitudinal scans would appear to cut through the transverse scans. A realistic 'solid' 3D image could be presented by viewing a stereo pair of images [33].

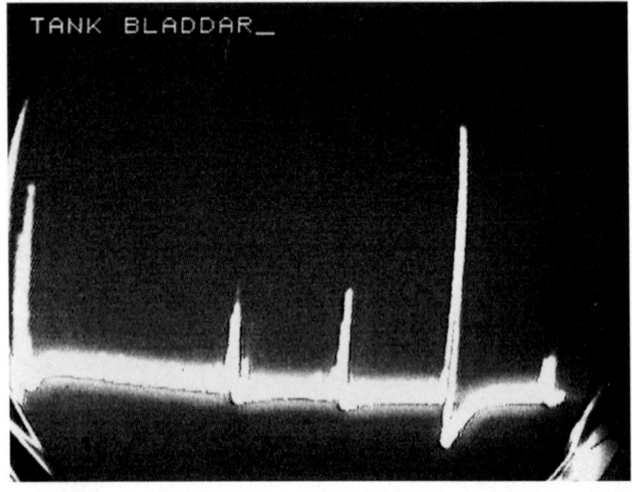

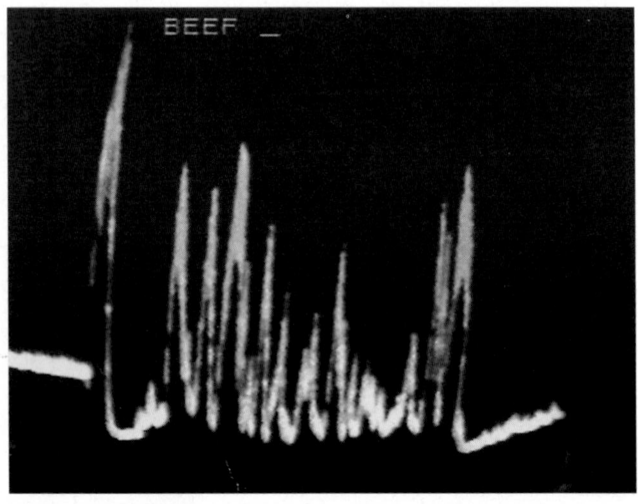

Fig. 1.19 A-scan traces made during the re-enactment of Professor Ian Donald's earliest ultrasound experiments (see footnote on p. 5). (a) Echoes from a water-filled animal bladder; (b) a sample of muscle tissue.

1943 D.O. Sproule (Henry Hughes, UK), first demonstration of supersonic apparatus.

1945 F.A. Firestone (Sperry Inc., USA), supersonic reflectorscope (A-scan).

1946 C.H. Desch, D.O. Sproule, W.J. Dawson (UK), 'The detection of cracks in steel by means of ultrasound waves'.

1948 D. Howry (USA), started experimental work.

1949 G.D. Ludwig, F.W. Struthers (USA), detection of gallstones and foreign bodies.

J. Wild (USA), started experimental work.

J.R. Uchida (Japan), built an A-scan instrument.

1950 J.J. Wild, D. Neal (USA), first paper detecting changes of texture in living tissue.

L.A. French, J.J. Wild, D. Neal (USA), detection of cerebral tumours.

1953 I. Edler, H. Hertz (Sweden), first recording of an echocardiogram.

1954 K. Tanaka (Japan), started using contact scanning for neurology.

Ian Donald (UK), started experimental work.

I. Edler, H. Hertz (Sweden), first paper on echocardiology.

J.J. Wild, J.M. Reid (USA), visualization of breast lesions.

D. Howry, J. Holmes *et al.* (USA), papers on visualization of soft tissues.
H.P. Kalmus *et al.*, papers on acoustic flow meter systems.
1956 T.G. Brown joined ID (UK) and improved A-scan.
Denver group (USA), paper on 3D and stereo methods.
S. Satomura (Japan), studying heart with Doppler.
G. Baum/J.G. Henry *et al.* (USA), papers on ophthalmic ultrasound.
T. Cieszynski (Czechoslovakia), first intraluminal transducer.
1957 T.G. Brown (UK), built contact scanner for Ian Donald.
E.J. Baldes *et al.* (USA), 'Forum on ultrasonic measurement of blood velocity'.
1958 I. Donald, J. MacVicar, T. Brown (UK), first paper on diagnostic ultrasound from Glasgow.
1959 T.G. Brown (UK), started work on automatic contact scanner.
D.L. Franklin, D.W. Baker *et al.* (USA), pulsed Doppler flow meter.
1962 B. Sunden (Sweden), started using the first B scanner sold by Kelvin Hughes.
K. Kato showed that RBC were source of Doppler shift signals.
1963 Kelvin Hughes (later Smiths) (UK), first Diasonograph manual contact scanners sold.
Denver (USA), contact scanner in use.
1964 Denver (USA), group's first publication on obstetric use of contact scanner.
Physionic Inc. (USA), Porta-Arm scanner delivered to Denver group.
1965 W. Buschmann (GDR), showed 10 element array for the eye.
First International Congress, Pittsburgh, 33 papers from nine countries.
SKI Doptone (USA), fetal heart detector on market.
1966 K. Kato (Japan), described directional Doppler.
Postgraduate course on diagnostic ultrasound started in Denver (USA).
1967 W. Krause, R. Soldner (FRG), Siemens 'Vidoson' real-time scanner.
Cardiac scanning by Y. Kikuchi and K. Tanaka (Japan).
1968 J.C. Somer (Netherlands), electronic phased array sector scanner.
D.A. Lobdell (USA), annular array.
1969 P. Peronneau (France), flow profiles with multi-gate Doppler.
Kretztechnik AG (Austria), built vaginal transducer for A. Kratochwil
1970 Courses on diagnostic ultrasound started in Glasgow (UK).
1971 N. Bom (Netherlands), linear array 'for moving cardiac structures'.
1972 First commercial linear array scanner from ADR Inc. (USA).
1973 D.L. King (USA), first paper on use of linear array; referred only to cardiac use.
1974 F.E. Barber, D.W. Baker *et al.* (USA), duplex echo Doppler scanner.
B.A. Coglan *et al.* (UK), time compression spectrum analyser.
1977 T.G. Brown (Sonicaid, UK), multiplanar 3D scanner in production.
1982 K. Namekawa, C. Kasai *et al.* (Aloka, Japan), described colour Doppler at WFUMB-82.
Acuson (USA), delivered first 'computed sonography' system.
1983–96 The performance of ultrasound systems improved rapidly, Colour Doppler imaging, both giving velocity and 'power' displays has became commonplace and 3D arrived on the scene. It has been estimated that ultrasound now accounts for 40% of all medical imaging.
1997 First World Congress on 3D Ultrasound in Obstetrics and Gynaecology, Mainz, Austria.

Appendix 2: Ultrasound collections

American Institute of Ultrasound in Medicine

American Institute of Ultrasound In Medicine (AIUM), 14750 Sweitzer Lane, Laurel MD 20707-5906, USA. The large collection and archive is the result of the work of Professor Barry Goldberg who organized a symposium on the history of medical ultrasound in Washington in 1988; included are five large filing cabinets (a total of 25 drawers) of papers, audio- and videotapes, images and photographs, and a considerable number of pieces of hardware including Howry's early scanners.

German Society of Ultrasound in Medicine

In 1995 an ultrasound museum was established in Dresden by the German Society of Ultrasound in Medicine (DEGUM). The collection is housed in the Hygiene Museum, Dresden which underwent reconstruction during 1997. It is intended that the principal focus, will be on the development of ultrasound in the German-speaking countries of central Europe [36,37] (H. Lutz, 1997, personal communication).

British Medical Ultrasound Society

The British Medical Ultrasound Society (BMUS) Historical Collection was established in 1984. Currently it contains over 60 items of hardware, scanners and associated equipment, a wide range of manufacturer's literature and a substantial and increasing archive of unique documents. Many items of hardware are on display in the Department of Obstetrics and Gynaecology, University of Glasgow, Queen Mother's Hospital, Yorkhill, Glasgow G3 8SJ, UK. The archive material is also available for viewing and study. In the long term the collection will pass into the care of the Hunterian Museum, University of Glasgow. Glasgow G12 8QQ, UK.

Science Museum, London

A Kelvin Hughes Mk2 flaw detector (see Fig. 1.4) of the type used by Ian Donald in his early experiments is in the Science Museum, London. There are also a few other ultrasound items in store including the Smiths Diasonograph used by Professor Stuart Campbell when working at Queen Charlotte's Hospital.

Other collections

As industrial non-destructive test equipment supplied much of the equipment used by the early experimenters it is of interest that the British Institute of Non-Destructive Testing is establishing a collection. Also a few items of medical ultrasound equipment are in store at the Royal Scottish Museum, Edinburgh, UK.

Note added in proof

Since writing this chapter a further article in a series on the history of medical ultrasound has been published in *Ultrasound in Medicine and Biology* [43].

References

1 Edler, I., Lindstrom, K. The history of echocardiography. *Ultrasound in Medicine and Biology* (in press).
2 Coste, P. (1989) *Diagnostic ultrasound: an historical industry analysis*. PhD dissertation, Claremont Graduate School, California.
3 Blackwell, G. (1995) *The World Market for Ultrasound Imaging Systems*. Clinica Reports. PJB Publications Ltd, Richmond, UK.
4 Nicolson, M., Spencer, I.H., Fleming, J.E.E. (1996) Ultrasound and the construction of the fetal image. Presented at the Conference of the Medical Sociology Group of the British Sociological Association, September 1996, Edinburgh.
5 Spencer, I.H., Fleming, J.E.E., Nicolson, M. (1996) Clinical ultrasound and interprofessional rivalries. Presented at the Society for the History of Technology Annual Meeting, August 1996, London.
6 Spencer, I.H., Fleming, J.E.E., Nicolson, M. (1996) The role of medical ultrasound in the abortion debate in Scotland. Presented at Scottish Medical Sociology Group of the British Sociological Association, May 1996, Pitlochry.
7 Donald, I. (1974) Sonar—the story of an experiment. *Ultrasound in Medicine and Biology* **1**, 109–117.
8 Goldberg, B.B., Gramiak, R., Freimanis, A.K. (1993) Early history of diagnostic ultrasound: the role of American radiologists. *American Journal of Roentgenology* **160**, 189–194.
9 Hertz, C.H. (1973) The interaction of physicians, physicists and industry in the development of echocardiography. *Ultrasound in Medicine and Biology* **1**, 3–11.
10 Thijssen, J.M. (1993) The history of ultrasound techniques in ophthalmology. *Ultrasound in Medicine and Biology* **19**, 599–618.
11 Wells, P.N.T. (1993) Milestones in cardiac ultrasound: echoes from the past. *International Journal of Cardiac Imaging* **9**(suppl. 2), 3–9.
12 White, D.N. (1988) Neurosonology pioneers. *Ultrasound in Medicine and Biology* **14**, 541–561.
13 White, D.N. (1992) The early development of neurosonology. I. Echoencephalography in adults. *Ultrasound in Medicine and Biology* **18**, 115–165.
14 White, D.N. (1992) The early development of neurosonology. II. Fetal and neonatal echoencephalography. *Ultrasound in Medicine and Biology* **18**, 227–247.
15 White, D.N. (1992) The early development of neurosonology. III. Pulsatile echoencephalography and Doppler techniques. *Ultrasound in Medicine and Biology* **18**, 323–376.
16 Koch, E.B. (1990) *The process of innovation in medical technology: American research on ultrasound, 1947 to 1962*. PhD dissertation in history and technology of science, University of Pennsylvania.
17 Kodak (1988) *Medical Diagnostic Ultrasound: A Retrospective on its 40th Anniversary*. Eastman Kodak Company.
18 White, D.N., Clark G., Carson, J., White, E. (1982) *Ultrasound in Biomedicine: Cumulative Bibliography of the World Literature to 1978*. Pergamon Press, Oxford.
19 Ackerstaff, R.G.A., Mess, W.H. (1997) 11th International Symposium on Cerebral Hemodynamics/ 2nd Meeting of the European Society of Neurosonology with Cerebral Hemodynamics. *European Journal of Ultrasound*, **5**(suppl. 1), s1–s66V (abstracts).
20 Wild, J.J., Neal, D. (1951) Use of high-frequency ultrasound waves for detecting changes of texture in living tissue. *Lancet* **i**, 655–657.
21 Brown, T.G. (1988) Ultrasound in Glasgow. Text of talk at HMUS 1988, Washington, BMUS Collection and Archives.
22 Donald, I., MacVicar, J., Brown, T.G. (1958) Investigation of abdominal masses by pulsed ultrasound. *Lancet* **1**, 1188–1195.
23 Howry, D.H. (1957) Techniques used in ultrasonic visualisation of soft tissues. In: Kelly, E. (ed.) *Ultrasound in Biology and Medicine*, publication no. 3, Symposium Illinois, 20–22 June 1955. American Institute of Biological Sciences, Washington, pp. 49–65.
24 Sunden, B. (1964) On the diagnostic value of ultrasound in obstetrics and gynaecology. *Acta Obstetrica et Gynecologica Scandinavica*, **63**(suppl. 6), 1–191.
25 Kratocwil, A. (1988) Video recording of interview by Barbara Kimmelman, Washington, DC. Tape no. 2, History of Ultrasound Project, AIUM Archives.

26 Garrett, W. (1988) Video recording of interview by Barbara Kimmelman, Washington, DC. Tape no. 2, History of Ultrasound Project, AIUM Archives.

27 Hansmann, M., Hackeloer, B.J., Staudach, A., Wittmann, B.K. (1986) *Ultrasound Diagnosis in Obstetrics and Gynaecology*. Springer-Verlag, Berlin.

28 Bom, N., Lancee, C.T., Honkoop, J., Hugenholtz, P.G. (1971) Ultrasonic viewer for cross-sectional analysis of moving cardiac structures. *Biomedical Engineering* **6**, 500–503, 508.

29 Donald, I. (1976) The ultrasonic boom. *Journal of Clinical Ultrasound* **4**, 323–328.

30 Satomura, S. (1957) Ultrasonic Doppler method for the inspection of cardiac function. *Journal of the Acoustics Society of America* **29**, 1181–1185.

31 Kaneko, Z., Kotani, H., Komuta, K., Satomura, S. (1961) Studies on peripheral circulation by ultrasonic blood-rheograph. *Japanese Circulation Journal* **25**, 203–213.

32 Namekawa, K., Kasai, C., Tsukamoto, M., Koyano, A. (1982) Realtime bloodflow imaging system utilising auto-correlation techniques. Presented at the Third Meeting of the World Federation for Ultrasound in Medicine and Biology, Brighton, UK, 26–30 July 1982, pp. 203–208.

33 Brown, T.G., Younger, G.W., Skrgatic, D., Fortune, J. (1977) Multiplanar B-scanning—using the third dimension. In: White, D.N., Brown, R.E. (eds) *Ultrasound in Medicine*, vol. 3B. Plenum Publishing, New York, pp. 1797–1799.

34 Merz, E. (1997) Preliminary program for First World Congress on 3D Ultrasound in Obstetrics and Gynaecology, Mainz, September 1997.

35 Koch, E.B. (1988) Historical overview, video recording of talks at HMUS, Washington, October 1988. AIUM Archives.

36 Hofmann, V. (1996) Ultrasound Museum. *EFSUMB Newsletter* **10**, 9.

37 Hofmann, V. *et al*. (eds) (1996) Symposium anlaBlich der Eroffnung des US-Museums in Dresden 10–12 October 1995. *Ultraschal in Klinik Und Praxis* **10**, 165–206. Springer-Verlag, Berlin.

38 Fleming, J.E.E., Spencer, I.H., Nicolson, M.A. (1997), 40 years of ultrasound. In: Cockburn, F. (ed.) *Advances in Perinatal Medicine*. Proceedings of XVth European Congress of Perinatal Medicine, Glasgow, September 1996. Parthenon Publishing, New York, pp. 92–99.

39 Spencer, I.H., Fleming, J.E.E., Nicolson, M. (1996) A-scan through the history of ultrasound, video. AV Services, University of Glasgow.

40 Howry, D.H. (1948) Unpublished material obtained by ultrasonic diagnostic methods, April 1954, C-2423, no. SS, AIUM Archives.

41 Kossof, G., Robinson, D.E., Garrett, W.J. (1966) Two dimensional ultrasonography in obstetrics. In: Grossman, C.C., Holmes, J.H., Joyner, C., Purmell, E.W. (eds) *Diagnostic Ultrasound*, Proceedings of the 1st International Conference, University of Pittsburgh. Plenum Press, New York, pp. 333–347.

42 Kossof, G., Garrett, W.J. (1972) Ultrasonic film echography in gynecology and obstetrics. *Obstetrics and Gynecology* **40**, 299–305.

43 McNay, M.B., Fleming, J.E.E. (1999) Forty years of obstetric ultrasound 1957–1997: from A-scope to three dimensions. *Ultrasound in Medicine and Biology* **25**, 3–56.

Part 1
Instrumentation

Chapter 2: Grey-scale imaging

S.D. Pye & P.R. Hoskins

The term ultrasound applies to any sound above the range of human hearing, which is greater than 20 kHz (1 Hz = 1 cycle s^{-1}). Commonly used ultrasound imaging frequencies range from 2 to 15 MHz. The very earliest ultrasound systems used on patients were adapted from industrial flaw detectors. Now ultrasound techniques are used throughout the world and are an essential tool in the diagnostic armoury. There are several reasons for this widespread use. Probably the most important is that ultrasound provides high quality information on soft tissue. Visualization of soft tissue using traditional plane radiographic techniques is restricted to particular areas such as mammography or investigation of the lining of the gastrointestinal (GI) tract using barium contrast. Diagnostic ultrasound is a procedure involving in the majority of examinations no risk to the patient, compared with imaging techniques involving ionizing radiations, which have known quantifiable risks. Ultrasound is an inexpensive modality with low capital costs of 5–50% of that of a computed tomography (CT) scanner, and low operator costs as examinations are usually performed and reported by a single operator. Ultrasound does have some limitations. Gas and bone block the ultrasound beam and so restrict the ability to image a number of body sites. Good image quality can be difficult to obtain in obese patients. Interpretation of ultrasound images can be difficult: they are non-quantitative in the sense that the image pixel brightness does not correspond to a single tissue property, but is a complex mixture of many things.

This chapter describes the physics and instrumentation of ultrasound applicable to imaging of soft tissue. Chapters immediately following describe the complementary technique of Doppler ultrasound which is concerned with measurement and display of blood flow. More extensive descriptions of some of the issues raised are covered in the standard texts by Fish [1] and McDicken [2].

Pulse–echo technique

Diagnostic ultrasound systems for imaging soft tissue rely on the transmission and reception of ultrasound pulses in order to obtain information about the tissue content along the path of the pulse. In this section the basic physics of this process will be described.

Generation of ultrasound

Ultrasound is generated using a transducer (often referred to as a crystal) mounted in a hand-held probe. The transducer is piezoelectric which means that it converts electrical energy into mechanical energy. Vibration of the transducer is produced by connecting the transducer to an electrical source, which may either be an alternating voltage or a voltage spike. The ultrasound pulse which is produced is short, consisting of just two or three wavelengths. When a hand-held probe is coupled to the skin the transducer vibrations are transmitted into the tissue as waves of high and low pressure (Fig. 2.1), and individual particles move microscopically backwards and forwards about their rest position.

Reflection, scattering and absorption

Ultrasound passes through tissue along a well-defined path or beam (Fig. 2.2) and undergoes interactions with the tissue. An important quantity affecting the propagation of waves within the tissue or material is the acoustic impedance, which is related to the elasticity and density of the material. Reflection of the incident ultrasound arises when there is a difference in the acoustic impedance between different organs or tissues, such as liver and kidney, or fat and muscle. Reflected ultrasound is highly directional; that is, most of the energy within the reflected wave travels in a single direction. Scattering of ultrasound occurs from the tissue parenchyma, where there are changes in acoustic impedance over a microscopic level within the tissue. Scattered ultrasound consists of low amplitude waves which travel in all directions. Ultrasound which returns in the direction of the probe is said to be backscattered.

In addition to scattering and reflection, energy is lost from the pulse by absorption of ultrasound in tissue. In

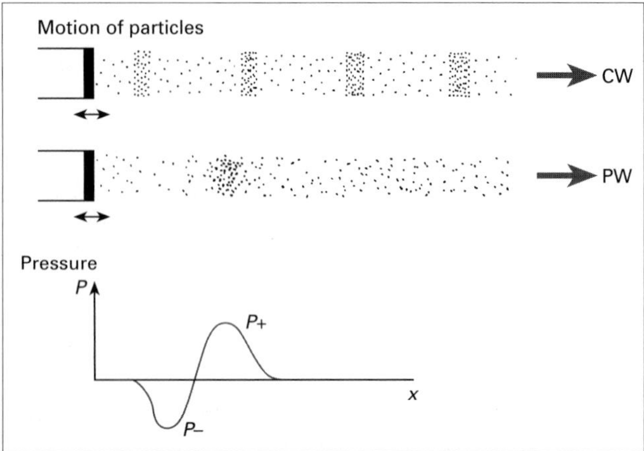

Fig. 2.1 The vibrations of the transducer are transmitted into the patient as longitudinal waves of high and low pressure. On a microscopic scale individual particles move to and fro about their rest position as the wave passes. CW, continuous wave excitation; PW, pulsed wave excitation.

most soft tissues, the fraction of energy lost by absorption is much greater than that lost by scattering. The energy absorbed is converted into heat, resulting in small increases in temperature of the tissue. The overall process of energy loss involving absorption, reflection and scattering is referred to as attenuation. Attenuation increases with depth and frequency. A typical attenuation coefficient for soft tissue is $0.6\,dB\,cm^{-1}\,MHz^{-1}$.

Measurement of depth

The first echoes received by the probe come from the tissues nearest to the probe. Later echoes will come from deeper tissue. An ultrasound scanner assumes that ultrasound travels with a constant value of $1540\,m\,s^{-1}$. The depth of returning echoes is then calculated purely from the time delay between pulse transmission and echo reception; this is referred to as the pulse–echo technique. The speed of sound in tissues actually varies from approximately 1480 to $1580\,m\,s^{-1}$. This results in errors in the depth and calculated linear dimensions of tissues of up to about 3.5%.

Detection of ultrasound

Immediately after transmission of the ultrasound pulse, the transducer switches into reception mode. The backscattered ultrasound hits the transducer, causing mechanical motion of the transducer on a microscopic level. An electrical voltage signal is produced whose amplitude is proportional to the amplitude of the ultrasound pressure wave at the transducer face.

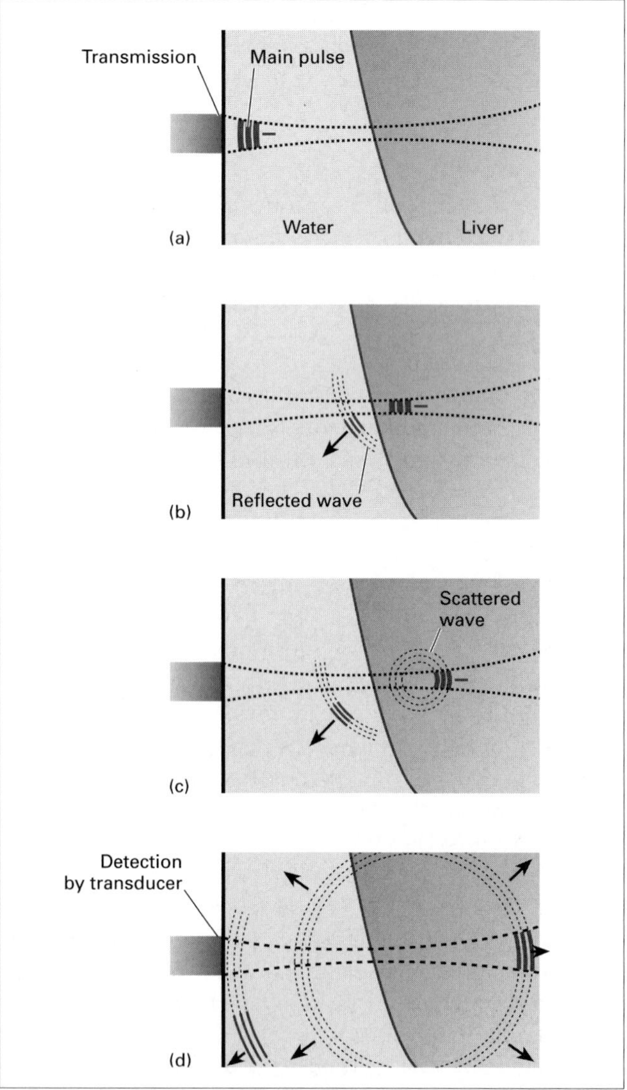

Fig. 2.2 Propagation of an ultrasonic pulse through a simplified tissue model consisting of liver and water. (a) The ultrasound pulse travels along a well-defined beam; (b) reflection occurs at the boundary between the liver and water; (c) scattering occurs from the parenchyma of the liver (for the purposes of clarity only one region of scattering has been shown); (d) the reflected wave is detected by the transducer. (Redrawn from Reed *et al.* 1995 [14].)

Scanning modes

The pulse–echo ultrasound technique may be incorporated into several different types of ultrasound system. These are described below.

A-scan

The amplitude (A) of the returned echo signal is displayed against time for each transmitted pulse. The technique was widely used in the early days of ultrasound, but is now restricted to specialist uses such as ophthalmology in order to perform very accurate measurement of distance.

B-scan

The vast majority of diagnostic ultrasound scans are carried out in this way. A large number of A-scan lines are acquired and high/low echo amplitudes are displayed as bright/dark spots. A two-dimensional (2D) image is formed of a slice through the body, which is known as a brightness-mode scan, or simply B-scan. Modern scanners acquire and display echo information fast enough to enable tissue motion to be followed, and are referred to as real-time B-scanners or just real-time scanners.

M-mode

This was originally developed, and is still widely used, in cardiology. The A-scan is displayed as a single vertical line with the brightness at each point corresponding to the echo amplitude. The M-mode consists of a display of consecutive lines plotted against time. Using this mode, detailed information may be obtained about various cardiac dimensions, and also the accurate timing of valvular motion.

Volume scan

In this mode a three-dimensional (3D) dataset is acquired. A small number of commercial systems provide this facility by the sequential acquisition of 2D scans with storage of the data in digital memory. A 3D perspective may be displayed using surface shading techniques. Where there is sufficient contrast between different tissues the volume of organs may be estimated.

Components of a real-time B-scanner

The most widely used mode in modern commercial machines is the real-time B-scan. For many operators it is the starting point of their training, and it is appropriate to describe the instrumentation involved. Figure 2.3 shows the components of the imaging system. The B-scan image is built up line by line using the information acquired by the probe, hence the details of probe design and the mechanisms by which the beam is scanned through the tissue are important. These are discussed below.

Transducer and probe

The piezoelectric transducer in the hand-held probe transmits and receives the ultrasound signals. Using traditional

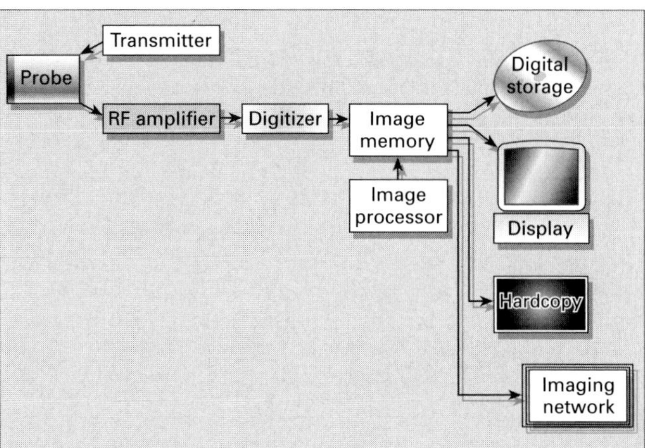

Fig. 2.3 Components of a 2D B-scanner.

piezoelectric materials such as PZT (lead zircorate titrate) the probe sensitivity has a strong frequency dependence, and it is necessary to use a range of probes each with a different centre frequency (e.g. 3.5, 5 or 10 MHz). The use of modified piezoelectric materials means that the sensitivity of modern probes is less dependent on frequency; these are referred to as wide-band probes. It is possible to drive such probes at different frequencies for different applications. The design of probes is discussed further by Shung and Zipparo [3] and Whittingham [4].

The probe is connected to the scanner by a cable which carries the transmit pulses from the scanner to the probe and the echo signals from the probe back to the scanner. The received echoes have a range of 80–100 dB in amplitude. On reception by the probe the ultrasound echoes are converted into voltage signals. These are called radiofrequency, or RF, signals as they are within the frequency band used for radio transmission. Amplification is carried out as soon as the signals from the probe reach the scanner.

Time gain compensation

Ultrasound is strongly attenuated by soft tissue. Electronic correction for the progressive decrease in echo amplitude is required and is referred to by terms such as time gain compensation (TGC), depth gain compensation and swept gain. TGC is achieved by progressively increasing the amplification (gain) which is applied to echo signals as they arrive from deeper in the body. There are a number of front panel controls on a scanner which give the operator a degree of choice over the way the echoes in the image are emphasized by this correction. The most commonly used method is to divide the imaged depth range into several (perhaps five to eight) equally spaced regions whose gain is controlled by one of a series of slider controls.

Adaptive or automatic time gain control (ATGC or AGC) is also available on some systems [5]. With adaptive correction of each individual scan line, the image can be optimized automatically.

Digitizer

The digitizer converts the electrical signal from an analogue signal to a digital signal. The exact position of the digitizer in the signal processing chain will vary between scanners, and the position shown is typical of many scanners currently available. The most expensive scanners will digitize as early as possible in the signal processing chain in order that the highest image quality may be displayed.

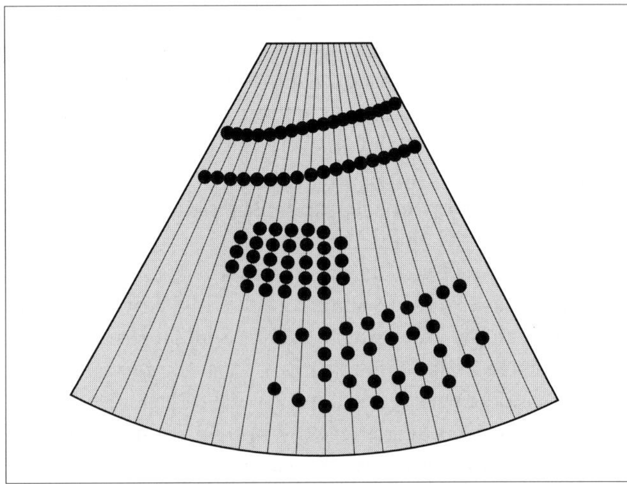

Fig. 2.4 The raw B-scan data has gaps between the scan lines which must be filled by interpolation of image values between adjacent lines.

Image memory

The image memory, sometimes called the scan converter, is a temporary image store capable of holding at least one complete TV image in digital form. Many modern machines can hold several hundred images at once. Echo data is digitized and read into the image memory line by line as it arrives from the probe and TGC amplifier. Data is read out of the image memory in the horizontal raster format appropriate for the TV display.

Image processor

Several operations are carried out on the image data while it is in the image memory, and these are as follows.

1 Logarithmic (log) compression. If the ultrasound signal after TGC were displayed then the image would be dominated by the very high amplitude signals from tissue boundaries, with the low amplitude signals from tissue parenchyma being lost. In order to boost the signal amplitude from the low level signals and enable these to be displayed the ultrasound signal is 'log-compressed'.

2 Interpolation between scan lines. This is necessary as there are often blank pixels in the gaps between adjacent scan lines (Fig. 2.4).

3 Postprocessing. As the data is held in digital form image enhancement may be performed in real-time in order to improve the image. This involves spatial filtering which is the combination of adjacent pixel values within a single frame, and temporal filtering which is the combination of pixel values from consecutive frames. Spatial filtering may be used to reduce noise and enhance edges. Some sophisticated filtering regimes manage to perform both of these tasks at the same time. Temporal filtering is also referred to as frame averaging or persistence, and it is used to reduce image noise. All scanners utilize frame averaging to some extent, even if this is not indicated on the front panel.

4 Frame freeze. The last image acquired is displayed on the TV enabling measurements to be performed or hard copy to be taken.

5 Measurements and graphics. The digital ultrasound image is combined with a graphics/text overlay to allow measurements to be made, or to allow the display of demographic information.

Display

Video monitors are widely available which have low distortion, are inexpensive and are designed to generate a large range of grey tones in the image. The image can also be transmitted to remote slave monitors for teaching purposes or to obtain advice from more experienced colleagues. Domestic TV sets in the UK have 625 horizontal lines. A modern top-of-the-range ultrasound scanner uses so-called hi-line monitors with 1049 lines so as not to degrade the spatial resolution of the image.

Digital storage

Archiving of digital image data is gaining in popularity, and in the future the digital storage of ultrasound data will be increasingly used. Various digital storage devices are available, and the criteria used for selection are cost and data access time. Three commonly used devices are the hard disc, the optical disc and magnetic tape. Fastest retrieval time is provided when images are stored on the hard disc, and this is also the most expensive. Storage on optical disc provides rapid retrieval once the appropriate disc has been found and loaded. Magnetic tape is the least expensive option but the access time is slow due to the necessity of winding the tape to the correct point. Digitally stored images are usually compressed, either in a form which enables full retrieval of the raw data, or in a form in which some of the image information is lost. The advantage of the latter approach is that much higher compaction may be achieved than for the loss-less methods, which currently afford two times reduction in size. Full retrieval of raw data is desirable when it is possible that analysis of the images may be required for research projects. Some minor loss in image quality is usually acceptable for non-research images.

Many modern ultrasound scanners come equipped with an optical disc drive, and can be connected to a local or hospital imaging network.

Hard copy devices

There are a number of different hard copy devices in common use. Transparency film has a higher image quality than paper hard copy. However, in ultrasound scanning the diagnosis is not generally made from the hard copy but is made in real-time while scanning the patient. The hard copy is then used as a record of the examination, for which it is acceptable to use a medium, often paper based, which does not necessarily have the highest image quality. Below are listed several hard copy devices in order of increasing image quality.

1 Thermal printer. Heat-sensitive paper is used allowing a black and white image to be produced within a few seconds.

2 Colour video printer. Most modern ultrasound machines, especially those with colour Doppler, come equipped with an in-built colour video printer. Processing times are typically 0.5–2 min.

3 Multiformat camera. Grey tone transparency film is used which is then developed in a film processor.

4 Laser printer. The ultrasound scanner may be linked via a local or hospital network to a remote laser printer to produce grey tone transparency film of comparable image quality to the multiformat camera.

In addition to static pictures it may be useful to record a dynamic sequence. The most cost-effective method is the videotape recorder. All videorecorders degrade the image; VHS recorders more so than super-VHS recorders, and most clinical users prefer the latter. Playback of digitally stored data will probably become routinely used in the future.

Probes and beam steering

General principles

The ultrasound image is built up by scanning the beam through the tissue in a controlled manner. In the original B-scan devices this action was performed by the operator who moved the probe over the skin of the patient. These so-called static B-scanners have not been commercially available for over a decade. Modern B-scanners sweep the beam automatically through the tissue. The spatial resolution of the image is critically dependent on the probe frequency, number of scan lines and beam shape. The production of a focused beam which is uniformly narrow over the whole field of view is most desirable in optimizing spatial resolution.

There are therefore three aspects of design which are important for the modern B-scanner; the transducer, the system used for focusing the beam and the system used for steering the beam.

DESIGN OF MODERN PROBES

Older designs of probes consist of single disk-shaped transducers whose diameter varied from 1 to 2 cm depending on transmit frequency. The use of multi-element probes enables superior focusing and beam steering, and these are more commonly used than single element probes in mid- and high-end machines. With modern construction techniques the number of elements can be as high as 1000 in a single probe.

FOCUSING THE BEAM BY USING AN ACOUSTIC LENS

The disk-shaped PZT transducer used in lower-end machines must have a diameter small enough to allow it to fit into a hand-held probe. If the PZT disk has no arrangement for focusing at all, the ultrasound beam gradually diverges as it travels away from the probe. This results in a poor spatial resolution. An acoustic lens made from suitable material may be positioned in front of the transducer in order to provide weak focusing of the beam. The lens acts in the same way that a glass lens does for visible light. The focal depth for such a lens is fixed. Circular acoustic lenses are used for single element transducers producing a beam which is symmetrically narrowed (Fig. 2.5a). For a linear array focusing in the plane perpendicular to the scan plane is usually effected by the use of an acoustic lens (Fig. 2.5b). In this case the lens itself only produces focusing perpendicular to the scan plane.

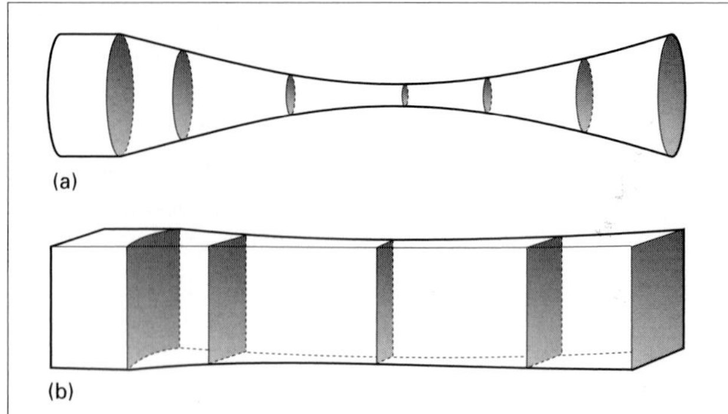

Fig. 2.5 Focusing a beam using an acoustic lens: (a) for a single transducer the beam is symmetrically narrowed, and (b) for a linear or phased array the beam is narrowed in the elevation plane.

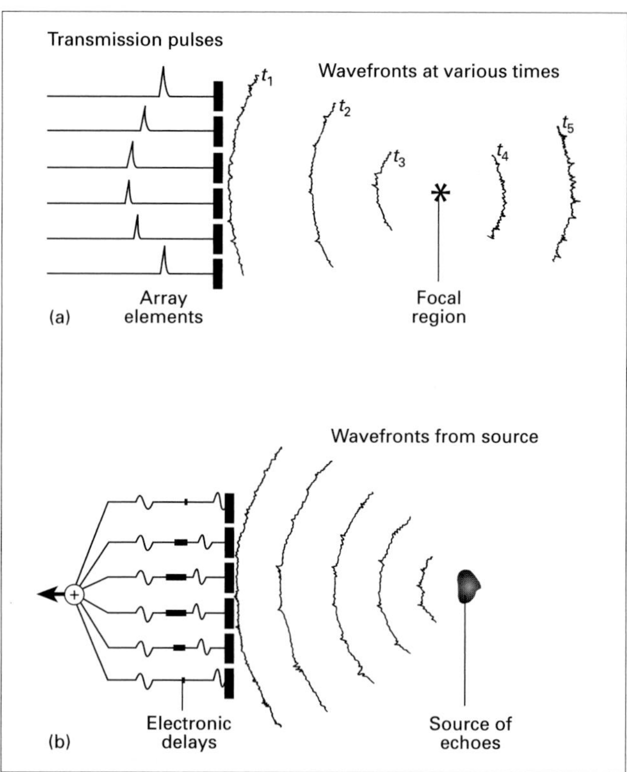

Fig. 2.6 Electronic focusing: (a) on transmit, and (b) on receive.

FOCUSING THE BEAM ELECTRONICALLY

If the transducer is composed of several elements the beam may be focused electronically. This is illustrated in Fig. 2.6a. The firing of the central element is delayed compared with the outer elements, producing a curved wavefront, and a beam with a single focal region.

Echoes from a particular depth will arrive at the transducer with a curved wavefront, so that different parts of the wavefront will hit the transducer at different times. Optimum spatial resolution is achieved by ensuring that different parts of the wavefront are detected at the same time. This is done by delaying the echoes received from the central element compared to the outer elements (Fig. 2.6b). This is called focus-on-receive. In practice the delays may be adjusted continuously with time to move the reception focus from near to the transducer immediately after transmission, to deeper depths later after transmission. This is called dynamic focusing.

STEERING THE BEAM MECHANICALLY

Transducers in which the beam direction from the transducer is fixed must either be moved manually (as in static B-scanners) or mechanically in order to generate different beam directions. Mechanical steering can be achieved by rotating or oscillating the transducer.

STEERING THE BEAM ELECTRONICALLY

If the transducer is composed of a line of very narrow rectangular elements then it is possible to steer the beam electronically. Progressive delay in the firing of elements produces a wavefront whose direction may be controlled (Fig. 2.7).

Types of probe

PROBES WITH MECHANICALLY ROTATING TRANSDUCERS

In this type of probe, one to four circular piezoelectric transducers are mounted on a wheel which is contained within an oil-filled bath with an acoustically transparent window (Fig. 2.8a). Sweeping of the beam through the tissue is performed by simply rotating the wheel, producing a circular or sector-shaped image. The transducers may all transmit at the same frequency, with all of them contributing scan lines to the image, or they may be of different frequency with only one operational at any one time. These devices are relatively inexpensive. However, as the probe contains single element transducers the beam focus is fixed and the image quality is generally inferior to more versatile multi-element transducers. Rotating transducers used to be common in low- and mid-range machines for obstetric and abdominal scanning.

PROBES WITH MECHANICALLY OSCILLATING TRANSDUCERS

These consist of a single transducer housed in an oil-filled bath with an acoustically transparent window (Fig. 2.8b). The transducer oscillates about a pivot point so that the

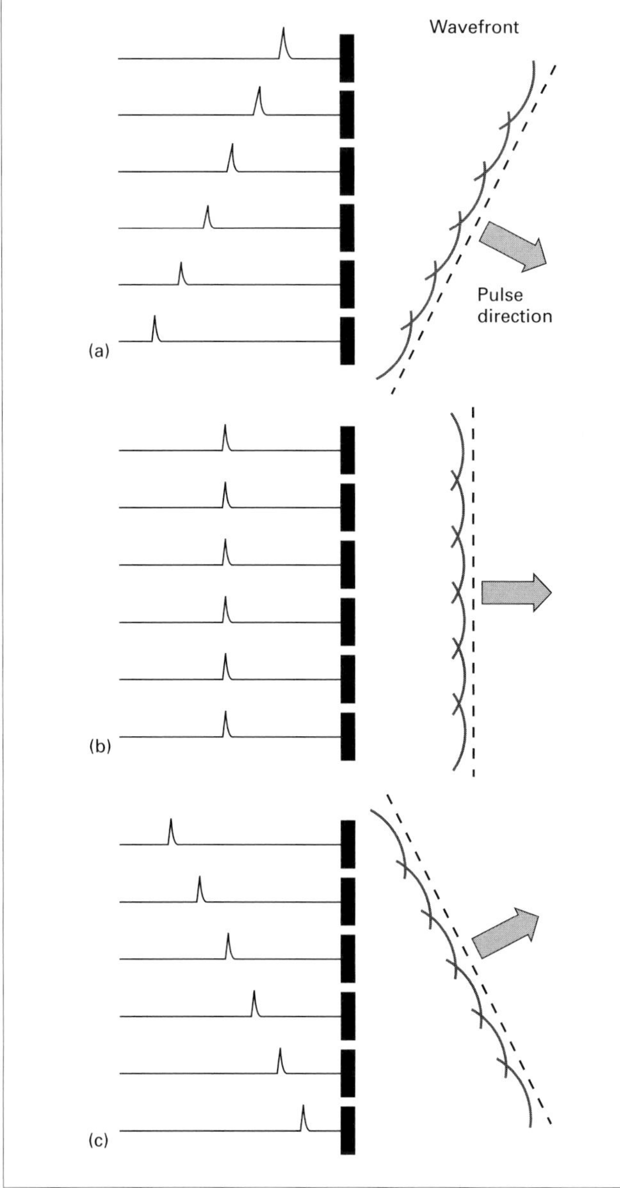

Fig. 2.7 Progressive delay in the firing of elements may be used to alter beam direction. (a) The top element fires first followed by the elements below in turn and the beam is steered downward; (b) all elements fire at the same time and the beam is directed ahead; (c) the bottom element fires first followed by the others above in turn and the beam is steered upward.

beam is swept to and fro producing a sector image. These probes are sometimes referred to as 'wobblers' for obvious reasons. Single element oscillating transducer probes are inexpensive and provide the same basic image quality as single element rotating transducer probes. Multi-element annular array probes may be made in which the single transducer consists of several concentric rings (annuli), usually five to eight in number. Electronic focusing may be applied to annular arrays, and in principle the image quality should be high as there is focusing in the scan plane and also in the plane perpendicular to the scan. In practice there are significant technical problems which restrict image quality. These are concerned with multiple reflections within the large oil bath in which the transducer sits, and the difficulty of mechanically steering a large, heavy transducer.

LINEAR AND CURVILINEAR ARRAY PROBES

Modern linear array probes consist of a line of narrow, rectangular transducer elements whose number varies typically from 64 to 500, and where the overall length of the array varies from 5 to 20 cm (Fig. 2.8c). Electronic focusing is possible and the resolution can be very good. The beam is swept through the patient by firing overlapping groups of elements in turn. The wavefronts from the linear array are generated parallel to the transducer face, and the image is thus rectangular. This image format has a wide field of view near to the transducer face and is suitable for imaging superficial structures. Applications requiring a very wide field of view must use a very wide linear array. The modern approach to this problem is to bend the linear array to form a curvilinear array (Fig. 2.8d). A large field of view at depth may then be obtained using a relatively small transducer. Curvilinear arrays are often used in abdominal and obstetric imaging.

In most linear arrays electronic focusing is active within the scan plane. Elevation focusing is performed by use of an acoustic lens, which as discussed above has a fixed focus. At the time of writing the linear arrays built by a few manufacturers consist of three rows of elements rather than one (Fig. 2.8e). This allows a degree of electronic focusing in the elevation plane, and hence improved image quality. These are called 1.5D arrays; this is to distinguish these from true 2D arrays which have many rows of elements. Clinically usable 2D arrays have proved very difficult to construct and have so far only been described in a small number of research publications.

PHASED ARRAY PROBES

Phased array probes consist of a line of rectangular elements sliced much thinner than those of linear arrays (Fig. 2.8f). These probes have a small footprint, typically they are 2–3 cm long. They are especially used where access is difficult, such as imaging of the heart or the liver through the intercostal spaces. Steering and focusing of the beam is performed electronically.

ENDOLUMINAL PROBES

All of the above probes may be used to image the patient through the external surface, usually the skin. In addition

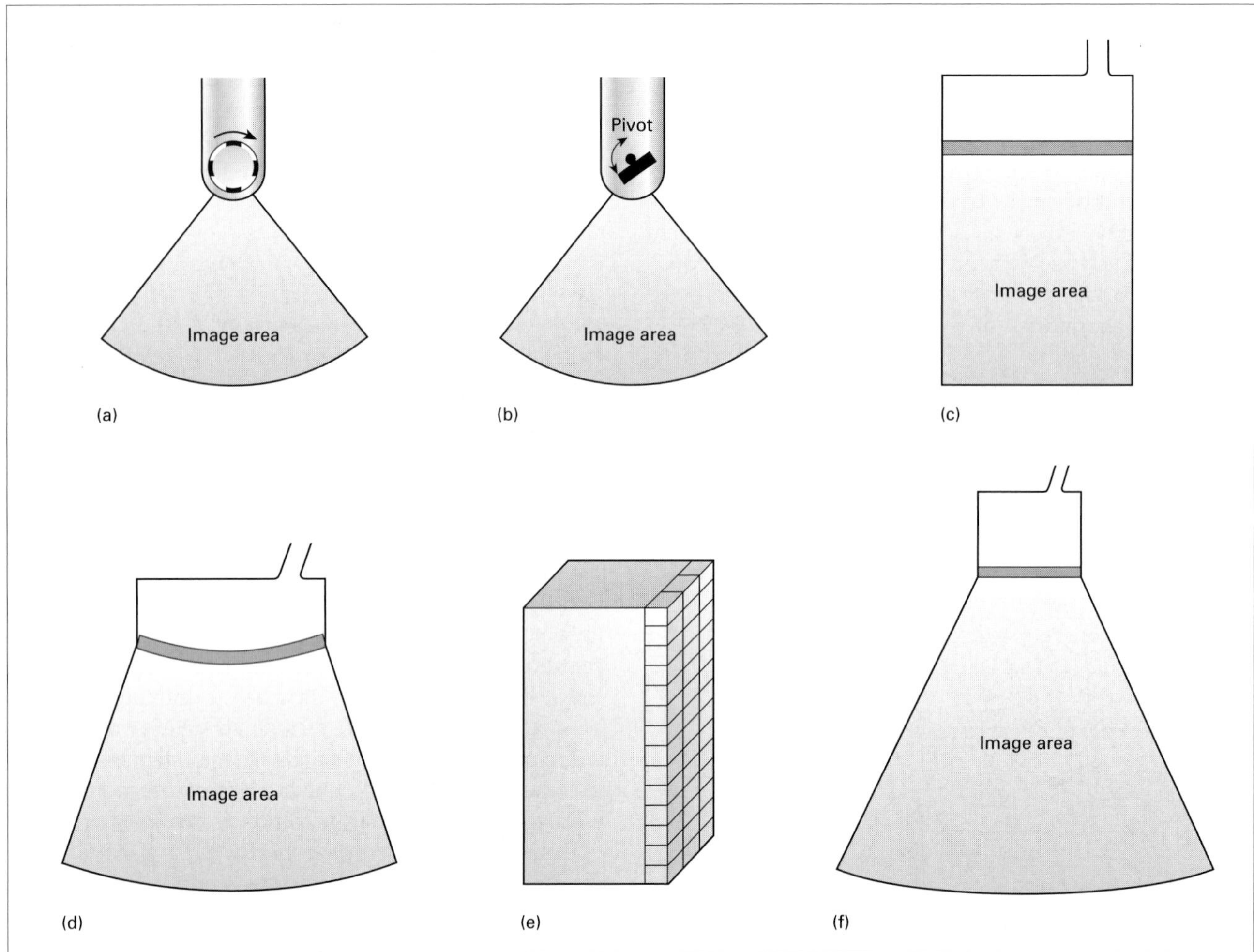

Fig. 2.8 Types of probe. (a) Mechanical rotating scanner, and field of view. (b) Mechanically oscillating scanner and field of view. (c) Linear array and field of view. (d) Curvilinear array and field of view. (e) A 1.5D array enables some degree of focusing in the elevation plane. (f) Phased array and field of view.

configurations of probe are available which may be inserted into body orifices and used to scan the patient from the inside. Such probes are termed endoluminal and include endorectal probes for imaging the rectum and prostate, intraoesophageal probes for imaging the heart and upper GI tract, transvaginal probes for imaging the cervix, uterus, ovaries, fetus and placenta, and intravascular probes for insertion into vessels, usually through arterial puncture, for imaging of vessel wall. The organ of interest for these probes is very close to the probe surface enabling the use of high frequencies, in the range 5–40 MHz, with the highest frequencies used by intravascular probes for coronary artery imaging. Simple rotating or oscillating transducer assemblies are still used in many endoluminal probes, where the restriction on size makes multi-element probes difficult to manufacture.

Image quality

Image quality is extremely important in ultrasound imaging. Considerable effort and resources have been devoted by manufacturers over the years to improve the image quality in order to be more competitive. Various aspects of image quality relevant to ultrasound scanning are covered in this section.

Lesion detection

Detection of small lesions, such as a small metastasis in the liver, is desirable. The influence of the physical properties of the lesion on detection may be illustrated using a simple test object (Fig. 2.9) [6]. Figure 2.10 shows a composite B-scan image taken of this phantom. The lesions which are most easily seen are those which are large, and whose brightness is very different compared to the surrounding background. Very small lesions are not seen as their imaged size is comparable with the pattern of noise and hence indistinguishable from the noise. Lesions which have the same brightness as the surrounding background are also not seen, regardless of their size. This simple illustration emphasizes that the ability of the operator to see the lesion of interest is fundamentally influenced by the size and acoustic properties of the lesion.

True tissue background is structured and the detection of lesions is more difficult than would be the case if the background were uniform. The ability of the observer to detect lesions improves as the lesion size increases.

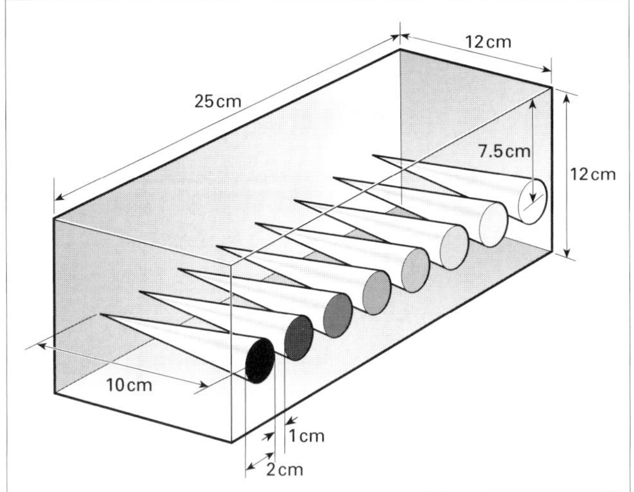

Fig. 2.9 Contrast resolution test object as described by Smith *et al.* [6].

However, when the lesion is so large that there is very little normal tissue then the observer has nothing to compare the lesion against, and the lesion may be undetected.

Perception of images is a complex procedure involving several different tasks [7].

1 Detection—the object may be observed but its shape and details within the structure cannot be distinguished. For example small specks of calcification give rise to strong echoes that can be easily observed even though the shape of the calcification cannot be made out.

2 Observation of shape—the structure is seen in sufficient detail to enable the object's shape to be seen.

3 Assessment of detailed features and texture variation within the object—for example assessment of intraplaque contents.

4 Interpretation—the operator combines the image features with his or her own knowledge of the anatomy and pathology, the end result of which is a report on the findings and their significance.

The first three of the detection tasks can be considered to be machine dependent, emphasizing that the design of a machine with high image quality is extremely desirable. The last task is operator dependent. For the inexperienced operator structures will be there to be seen, but the operator does not have sufficient knowledge to recognize them, emphasizing that training and experience are both essential.

Descriptors of image quality

A number of standard terms are used in describing images, which are defined and discussed below.

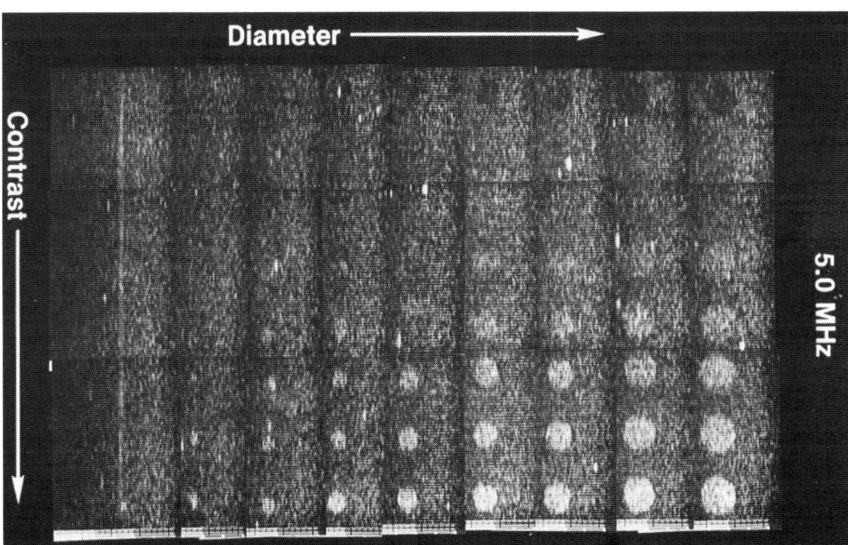

Fig. 2.10 Composite picture of B-scan images of the test object of Fig. 2.13. Along a single row all lesions are of the same contrast, and along a column all lesions are of the same size. The most easily seen lesions are those of high contrast and high diameter. Lesions which are small, or which have low contrast, are not distinguishable from the image noise.

CONTRAST

In order to be seen on an ultrasound image the ultrasound backscattered from an object must in some way be different to the ultrasound backscattered from the surrounding tissue. The image contrast refers to the difference in brightness levels between the image of the tissue of interest and the image of the surrounding tissue.

CONTRAST RESOLUTION

This is the ability of the observer to distinguish between regions of different average brightness; for example between liver and focal lesions. In ultrasound imaging, there is an important distinction to be made between objects which are high contrast relative to surrounding tissues, and those which are low contrast. Images of small low contrast objects (for example, cysts or some metastases) may fill in with echoes from surrounding tissues due to the finite width of the ultrasound beam. This may make them totally undetectable. Conversely, the image of a small high contrast lesion (for example, calculi or gas bubbles) will always be visible.

SPATIAL RESOLUTION

Many structures of interest in the body are small, such as fetal vessels and regions of arterial plaque, and it is desirable to be able to assess these using ultrasound scanning. All imaging systems lose detail to some extent. This may be most easily understood with respect to a very small reflective point object. The image of this is not a point, but is larger (Fig. 2.11). The size of the image of the point target is a measure of the spatial resolution of the ultrasound scanner. The spatial resolution along the beam axis is termed axial resolution. At 90° to the beam axis the resolution within the scan plane is termed lateral resolution, and at 90° to the scan plane is termed the azimuthal or elevation resolution.

TEMPORAL RESOLUTION

This is the ability to distinguish between different events in time.

RANDOM NOISE

Random noise refers to any signal that causes random variations in brightness level at any point in the image. These tend to obscure the detection of structures of interest. In ultrasonic imaging there are two sources of noise, acoustic and electronic. The acoustic noise varies with position in the image and is referred to as speckle. Electronic noise varies randomly with position in the image and with time.

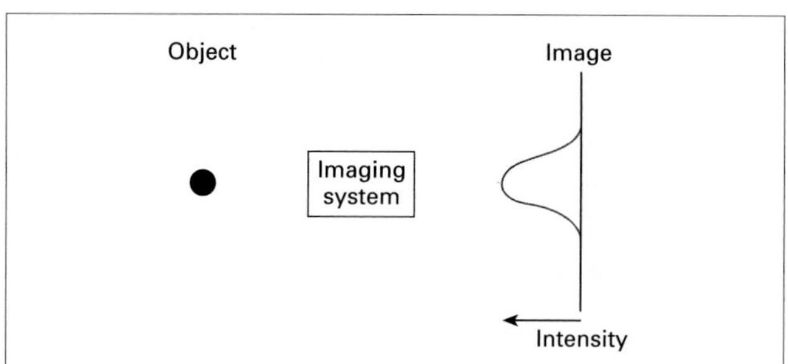

Fig. 2.11 Spatial resolution; a point object will produce a disc-shaped region on the image, the same shape as the ultrasound pulse.

Physical factors affecting image quality

Image quality is determined by several fundamental physical limitations as well as the design of the machine. These factors are considered in this section.

FREQUENCY

The width and length of the ultrasound pulse may be made shorter by the use of higher frequencies of ultrasound, which leads to improved spatial resolution. However, ultrasound is strongly attenuated in tissue and the attenuation increases as the frequency of the ultrasound increases. At the limit of viewing the echoes will have been attenuated by more than 100 dB relative to echoes from very superficial structures. Beyond this point the acoustic echoes returning to the probe give rise to voltage signals whose size is smaller than the electronic noise level within the circuitry of the scanner, and hence no sensible ultrasound image may be seen. A compromise must therefore be reached between spatial resolution and the maximum depth from which echoes can be obtained. In practice, a probe with a centre frequency of 3.5 MHz might be expected to have a useful field of view down to 20–25 cm, a 5 MHz probe to 10–15 cm and a 10 MHz probe to 3–4 cm.

PULSE LENGTH AND BEAM SHAPE

The highest spatial resolution will be obtained when the pulse length is short (to give best axial resolution), and when the beam width in the scan plane and the slice thickness are narrow (to give best lateral resolution and elevation resolution). There is blurring of images caused by finite spatial resolution, and also loss of tissue contrast.

FRAME RATE AND PERSISTENCE

The temporal resolution is determined by the frame rate and the amount of frame averaging. Maximum imaging frame rates are now greater than 100 s^{-1}; without frame averaging this gives a temporal resolution of 10 ms. Frame rate is highest when the depth and width of the field of view used are minimum. For most real-time scanning in abdominal and obstetric work, a frame rate of 20–30 s^{-1} is adequate. If measurements are to be made of the motions of cardiac valves then a much higher frame rate is needed, and the use of M-mode ultrasound is preferable. In M-mode ultrasound all the pulses are directed along one scan line. This gives very good temporal resolution of down to about 0.1 ms for the smallest depth of field in paediatric examinations.

Frame averaging is a very effective way of reducing image noise. However, it results in a reduction in the temporal resolution. To the operator the image will demonstrate a distinct lag. For some applications such as early fetal heart detection even relatively small amounts of frame averaging may be unacceptable. Many scanners do have a control that allows the amount of frame averaging to be adjusted.

ACOUSTIC NOISE

On all ultrasound images there is a spatially fluctuating signal known as speckle. This is similar in some ways to laser speckle, and results from sound being scattered by many very small scatterers within the ultrasound pulse volume. Within uniform parenchyma ultrasound is scattered from many small inhomogeneities in density and elasticity. It is not known in any biological detail what these are. The tiny echoes from the many scatterers within the volume of the ultrasound pulse undergo constructive and destructive wave interference when they arrive at the transducer. The speckle pattern which is produced reduces the contrast resolution of the image. The appearance of speckle is affected by the wavelength of the ultrasound, the aperture of the transducer and the position of the transducer. Because the speckle pattern does not alter with time if the transducer and tissue remain stationary, the tissue appears to have a cellular structure. The speckle dimensions are similar to those of the ultrasound pulse. The speckle artefact is hard to remove, although some scanners do have effective techniques for speckle reduction.

ELECTRONIC NOISE

This is generated by sources that are both internal and external to the scanner. The high gain required to amplify very small, deep echo signals also amplifies the small amounts of electrical thermal (and other) noise present in any electronic circuit. A fuzz of electronic noise can almost always be seen in the deepest parts of an ultrasound image. Because blips of internal electronic noise occur randomly in time (and therefore in random positions on the ultrasound image), the signal-to-noise ratio of the image can be improved by frame averaging.

Ultrasound scanners are very sensitive detectors of radiofrequency signals. Unfortunately, such signals are generated in abundance by many modern devices; computers and networking cables, faulty fluorescent lights, digital telephone exchanges, mobile phones, radio broadcasts, electromechanical pumps, switches and motors. This type of noise can be very intrusive. There is little that can be done to remedy this, except to distance the scanner from the source of noise, or to eliminate the source. Some scanners are more sensitive to external noise than others, so wherever possible, it is worth testing a scanner in the location in which it will be used.

Artefacts

An artefact may be defined as any image appearance which is not a genuine representation of a physical structure. In this respect noise may be considered to be an artefact. In general, noise in imaging systems is related to the random variations in image values, and hence their temporal or spatial behaviour may be characterized statistically. Other forms of artefact cause more defined local appearances. In addition to acoustic and electronic noise, there are a number of other artefacts of ultrasound imaging, the most common of which are listed below.

REFRACTION

If there is a difference in the velocity of sound between two adjacent tissues then the direction of travel of the ultrasound pulse will be deviated at the boundary (Fig. 2.12). The only situation where this effect is not apparent is when the pulse travels perpendicular to the boundary. The scanner assumes that the pulse moves in a straight line at a constant speed of 1540 m s^{-1}. Variations in the speed of sound in tissue and subsequent refraction of the pulse will cause some structures to be displayed at incorrect positions in the image. This effect is usually only slight. It is most severe at bone/soft tissue interfaces where deviations as large as 20° can occur.

ACOUSTIC ENHANCEMENT

This is the increase in brightness seen behind a low attenuation region (often a fluid-filled structure; Fig. 2.13). It

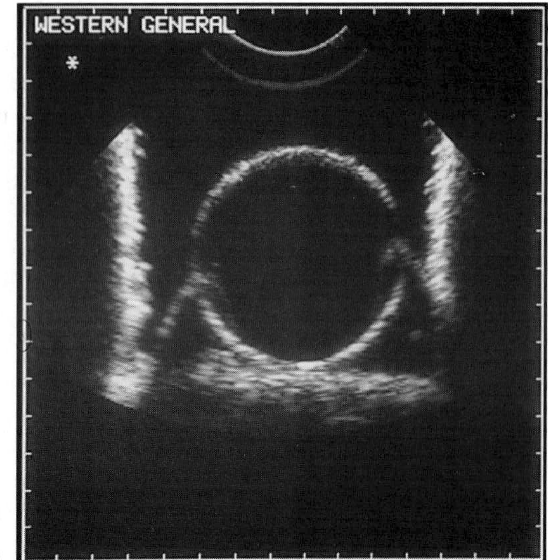

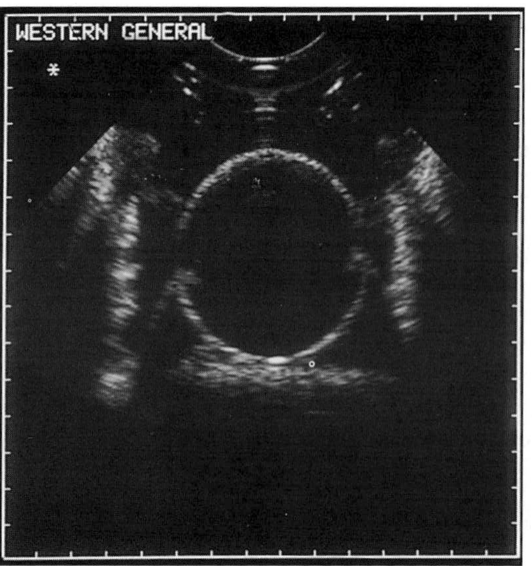

Fig. 2.12 Refraction artefact. (a) Undistorted image of a cylinder in a water tank; and (b) cylinder scanned through a perspex plate at which there has been refraction of the beam causing a shift in the beam direction, resulting in the cylinder appearing squashed in the horizontal direction.

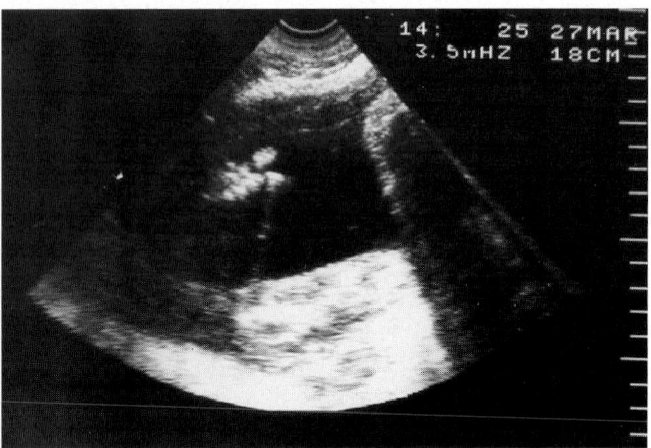

Fig. 2.13 Acoustic enhancement distal to a pool of liquor.

occurs because the TGC is set to compensate for attenuation in surrounding tissue, so that echoes returning from behind a low attenuation region are amplified more than necessary. In fact, this can be a useful way of detecting fluid-filled structures. Enhancement occurs behind large blood vessels, amniotic fluid, cerebrospinal fluid and urine.

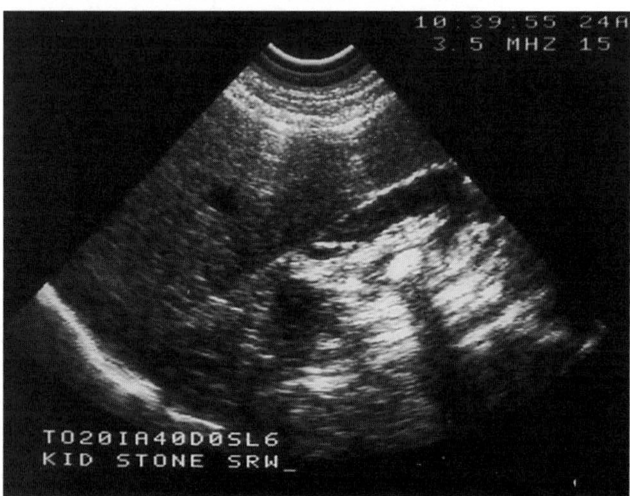

Fig. 2.14 Acoustic shadowing distal to a renal calculus.

ACOUSTIC SHADOWING

This is the converse of acoustic enhancement. When a highly attenuating object is encountered by the ultrasound beam, smaller echoes are produced from greater depths. The TGC is set to compensate for attenuation in surrounding tissue. Echoes returning from behind the high attenuation region are not amplified enough. The object appears to cast a shadow behind itself (Fig. 2.14).

MULTIPLE REFLECTION

When two strongly reflecting surfaces lie parallel to each other, and the ultrasound beam is incident at 90° to these

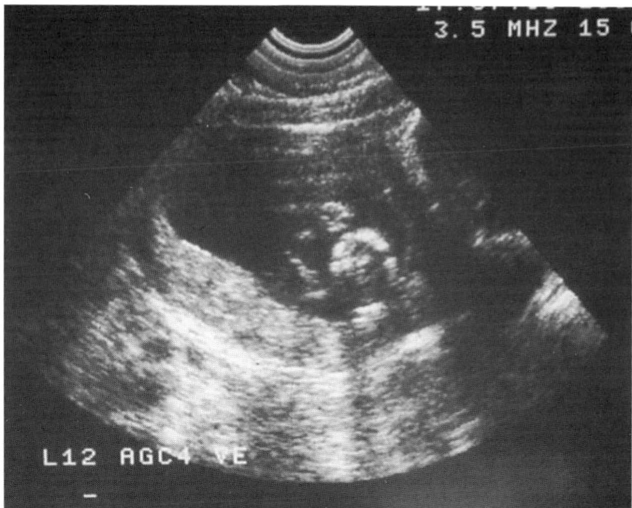

Fig. 2.15 Multiple reflection artefact between layers of tissue visible in the liquor.

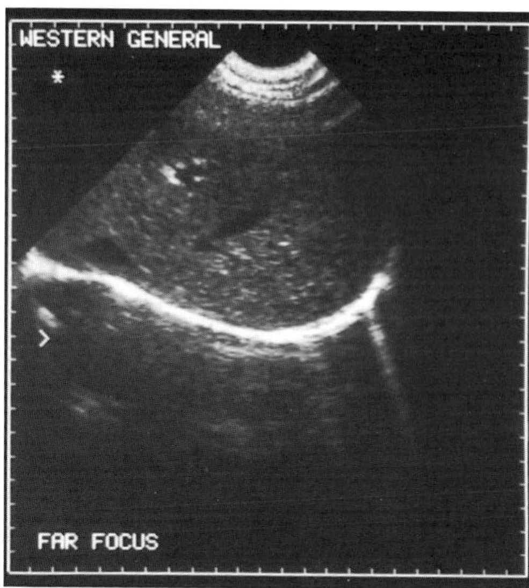

Fig. 2.16 Mirror artefact behind the diaphragm.

surfaces, the sound can bounce back and forth between the layers. Echoes from these multiple reflections return to the transducer later than the direct echoes, and appear in the image as interfaces deeper in the body (Fig. 2.15). Multiple reflections can also occur between the transducer face and one strongly reflecting interface in the body.

MIRROR EFFECT

A strongly reflecting interface such as the diaphragm can act like a mirror—the vessels and ducts in the liver (in front of the diaphragm) appear also in the mirror image behind the diaphragm (Fig. 2.16).

SIDE LOBE AND GRATING LOBE SIGNALS

In addition to the strong main beam (also called the main lobe), a transducer transmits two or more much weaker beams, on either side of the main beam. These are the result of diffraction and interference effects, either between different parts of a single element transducer (side lobes) or between the different elements of a transducer array (grating lobes). A number of techniques are employed by manufacturers to minimize the amplitude of side lobes and grating lobes. Strong side or grating lobes result in spurious multiple echoes in the image on either side of the true echo position (Fig. 2.17). Some phased arrays and annular arrays are prone to this.

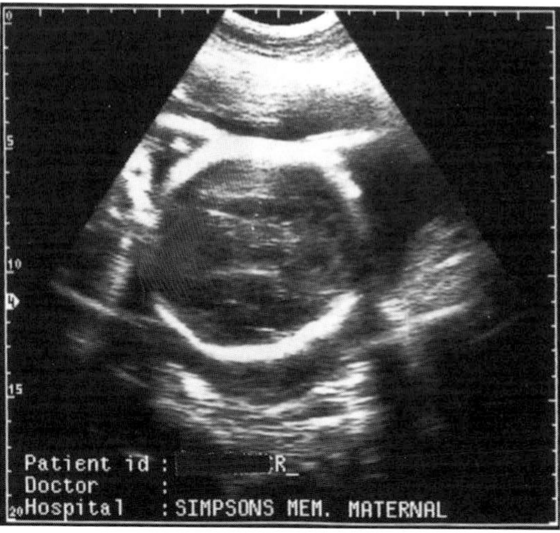

Fig. 2.17 Side lobe artefacts, visible on either side of the fetal skull.

Using a scanner

Before beginning to scan there are a number of parameters which must be considered by the operator.

WHICH PROBE?

A modern machine may have a choice of up to 20 probes for purchase. Typically one to four probes may have been purchased dependent on the types of examinations regularly performed. Specialist probes are available for applications such as transvaginal, rectal and intravascular scanning. For these probes the choice is more restricted. In transcutaneous scanning the choice of footprint and probe frequency are important. A small footprint is needed where access is difficult, such as in imaging the heart, whereas in other applications such as fetal scanning it is important to have a broad field of view from the skin surface downwards. The probe's frequency range dictates the useful depth of the field of view. From the available probes the operator selects the one suitable for the examination to be performed.

SCANNING FREQUENCY

For probes incorporating unmodified PZT the probe is designed to be sensitive over a restricted range of frequencies, and different probes must be used for different frequencies (see above). For wide-band probes, after selecting the probe, the user may also be able to select the transmit frequency. The general rule is to use the highest possible frequency for the penetration depth required in order to obtain an image with the greatest spatial resolution.

Typical probes incorporating unmodified PZT operate at centre frequencies of 3.5, 5 or 7.5 MHz. Broad-band probes deliver frequencies between 2–5 MHz and 4–8 MHz.

FIELD OF VIEW

The depth of the field of view may be altered as desired. Some machines offer a zoom facility. This can be useful if detailed examination of a particular region is required. The zoom may be passive in that zooming produces no change in the scan line density: there is simply a magnification of the image already stored in the image memory. In this case the zoom is an image zoom only and there will be scanning outside of the viewed area. Other machines offer active zoom in which the scanned area is restricted to the zoomed region and there is an increase in line density with a commensurate improvement in image quality.

TRANSMIT FOCUS POSITION AND NUMBER OF TRANSMIT FOCUSES

For those probes using electronic focusing the transmission focal depth should be adjusted as required. If a high frame rate is not important several focal zones may be placed to give optimum focusing over a range of depths.

OUTPUT POWER AND OVERALL RECEIVER GAIN

In general to avoid the use of high ultrasound intensities it is recommended that the overall receiver gain be set to its maximum value, and the power increased until the image quality is satisfactory. Operators should familiarize themselves with the acoustic output information contained in the scanner's user manual, or displayed in real-time on the screen. This will help to minimize patient exposure without compromising the diagnostic quality of the image.

TGC

The TGC controls (usually a series of sliding controls) should be adjusted to provide an evenly balanced image in which similar tissues have similar brightness at different depths. For uniform tissue this will mean that the gain is low near to the surface and increases with depth. If there are fluid-filled areas, such as the bladder or ventricles in which there is little ultrasound attenuation, it is better to leave the gain unchanged over the relevant depths. Operators should be aware of the difference between the two commonly used types of TGC control. In systems with a preprogrammed TGC curve all the sliders are initially centrally positioned. In other systems there is no preprogrammed TGC curve and the top slider must be positioned at the extreme left, and the bottom slider much further to the right.

SOFTWARE APPLICATION MENU

The initial settings for most scan parameters are often incorporated into an application menu. Usually a series of preset applications are provided by the company, and further applications can be set up by the operator. This is a useful feature and comes into its own for colour flow and spectral Doppler where there are a very large number of machine factors affecting the image. After selection of the appropriate application the user must then alter relevant controls if necessary for individual patients.

OTHER CONTROLS

Some modern machines allow a very high degree of operator control over the image parameters using software-driven menus. Frame averaging, line density, sector size and grey-scale mapping may all be controlled. These controls usually come preset for particular applications as discussed above, and it is not usually necessary to alter them during routine clinical use.

Measurements

Measurements made

As B-scan images are 2D in nature, the most widely used measurements are those of distance and area. As 3D imaging becomes more popular it is likely that measurements of volume may also become common. At present estimation of volume relies on measurements of 2D images; volume is then estimated by assuming that the organ has a regular shape. In routine practice measurements are compared against the range of values normally encountered, accounting for relevant factors such as age and sex.

Systems used for measurements

MANUAL MEASUREMENT

The preferred method at present is manual placement of graphical cursors on the frozen B-scan image. Placement of two cursors at the extreme ends of the object allows distance to be measured (Fig. 2.18). For circumference and area measurements there are two widely used methods. The first is for the operator to manually mark multiple points around the perimeter of the object (Fig. 2.19). The machine automatically joins adjacent points with straight lines. The circumference is calculated from the sum of the individual lines, and the area from the number of pixels within the enclosed region. The second method which is commonly used is for the machine to assume that the structure of interest is an ellipse. The ellipse may be anchored at two fixed points, defined by the operator. The line joining these points then forms one axis of the ellipse. The second axis is then adjusted by the operator until the ellipse coincides as closely as possible with the perimeter of the structure of interest.

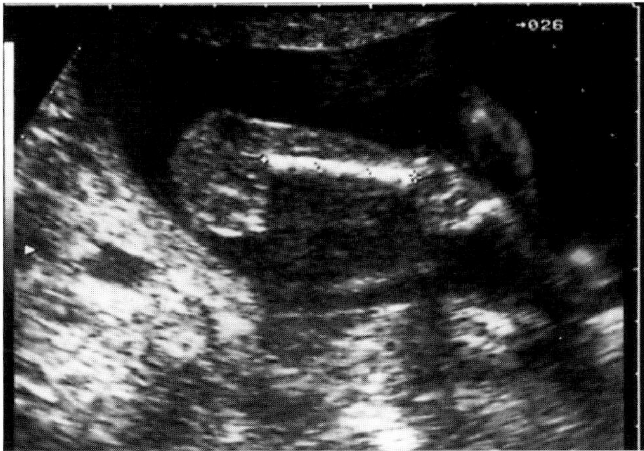

Fig. 2.18 Measurement of fetal limb length by placement of cursors at the extreme ends of the limb.

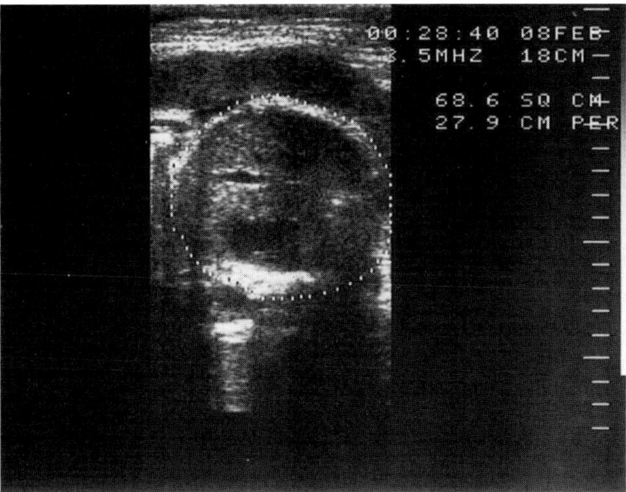

Fig. 2.19 Multiple points placed around the fetal head.

AUTOMATIC MEASUREMENT

Although most measurements which are currently performed use manual cursor placement, it is likely that the future will see more widespread use of systems which automatically measure organ dimensions. The advantage to the operator is that the measurements will be made more rapidly and with greater accuracy than is possible using manual systems. The first steps in this direction have been taken with 3D ultrasound of the heart, in which sequential 2D images are acquired by rotating the transducer through 180°.

Measurement accuracy and precision

A number of factors will influence accuracy and precision; not all of these will be under the control of the operator.

1 Measurement system. For irregularly shaped structures it is most appropriate to use a tracing algorithm rather than one which assumes a particular shape (such as the ellipse method described above). The accuracy and precision improve as the number of points marked increases. Most machines will calculate the distance as the distance between points; however, some have been reported to calculate the distance as a pixel-by-pixel distance, resulting in overestimation of circumference by 15% [8].

2 Spatial resolution. Images of small objects taken on machines with poor spatial resolution will appear to be larger than on machines with good spatial resolution. Measurements in the fetal femur suggest that this is a small effect causing a change in dimension of 1 mm or so [9].

3 Image registration. The direction of transmission of the beam must be correctly registered on the screen.

4 Acoustic velocity. There are always small errors introduced into clinical ultrasound images because of small differences in the speed of sound in different soft tissues. The scanner assumes a speed of sound of $1540\,m\,s^{-1}$. Deviations from this in most tissues of interest are less than $60\,m\,s^{-1}$ (Table 2.1). This may cause an error in measurements along the beam axis of about 4%. A larger effect may occur in the measurement of fetal femur length. If the femur is aligned with the beam then it will appear to foreshorten due to the high acoustic velocity within the fetal bone. Refraction at tissue boundaries may also cause errors of measurement in the lateral direction of typically 1 or 2%.

Table 2.1 Accuracy and precision of measurements

Measurement	Accuracy	Precision
Linear distance (based on a true value of 10 cm)	±1.5 mm (1.5%)	0.5 mm (0.5%)
Circumference (based on a true value of 30 cm)	±9 mm (3%)	1 mm (0.3%)
Area (based on a 10 cm diameter object)	±3 cm^2 (4%)	1 cm^2 (1%)

Table 2.1 summarizes the accuracy and precision which can be expected using careful techniques. These values ignore the errors produced by minor differences in acoustic properties of different tissues.

Quality assurance

Quality and the operator

In its widest sense quality assurance is a procedure carried out in order to ensure that a certain outcome is achieved to a particular standard. For ultrasound scanning this implies that there is an appropriate quality strategy in place at all levels in the ultrasound department, involving all relevant staff.

The operator should adopt the following practices to help maintain standards.

1 Take care to drive the scanner correctly. Proper training is essential and this involves both clinical knowledge and a thorough understanding of the function and operation of the scanner controls.

2 Awareness of skill level. The operator should never attempt to offer supposed expertise in an area where they have not been adequately trained.

3 Awareness of the limitations of the machine. Machines differ significantly in image quality; usually there is a proportional relationship with machine price.

4 Be sceptical when interpreting quantitative results. The user should ensure that the measurements made are sufficiently accurate and precise.

5 Ensure that reference ranges used in the interpretation of quantitative results are appropriate for the locally used methodologies and the local population.

Quality and the machine

It is common to perform testing of machines using dedicated test objects. Various levels of testing can be defined.

FULL OBJECTIVE COMPARISON BETWEEN MACHINES

This can be a difficult area as it is not possible to test all aspects of ultrasound machine performance using test objects. In practice some quantities may be measured using well-established procedures and techniques. Such work needs the expertise of a specialist centre, who have knowledge of the test objects and in some cases can alter the machine settings internally. Comparison of machines has been performed using the results of test object assessment [10], where the measured quantities such as spatial resolution did not correlate well with the clinically perceived image quality. The use of test objects to compare the image quality of machines is a subject still under development.

LIMITED TESTING OF MACHINE ACCURACY

In some cases the test objects and procedures have been developed sufficiently to allow objective measurements of machine parameters to be made in the hospital setting. This usually means that the local medical physics department will be involved in providing the appropriate level of expertise, either to perform the tests themselves or to assist operators in establishing their own procedures. Examples of limited testing are: the checking of calliper accuracy for distance and area measurements using a test object containing parallel wires at known separations immersed in a medium with a velocity of 1540 $m\,s^{-1}$.

MONITORING

A change in performance can often be monitored in situations where absolute measurements are not possible. This may be useful in picking up machine faults. As the question of comparison with other machines is not of interest, the test objects and procedures which are used tend to be simpler. Commonly, baseline values are established at purchase and then routine tests are made on a regular basis. An example might be imaging a uniform block of tissue mimicking material, looking for penetration depth and image uniformity.

Test objects and tests

Several test objects are used routinely. These may be divided into those which assess some aspect of image quality, and those which test the accuracy of quantitative measurements. It is not the purpose of this book to go into great detail about test object design features and tests which may be performed. This is covered in Price *et al.* [11]. Table 2.2 lists those tests considered useful, along

Table 2.2 Test objects for testing B-scan systems

Test	Principle	Design	Commercial test objects
Penetration depth	Maximum penetration depth in tissue equivalent material	Tissue equivalent block of material	Cardiff test object; Gammex-RMI; ATS
Spatial resolution	Width of image of single line target, or separation of two line targets	Nylon or steel wires (single or pairs) at different depths, in water or tissue equivalent material	Cardiff test object; Gammex-RMI; ATS
Low contrast resolution	Observer's ability to detect lesions of different contrast and area	Discs of material of differing backscatter to surrounding medium	ATS; Gammex-RMI
Calliper accuracy	Comparison between true and measured distance/circumference/area between targets	Wire or fibre targets of known separation in medium with a sound velocity of $1540\,m\,s^{-1}$	Cardiff test object; Gammex-RMI; ATS

with the test objects which may be used to make the measurements.

Acknowledgements

Thanks to Dr H. Lopez (FDA, Rockville, USA) for providing the image of the contrast-detail test object shown in Figs 2.14 and 2.15. Thanks are due to the following people for helpful discussions and comments on drafts of this chapter: Mr N. Dudley, Dr S. Chambers and Ms V. Elliott.

Appendix: Historical perspective

1950s

The first attempt to produce A-scan devices were made and the first clinical trials took place using these devices.

1960s

Early imaging machines in the 1960s were quite primitive in that the image was formed by the operator moving a single transducer by hand over the body, so that a single image took several seconds to build up. The images depicted structure, but not movement. Indeed, movement occurring while the image was being formed would cause severe blurring—a real problem with cardiac and obstetric work. The images were black and white (bistable), showing only major organ boundaries. These are the machines from which modern scanners have developed. It is now common to refer to early machines as static B-scanners and to modern machines as real-time B-scanners or just real-time scanners. The quality of ultrasound images has improved dramatically since the 1960s.

1970s

During the 1970s real-time scanning was developed, in which the ultrasound beam from a hand-held probe was swept quickly and repetitively through the body by mechanical or electronic means. This allowed large volumes of tissue to be scanned in a short time and for tissue movement to be studied. Although designed to be hand-held, probes were large and often heavy.

During this period it was realized that low level signals which had previously been rejected as noise were in fact small echoes scattered back from parenchymal tissue. Modern scanners are designed to preserve and emphasize these low level signals.

1980s

During the 1980s advances in digital technology meant that scanners could be made smaller, more portable and relatively low cost. It became possible to use digital memory as a temporary image store (the scan converter) enabling improved stability and low noise. A much better understanding was gained of the propagation of sound in tissue, and sophisticated electronic focusing techniques were developed. Improvements in probe design made them much smaller and lighter and easier for the operator to handle during long scanning sessions.

1990s

The large leaps in B-scan technology which were a feature of the 1960s, 1970s and early 1980s have been replaced with smaller steps [4]. Commercial systems are beginning to look similar, both in design and in image quality. New transducer materials and engineering techniques have been developed, allowing the use of much wider frequency bandwidths and higher sensitivity than was previously available. This makes possible genuine multi-frequency transducers, improved contrast resolution and the display of harmonic images. Improvements in spatial resolution have been made by increasing the number of transducer elements and scan lines, increasing the computer processing power of the scanner, the use of sophisticated signal processing algorithms and the use of arrays with three or more parallel rows of elements (1.5D arrays) which enable improved elevation focusing. Increases in frame rate have been brought about by the use of complex pulse timing sequences. 3D display of ultrasound data starts to become commercially available.

One of the main features to date in this decade is the introduction of endoluminal devices. The highest frequency devices, about 40 MHz, are used to provide images of vessel wall structure from within the vessel. At present such intravascular transducers are mostly crude single transducer devices, as there are technical problems associated with the use of miniature multi-element arrays which would be required for high spatial resolution.

The future

Not all of the innovations developed to date are available on machines from every manufacturer. The future will probably see increasing consensus and convergence on the design which provides the best spatial resolution and clinical performance. The mainstay of ultrasound is the 2D scan. The display of ultrasound images in 3D has been attempted for many years. The speed of digital processing has now reached the stage where real-time display of 3D datasets is possible using surface shading and other techniques. The acquisition of real-time 3D ultrasound datasets represents a challenge for the design of transducers [12]; however, it is unclear whether this technology will have a major impact on the clinical use of ultrasound. The spatial resolution of high frequency intravascular devices should improve as the problems associated with miniature multi-element arrays are solved [13].

References

1 Fish, P.J. (1990) *Physics and Instrumentation of Diagnostic Medical Ultrasound.* Wiley, New York.
2 McDicken, W.N. (1991) *Diagnostic Ultrasonics. Principles and Use of Instruments.* Churchill Livingstone, New York.
3 Shung, K.K., Zipparo, M. (1996) Ultrasonic transducers and arrays. *IEEE Engineering in Medicine and Biology Magazine* **15**, 20–30.
4 Whittingham, T.A. (1995) Modern developments in diagnostic ultrasound I. Transducer and signal processing developments. *Radiography* **1**, 61–73.
5 Pye, S.D., Wild, S.R., McDicken, W.N. (1992) Adaptive time gain compensation for ultrasonic imaging. *Ultrasound in Medicine and Biology* **18**, 205–212.
6 Smith, S.W., Lopez, H., Bodine, W.J. (1985) Frequency independent ultrasound contrast-detail analysis. *Ultrasound in Medicine and Biology* **11**, 467–477.
7 Sharp, P.F. (1993) Display and perception of ultrasound images. In: Wells, P.N.T. (ed.) *Advances in Ultrasound Techniques and Instrumentation.* Churchill Livingstone, New York, pp. 1–18.
8 Dudley, N.J., Griffith, K. (1996) The importance of rigorous testing of circumference measuring callipers. *Ultrasound in Medicine and Biology* **22**, 1117–1119.
9 Jago, J.R., Whittingham, T.A., Heslop, R. (1994) The influence of ultrasound beam width on femur length measurements. *Ultrasound in Medicine and Biology* **20**, 699–703.
10 Metcalfe, S.C., Evans, J.A. (1992) A study of the relationship between routine ultrasound quality assurance parameters and subjective operator image assessment. *British Journal of Radiology* **65**, 570–575.
11 Price, R. (ed.) (1995) *Routine Quality Assurance of Ultrasound Imaging Systems.* IPSM, York.
12 Fenster, A., Downey, D.B. (1996) 3-D ultrasound imaging: a review. *IEEE Engineering in Medicine and Biology Magazine* **15**, 41–51.
13 Lockwood, G.R., Turnbull, D.H., Christopher, D.A., Foster, F.S. (1996) Beyond 30 MHz. *IEEE Engineering in Medicine and Biology Magazine* **15**, 60–71.
14 Reed, G.B. *et al.* (eds) (1995) *Disease of the Fetus and Newborn*, 2nd edn. Chapman and Hall, London.

Chapter 3: Spectral Doppler systems

P.R. Hoskins

Principles of spectral Doppler

What is Doppler?

Doppler ultrasound is concerned with the detection of moving blood or tissue by the use of the Doppler effect. In medical ultrasound use is made of a fixed transmitting and receiving transducer and the Doppler effect arises as a result of the motion of the blood or tissue. For blood the Doppler shift signal arises from the red cells. The Doppler effect is the change in observed frequency when there is a progressive change in path length between the transmitter and receiver of an ultrasound signal. The Doppler effect in medical ultrasound is actually composed of two steps. In the first step the probe emits ultrasound which hits the moving target (Fig. 3.1a). As the target moves towards the probe a larger number of complete waves are encountered than would be the case if the target were stationary; that is, the frequency increases. Ultrasound is scattered from the target, so in the second step the probe can be considered as a source which is moving with respect to the target (Fig. 3.1b). The same rationale applies and the probe encounters a larger number of complete waves than it would do if were stationary.

The frequency (δF) of the Doppler signal from blood moving with velocity (v) is proportional to the scatterer velocity (Fig. 3.2). Specifically:

$$\delta F = 2F\frac{v}{c}\cos\theta \qquad (1)$$

where F is the transmitted frequency, c is the speed of ultrasound and θ is the angle between the ultrasound beam axis and the direction of movement. There is no Doppler shift ($\delta F = 0$) if $\theta = 90°$ ($\cos\theta = 0$) and the Doppler shift increases as θ decreases from 90 to 0°. Using ultrasound in the frequency range 2–10 MHz, typical velocities give rise to Doppler shifts in the audible range of frequencies (50 Hz to 20 kHz).

Why use Doppler?

Many disease processes in the body result in alterations in the circulatory system. There may be gross tissue changes such as proliferation of new vessels, deposition of atheroma, plaque development in arteries and regions of infarction. Many of these changes alter the motion of the tissue, the overall blood flow and also local blood flow patterns in vessels.

The general features of ultrasound described in Chapter 2 also apply to Doppler ultrasound; the examinations are usually non-invasive, rapid, inexpensive and in general there is little risk of harm. The motion of blood is three dimensional (3D), whereas Doppler ultrasound provides information only on the component of velocity in the direction of the Doppler beam. Accurate quantitative information on true blood velocities and of volumetric blood flow is therefore difficult to obtain.

Doppler modes

A variety of Doppler systems and types of display are commonly used. Some varieties of systems to date have not been popular, such as dedicated instruments showing velocity profiles.

1 Spectral Doppler. General term referring to the display of Doppler frequency shift data in the form of a time–frequency plot.

2 Continuous wave (CW) system. Device in which ultrasound is transmitted and received continuously.

3 Pulsed wave (PW) system. Device in which ultrasound is transmitted in pulses enabling depth discrimination.

4 Duplex scanner. Device consisting of a real-time B-scanner and a pulsed wave or continuous wave Doppler; the Doppler beam direction and sample volume location are displayed on the screen.

Doppler detection

The ultrasonic signal picked up by the receiving transducer consists of the backscattered ultrasound from blood

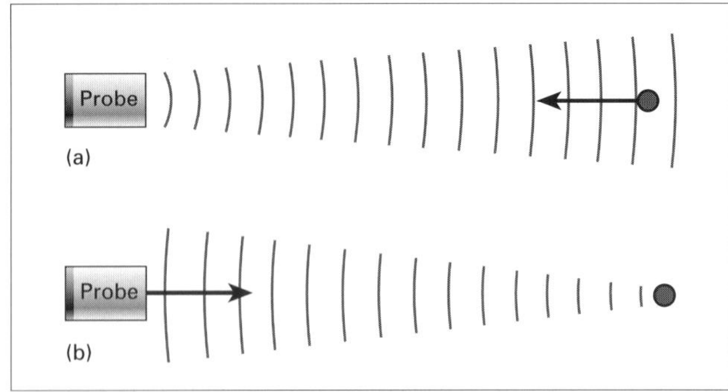

Fig. 3.1 (a) Motion of the target towards the probe causes an increase in frequency as perceived by the target; and (b) motion of the probe towards the target causes an increase in frequency as perceived by the probe.

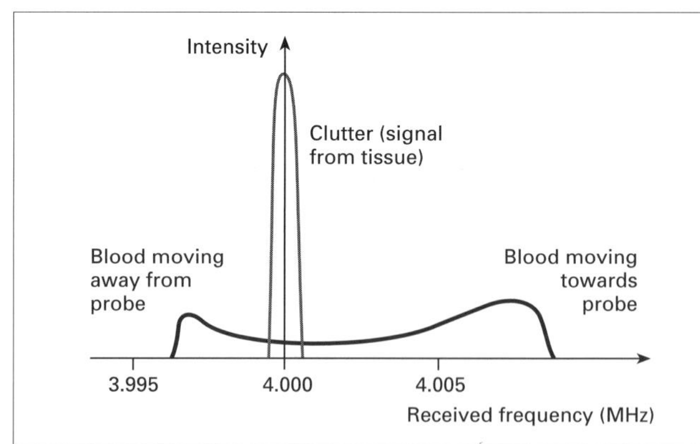

Fig. 3.3 Frequency spectrum of received ultrasound signal from a CW system.

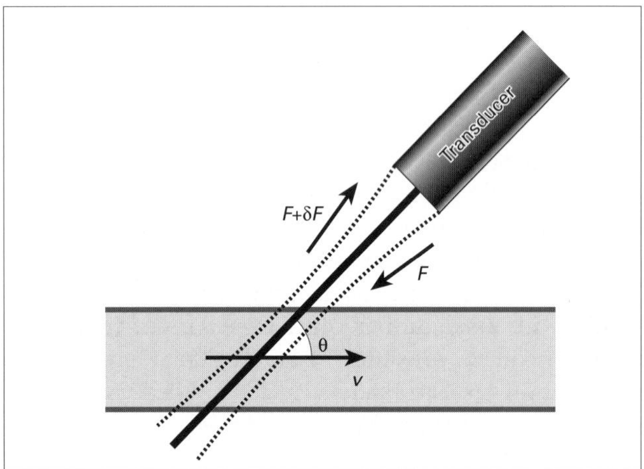

Fig. 3.2 Blood of velocity (v) moves at an angle θ with respect to the Doppler beam. The transmitted frequency is F and the received frequency is $F + \delta F$.

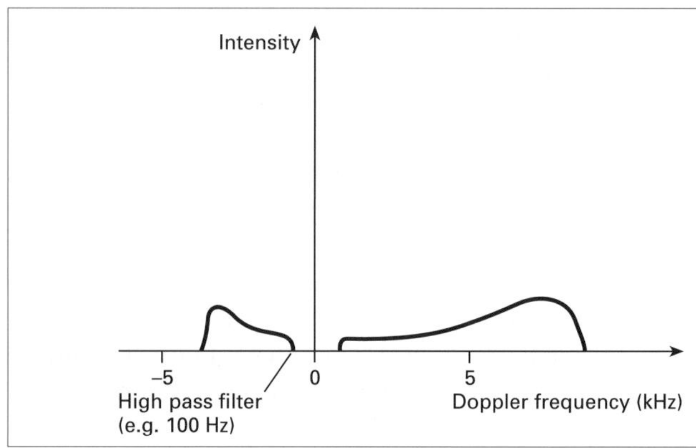

Fig. 3.4 Audio spectrum after Doppler detection and high pass filtering from a CW system.

cells, and ultrasound of much greater amplitude from other tissues (Fig. 3.3). These tissues are either stationary with respect to the transducer, such as skin, muscle and fat, or are slowly moving, such as arterial walls which pulsate, the heart and the moving fetus. Such signals are called 'clutter' and are typically 40 dB greater than those from blood. The high intensity signals from tissue, useful for formation of the B-scan image, are of no use in spectral estimation, and must be removed. The second function of the Doppler detector is to provide directional discrimination; that is, the Doppler frequency components arising from motion towards and away from the transducer must be separated.

A variety of techniques may be used for directional discrimination, of which the most commonly used method is the 'phase-quadrature' technique. The details of this are unimportant for this book, but are described in other sources such as Evans *et al.* [1].

The clutter signal is removed by the 'wall thump filter'. An unavoidable side-effect of this process is the loss of low frequency Doppler signals from slowly moving blood (Fig. 3.4). This is particularly relevant in obstetrics where the degree of diastolic flow of the umbilical artery is used as an indicator of fetal well-being. In this case typical filter levels are 50–100 Hz. In peripheral vascular applications higher filter levels of 100–200 Hz may be necessary, and in cardiology levels of 300 Hz are not uncommon.

Doppler feature estimation

The Doppler frequency shift data consists of a range of frequencies related to the range of velocities present. The amplitude of individual frequency components is related to the volume of blood moving at the corresponding velocity. There are in principle two types of data which

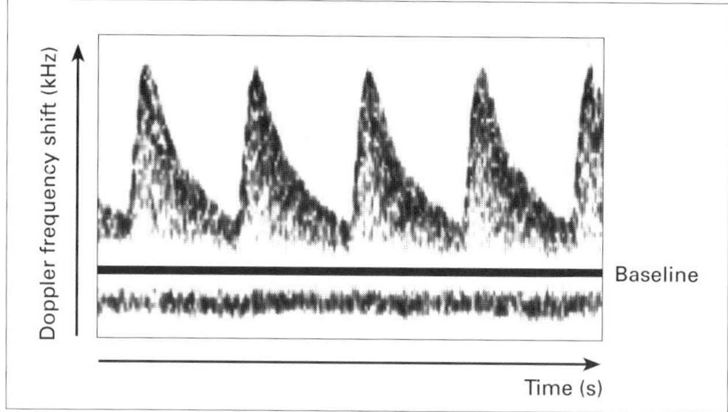

Fig. 3.5 Spectral display from the umbilical cord obtained using a 4 MHz CW system and showing arterial waveforms shown above the baseline and venous waveforms below the baseline.

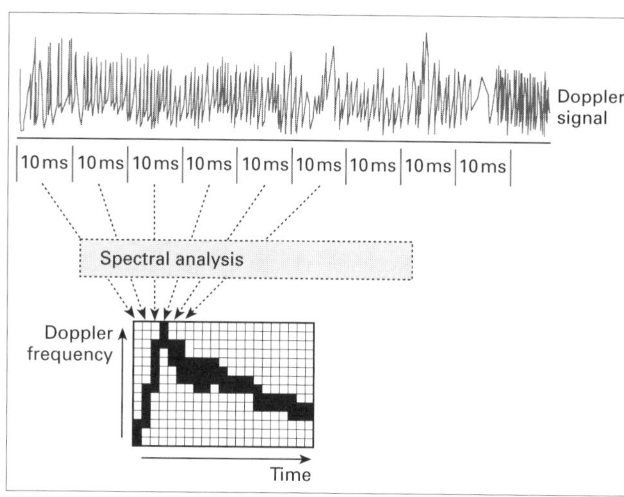

Fig. 3.6 Spectrum analysis of the audio Doppler signal.

may be extracted from the Doppler shift signal: power and frequency shift.

1 Frequency shift. Where detailed information is required concerning alterations in velocity values with time, then the Doppler shift information is analysed to give a display of frequency shift versus time.

2 Power. Typical blood flow patterns change in velocity during the cardiac cycle but not much in detected Doppler power. It was only with the advent of colour systems, in which the spatial distribution of received power could be displayed, that this feature became of interest; this is considered in Chapter 4.

The frequency content of the Doppler signal is displayed using a real-time spectrum analyser as shown in Fig. 3.5. Flow towards the probe is displayed above the baseline, and flow away from the probe below the baseline. To form the display (Fig. 3.6), the frequency spectrum of the Doppler signal within sequential or overlapping time segments of duration 2–40 ms is calculated by means of a fast Fourier transform (FFT) algorithm. The brightness of the spectral display at any time and frequency indicates the power of the Doppler signal component at that particular frequency and time. Changes in the number and location of red cells in the ultrasound beam produce fluctuations in the amplitude of the received ultrasound. This results in the structured noise seen on the Doppler spectral display, called Doppler speckle. The observer must 'edit' the noise to reveal the underlying brightness level.

It is generally accepted that examination of blood velocity waveforms is best performed by spectral display of the Doppler information. It is possible to display a single quantity related in some way to the Doppler shift frequencies as a function of time. In the early days of Doppler ultrasound it was common to use the zero-crossing detector. The output is proportional to the root mean square of the Doppler frequencies, but the exact relationship with mean frequency is dependent on the velocity profile in the vessel of interest. This is a very simple method to implement; however, the limitations, have been well documented in the literature [2–4], and these devices were discontinued. Other quantities which may be estimated from the Doppler signal and presented as a real-time trace include the maximum frequency and mean frequency. Doppler signals are often contaminated by electronic noise, high intensity signals from moving tissue, and signals from unwanted vessels. Their effect on the waveform of interest may easily be seen using real-time spectral display; however, this is much more difficult when a single trace display is used.

Other methods of spectral estimation have been attempted [5]. In practice the limitations of FFT-based spectral analysis do not appear to be great. FFT estimation of the Doppler spectrum has been widely accepted, and there is no move on the part of manufacturers to use other spectral estimation methods.

PW or CW Doppler

Comparison between CW and PW Doppler may be done by considering a single detected frequency. For a CW device the output from the Doppler detector is a single sine wave as shown in Fig. 3.7a. For a PW system the output is a series of pulses (Fig. 3.7b) which are a sampled version of the sine wave. A smooth sine wave signal is obtained by appropriate filtering. This demonstrates that the detected Doppler signals from CW and PW systems are of the same nature. In the example of Fig. 3.7b there are a large number of samples for one cycle of the sine wave which enables the underlying sine wave structure to be

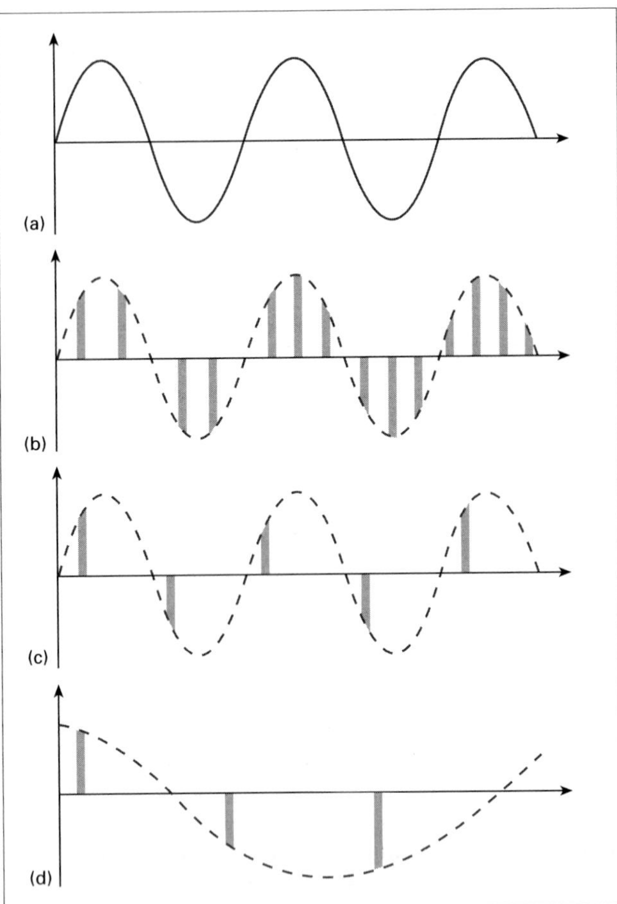

Fig. 3.7 Detected signals from a target with a single velocity under ideal conditions: (a) sine wave from CW system; (b) sampled and smoothed signal from PW system; (c) sampled and smoothed signal from a PW system in which the sampling rate is set to be at the borderline to allow proper estimation of the Doppler signal; and (d) sampled and smoothed signal from a PW system in which the sampling rate is set to be too low to allow accurate calculation of the underlying signal. (The Doppler signal is in fact sample-and-held; however, for the purposes of clarity the case for just sampling is shown.)

seen. If the number of samples falls then a point is reached where Doppler detection circuitry is unable to calculate the correct underlying frequency (Fig. 3.7c, d). The incorrect estimation of Doppler frequency for undersampled signals is called 'aliasing' and is an important limitation of PW systems; this is explored further in the section on PW devices.

Probes

In principle any of the probes used for B-scan imaging can be used for spectral Doppler. Simultaneous display of real-time B-scan and spectral data is desirable but not essential. The main limitation in this respect is the pick up of mechanical vibration. The choice of sector, convex or linear array is governed by similar considerations to those of grey-scale two-dimensional (2D) imaging—leading to the use of sector probes for cardiac and some abdominal work, convex/linear array for abdominal and small linear arrays for peripheral vascular work.

Mechanical sector probes

Vibration of the transducers is detected as an artefactual Doppler shift signal. Most mechanical sector probes freeze the motion of the probe while acquiring the Doppler spectrum, and suspend spectral analysis while updating the B-scan display. This type of updated display, with regular gaps in the spectrum is disconcerting and generally not preferred. It is possible to produce a mechanical sector probe in which the movement of the probe produces a sufficiently low intensity signal to allow simultaneous display of the B-scan image and the Doppler spectrum; however, this is not the case for most commercial systems.

Phased arrays

As there is electronic beam steering there is no vibration artefact and simultaneous display of the B-scan image and Doppler spectrum is possible, making this the probe of choice if a sector image is required. Both the B-scan and Doppler beam directions are perpendicular to the transducer face. In vessels optimum B-scan image quality is obtained with the beam perpendicular to the vessel axis, whereas optimum Doppler signals require the Doppler beam to be angled with respect to the vessel axis. Use of phased array probes therefore leads to a compromise between image quality and Doppler spectral quality. These probes are most used in cardiac and abdominal imaging, but less so in peripheral vascular imaging.

Curvilinear array

The region of interest of the curvilinear array is similar to that of the phased array and the same limitations apply.

Linear array

Linear arrays are particularly suitable for peripheral vascular scanning because they enable imaging of a reasonable length of vessels which are often running roughly parallel to the skin surface. Some linear arrays from low and mid priced machines do not steer the Doppler beam and a fluid-filled or rubber wedge is used to provide angulation with respect to the vessel. The same limitations as for phased array probes applies in that the image quality is no longer optimal. Most modern linear array probes now allow the operator to select angled beams using the same beam steering techniques used in a phased array probe, but maintaining the grey-scale imaging beams perpendicular to the probe surface. Typically, the Doppler beams may be angled at +20, 0 and −20° to the grey-scale imaging beams. The Doppler beam shape for a steered beam is usually not of the same quality as for the equivalent phased array as the width of the array elements is much larger for linear arrays than for phased arrays; the increased width will produce large grating lobes which give rise to Doppler signals from unexpected directions.

Instruments

CW Doppler instrument

The simplest ultrasonic Doppler instrument, the CW device, is shown in block diagram form in Fig. 3.8. Two transducers—one used for transmitting and the other for receiving—are mounted, as shown, in a probe. The ultrasound beams from the two transducers are arranged to overlap such that the instrument is sensitive to movement within the region of overlap, known as the sensitive beam. Focusing may be applied by shaping the end of the probe to form an acoustic lens.

Since flow direction is often important, and indeed, in many arteries the blood velocity changes direction at least once during the cardiac cycle, flow direction discrimination is incorporated in all but the simplest devices.

A major limitation of the CW instrument is that it is sensitive to flow in the whole region of overlap of the two ultrasound beams. Within the beam there is no separation of Doppler signals from two or more vessels in the beam or of signals from different points in a single vessel. The use of CW devices is therefore restricted to those vessels with well-defined velocity waveform shapes and/or well-defined locations. They are particularly suited to the detection of velocity waveforms from the peripheral vessels and umbilical arteries. Below is a summary of the features of a CW Doppler system.

1 Doppler shift cos θ dependence.
2 Ultrasound transmitted and received continuously.
3 No depth discrimination.
4 No aliasing (no upper limit to detected velocity).
5 No B-scan image for stand alone devices.
6 Stand alone systems are used for vessels with well-defined locations.
7 Stand alone systems are used for vessels with well-defined waveform shape.

PW Doppler instrument

PW Doppler systems are similar to CW Doppler systems (Fig. 3.9). The one main difference is that ultrasound is transmitted as a series of regularly spaced pulses. This allows depth discrimination in the same way that is performed for B-scan imaging; by measurement of the time between transmission of the ultrasound pulse and reception of echoes. The Doppler signal arises from a small region along the beam called the sample volume, the depth of which is selectable by the operator. The range of depths for which ultrasound signals are received may also be set by the operator. This is generally referred to as the 'gate', and refers to the electronic implementation whereby, from the point of transmission, the received ultrasound signal is blocked (gate closed), until the appropriate depth has been reached, when the gate is opened. The length of time the gate is open is the main factor which

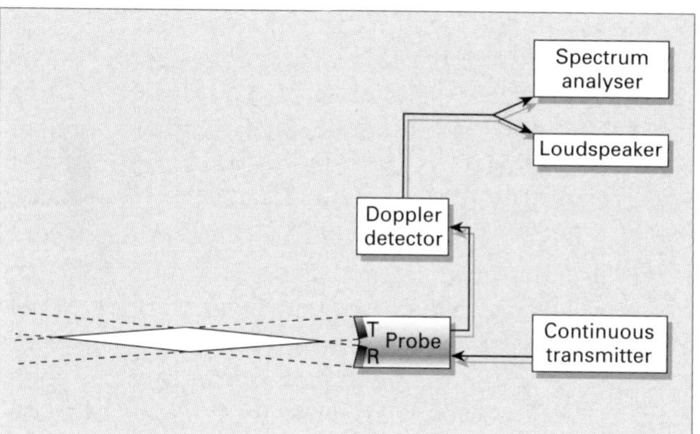

Fig. 3.8 Continuous wave instrument. R, receive; T, transmit.

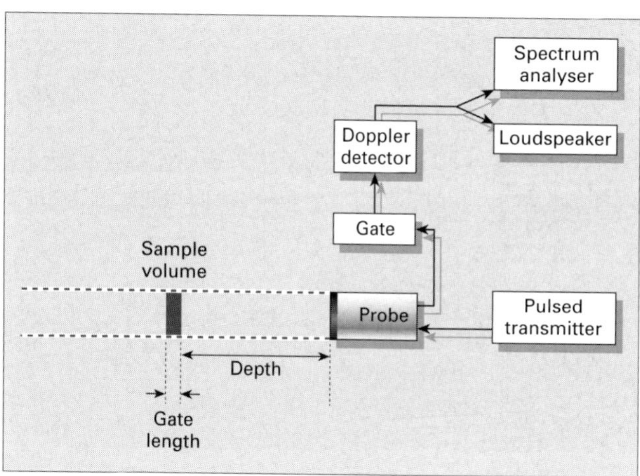

Fig. 3.9 Pulsed wave instrument.

dictates the range of depths from which Doppler signals are received. Typical gate lengths vary from 1 to 15 mm. The sample volume length is also dependent on the length of the ultrasound pulse; because of this the sample volume length is larger than the gate length. In the PW device the same transducer may be used for transmission and reception as the two processes are separated in time.

The main advantage of the PW Doppler instrument is depth discrimination. The main disadvantage is that the use of PW (rather than CW) places an upper limit on the maximum detectable Doppler shift δF_{max}. The pulse repetition frequency (prf) is the number of pulses that are transmitted per second. The maximum detectable Doppler frequency shift is

$$\delta F_{max} = prf/2 \quad (2)$$

This is a general feature of sampled signals. Frequencies above half of the prf are estimated incorrectly, and there is 'aliasing'. This is demonstrated in Fig. 3.10, which shows the spectra obtained from the same vessel at two different prf values. Doppler shift frequencies greater than prf/2 are displayed in the incorrect channel of the spectral display.

For a PW system the aliasing frequency will decrease for greater depths. This follows from the fact that a greater time must elapse for the capture of ultrasound signals from greater depths, and hence the prf must fall. There are two methods of pulse transmission commonly used. In the first the prf is fixed, and is determined by the greatest depth which may be of interest. In these systems the maximum detectable Doppler frequency is very limited. In 'high prf' systems the next pulse is transmitted as soon as the echo information from the depth of interest is received. This has the advantage of allowing the use of a higher prf, and hence of detecting higher Doppler frequency shifts, but has the disadvantage of generating multiple sample volumes within the image. Attempts to overcome the aliasing limit by signal processing are in an early stage of development, and are not yet commercially available. Below is a summary of the features of a PW Doppler system.

1 Ultrasound transmitted as pulses (prf = 1–20 kHz).
2 Depth discrimination.
3 Gate length depth and size set by user.
4 Aliasing.
5 Doppler shift $\cos\theta$ dependence.
6 Stand alone systems are used for vessels with well-defined locations.
7 Stand alone systems are used for vessels with well-defined waveform shape.

(a)

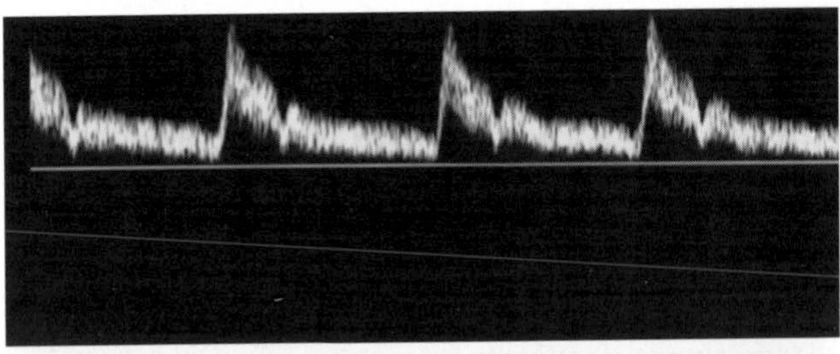

(b)

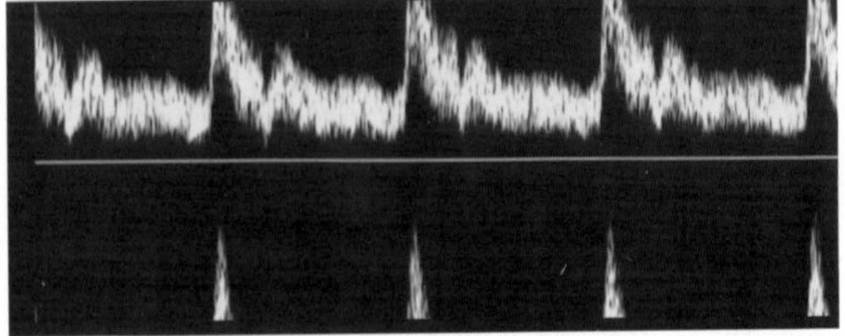

Fig. 3.10 Waveforms from the common carotid artery obtained (a) without aliasing, and (b) at a lower prf with aliasing.

Duplex instruments

A duplex system usually consists of a real-time B-scanner combined with a PW Doppler. Some duplex systems also incorporate a CW Doppler in order that high velocity signals may be acquired without aliasing. Usually the same probe is used for the B-scan image and for Doppler spectral acquisition. In addition to enabling the operator to monitor flow at specific sites in imaged blood vessels (Fig. 3.11), the instrument also enables measurement of the angle between the blood vessel and the ultrasound beam, thereby allowing a conversion from measured Doppler shift frequencies to velocities. Doppler instruments usually have a means of measuring this angle conveniently—an electronically generated marker line at the position of the sample volume may be rotated by the operator until it is lined up with the axis of the blood vessel, in which case the instrument knows the relative orientations of blood vessel and ultrasound beam and can calculate the angle between them. Flow volume may be estimated by incorporating a measurement of a blood vessel cross-sectional area using the electronic callipers of the B-scan instrument. Usually estimates are made by measuring a diameter of the blood vessel and assuming a circular cross-section.

The transmission of ultrasound pulses is time shared between the Doppler spectral display and the B-scan image. In order to produce a single spectral line 50–100 pulses are needed, whereas typically one to four pulses are required for a B-scan line. In duplex mode the majority of pulses are used for production of the Doppler spectrum. The line density and frame rate of the B-scan image may be reduced in order to obtain the largest possible prf for the Doppler spectrum. Switching off the B-scan image

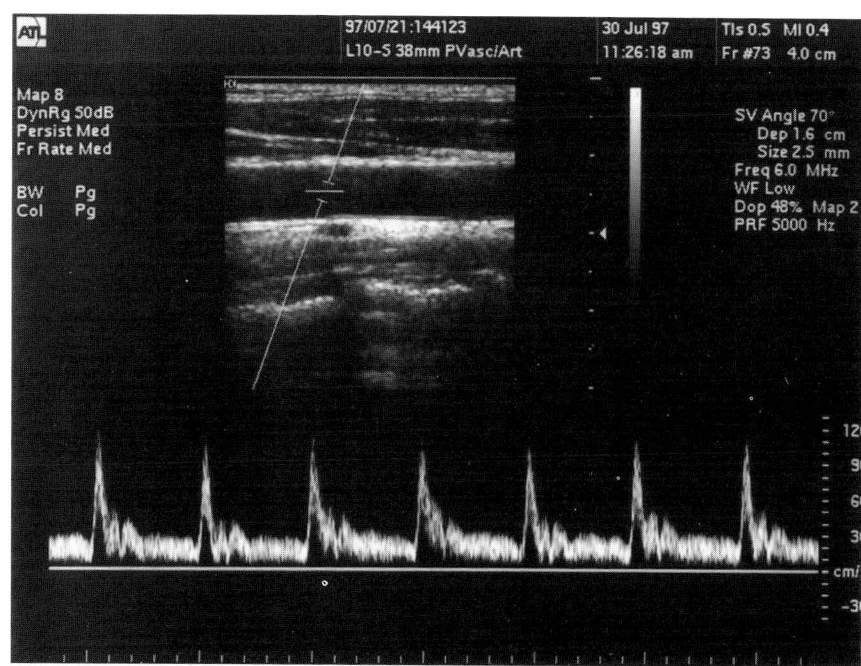

Fig. 3.11 Duplex display.

allows all pulses to be used for spectral Doppler, and may sometimes be useful. The features of a duplex system may be summarized as follows.

1 Real-time B-scan and PW and/or CW Doppler.

2 Spectral display from known vessel and location with vessel.

3 Use angle correction to convert to velocity.

Controls

Gate position. The gate position is usually controlled using a trackerball, but on some stand alone instruments the gate position is controlled by a simple dial. In high prf mode there may be more than one gate present on the image.

Gate length. The gate length is usually adjustable between about 1 and 15 mm. The usual rule, when the vessel is large, is to set the gate length to be less than the vessel diameter in order to avoid as far as possible the pick-up of wall thump signals. There are no hard and fast rules about setting gate length size, and nothing in the literature to support any one procedure, so that a common procedure is to set the gate length to about half of the vessel diameter. For small vessels this is not practical and the gate is set to encompass the vessel.

Beam steering angle. The angle between the beam and vessel may be altered by adjusting probe orientation as well as by changing the beam steering angle. For some linear array probes the point of origin of the Doppler beam from the array may be adjusted. In such systems the number of elements used to produce the beam is not constant with beam position, but is usually less when the beam is steered from the edge of the array. This results in a reduced sensitivity as well as altering the estimated velocity (as the degree of geometric spectral broadening is changed as explained in the next section).

Focal depth. There is usually only one focal depth operational when spectral Doppler is used. Some machines will automatically set the focal depth at the level of the indicated gate. If this is not performed automatically it is best to achieve this by manual adjustment of the focal depth to obtain maximum sensitivity.

Filter. The general rule is to use as low a filter level as possible in order to visualize low blood velocities. If the filter level is too high then signals from slowly moving blood will be removed. If the filter level is too low then the large amplitude signals from tissue will swamp the Doppler detector and prevent proper visualization of the true Doppler signal from blood.

Doppler gain. The gain should be adjusted so that the Doppler signal uses the full grey-scale range of the display (Fig. 3.12). If the gain is too low then the Doppler signal will not be seen, and if it is too high then saturation of the Doppler detector may cause spurious ghost signals to be produced. It should also be noted that the estimated

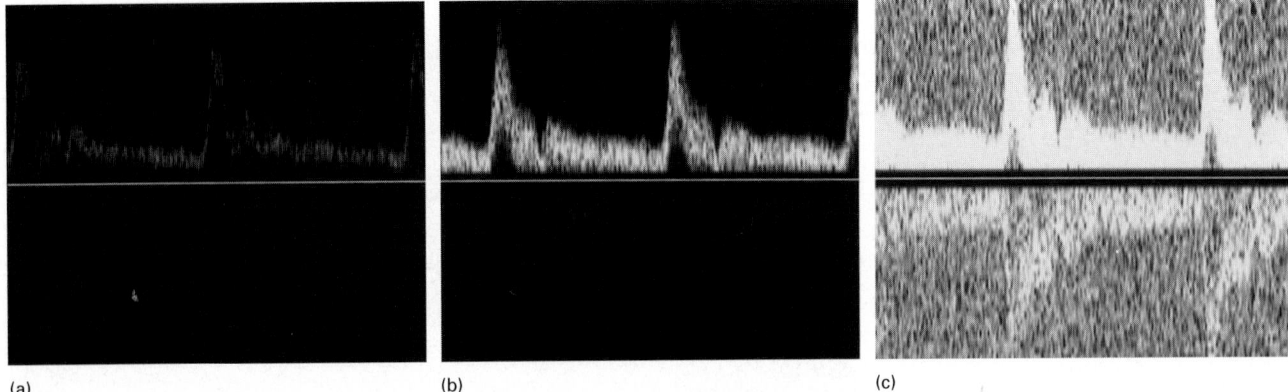

Fig. 3.12 Effect of Doppler gain on the spectral display: (a) gain too low, the waveform is hardly seen; (b) gain correct, the distribution of grey levels within the waveform is seen; and (c) gain too high, there is saturation of grey level and background noise.

velocity will be dependent on the gain setting, so that standardization of gain settings is required for reproducible velocity measurements.

Transmit power. As far as possible an adequate Doppler signal should be displayed by increasing the Doppler gain rather than increasing the transmit power.

Invert. This allows display of the spectrum in an orientation which suits the operator; usually with the forward velocity components of arteries on the upper channel, and venous signals displayed on the lower channel.

Velocity range and baseline shift. These two controls may be adjusted to obtain a spectral trace with a large enough excursion on the display; if the excursion is too small then the characteristics of the waveform may not be fully seen, and measurements obtained on tiny traces will not be of the highest accuracy.

Grey map. The grey map is usually set to linear. Alterations in the appearance of the spectral display may be produced by alteration of the grey map, e.g. by accentuating the higher amplitude signals; in practice there should be no need to alter the grey map controls.

Angle cursor. The angle cursor should be aligned with the vessel wall. In modern machines the angle cursor increments every 1 or 2°. Larger increments of 5° or so were used in older machines but do not provide adequate accuracy.

Uses of spectral Doppler

There may be a tendency to treat the spectral display as one showing only the variation in the maximum velocity with time; however, the spectral display has a grey-scale and the information below the maximum frequency outline is also useful. There are three basic types of information which can be derived from the spectral display.

1 Measurements of velocity. Usually made at particular points such as at peak systole or end diastole.
2 Measurement of waveform shape. Indices are calculated, usually from the maximum frequency trace, to provide information on the degree of diastolic flow and other waveform features.
3 Analysis of spectral broadening. The width of the displayed spectrum provides useful information.

Spectral broadening

According to the Doppler shift equation (1) shown above, a single velocity will give rise to a single Doppler frequency shift, so that if the velocities within the sample volume are all the same then the spectral display should consist of a single line at the relevant Doppler frequency. In practice the spectrum is broadened for a number of reasons as listed below.

Transducer size. The transducer producing the Doppler beam has a finite width, and therefore the single velocity subtends a range of angles (Fig. 3.13). According to equation (1) there will be a range of Doppler frequencies produced. This effect is called geometric spectral broadening and its effect is large, especially for angles near to 90° as seen in Fig. 3.14 [6].

Variation in blood motion direction. Within the sample volume the blood may be flowing at different angles with respect to the Doppler beam. Regardless of any variation in velocity the variation in angle in itself will produce

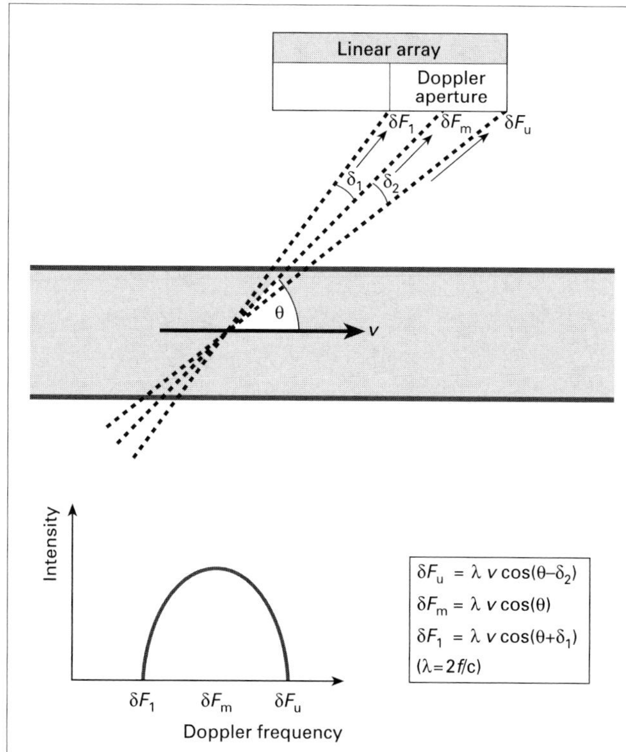

Fig. 3.13 Geometric spectral broadening. The transducer (or aperture) size is large and the velocity vector (v) subtends a range of angles at the display.

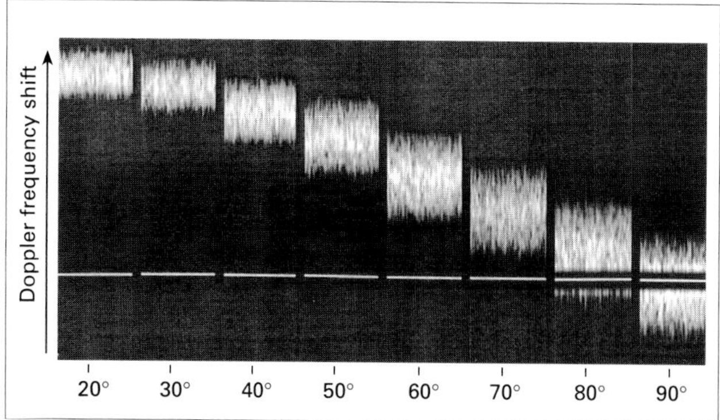

Fig. 3.14 Doppler spectra obtained at different angles from a string phantom with a single velocity. Geometric spectral broadening is seen whose magnitude increases as the angle approaches 90°.

spectral broadening. This occurs in regions of vortex shedding and turbulence.

Variation in velocities within the sample volume. If there is a velocity gradient then this will produce spectral broadening. This effect may be large, for example in a stenosis with a residual lumen of 2 mm and a maximum velocity of $5\,\mathrm{m\,s^{-1}}$, the velocity gradient is about $5\,\mathrm{m\,s^{-1}\,mm^{-1}}$. This also occurs in regions of vortex shedding and turbulence.

Other effects. Spectral broadening is also produced when velocities are changing rapidly during the period of 10 ms or so when the spectrum is being calculated; this typically occurs when blood is being rapidly accelerated or decelerated, such as in the systolic leading-edge region of Doppler waveforms [7].

It can be seen that the degree of spectral broadening depends on a large number of factors, some of which are machine dependent. This makes the quantitative use of spectral broadening as an indicator of disease difficult.

The main area in which increased spectral broadening is used as an indicator of disease is in the assessment of the degree of arterial stenosis. In the poststenotic region the flow field is complex with recirculation, vortex shedding and turbulence. These effects tend to increase the degree of spectral broadening as within the sample volume the velocity gradient is large, and there is variation in the direction of motion of different elements of blood. As the size of an intrusive lesion increases, increased spectral broadening resulting from flow disturbance usually occurs, first during the decelerative phase of systole and then spreading to the whole of the cardiac cycle.

Velocity estimation

Maximum velocity is probably the most widely estimated index using Doppler ultrasound systems. It is common to use the maximum frequency in preference to the mean frequency as it is not critically dependent on beam–vessel alignment. Knowledge is required of the angle between the beam and the direction of motion of the blood in order that the Doppler frequency shift may be converted to velocity using equation (1). The angle is measured by manual alignment of a cursor with the vessel wall; and as noted above, it is common to refer to this as the beam–vessel angle. Atherosclerosis results in narrowing of the vessel lumen, the degree of which can be estimated using the measured increase in velocity using standard tables [8,9]. There are two sources of error in velocity, both concerned with the measurement of angle.

Geometric spectral broadening. The origins of geometric spectral broadening are discussed above. Virtually all Doppler machines correct the detected Doppler shift using the angle to the centre of the Doppler aperture, whereas the maximum Doppler frequency shift is detected at the edge of the Doppler aperture (see Fig. 3.13). This leads to an overestimate in maximum velocity whose

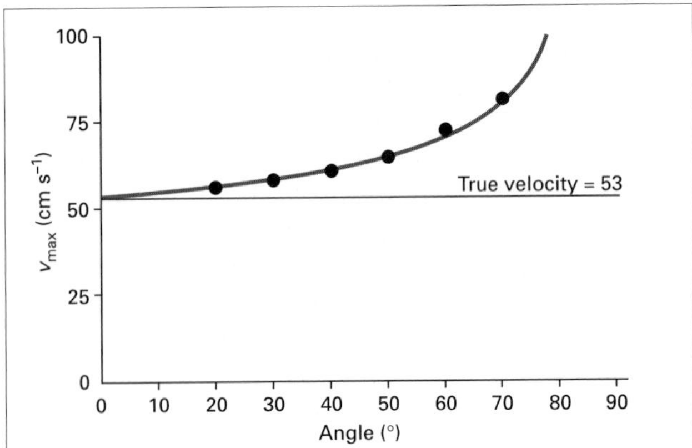

Fig. 3.15 Estimated maximum velocity as a function of beam–string angle for the waveforms shown in Fig. 3.14.

size is typically 10–60%; however, if the angle is near to 90° errors of over 100% may be easily produced (Fig. 3.15).

Measurement of true beam–vector angle. The second source or error in estimation of maximum velocity is concerned with knowledge of the angle between the direction of motion of the blood and the beam, which can be called the beam–vector angle. Conventional Doppler systems assume that the beam–vector and the beam–vessel angles are equal. However, the blood velocity will change direction as it passes through the stenosis, and this assumption cannot be made (Fig. 3.16). All current Doppler systems derive Doppler frequency shift information only from the component of velocity in the direction of the beam, and therefore these systems cannot be used to obtain accurate estimates of true beam–vector angle. Correct estimation of the magnitude and direction of blood velocities would require a system capable of measuring all three components of blood velocity (along the x, y and z axes). These are called vector Doppler systems and are not commercially available at the time of writing.

The best current advice that can be given is to use a fixed angle of 60°. This should reduce the intramachine variability, but this will not solve the problem of variation in values between machines.

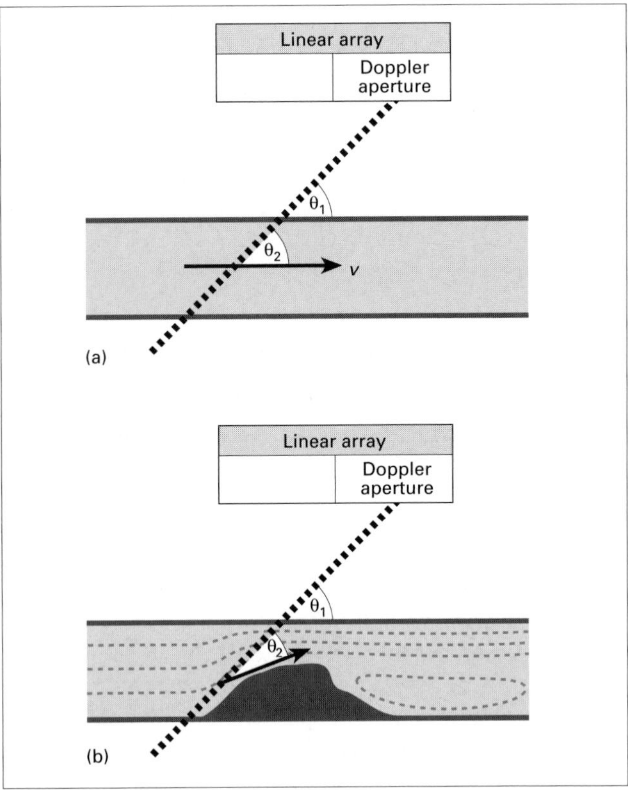

Fig. 3.16 (a) Flow is a straight tube, in which the beam–vector angle is equal to the beam–vessel angle; and (b) flow in a vessel with a stenosis in which case the beam–vector angle is not equal to the beam–vessel angle.

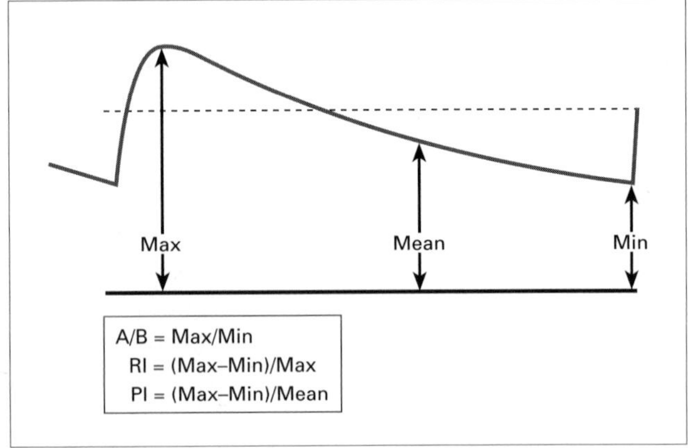

Fig. 3.17 Indices used to describe the waveform shape.

Waveform shape analysis

Analysis of the shape of the waveform can be used to provide information on disease. The simplest quantitative approach is to use indices which are related to the degree of waveform pulsatility; that is, the degree of diastolic flow. Two common indices (Fig. 3.17) are the resistance index (RI; [12]) and pulsatility index (PI; [13]). These indices are related to the degree of distal resistance to flow in some circumstances; for example this is true for arteries supplying normal musculature. In this case vasodilatation, occurring during exercise or reactive hyperaemia, produces a marked decrease in waveform pulsatility. In the fetal placental circulation there is good evidence to suggest that the increase in RI and PI of umbilical artery waveforms is related to increased placental resistance [14,15]. Advanced methods of waveform analysis have been attempted based on feature extraction (principal component analysis; [16]) or mathematical modelling (Laplace transform analysis; [17]). These methods have never passed into routine use, possibly because they do not add any more useful information than very simple indices.

Automatic and manual measurements systems

Measurements on the maximum frequency outline may be made manually or automatically. Manual methods usually involve tracing using a cursor controlled by a trackerball. This can be time-consuming and in a busy clinical setting the operator usually obtains only a few waveform values. Automatic tracing of the maximum frequency outline is attractive as it is potentially less time-consuming. Such systems present real-time values of the relevant waveform index averaged over several cardiac cycles, typically five to 15, and these systems are most popular in transcranial Doppler and obstetrics. Automatic maximum frequency estimators work reasonably well provided there is no noise of any kind above the maximum frequency (Fig. 3.18). Any kind of noise, such as random background noise, spurious electronic signals, and signals from overlying vessels, upset the algorithm and under these conditions the estimated maximum frequency is inaccurate, and the displayed index is also inaccurate.

It is best using these devices to have simultaneous displays of the Doppler spectrum and the estimated maximum frequency. Good spectral waveforms and a representative maximum frequency trace should be obtained by adjustment of the probe position and Doppler gain. Possibly the least desirable implementation is that of a real-time spectral display and waveform index values, but not the estimated maximum frequency trace. With this type of system it is not possible to see if the estimated maximum frequency trace is accurate, and hence whether or not the displayed index is reliable. Provided that care is taken in the acquisition of noise-free waveforms with good maximum frequency outlines, good results may be obtained using automated estimation of waveform indices. A summary of points concerning the use of spectral Doppler is given below.

1 Atheromatous disease is associated with increases in Doppler frequency shift and spectral width.

2 Velocity measurement:
- (a) there is no perfect beam–vessel angle below which velocity errors are small;
- (b) best current advice is to use a fixed angle of 60°;
- (c) do not expect to get the same measured velocities using different machines.

3 Waveform indices:
- (a) use the maximum frequency envelope as this is relatively independent of beam–vessel geometry;
- (b) get waveforms with a clearly defined outline;
- (c) do not always believe automatic index estimators.

Artefacts

Some of the artefacts observed in spectral Doppler are similar to those found in 2D grey-scale imaging—the shadowing arising from bowel gas in abdominal scanning or from calcified plaque in the blood vessel, for example. There are other artefacts which are specific to

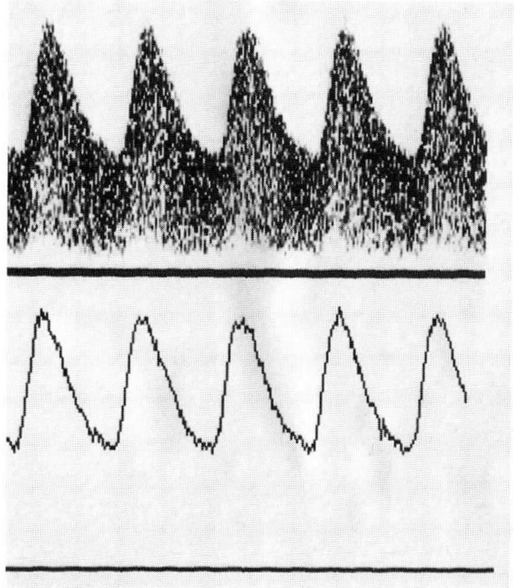

(a)

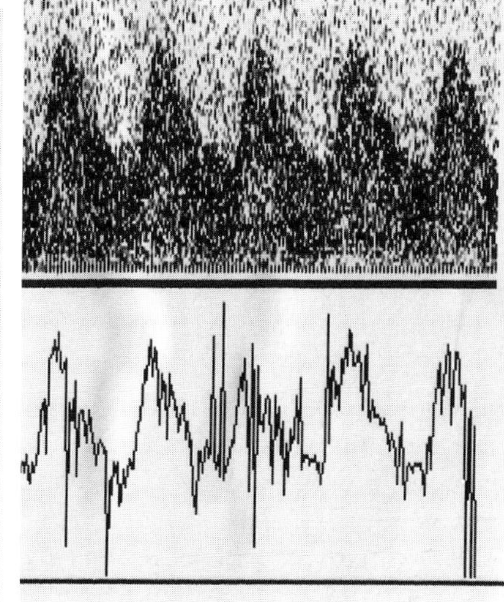

(b)

Fig. 3.18 Estimation of the maximum frequency envelope: (a) when there is no noise; and (b) when there is a lot of noise.

spectral Doppler and which, with care, can be reduced or eliminated.

Shadowing. As in 2D imaging highly reflecting and/or attenuating structures between the transducer and blood vessel will reduce signal strength. A fairly common problem is the shadowing caused by hard plaque in the vessel under examination.

Reflection. Again, as in 2D imaging, reflection of the ultrasound beam from a highly reflecting interface can lead to Doppler signals being detected when the sample volume is outside a blood vessel. For example, reflection at the calcified distal wall of an artery can give rise to Doppler signals when the sample volume is positioned distal to the vessel.

Refraction. The ultrasound beam is bent when passing across a boundary between media with differing propagation speeds. This can lead to displacement of vessel images in duplex measurements and, potentially, displacement and distortion of sample volumes within blood vessels containing plaque.

Angle dependence. Possibly the most obvious artefact in spectral Doppler is that resulting from the dependence of the measured component of velocity along the ultrasound beam on the angle between the beam and the flow orientation.

Range ambiguity. This occurs if the prf is too high, and multiple sample gates are produced along the beam.

Aliasing. Aliasing and its effect has already been described. It may be alleviated by the use of the baseline control, increasing the prf if possible and increasing the beam–vessel angle by altering the probe orientation. In practice, aliasing may not be a great problem as it is usually easily identified and can be used diagnostically as an indication of high velocities in poststenotic jets.

Wall thump filter artefact. Low velocities are lost if the filter is too high (Fig. 3.19).

Interference from other vessels. The spectral display may be confusing when there is more than one vessel in the beam; this mostly happens with stand alone CW devices, but may also happen when PW devices are operating in high prf mode (Fig. 3.20).

Beam–vessel geometry. The spectral content of the Doppler signal is critically dependent on the orientation and position of the sample volume within the vessel. When there is gross movement of the vessel, such as the motion of the umbilical artery due to maternal breathing, then the Doppler signal may disappear altogether (Fig. 3.21). Loss of clarity of the maximum frequency outline of the waveform may result from misalignment of the beam and vessel (Fig. 3.22), and the degree of spectral broadening will change markedly with different sample volume positions within the vessel.

The term sample volume is a convenient term to give to a region of sensitivity to flow but it does not denote a region inside of which the instrument has constant sensi-

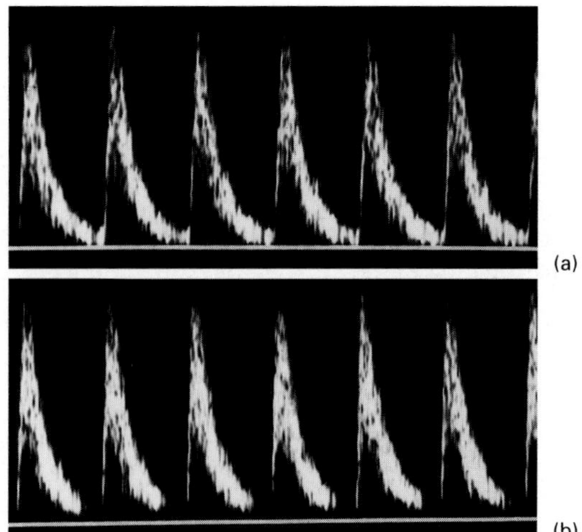

Fig. 3.19 Umbilical artery waveforms: (a) the high pass filter set to a low value of 50 Hz and the end-diastolic flow is clearly seen; and (b) the high pass filter is set to a higher value of 200 Hz causing apparent loss of end-diastolic flow.

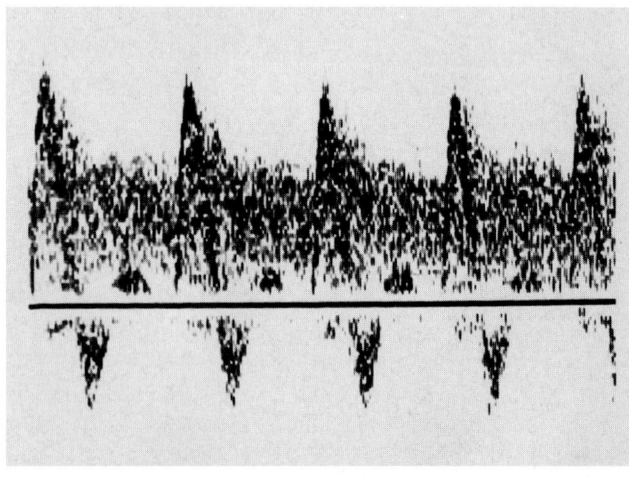

Fig. 3.20 Waveforms from two arteries are seen, an arcuate artery waveform and an iliac waveform. Data was acquired using a 4 MHz CW unit.

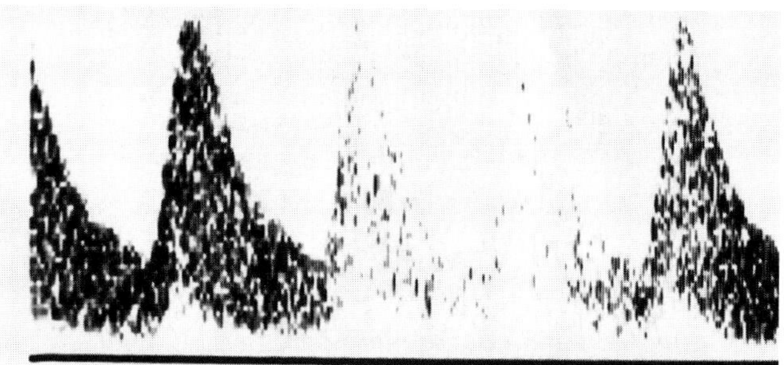

Fig. 3.21 Umbilical artery waveforms obtained using a 4 MHz CW system during maternal breathing; the motion of the vessel is sufficient to produce complete misalignment of beam and vessel and complete loss of signal.

(a)

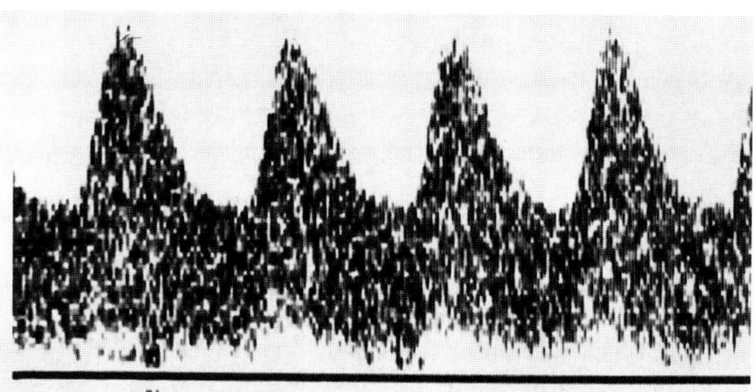

(b)

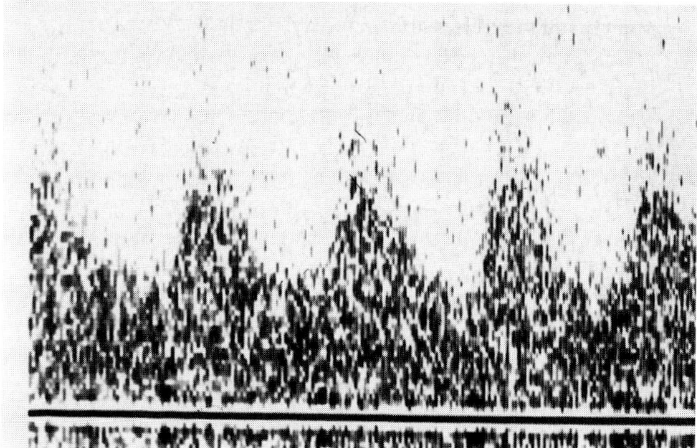

Fig. 3.22 Umbilical artery waveforms obtained using a 4 MHz system (a) with alignment of the beam and vessel, and (b) with misalignment of the beam and vessel.

tivity to flow and outside of which there is zero sensitivity. The markers on the screen of a duplex scanner simply indicate the distances along the beam at which the sensitivity has dropped to a certain fraction of its maximum. A long tail on the axial sensitivity variation in a pulsed Doppler instrument may lead to significant contamination of the desired Doppler signal from parts of the vessel or even a different vessel outside the indicated limit of the sample volume.

Non-axial flow. It is possible for the direction of flow, for example within the jet at the exit of a non-symmetrical stenosis, to be at an angle to the vessel axis. Assuming the flow to be parallel to the vessel axis and setting the flow direction indicator appropriately leads to an error in the velocity estimated from the Doppler shift frequency.

Acknowledgements

Thanks to Mr P.J. Fish for helpful comments and discussions.

Appendix: Historical perspective

1950s

The earliest published work is performed using a CW device by Satomura in Japan, first detecting the large amplitude signals from the moving myocardium and valves and then for the lower intensity signals from blood.

1960s

Doppler ultrasound devices in this decade were simple CW hand-held probes with an audio output. In 1969 the first PW devices were reported.

1970s

Doppler ultrasound devices capable of producing off-line display of spectra were developed, and the first duplex systems became available. At the end of the decade the first systems with real-time display of spectra were introduced. The first vector Doppler systems were described.

1980s

Other forms of spectral estimation were attempted in order to improve the temporal resolution and reduce Doppler speckle. To date these have not passed into commercial use. Commercial systems were released which provided automatic estimation of waveform indices.

1990s

No major developments in commercial spectral Doppler systems have taken place in recent years other than improvements in sensitivity through the use of low noise circuit design and new transducer materials. The accuracy of quantitative measurements, especially velocity, is discovered to be low through the use of suitable test objects.

The future

Future improvements are likely to be concerned with improvements in sensitivity, in the use of other forms of spectral estimation, in the accuracy of calculated waveform indices and in the reliability of automatic waveform index estimators. Real-time vector Doppler systems may become commercially available; these devices have the potential of automatically estimating the true angle between the beam and direction of blood motion. This has the advantage of disposing of the need for the operator to measure the beam–vessel angle manually, and provides for improvements in velocity estimation.

References

1 Evans, D.H., McDicken, W.N., Skidmore, R., Woodcock, J.P. (1989) *Doppler Ultrasound: Physics, Instrumentation and Clinical Applications*. Wiley, Chichester.

2 Flax, S.W., Webster, J.G., Updike, S.J. (1970) Statistical evaluation of the Doppler ultrasonic blood flowmeter. *Biomedical Sciences Instrumentation* 7, 201–222.

3 Lunt, M.J. (1975) Accuracy and limitations of the ultrasonic Doppler blood velocimeter and zero crossing detector. *Ultrasound in Medicine and Biology* **2**, 1–10.

4 Johnston, K.W., Maruzo, B.C., Cobbold, R.S.C. (1977) Errors and artefacts of Doppler flowmeters and their solutions. *Archives of Surgery* **112**, 75–76.

5 Schlindwein, F.S., Evans, D.H. (1989) A real time autoregressive spectrum analyser for Doppler signals. *Ultrasound in Medicine and Biology* **15**, 263–272.

6 Newhouse, V.L., Furgason, E.S., Johnson, G.F., Wolf, D.A. (1980) The dependence of ultrasound Doppler bandwidth on beam geometry. *IEEE Transactions in Sonics and Ultrasonics* **27**, 50–59.

7 Fish, P.J. (1991) Non-stationarity broadening in pulsed Doppler spectrum measurements. *Ultrasound in Medicine and Biology* **17**, 147–155.

8 Bluth, E.I., Stavros, A.T., Marich, K.W., *et al*. (1988) Carotid duplex sonography: a multicenter recommendation for standardised imaging and Doppler criteria. *Radiographics* **8**, 487–506.

9 Robinson, M.L., Sacks, D., Perlmutter, G.S., Marinelli, D.L. (1988) Diagnostic criteria for carotid duplex sonography. *American Journal of Roentgenology* **151**, 1045–1049.

10 Thrush, A.J., Evans, D.H. (1995) Intrinsic spectral broadening: a potential cause of misdiagnosis of carotid artery disease. *Journal of Vascular Investigation* **1**, 187–192.

11 Hoskins, P.R. (1996) Measurement of maximum velocity using duplex ultrasound systems. *British Journal of Radiology* **69**, 172–177.

12 Pourcelot, L. (1974) Applications cliniques de l'examen Doppler transcutane. In: *Velocimetrie Ultrasonore Doppler*. Seminaire INSERM, Paris, pp. 213–240.

13 Gosling, R.C., King, D.H. (1974) Continuous wave ultrasound as an alternative and complement to X-rays. In: Reneman, R.S. (ed.) *Cardiovascular Applications of Ultrasound*. North-Holland, Amsterdam, pp. 266–282.

14 Adamson, S.L., Morrow, R.J., Langille, B.L., *et al*. (1990) Site dependent effect of increases in placental vascular resistance on the umbilical arterial velocity waveform in fetal sheep. *Ultrasound in Medicine and Biology* **16**, 19–27.

15 Thomson, R.S., Stevens, R.J. (1989) Mathematical model for interpretation of Doppler velocity waveform indices. *Medical and Biological Engineering and Computing* **27**, 269–276.

16 McPherson, D.S., Evans, D.H., Bell, P.R.F. (1984) Common femoral artery Doppler waveforms: a comparison of three methods of objective analysis with direct pressure measurements. *British Journal of Surgery* **71**, 46–49.

17 Skidmore, R., Woodcock, J.P. (1980) Physiological interpretation of Doppler shift waveforms. I. Theoretical considerations. *Ultrasound in Medicine and Biology* **6**, 7–10.

Chapter 4: Flow imaging

P.J. Fish

The detection of blood flow within the scan plane of an ultrasound scanner and the colour display of haemodynamic parameters such as flow velocity (magnitude and direction), turbulence or simply the presence of flow is known as colour flow imaging. The clinical need driving its development was a requirement for flow information in an easily assimilated form in combination with the grey-scale anatomical information of the normal B-scan display. While a duplex system enables the operator to interrogate the grey-scale image one point at a time in order to determine flow conditions, colour flow imaging presents an overall, if rather less detailed, picture in an easily assimilated form within a colour box set by the operator. The operator is then able to look at specific points in the displayed vessels to obtain the more detailed information that the pulsed (spectral) Doppler section of the instrument can provide.

Colour flow imaging can be considered a natural development of the manually scanned continuous wave imager [1–3] described in the first edition of this book which gave a projection view of the vessels underlying the scanned skin surface, and the multi-channel pulsed Doppler instrument [4,5] which enabled views requiring depth information to be generated. These devices were limited because the image took several minutes to generate and there was no simultaneous display of anatomical information. The detection and quantification of flow in real-times over a comparatively wide field of view required a degree of computing power which has only recently become available.

There are two colour flow modes which are widely used in current instruments—velocity imaging which displays the component of velocity in the direction of the Doppler beam, and power imaging which displays the power of the signal backscattered from the blood and is independent of blood velocity.

The most commonly used technique for deriving velocity and power information for display is the autocorrelation method [6,7] which derives the velocity from the Doppler shift frequency, which is derived in turn from the rate of change of phase of the echo signal. A second technique measures velocity more directly by noting the movement of echoes from blood over the time interval between transmission pulses [8]. This latter technique is sometimes called the time domain method. Both methods make comparisons between echo signals from a small number or ensemble of pulses transmitted along each scan beam and measure the velocity component along the line of the beam thereby requiring, as in spectral Doppler measurements, an angulation of the beam with respect to the vessel of interest.

Principles

Components of a colour flow imaging system

A block diagram of the most common type of colour flow imager using a measurement of Doppler frequency shift in the received signal is shown in Fig. 4.1.

In some instruments the same transmitted pulses are used for both B-scan and colour flow imaging in which case the same received signals from the scanner probe are processed to generate both images. However, longer pulses are preferred for colour flow imaging in order to give the increased sensitivity required to register the weak signals backscattered from blood and most instruments use separate colour flow and B-scan imaging pulses [9].

The functions of the various components are described below.

Transmission and reception

The instrument extracts information on scatterer movement by transmitting a small number of pulses (typically 10) along each beam in the scan. The received signal is effectively range-gated to enable the echoes from a number (typically 256) of small sample volumes along the beam to be processed individually.

Clutter filter

As in continuous wave or pulsed Doppler instruments,

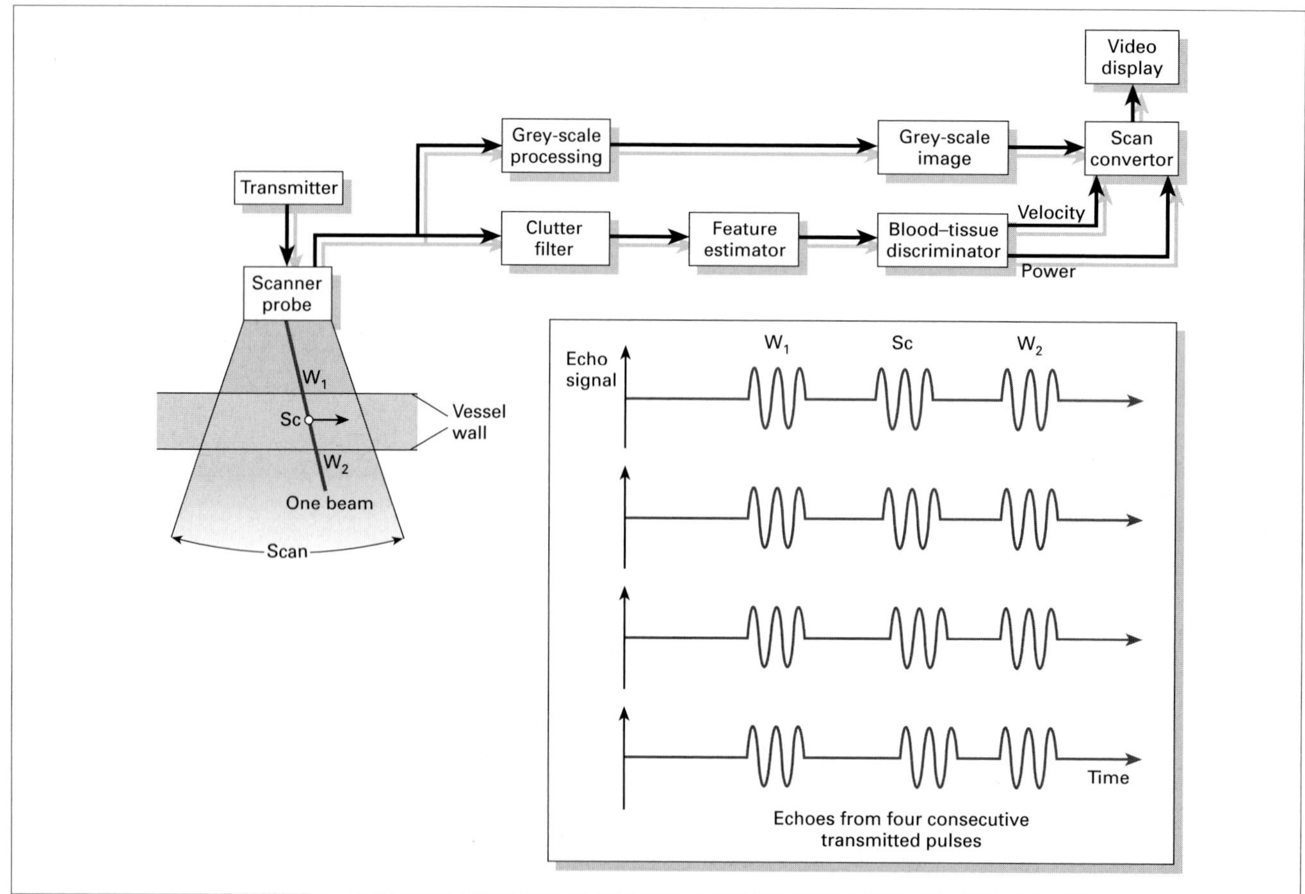

Fig. 4.1 Block diagram of colour flow scanner and echoes from vessel wall (W_1 and W_2) and scatterer (Sc) following four sequential transmitted pulses.

the high amplitude signals from stationary or slowly moving tissue structures (e.g. vessel walls) are removed as these would otherwise swamp the low level signals from blood during the subsequent processing [10–13]. This is achieved by comparing the echo signals received after each transmitted pulse and eliminating those which do not change location from pulse to pulse (W_1 and W_2 in Fig. 4.1). This filtration process can be achieved by subtracting the echo signals from alternate transmitter pulses. This simple process, however, does have a very marked effect on the Doppler frequency response, leading to a gradual increase in sensitivity from zero at zero Doppler shift to a maximum at the highest frequency shift in the range [14]. It is preferable to have a more rapid increase in sensitivity at a cut-off frequency which can be selected to suit a particular examination and this can be achieved using a more complex filter requiring echoes from a number of transmitter pulses, typically four [15].

Feature estimation

As illustrated in Fig. 4.1 the echo from a moving scatterer (Sc in Fig. 4.1) changes position between transmitter pulses, arriving progressively later if the scatterer is moving away from the probe. This movement may be quantified by measuring the phase difference between successive echoes using the autocorrelation method. The rate of change of phase, calculated from the phase difference and the interval between transmission pulses, is proportional to the Doppler shift frequency which is in turn proportional to the velocity component along the beam. In the power mode [16] the total power of the signal passing through the clutter filter, and therefore arising from moving targets, is measured—again using a property of the autocorrelation function.

The ultrasound echoes from blood are random and the measured phase difference therefore has a random estimation error which leads to a random variation (speckle) in the displayed colour image. This speckle is reduced by averaging the measured phase shift over a number of pulses; the variation decreases as the number of pulses used for the estimation increases. If the flow within a sample volume is disturbed then the variation of phase shift between echo pulses and thus the estimated velocity variance increases. This variation may be measured and represented on the colour image as an indication of velocity variance or disturbed flow.

Blood–tissue discriminator

The function of the blood–tissue discriminator is to write colour to regions of true blood flow. This is usually done on the basis of the detected signal amplitude and frequency shift, with signals from tissue having high amplitude and low Doppler frequency, and true blood flow having low amplitude and higher Doppler frequency. At least one manufacturer has an additional filter arrangement, commonly called a 'flash filter' which removes the abnormally high amplitude signals above the clutter frequency cut-off which arise if the probe or the patient moves suddenly.

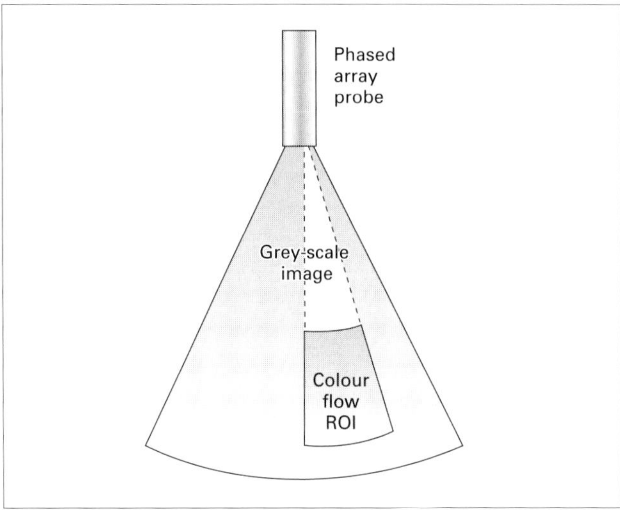

Fig. 4.2 Colour flow region of interest (ROI) in phased array scan.

Scan convertor

As in the grey-scale imagers the scan convertor stores echo information as it is acquired, with data arriving in a sequence dictated by the scanning pattern, and sends the information out in the standard video raster form required by the video display monitor. In colour flow imaging the scan convertor performs the additional task of storing velocity or power information at store locations assigned to areas of the scan plane where flow has been detected.

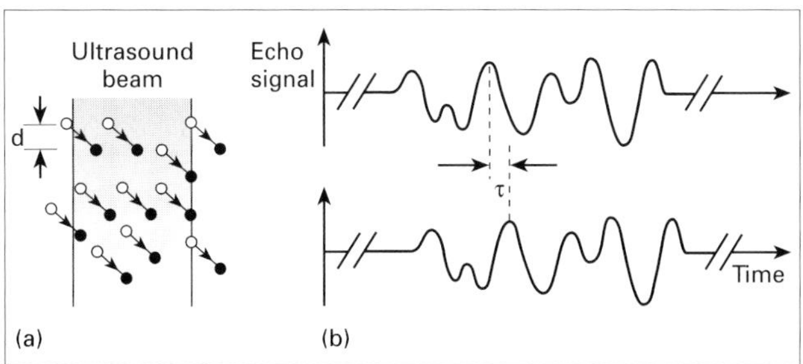

Fig. 4.3 Velocity component estimation using time domain processing. (a) Beam/scatterer geometry. Open and closed circles show scatterer positions during backscatter of two sequential transmitted pulses. (b) Received signal from region shown in (a) following two sequential transmitted pulses.

Display

The combined grey-scale anatomical image and colour flow image is displayed on a standard colour video monitor. In order to limit the number of channels (sample volumes) required for colour flow processing it is usual to limit the length of the beam used for flow analysis. In addition, since transmitting a number of pulses along each beam reduces the frame rate it is usual to limit the number of scan lines, and therefore the width of the colour flow scan, to less than that of the B-scan grey-scale display. The colour flow image is therefore limited to a defined region of interest called a colour box whose position and dimensions are under operator control (Fig. 4.2).

Time domain colour flow system

An alternative method of colour flow imaging used in at least one commercial instrument at present is shown in Fig. 4.3. Successive echo signals from a short section of the beam in a region of moving blood are similar in shape (altered only by the comparatively small number of cells leaving and entering the section) but delayed by $\tau = 2d/c$, where d is the distance moved by the blood, between transmitted pulses, in the direction of the beam axis and c is the speed of ultrasound in blood. The velocity of blood flow can then be calculated from this distance and the delay time between transmitted pulses. The time shift τ in the pulse–echo delay time can be measured using a cross-correlation technique using echo signals from alternate transmitted pulses [8]. For a substantial part of the signal processing chain the signal processing is performed on the radiofrequency data, which is computationally time-consuming and hence expensive to implement. This is probably the reason that time domain systems to date have not been widely adopted commercially.

Probes

In principle any of the probes used for B-scan imaging can be used for colour flow imaging. However, the problems associated with transducer movement in mechanical probes mean that, in practice, its use is mainly limited to electronically steered beam probes. The choice of sector, convex or linear array is governed by similar considerations to those of grey-scale B-scan imaging—leading to the use of sector probes for cardiac and some abdominal work, convex/linear array for abdominal and small linear arrays for peripheral vascular work.

Mechanical sector probes

Systems using continually swept transducers suffer since, ideally, the ensemble of pulses required to detect flow should be transmitted along the same beam direction and when using these probes the beam moves slightly between pulses. In addition, any vibration of the transducers is a movement with respect to stationary tissue and will lead to apparent movement being detected in this tissue. Rocking transducers require sufficient time to decelerate and accelerate at the extremes of their movement, thereby slowing the frame rate.

Phased arrays

Normally this is the probe of choice if a sector scan pattern is required. The beam can be held in each position for sufficient time for the transmission and reception of the colour flow pulse ensemble before switching to the next position. The shape of the colour box is shown in Fig. 4.2, it may be positioned anywhere within the grey-scale scan and the length and width may be varied. Angulation of the beam with respect to the vessel of interest is achieved by movement of the probe and colour box.

Since the colour flow and grey-scale imaging beams are both radial, the optimum beam orientation for vessel imaging—perpendicular to the vessel axis—results in a very low or absent component of flow along the beam and, therefore, no colour flow image. This leads to a compromise between colour flow and grey-scale image quality—small angles lead to poor images of the vessel but relatively high velocity component and a low variance colour flow image; angles approaching 90° produce good images of the vessel but low velocity components and high variance (noisy) colour flow images.

Convex array

The colour box of the convex array is similar to that of the phased array and the same limitations apply.

Linear array

Linear arrays are particularly suitable for peripheral vascular scanning because they enable imaging of a reasonable length of vessels which are often running roughly parallel to the skin surface. In order to provide significant angulation between the beam and vessel early colour flow scanners sometimes used a removable fluid-filled wedge (Fig. 4.4). This meant that the beams were no longer in the optimum orientation for grey-scale vessel imaging and it was therefore necessary to accept either an inferior grey-scale image or to obtain a grey-scale image separately without the wedge in place.

Scanners using a linear array now allow the operator to select angled colour flow beams using the same beam steering techniques used in a phased array probe, but maintaining the grey-scale imaging beams perpendicular to the probe surface. Typically, the colour flow beams may be angled at +20, 0 and −20° to the grey-scale imaging beams giving the colour boxes shown in Fig. 4.5.

Display modes

Both velocity and power can be displayed superimposed on the grey-scale image within the colour box. For power an alternative is to display only colour within the colour box; low level power signals constituting mainly noise from regions containing tissue are displayed in one colour, e.g. blue, whereas signals above the noise floor are displayed in a different colour, usually shades of yellow. Doppler spectra may be acquired and displayed in the usual way. If there is simultaneous real-time B-mode, colour flow and spectral display, this is referred to as triplex scanning (Fig. 4.6); in this mode, the colour flow and B-scan frame rates are significantly reduced.

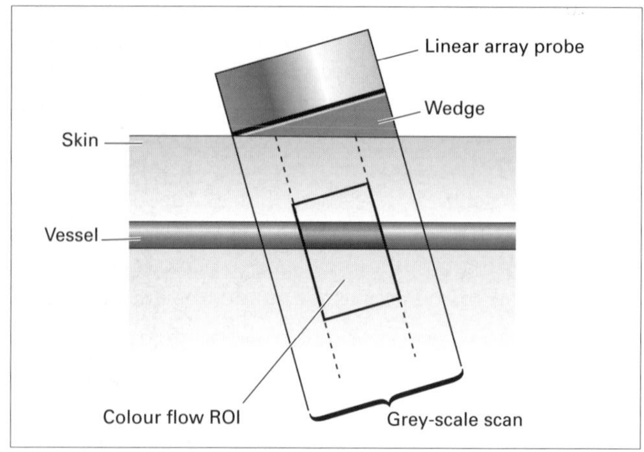

Fig. 4.4 Beam angulation using fluid-filled wedge. ROI, region of interest.

Mean frequency

In this mode the mean frequency shift is estimated and colour coded. This was the first colour mode to be widely adopted for clinical use. Spectral Doppler was concerned with the variation in velocity with time, so it was logical for the first colour flow systems to display an image of the spatial variation of velocity. It is usual practice to convert the mean frequency to velocity assuming that the angle between the beam and direction of motion is zero.

In most scanners a number of colour scales are available to the operator. Probably the most common is that shown in Fig. 4.7a in which the direction of flow is indicated by red or blue and increasing velocity magnitude by decreasing colour saturation (increasing addition of white).

A green tag can be used in some instruments to indicate the position of flow at an operator-selected velocity, or to indicate velocities above a selected figure. This can be useful in illustrating poststenotic jets.

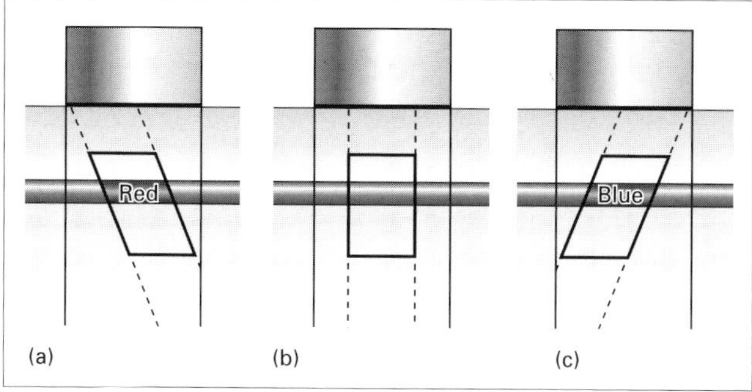

Fig. 4.5 Example of beam angulation using electronic beam steering with vessel parallel to skin surface. (a) −20°, negative flow velocity component along beam. (b) 0°, zero flow velocity component along beam. (c) +20°, positive flow velocity component along beam.

Variance

Increased velocity variance can be indicated by the addition of another colour (e.g. green) to the velocity image or alternatively an image just of velocity variance may be displayed in order to more clearly locate regions of flow disturbance.

Power

In this mode the power of the Doppler signal is colour coded. This mode was available in early machines; however, it was not adopted clinically until recently, following alteration of machine settings [16]. In spectral Doppler there is little variation in Doppler power through the cardiac cycle so that the market was perhaps not used to this mode; however, there is better visualization of small vessels using this mode and it is now widely used [17–19].

In the power mode flow is shown wherever the Doppler power is above a selected threshold, and no flow direction or velocity information is displayed. As with colour

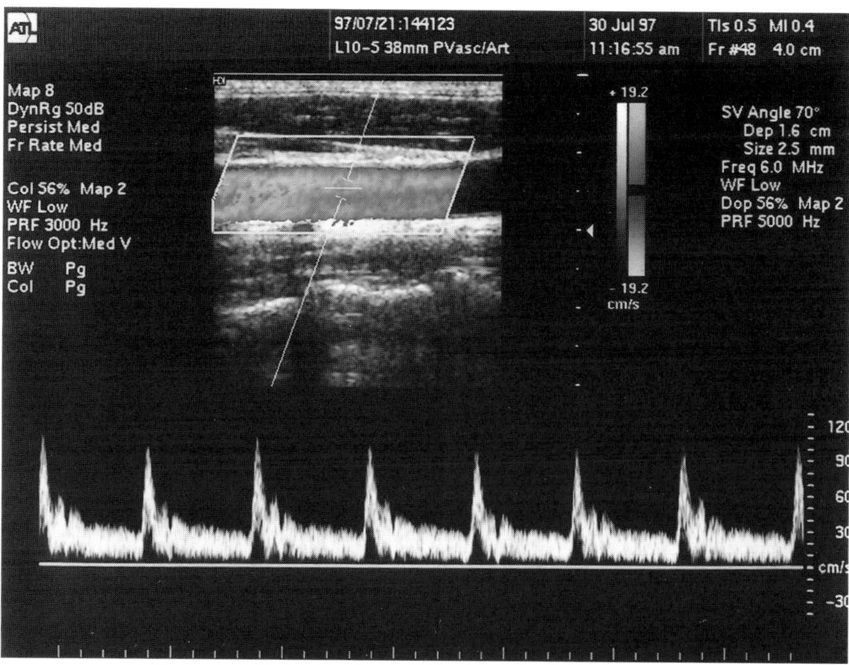

Fig. 4.6 Triplex display of carotid artery with spectral display. For colour, see Plate 4.6 (between pp. 308 and 309).

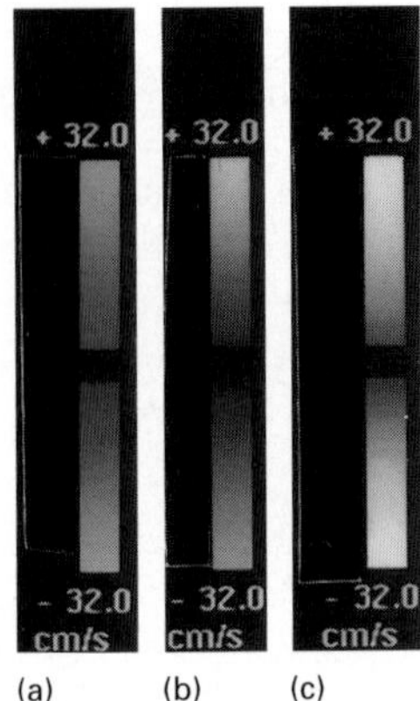

Fig. 4.7 Velocity colour maps. (a,b) Broad range maps. (c) Rapidly saturating map. For colour, see Plate 4.7 (between pp. 308 and 309).

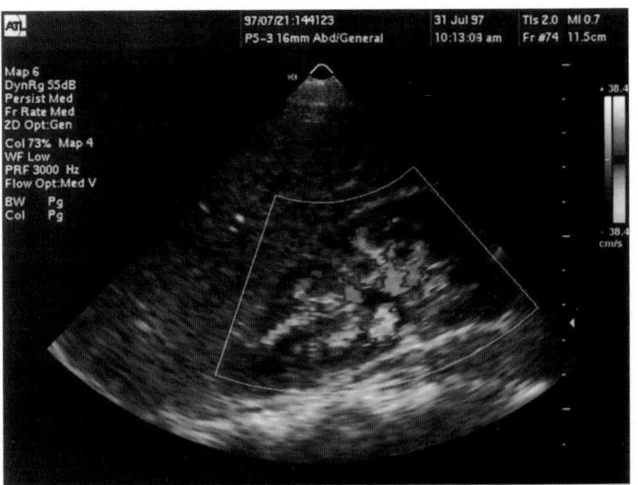

(a)

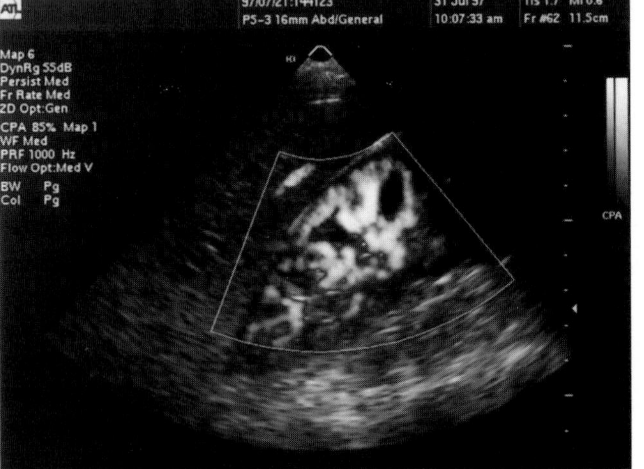

(b)

Fig. 4.8 (a) Velocity and (b) power colour flow images of a normal kidney. For colour, see Plate 4.8 (between pp. 308 and 309).

Doppler a number of colour scales are available which indicate the level of signal power. This level is determined by the volume of blood within the sample volume and is also affected by flow conditions—indicating low power at low velocity as a result of the action of the clutter filter and high power from turbulent flow as a result of increased backscatter. Signals from flow in small vessels and at the edges of vessels will be displayed as having low power as a consequence of low velocity and partial occupancy of each sample volume. The power map of flow in a normal kidney compared with a velocity map is shown in Fig. 4.8.

Controls

The performance of the colour flow instrument is determined by a number of design parameters some of which can be altered to suit the conditions of particular examinations. An appreciation of their effect on performance is necessary in order to aid the selection and purchase of an instrument and the choice of available parameter values in use. It should be noted that many of the parameters discussed are not adjustable using front panel controls but by means of software menus. These parameters will have default values determined as optimum for given examinations and preset by the manufacturer. In addition, parameter profiles may be set and stored by the user in many systems.

Clutter

Some of the most important operations in the colour flow device are those which remove or reduce the effect of clutter—those echoes from stationary or slowly moving tissues which are used to generate the grey-scale display but can interfere with the colour flow image.

CLUTTER FILTERS

The cut-off frequency of the filters used to remove or reduce signals from stationary or slowly moving tissues may be set by the operator. Generally this should be set, as with the wallthump filter in the pulsed Doppler mode, to a high frequency when monitoring flow in the vicinity of rapidly moving tissues (e.g. cardiac work) and to low values when attempting to detect slow flow in small vessels with little tissue movement (e.g. peripheral venous work). Too high a value will lead to slowly moving blood close to the vessel wall not being imaged and too low a value will lead to tissue movement being displayed as a spurious image on the flow display.

FLASH FILTER

The flash filter removes the colour flash artefacts produced from tissue or probe movement. There is no commonly accepted name for this control. The filter can usually either be set on or off.

GREY-SCALE/COLOUR PRIORITY

Since the axial resolution of the colour flow display is poorer than that of the B-scan display the colour flow vessel image will usually spread outside the vessel lumen and overlap the grey-scale image of the vessel walls. Since the scan converter will be presented with both grey-scale and colour flow data in the vicinity of the vessel wall it is necessary to decide which is displayed in a particular pixel when both types of data are present, and this is the function of the blood–tissue discriminator. In order to maintain the benefit of the higher resolution of the B-scan image it is usual to arrange for the B-scan grey-scale image to have priority and to be displayed where there is a conflict. The priority level is the grey-scale threshold which the B-scan echo amplitude has to exceed in order to be written into a pixel if both B-scan and colour flow data are present. Below that threshold the colour flow data will be displayed.

If this threshold is set too high then some wall echoes will not exceed it and the colour image will spill out beyond the vessel lumen image. If the threshold is set too low then small spurious echoes such as those arising from vessel walls outside the scan plane but within a slice width will register within the vessel lumen instead of the colour flow image.

Velocity

There are a number of instrument controls which primarily affect the mapping of blood velocity-to-colour display. Their setting will affect the visibility of the particular vessel or flow disorder being examined.

COLOUR SCALE

Normally a number of colour scales are available to the operator in addition to the standard red/blue plus white scale. A few are shown in Fig. 4.7. The broad range maps (Fig. 4.7a,b) are suitable for general work when it is required to visualize and discriminate over as wide a range of blood velocities as possible. The rapidly saturating map (Fig. 4.7c) can be used to indicate more clearly the location of fast flow—in jets for example.

It is possible to indicate turbulent flow by mixing in a velocity variance indicator such as green, or even to visualize velocity variance alone. This facility does not appear to have been adopted widely in clinical practice. Tagging a particular velocity with a colour (e.g. green) has found some application in research and tagging all velocities above a selected value can be used as an alternative method for indicating high velocity (e.g. poststenotic jets).

VELOCITY RANGE/PULSE REPETITION FREQUENCY

The range of velocities displayed by the instrument is governed by the pulse repetition frequency (PRF) of the instrument. The Doppler shift frequency is limited to the range ±PRF/2 (the Nyquist limit). If the Doppler shift exceeds these limits then aliasing occurs just as in the pulsed (spectral) Doppler mode and flow velocities will be indicated in the wrong direction. The implications for setting the PRF for temporal resolution and sensitivity are addressed below; here we note that in order to detect high velocities unambiguously (that is without aliasing) it is necessary to have a high PRF but this reduces the resolution of low velocities, such as are found in lower limb venous studies, for example.

The PRF is often limited by depth considerations. As in B-scan imaging it is necessary to wait until the echoes from one transmitted pulse to return before transmitting the next which leads to a low PRF requirement for deep vessels. It is therefore sometimes difficult to avoid aliasing when examining high velocity flow (e.g. cardiac) at depth.

When imaging low flow velocities a low PRF should be selected since the instrument reduces its bandwidth to suit and thereby reduces the background noise.

BASELINE SHIFT

As in pulsed Doppler, shifting the velocity display baseline is one method of increasing the highest measurable velocity if the flow is all or mostly in one direction. The ranges available for forward and reverse flow can be altered provided that the total range available for non-aliased display is not exceeded. Potentially this can increase the maximum non-aliased velocity by a factor of 2 if the whole of the range is used for flow in either the forward or reverse direction.

COLOUR BOX ANGLE

The colour flow instrument assigns a colour on the basis of a measurement of the component of blood velocity along the ultrasound beam. This component is equal to the blood velocity multiplied by the cosine of the angle between the direction of flow and the beam axis. It is zero if this angle is 90° and is a maximum at an angle of 0°. It is necessary, therefore, to avoid attempting colour flow imaging with the beam at or near to perpendicular to the vessel of interest and the facility for altering the angle of the colour box to improve the angle of insonation should be used.

ANGLE CORRECTION

The instrument may simply indicate the velocity component along the beam against the displayed colour bar, in which case it is important to note that the displayed colour does not correspond to the velocity within the vessel. However, some instruments enable the operator to position an on-screen marker indicating the flow orientation and in this case the instrument will correct the velocity indication and the colour display will represent the true blood velocity.

Power

Although the power mode is intrinsically simpler than velocity mode there are still several controls and options which influence the power image.

COLOUR SCALE

Most systems choose a yellow-based scale for display of power. Most machines offer a variety of other colour scales which the operator can select.

VELOCITY RANGE/PRF

The power mode does not suffer from aliasing and a low PRF is usually selected since this reduces the background noise.

COLOUR BOX STEERING ANGLE

The power image is much less dependent on angle than the velocity image; however, at 90° there may be loss of colour due to the low Doppler frequencies falling below the clutter filter. In most situations the influence of the colour box steering angle on the power image is not important; however, the loss of signal at 90° may be a problem for vessels aligned perpendicular to the beam.

Resolution and sensitivity

There is a general requirement in medical imaging for both good spatial and temporal resolution and high sensitivity. Unfortunately, many measures taken to improve sensitivity decrease resolution and vice versa and it is therefore necessary to arrive at some compromise for the settings of some of the machine controls. The general principles outlined below apply to both velocity and power, except where stated.

TRANSMITTED FREQUENCY

The transmitted frequency used for colour flow may not be the same as for B-scan grey-scale imaging if separate pulses are used. The compromise required between increasing backscatter from blood, increased Doppler shift for a given velocity and decreased signal strength as a result of attenuation as the frequency increases may lead to a lower transmission frequency being appropriate in some situations; 3 MHz for colour flow with 5 MHz for grey-scale imaging, for example.

In general, however, as with grey-scale imaging, lower frequencies are selected in order to achieve adequate penetration for imaging deep vessels in abdominal and cardiac work and higher frequencies, with better resolution, can be used for more superficial work.

TRANSMITTED POWER

The ability to image deeper vessels is strongly affected by the transmitter power and as with other imaging modalities the ALARA principle ('as low as reasonably achievable') should be adopted so that the lowest power output consistent with an adequate examination is used.

COLOUR GAIN (SENSITIVITY)

The colour gain control adjusts the amplification of received signals and should be used in preference to the transmitted power, as far as possible, to increase the instrument penetration. If the gain is increased too far the background noise will give rise to random colour noise on the image, if it is too low then the small signals from deeper or smaller vessels will fail to register.

COLOUR THRESHOLD (REJECT)

To avoid background noise giving rise to a colour image a threshold is set in the instrument and only signals with an amplitude above this level are used to create an image. This may not be adjustable by the operator since sufficient control over the level of noise suppression is afforded by the use of the colour gain control. It may be used deliberately to remove signals from very small vessels.

In the power mode when colour is written throughout the colour box it may be possible to alter the threshold below which the low level signals are displayed.

AXIAL RESOLUTION

The axial resolution of the instrument is determined by the length of the transmitted pulses. The preference is for longer pulses for colour flow compared with those for B-scan imaging since longer pulses have smaller bandwidths which allow the use of narrow receiver bandwidths. Since background noise increases with receiver bandwidth this strategy reduces the overall noise and thereby increases sensitivity but at the expense of poorer axial resolution.

LATERAL RESOLUTION

Lateral resolution is determined by the beam width and is controlled by focusing. In order to avoid excessively slow frame rates it is usual to have only one focal zone on transmit rather than the multiple zones which are commonly used in grey-scale imaging.

ENSEMBLE LENGTH (DWELL TIME, PACKET SIZE)

Temporal resolution is strongly affected by the choice of the ensemble length—the number of pulses used for velocity determination along each scan line. The reason for increasing the number of pulses above the minimum required for the determination of a phase difference and the operation of the clutter filter is that an increase in the number of phase differences averaged decreases the random variation of the velocity estimation. This leads to a smoother, less random image, with reduced speckle but the price paid for the improved image quality is poorer temporal resolution. Increasing the dwell time at each line decreases the frame rate and the ability to respond to fast changes in velocity.

FRAME RATE

The frame rate is determined by a number of factors and does not have a separate control. It determines temporal resolution and thus the ability to respond to rapid changes in flow. Improving the frame rate by changing one or more of these determining factors is always at the expense of another performance measure. The frame rate increases with an increase in PRF (normally limited by the maximum depth of interest) and decreases with an increase in colour box width, line density and ensemble length.

COLOUR BOX WIDTH AND COLOUR LINE DENSITY

It is possible to increase the frame rate for a given ensemble length by reducing the width of the colour box and so reducing the number of lines scanned. Alternatively, frame rates can be increased and colour box width maintained by increasing the spacing between scan lines—decreasing the colour line density and leading to a drop in lateral resolution.

INTERPOLATION

Many instruments will automatically maintain displayed line density if the frame rate is increased and colour box width maintained by providing alternate lines along which the pixel colours are derived by interpolation from the pixel colours in the lines on either side. Note that this is purely cosmetic and the lateral resolution determined by the density of (true) data lines is unaffected.

NON-SEQUENTIAL SCANNING

Some manufacturers have increased the frame rate for a given PRF by using non-sequential scanning. Instead of transmitting all the pulses in the colour flow ensemble along a scan line before moving to the next line the instrument sends the first pulse of an ensemble along a scan line followed by the first pulse along another scan line followed by the first pulse along a third scan line before returning to the first scan line in order to transmit the second pulse in the ensemble, and so on. By effectively imaging along a number of beams (three in the example above) simultaneously the frame rate can be increased by the same factor. There is no penalty other than increase in instrument complexity and, therefore, presumably cost.

COLOUR PERSISTENCE

As in B-scan grey-scale imaging the image to noise ratio can be increased and the colour Doppler or power Doppler image variability decreased by averaging a number of successive frames. The averaging is achieved by adding a proportion of the previously displayed image to the latest acquired frame. The influence of any one frame gradually decreases as time progresses and the temporal averaging time increases with the proportion of the old image used. A high colour persistence decreases the ability to follow the rapid changes in flow patterns and may lead to difficulties in monitoring changes in cardiac work Conversely, some cardiac events are so rapid that they can only be seen if the persistence is set to be non-zero. In practice for vascular applications it is often not necessary for the velocity image to follow in detail the variations in velocity with time through the cardiac cycle; this is the role of spectral Doppler, and a degree of frame averaging is desirable. For power Doppler no information is available concerning variation of velocities, and a high persistence is commonly used.

SPATIAL FILTERING

The colour flow image speckle can be decreased by spatial averaging—replacing the pixel colour by an average of its own value and those of the surrounding pixels. The image will appear smoother but the spatial resolution is poorer.

Artefacts

Some of the artefacts observed in colour flow are similar to those found in B-scan grey-scale imaging—the shadowing arising from bowel gas in abdominal scanning or arising from calcified plaque in the blood vessel, for example. There are other artefacts which are specific to colour flow and which, with care, can be reduced or eliminated.

Angle dependence

For colour Doppler possibly the most obvious artefact is that resulting from the dependence of the measured component of velocity along the ultrasound beam on the angle between the beam and the flow orientation. This means that a particular blood velocity does not necessarily give rise to a particular colour. For example, in the radial scan pattern from a sector or convex probe a constant velocity in a straight vessel can lead to a wide range of displayed colours—even an apparent change in direction as the angle changes from acute to oblique across the scan plane (Fig. 4.9a). This particular problem is not found with the linear array since the beam orientation is constant within the colour box. However, changes in vessel orientation within the colour box leads to a change in colour for a constant velocity.

In the power mode there is little variation in displayed colour with angle, except near to 90° where there may be no colour displayed due to the low frequencies falling below the clutter filter (Fig. 4.9b).

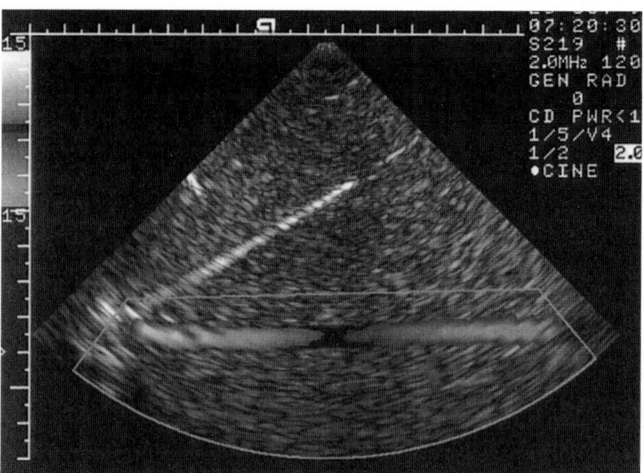

(a)

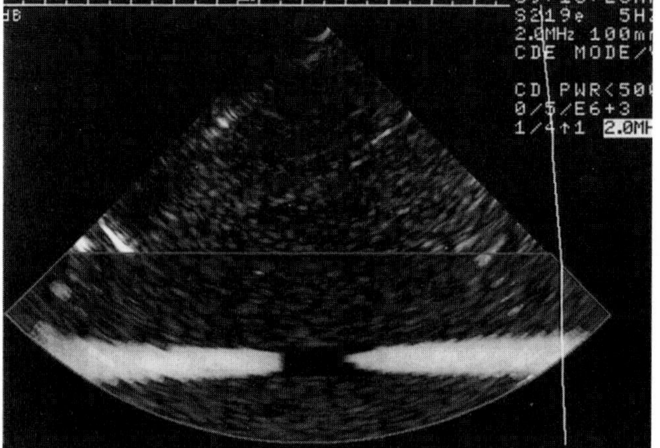
(b)

Fig. 4.9 Images from a flow phantom using a convex probe showing (a) colour Doppler images showing variation in colour with beam–vessel angle across scan; and (b) a power Doppler image showing no variation except near to 90°. For colour, see Plate 4.9 (between pp. 308 and 309).

Aliasing

The appearance and cause of aliasing have already been discussed. In practice aliasing in the colour Doppler image may not be a great problem as it is usually easily identified and can be used diagnostically as an indication of high velocities in poststenotic jets. It may be alleviated by the use of the baseline control, increasing the PRF if possible and increasing the beam–vessel angle by altering the probe orientation. The power mode does not suffer from aliasing.

Clutter breakthrough

The clutter filters used in colour flow are not perfect filters which would remove all signals with a Doppler frequency below the cut-off. They have a relatively gradual decrease in sensitivity as the frequency falls and it is sometimes difficult to arrive at a suitable compromise value for the cut-off such that low flow velocities are imaged but vessel wall movement is excluded. This may be a problem when attempting to discover whether there is slow flow through a very tight stenosis or if the vessel is completely occluded. Clutter breakthrough is displayed as a colour image generated by tissue movement rather than blood flow. It can be removed by increasing the clutter filter cut-off frequency.

Low frame rate

For colour Doppler low frame rates can lead to an artefact whereby flow at different phases of the cardiac cycle are displayed in one image. The appearance depends on whether a sequential or non-sequential scan pattern is used.

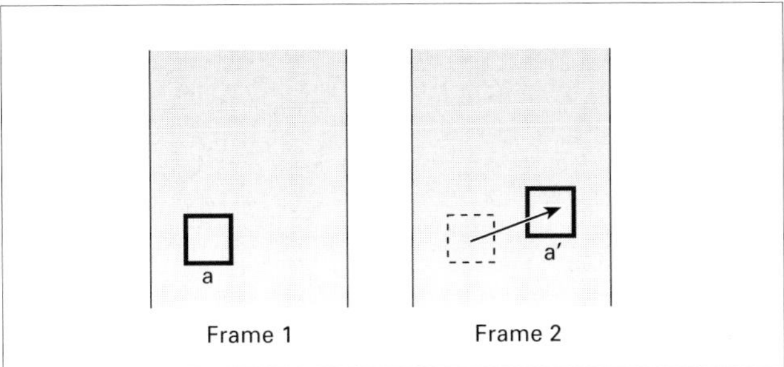

Fig. 4.10 Speckle tracking relies on the echo pattern within a region remaining sufficiently unchanged to allow correlation algorithms to track speckle between successive frames. The blood velocity and direction may then be measured.

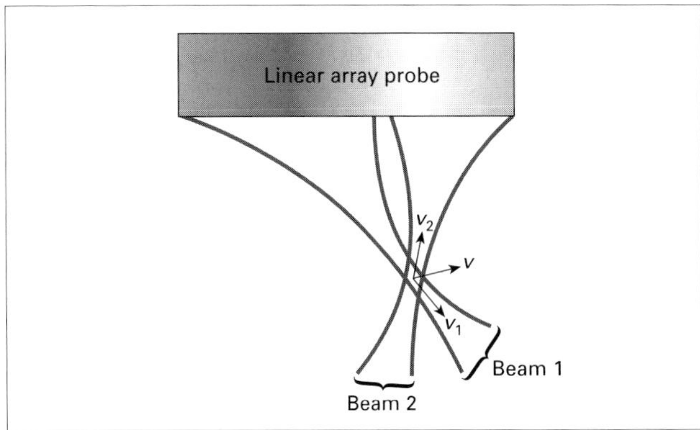

Fig. 4.11 Vector Doppler system using two transmit–receive beams generated from different parts of the linear array. Each beam measures a different velocity component which may be combined to allow estimation of the velocity magnitude and direction within the scan plane.

Developments

Angle-independent methods

One of the major limitations of current colour flow imaging systems is the dependence of the image colour on beam and flow direction orientation in addition to velocity magnitude. Two methods have been proposed to overcome this. The first of these is an extension of the time domain method whereby the echoes from a region of blood are tracked in two dimensions (2D) [20–22]. For each small region of flow image in one frame a search is performed in order to find a region having the greatest similarity of echo pattern in the succeeding frame. The line joining the centres of the regions has a length proportional to the velocity magnitude and its orientation shows the local flow direction (Fig. 4.10).

The alternative method depends on making measurements of blood velocity components along two beams steered through different angles to each region of flow (Fig. 4.11). The flow velocity magnitude and direction can be calculated from these two velocity component measurements and the known angle between the two beams [23–25].

Three-dimensional imaging

Three-dimensional (3D) data acquisition and display is currently under investigation [26]. A volume of tissue is scanned, for example, sweeping a sector scan through a sector in a perpendicular direction. The display is an operator-selected 2D view of the stored 3D image.

Aliasing removal

Methods of removing the effect of aliasing also are under investigation. These include methods for reversing the spurious change in indicated flow direction when the blood velocity increases, by temporal or spatial variation [27,28], through the Nyquist limit. A third possible method uses transmitted pulses at two frequencies and makes use of the fact that the Nyquist limit frequency corresponds to two different velocities [29].

Combination method

In each of the autocorrelation and time domain methods of velocity estimation the information used by the other method is ignored. A method effectively combining the two methods and therefore making use of both pieces of information in the echo signal has been investigated [30,31]. The extra computational complexity may limit the application in the near future.

Conclusion

The rapidity with which the colour flow technique has been adopted is a measure of the attractiveness and utility of this new imaging method. No doubt the incremental changes in sensitivity and clutter rejection in addition to the possibilities of overcoming aliasing, 3D display and the removal of angle dependence will ensure that this imaging technique will continue to grow.

References

1 Reid, J.M., Spencer, M.P. (1972) Ultrasonic Doppler technique for imaging blood vessels. *Science* **176**, 1235–1236.

2 Spencer, M.P., Reid, J.M., Davis, D.L., Paulson, P.S. (1974) Cervical carotid imaging with a continuous-wave Doppler flowmeter. *Stroke* **5**, 145–154.

3 Curry, G.R., White, D.N. (1978) Color coded ultrasonic differential velocity arterial scanner. *Ultrasound in Medicine and Biology* **4**, 27–35.
4 Fish, P.J. (1975) Multichannel, direction-resolving Doppler angiography. *Excerpta Medica International Congress Series* **363**, 153–159.
5 Hokanson, D.E., Mozersky, D.J., Sumner, D.S., McLeod, F.D., Strandness, D.E. (1972) Ultrasonic arteriography: a noninvasive method of arterial visualization. *Radiology* **102**, 435–436.
6 Namekawa, K., Kasai, C., Tsukamoto, M., Koyano, A. (1982) Imaging of blood flow using auto-correlation. *Ultrasound in Medicine and Biology* **8**, 138.
7 Kasai, C., Namekawa, K., Koyano, A., Omoto, R. (1985) Real-time two dimensional blood flow imaging using an autocorrelation technique. *IEEE Transactions in Sonics and Ultrasonics* **32**, 458–463.
8 Bonnefous, O., Pesque, P. (1986) Time domain formulation of pulse-Doppler ultrasound and blood velocity estimation by cross correlation. *Ultrasonic Imaging* **8**, 73–85.
9 Hedrick, W.R., Hykes, D.L., Starchmann, D.E. (1995) *Ultrasound Physics and Instrumentation*, 3rd edn. St Louis, Mosby.
10 Evans, D.H. (1993) Techniques for color-flow imaging. In: Wells, P.N.T. (ed.) *Advances in Ultrasound Techniques and Instrumentation*. Churchill Livingstone, New York.
11 Herment, A., Guglielmi, J.P. (1994) Principles of colour imaging of blood flow. *European Journal of Ultrasound* **1**, 197.
12 Herment, A., Dumee, P. (1994) Comparison of blood flow imaging methods. *European Journal of Ultrasound* **1**, 345.
13 Routh, H.F. (1996) Doppler ultrasound, *IEEE Engineering in Medicine and Biology* **15**, 31–40.
14 Nowicki, A., Reid, J.M. (1981) An infinite gate pulse Doppler. *Ultrasound in Medicine and Biology* **7**, 41–50.
15 Willemetz, J.C., Nowicki, A., Meister, J.J., De Palma, F., Pante, G. (1989) Bias and variance in the estimate of the Doppler frequency induced by a wall motion filter. *Ultrasonic Imaging* **11**, 215–225.
16 Rubin, J.M., Bude, R.O., Carson, P.L., Bree, R.L., Adler, R.S. (1994) Power Doppler US: a potentially useful alternative to mean frequency-based color Doppler US. *Radiology* **190**, 853–856.
17 Bude, R.O., Rubin, J.M., Adler, R.S. (1994) Power versus conventional colour Doppler sonography: comparison in the depiction of normal intrarenal vasculature. *Radiology* **192**, 777–780.
18 Kenton, A.R., Martin, P.J., Evans, D.H. (1996) Power Doppler: an advance over colour Doppler for transcranial imaging. *Ultrasound in Medicine and Biology* **22**, 313–317.
19 Griewing, B., Morgenstern, C., Driesner, F., *et al.* (1996) Cerebrovascular disease assessed by color-flow and power Doppler ultrasonography: comparison with digital subtraction angiography in internal carotid artery stenosis. *Stroke* **27**, 101–104.
20 Bohs, L.N., Friemel, B.H., McDermott, B.A., Trahey, G.E. (1993) Real-time system for angle-independent ultrasound of blood flow in two dimensions: initial results. *Radiology* **186**, 259.
21 Bohs, L.N., Trahey, G.E. (1991) A novel method for angle independent ultrasonic imaging of blood flow and tissue motion. *IEEE Transactions in Biomedical Engineering* **38**, 280–286.
22 Trahey, G.E., Hubbard, S.M., von Ramm, O.T. (1988) Angle independent ultrasonic blood flow detection by frame-to-frame correlation of B-mode images. *Ultrasonics* **26**, 271–276.
23 Vera, N., Steinman, D.A., Ethier, C.R., Johnston, K.W., Cobbold, R.S.C. (1992) Visualisation of complex flow fields, with application to the interpretation of colour flow Doppler images. *Ultrasound in Medicine and Biology* **18**, 1–9.
24 Overbeck, J.R., Beach, K.W., Strandness, D.E. (1992) Vector Doppler: accurate measurement of blood velocity in two dimensions. *Ultrasound in Medicine and Biology* **18**, 19–31.
25 Hoskins, P.R., Fleming, A., Stonebridge, P., Allan, P.L., Cameron, D. (1994) Scan-plane vector maps and secondary flow motions in arteries. *European Journal of Ultrasound* **1**, 159–169.
26 Fenster, A., Downey, D.B. (1996) 3-D ultrasound imaging: a review. *IEEE Engineering in Medicine and Biology* **15**, 41–51.
27 Baek, K.R., Bae, M.H., Park, S.B. (1989) A new aliasing extension method for ultrasonic 2-dimension pulsed Doppler systems. *Ultrasonic Imaging* **11**, 233.
28 Hartley, C.J. (1981) Resolution of frequency aliases in ultrasonic pulsed Doppler velocimeters. *IEEE Transactions in Sonics and Ultrasonics* **28**, 69–75.
29 Fehr, R., Dousse, B., Grossniklaus, B. (1991) New advances in color mapping: quantitative velocity measurement beyond the Nyquist limit. *British Journal of Radiology* **64**, 651.
30 Ferrara, K.W., Algazi, V.R. (1991) A new wideband spread target maximum likelihood estimator for blood velocity estimation. 1. Theory. *IEEE Transactions in Ultrasonics, Ferrolectrics and Frequency Control* **38**, 1–16.
31 Ferrara, K.W., Algazi, V.R. (1991) A new wideband spread target maximum likelihood estimator for blood velocity estimation. II. Evaluation of estimators with experimental data. *IEEE Transactions in Ultrasonics, Ferrolectrics and Frequency Control* **38**, 17.

Chapter 5: The physics of blood flow

P.R. Hoskins

This chapter describes the relevant physics useful to sonographers in their daily practice. Further details of the physics is available in a number of sources including texts by McDonald [1], Caro *et al.* [2], Strackee and Westerhof [3], and chapters in the Doppler ultrasound books by Evans *et al.* [4] and Taylor *et al.* [5].

Vessel structure

The normal artery is a three-layered structure consisting of the intima which is a thin membrane of squamous epithelium in contact with the blood, the media which consists of smooth muscle and elastic tissue, and the adventitia which is the outer layer consisting of fibrous tissue. In superficial arteries such as the carotid and femoral arteries the thickness of the medial layer is 0.5–1 mm in health which can be resolved by modern ultrasound scanners using transcutaneous probes. Using intravascular ultrasound systems with their higher frequency and superior axial resolution the three-layered structure is easily seen. Changes to the composition of the arterial wall which occur in disease include thickening of the intimal layer in early disease, with calcification and plaque formation occurring as the disease progresses (Fig. 5.1).

The vein has the same three-layered structure; however, the thickness of the media is less. Some veins possess a series of valves which help ensure that blood flows towards the heart. The most common venous diseases are venous thrombosis and valvular incompetence.

The spatial resolution of linear array systems for peripheral vascular scanning is in the region of 0.5 and 1.5 mm for axial and lateral resolution, respectively. In practice the smallest vessels which can be observed on the B-scan image are digital arteries which have a diameter of approximately 1 mm. The ability to distinguish individual vessels improves every year as the technology improves. For intravascular ultrasound scanners the ability of the scanner to visualize the vessel is limited not by the spatial resolution of the imaging device, but by the size of the catheter and its ability to pass through the vessel. Currently catheters have a diameter of 1 mm.

Blood

Blood is not a fluid; it is a suspension of mainly red cells. The Doppler signal arises from scattering of the ultrasound by the red cells. The backscattered ultrasound power depends on a number of variables. It increases as the scatterer size increases and also as the difference between the elasticity of the particle and the surrounding fluid increases. The power also depends on the scatterer concentration; however, this is not a linear behaviour. For blood a peak power is reached at approximately 15–20% haematocrit [6,7]. At very low velocities the red cells aggregate to form 'rouleaux', whereas at higher velocities the rouleaux are broken down and the red cells behave independently. The increase in size of the scattering components which occurs at low velocity therefore leads to enhanced power. The blood on B-scan images of arteries is normally invisible. However, when the velocity is very low rouleaux are formed and the blood is seen more easily. The backscattered ultrasound power also increases when there is turbulence [7], but, although this effect can be measured in the laboratory it does not generally impact on the clinical application of Doppler techniques or colour flow images.

Flow states

Concepts of flow states originally arose from experiments performed in long straight tubes during steady flow. At low velocities the flow is laminar (Fig. 5.2a), and there is little mixing of adjacent layers of fluid. Components of the fluid travel in well-defined paths along the vessel and the velocity magnitude and direction at each point do not change. At high velocities the flow is turbulent; there is a random element to the motion of the fluid, with much more mixing of the fluid between adjacent layers (Fig. 5.2b). The velocity magnitude and direction at each point vary in a random manner. Energy losses are high in turbu-

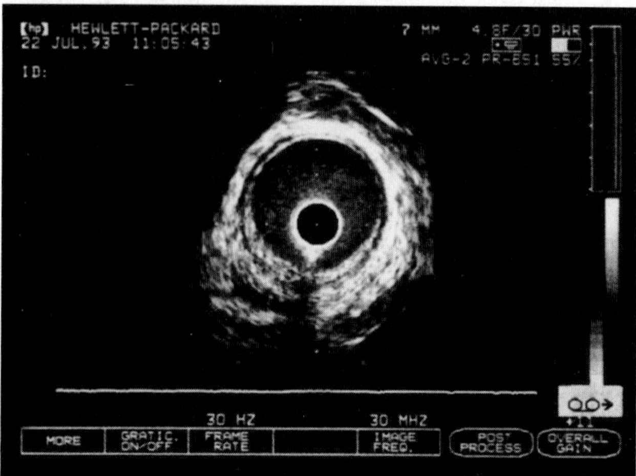

Fig. 5.1 Intravascular ultrasound B-scan image. The junction between the intima and media is seen as a bright layer adjacent to the blood. The junction between the adventitia and the media is also seen clearly. The localized increase in thickness of the media is clearly seen is this example.

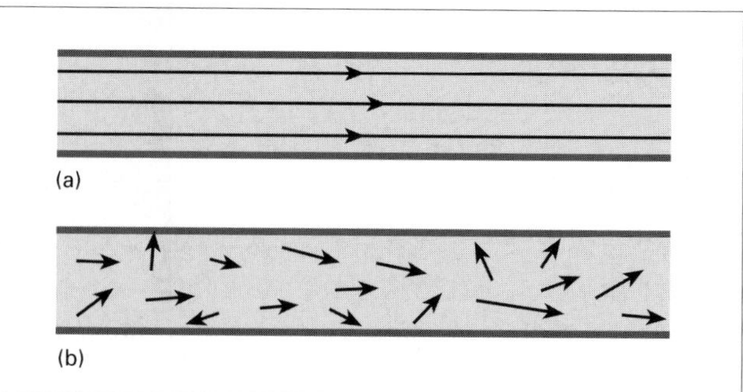

Fig. 5.2 (a) Laminar flow consist of the movement of blood along well-defined pathways called stream lines. (b) At very high velocities there is turbulence consisting of random motions of the blood.

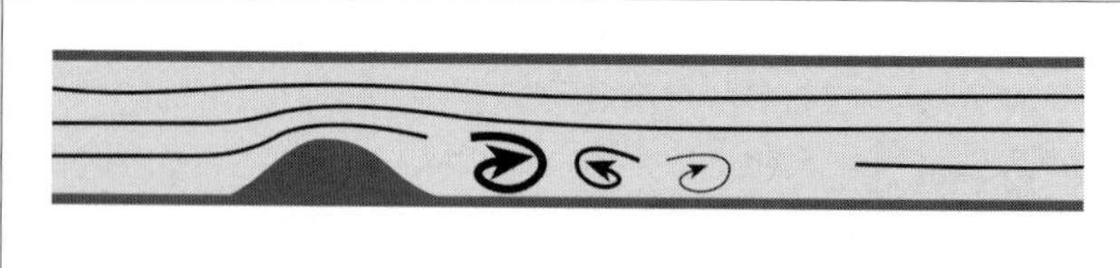

Fig. 5.3 In the poststenotic region there is vortex production. At low velocities and for minor degrees of stenosis the vortex is stable and confined to the immediate poststenotic region, but at higher velocities the vortex is propagated downstream.

lent flow. The fluid is properly described by a dimensionless number called the Reynolds number (*Re*). This is defined as $Re = \rho Lv/\mu$ where ρ is the fluid density, L is the vessel diameter, v is the mean velocity and μ is the fluid viscosity. For a wide variety of fluids the transition to turbulence in a long straight pipe takes place at a value of *Re* of about 2000. For flow in which *Re* is about 2000 the fluid flow will alternate between turbulent and laminar. When velocity is increased so that *Re* is above the critical value turbulence will take a small amount of time to develop. It is possible during pulsatile flow for the flow to be laminar at values of *Re* higher than the critical value; turbulence does not have time to develop before the blood velocity has decreased. The only vessel in which turbulence exists in the normal circulation is the aorta for a brief period during the cardiac cycle. There is also a third flow state known as disturbed flow. This is concerned with situations where there will be variation in velocity magnitude and direction with time at values of *Re* much less than the critical values of 2000. Disturbed flow is mostly concerned with the production of vortices, or eddies. These are circulating regions of flow which are produced when there is some obvious change in vessel cross-sectional area, caused most commonly in the circulation by arterial stenoses. The characteristics of vortices are dependent on the degree of stenosis and the blood velocities. At low *Re* values the vortex is confined to the immediate poststenotic region. At higher *Re* values the vortex will be shed. It will travel several diameters downstream and die out (Fig. 5.3) losing its energy in the form of heat due to friction between adjacent layers of fluid within the vortex.

The practical consequences of different flow types on the Doppler waveform may be illustrated using waveforms from the femoral artery. Figure 5.4a shows Doppler waveforms from the normal femoral artery in which flow is laminar. Within the sample volume the blood velocity magnitude and direction are all similar, hence the waveform outline is smooth and the spectral width is low. Figure 5.4b shows Doppler waveforms downstream from a stenosis. The upslope of the waveform is clearly defined, and this corresponds to the passage through the Doppler sample volume of the blood which was at rest in the poststenotic region during diastole. Blood which was at rest during diastole in the prestenotic region is accelerated through the stenosis producing disturbed and turbulent flow within the Doppler sample volume. The downslope of the waveform demonstrates considerable spectral broadening, high Doppler shift frequencies and a generally ragged appearance to the waveform outline. This is caused by variation of velocity magnitude and direction within the sample volume and with time as the vortex passes through the stenosis.

In clinical practice little if any distinction is made between disturbed and turbulent flow; both produce spectral broadening.

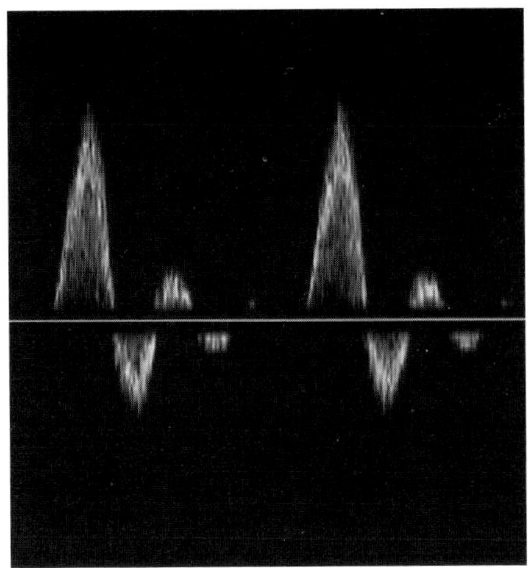
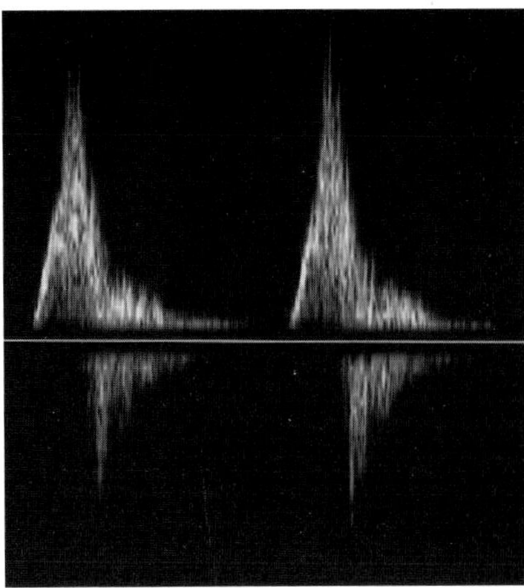
(a),(b)

Fig. 5.4 Femoral artery Doppler waveforms: (a) from the non-diseased circulation; the waveform has a smooth outline and the spectral width is low; and (b) from the poststenotic region; in the early systolic phase the waveform has a clearly defined outline associated with passage of the blood which was at rest in the poststenotic region during diastole past the insonation site. Blood which was initially in the prestenotic region passes through the stenosis, increases in velocity and enters the turbulent poststenotic region. This appears as a region in which there is spectral broadening and high frequency spikes.

A simple flow model

The creation of a pressure gradient within the arterial system is performed by ejection of blood into the arterial tree by the heart. The resistance (R) to flow of a vessel segment may be defined as $R = (P_1 - P_2)/Q$, where Q is the flow rate through the vessel, and P_1 and P_2 are the pressures at the entrance and exit points of the vessel. The implication of this equation is that in order to maintain a constant flow value, the pressure difference must be greater when the resistance to flow increases. This formula only strictly applies for steady flow. For pulsatile flow a more complex version of this equation must be used. The resistance to flow for a long straight vessel depends on the fourth power of the diameter. A segment of vessel 2 mm in diameter will therefore have a resistance 16 times that of a similar segment of 4 mm diameter.

Figure 5.5 shows a simple model of the flow to an organ. The net flow is controlled by a combination of the small vessel (arteriolar) resistance and the large vessel (arterial) resistance. The large arteries have a large diameter in the non-diseased circulation, and hence their resistance to flow is small. The main resistance vessels in the non-diseased circulation are the arterioles. The essential clinical manifestations of atherosclerosis may be understood with the aid of this model. Increase in resistance in a large distributing artery because of atheroma is compensated by a decrease in the resistance of the arteriolar bed in order to preserve flow to the organ. As the disease progresses, organ flow is maintained by further arteriolar dilatation until the point is reached where there is full arteriolar dilatation. Further progression of the proximal disease results in a reduction in organ flow with development of ischaemia because no further compensatory dilatation is possible.

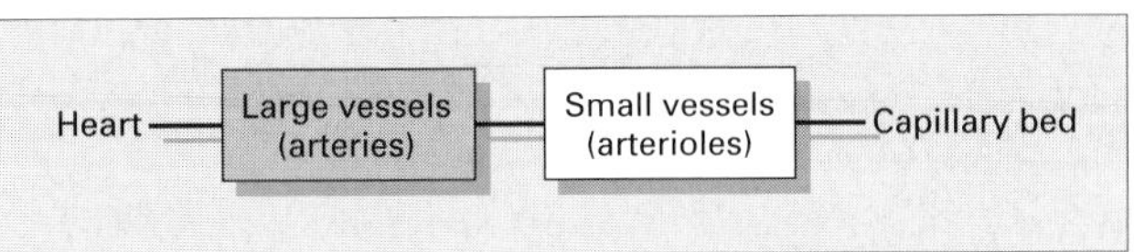

Fig. 5.5 Simple model of flow to an organ consisting of a large vessel (arterial) resistance and a small vessel (arteriolar bed) resistance.

As the degree of narrowing at a single, isolated stenosis increases, a point is reached where the distal arteriolar dilatation is maximum, and any increase in the degree of stenosis beyond this point leads to reduction in flow. The degree of stenosis at which this occurs is called the critical stenosis. Animal experiments suggest that critical stenosis is reached with 75% area reduction (50% diameter reduction). Two quantities of interest in Doppler ultrasound are volumetric flow rate and velocity; the relationship between these two parameters, according to the model developed above is shown in Fig. 5.6. With increase in the degree of stenosis, the volume of blood flowing along the vessel is maintained by increasing the velocity. Above the point of critical stenosis, there is reduction in flow rate.

As atherosclerosis develops various other compensatory mechanisms come into play in an attempt to preserve perfusion, these include the development of a collateral circulation and increase in the extraction efficiency of oxygen from blood. This implies that the concept of critical stenosis should not be taken too far.

Flow and pressure waves in arteries

For a particular element of blood it is the pressure gradient, not the actual pressure, which accelerates the blood.

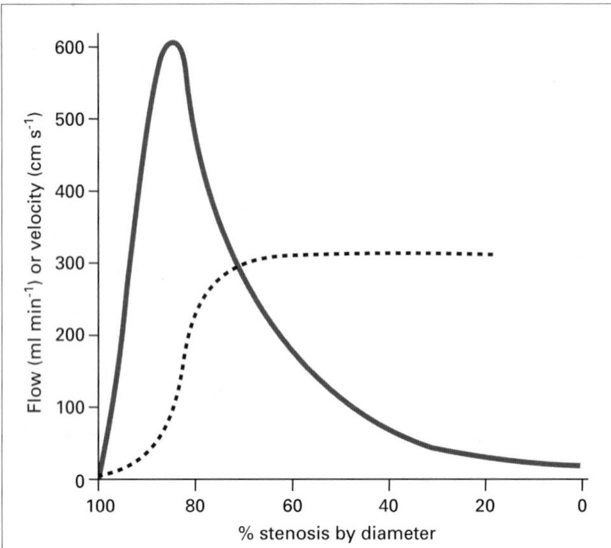

Fig. 5.6 Flow rate (--) and velocity (—) based upon a single arterial stenosis inserted into an otherwise normal circulation. (Redrawn from Spencer & Reid [10] with permission; © 1979 American Heart Association.)

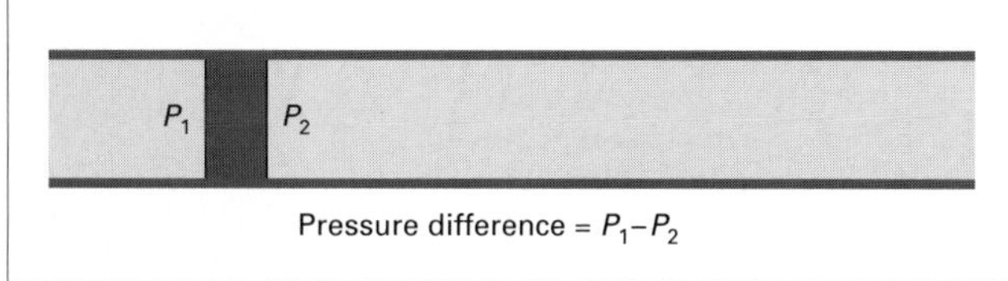

Fig. 5.7 The force acting on the element of blood is related to the difference in pressures on either side of the element.

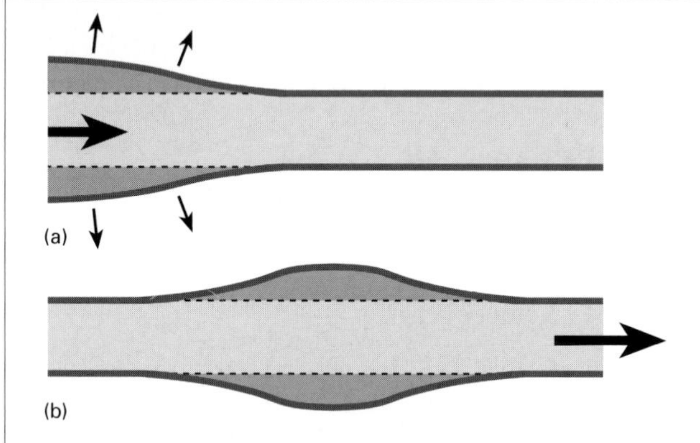

Fig. 5.8 Formation and propagation of the pressure pulse: (a) the cardiac output is ejected into the major arteries including the aorta, causing expansion of the arteries and increase in the blood pressure; and (b) the arterial expansion and subsequent recoil pass down the vessel as a wave whose velocity (pressure pulse wave velocity or PWV) is 5–15 m s^{-1}.

The pressure gradient is related to the difference between the pressures on either side of the element of blood (Fig. 5.7). When the pressure gradient is positive the blood will be accelerated downstream, and when the gradient is negative the blood will be decelerated. In the discussion below the pressure will be considered as it is a familiar quantity. The corresponding flow waveform is found by detailed calculation of the pressure gradient at the site of interest.

The medial layer of arteries has a high proportion of an elastic material called, appropriately, elastin. When the heart ejects blood into the aorta and other major vessels during the systolic phase these arteries quickly expand, and the blood pressure increases. There is then a pressure difference between the blood in arteries near to the heart and the more distal arteries. The momentum of the blood ejected from the heart and the pressure difference force the blood downstream. A more detailed examination of events demonstrates that the expanded region and the blood pressure pass down the arterial tree in the form of a wave (Fig. 5.8). Typical pulse pressure wave velocities are 5 m s^{-1} in the aorta, and 10–15 m s^{-1} in the peripheral circulation.

In a long straight vessel a single heart beat would produce a pressure wave which propagates down the artery, causing blood to flow. This situation can be modelled using a long elastic pipe connected to a large syringe. Ejection of fluid into the pipe gives rise to the waveform shown in Fig. 5.9. There is an initial phase in which the velocity increases rapidly followed by a later phase in which the velocity returns slowly to zero. This example is consistent with the above description whereby the vessel has been stretched as a result of the injection of the fluid, and returns slowly to its original dimensions under elastic recoil, and in doing so pushes the fluid down the vessel. The flow waveform in this simple example is monophasic. In human arteries the flow often demonstrates a

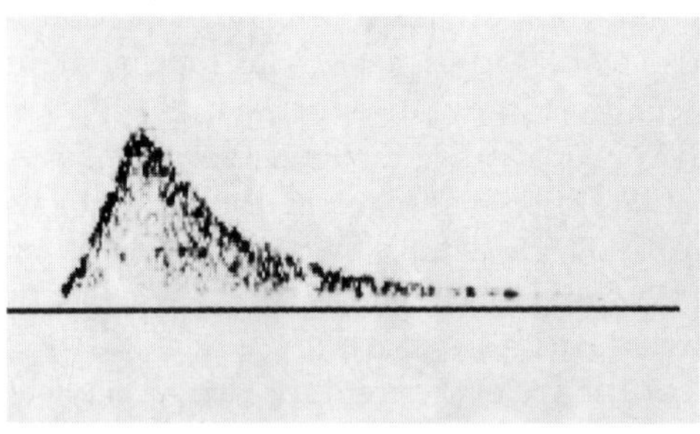

Fig. 5.9 Doppler waveform from a long straight tube; there is an initial phase in which the velocity increases rapidly followed by a later phase in which the velocity returns slowly to zero.

reverse component. It can be observed (Fig. 5.10) using a Doppler system that after a period of exercise or reactive hyperaemia the flow waveform loses the reverse flow component, and in fact there is flow throughout the cardiac cycle. Initially after exercise the arteriolar bed is fully dilated in order to maximize flow. During the recovery period lasting 1–2 min the arteriolar bed dilatation decreases as the flow requirements of the muscles decrease, and simultaneously the degree of diastolic flow reduces until, when recovery is complete, the reverse flow component is restored. These observations suggest that in some circumstances there is a relationship between the degree of downstream resistance to flow and the pulsatility of the flow waveform. It is thought that the key to understanding this observation lies in the presence of reflected pressure waves produced by the arteriolar bed (Fig. 5.11). At this region there is an alteration, or mismatch, in the resistance to flow, with the arteriolar network demonstrating a higher resistance than the proximal arteries. The reflected pressure waves travel up the arterial tree and the resultant pressure wave will be a combination of the forward going and the reflected pressure waves. The resulting pressure gradient causes the flow waveform to have a reverse flow component (Fig. 5.12). The effect is maximum when the resistance mismatch is greatest, giving rise to reverse flow, and is minimum when the arterioles are fully dilated, producing minimum flow waveform pulsatility. This simple model has been shown to be effective for certain vascular areas, especially in the fetal placental circulation where the pulsatility of the umbilical artery waveform (Fig. 5.13) is related to the impedance to flow of the fetal placenta [8], and measure-

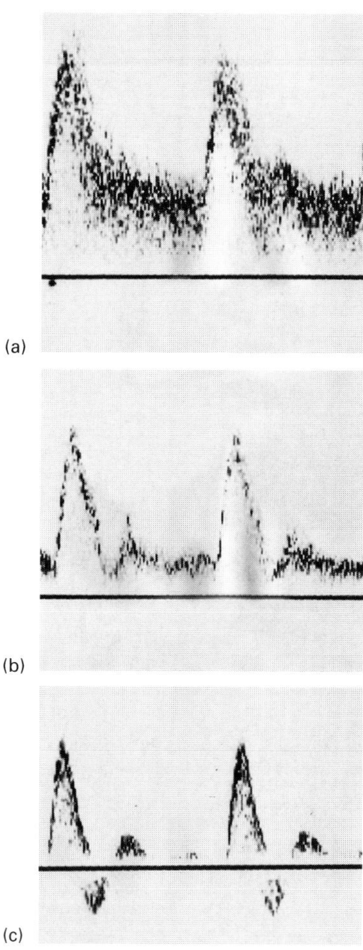

Fig. 5.10 Doppler waveforms after reactive hyperaemia from the common femoral artery: (a) initially there is substantial flow throughout the cardiac cycle; (b) during recovery the degree of diastolic flow decreases, with reverse flow present when recovery is almost complete (c).

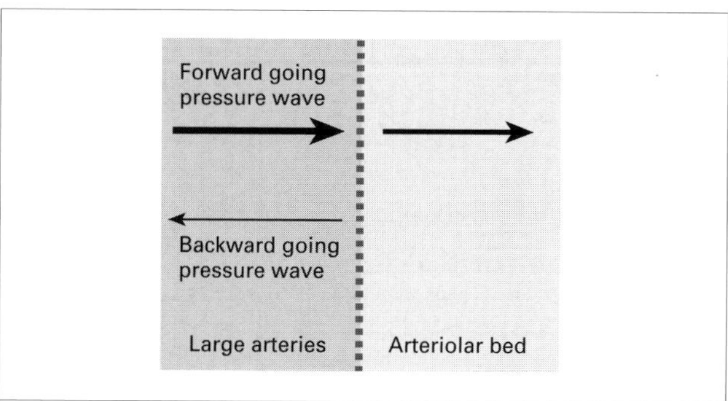

Fig. 5.11 Pressure waves are reflected at the arteriolar bed, causing a pressure wave which travels back up the arterial tree.

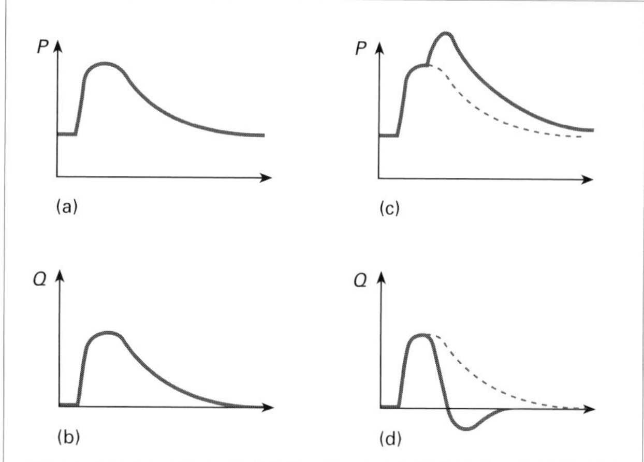

Fig. 5.12 (a,b) Pressure and flow waves in the absence of distal reflection; (c,d) pressure and flow waves when there is distal reflection; the reflected waves combine with the forward going waves as shown. (Redrawn from Murgo *et al.* [11] with permission; © 1981 American Heart Association.)

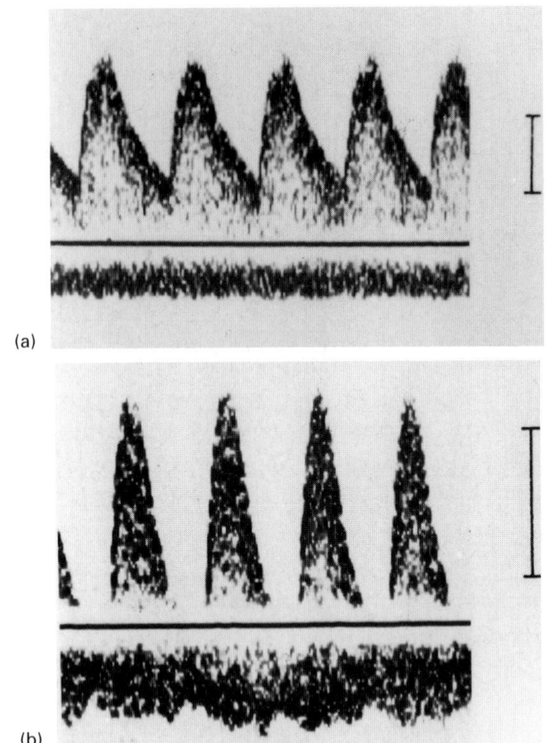

Fig. 5.13 Umbilical artery Doppler waveforms: (a) normal showing flow throughout the cardiac cycle; and (b) abnormal showing absent end-diastolic flow. Venous flow is seen below the line. The bar represents an excursion of 1 kHz.

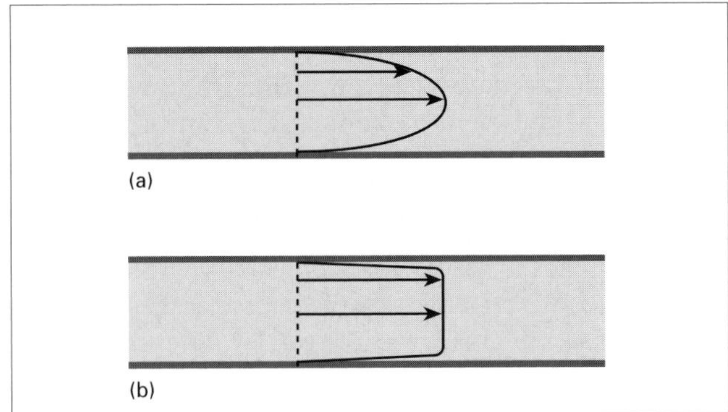

Fig. 5.14 Velocity profiles in a long straight tube: (a) parabolic profile during laminar flow; and (b) blunted profile during turbulent flow.

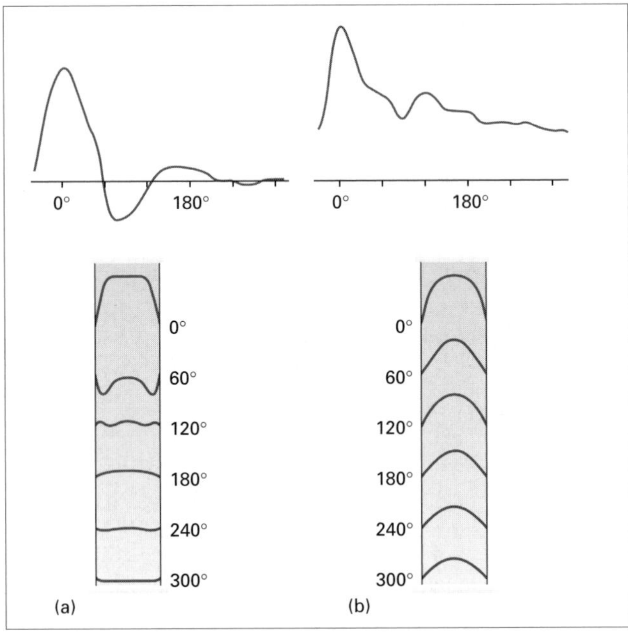

Fig. 5.15 Mean velocity waveforms and velocity profiles at various times during pulsatile flow: (a) femoral artery; and (b) carotid artery. (Redrawn from Evans *et al.* [4] with permission; © 1989 John Wiley and Sons Ltd.)

ments of the pulsatility of the Doppler waveform are used as a measure of placental insufficiency [9].

Velocity profiles

The velocity profile is the variation of velocity as a function of the vessel diameter. In steady laminar flow in a long straight tube the velocity profile is parabolic (Fig. 5.14a). The maximum velocity occurs at the centre of the vessel and there is zero flow at the vessel wall. When there is turbulence the time-averaged profile becomes more blunt (Fig. 5.14b). In conditions of pulsatile flow the velocity profile is no longer parabolic (Fig. 5.15), and in fact changes throughout the cardiac cycle. During periods of forward flow the maximum velocity is at the centre of the tube; however, this may not be the case during reverse flow.

The Doppler spectral display is critically related to the manner in which the sample volume is placed within the vessel. Usually Doppler spectra are required in which the maximum velocity is clearly demonstrated. Optimum display occurs when the region of maximum sensitivity within the beam is coincident with the region of maximum velocity in the vessel. For a straight tube this normally corresponds to alignment of the beam axis and vessel axis. If there is severe misalignment then the maximum frequency lies in a less sensitive part of the Doppler beam, and may not be adequately visualized. Doppler waveforms in this case demonstrate a noisy waveform outline. In practice using a stand alone continuous wave Doppler probe the operator will search for waveforms with a clear waveform outline; making small adjustments of the probe position in order to align the beam axis and the vessel axis. Using a duplex or colour flow system visualization of the vessel assists in this process.

The effect of sample volume size and position on the Doppler spectrum can easily be demonstrated using the long straight tube model (Fig. 5.16) in which the sample volume is positioned centrally and the gate length steadily increased. Figure 5.17 shows spectra obtained from a 10 mm diameter vessel in which the gate length has been increased from 1.5 to 12 mm. For small gate lengths there is little variation in velocity magnitude and the spectrum is concentrated around the maximum frequency outline. At the other extreme for large gate sizes the sample volume incorporates the low velocity components at the edge of the beam and the spectrum is broadened.

The long straight tube model is useful for outlining principles; however, there are few arteries in the body which are long and straight. Possibly the artery that comes closest to this is the non-diseased superficial femoral. Change in vessel geometry causes several effects; for example, skewing of the velocity profile, whereby the point of maximum velocity is no longer located at the centre of the vessel; secondary flow motions which are motions at 90° to the vessel axis, resulting in the flow down the vessel travelling in a helical fashion, and vortex production which has already been discussed. Several specific idealized examples are given below to illustrate the range of possible effects.

1 Entrance region of a vessel. Figure 5.18 shows the profiles at various distances after the entrance to a vessel from a large reservoir during steady flow. The velocity profile is flat near the entrance to the vessel, and assumes a stable parabolic shape at a distance beyond the vessel called the entrance or inlet length. Values may be calculated for the entrance length [1] which suggest that for the larger arteries most of the arterial length is in the inlet region.

2 Vessel narrowing. For steady flow a gradual narrowing taper will tend to sharpen the velocity profile.

3 Vessel expansion. At regions where the cross-sectional area of the vessel increases an adverse pressure gradient is created; that is, there is a pressure decrease in the direction of flow which retards the flow. For the central high velocity region the high momentum opposes this, but at the edge of the vessel the velocities are low, and the direction of motion near the wall will reverse if there is sufficient rapid increase in vessel cross-sectional area with distance. The phrase 'flow separation' is often used to describe this phenomenon; that is, the high velocity central jet is located next to a region in which the flow is of low velocity and recirculating. The production of vortices was noted above; both the central jet and vortices die out after a few diameters and laminar flow is re-established. Figure 5.19 shows the velocity profiles in the region of a small stenosis. When the expansion is less severe, such as a gradually widening taper, the velocity profile simply becomes more blunted.

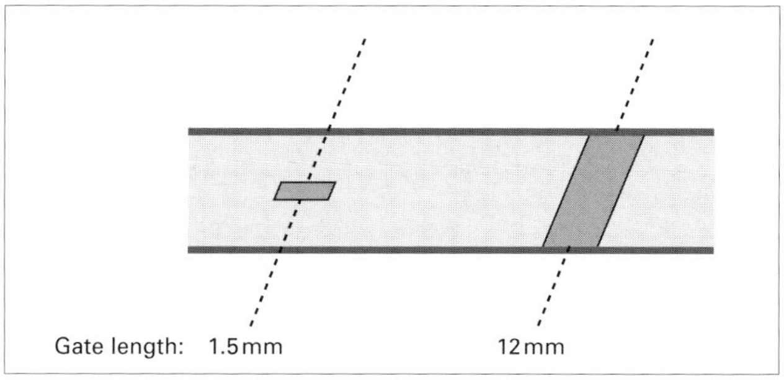

Fig. 5.16 Geometry for acquisition of Doppler spectra from a 12 mm diameter tube. The gate is positioned centrally and the gate length increased from 1.5 to 12 mm, where it encompasses the whole diameter. At low gate lengths the sample volume contains only the high velocities in the centre of the vessel, whereas for larger sample volumes lower velocity components also contribute to the Doppler signal giving increased spectral broadening.

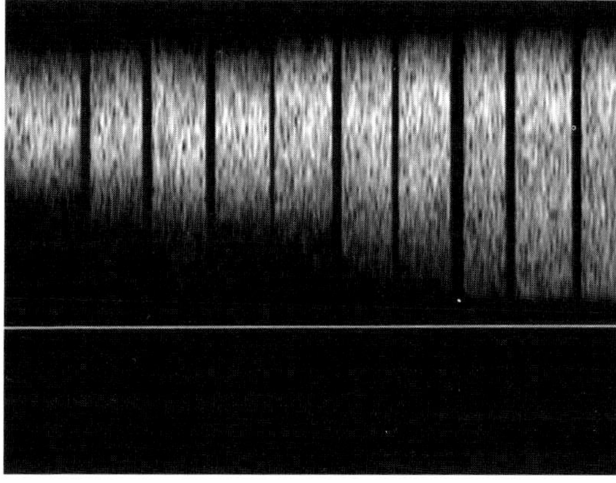

Fig. 5.17 Doppler waveforms from an 8 mm vessel during pulsatile flow with gate length varying from 1.5 to 10 mm. The degree of spectral broadening increases with gate length.

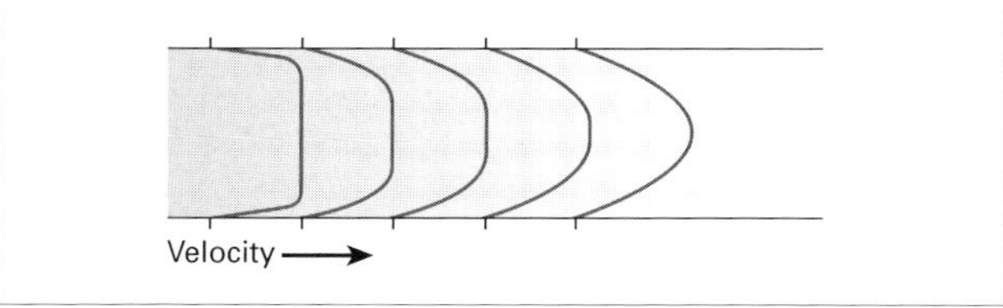

Fig. 5.18 Velocity profiles at various distances from the entrance to a long straight tube during steady flow. The parabolic velocity profile is restored at a distance from the entrance. (Redrawn from Caro *et al.* [2] with permission; © 1978 Oxford University Press.)

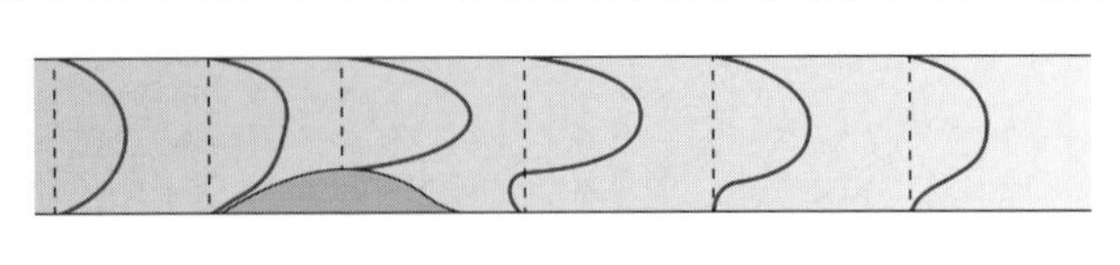

Fig. 5.19 Velocity profiles from a stenosis model; the region of recirculation in the poststenotic region can be seen.

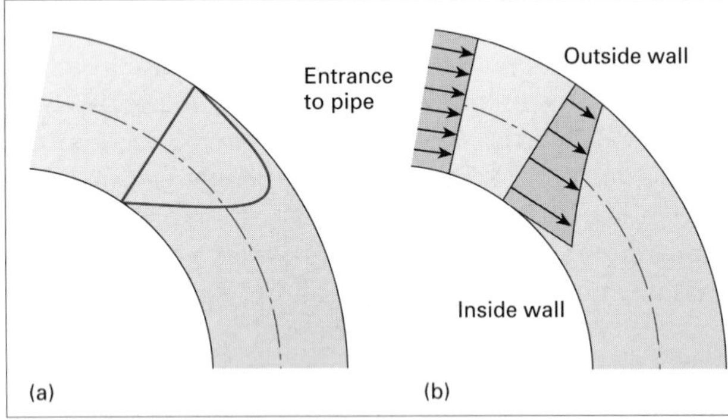

Fig. 5.20 Velocity profiles within a curved vessel during steady flow: (a) parabolic velocity profile at the entrance; and (b) blunt velocity profile at the entrance. (Redrawn from Caro *et al.* [2] with permission; © 1978 Oxford University Press.)

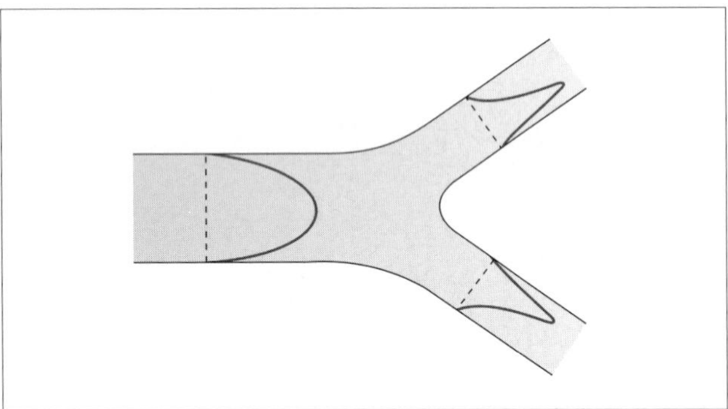

Fig. 5.21 Velocity profiles in the branches of a Y-shaped junction during steady flow.

4 Curved vessel. The velocity profile is skewed (Fig. 5.20).
5 Y-shaped junction. In the branches the flow profiles are skewed (Fig. 5.21).

The factors associated with deviation of the artery from the ideal do not much affect the day-to-day collection and interpretation of Doppler spectra and colour flow images. They are of concern mainly in research programmes which attempt to perform, for example, quantification of blood flow and accurate measurement of blood velocity.

Conclusion

The detailed composition of the Doppler signal is critically dependent on several factors including flow type, vessel geometry, and the blood flow pulsatility. For routine clinical use a basic understanding of haemodynamics is important in order to interpret the Doppler spectral and colour flow displays. For research use detailed analysis of the frequency and intensity of Doppler signals must take the factors described in this chapter into account.

Acknowledgements

Thanks to Mr Peter Fish, School of Electronic Engineering Science, University of Wales, and Professor Clive Greated, Physics Department, Edinburgh University, for helpful discussion and comments.

References

1 McDonald, D.A. (1974) *Blood Flow in Arteries*. Edward Arnold, London.
2 Caro, C.G., Pedley, T.J., Schroter, R.C., Seed, W.A. (1978) *The Mechanics of the Circulation*. Oxford University Press, Oxford.
3 Strackee, J., Westerhof, N. (1993) *The Physics of Heart and Circulation*. IOP, Bristol.
4 Evans, D.H., McDicken, W.N., Skidmore, R., Woodcock, J.P. (1989) *Doppler Ultrasound: Physics, Instrumentation and Clinical Applications*. Wiley, Colchester.
5 Taylor, K.J.W., Burns, P.N., Wells, P.N.T. (1995) *Clinical Applications of Doppler Ultrasound*. Raven Press, New York.
6 Yuan, Y.W., Shung, K.K. (1988) Ultrasonic backscatter from flowing whole blood. I: dependence on shear rate and hematocrit. *Journal of the Acoustics Society of America* **84**, 52–58.
7 Shung, K.K., Cloutier, G. (1992) The effects of hematocrit, shear rate, and turbulence on ultrasonic Doppler spectrum from blood. *IEEE Transactions on Biomedical Engineering* **39**, 462–469.
8 Adamson, S.L., Morrow, R.J., Langille, B.L., Bull, S.B., Ritchie, J.W.K. (1996) Site-dependent effects of increases in placental vascular resistance on the umbilical arterial velocity waveform in fetal sheep. *Ultrasound in Medicine and Biology* **16**, 19–27.
9 Alfirevic, Z., Neilson, J.P. (1996) The current status of Doppler sonography in obstetrics. *Current Opinion in Obstetrics and Gynecology* **8**, 114–118.
10 Spencer, M.P., Reid, J.M. (1979) Quantitation of carotid stenosis with continuous wave (C-W) Doppler ultrasound. *Stroke* **10**, 326–330.
11 Murgo, J.P., Westerhof, N., Giolma, J.P., Altobelli, S.A. (1981) Manipulations of ascending aortic pressure and flow wave reflections with the Valsalva maneuver: relationship to input impedance. *Circulation* **63**, 122–132.

Chapter 6: Safety issues in diagnostic ultrasound

P.N.T. Wells

Although it is in its diagnostic applications that medical ultrasound is perhaps at its most visible, ultrasonic energy is widely used in physiotherapy and for the functional modification and even the selective ablation of tissue. It is also used for lithotripsy and in applications such as phacoemulsification and dental scaling. Examples of some of these procedures are illustrated in Fig. 6.1. Thus, it has to be accepted that ultrasound can produce biological effects and that, under some circumstances, these effects may be damaging to tissue and, consequently, potentially hazardous.

Safety considerations in the use of diagnostic ultrasound can logically follow the pattern familiar in radiation protection for ionizing radiation. As with ionizing radiation, individuals potentially needing protection against ultrasonic radiation can be categorized as patients being investigated by ultrasound, operators of ultrasonic equipment and, theoretically at least, passers-by including members of the public.

Measurement of exposure conditions

Ultrasonic power

At the outset, it is necessary to have details of the ultrasonic power emitted by the diagnostic transducer. Ultrasonic power can be measured by several different instruments, including calorimeters, radiation force balances and calibrated hydrophones.

When an ultrasonic beam is absorbed, the ultrasonic energy is converted to heat. For example, a simple calculation (based on the facts that $1\,W = 1\,J\,s^{-1}$ and $1\,J = 0.24\,cal$) reveals that complete absorption of a wave carrying a power of 1 W in a calorimeter with a water equivalent of 0.1 kg results in a rise in temperature of $0.0024\,K\,s^{-1}$. Although calorimetry is an absolute method of measurement, the temperature rise in an instrument of reasonable size is quite small even for moderately high ultrasonic powers. There is the added problem that there may be an error in the measurement due to the direct transfer of heat resulting from the inefficiency of the probe. For these reasons, calorimetry is seldom used to measure diagnostic ultrasonic power levels.

In addition to the heat that is produced when ultrasound is absorbed, a force is also created at the surface of the absorber where it is entered by the wave. Although the theory is complicated, the actual relationship is quite simple. The radiation force is equal to the ultrasonic power divided by the speed of ultrasound. For example, complete absorption of a wave travelling in water and carrying a power of 1 W produces a force of $6.7 \times 10^{-4}\,N$. This is equal to the force of gravity acting on a weight of 69 mg. Although this is not a very large force, it can easily be measured with a suitable balance. Of course, the absorbing target has to be immersed in the water supporting the ultrasonic beam. Various ingenious designs have been adopted, ranging from simple submerged beam balances to complicated electronic servosystems; an example is illustrated in Fig. 6.2. Although the situation in which the target is a perfect absorber is the one which is theoretically easier to consider, the target can be a reflector; in the case of a perfect reflector, the radiation force is doubled.

Hydrophones are, in effect, microphones designed to operate under water at ultrasonic frequencies. There are two main kinds of hydrophones. Needle- or catheter-mounted hydrophones, such as those illustrated in Fig. 6.3a, are as small as possible in relation to the wavelength and consist of a small rigid or flexible tube at the tip of which is mounted a piezoelectric element. A membrane hydrophone, shown in Fig. 6.3b, is a thin piezoelectric plastic film stretched over a supporting ring, with one or more small electroded areas sensitive to ultrasound passing through the membrane. A hydrophone can be calibrated so that the measured output voltage has a known relationship to the amplitude of the ultrasonic wave and hence, to the ultrasonic power carried by the wave. Usually, measurements are made in a water tank but it may be possible to introduce the device into tissue to determine *in situ* values.

(a)
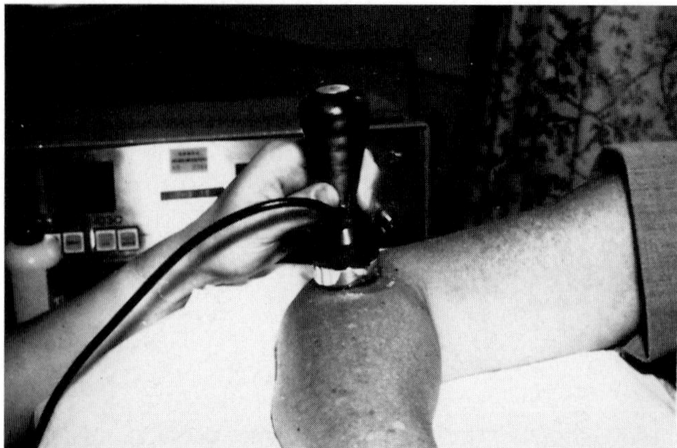

(b)
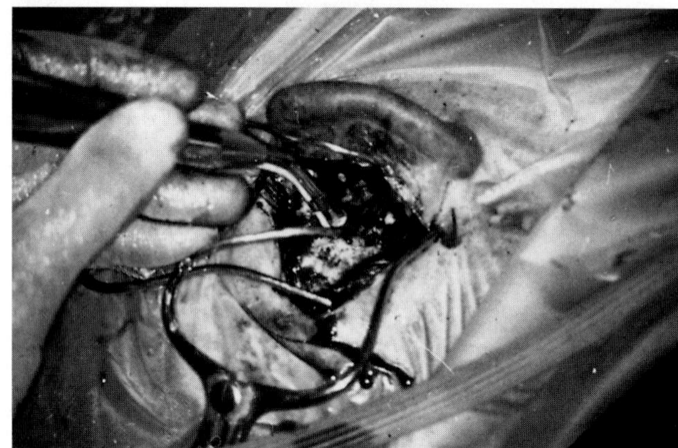

Fig. 6.1 (a) Ultrasonic physiotherapy. The hand-held probe contains a 3 MHz transducer with a diameter of 25 mm. Typically, the ultrasonic intensity is a few watts per square centimetre and the treatment lasts for 5–10 min. (b) Ultrasonic surgical treatment of Ménière's disease. The tip of the ultrasonic probe contains a 3 MHz transducer with a diameter of 5 mm, in front of which there is a small water-filled cone reducing the beam diameter to 2 mm. Ultrasound is applied directly to the lateral semicircular canal through a surgically prepared bone window a fraction of a millimetre in thickness. Typically, the treatment lasts about 15 min.

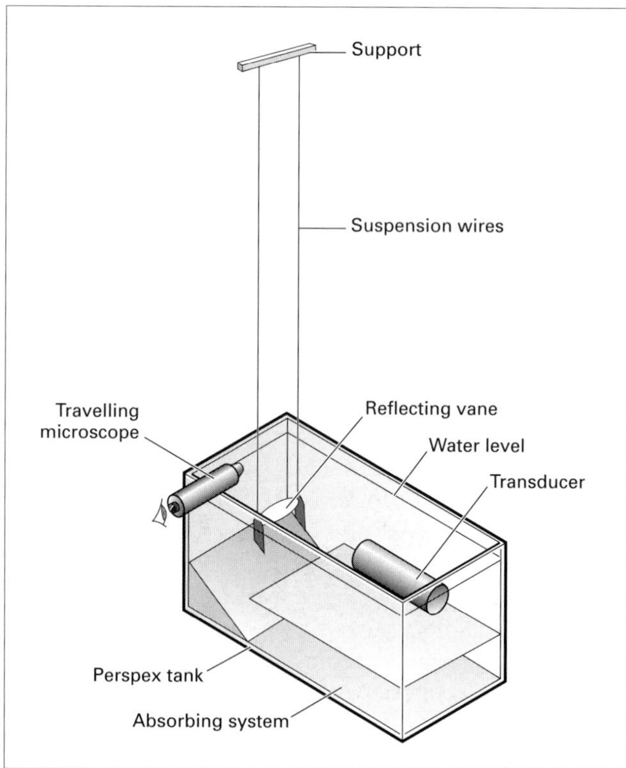

Fig. 6.2 Irradiation force balance. The force due to the ultrasound is sensed by the reflecting vane, the deflection of which is measured by the travelling microscope. The balance is sensitive enough to measure powers of a few milliwatts.

Continuous wave and pulsed ultrasound

In simple ultrasonic Doppler instruments, such as those used for fetal heart motion detection and some peripheral vascular studies, continuous wave ultrasound is used. This means that the transmitting transducer in the probe operates continuously; a separate transducer, in the same probe, is usually used for reception. In other ultrasonic diagnostic instruments, the ultrasound is pulsed. For imaging, it is usually desirable for the pulse to be as brief as possible. In some pulsed Doppler applications, however, a somewhat longer pulse may be used. Figure 6.4 is an example of a typical pulse used for grey-scale real-time imaging. Most of the energy in the pulse is contained within two cycles of oscillation, although the decay of the pulse, in particular, is slightly extended and followed by a rather persistent ripple.

In considering a train of sequential pulses, such as is used in an imaging instrument and illustrated in Fig. 6.5, three important quantities can be identified.

1 The 'on-time', which is the time during which the ultrasound is switched on during an exposure time and which is equal to (pulse duration) × (pulse repetition rate) × (total exposure time).

2 The 'on-power', which is equal to the power whilst the ultrasound is switched on.

3 The 'average power', which is equal to (on-power) × (on-time) ÷ (total time).

Beam shape and ultrasonic intensity

Because the ultrasonic beam carrying the power has a definite cross-sectional area, the concept of 'intensity' has to be introduced. In its simplest form, the intensity can be defined as (power) ÷ (beam area). In practice, the beam has a complicated shape; it is likely to be focused so as to optimize the imaging resolution, to converge towards the

(a)
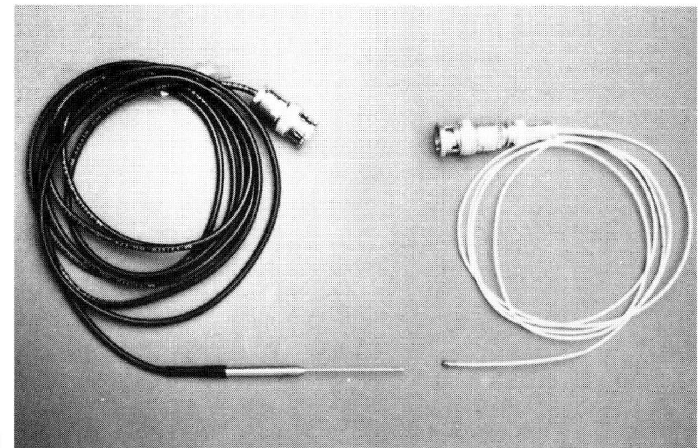

(b)
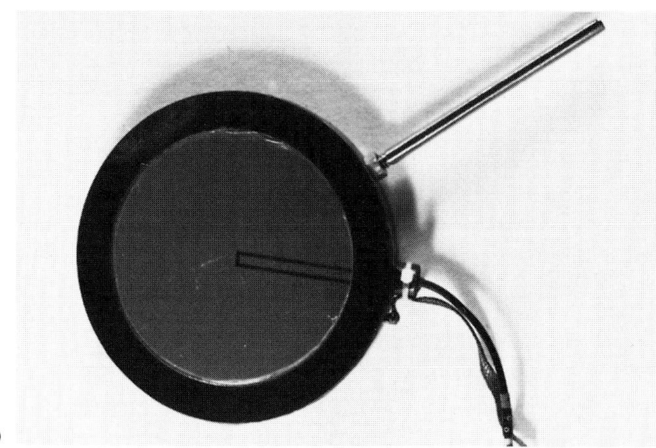

Fig. 6.3 (a) Examples of miniature hydrophones. (Left) A needle-tip hydrophone for water-tank measurements; (right) a hydrophone mounted on a flexible tube, for *in situ* tissue measurements. (b) A membrane hydrophone. The sensitive element is the small area at the centre of the membrane.

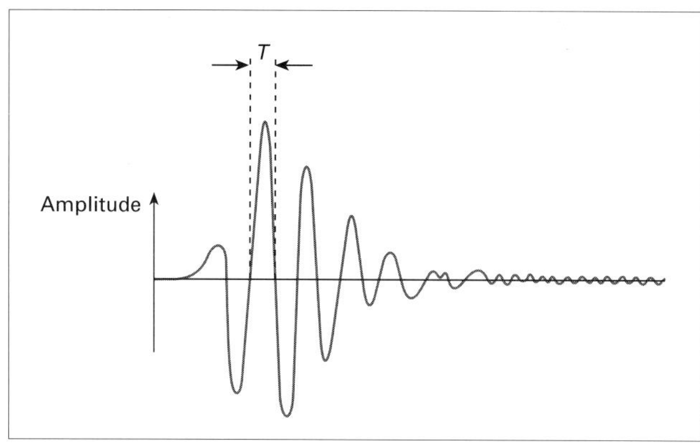

Fig. 6.4 Typical pulse–echo waveform as used in ultrasonic imaging. The time *T* is the duration of half a cycle of ultrasonic vibration.

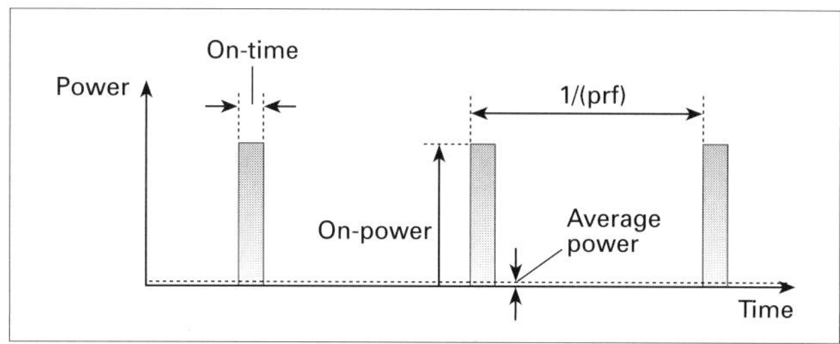

Fig. 6.5 A sequence of pulses, as transmitted into the patient during pulse–echo imaging. The stippled areas indicate the power and duration of the pulses; the interval between the pulses is the reciprocal of the pulse repetition frequency (prf).

focus and to diverge beyond it. A typical ultrasonic beam shape is represented in Fig. 6.6. Moreover, the beam does not have sharply defined edges but, in the same way that the pulse grows and decays in time, so the beam has a maximum amplitude along its central axis about which it decays (usually symmetrically) on both sides. The actual duration of the pulse and width of the beam are often defined in relation to some arbitrarily chosen level such as, for example, −10 dB relative to the maximum amplitude of the pulse. If this is done, it becomes possible to define spatial peak and spatial average, as well as temporal peak and temporal average, intensities for the ultrasonic beam. Thus, the spatial peak intensity is the maximum instantaneous value (usually at the centre of the beam) during the passage of the pulse. The spatial average intensity is the intensity averaged over the whole of the useful beam cross-section (for example, the area of the beam within which the intensity is greater than −10 dB with respect to the spatial peak intensity). The temporal peak intensity is the instantaneous maximum intensity of the pulse and the temporal average intensity is the intensity averaged over time.

These various intensities are generally abbreviated to SP (spatial peak), SA (spatial average), TP (temporal peak) and TA (temporal average). The abbreviation I is used for intensity. Thus, for example, I_{SPTA} means the spatial peak temporal average intensity.

Exposure conditions used in medical applications of ultrasound

Most surgical applications of ultrasound, such as in the production of trackless focal lesions in soft tissues, use intensities (I_{SPTP}) of between 1 and 100 W cm^{-2}. Exposure times are in the range of a few tenths to a few tens of seconds. For extracorporeal shockwave lithotripsy, intensities (I_{SPTP}) of between 100 and 1000 W cm^{-2} are commonly employed with perhaps 100–1000 very brief pulses (a few microseconds) applied at rates of 1–10 s^{-1}. For physiotherapy, ultrasonic intensities (I_{SPTA}) of 1–5 W cm^{-2}

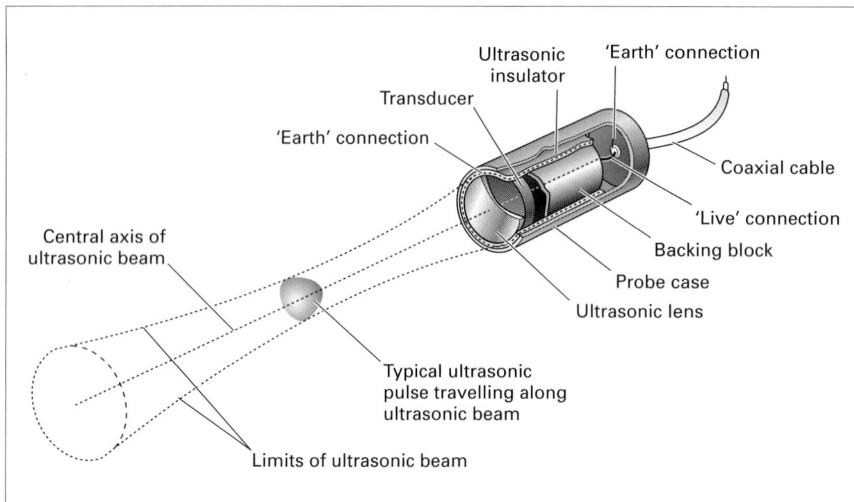

Fig. 6.6 Construction of a typical pulse–echo ultrasonic probe and diagrammatic representation of the focused ultrasonic beam and pulse shapes.

are used and pulsed operation is common, pulses typically having a mark-space ratio of 1 : 1 at a repetition rate of 50 s^{-1}.

The I_{SPTA} employed in ultrasonic diagnosis typically lies in the range 5 mW cm^{-2} to 5 W cm^{-2}. Thus, the range extends over three orders of magnitude and may reach levels equal to those used in physiotherapy. Moreover, there are diverse pulsing and scanning conditions which need to be taken into account when considering biological effects and the possibility of hazard.

Exposure and dose

Just as with ionizing radiation, ultrasonic irradiation can be considered both in terms of exposure and of dose (and dose rate). The exposure describes the ultrasonic field quantities such as the shapes of the pulse and the beam, the intensity and the wave pressure. The dose is the quantity of energy absorbed; its calculation requires information about the properties of the biological material being irradiated.

There are some aspects of the physical exposure conditions which are of particular relevance to biological effects of ultrasound. These are I_{SPTA} (because it is an index of ultrasonic heating), peak negative pressure (which relates to the possibility of cavitation as discussed below), beam shape (which controls the volume of irradiated tissue), working frequency (which affects the possibility of cavitation and the rate of heat deposition), pulse repetition frequency (which is important if there is a period of recovery following each pulse) and the total exposure time (which determines the dose). In addition, account needs to be taken both of the beam scanning format and the attenuation in tissues between the transducer and the site at which the possibility of damage is being considered.

Biological effects of ultrasound

Thermal effects

There are two principal mechanisms by which it has been established that ultrasound can produce biological effects—thermal and mechanical. The thermal mechanism results from the rise in the temperature of ultrasonically irradiated tissue due to the absorption of ultrasound within it. The attenuation coefficient for soft tissues is generally in the range 0.5–1.0 dB cm^{-1} MHz^{-1}. Assuming a value of 1.0 dB cm^{-1} MHz^{-1}, the half-power distance (the thickness of tissue travelling through which an ultrasonic beam loses half its power) is 30 mm at 1 MHz, 10 mm at 3 MHz, and so on. Again, assuming that the specific heat of tissue is the same as that of water, an intensity of 1 W cm^{-2} results in an initial time rate of rise of temperature of 0.05 °K s^{-1} at 1 MHz and 0.5 °K s^{-1} at 10 MHz. Of course, the initial time rate of rise of temperature is not usually maintained because of the cooling effects of conduction and local blood flow. At the typical ultrasonic intensity of 20 mW cm^{-2}, the initial time rate of rise of temperature is only 0.01 °K s^{-1} even at the rather high frequency of 10 MHz and so thermal mechanisms can often be discounted as a source of hazard in diagnostic applications. This is not always the case, however, since some diagnostic applications involve the use of much higher intensities. Furthermore, if bone is present in the beam, very high local temperatures can be produced because of the high attenuation coefficient of bone.

Mechanical effects: cavitation

The other established mechanism for ultrasound to produce biological effects is that of direct mechanical interaction. This may arise either through streaming, which is induced in liquids by radiation force when there is attenuation of the beam, or through bubble-associated activity. Bubble-associated activity is known as cavitation and it may be either stable or transient. Stable cavitation occurs when there is a pre-existing bubble in an ultrasonic field. It is most effective when the bubble is of resonant size, so that it vibrates with maximum amplitude; the bubble acts as the elastic member and the oscillating mass is provided by the surrounding liquid or tissue. The actual relationship is that resonance occurs when the product of the ultrasonic frequency (in Hz) multiplied by the bubble radius (in m) is equal to about 3.3. Thus, a bubble with a radius of 1.1 μm resonates at a frequency of 3 MHz. In the liquid in the neighbourhood of a resonating bubble, there is amplification of the streaming field which occurs in liquids in which radiation force develops as the result of absorption.

However the streaming is caused, it results in velocity gradients which may be large enough physically to break biological macromolecules or to cause other kinds of mechanical damage. Figure 6.7 shows the relationship between the number of breaks per original average DNA molecule suspended in liquid, plotted against irradiation time, for three different velocity gradients in the liquid. During the early stages of irradiation, there is a rapid increase in the breakage rate as the larger macromolecules move through the ultrasonic field. After some time, however, a plateau is reached because, at any particular value of velocity gradient, the macromolecules have all been broken down so that their length is just below that at which the shearing force is sufficient to cause further breakage.

The other kind of cavitation, transient cavitation, occurs when the negative pressure in the ultrasonic field is sufficient to rupture the liquid so that a cavity appears which collapses during the following positive pressure half-cycle. Besides the commotion that accompanies the phenomenon, the collapse of the cavity leads to very high temperatures (in the order of 10^4 K) for extremely short periods. These high temperatures can, theoretically, produce effects akin to those of ionizing radiation and their presence can be detected by the brief flashes of light (sonoluminescence) to which they give rise.

Although there is no evidence that diagnostic ultrasonic exposures can create the conditions necessary for transient cavitation, it is reasonable to suppose that stable cavitation does take place when pre-existing gas bubbles of resonant size are present in the tissue. Although normally this is not the case, encapsulated microbubbles administered as ultrasonic contrast agents, which coincidentally are most effective when they are of resonant size, are an obvious potential source of hazard.

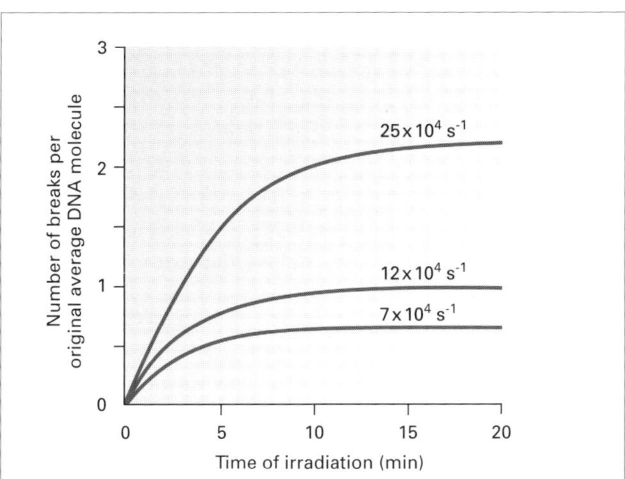

Fig. 6.7 Results of a typical experiment in which a suspension of DNA is exposed to ultrasound producing various levels of shear. With increasing shear, the DNA is broken into smaller elements but there is a plateau in the number of breaks for each level of shear.

Possibility of direct effects of ultrasound

Although there is no firm evidence to support the idea, occasionally it has been suggested that ultrasound may interact with biological tissues in a direct way not dependent on thermal or mechanical effects. It is prudent, however, that the search for such interactions should continue; if they do occur, they are likely to be subtle in nature.

Comparison with biological effects of ionizing radiation

The damage that ionizing radiation causes in biological tissues is stochastic, depending on the statistical probability of an interaction occurring between an ionization event and a biologically sensitive target. Thus, the effect of ionizing radiation is cumulative and, moreover, there is a time delay between the exposure and the manifestation of the biological damage.

As a general rule, ultrasonic bioeffects are all-or-none phenomena not associated with a latent period; moreover, exposures separated in time are not cumulative in effect. Thus, it is reasonable to assume that there is an exposure threshold below which no biological damage occurs, even though there may be innocuous biological effects during irradiation resulting from slightly raised temperature or increased metabolic activity due to streaming.

Biological effects of possible relevance to safety

Where ultrasound affects biological systems, it can do so at various levels of structural complexity. Thus, there may be effects on chemical systems (such as increased rate constants resulting from increased temperature), macromolecules (breakage due to liquid streaming velocity gradients, or thermal denaturation), isolated cells and cell cultures (for example, lysis due to cavitation) and tissues and multicellular organisms (or cavitational effects on solid organs or whole animals). Moreover, indirect evidence of biological effects in humans, if indeed they do occur, could be provided by appropriately designed epidemiological studies.

Biological effects may be genetic or somatic in nature. Generally, genetic effects are the least desirable but there is little if any evidence that they can be caused by ultrasound. Somatic effects can be of importance to the individual; the degree of importance depends on the differential susceptibility of different tissues and on the lifestyle relevance of any resultant detriment. Important detriments would include teratogenesis and carcinogenesis (although there is no evidence that the latter occurs with ultrasound). Of course, the target tissue is also very relevant. It is, for example, clearly much more important to avoid the damage to an embryo or a fetus than it is to be careful not to expose a peripheral vein in an adult to a hypothetical hazard.

As the risk of damage increases, so measurements of exposure and dose conditions need to be made with increasing accuracy. Thus, if there is no real risk of hazard, it is obviously not important to know exactly what the ultrasonic intensity is. If, however, the intensity is approaching the threshold above which damage can occur, and it is desired to operate as close as possible to the threshold, the measurement of exposure has to be quite precise.

Benefits and risks in ultrasonic diagnosis

Diagnostic accuracy and the possibility of misdiagnosis

The benefits of ultrasonic diagnosis are usually self-evident or, at least, they are perceived (at least by special-interest groups) to be so. Wherever ultrasonic diagnosis as currently practised results in advantageous modification of clinical management, or leads to an improvement in clinical practice, the only cost that needs to be taken into account is the financial one of carrying out the test. Of course, this includes the opportunity cost, since carrying out an ultrasonic investigation means that, in an environment in which total resources are fixed, something else (possibly otherwise unrelated) cannot be done.

The risks of ultrasonic diagnosis include the possibility of inducing some adverse biological consequence. In common with many other diagnostic tests, however, the principal risk is currently perceived to be that of misdiagnosis. In considering the risk of misdiagnosis, it is important to grasp the concept that there is a spectrum of disease and that any diagnostic test is subject to error. Figure 6.8 illustrates how the position of the detection threshold of the test within the clinical distribution of some particular disease affects the rate of true positive and false negative classification. Shifting the detection threshold, perhaps by changing the criteria used by the diagnostician in interpreting an image, can increase the true positive rate but only at the expense of an increase in false negatives (and vice versa). Patients for whom a true positive diagnosis is obtained receive the appropriate treatment, whereas those for whom the result of the test is a false negative are likely to be denied treatment. Generally, this is the most serious outcome for any individual patient. False positive results may lead to inappropriate treatment but diagnostic tests are seldom considered in isolation and, in any case, unnecessary treatment is not usually serious although the possibility of iatrogenic disease has to be taken into account.

An example of ultrasonic misdiagnosis

Figure 6.9 illustrates the clinical outcome of managing patients with suspected appendicitis using protocols with and without ultrasonic diagnosis. The hypothetical example is for 1000 patients with suspected appendicitis. It is reasonable to assume that 800 of these symptomatic patients actually have appendicitis requiring surgical treatment, whereas 200 have symptoms mimicking those of appendicitis but not requiring appendectomy. Figure

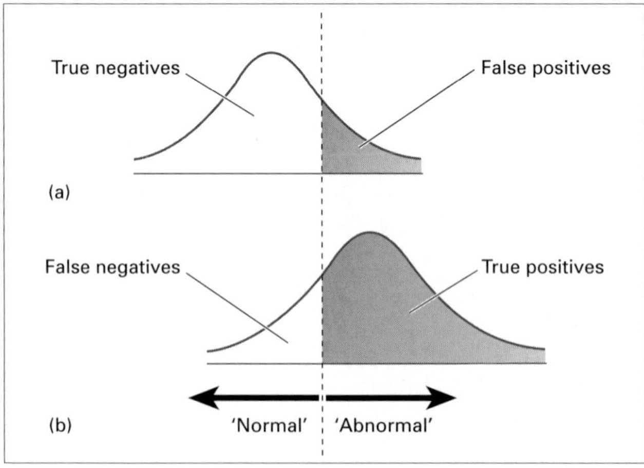

Fig. 6.8 The position of the detection threshold of a diagnostic test on the resultant classification of individuals (a) without and (b) with disease. The vertical dotted line represents the position of the detection threshold within the distributions of normal and abnormal cases.

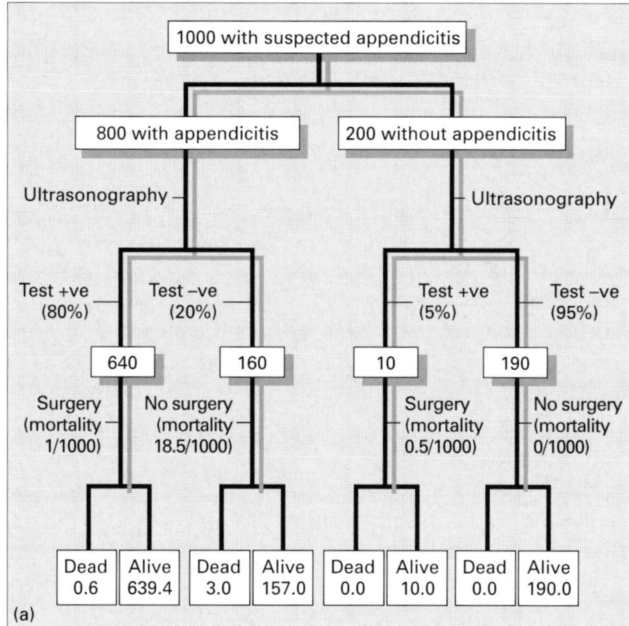

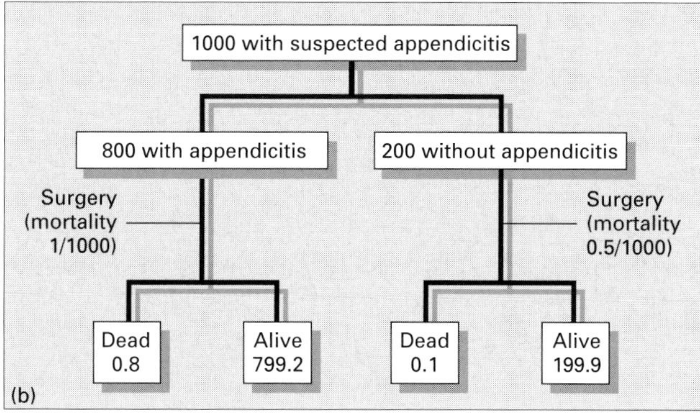

Fig. 6.9 Mortality in patients with suspected appendicitis. (a) Initial management determined by the results of ultrasonography; the overall mortality is 3.6 in 1000. (b) Traditional management based on surgery for all patients; the overall mortality is 0.9 in 1000.

6.9a illustrates the result of basing management on the result of ultrasonography, a test which typically has a true positive rate of 80 per cent and a false positive rate of 5 per cent. Moreover, surgery for needed appendectomy has a mortality rate of 1 in 1000 whereas when needed surgery is inappropriately postponed, the mortality rate rises to 18.5 in 1000. Operating on a patient with false symptoms of appendicitis results in a mortality of 0.5 in 1000. The outcome of using ultrasonography is that 650 in 1000 patients have immediate surgery and the overall mortality rate is 3.6 in 1000. Figure 6.9b shows, and this may at first seem surprising, that, when ultrasonography is not used but the 1000 patients with suspected appendicitis all have surgery, the mortality rate falls to 0.9 in 1000! Thus, in this example, the delay due to ultrasonic misdiagnosis results in a fourfold increase in mortality.

It is easy to think of numerous other undesirable consequences resulting from ultrasonic misdiagnosis. For example, a healthy fetus may be aborted, a normal gallbladder may be removed and hepatic metastases may be missed. All these are highly undesirable outcomes for the patient.

Thermal and mechanical acoustic output indices

As far as relative exposure levels are concerned, it is generally the case that the I_{SPTA} intensities are highest with pulsed Doppler studies, lowest with grey-scale real-time imaging and of an intermediate level with colour flow imaging. Indeed, it is recommended that pulsed Doppler studies should not be carried out in the first trimester of pregnancy.

In order to help the operator to make a judgement about the possibility that particular instrument settings may be potentially hazardous, some manufacturers have developed on-screen displays of quantities called the thermal index (TI) and the mechanical index (MI) of acoustic output.

The TI is defined as the ratio of the actual acoustic power to acoustic power estimated to be necessary to raise the temperature of the target tissue by 1 °K. Thus, it is numerically equal to the likely temperature rise of the target tissue during prolonged ultrasonic study.

The MI is defined as the estimated maximum negative ultrasonic pressure in the target tissue divided by the square root of the frequency; pressure is expressed in MPa and the frequency in MHz. By using this choice of units, TI and MI can be given equal weight in the assessment of risk. Different tissue models are used for the calculations relating to different kinds of examinations (soft tissue, unscanned, large transducer aperture; soft tissue, unscanned, small transducer aperture; soft tissue, scanned; soft tissue, unscanned, bone at focus; bone at surface, scanned or unscanned) and the operator has to select the one that is appropriate. If either index falls below 0.4, the associated risk is considered to be negligible and the value of the index is not normally displayed.

Consequences of inappropriate estimation of the risk of ultrasonic diagnosis

Only when the cost (including the risk) of ultrasonic diagnosis is properly shown to be less than the value of the benefit of the diagnostic test is the method appropriately used. This is still a matter of clinical judgement and it is best to leave it to the clinicians. Nevertheless, clinicians need to be properly informed in order to make the right judgements.

If a clinician makes too high an estimate of the risk of using ultrasonic diagnosis, either in terms of its resource cost or the possibility of causing some adverse biological effect, another diagnostic test is likely to be used. There is a risk that this test may actually be more dangerous than the ultrasonic study, or it may be inappropriate for some other reason, for example, it may actually have a greater risk of misdiagnosis. Conversely, if the clinician makes too low an estimate of the risk of ultrasonic diagnosis, ultrasound may be used inappropriately or there may be a failure to use a more appropriate test.

Guidelines and regulations

Radiation protection against ionizing radiations has undergone a shift of emphasis from the specification of safe maximums and the concept of permissible dose to the exercise of clinical judgement based on the principle that the dose should be 'as low as reasonably achievable' (ALARA). This change has been in response to the recognition that there is no threshold below which exposure to ionizing radiation is safe. The application of the ALARA principle requires the measurement of personal doses of radiation, bearing in mind the possibility of legal sanctions.

Although there may be some argument concerning the reality of safe threshold exposure conditions for ultrasound, it is now generally accepted that ultrasonic irradiation for diagnostic purposes should be guided by the ALARA principle. There remain, however, continuing hints from the regulatory authorities that ALARA should be complemented by thresholds above with ultrasonic diagnosis would be difficult to justify under foreseeable clinical conditions. Such pressures probably arise from guidelines such as those issued in the 1980s by, for example, the American Institute of Ultrasound in Medicine, whose Safety Statement led to a widespread understanding—or, perhaps more correctly, misunderstanding—that intensities below $100\,mW\,cm^{-2}$ could be taken to be 'safe'. Later, when account was taken of attenuation in overlying tissues, the acceptable maximum intensity was derated but the concept remained the same. Similarly, some regulatory authorities have debated the possibility of categorizing diagnostic instruments according to maximum ultrasonic output intensities, with the idea that categories with outputs below some threshold should be free from regulatory constraint.

Guidelines are influenced by socioeconomic conditions and the medicolegal climate. For example, conclusions reached by policy-forming organizations concerning the use of routine ultrasound in pregnancy have differed widely, apparently depending as much on vested interests and the risks of litigation as on scientific data. This is something that needs to be remembered when trying to come to a balanced conclusion about the safety of diagnostic ultrasound in any particular clinical situation.

Conclusion

The safe use of diagnostic ultrasound is the subject of continuing debate. There are many unanswered questions, concerning both the specification of exposure and dose, the mechanisms and kinds of biological effects, and the balance of risk against benefit. In the meanwhile, there are some obvious sensible measures that should be adopted.

1 Minimize exposure by minimizing ultrasonic intensity and examination time.

2 Maximize efficacy by employing skilled personnel and by using appropriate equipment with good quality assurance.

3 Insist on having exposure data, so that the judgement of risk and benefit can be as well informed as possible.

Before embarking on an individual ultrasonic study, the clinician would be well advised to ask the question 'Do I need to be concerned about hazardous ultrasonic bioeffects in this case?' The answer could be 'No', 'Probably not', 'Perhaps', 'Probably' or 'Yes'. Usually, the answer is likely to lie between 'Probably not' and 'Perhaps', with a slight preference for 'Probably not'. This is not intended to encourage complacency; clinicians should be constantly alert for new advice and the results of research which might affect their judgement of what is best for their patients.

Further reading

Barnett, S.B., Kossoff, G. (eds) (1992) WFUMB symposium on safety and standardisation in medical ultrasound. *Ultrasound in Medicine and Biology* **18**, 731–814.

Barnett, S.B., Kossoff, G., Edwards, M.J. (1994) Is diagnostic ultrasound safe? Current interventional consensus on the thermal mechanism. *Medical Journal of Australia* **160**, 33–37.

Docker, M.F., Duck, F.A. (eds) (1991) *The Safe Use of Diagnostic Ultrasound*. British Medical Ultrasound Society/British Institute of Radiology, London.

Duck, F.A., Martin, K. (1991) Trends in diagnostic ultrasound exposure. *Physics in Medicine and Biology* **36**, 1423–1432.

European Committee for Ultrasound Radiation Safety—the Watchdogs (1996) Epidemiology of diagnostic ultrasound exposure during human pregnancy. *European Journal of Ultrasound* **3**, 69–73.

European Committee for Ultrasound Radiation Safety—the Watchdogs (1996) Clinical safety statement for diagnostic ultrasound (1995). *European Journal of Ultrasound* **3**, 283.

Hedrick, W.R., Hykes, D.L. (1993) An overview of thermal and mechanical output indices. *Journal of Diagnostic Medical Sonography* **9**, 228–235.

Henderson, J., Willson, K., Jago, J.R., Whittingham, T.A. (1995) A survey of the acoustic outputs of diagnostic ultrasound equipment in current use. *Ultrasound in Medicine and Biology* **21**, 699–705.

Preston, R.C. (ed.) (1991) *Output Measurements for Medical Ultrasound*. Springer, London.

Wells, P.N.T. (1986) The prudent use of diagnostic ultrasound. *British Journal of Radiology* **59**, 1143–1151.

Wells, P.N.T. (ed.) (1987) The safety of diagnostic ultrasound. *British Journal of Radiology* (suppl. 20).

Whittingham, T.A. (1994) The safety of ultrasound. *Imaging* **6**, 33–51.

Williams, A.R. (1983) *Ultrasound: Biological Effects and Potential Hazards*. Academic Press, London.

Ziskin, M.C., Lewin, P.A. (eds) (1993) *Ultrasonic Exposimetry*. CRC Press, Boca Raton.

Chapter 7: Ultrasound contrast agents and recent developments

C.M. Moran, W.N. McDicken & G.R. Sutherland

Echo enhancement using a contrast agent was first reported in 1968 by Gramiak and Shah [1] who observed a striking enhancement in the reflectivity of blood in the left atrium when indocyanine green was injected into it. The same phenomena was observed using saline and dextrose and indeed the patient's own blood [2]. Over the next 20 years contrast agents were used mainly to determine the presence of cardiac shunts and to validate cardiac anatomy. Ophir and Parker [3] have reviewed these early contrast agents and it is evident from this review and subsequent work that agents working on the principle of scattering from microbubbles were most likely to be successful in future clinical applications. In the mid-1980s clinical interest in contrast agents re-emerged. The reason behind this interest was primarily due to the development of processes capable of manufacturing more stable contrast agents which could be injected intravenously and survive passage through the pulmonary circulation. In addition, there existed an increasing clinical demand for the development of an ultrasonic technique that was capable of measuring myocardial perfusion. A more recent longer term interest in microbubbles is related to their potential use as carriers of pharmaceuticals to specific sites where they would be destroyed on arrival by an ultrasound beam. Some specific microbubble agents are discussed in this chapter; they should be considered as early examples in a field which is growing, and will continue to grow, rapidly in the future. In addition a brief consideration of non-microbubble types of agents is worthwhile to illustrate the range of phenomena which produce contrast effects, although to date these agents appear to have a performance well short of that required for clinical studies. Nevertheless, although at present no routine, accepted, clinical uses of contrast agents exist, improvements in scanning technology and an increasing understanding of the optimal methods of imaging the agents suggest that contrast agents will provide a major advance in ultrasonic diagnostic imaging capabilities.

Types of contrast agents

Free microbubbles

Microbubbles have been investigated in both a free unencapsulated form and encapsulated by a thin shell. The low acoustic impedance of the gas and the fact that bubbles of diameter around 5 μm resonate when insonated with ultrasound in the low megahertz frequency range result in a very high level of backscatter. The intensity of ultrasound received by a scanning transducer from such microbubbles is more than a million times higher than that which would be received from solid particles of similar dimensions. Free gas bubbles are very efficient scatterers of ultrasound; however, they either dissolve quickly in the blood or are too big to pass through the lungs and are therefore unsuited to intravenous injection. These were the first type of contrast agent to find clinical application when injected into the aorta [1,2]. Such free bubble contrast agents were initially made by agitating the carrier liquids; however, the range of bubble size was large. By a process called 'sonication', in which a fairly intense low frequency sonic field (20 kHz) is applied to liquids, small cavitation bubbles of a more limited size range (<10 μm) were created [4].

Phase change agents

Free bubbles may also be created in the blood stream by injecting a liquid which changes into the gas phase by boiling at, or slightly below, body temperature. An early example of such a phase change agent was the use of ether [5]. More recently a commercial agent called Echogen made by Sonus Pharmaceuticals (Bothell, Washington, USA) has been introduced. The size of bubbles which result from the phase change of the injected liquid (dodecafluoropentane) are between 2 and 5 μm in diameter. Surfactants are used to ensure stable and reproducible bubble size.

Encapsulated bubbles

In 1980 stable bubbles encapsulated in gelatin were reported [6] although these bubbles were too large to pass through the lungs. By 1987 bubbles smaller than 5mm were produced by sonicating albumin at high intensity and low frequency [7]. The encapsulating shell consisted of the denatured albumin protein. Another practical approach to making small encapsulated microbubbles was to support the small bubbles in a saccharide crystal structure which dissolved in the blood [8,9]. It has been shown that the size of the gas molecules within the encapsulated microbubble is related to the rate of diffusion from the bubble and hence its lifetime [10]. These breakthroughs in the production of encapsulated bubbles which pass through the lung and last for several minutes in blood, have opened up the possibility of a wide range of clinical applications. Microbubbles have a spread of diameters, typically 2–10 μm and have an outer shell between 10 and 100nm. The oscillation in size of encapsulated bubbles under the influence of an ultrasonic wave is damped compared to a free bubble. de Jong [11] has shown that a free bubble of diameter 3.4 μm driven at its resonance frequency shows a change in diameter which varies between 60% of its initial diameter in the expanding phase and about 40% in the compression. For an encapsulated bubble there is less than 5% change in diameter in either phase. However, the resonant oscillation still adds significantly, say 1000-fold increase for free bubbles, to the magnitude of the backscattered intensity.

It is a happy coincidence that microbubbles of size similar to red blood cells resonate at low megahertz frequency, e.g. 4mm at 4MHz. The resonance frequency f_0 is given by:

$$f_0 = \frac{1}{2\pi a}\sqrt{\frac{3\gamma p_0}{\rho_0}} \qquad (1)$$

where a is the bubble radius, γ is the adiabatic ideal gas constant and p_0 and ρ_0 are the ambient fluid pressure and density, respectively [12]. Substituting appropriate values into this formula shows that bubbles of the order of 5mm or less have resonances in the range 1 to 10MHz as used in medical imaging.

Miscellaneous agents

The early search for ultrasonic agents explored the use of other types apart from microbubbles. For example an agent consisting of a colloidal suspension of dense 1mm iodipamide ethyl ester particles is reported to enhance backscatter and attenuation in rat liver [13]. Recently these particles have been developed further to encapsulate microbubbles and go by the name of 'bubbicles'. Another contrast agent, a suspension of perfluoro-octyl bromide (perflubron or PFOB) with particle sizes less than 0.5mm is reported to enhance tumour rim in rabbit liver. This enhancement is related to agglomeration of the particles in the Kupffer cells [14]. Due to this mechanism interest remains in this type of agent. Aqueous solutions with speed of sound different from that of tissue have been shown to enhance backscatter when injected into kidney tissue [15]. However, the steady improvement in microbubble agents with their dramatic scattering properties and ability to pass through lungs has resulted in almost all effort in the field being devoted to them. It is forecast that a range of agents will be available for specific applications as in nuclear medicine, for example to target specific organs, to adhere to thrombi or to lodge in the myocardium and eventually permit quantification of perfusion.

Recommended preparation and concentration of agents

Some specific microbubble agents are described to provide insight into their preparation and properties (Table 7.1).

Albunex

Albunex, which is marketed in Europe under the name Infoson, is manufactured by Molecular Biosystems Inc. (San Diego, CA). It is an air-filled encapsulated bubble, the shell of which is made of albumin. Albunex is supplied in vials containing approximately 4.5ml of solution. The vial is inverted and swirled for about 3min to resuspend the microbubbles and the solution turns milky white. The solution is then drawn up into a syringe and injected intravenously.

Echovist (SHU 454)

Echovist is manufactured by Schering (Berlin, Germany) and is commercially available in Europe. The median diameter of the microparticles is 3 μm with 97% of the diameters below 7 μm. Echovist is supplied in two vials: one containing either 8.5 or 13.5ml of a galactose solution and the second containing granules of approximately 1mm diameter. These granules are composed of clumps of galactose microparticles. After injection of the galactose solution into the vial containing the galactose granules and vigorous shaking of the vial for 5s, the granules break down into the constituent microparticles and air microbubbles become trapped on their surface (Fig. 7.1). The size of the microparticles ensures that the air bubbles which are trapped are of a consistent size. After injection

Table 7.1 Properties of some common intravenous, lung-crossing contrast agents

Left heart agent	Manufactured by	Type of agent	Capsule	Gas	Bubble size (μm)	Dose/concentration
Levovist (SHU 508A)	Schering	Lipid-stabilized bubble	Palmitic acid	Air	3–5	0.8–3.2 g
Sonovist (SHU 563A)	Schering	Solid microspheres	Cyano-acrylate	Air	Mean 2	0.1–1 μl kg^{-1} (200 × 10^8 μbubbles ml^{-1})
Definity (DMP-115)	ImaRx/Du Pont	Encapsulated bubble	Lipid	Perfluoropropane	Mean 2.5	3–5 μl kg^{-1} (10 × 10^8 μbubbles ml^{-1})
Quantison™	Quadrant Healthcare	Rigid microsphere	Albumin	Air	Mean 3.2; range (<2% > 6 μm)	To be infused at 1 ml min^{-1} (5 × 10^8 μbubbles ml^{-1})
Optison	Mallinckrodt	Encapsulated microsphere	Albumin	Octafluoropropane	Mean 3.7 μm	1 ml at fundamental 0.5 ml at second harmonic ((5–8) × 10^8 μbubbles ml^{-1})
Sonovue (BR1)	Bracco	Stabilized bubble	Phospholipid	SF_6	2–3 (90% < 8 μm)	(1–5) × 10^8 μbubbles ml^{-1}
Albunex (Infoson in Europe)	Nycomed (Europe); Mallinckrodt (USA)	Encapsulated bubble	Albumin	Air	Mean 4; range 2–10	0.025–1.0 ml kg^{-1} of 3–5 × 10^8 μbubbles ml^{-1}

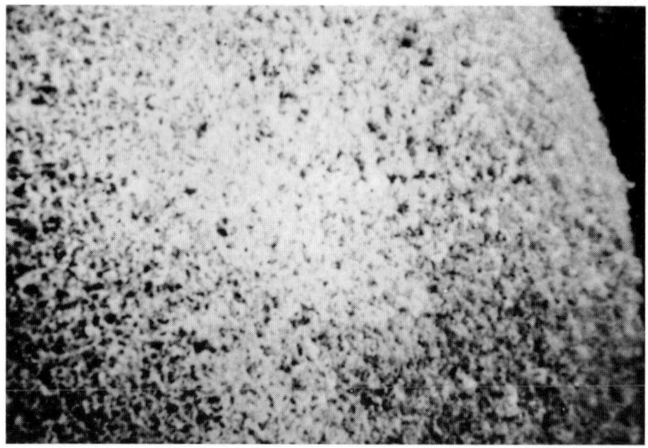

Fig. 7.1 Micrograph of a galactose granule (×250). Note the granule is composed of clumps of microparticles. (Courtesy of Schering Health Care.)

of the solution the microparticles dissolve releasing the air microbubbles. However as these microbubbles are not encapsulated they are not capable of passing through the lungs and consequently this agent is only suitable for investigations where it may be injected near the region to be ultrasonically scanned.

Levovist (SHU 508A)

Levovist is also manufactured by Schering (Berlin, Germany) and is also commercially available in Europe. It is an air-filled encapsulated bubble, the shell of which is palmitic acid. The diameter of the microbubbles lies between 3 and 5 mm. The agent is supplied in vials containing 4 g of dry galactose granules and 0.1% palmitic acid. Sterile water is injected into the vials, the quantity of water determining the concentration of the agent. Recommended concentrations are 200 mg ml^{-1} (17 ml injection of water into vial), 300 mg ml^{-1} (11 ml injection of water into vial) or 400 mg ml^{-1} (8 ml injection of water into vial). Once the water is injected the granules are vigorously shaken for 5–10 s and then allowed to stand for a further 2 min prior to injection. By this stage the solution will be milky white. Care must be taken to avoid excessive increases in temperature by holding the vials tightly in the hands or strong negative pressure when drawing up the solution.

Sonovist (SHU 563A)

This is a relatively new agent which has also been developed by Schering (Berlin, Germany). It is composed of air-filled cyanacrylate-encapsulated microspheres with a

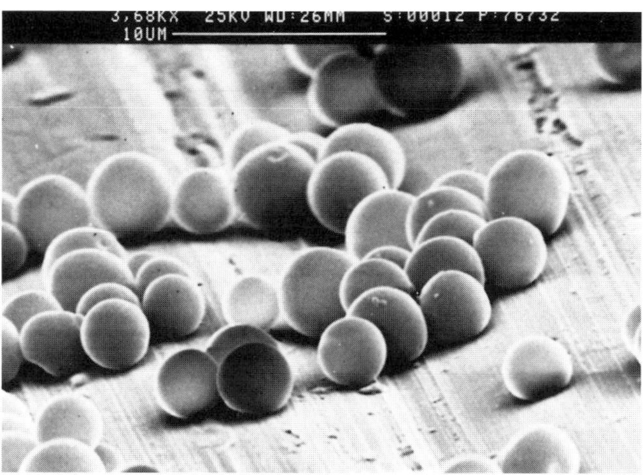

Fig. 7.2 Electron micrograph of Quantison™. (Courtesy of Quadrant Healthcare, Nottingham, UK.)

mean diameter of 2 μm. The agent is supplied as a dry powder and resuspended by shaking in saline prior to injection. Optimum dose has yet to be established.

Definity (MRX-115, DMP-115)

Aerosomes are manufactured by ImaRx Pharmaceuticals (Tuscon, AZ) in association with DuPont Pharmaceuticals and are lipid-coated microbubbles containing a perfluoropropane gas. The agent is supplied in 1.5 ml vials of a clear solution which is shaken vigorously for 60 s in a shaker which is supplied with the samples.

Quantison™

Quantison is manufactured by Quadrant Healthcare (Nottingham, UK). This is another air-filled, albumin-encapsulated microbubble. Slight variations during manufacturing processes, permit the thickness of the shell to be varied between 100 and 200 nm. The agent is distributed in vials containing a dry, white powder. The powder is resuspended in 5 ml of sterile water which is supplied in ampules (Fig. 7.2).

Myomap™ (formerly AIP 201)

AIP 201 is also manufactured by Quadrant Healthcare and is similar in composition to Quantison™ except that the capsules have a mean diameter of 10 μm. Due to the size of the particles they do not pass through the lungs, but when injected into the left atrium or directly into the coronary arteries of a pig model, the agent has been shown to give pronounced myocardial enhancement which can persist for over 30 min (Fig. 7.3).

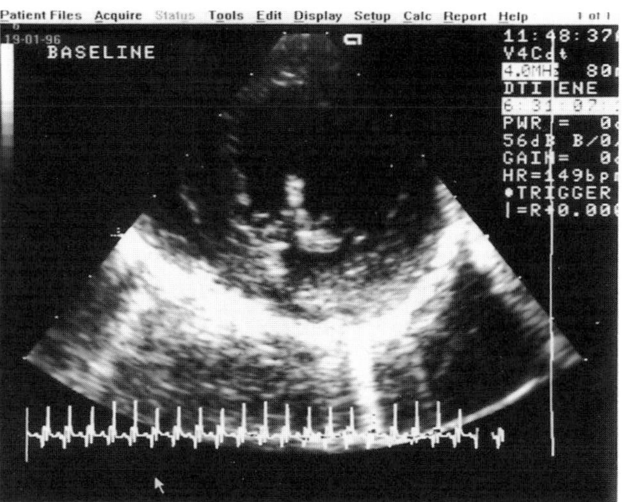

(a)

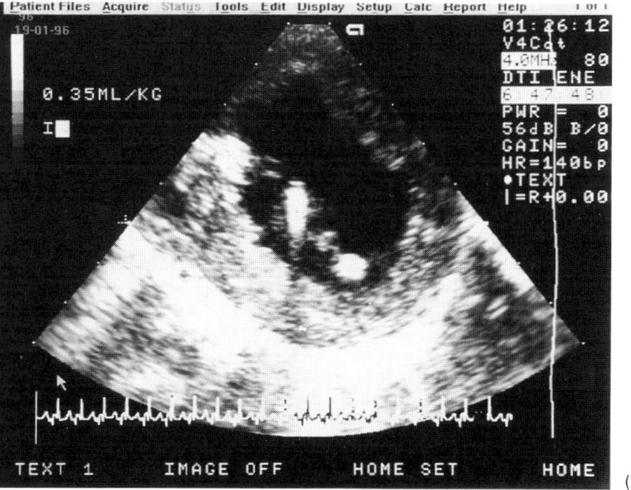

(b)

Fig. 7.3 (a) Precontrast ultrasound image of open-chest pig. (b) Same image after 0.35 ml kg^{-1} injection of Myomap™ into left atrium of pig. Note marked enhancement of all walls.

Optison

This contrast agent is manufactured by Mallinckrodt and is presented as a vial containing 3 ml of a clear liquid with an upper white layer. By inverting the vial several times, the solution turns a milky white. The vial must be vented before withdrawing the Optison suspension. The agent is marketed for improvement in endocardial border visualization for use both in fundamental and second harmonic imaging modalities (Fig. 7.4).

Sonovue (BR1)

BR1 is manufactured by Bracco (Switzerland) and consists of microbubbles of sulphur hexafluoride (SF_6) encapsulated in a phospholipid shell. The agent is presented as 25 mg of powder in a vial. Sterile saline (5 ml) provided in an

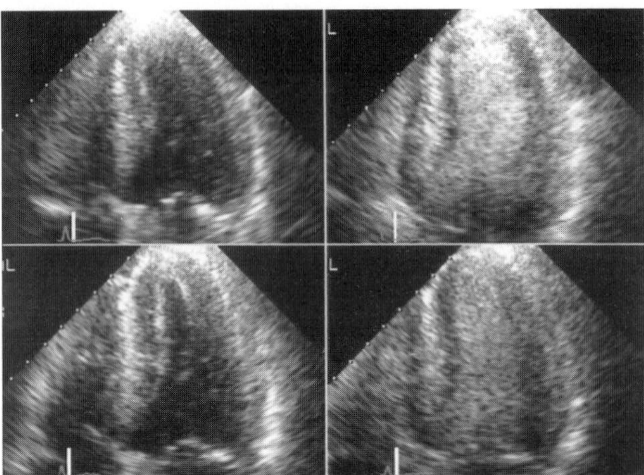

Fig. 7.4 Enhanced endocardial border definition in an apical four-chamber view using Optison in fundamental imaging mode during a stress-echo study. Top left: baseline apical four-chamber view. Top right: contrast-enhanced apical four-chamber view at baseline. Botton left: peak stress apical four-chamber view. Bottom right: contrast-enhanced, peak-stress apical four-chamber view.

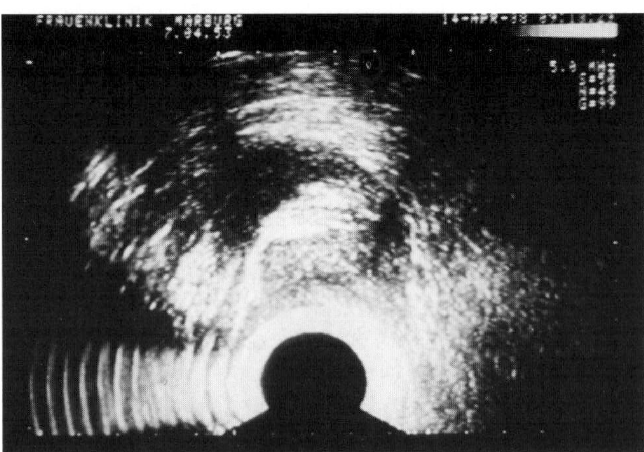

Fig. 7.5 Grey-scale image obtained during hysterosalpingo-contrast sonography. Note the contrast-enhanced uterine cavity and fallopian tube. (Courtesty of Schering Health Care.)

ampoule is injected and the vial shaken for 30 s. The required dose is then withdrawn. Unlike the majority of other contrast agents, this agent must be stored at room temperature.

Quantification of contrast effects

To date, methods for assessing organ perfusion have largely been centred on the analysis of time sequences of contrast-enhanced images acquired from an ultrasound machine. Whether this analysis is performed qualitatively or quantitatively is largely dictated by the information required from the contrast study and the resources available for image manipulation and analysis. In many instances, a qualitative assessment, either by visually interpreting the grey-scale images as they are acquired or retrospectively from a videotape, provides sufficient information for diagnosis. An example of this is in the assessment of fallopian tube patency (hysterosalpingo-contrast sonography), where the patency of the tubes can be determined by the passage of the contrast agent and a constriction within the tube will reduce or completely block the passage of the agent (Fig. 7.5).

For quantitative analysis, the earlier in the ultrasonic signal processing path that access is gained to the data, the more accurate the subsequent analysis. Unfortunately, in many instances gaining access to the ultrasound digital data early in the processing path is dependent, to a large extent, on the goodwill of the machine manufacturer. In addition, some manufacturers work with the analogue signal till late in the processing path, so access to the ultrasound signal earlier necessitates the use of a high speed digitizer. Without access to this unprocessed digital data, it is still possible to perform limited quantitative studies using a video frame-grabber attached to the scanner via the video output. The analogue video signal from the scanner is digitized and the data downloaded to a computer. Alternatively, it is possible to utilize the images from a videotape but these images will have significantly degraded quality.

Having stored a sequence of images, various image manipulation packages exist which permit single or multiple regions of interest (ROIs) within blood pools or organs to be selected and the mean grey-scale intensity within these regions to be plotted versus time. Dependent on the sophistication of the image processing packages the ROIs may be automatically or manually aligned throughout the sequence to account for displacement of the region over time. In cardiac sequences compensation for the movement of the heart and consequently movement of the ROI throughout the cardiac cycle can be incorporated within the analysis program, but in general such image sequences are triggered so that frame acquisition occurs only at one position in the cardiac cycle. Many packages permit up to 64 frames to be collected, with up to six ROIs selected, with contrast wash-in, wash-out curves plotted for the ROIs. In recent years, an increasing number of manufacturers are entering the market of image manipulation with software dedicated to the acquisition, storage and manipulation of video ultrasonic images.

For many applications the variation in the grey-scale intensity values versus time can be fitted to a curve. From such curves, parameters such as time to maximum intensity, half-life of contrast and total wash-out time of the contrast agent may be estimated. Such parameters reflect information on perfusion of the ROI. The accuracy of this information is reliant upon how 'perfect' the contrast agent is. Such a 'perfect' contrast agent should resemble blood as closely as possible in haemodynamic and physiological terms. Consequently, the agent should not alter or impede blood flow. The microparticles should be of comparable or smaller size than red blood cells, should pass through the lungs and be readily detectable in injectable concentrations. Their lifetime should be sufficient for them to be observed clearly and for them to pass through the biological system without any adverse reactions. In addition, the agents must not be destroyed by the ultrasound beam.

Quantitative videodensitometric analysis from videotape

The main advantage of using images digitally acquired from a videorecording for contrast analysis is that the ultrasonic data can be digitized and analysed off-line avoiding an elongation of the study period generally required for downloading digital images. Also, for studies using contrast agents with an extended wash-out time, recording the complete study on videotape is the least expensive method of storing the complete contrast study.

However, ultrasonic data digitized from videotape has been subjected not only to the non-linear compressions within the ultrasound machine but also to the limited dynamic range of the videotape (20 dB). Consequently, dependent on the set-up of the machine small changes in grey-scale intensity may be missed. Rovai *et al.* [16] has shown that analysis of the mean transit time of a contrast agent estimated from videodensitometric analysis compared to unprocessed radiofrequency (RF) echo data can be significantly over- or underestimated depending on the initial set-up of the scanner.

Quantitative videodensitometric analysis with a frame-grabber

Using this option, the frames displayed on the ultrasonic scanner are digitized directly by an image frame-grabber at the time of scanning or from the frozen cine-loop sequence on the ultrasound machine. The time and memory required to digitize and store these image frames is dependent on the temporal and spatial resolution required. Most frame-grabbers currently on the market offer 512 × 512 × 8 bit resolution images with up to 64 frames being stored in each acquisition. As with images digitized directly from videotape the images have still undergone non-linear processes within the ultrasound machine, but the overall dynamic range of the signal is in this instance limited by the ultrasound machine rather than the videotape. If the non-linear processes within the ultrasound machine are known it is possible to compensate the data for these internal processes. Unfortunately, as stated previously, many ultrasound manufacturers consider this information confidential and it is left to the individual user to determine the processes which constitute the 'black box' between transducer and output screen.

Quantitative RF analysis

For analysis of the basic RF ultrasonic echo signals, access is required to the echo data at an early stage in the processing path within the ultrasound scanner before non-linear processing such as demodulation and log compression. Consequently, the entire signal range (60 dB) may be analysed. Depending at what stage in the path access is gained to the RF data, it may be necessary to compensate the images for gain and time gain compensation (TGC) settings. After such compensation, a direct linear relationship exists between the amplitude of the signal backscattered to the transducer and the RF digital data output. Such a relationship allows a quantitative approach to the evaluation of organ perfusion.

However, the acquisition of RF data, does have several distinct drawbacks. In a typical sector scan, there are 128 lines, 4096 samples in each line and two bytes per sample. Hence each frame of data collected can occupy up to 1 MB of memory. Collection of all frames within a contrast study has the potential to generate vast amounts of data. To reduce the amount of data from such studies, acquisition of image frames may be triggered either from the cardiac cycle or at a fixed time interval set prior to the study. Alternatively, if a ROI can be selectively chosen from within the sector scan in real-time, this reduces the amount of memory required for storage and increases the number of frames that may be analysed.

Quantitative analysis of Doppler signals

Contrast agents have been used to enhance weak Doppler signals from small vessels and although this need has diminished due to improvements in Doppler colour flow imaging there is always a desire to study flow in smaller and smaller vessels. Consequently, contrast agents are of specific importance in vascular imaging for detecting vessels where the strength of the backscatter signals from the moving blood are very weak either because the vessels lie deep within the body, have strong attenuating layers around them or are very small such as neovascularization associated with tumour growth. Injection of contrast increases the backscatter of the blood, increasing the signal to noise ratio of the Doppler signal from these vessels by approximately 20 dB [17].

It is surprising that to date, the use of contrast agents to enhance the Doppler signal has been used on a qualitative basis rather than as a method of acquiring more quantitative information from an ultrasound study [18]. It is only in more recent years that attempts have been made to correlate the increase in Doppler signal with the amount of contrast present. Schwarz *et al.* [19] outline several distinct advantages to using an audio or spectral Doppler signal to quantitate the presence of contrast. Firstly, the Doppler signal has a large dynamic range (100 dB) and is accessible on any ultrasound machine whereas access to the RF data is not currently commercially available. Secondly, processing of the RF data requires relatively sophisticated equipment due to the high digitizing frequencies required, whereas the Doppler signal is in the audiofrequency range and can be easily digitized and recorded. In addition, with the advent of colour Doppler energy mapping (power Doppler), where the power of the Doppler signal is encoded rather than the frequency shift, it may become increasingly possible to directly correlate an increase in signal with a known injection of contrast.

Second harmonic imaging

When the radius of a bubble changes its size in direct proportion to the pressure variations of the ultrasonic wave it is said to be responding in a linear fashion. In this case the frequency of the scattered wave is the same as that of the incident wave. However, for larger pressure fluctuations, i.e. larger intensities, the change in radius is not in proportion and the bubble is said to be responding in a non-linear way. It is analogous to a spring moving readily for a certain increase in length when it is near its rest position but requiring a larger pull for the same increase in length when it is already in a stretched state. When a bubble responds in a non-linear fashion, the scattered ultrasound wave is distorted and contains additional frequency components over and above the frequency of the incident wave. These additional components are called harmonics and there is particular interest in the second harmonic which can be as strong as the ultrasound scattered at the incident frequency, i.e. the first harmonic (fundamental frequency). A technique has been developed which only detects the second harmonic in the scattered ultrasound. This second harmonic ultrasound has come largely from the microbubble contrast agent and can be distinguished from that from tissue or blood which does not have significant amounts of second harmonic component in it. The indications are that by using this second harmonic technique the signal from the microbubbles can be enhanced by as much as 30 dB relative to the surrounding tissue [20]. Agents with thin shells (tens of nanometres) exhibit second harmonic generation but thicker shells reduce this frequency component rendering such agents unsuitable for the second harmonic technique. The thin-shelled agents used at present have not been specifically designed to generate a large second harmonic component. A further increase in sensitivity may be achieved if current research to make specialized second harmonic agents is successful.

If the microbubbles are moving, the ultrasound scattered from them suffers a Doppler shift and just as for blood cells this enables their motion to be detected and their velocity to be measured. Agents have been used to enhance the sensitivity of duplex Doppler, colour velocity imaging and power Doppler imaging. It is also possible to detect a Doppler shift in the second harmonic and since it is enhanced relative to the tissue (clutter) signal the motion of the agent can be detected in regions where there is not much of it present, for instance in small blood vessels [21,22].

Imaging artefacts associated with contrast agent studies

There are several artefacts which must be taken into consideration when making clinical ultrasound measurements after the injection of a bolus of contrast. These may be subdivided into propagation artefacts and Doppler artefacts.

Propagation artefacts

When contrast is injected into the body, although it scatters ultrasound strongly it also strongly attenuates and consequently as the bolus of contrast passes through a vessel or through the heart, organs distal to the vessels will temporarily disappear from the screen until the bolus clears through the system. This is readily observed in cardiac scanning where a large amount of the contrast agent can build up within the ventricles and obscure the posterior walls. Shadow artefacts are commonly helpful in making a diagnosis in ultrasonic imaging; however, those created by contrast agents have not been used in that way.

Although a single bubble can be detected as a single spot in an image, when there are a large number of bubbles the spots in the image cannot be directly related to individual bubbles. The echo signals from bubbles in this situation interfere to form a speckle pattern, just as in the familiar case of echoes from the scattering centres in the parenchyma of organs forming a speckle pattern. It is worth noting that the motion of the speckle pattern does not necessarily relate directly to the motion of the bubbles.

Where strong scatterers are present, such as gas bubbles, the echo signals may not travel directly back to the transducer, instead the path may involve multiple scattering events. The multiple scattering delays the return time of an echo and hence it is depicted deeper than the actual position of the original source of the echo. The distal aspect of the region containing bubbles may therefore be displayed beyond its true boundary.

Doppler artefacts

After the injection of a bolus of contrast agent an artefact known as colour blooming may be observed during colour Doppler studies. When contrast agent enters a vessel the magnitude of the signal scattered from within the vessel increases giving a corresponding increase in the Doppler signal. This effectively broadens the width of the scanning beam allowing flow to be detected in the weaker regions of the beam. The resulting degradation of the lateral resolution causes the colour-coded flow region in the image to 'bloom'. The effect is similar to having the Doppler gain too high and may be compensated by reducing the gain.

On a similar issue, injection of contrast must be taken into consideration when assessing the viability of heart valves. Patency of mitral and tricuspid valves is assessed by the depth into the atria that the regurgitant jet is propelled. The presence of contrast within the blood will appear to enhance the distance that the regurgitant jet is propelled back into the atria as the contrast agent increases the backscatter from blood signals which were previously too weak to be colour encoded. Thus if the same criteria for the assessment of patency of these valves is used when contrast is injected as when it is not the severity of the valvular disease will be overestimated. Studies by von Bibra *et al.* [23] suggest that a new system of classification of regurgitant jets is necessitated by the use of contrast. On an encouraging note, however, several studies have shown that such enhancement effects are not associated with significant mean velocity changes within the jet [9,24,25].

In vascular studies, Forsberg *et al.* [26] have shown that an increase in maximum Doppler shift can be expected between pre- and postcontrast peak measurements. This is as a result of the limited dynamic range of the Doppler spectral display which places a lower limit threshold on the Doppler signal strength. After the injection of the contrast more high frequency Doppler signals exceed the signal strength threshold.

Toxicity

The safety of using contrast agents can be considered in two parts: the possible effects of cavitation of the bubbles when insonated by ultrasound and the possible toxicity effects of the contrast agents. Initial work on the safety of contrast agents by the American Society of Echocardiography stated that contrast echocardiography appeared to carry minimal risk to the patient with little residual or complicating side-effects [27]. More recent work by Holland and Apfel [28] have shown that Albunex microbubbles, upon injection into an *in vitro* model, appeared to be very efficient cavitation nuclei. Furthermore, Miller *et al.* [29] found that the addition of small amounts of Levovist or Albunex into a non-cavitating system initiated hydrogen peroxide production suggesting that the presence of contrast agents provided nuclei for cavitation. Indeed Williams *et al.* [30] demonstrated that the addition of Echovist enhanced haemolysis induced by cavitation *in vitro* while Dalecki *et al.* [31] indicated that haemolysis could be induced *in vivo* in murine hearts after an injection of Albunex. Nevertheless there is little conclusive evidence to suggest that any significant risk factors are associated with diagnostic injections of contrast. However, as with all diagnostic ultrasonic examinations, the output power of the scanner should be kept as low as reasonably possible when imaging contrast agents *in vivo*.

Cosgrove [32] and Nanda [33] have addressed the issue of the possible toxic effects of contrast agents from two perspectives. Cosgrove has examined the risk associated with the injection of gas-filled microspheres into the microcirculation and has suggested that since the volume of gas injected is relatively small, it would be extremely unlikely that any ischaemic damage would result even if all the gas from the injection embolized in one site. In addition because the bubbles are manufactured to be sufficiently small to travel through capillaries it would be unlikely that they would embolize. Nanda [33] has addressed the issue of toxic effects actually caused by the constituents of the contrast agent. He has suggested that the osmolarity, viscosity and surfactant properties of the carrier solution are as important to consider as the contrast microcapsules. Side-effects such as vasodilation, injection site pain, paraesthesia, pain, taste perversion and transient changes in left ventricular haemodynamics have all been experienced by some patients after injection, but the reported numbers experiencing these effects are small and the effects transitory in nature.

Clinical applications

Many of the contrast agents discussed in this chapter, are still at the developmental stage and consequently are still undergoing clinical trials. At present, the three agents which are nearest to completing their safety and toxicity studies are Infoson which has already received Food and Drug Administration (FDA) approval in the States, Levovist which has been approved for use in Germany and the UK, and Echovist which has been approved for use in Europe. These three agents have been studied most widely in clinical diagnostic applications. Other agents such as Quantison is undergoing phase II European trials and BR1 combined phase II and III clinical trials. Diagnostic applications for which contrast agents have been shown to be of benefit include the following.

1 Transcranial sonography. Large intracranial vessels can be easily identified and slow flow vessels imaged clearly with colour Doppler [34,35] (Figs 7.6, 7.7).

2 Assessment of patency of fallopian tubes. Hysterosalpingo-contrast sonography is performed where the contrast is injected into the uterine cavity and the patency of the tubes is assessed by the passage of contrast [36,37] (see Fig. 7.5).

3 Ultrasound detection of tumours. The injection of a contrast agent helps to identify the complex blood vessel network associated with tumours using either spectral Doppler or power Doppler [38,39].

(a)

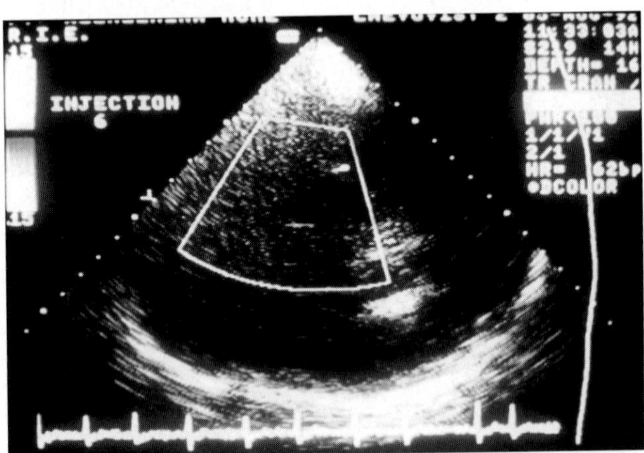

(b)

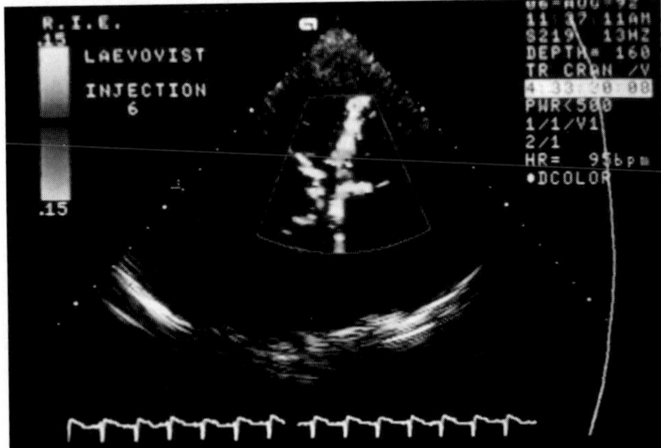

Fig. 7.6 (a) Transcranial colour Doppler scan prior to injection of Levovist. (b) Same scan after injection of Levovist. Notice the circle of Willis clearly enhanced. (Courtesy of P. Allan, Edinburgh.) For colour, see Plate 7.6 (between pp. 308 and 309).

4 Assessment of myocardial perfusion. Several agents currently on the market, are reputed to give myocardial enhancement when injected intravenously but the mechanism by which these contrast agents remain in the myocardium is as yet unclear. Measurement of the degree of signal enhancement within the myocardium either by grey-scale or power Doppler has yet to be quantitatively correlated with myocardial perfusion [40,41] (Fig. 7.8).

New technology

As mentioned above the application of contrast agents in medical ultrasound is in an initial phase and hence new developments are occurring in all aspects of the subject. Probably the main area of development of new technology is in the actual agents themselves. Many laboratories and at least 12 companies are very active in this area. Fortunately the point has now been reached where contrast agents are becoming available to researchers and clinical users which is helping to reduce the frustration of recent years. Apart from the usual delays associated with safety studies it has taken time for manufacturers to produce agents which give reproducible results. The variability of results which has dogged the field is also due in part to lack of exact specification on how users should handle the agents and to less than rigorous practice by the users. Novel agents may lead to completely new applications, for example drug transport and deposition when the agent is degraded at a specific site by an ultrasound beam, and agents tagged with radiopharamaceuticals for ultrasound/nuclear medicine comparison studies.

It is fortunate that no new technological hardware is required for the implementation of second harmonic imaging. Broadband transducers, which can for instance transmit at a fundamental frequency f_0 and receive at the second harmonic f_1, have already been developed. They were developed initially to enable users to generate short pulses or to switch quickly from one frequency to another during conventional scanning. Only additional software to control the functioning of the machine is required.

Another technique for imaging contrast agents, called 'intermittent scanning', also only requires additional software within the scanner [42]. It is reported that for some agents, the acoustic pressure generated by the scanning beam may be destroying the contrast microcapsules. For some agents this results in the release of free gas bubbles which, although having a much shorter lifetime, scatter more efficiently than when encapsulated resulting in increases of up to 20 dB in echo amplitude from perfused regions. This phenomena is known as 'enhanced backscatter' and intermittent scanning takes advantage of this phenomena, whereby the scanning is switched off for some time (triggered) to allow the agent to accumulate

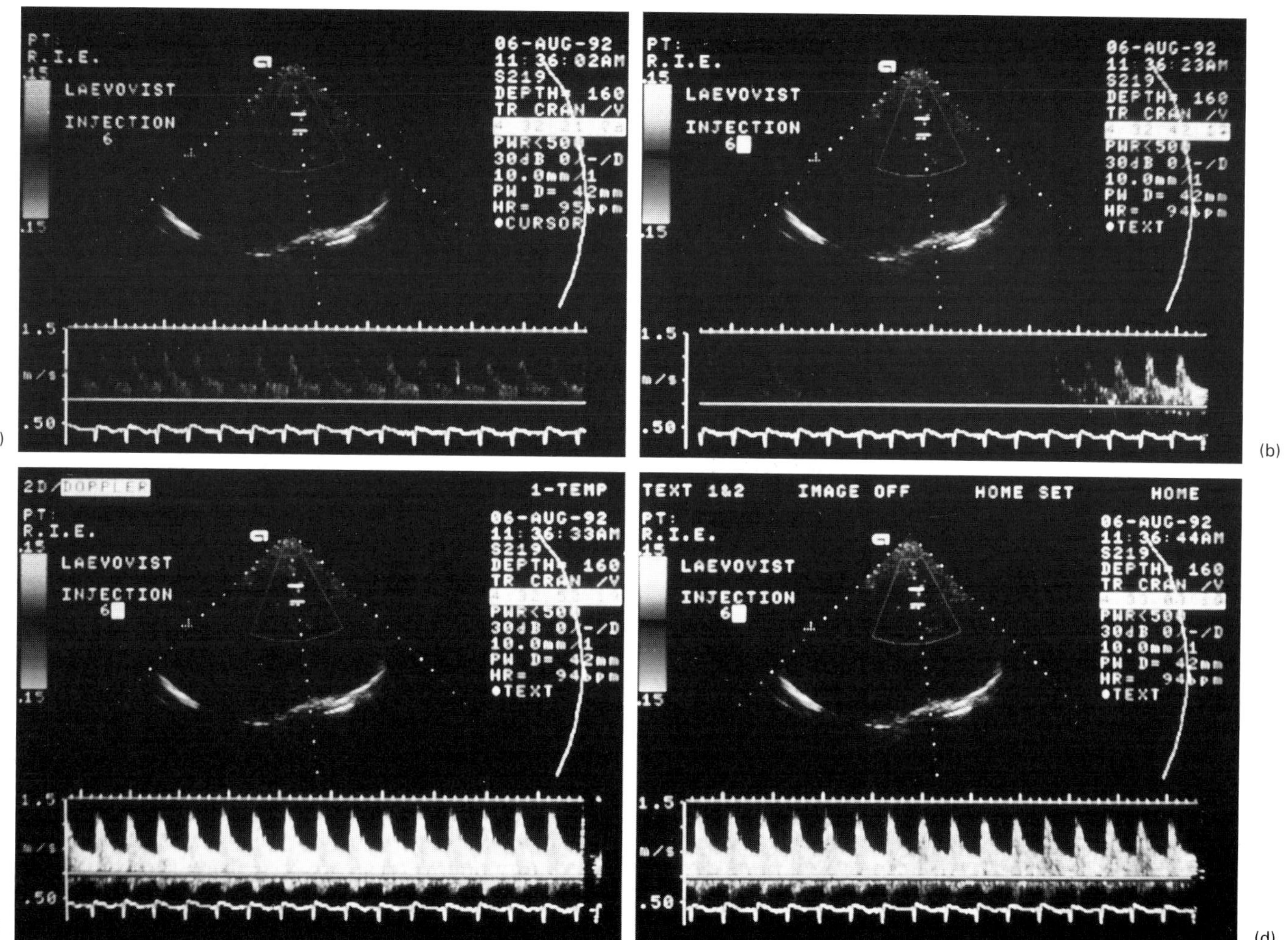

Fig. 7.7 Transcranial colour Doppler M-mode (a) prior to, (b,c) during, and (d) alter an injection of Levovist. (Courtesy of P. Allan, Edinburgh.) For colour, see Plate 7.7 (between pp. 308 and 309).

before it is then scanned. A further imaging technique which relies upon the interaction of the contrast agent with the acoustic beam is referred to as 'acoustically stimulated acoustic emission'. Using this technique, the microcapsules of a contrast agent when exposed to an ultrasound beam of sufficient magnitude, break up causing the microspheres to produce a strong acoustical signal. When insonated in colour Doppler mode this causes a random generation of colour velocities but allows visualization of perfused regions. Both techniques are very new and have still to be further explored.

At present most quantitation processes are still performed off-line on a separate PC computer plus frame-grabber and the manual tracing of the regions of interest is tedious and time-consuming. New systems, some incorporated in clinical scanners, are appearing which are semi-automatic in that the operator roughly identifies the ROI and the computer determines it exactly excluding boundary echoes which would upset the calculation of the echogenicity of the perfused region. These automatic systems have been greatly improved by more reliable boundary detecting computer programs which are now available. ROIs can also be segmented for more detailed study. The capacity of computer systems to store increasing numbers of images is also very beneficial particularly in cardiology since different phases of the heart cycle can be studied and averaging over several cycles gives more accurate results. Being able to store a limited number of images, say only 16, is surprisingly limiting in cardiac work. A cine-loop facility for review of fast moving events is of value.

The noise in ultrasonic images affects the accuracy of quantitation of backscatter from the parenchyma of tissue.

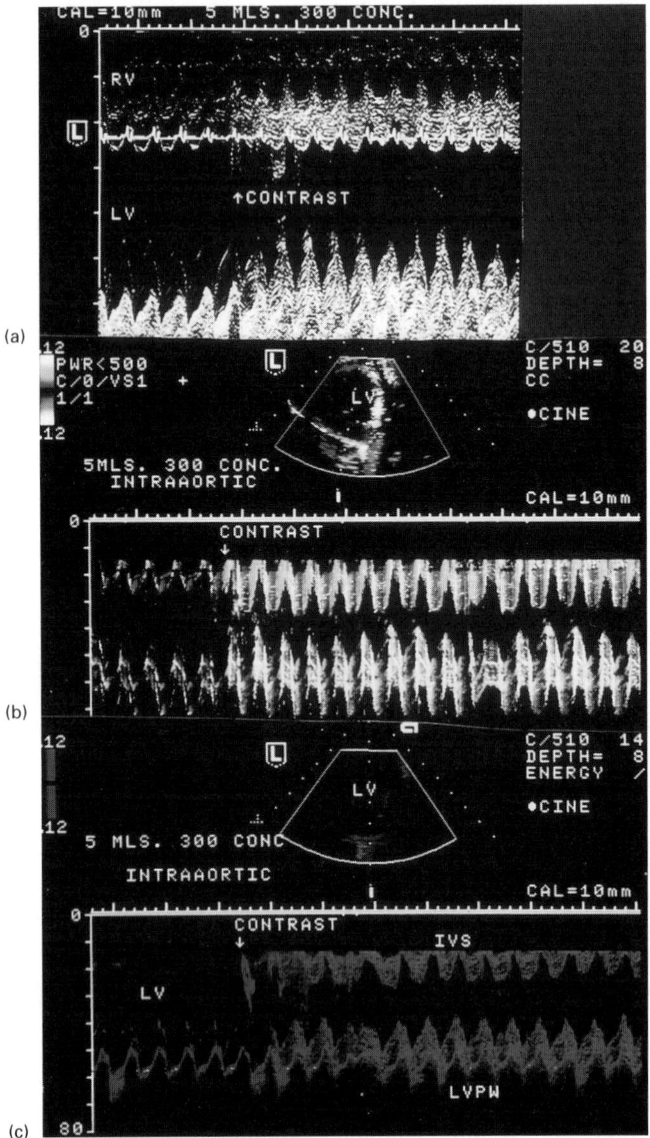

Fig. 7.8 Open-chest pig study after intra-aortic injection of Levovist. (a) Standard grey-scale M-mode through the left ventricle; (b) the same M-mode using Doppler tissue velocity imaging, and (c) an M-mode using the Doppler energy map. For colour, see Plate 7.8 (between pp. 308 and 309).

This noise is predominantly speckle noise arising from interference of the ultrasound waves from the many small scattering centres in the tissue. Techniques are available for smoothing this noise and may find application in the quantitation of backscatter intensity [43,44]. Alternatively, changes in the speckle pattern may be employed to observe regions of perfusion.

Currently there is considerable activity in the field of three-dimensional (3D) ultrasonic imaging. To some extent this is taking place since suitable computer technology is now available. However, although in many cases

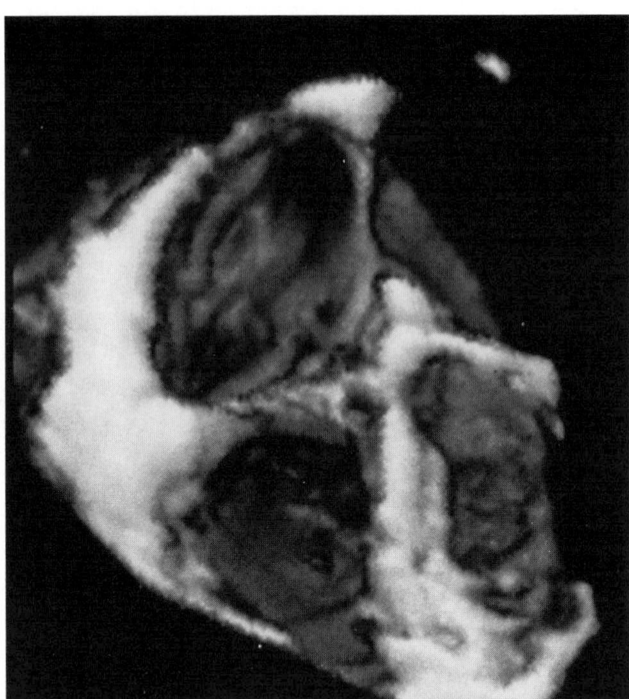

Fig. 7.9 Three-dimensional reconstruction of heart. Notice the superior vena cava, coronary sinus and inferior vena sava. (Courtesy of A. Lange, Edinburgh.)

the clinical value of 3D has still to be established and the optimum scanning systems have to be developed, interest in fields such as cardiology, obstetrics and vascular imaging is strong. The desire for full identification of tissue volumes perfused by contrast agents is perhaps one of the strongest reasons for research into 3D techniques. At present 3D scanners build up the 3D image by gathering a number of neighbouring 2D B-scan images. Typically this takes several seconds to produce one 3D image, in other words 3D scanning is not real-time (Fig. 7.9). Real-time 3D scanning is theoretically possible but the availability is some distance into the future [45]. For the present relatively slow 3D systems it is evident that the contrast agents must remain in the tissue of interest for several seconds. Such agents exist, e.g. Myomap™. 3D imaging will allow studies analogous to those which have been carried out in nuclear medicine for many years and the ultrasonic approach should be able to benefit a great deal from experience in that speciality.

Conclusion

While at present there are no accepted routine clinical uses of contrast agents, it is likely that within the next few years, injection of contrast media pervenously will become a routine method of increasing the diagnostic capabilities of ultrasonic scans. In addition, improvements in methods of detecting and quantifying the presence of contrast *in vivo* suggest that a quantitative assessment of perfusion may now be attainable.

References

1 Gramiak, R., Shah, P.M. (1968) Echocardiography of the aortic root. *Investigative Radiology* **3**, 356–366.

2 Gramiak, R., Shah, P., Kramer, D. (1969) Ultrasound cardiography: contrast study in anatomy and function. *Radiology* **92**, 939–948.

3 Ophir, J., Parker, K.J. (1989) Contrast agents in diagnostic ultrasound. *Ultrasound in Medicine and Biology* **15**, 319–333.

4 Feinstein, S.B., ten Cate, F.J., Zwehl, W., *et al*. (1984) Two-dimensional contrast echocardiography. I. *In vitro* development and quantitative analysis of echo contrast agents. *Journal of the American College of Cardiology* **3**, 14–20.

5 Ziskin, M.C., Bonakdapour, A., Weinstein, D.P., Lynch, P.R. (1972) Contrast agents for diagnostic ultrasound. *Investigative Radiology* **7**, 500–505.

6 Carroll, B., Turner, R., Tickner, E., Boyle, D., Young, S. (1980) Gelatin encapsulated nitrogen microbubbles as ultrasonic contrast agents. *Investigative Radiology* **15**, 260–266.

7 Keller, M., Feistein, S.B., Watson, D.D. (1987) Successful left ventricular opacification following peripheral venous injection of sonicated contrast agent: an experimental evaluation. *American Heart Journal* **114**, 570–575.

8 Schlief, R., Deichert, U. (1991) Hysterosalpingo-contrast sonography of the uterus and fallopian tubes: Results of a clinical trial of a new contrast agent in 120 patients. *Radiology* **178**, 213–215.

9 Schlief, R., Schurmann, R., Balzer, T., Zomack, M., Niendorf, H.-P. (1993) Saccharide based contrast agents. In: Nanda, N.C., Schlief, R. (eds) *Advances in Echo Imaging Using Contrast Enhancement*. Kluwer Academic, The Netherlands, pp. 71–96.

10 Correas, J.M., Kessler, D., Worah, D., Quay, S.C. (1996) Echogen emulsion: current clinical status in the development of the first fluorocarbon gas-based contrast agent. Presented at First European Symposium on Ultrasound Contrast Imaging, Rotterdam, January 1996.

11 de Jong, N. (1993) Acoustic properties of ultrasound contrast agents. PhD thesis, Erasmus University, Rotterdam.

12 Kinsler, L.E., Frey, A.R., Coppens, A.B., Sanders, J.V. (1982) *Fundamentals of Acoustics*, 3rd edn. Wiley, New York.

13 Parker, K.L., Tuthill, T.A., Lerner, R.M., Violante, M.R. (1987) A particulate contrast agent with potential for ultrasound imaging of liver. *Ultrasound in Medicine and Biology* **13**, 555–566.

14 Mattrey, R.F., Scheible, F.W., Gosink, B.B., Leopold, G.R., Long, D.M., Higgins, C.B. (1982) Perfluoroctyl bromide: a liver–spleen specific and tumor-imaging ultrasound contrast material. *Radiology* **145**, 759–762.

15 Ophir, J., McWhirt, R.E., Maklad, N.F. (1979) Aqueous solutions as potential ultrasonic contrast agents. *Ultrasonic Imaging* **1**, 265–279.

16 Rovai, D., Lombardi, M., Marzzarisi, A. (1993) Quantification by radiofrequency analysis of contrast echocardiography. *Cardiac Imaging* **9**, 17–19.

17 Becker, H., von Bibra, H., Walther, M., Glazer, K., Vetter, H. (1993) Contrast enhanced color Doppler—basics and potential clinical value. In: Nanda, N.C., Schlief, R (eds) *Advances in Echo Imaging Using Contrast Enhancement*. Kluwer Academic, The Netherlands, pp. 253–273.

18 Burns, P.N. (1995) Contrast agents for Doppler ultrasound. In: Taylor, K.J., Burns, P.N., Wells, P.N.T. (eds) *Clinical Applications of Doppler Ultrasound*, 2nd edn. Raven Press, New York, pp. 369–372.

19 Schwarz, K.Q., Bezate, G.P., Che, X., Schlief, R. (1993) Quantitative echo contrast concentration measurement by Doppler sonography. *Ultrasound in Medicine and Biology* **19**, 289–297.

20 Burns, P.N., Powers, J.E., Hope Simpson, D., Uhlendorf, V., Fritzsch, T. (1994) Harmonic imaging and Doppler using microbubble contrast agents: a new method for contrast imaging. *Ultrasound in Medicine and Biology* **20**(suppl. 1), S73.

21 Schrope, B., Newhouse, V.L., Uhlendorf, V. (1992) Simulated capillary blood flow measurement using a nonlinear ultrasonic contrast agent. *Ultrasonic Imaging* **14**, 134–158.

22 Chang, P.H., Shung, K.K., Levene, H.B. (1996) Quantitative measurements of second harmonic Doppler using ultrasound contrast agents. *Ultrasound in Medicine and Biology* **22**, 1205–1214.

23 von Bibra, H., Hartmann, F., Petrik, M. (1989) Contrast-color Doppler echocardiography. Improved right heart diagnosis following intravenous injection of Echovist. *Zeitschrift fur Kardiologie* **78**, 101–108.

24 Becker, H., Mintert, C., Grube, E., Luderitz, B. (1989) Classification of mitral regurgitation by colour flow mapping. *Zeitschrift fur Kardiologie* **78**, 764–770.

25 von Bibra, H., Stempfle, H.U., Poll, A., Scherer, M., Bluml, G., Blomer, H. (1991) Limitations of flow detection by colour Doppler; *in vitro* comparison to conventional Doppler. *Echocardiography* **8**, 633–642.

26 Forsberg, F., Liu, J.B., Burns, P., Merton, D.A., Goldberg, B.B. (1994) Artifacts in ultrasonic contrast studies. *Journal of Ultrasound in Medicine* **13**, 357–365.

27 Bommer, W.J., Shah, P.M., Allen, H., Meltzer, R., Kisslo, J. (1984) The safety of contrast echocardiography. Report of the Committee on Contrast Echocardiography for the American Society of Echocardiography. *Journal of the American College of Cardiology* **3**, 6–13.

28 Holland, C.K., Apfel, R.E. (1990) Thresholds for transient cavitation produced by pulsed ultrasound in a controlled nuclei environment. *Journal of the Acoustic Society of America* **88**, 2059–2069.

29 Miller, D.L., Thomas, R.M. (1995) Ultrasound contrast agents nucleate inertial cavitation *in vitro*. *Ultrasound in Medicine and Biology* **21**, 1059–1065.

30 Williams, A.R., Kubowicz, G., Cramer, E., Schlief, R. (1991) The effects of the microbubble suspension SHU 454 (Echovist) on ultrasonically induced cell lysis in a rotating tube exposure system. *Echocardiography* **8**, 423–433.

31 Dalecki, D., Raeman, C.H., Child, S.Z., *et al*. (1997) Hemolysis *in vivo* from exposure to pulsed ultrasound. *Ultrasound in Medicine and Biology* **23**, 307–313.

32 Cosgrove, D. (1995) Echo enhancers—'contrast' agents for ultrasound. *British Medical Ultrasound Society Bulletin* **3**, 34–38.

33 Nanda, N.C. (1993) Echocontrast enhancers—how safe are they? In: Nanda, N.C., Schlief, R. (eds) *Advances in Echo Imaging Using*

Contrast Enhancement. Kluwer Academic, The Netherlands, pp. 97–110.

34 Becker, G., Perez, J., Krone, A., *et al*. (1992) Transcranial colour-coded real-time sonography in the evaluation of intracranial neoplasms and arteriovenous malformations. *Neurosurgery* **31**, 420–428.

35 Bauer, A., Becker, G., Jachimczak, P., Krone, A. (1995) Contrast-enhanced transcranial duplex sonography. *British Medical Ultrasound Society Bulletin* **3**, 26–29.

36 Deichert, U., Schlief, R., van de Sandt, M., Daume, E. (1992) Transvaginal hysterosalpingo-contrast sonography for the assessment of tubal patency with gray scale imaging and additional use of pulsed Doppler. *Fertility and Sterility* **57**, 62–67.

37 Schlief, R. (1991) Ultrasound contrast agents. *Current Opinion in Radiology* **3**, 198–207.

38 Allen, C.M., Lees, W.R. (1995) Contrast enhanced ultrasound in tumour detection. *British Medical Ultrasound Society Bulletin* **3**, 30–32.

39 Kedar, R.P., Cosgrove, D.O., McCready, V.R., Bamber, J.C., Carter, E.R. (1996) Microbubble contrast agent for color Doppler US: effect on breast masses. Work in progress. *Radiology* **198**, 679–686.

40 Wiencek, J.G., Feinstein, S.B., Walker, R., Aronson, S. (1993) Pitfalls in quantitative contrast echocardiography: the steps to quantitation of perfusion. *Journal of the American Society of Echocardiography* **6**, 395–416.

41 Lindner, J.R., Kaul, S. (1995) Insights into the assessment of myocardial perfusion offered by different cardiac modalities. *Journal of Nuclear Cardiology* **2**, 446–460.

42 Porter, T.R., Xie, F. (1995) Transient myocardial contrast after initial exposure to diagnostic ultrasound pressures with minute doses of intravenously injected microbubbles. *Circulation* **92**, 2391–2395.

43 Bamber, J.C., Phelps, J.V. (1991) Real-time implementation of coherent speckle suppression in B-scan images. *Ultrasonics* **29**, 218–224.

44 Loupas, T., McDicken, W.N., Anderson, T., Allan, P.L. (1994) Development of an advanced digital image processor for real-time speckle suppression in routine ultrasonic scanning. *Ultrasound in Medicine and Biology* **20**, 239–249.

45 von Ramm, O.T., Smith, S.W., Pavy, H.G. (1991) High-speed volumetric imaging system. 1. Transducer design and beam steering. *IEEE Transactions on Ultrasonics, Ferroelectrics and Frequency Control* **38**, 100–108.

Part 2
Echocardiology

Chapter 8: Congenital heart disease

A. Houston & S. Lilley

Congenital heart disease is the most common congenital abnormality, with an incidence of about 8 in 1000 live births. The relative frequency of the different lesions is summarized in Table 8.1 [1]. Acyanotic lesions may be minor and not require intervention while cyanotic ones are always serious.

Imaging ultrasound provides a detailed assessment of the basic intracardiac anatomy and a limited amount of information on the arterial and venous connections. Colour Doppler demonstration of flow is necessary to show small defects and can improve the identification of the veins or great arteries, and spectral Doppler is used to infer valve gradients and pulmonary artery pressure.

Determination of the connections and relations of the cardiac structures

The classification and morphology of congenital heart defects has been the subject of much study. The terminology most accepted is that of sequential chamber analysis which has been developed and advocated by Anderson and his colleagues [2–4] and ultrasound assessment of complex cardiac disease should be based on this.

The detailed echocardiographic assessment of congenital heart disease requires the determination of the:

1 atrial arrangement (or situs);
2 venous connections;
3 pulmonary venous drainage;
4 atrioventricular connections;
5 ventricular morphology;
6 ventriculoarterial connections;
7 great artery position and relations; and
8 associated defects.

In the majority of cases the heart is assembled normally with normal position, connections and relations and the echocardiographic examination is directed only at determining the presence of an associated defect. Much of this chapter will consider this group of lesions with the more complex and less common forms being dealt with in less detail. More detailed descriptions of ultrasound in paediatric heart disease can be obtained from books devoted to paediatric echocardiography [5] or to general cardiac ultrasound [6,7].

Atrial arrangement

The description as 'right atrium' or 'left atrium' is based on atrial morphology and makes no inference as to the side of the body on which the atrium is placed. The atria can most accurately be identified by the morphology of the appendages: the left has a narrow junction with the atrium and is relatively long and narrow while the right has a wide junction and is relatively short and broad. The atrial arrangement or 'situs' can be situs solitus (left atrium on the left and right atrium on the right), situs inversus (left atrium on the right and right atrium on the left) or atrial isomerism (two morphologically right or left atria).

It is difficult to obtain good images of the atrial appendage morphology and the atrial arrangement can be inferred from the relationships of the aorta and inferior vena cava (IVC) at the level of the 12th vertebra [8]. In a transverse section just below the diaphragm the aorta and IVC should be on opposite sides of the spine and the morphological right atrium will be on the same side as the IVC which drains into it. Thus in situs solitus the IVC will be on the right of the spine and the aorta to the left though it may be quite near the midline (Fig. 8.1a). With right atrial isomerism the aorta and IVC are usually on the same side of the spine with the vein just anterior to the aorta (Fig. 8.1b). With left atrial isomerism commonly the IVC cannot be identified in the subhepatic area and tilting the scanning plane upwards to the junction of the liver and the atrium will show the hepatic veins entering the atrium directly or by a common confluence; the aorta usually will be in the midline and below the diaphragm the azygous vein should be apparent and seen to pass up to join the superior vena cava (SVC).

Table 8.1 The most common congenital cardiac lesions as a percentage of the total, modified from a study in Liverpool, UK, of children born in the decade 1960–69 [1]

	% of total
Acyanotic lesions	
ventricular septal defect	32
arterial duct	12
pulmonary stenosis	8
coarctation of the aorta	6
atrial septal defect	6
aortic stenosis	5
atrioventricular septal defect	2
Total	71
Cyanotic lesions	
tetralogy of Fallot	6
transposition of the great arteries	5
single ventricle (including tricuspid atresia)	4
hypoplastic left heart syndrome	3
total anomalous pulmonary venous drainage	1
truncus arteriosus	1
Total	20

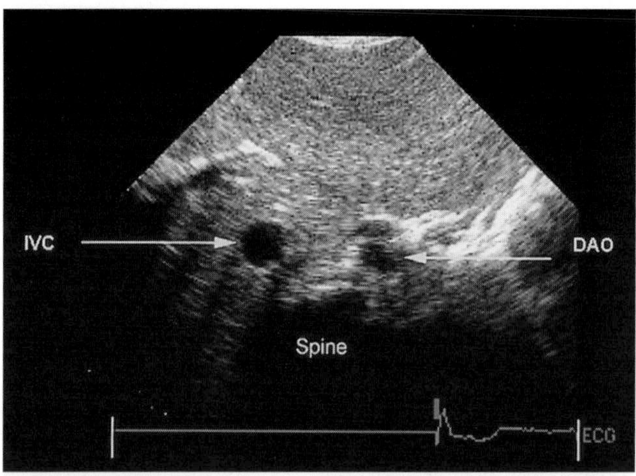

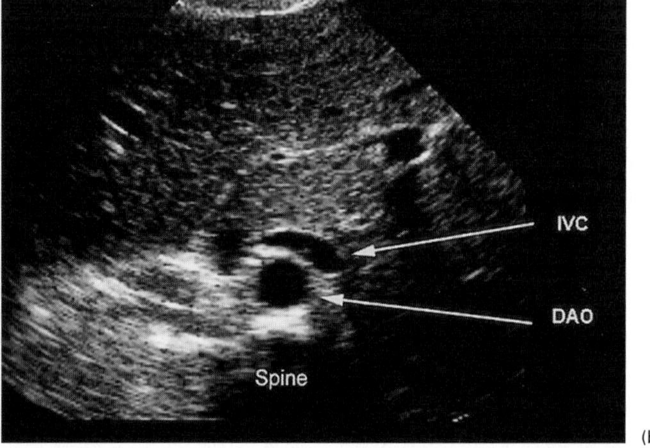

Fig. 8.1 Transverse views through the liver of patients with (a) situs solitus and (b) right atrial isomerism. In (a) the inferior vena cava (IVC) lies to the right of the spine and descending aorta (DAO) to the right while in (b) the descending aorta lies just to the left of the spine with the inferior vena cava just anterior to it.

Systemic venous connections

The IVC is shown coming upwards from below the diaphragm, where the hepatic veins join it, and entering the right atrium. The superior vena cava can be shown entering the right atrium if a four-chamber view (often subcostal) is used and angled anteriorly and upwards or a high parasternal view is used.

The most common variation of the superior caval system is a persistent left SVC draining to the coronary sinus. This is suggested in a long axis view when a dilated coronary sinus is seen posterior to the left atrium. A parasagittal plane can show the left-sided vein draining inferiorly to the coronary sinus.

Pulmonary venous connection

The connection of the pulmonary veins to the left atrium can be shown using a subcostal four-chamber view or a suprasternal paracoronal section angled relatively posteriorly to show the veins just below the pulmonary arteries. Colour Doppler, and particularly the power mode, can be helpful in demonstrating flow and outlining a vein. All four veins may not be seen with certainty, but in the context of the neonate with cyanotic heart disease the presence of even one vein draining normally excludes the diagnosis of total anomalous pulmonary venous drainage.

Atrioventricular connections and ventricular morphology

The morphology of the ventricles can be inferred by identifying the inlet valves since the tricuspid enters the morphological right ventricle and the mitral the left. This is most readily determined from the offsetting of the atrioventricular valves, the tricuspid being attached to the septum nearer the apex than the mitral. In addition the left ventricle usually has two almost symmetrical papillary muscles and a smooth trabecular pattern with the mitral chordae attached to the papillary muscles and only rarely to the ventricular walls. The right ventricle has papillary muscles of unequal size and a more coarse trabecular pattern with the tricuspid chordae connecting to the right side of the ventricular septum. The mitral valve is generally continuous with the artery arising from the left ventricle, while an infundibulum separates the tricuspid from the great artery.

Ventriculoarterial connections and relations

The aorta is identified in a high parasternal or suprasternal long axis view by its long upward course and the origin of the head and neck vessels from the superior aspect. The pulmonary artery turns posterior at a lower level and in a short axis view can be seen to bifurcate to give the left and right branches. With normally related great arteries a short axis view shows the aorta as a circular structure with the right ventricular outflow crossing it anteriorly from right to left then passing posteriorly to its left and branching. In the transposition complexes the great arteries do not cross and the short axis view will show them as two parallel circular structures.

A ventricle is considered to connect with an artery when more than half of the artery takes origin from it. This may be apparent in a long axis view or short axis sweep upwards from the ventricle to artery but echocardiographic assessment may not be certain since the relationship varies as the heart beats.

Ventricular septal defect

The ventricular septal defect accounts for about one-third of all congenital cardiac lesions. In the majority it is small, is recognized by the incidental finding of a murmur and does not require closure. Surgical closure is deemed necessary in infancy for intractable cardiac failure or pulmonary hypertension. Knowledge of the site of a ventricular septal defect is necessary if surgery is required or with a small defect to give information on the likelihood of the defect closing or causing later problems. Since decisions on the need for surgical closure are largely based on the shunt size and pulmonary pressure the assessment of these is most important in the management of the infant with a ventricular septal defect.

A ventricular septal defect can be present at any site and the detailed anatomy and relationship of this to the echocardiographic assessment of the site of the ventricular septal defect has been well described [9–11]. For practical echocardiographic purposes it is useful to classify the site as being perimembranous or muscular, the latter being in the inlet, trabecular, apical or outlet areas.

Perimembranous defects

Defects in the membranous septum usually extend into the surrounding muscular septum. They are recognized in a four-chamber view (apical or subcostal) which shows the defect at the crux of the heart directly adjacent to the tricuspid valve. There is often an aneurysm round the defect formed of tissue which appears to be part of the tricuspid valve. Extension downwards into the muscular septum (Fig. 8.2) can be appreciated in this view. An upward tilt towards a five-chamber view can show extension into the outlet septum. Outlet extension can also be seen in a high short axis view and when the defect is large this may be apparent extending up to the right coronary cusp. Extension into the outlet septum can also be shown in a parasternal long axis view (Fig. 8.3), often by tilting the scanning plane slightly towards the right. With outlet extension, prolapse of the right coronary cusp and aortic regurgitation should be sought and may be an indication for surgical closure.

Muscular defects

A muscular defect is recognized by the presence of muscular tissue round its margins. The view which best shows this depends on the site and may be a four-chamber view, long axis view either standard or with tilt to the left or right, or short axis view as the transducer is swept down from the aortic root towards the apex. It may be situated in the inlet, mid (trabecular) (Fig. 8.4), apical or outlet septum. There can be multiple defects and trabecular and apical ones are often small in which case colour Doppler is helpful in determining their presence and site (Fig. 8.5).

Outlet defects can be subaortic, subpulmonary or doubly committed. Subaortic defects usually occur as part of a more complicated lesion (such as tetralogy of Fallot)

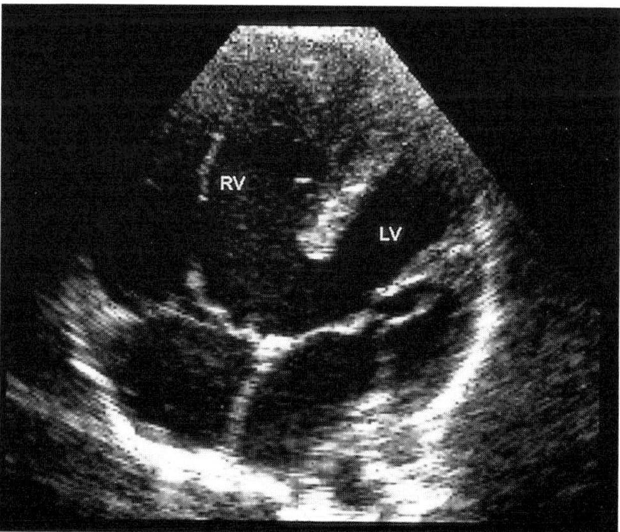

Fig. 8.2 Four-chamber view of a patient with perimembranous inlet ventricular septal defect which extends from the crux of the heart well into the muscular septum. LV, left ventricle; RV, right ventricle.

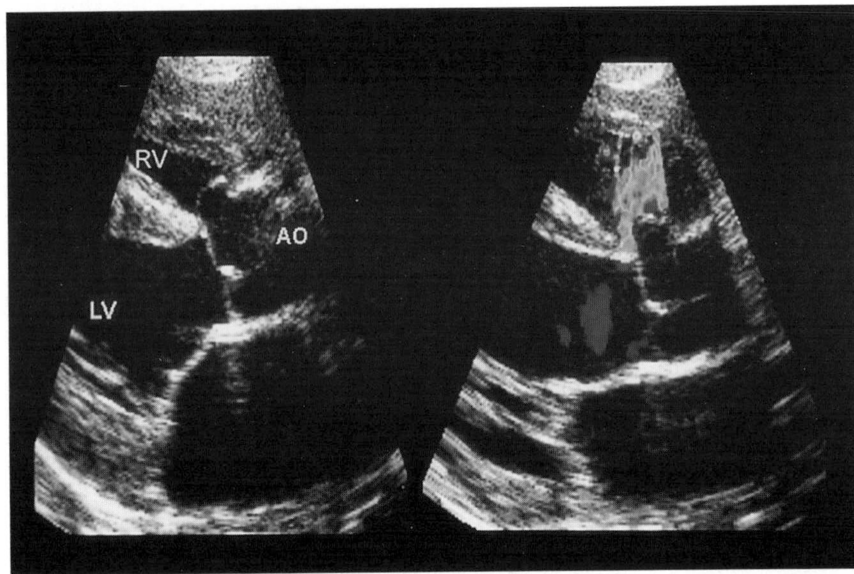

Fig. 8.3 Long axis views with and without colour of a patient with a subaortic ventricular septal defect and aortic valve prolapse. The defect is between the upper edge of the septum and the aortic margin. In this diastolic frame it is partially closed by the prolapsed right coronary cusp. AO, aorta; LV, left ventricle; RV, right ventricle. For colour, see Plate 8.3 (between pp. 308 and 309).

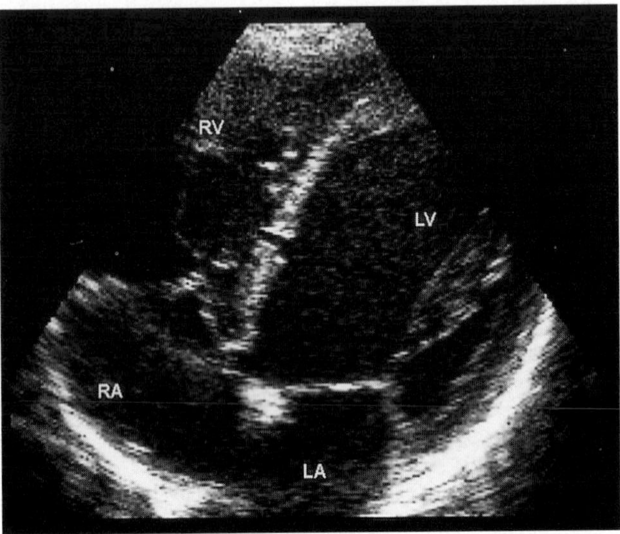

Fig. 8.4 Four-chamber view of a patient with a small muscular ventricular septal defect in the mid septal region. LA, left atrium; LV, left ventricle; RA, right atrium; RV, right ventricle.

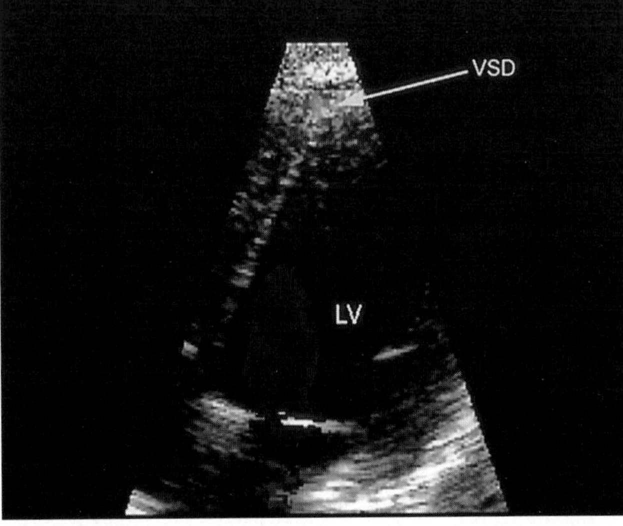

Fig. 8.5 Apical view in systole of a child with a very small apical ventricular septal defect (VSD) which is so small and anterior it is difficult to image, but colour Doppler highlights its position. LV, left ventricle. For colour, see Plate 8.5 (between pp. 308 and 309).

and can be recognized in a long axis or five-chamber view as discontinuity between the aorta and upper septum with a degree of aortic over-ride of the ventricular septum. Subpulmonary defects are shown in a short axis view or subcostal view tilted up to show the right ventricular outflow tract and pulmonary artery. The doubly committed subarterial defect lies in the highest part of the outflow tract and results in continuity of the aortic and pulmonary valves. This defect is seen in a short axis view as a deficiency in the area of the left coronary cusp and reaches to the pulmonary ring, with no tissue inferior to the site at which the aortic and pulmonary valves are seen to join.

Haemodynamic information

Initial reports of the use of Doppler suggested that quantitation of the pulmonary systemic flow ratio was possible by measuring mean velocities with spectral Doppler and valve area with imaging ultrasound [12]. However, these are subject to potential errors and it is not recommended that these calculations are used for clinical purposes. M-mode echocardiographic measurement of the sizes of the left ventricle or atrium can provide a simple guide to whether there is a significant shunt, the larger the shunt the larger the left-sided chambers are likely to be.

Spectral Doppler can provide an assessment of the pulmonary artery pressure. The maximum velocity of flow through the defect is measured and converted to a pressure gradient between the ventricles using the modified Bernoulli equation [13,14]. The left ventricular systolic pressure should equal the systemic blood pressure so the right ventricular pressure can theoretically be estimated by subtracting the interventricular pressure gradient from systolic blood pressure (i.e. the left ventricular pressure). In the absence of pulmonary stenosis the right ventricular systolic pressure equals the pulmonary artery pressure. There are potential inaccuracies in measuring the systolic blood pressure and the ventricular gradient so it is not recommended that the calculation be performed. Rather the velocity should be taken into consideration with other factors in deciding if the pulmonary pressure is raised. Thus a low velocity or bidirectional (Fig. 8.6) signal will be consistent with pulmonary hypertension while a high velocity (Fig. 8.7) will indicate low pulmonary pressure.

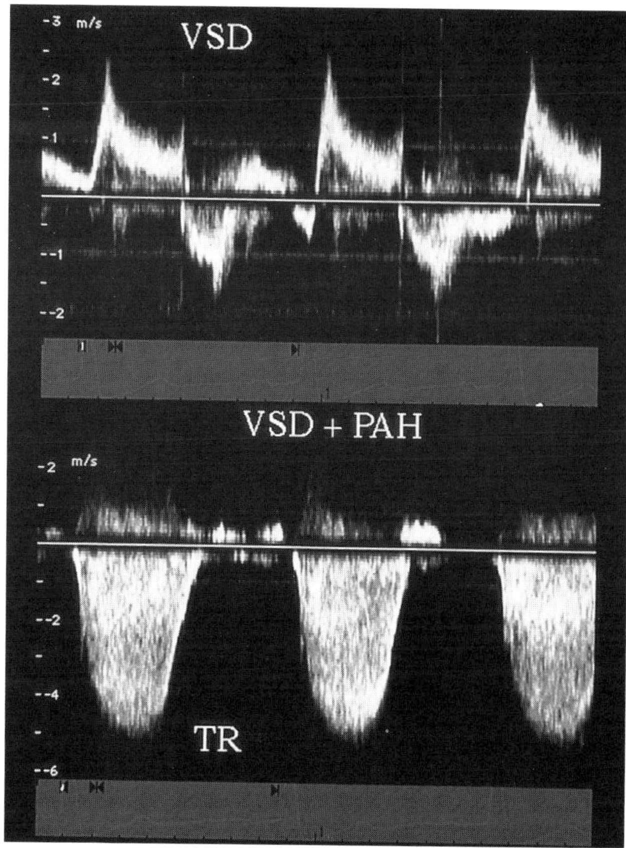

Fig. 8.6 Spectral signals of a patient with a ventricular septal defect (VSD) and pulmonary hypertension (PAH) at systemic level. The upper signal shows flow through the ventricular septal defect which is bidirectional, from left to right ventricle in systole and right to left ventricle in diastole. The signal of tricuspid regurgitation (TR) is over 5 m s^{-1}, indicating a right ventricular pressure of over 100 mmHg.

Atrial septal defect

Children with an atrial septal defect are usually asymptomatic, the possibility of a cardiac anomaly being raised by the finding of a murmur. This murmur is often unimpressive and many defects are not detected in childhood and present with a murmur, arrhythmia or right heart failure in later life.

The most common is the ostium secundum defect which occurs in the centre of the septum. The ostium primum defect lies lower and impinges on the crux of the heart and is a variant of the atrioventricular septal defect discussed below. The sinus venosus defect is in the upper aspect of the septum related to the SVC and is usually associated with anomalous drainage of the right upper pulmonary vein to the SVC.

The possibility of a significant atrial shunt is initially suggested by right ventricular volume overload recognized from the presence of a large right ventricular chamber and paradoxical septal motion. The latter is manifest on M-mode study by an abnormal pattern of septal systolic motion, either flat with little movement or paradoxical and moving anteriorly in parallel with the posterior wall rather than towards it (Fig. 8.8). This appearance occurs with any cause of right ventricular volume overload, such as tricuspid or pulmonary regurgitation, anomalous pulmonary venous drainage or a fistula to the right atrium. The size of the left-to-right shunt through the atrial septal defect is reflected in the right ventricular dimension [15]. If the right ventricular size is normal or only slightly increased and the septal motion normal the shunt will be small and closure is not warranted on this basis.

If right ventricular volume overload is apparent it is necessary to determine the underlying cause and, in the case of an atrial septal defect, demonstrate its presence. The atrial septum is imaged optimally in a four-chamber view but since an apical one provides a plane parallel to the septum it is not ideal for showing an atrial septal defect. A subcostal view should be employed to bring the septum into a plane at right angles to the ultrasound beam [16] and optimally show the defect. The normal atrial septum shows a relatively thin central area representing the fossa ovale. A secundum defect occurs in this position

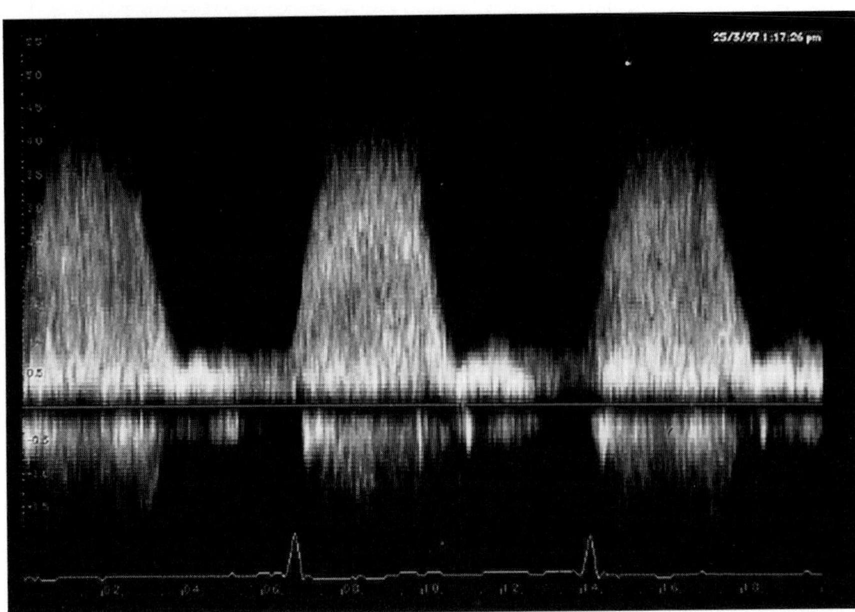

Fig. 8.7 Spectral signal from a child with a ventricular septal defect and low right ventricular pressure showing a high velocity (about 4 m s^{-1}) flow signal from the left to right ventricle indicating a pressure difference of over 60 mmHg and thus a low right-sided pressure.

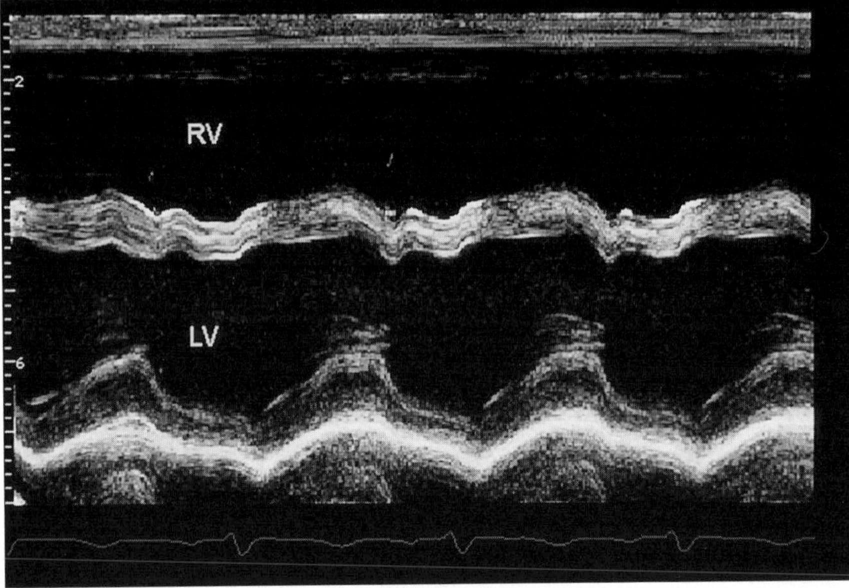

Fig. 8.8 M-mode recording through the right and left ventricles (RV and LV) in a patient with a large atrial septal defect. The right ventricle is enlarged and there is paradoxical septal motion, the septum moving anterior in systole.

(Fig. 8.9) while a sinus venosus defect is imaged from the subcostal position by tilting the scanning plane upwards when the defect will become apparent at the junction of the septum and the SVC (Fig. 8.10). This is usually associated with an anomalous pulmonary vein draining into the SVC but it may be difficult to show this vein with echocardiography.

In children there is generally no difficulty in deciding that there is a defect but on occasions there can be some uncertainty and in adults the distance from the transducer can make this difficult. In all cases it is appropriate to use colour Doppler to show that there is flow through the area and a definite defect [17]. With colour Doppler flow through the normal foramen ovale can be apparent for weeks or even months.

In adult patients it can be difficult to image the septum well and the distance from the transducer can limit the sensitivity of colour Doppler. In this situation transoesophageal echocardiography will provide extremely clear demonstration of the anatomy of the atrial septum and simply identify the presence of the type of atrial defect [18].

Atrioventricular septal defect

In the normal heart the atrial and ventricular septa are continuous and the mitral and tricuspid valves inserted into them at different levels, the tricuspid being more apical.

In an atrioventricular septal defect the two septa do not join but leave a confluent defect produced by absence of part of both the ventricular and atrial septa. There is a common atrioventricular valve and the atrioventricular defect can be classified on the basis of the relationship of the valve to the defect [19], this being readily apparent on echocardiography [20,21]. In the lesion known as a partial atrioventricular septal defect (or a primum atrial septal defect) echocardiography shows the anterior leaflet to be divided into left and right components inserted directly into the rim of the ventricular septum, and there is no direct ventricular communication (Fig. 8.11). In a complete atrioventricular septal defect there is a communication between the ventricles (Fig. 8.12) and there may be chordal attachments directly to the rim of the ventricular septum or passing through the septal defect.

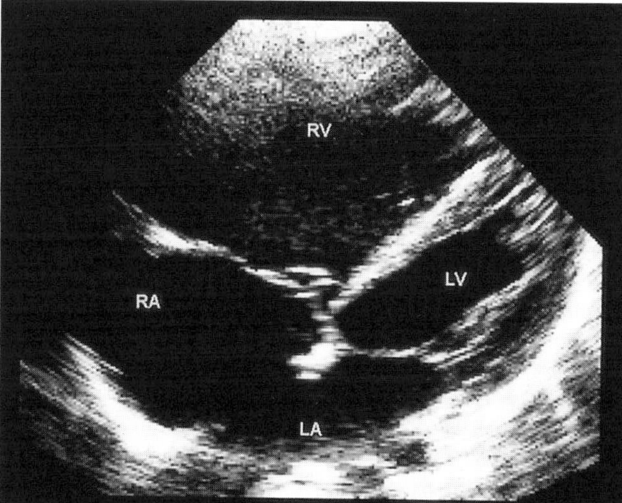

Fig. 8.9 Parasternal four-chamber view in a patient with a large secundum atrial septal defect. LA, left atrium; LV, left ventricle; RA, right atrium; RV, right ventricle.

In patients with an atrioventricular septal defect the left (mitral) component of the valve is different from a normal mitral, with an apparent anterior cleft being formed between the central and lateral leaflets. Detailed anatomy of the valve can be ascertained from a subcostal short axis view [22]. The practical importance of this is related to the degree to which this valve is regurgitant and colour Doppler frequently shows multiple regurgitant jets, these passing in a variety of directions including left ventricle to right atrium.

If there is a ventricular septal defect spectral Doppler can be used to assess the pulmonary artery pressure from the velocity of the jet (p. 101). If an attempt is made to assess right ventricular pressure from the signal of tricuspid regurgitation care must be exercised to ensure that the

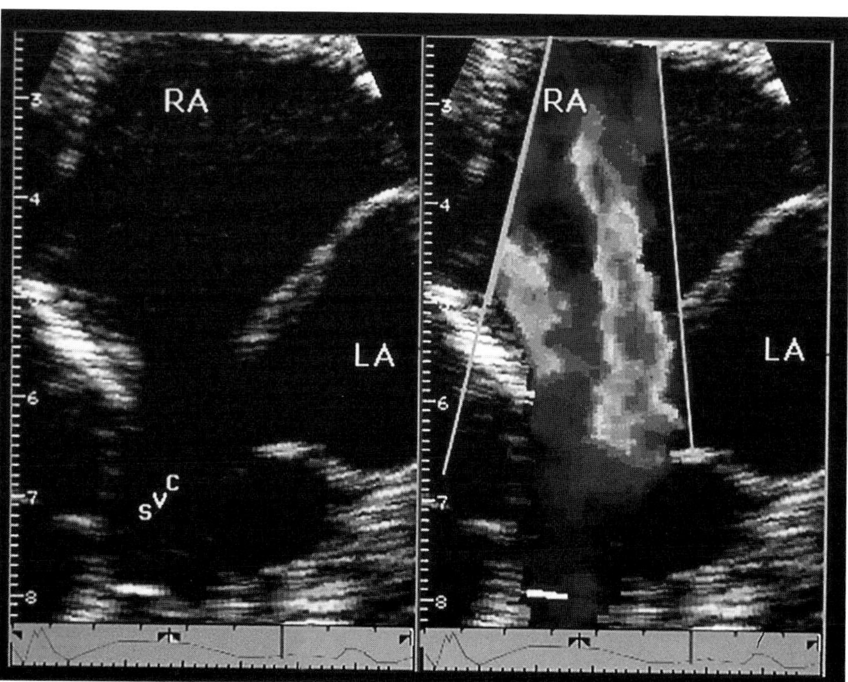

Fig. 8.10 Subcostal images of a patient with sinus venosus atrial septal defect. The scanning plane is tilted up from a subcostal position to show the upper margin of the right atrium and the sinus venosus defect with apparent overriding of the superior vena cava (SVC). The right image shows flow from both the SVC and left atrium (LA) into the right atrium (RA). For colour, see Plate 8.10 (between pp. 308 and 309).

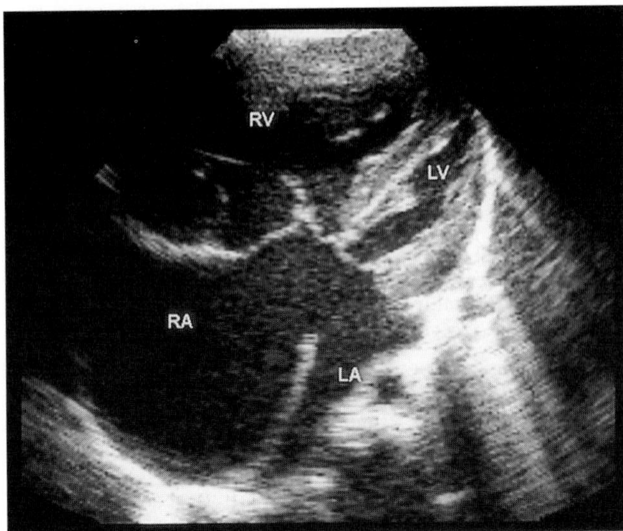

Fig. 8.11 Parasternal view of a patient with a partial atrioventricular septal defect. The anterior valve leaflets are attached directly to the crest of the ventricular septum and there is a large gap low in the atrial septum (primum atrial septal defect). The left ventricle (LV) and atrium (LA) are foreshortened in this view. RA, right atrium; RV, right ventricle.

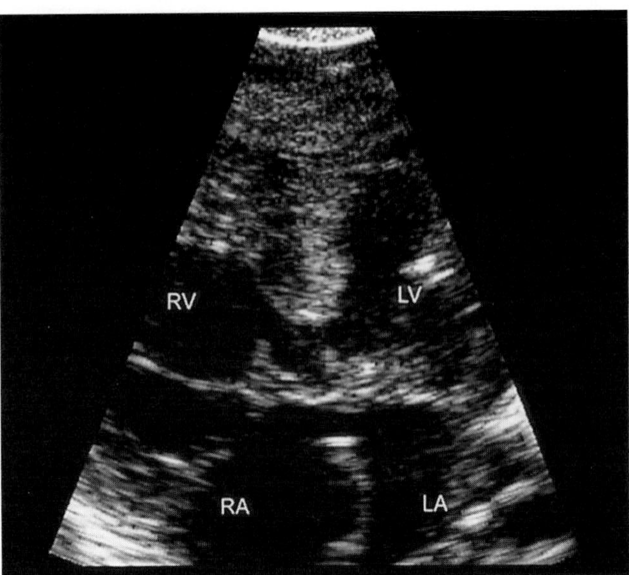

Fig. 8.12 Four-chamber view of a patient with a complete atrioventricular septal defect. The margins of the atrial septum and ventricular septum shows bright echoes, and there is an apparently single anterior valve leaflet passing through the defect leaving a left-to-right communications at atrial and ventricular levels. LA, left atrium; LV, left ventricle; RA, right atrium; RV, right ventricle.

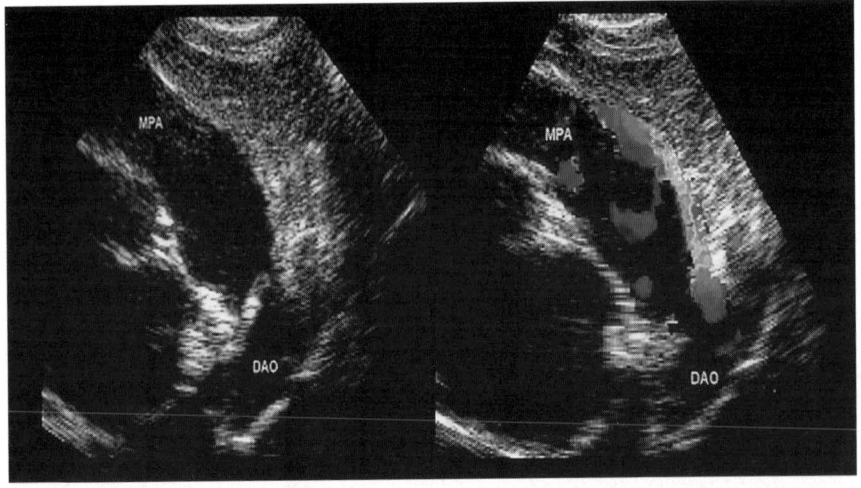

Fig. 8.13 Left parasagittal images of a patient with an arterial duct. The colour image shows acceleration into the mouth of the duct with the jet passing along the superior wall of the main pulmonary artery (MPA). DAO, descending aorta. For colour, see Plate 8.13 (between pp. 308 and 309).

jet recorded is not that from the left ventricle to the right atrium.

Arterial duct

In the fetus the arterial duct (ductus arteriosus) is an essential communication allowing blood to flow from the pulmonary artery to the descending aorta. It usually closes in the first days of life, and though colour Doppler can show that it may subsequently reopen briefly, functional closure occurs by the sixth day of life [23]. In some cyanotic lesions without normal flow to the pulmonary artery, its patency is essential to maintain postnatal life.

The duct can be shown in a variety of views as a continuation of the pulmonary artery into the descending aorta. It is often best shown in a parasagittal view from the left upper sternal edge by tilting the plane inferiorly and moving the transducer from left to right with some rotation as required (Fig. 8.13). A similar view is obtained from the suprasternal notch or even the right upper sternal edge in a view which shows it in relation to the aortic arch and descending aorta [24]. A short axis view of the great arteries can be adjusted to show the pulmonary artery continuing into the descending aorta but care should be taken to ensure that the duct is not confused with the left pulmonary artery. Colour Doppler is most useful when imaging is inconclusive and characteristically shows ductal flow as a flame-shaped jet arising at the mouth of the duct and directed along the superolateral wall of the main pulmonary artery [25]. With some congenital cardiac abnormalities the ductus may be of unusual shape and follow an abnormal course. As necessary the scanning plane has to be adjusted but colour mapping will simplify the process.

Colour Doppler is so sensitive that it will show flow through a tiny ductus which is so small that there is no ductal flow murmur. The authors consider that this should be considered as a variant of normal, similar to physiological mitral regurgitation, and intervention or antibiotic prophylaxis against endocarditis is not necessary [26].

The left-to-right shunt is difficult to assess with ultrasound but in the neonate it seems that the size of the left atrium in relation to the aorta, first described in 1974 [27,28] still provides a clinically useful ultrasound technique. A ratio of the atrium to aorta greater than 1.3 is likely to be associated with a clinically significant shunt. Retrograde flow from the descending aorta in diastole indicates a large run-off back to the pulmonary artery and thus high flow [29].

The spectral Doppler record of the flow into the pulmonary artery allows some assessment of the pulmonary artery pressure. With normal low pulmonary pressure the signal is a continuous one of relatively high velocity, this being maximal in mid to late systole and falling to its lowest level at end diastole (Fig. 8.14). The velocity of the systolic signal can be used to provide an assessment of the pulmonary artery systolic pressure by subtracting it from the aortic pressure but the value obtained is not clinically reliable [30]. In the newborn where the pulmonary pressure is elevated at systemic levels the ductal flow signal will show a variety of patterns, often with bidirectional shunting, usually right to left in systole and left to right in diastole (Fig. 8.14) [30]. Even in situations such as left heart hypoplasia where the aorta fills only from the pulmonary artery through the duct this bidirectional appearance is maintained because, although the pulmonary pressure is higher than the aorta in systole, it is lower in diastole. Only rarely with very high pulmonary resistance is the ductal flow entirely right to left throughout the cardiac cycle.

Aortic stenosis

Congenital aortic stenosis most commonly occurs at valve level but in about one-quarter of cases it is at subvalve and rarely at supravalve level. The valve may be mor-

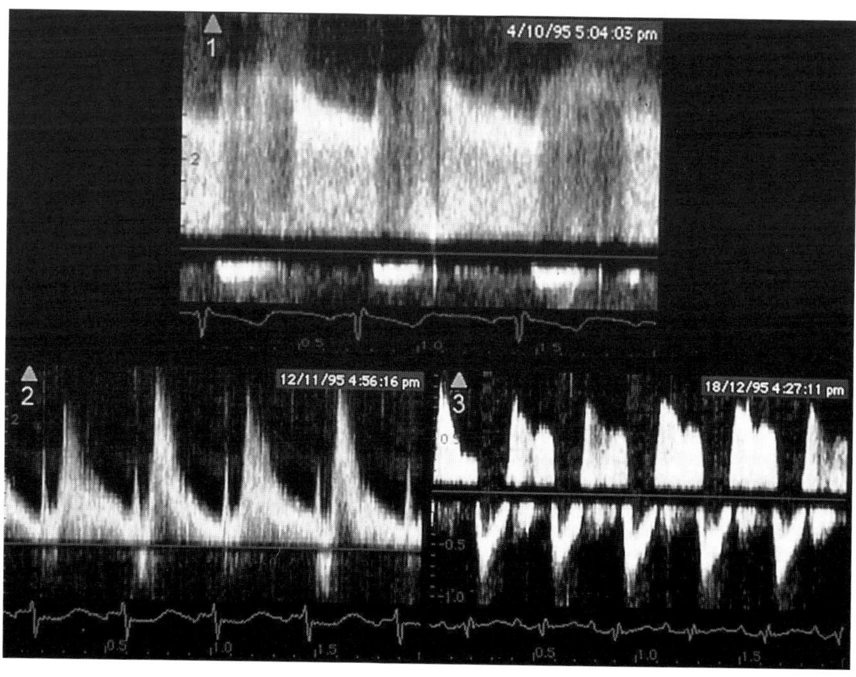

Fig. 8.14 Spectral signals of patients with an arterial duct (1) Low pulmonary pressure with a high velocity signal maximal in mid to late systole, but remaining of high velocity throughout the cardiac cycle. The signal appears weaker in systole due to the effect of the automatic gain control. (2) Pulmonary hypertension showing a maximum velocity of only about 2.5 m s^{-1} and very low diastolic velocity. (3) Pulmonary hypertension at systemic levels showing bidirectional flow from the pulmonary artery to the aorta (below the baseline) in systole and diastole.

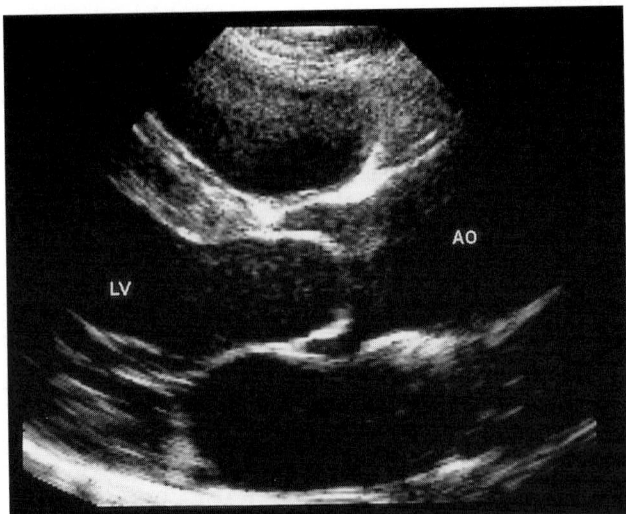

Fig. 8.15 Systolic frame of a patient with aortic valve stenosis showing doming of the aortic valve. AO, aortic root; LV, left ventricle.

phologically abnormal, most commonly bicuspid (1–2% of the population) but occasionally unicuspid or quadricuspid.

The short axis view of the normal aortic valve in diastole shows the three cusps of approximately equal size, with the right and left coronary cusps anteriorly and the non-coronary cusp posteriorly. In systole the open cusps can be seen against the aortic wall. A functionally bicuspid valve may appear to be normal in diastole but in systole only two cusps are shown, one being formed from what appears in diastole as two separate ones with a fused raphe between them [31] but clear demonstration of this is not always possible in older subjects [32].

In aortic valve stenosis in children the leaflets are generally pliable and dome (Fig. 8.15) in systole [33]. Subaortic stenosis can be fibromuscular or membranous (Fig. 8.16) and it is not always possible to show the complete margins of this in a long axis view. An apical view [34] will provide more detail of its structure. Transoesophageal imaging provides very clear images of the left ventricular outflow tract [35,36]. Subaortic stenosis is almost invariably associated with mild aortic regurgitation which can be demonstrated with colour Doppler. Supravalve narrowing usually occurs just at or above the sinus of Valsalva and may be discrete or tubular (Fig. 8.17). M-mode echocardiography may show thickening of the septal and posterior left ventricular walls. In subaortic stenosis the aortic valve will show early closure and coarse fluttering during systole [37].

Colour Doppler is of little practical value in the assessment of aortic stenosis but the presence of aliasing will usually confirm the site of obstruction. Spectral Doppler

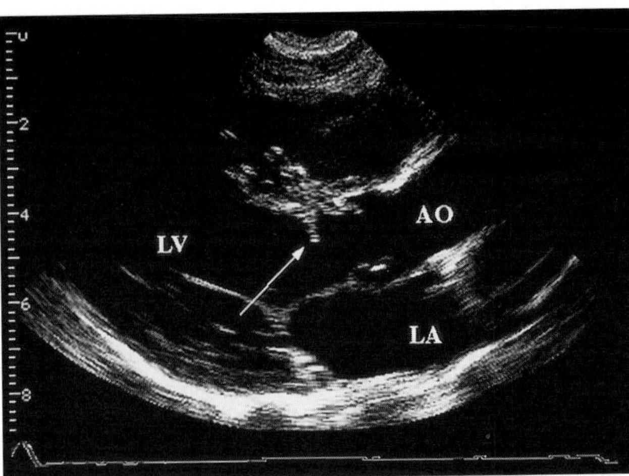

Fig. 8.16 Long axis view of a patient with subaortic stenosis showing the subaortic membrane (arrow). AO, aorta; LA, left atrium; LV, left ventricle.

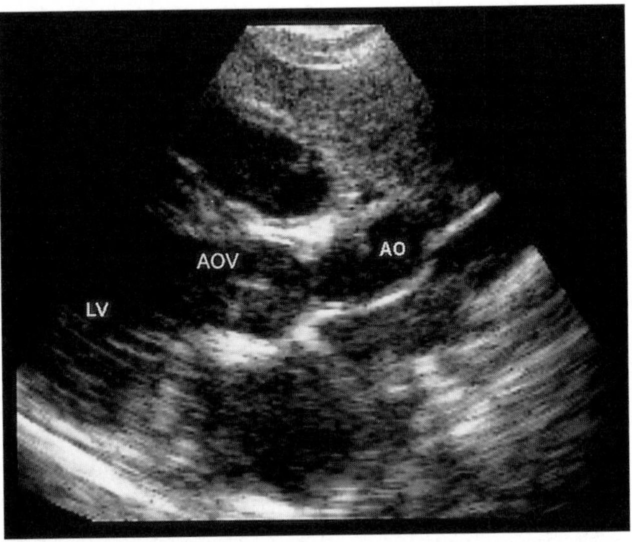

Fig. 8.17 Long axis view of a patient with supravalve aortic stenosis showing the obstruction just above the sinus of Valsalva. AO, aorta; AOV, aortic valve; LV, left ventricle.

provides a means of estimating the gradient across the obstruction by applying the modified Bernoulli formula. The problems involved in the application of this formula to predict the severity of stenosis in the clinical situation are similar to those in adult practice. In children it is usually more easy to obtain a signal from all the appropriate sites including the right upper sternal edge and right subclavicular position [38]. There are particular difficulties in predicting the gradient in subaortic stenosis where both under- and overestimation can occur. Because of the uncertainty in relating Doppler maximum gradient to severity of obstruction some would rather use the

Doppler information to estimate the valve area using the continuity equation [39] or the mean valve gradient [40].

Coarctation of the aorta

In coarctation of the aorta the narrowing can take the form of a discrete membrane, hour-glass shape, long segment narrowing or general hypoplasia of the aortic isthmus but this has little influence on the clinical situation. It is usually diagnosed clinically but in the newborn the clinical diagnosis may be difficult if the ductus is wide open or there is hypotension. The main role of ultrasound is in demonstration of its site.

The effect on the ventricles depends on the age and nature of the lesion: in the newborn right ventricular enlargement and a small left ventricle with decreased function is common, while in older infancy there may be an enlarged poorly contracting left ventricle. Left ventricular size and function are generally normal in older patients though there may be some thickening of its walls.

The aorta may be imaged in a view showing the aortic arch and its continuation as the descending aorta which can be obtained from a suprasternal [41] or high parasternal (right or left) position [42]. The transducer should be placed in a sagittal plane and then rotated somewhat clockwise and tilted as necessary to show the ascending aorta, arch and descending aorta. From the left upper sternal edge the coarctation may be best seen in a variation of the ductal view which shows the distal arch and descending aorta but not the whole arch (Fig. 8.18). When the coarctation is well seen the appearance will depend on the nature of the narrowed site and may be a membrane-like structure, or a more diffuse or a long segment narrowing. The area of the coarctation may not be well seen with imaging, particularly in older subjects [43] and then colour Doppler will often allow the narrowed area to be identified when this is not visible on the image.

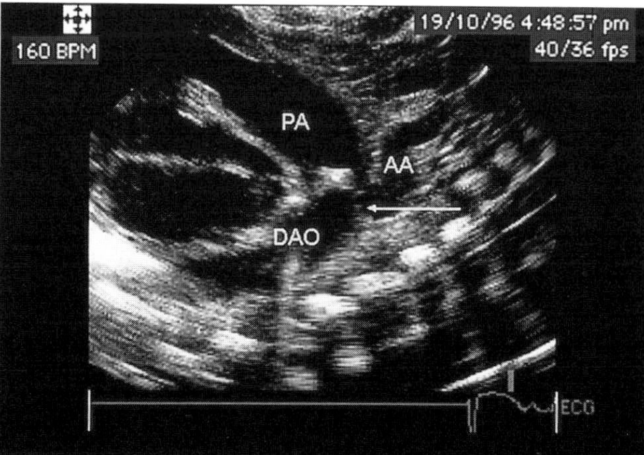

Fig. 8.18 Parasagittal view in an infant with periductal coarctation (arrow). This view shows the distal aortic arch (AA) and the descending aorta (DAO) with a duct still apparently patent leading into the pulmonary artery (PA).

The spectral Doppler signal of descending aorta flow will show increased velocity, this being typically continuous with highest velocity in mid systole, then falling but continuing with lower velocity throughout diastole. The diastolic signal reflects the continuing diastolic pressure drop across the obstruction and bears no clear relation to the maximum velocity. A signal showing no diastolic flow is usually associated with less severe obstruction even when the maximum velocity is relatively high. The maximum Doppler gradient and measured one show poor correlation with both over- and underestimation [44,45]. Difficulties in obtaining the correct alignment to the flow jet or use of the simplified Bernoulli formula do not fully explain this poor correlation and since the severity of the narrowing is not necessarily related to the gradient across it , the maximum velocity is of limited practical value in assessing coarctation. A similar poor correlation with measured gradient is found in the postoperative situation [46].

Pulmonary stenosis

Right ventricular outflow tract obstruction commonly occurs at valve level but subvalvar or supravalvar narrowing can be an isolated defect or part of a more complex lesion.

Pulmonary valve images are best obtained using a parasternal short axis great artery view or low parasternal or subcostal four-chamber view tilted upwards to show the right ventricular outflow tract anterior to the aorta. Doming of the pulmonary valve leaflets occurs but is of little diagnostic value.

Colour Doppler ultrasound will show acceleration of flow towards and aliasing at the site of obstruction. Spectral Doppler provides an accurate means of measuring the pressure gradient in pulmonary valve stenosis [47]. The maximum velocity may be recorded from either view. The signal of pulmonary stenosis is a systolic one with maximum velocity occurring at about mid systole. Measurement of gradient bears a close relation to the catheter measured figure. Although there is evidence that the formula is applicable in subpulmonary stenosis [48] there may be some difficulties in this and caution should be exercised in using this value clinically. A characteristic appearance is found with spectral Doppler where the subpulmonary obstruction is dynamic and increases throughout systole, as when there is secondary muscular right ventricular outflow tract hypertrophy. There is a concave

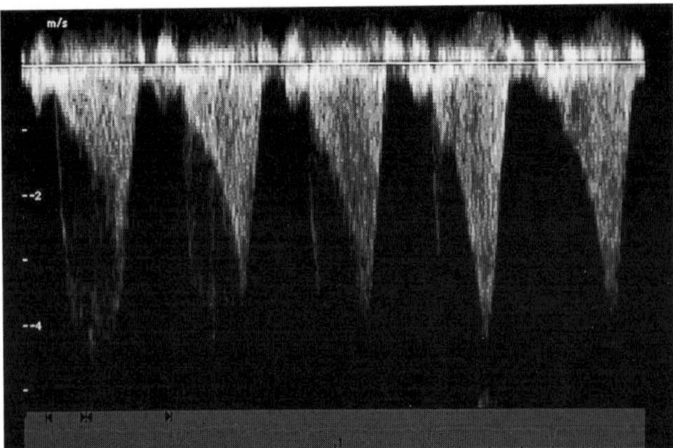

Fig. 8.19 Spectral signal from a patient with tetralogy of Fallot and obstruction at both valve and subvalve levels. The initial signals show both the rounded fixed signal and scimitar-shaped dynamic one, while alteration of the transducer position shows only the dynamic one in the last signal.

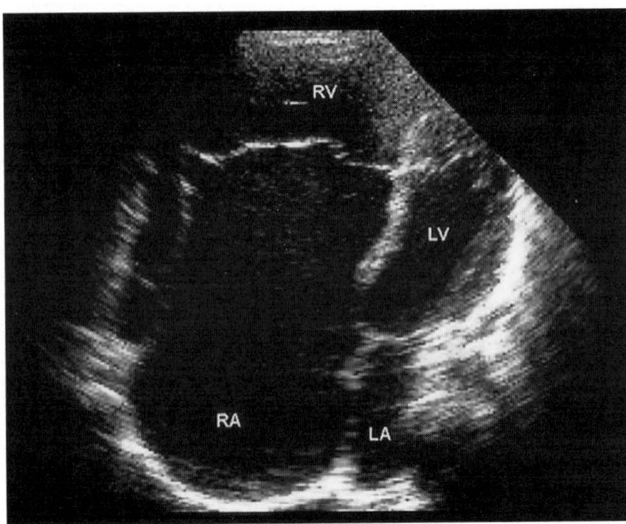

Fig. 8.20 Four-chamber view of a patient with Ebstein's anomaly showing marked apical displacement of the tricuspid valve. LA, left atrium; LV, left ventricle; RA right atrium; RV, right ventricle.

scimitar-shaped upstroke to the signal and after the peak a normal fall off. When this is associated with a distal fixed obstruction it is possible to show the superimposition of the fixed and dynamic patterns (Fig. 8.19).

Ebstein's anomaly

In Ebstein's anomaly there is apical displacement of the septal tricuspid leaflet which is frequently regurgitant. The less severe variants of this anomaly may not present until adult life. Symptoms are related to the severity of tricuspid regurgitation and on occasions the patient may become cyanosed from a right-to-left atrial shunt.

The diagnosis is readily reached with echocardiography using a four-chamber view [49] which shows the septal tricuspid leaflet is displaced apically, relatively far from the mitral valve (Fig. 8.20). Echoes from the tricuspid ring can be demonstrated in its normal position, and should not be mistaken for the tricuspid valve itself.

Corrected transposition of the great arteries

This lesion is characterized by discordant atrioventricular and ventriculoarterial connections. The morphological right atrium connects through the mitral valve to a right-sided morphological left ventricle which is connected to the pulmonary artery while the morphological left atrium connects through the tricuspid valve to a left-sided right ventricle and thence to the aorta. The ventricles lie relatively side by side and the great arteries are parallel at their origin with the aorta anterior and to the left of the pulmonary artery (and thus the term l-transposition).

A standard long axis view cannot be obtained. The anterior leaflet of the left inlet valve (the tricuspid) is separated by an infundibulum from the aorta which is positioned anteriorly and leftward. The septum may not be shown well because it lies in a more anteroposterior plane than in the normal heart. A four-chamber view shows the left-sided atrioventricular valve more apical than the right, identifying the left-sided tricuspid valve and right ventricle and right-sided mitral valve and left ventricle. Since the great arteries lie side by side and do not cross, a short axis view shows them as two circles, the aorta usually being anterior and to the left.

A ventricular septal defect and pulmonary or subpulmonary stenosis are commonly associated lesions and should be considered in making a full assessment. The systemic atrioventricular (tricuspid) valve may become regurgitant so long-term follow-up is necessary.

Cyanotic and complex defects

Transposition of the great arteries

In transposition of the great arteries the atria and ventricles are normally connected (atrioventricular concordance) and related but the pulmonary artery arises from the left ventricle and the aorta from the right (ventriculoarterial discordance).

The discordant ventriculoarterial connection can be identified using a long axis, short axis or four-chamber view. In the standard long axis view the great artery arising from the left ventricle is identified as the pulmonary artery by its posterior turn just above the valve, whereas the other vessel has a longer upward course, identifying it as the aorta (Fig. 8.21a) [50]. The aorta can also be identified in a high long axis or suprasternal view by the head and neck vessels arising from its superior surface and the pulmonary artery by its bifurcation seen in a short axis view or by a superior tilt from a five-chamber view [51]. A characteristic feature of complete transposition (and other related conditions) is that the great arteries do not cross and lie parallel at their origin where the short axis view shows them as two circular [52] rather than crossing structures (Fig. 8.21b). Most commonly the aorta is anterior and to the right of the pulmonary artery (hence the term d-transposition) but it can be anterior and in rare cases in other positions.

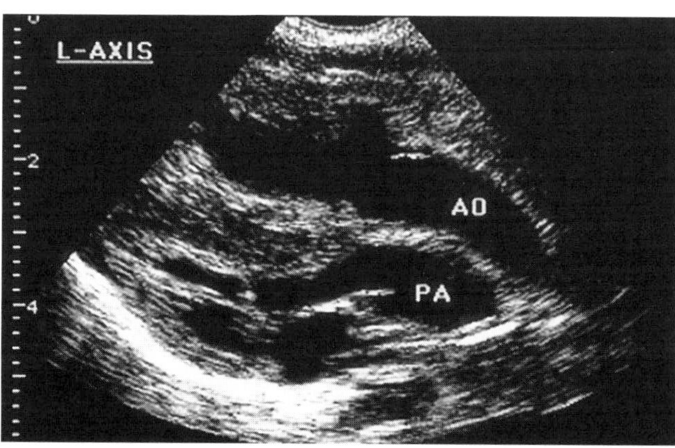

(a)

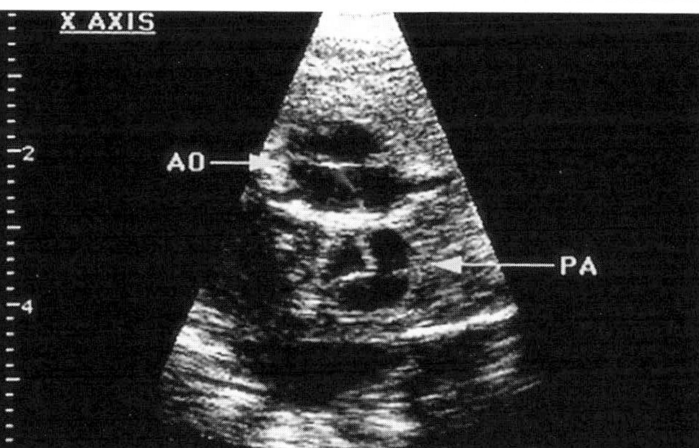

(b)

Fig. 8.21 Views of a patient with transposition of the great arteries. (a) A long axis view with the pulmonary artery (PA) arising from the left ventricle and turning posteriorly, while the aorta (AO) arises anteriorly from the right ventricle and continues further superiorly. (b) A short axis view at outlet valve level showing the arteries as two circles with the aorta (AO) anterior and slightly to the right of the pulmonary artery (PA). Note the coronary artery origins are seen from the aorta.

Cross-sectional echocardiography provides an ideal means of monitoring catheter position when performing a balloon atrial septostomy and the use of echocardiography and the umbilical vein simplifies this procedure in the neonatal unit in the first 48 h of life [53]. Ultrasound provides a relatively accurate means of follow-up of patients who have had surgical treatment for transposition of the great arteries, whether this be inflow or outflow redirection but details are outwith the remit of this chapter.

Tetralogy of Fallot

Tetralogy of Fallot is characterized by anterosuperior displacement of the infundibular septum [54]. The result is recognized by echocardiography as a ventricular septal defect with over-riding of the aorta, and narrowing of the right ventricular outflow which may affect the subpulmonary area, the valve or main and branch pulmonary arteries.

In the long axis or five-chamber view the ventricular septal defect and aortic over-ride is easily recognized. It is necessary to show the pulmonary outflow, and then to determine the site, nature and severity of the obstruction. A subcostal view tilted up and rotated anticlockwise (subcostal right coronal view) provides the best demonstration of the subvalve outflow tract where the narrowing is usually seen (Fig. 8.22). The anatomy and size of the main pulmonary artery and its branches is shown in a high parasternal short axis or suprasternal short axis view.

Spectral Doppler can be used to measure an outflow gradient and may show a fixed and a dynamic signal.

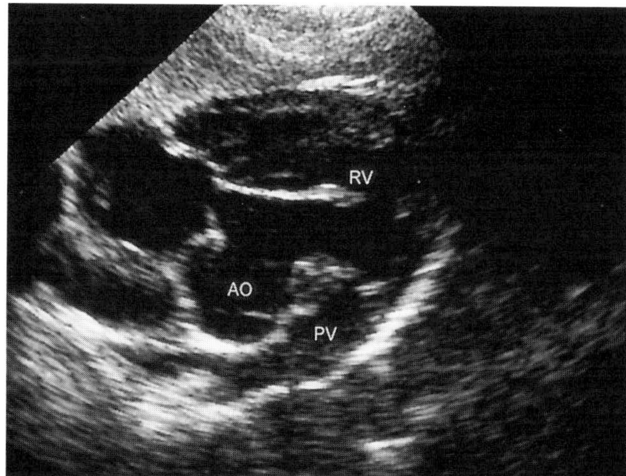

Fig. 8.22 Subxiphoid view tilted up to show the aortic root (AO) with the right ventricular (RV) outflow, pulmonary valve (PV) and main pulmonary artery passing round it from the left. The muscular obstruction below the pulmonary valve can be appreciated.

However, the gradient itself is of virtually no significance in management since the right ventricular pressure will not rise above the left and a rise in the gradient will reflect an increase in systemic pressure.

Pulmonary atresia

The anatomical abnormality in pulmonary atresia with a ventricular septal defect is similar to that in tetralogy of Fallot but there is atresia of the right ventricular outflow tract and the pulmonary arteries are small or absent. Much of the lung flow is from vessels (major aortopulmonary collateral arteries or MAPCAs) which arise from the descending aorta and supply individual lobes of the lungs.

Echocardiographic appearances are similar to those in tetralogy of Fallot but the outflow tract, main pulmonary artery or its branches will be atretic or absent [55]. The demonstration of the pulmonary branch size and confluence is essential in deciding on management and this may be best shown from a suprasternal view. MAPCAs should be sought using suprasternal long axis views or short axis views of the thoracic aorta, this being simplified by the use of colour Doppler to highlight their flow.

In pulmonary atresia with intact ventricular septum there may be a patent right ventricular outflow tract and main pulmonary artery with an imperforate valve or atresia of the right ventricular out flow tract or main pulmonary vein. The size of the right ventricle varies from tiny to normal [56] and is related to the function of the tricuspid valve: if there is significant regurgitation the cavity is usually of reasonable size, while if it is competent the right ventricle cavity will be small. The main and branch pulmonary arteries are almost always well developed and supplied by the ductus arteriosus without collaterals from the descending aorta.

An apical or subcostal four-chamber view [57,58] will show the size of the tricuspid ring and right ventricle cavity. The pulmonary valve may exhibit systolic doming, as in severe stenosis, and atresia can only be inferred if colour Doppler shows no flow.

Univentricular atrioventricular connection

The terminology for the defect in which there is physiologically a single ventricle has been much discussed and a variety of terms has been suggested. The most generally accepted is that of Anderson *et al.* [59] who suggest that the term univentricular atrioventricular connection be used for those variously called single or primitive ventricles, or even tricuspid atresia. The term covers the situation when both atria connect either directly or potentially to one ventricle. There can thus be a double inlet ventricle (both atria to the ventricle) (Fig. 8.23) or absent right or left connection (no atrioventricular outlet from an atrium to a ventricle) with the connection being to either a morphological left or right ventricle. The situation of absent connection most often occurs when there is no valve structure in the tricuspid position, the condition commonly termed

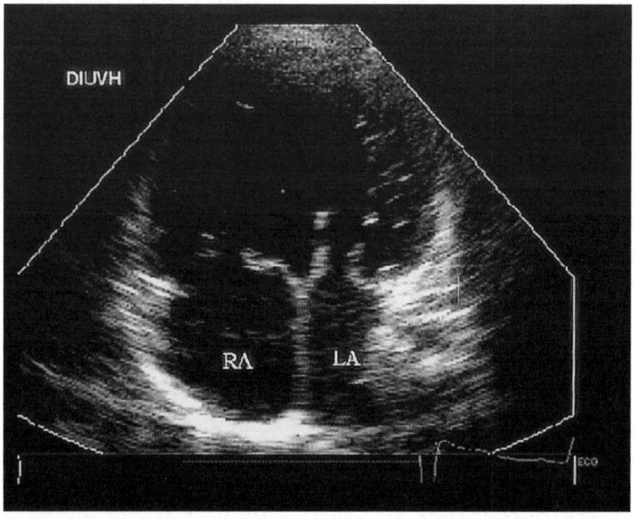

Fig. 8.23 Four-chamber view in a patient with double inlet univentricular heart. The atrioventricular valves enter the common ventricle and no ventricular septum apparent. LA, left atrium; RA, right atrium.

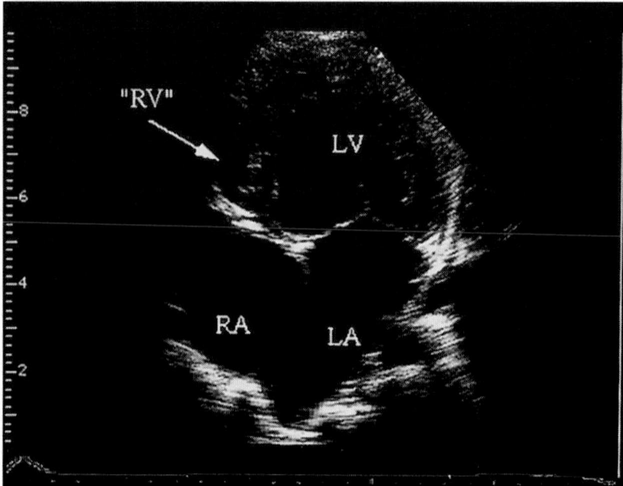

Fig. 8.24 Four-chamber view of a patient with a tricuspid atresia (or absent right connection). The left-sided valve is clearly seen, but the right is represented by immobile thick tissue. A rudimentary right ventricle (RV) is seen. LA, left atrium; LV, left ventricle; RA, right atrium.

tricuspid atresia (Fig. 8.24). On occasions there may be a single valve giving entry from both atria to the ventricle, similar to that of an atrioventricular septal defect.

Detailed diagnosis of such defects requires assessment of the situs and connections. The situs can be determined from echocardiography [8] (p. 97) or penetrated chest X-ray [60]. A four-chamber view is then used to show the atrioventricular valves and their connections to the ventricles [61,62] (see Figs 8.23, 8.24). There is usually another rudimentary ventricular chamber connected to the ventricle through a ventricular septal defect and which may give rise to a great artery (then called an outlet chamber) or have no outlet (termed a trabecular pouch). In the common situation where the ventricle is of left ventricular morphology the pouch is usually located in an anterosuperior position. Such chambers cannot always be shown with echocardiography [63].

Hypoplastic left heart syndrome

This term encompasses a spectrum of conditions with differing degrees of hypoplasia or the left atrium, ventricle and aorta with atresia or stenosis of the mitral and aortic valves. Infants with this present with circulatory collapse in the first few days of life when the ductus arteriosus closes, and without treatment usually die within a few days.

The diagnosis is readily made with echocardiography using standard long and short axis and four-chamber views to show the small left-sided chambers and hypoplastic aortic root and arch. The aortic valve is usually atretic and then colour Doppler will show retrograde flow in the aortic arch and ascending aorta from the ductus arteriosus. Ductal flow is from pulmonary artery to aorta in systole but there is usually some flow from aorta to pulmonary artery in diastole, reflecting a lower pulmonary than systemic resistance.

Truncus arteriosus

In truncus arteriosus a single great artery over-rides a large outlet ventricular septal defect. This vessel follows the course of an aorta but the pulmonary branch arteries take origin from it either separately or as branches from a single main pulmonary artery.

With echocardiography it is not sufficient to show a single artery but the pulmonary artery branches must be shown to arise from it. Long or short axis views of the ascending trunk will show the pulmonary artery branches [64]. The best view will depend on the site of origin of the branches and a subcostal view may be more helpful [65].

Origin of one pulmonary artery from the aorta is an uncommon condition usually presenting with cardiac failure in an acyanotic infant. The right ventricle and main pulmonary artery give origin to one of the main branches while the other arises from the aorta. This has been termed a hemitruncus. If the echocardiographer is not careful the pulmonary artery may be thought to be normal. However, only one branch from the main pulmonary artery can be imaged and the other will be shown to come from the aorta, using views similar to that in a truncus arteriosus.

Double outlet right ventricle

This term includes any condition in which both great arteries arise completely or predominantly from the right ventricle. The relative positions of the great arteries will determine how best to demonstrate this with echocardiography and may be using long axis, apical or subcostal five-chamber views or a short axis sweep. When the vessels are relatively anteroposterior a long axis view will clearly show the relationship of both to the septum. The great arteries are commonly parallel [66] with the aorta to the right of the pulmonary artery, either anterior or side by side.

Vascular ring

This is an uncommon abnormality but is worthy of mention since it is one which is often missed clinically although a careful history or examination indicates the presence of inspiratory difficulty or stridor. As the result of a developmental abnormality the trachea and oesophagus are trapped between the main arch and an embryonic remnant of the other arch, usually in the form of a fibrous cord but there may also be a double patent arch. A double arch may be shown with echocardiography [67] but when this is atretic echocardiography is unhelpful and a vascular ring cannot be excluded. A barium swallow and not echocardiography is the appropriate investigation. Tracheal compression from a pulmonary artery sling is recognized with ultrasound, which shows that the left pulmonary artery arises distally from the right pulmonary artery [68] and, in passing to the left chest, compresses the trachea.

Anomalous pulmonary venous drainage

In total anomalous pulmonary venous drainage all the pulmonary veins drain to a site other than the left atrium. In most cases they join together behind the left atrium in a chamber from which a vessel drains to the systemic venous circulation, either an ascending left vertical vein to the innominate vein, a descending vein to the portal system, or to the coronary sinus. Flow to the left heart is from the right atrium through the foramen ovale. In some there may be obstruction at the junction with the systemic circulation causing increase in the pressure in the common chamber and pulmonary veins and severe pulmonary hypertension and heart failure.

The left atrium and ventricle are small. The chamber of the venous confluence can often be recognized as an echo-free space immediately posterior to the left atrium (Fig. 8.25) [69,70] with no flow from it into the atrium. The draining vein must then be identified, often by turning the transducer to a more sagittal plane and identifying its passage upwards to the innominate vein or downwards and through the diaphragm. Colour Doppler can help to identify the vein. When the drainage is to the coronary sinus care should be exercised in a four-chamber view when the rim of the dilated mouth of the coronary sinus can show an appearance similar to that of an ostium primum atrial septal defect. Rarely the veins can return to the systemic venous circulation at different sites.

Cor triatriatum has different clinical findings from total anomalous pulmonary venous drainage but there are echocardiographic similarities. In the former the pulmonary veins join behind the heart in a venous confluence which enters the left atrium directly but this communication is of restricted size and pulmonary venous obstruction occurs. The echocardiogram will show the dilated confluence but its junction with the atrium will be apparent on imaging or flow through it will be apparent with colour Doppler.

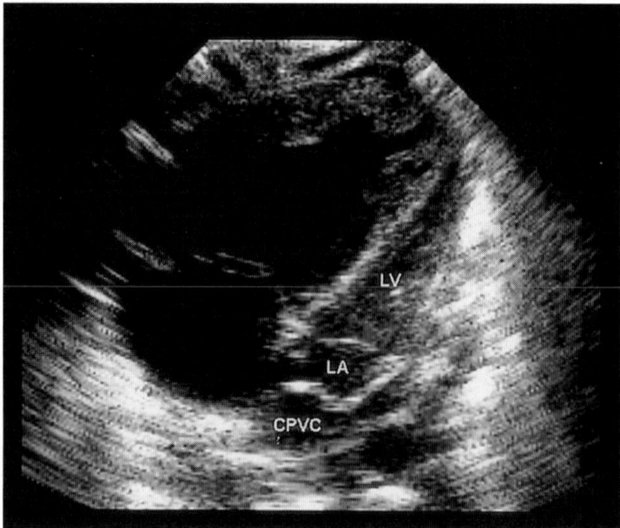

Fig. 8.25 Subxiphoid four-chamber view in a patient with total anomalous pulmonary venous drainage. The left atrium (LA) and left ventricle (LV) are very small compared to the right and an echo-free space, the common pulmonary venous chamber (CPVC) is seen posterior to the left atrium.

In partial anomalous venous drainage one or more of the pulmonary veins enters the systemic circulation while the others drain to the left atrium. The M-mode appearance of right ventricular volume overload is similar to an atrial septal defect. If an atrial septal defect cannot be shown the left atrium should be studied with colour Doppler for pulmonary veins and the systemic return examined for a vein entering the innominate vein, SVC or directly into the right atrium.

Coronary artery anomalies

KAWASAKI'S DISEASE

This is an acquired multisystem condition. The only serious consequence is the development of coronary artery aneurysms or stenoses with possible thrombosis and myocardial infarction. Most aneurysms occur proximally and can be imaged with echocardiography [71]. Since isolated distal aneurysms are rare [72] a study showing a normal origin and proximal portions of both the right and left coronaries virtually excludes coronary involvement.

ANOMALOUS ORIGIN OF A CORONARY ARTERY FROM THE PULMONARY ARTERY

This is an uncommon condition, usually affecting the left coronary artery. Patients commonly present at 3–4 weeks with cardiac failure, evidence of myocardial infarction and mitral regurgitation. Occasionally symptoms are not recognized and they present later in life with mitral regurgitation with or without left ventricular dysfunction. Initial echocardiographic examination may suggest the diagnosis from the presence of a dilated and poorly contracting left ventricle with mitral regurgitation and bright echoes from the papillary muscles. The origin of the right coronary will be seen to be dilated [73]. The anomalous left coronary follows an almost normal course and joins the pulmonary artery near the site where it would normally arise from the aorta. Colour Doppler should be used to demonstrate the flow is retrograde and the signal of flow into the pulmonary artery [74] (Fig. 8.26).

CORONARY ARTERY FISTULA

A coronary artery fistula may be suspected clinically from a continuous murmur in a relatively low position. On echocardiography the coronary artery affected is dilated

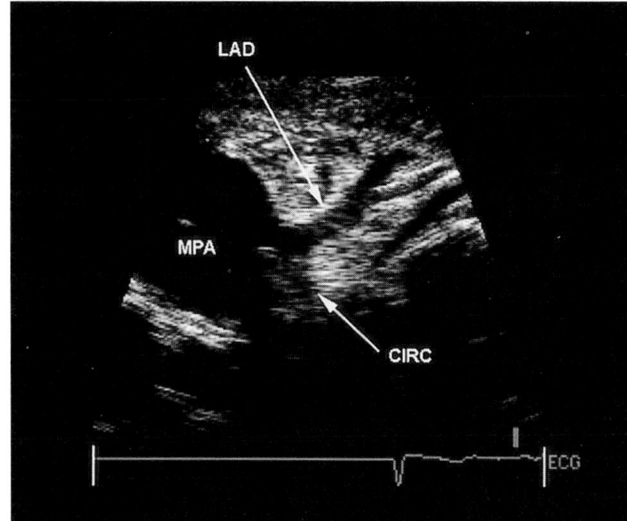

(a)

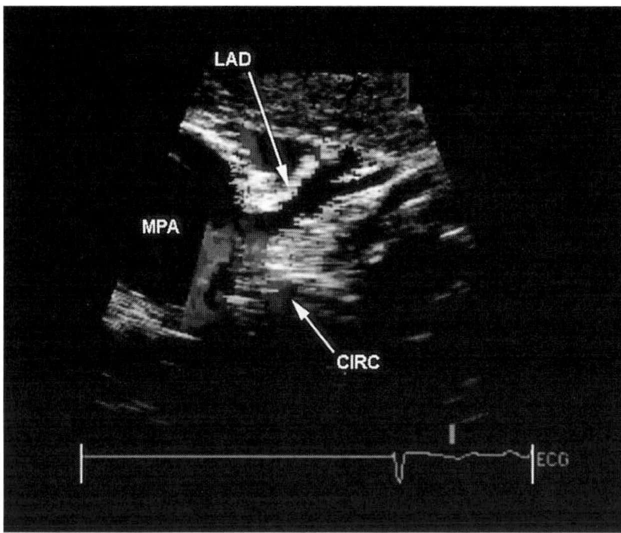

(b)

Fig. 8.26 Views from an infant with anomalous origin of the left coronary artery from the pulmonary artery. (a) The left anterior descending (LAD) and circumflex (CIRC) branches are seen, and (b) in the colour image retrograde flow is shown in the coronaries towards the main pulmonary artery (MPA). For colour, see Plate 8.26 (between pp. 308 and 309).

[75] and colour Doppler will show flow into the communicating chamber [76].

Pulmonary artery pressure assessment

An important contribution of ultrasound to the management of congenital heart disease has been the ability of spectral Doppler to provide an assessment of pulmonary artery pressure. As in adult practice this is possible using the velocity of tricuspid regurgitation to estimate the right ventricular pressure [77]. In infants with a normal heart and marked pulmonary hypertension, as in bronchopulmonary dysplasia, it is often difficult to obtain a signal adequate for making this measurement. In those with marked pulmonary hypertension in whom a tricuspid signal cannot be recorded some idea of the pressure can be obtained from pulmonary regurgitation. This does not readily translate to a systolic or diastolic pulmonary pressure but a high velocity will indicate high pulmonary pressure. The ventricular septal defect signal allows a relatively good assessment to be made (p. 101) but although that of the ductus is helpful (p. 105) it does not readily translate to a specific level.

References

1 Dickinson, D.F., Arnold, R., Wilkinson, J.L. (1981) Congenital heart disease among 160 480 liveborn children in Liverpool 1960–1969. Implications for surgical treatment. *British Heart Journal* **46**, 55–62.

2 Shinebourne, E.A., Macartney, F.J., Anderson, R.H. (1976) Sequential chamber localization—logical approach to diagnosis in congenital heart disease. *British Heart Journal* **38**, 327–340.

3 Tynan, M.J., Becker, A.E., Macartney, F.J. *et al.* (1979) Nomenclature and classification of congenital heart disease. *British Heart Journal* **41**, 544–553.

4 Anderson, R.H. (1991) Simplifying the understanding of congenital malformations of the heart. *International Journal of Cardiology* **32**, 131–142.

5 Snider, A.R., Serwer, G.A. (1997) *Echocardiography in Pediatric Heart Disease*, 2nd edn. Mosby-Year Book, St Louis.

6 Wilde, P. (ed.) (1993) *Clinical Ultrasound a Comprehensive Text. Cardiac Ultrasound.* Churchill Livingstone, Edinburgh.

7 Roelandt, J.R.T.C., Sutherland, G.R., Iliceto, S., Linker, D.T. (1993) (eds) *Cardiac Ultrasound.* Churchill Livingstone, Edinburgh.

8 Huta, J.C., Smallhorn, J.F., Macartney, F.J. (1982) Two dimensional echocardiographic diagnosis of situs. *British Heart Journal* **48**, 97–108.

9 Soto, B., Becker, A., Moulaert, A.J., Lie, J.T., Anderson, R.H. (1980) Classification of ventricular septal defects. *British Heart Journal* **43**, 332–343.

10 Sutherland, G.R., Godman, M.J., Smallhorn, J.F., Guiterras, P., Anderson, R.H., Hunter, S. (1982) Ventricular septal defects. Two dimensional echocardiographic and morphological considerations. *British Heart Journal* **47**, 316–328.

11 Hagler, D.J., Edwards, W.D., Seward, J.B., Tajik, A.J. (1985) Standardised nomenclature of the ventricular septum and ventricular septal defects, with applications for two-dimensional echocardiography. *Mayo Clinical Proceedings* **60**, 741–752.

12 Sanders, S.P., Yeager, S., Williams, R.G. (1983) Measurements of systemic and pulmonary blod flow and QP/QS ratio using Doppler and two-dimensional echocardiography. *American Journal of Cardiology* **51**, 952–956.

13 Murphy, D.J., Ludomirsky, A., Huhta, J.C. (1986) Continuous wave Doppler in children with ventricular septal defect: noninvasive estimation of interventricular pressure gradient. *American Journal of Cardiology* **56**, 428–432.

14 Houston, A.B., Lim, M.K., Doig, W.B., *et al.* (1988) Doppler assessment of the interventricular pressure drop in VSD. *British Heart Journal* **60**, 50–56.
15 Chen, C., Kremer, P., Schroeder, E., *et al.* (1987) Usefulness of anatomic parameters derived from two-dimensional echocardiography for estimating magnitude of left to right shunt in patients with atrial septal defect. *Clinical Cardiology* **10**, 316–321.
16 Shub, C., Dimopoulos, I.N., Seward, J.B., *et al.* (1983) Sensitivity of two-dimensional echocardiography in the direct visualization of atrial septal defect utilizing the subcostal approach. *Journal of the American College of Cardiology* **2**, 127–135.
17 Sherman, F.S., Sahn, D.J., Valdez-Cruz, L.M., *et al.* (1987) Two-dimensional Doppler colour flow mapping for detecting atrial and ventricular septal defects. *Herz* **12**, 212–215.
18 Gnanapragasam, J.P., Houston, A.B., Northridge, D.B., Jamieson, M.P.G., Pollock, J.C.S. (1991) Transoesophageal echocardiographic assessment of primum, secundum, and sinus venosus atrial septal defects. *International Journal of Cardiology* **31**, 167–174.
19 Rastelli, J.C., Kirkland, J.W., Titus, J.L. (1966) Anatomic observations on complete form of persistent common atrioventricular canal with special reference to atrioventricular valves. *Mayo Clinic Proceedings* **41**, 296–308.
20 Hagler, D.J., Tajik, A.J., Seward, J.B., *et al.* (1979) Real-time wide angle sector echocardiography: atrioventricular canal defects. *Circulation* **59**, 140–150.
21 Smallhorn, J.F., Tommasini, G., Anderson, R.H., Macartney, F.J. (1982) Assessment of atrioventricular defects by two-dimensional echocardiography. *British Heart Journal* **47**, 109–121.
22 Mortera, C., Rissech, M., Payola, M., *et al.* (1987) Cross sectional subcostal echocardiography: atrioventricular septal defects and the short axis cut. *British Heart Journal* **58**, 267–273.
23 Lim, M.K., Hanretty, K., Houston, A.B., *et al.* (1992) Intermittent ductal patency in healthy newborn infants: demonstration by colour Doppler flow mapping. *Archives of Disease in Childhood* **67**, 1217–1218.
24 Smallhorn, J.F., Huhta, J.C., Anderson, R.H., Macartney, F.J. (1982) Suprasternal echocardiography in assessment of patent ductus arteriosus. *British Heart Journal* **48**, 321–330.
25 Swensson, R.E., Valdes Cruz, L.M., Sahn, D.J., *et al.* (1986) Doppler colour flow mapping for detection of patent arterial ductus. *Journal of the American College of Cardiology* **8**, 1105–1112.
26 Houston, A.B., Gnanapragasam, J.P., Doig, W.B., *et al.* (1991) Doppler ultrasound and the silent ductus arteriosus. *British Heart Journal* **65**, 148–151.
27 Silverman, N.H., Lewis, A.B., Heymann, M.A., Rudolph, A.M. (1974) Echocardiographic assessment of ductus arteriosus shunt in premature infants. *Circulation* **50**, 821–825.
28 Sahn, D.J., Vaucher, Y., Williams, D.E., *et al.* (1976) Echocardiographic detection of large left-to-right shunts and cardiomyopathies in infants and children. *American Journal of Cardiology* **38**, 73–79.
29 Evans, N., Iyer, P. (1994) Assessment of ductus arteriosus shunt in preterm infants supported by mechanical ventilation: the effect of interatrial shunting. *Journal of Pediatrics* **125**, 778–785.
30 Houston, A.B., Lim, M.K., Doig, W.B., *et al.* (1989) Doppler flow characteristics in the assessment of pulmonary artery pressure in ductus arteriosus. *British Heart Journal* **62**, 284–290.
31 Fowles, R.E., Martin, R.P., Abrams, J.M., *et al.* (1979) Two-dimensional echocardiographic features of bicuspid aortic valve. *Chest* **75**, 434–440.
32 Zema, M.J., Caccuvano, M. (1982) Two-dimensional echocardiographic assessment of aortic valve morphology: feasibility of bicuspid valve detection. *British Heart Journal* **48**, 428–433.
33 Weyman, A.E., Feigenbaum, H., Hurwitz, R.A., *et al.* (1977) Cross-sectional echocardiographic assessment of the severity of aortic stenosis in children. *Circulation* **55**, 773–778.
34 Di Sessa, T.G., Hagan, A.D., Isobel-Jones, J.B., *et al.* (1981) Two-dimensional echocardiographic evaluation of discrete subaortic stenosis from the apical long axis view. *American Heart Journal* **101**, 774–782.
35 Mugge, A., Daniel, W.G., Wolpers, H.G., *et al.* (1989) Improved visualisation of discrete subvalvar aortic stenosis by transesophageal color coded Doppler echocardiography. *American Heart Journal* **117**, 474–475.
36 Gnanapragasam, J.P., Houston, A.B., Doig, W.B., Jamieson, M.P.G., Pollock, J.C.S. (1991) Transoesophageal echocardiographic assessment of fixed subaortic stenosis in children. *British Heart Journal* **66**, 281–284.
37 Davis, R.H., Feigenbaum, H., Chang, S., *et al.* (1974) Echocardiographic manifestations of discrete subaortic stenosis. *American Journal of Cardiology* **33**, 277–280.
38 Lima, C.O., Sahn, D.J., Valdes Cruz, L.M., *et al.* (1983) Prediction of the severity of left ventricular outflow tract obstruction by quantitative two dimensional echocardiographic studies. *Circulation* **68**, 348–354.
39 Skjaerpe, T.J., Hegrenaes, L., Hatle, L. (1985) Noninvasive estimation of aortic valve area in patients with aortic stenosis by Doppler ultrasound in two-dimensional echocardiography. *Circulation* **72**, 1106–1118.
40 Teien, D., Karp, K., Eriksson, P. (1986) Non-invasive estimate of the mean pressure difference in aortic stenosis by Doppler ultrasound. *British Heart Journal* **56**, 450–454.
41 Duncan, W.J., Ninimiya, K., Cook, D.H., *et al.* (1983) Noninvasive diagnosis of neonatal coarctation and associated anomalies using two-dimensional echocardiography. *American Heart Journal* **106**, 63–69.
42 Smallhorn, J.F., Huhta, J.C., Adams, P.A., *et al.* (1983) Cross-sectional echocardiographic assessment of coarctation in the sick neonate and infant. *British Heart Journal* **50**, 349–361.
43 Modena, M.G., Benassi, A., Mattiolo, G., *et al.* (1985) Computerised tomography and ultrasound in the noninvasive evaluation of coarctation of the aorta. *International Journal of Cardiology* **56**, 822–824.
44 Houston, A.B., Simpson, I.A., Pollock, J.C.S., *et al.* (1987) Doppler ultrasound in the assessment of severity of coarctation of the aorta and interruption of the aortic arch. *British Heart Journal* **57**, 38–43.
45 Rao, P.S., Carey, P. (1989) Doppler ultrasound in the prediction of pressure gradients across aortic coarctation. *American Heart Journal* **118**, 299–307.
46 Chan, K.C., Dickinson, D.F., Wharton, G.A., Gibbs, J.L. (1992) Continuous wave Doppler echocardiography after surgical repair of coarctation of the aorta. *British Heart Journal* **68**, 192–194.
47 Lima, C.O., Sahn, D.J., Valdes Cruz, L.M. (1983) Non-invasive prediction of transvalvular pressure gradient in patients

with pulmonary stenosis by quantitative two dimensional echocardiographic studies. *Circulation* **67**, 866–871.

48 Houston, A.B., Simpson, I.A., Sheldon, C.D., *et al.* (1986) Doppler ultrasound in the estimation of the severity of pulmonary infundibular stenosis in infants and children. *British Heart Journal* **55**, 381–384.

49 Shiina, A., Seward, J.B., Edwards, W.D., *et al.* (1984) Two-dimensional echocardiographic spectrum of Ebstein's anomaly: detailed anatomic assessment. *Journal of the American College of Cardiology* **3**, 356–370.

50 Houston, A.B., Gregory, N.L., Coleman, E.N. (1978) Echocardiographic characteristics of the aorta and main pulmonary artery in complete transposition. *British Heart Journal* **40**, 377–382.

51 Bierman, F.Z., Williams, R.G. (1979) Prospective diagnosis of d-transposition of the great arteries in neonates by subxiphoid two-dimensional echocardiography. *Circulation* **60**, 1496–1502.

52 Sahn, D.J., Terry, R., O'Rourke, R., *et al.* (1974) Multiple crystal echocardiography in the diagnosis of cyanotic heart disease. *Circulation* **50**, 230–238.

53 Ashfaq, M., Houston, A.B., Gnanapragasam, J.P., *et al.* (1991) Balloon atrial septostomy under echocardiographic control: six years' experience and evaluation of the practicability of the umbilical vein route. *British Heart Journal* **65**, 148–151.

54 Becker, A.E., Connor, M., Anderson, R.H. (1975) Tetralogy of Fallot: a morphometric and geometric study. *American Journal of Cardiology* **35**, 402–412.

55 Vargas Barron, J., Sahn, D.J., Attie, F. *et al.* (1983) Two-dimensional echocardiographic study of right ventricular outflow and great artery anatomy in pulmonary atresia with ventricular septal defects and in truncus arteriosus. *American Heart Journal* **105**, 281–286.

56 Zuberbuhler, J.R., Anderson, R.H. (1979) Morphological variations in pulmonary atresia with intact ventricular septum. *British Heart Journal* **41**, 281–288.

57 Marino, B., Franceschini, E., Ballerini, L., *et al.* (1986) Anatomical-echocardiographic correlations in pulmonary atresia with intact ventricular septum. Use of subcostal cross-sectional views. *International Journal of Cardiology* **11**, 103–109.

58 Andrade, J.L., Serino, W., de Laval, M., *et al.* (1984) Two-dimensional echocardiographic evaluation of tricuspid hypoplasia in pulmonary atresia. *American Journal of Cardiology* **53**, 387–388.

59 Anderson, R.H., Macartney, F.J., Tynan, M.J., *et al.* (1983) Univentricular atrioventricular connection: the single ventricle trap unsprung. *Pediatric Cardiology* **4**, 273–280.

60 Deanfield, J., Leanage, R., Stroobauat, J., *et al.* (1980) Use of high kilovoltage filtered beam radiography for detection of bronchial situs in infants and young children. *British Heart Journal* **44**, 577–583.

61 Rigby, M.L., Anderson, R.H., Gibson, D., *et al.* (1981) Two-dimensional echocardiographic categorization of the univentrucular heart. Ventricular morphology, type, and mode of artioventricular connection. *British Heart Journal* **46**, 603–612.

62 Freedom, R.M., Picchio, F., Duncan, W.J., *et al.* (1982) The atrioventricular junction in the univentricular heart: a two-dimensional echocardiographic analysis. *Pediatric Cardiology* **3**, 105–117.

63 Huhta, J.C., Seward, J.B., Tajik, A.J., *et al.* (1985) Two-dimensional echocardiographic spectrum of univentricular atrioventricular connection. *Journal of the American College of Cardiology* **5**, 149–157.

64 Houston, A.B., Gregory, N.L., Murtagh, E., Coleman, E.N. (1981) Two-dimensional echocardiography in infants with a persistent truncus arteriosus. *British Heart Journal* **46**, 492–497.

65 Sanders, S.P., Bierman, F.Z., Williams, R.G. (1982) Conotruncal malformations: diagnosis in infancy using subxiphoid two-dimensional echocardiography. *American Journal of Cardiology* **50**, 1361–1367.

66 Wilkinson, J.L. (1987) Double outlet ventricle. In: Anderson, R.H., Macartney, F.J., Shinebourne, E.A., Tynan, M. (eds) *Paediatric Cardiology*. Churchill Livingstone, Edinburgh, pp. 889–991.

67 Enderlein, M.A., Silverman, N.H., Stanger, P., Heyman, M.A. (1986) Usefulness of suprasternal notch echocardiography for diagnosis of double aortic arch. *American Journal of Cardiology* **57**, 359–361.

68 Gnanapragasam, J.P., Houston, A.B., Jamieson, M.P.G. (1990) Pulmonary artery sling. Diagnosis by colour Doppler flow mapping. *British Heart Journal* **63**, 251–252.

69 Smallhorn, J.F., Sutherland, G.R., Tommasini, G., *et al.* (1981) Assessment of total anomalous pulmonary venous connection by two-dimensional echocardiography. *British Heart Journal* **46**, 613–623.

70 Huhta, J.C., Gutgesell, H.P., Nihill, M.R. (1985) Cross sectional echocardiographic diagnosis of total anomalous pulmonary venous drainage. *British Heart Journal* **53**, 525–534.

71 Satomi, G., Nakamura, K., Narai, S., *et al.* (1984) Systematic visualization of coronary arteries by two-dimensional echocardiography in children and infants: evaluation on Kawasaki's disease and coronary arteriovenous fistulas. *American Heart Journal* **107**, 497–505.

72 Kato, H., Ichinose, E., Yoshioka, F., *et al.* (1982) Fate of coronary aneurysms in Kawasaki disease: serial coronary angiography and long-term follow up study. *American Journal of Cardiology* **49**, 1758–1766.

73 Koike, K., Musewe, N.N., Smallhorn, J.F., Freedom, R.M. (1989) Distinguishing between anomalous origin of the left coronary artery from the pulmonary trunk and dilated cardiomyopathy: role of the echocardiographic measurement of the right artery diameter. *British Heart Journal* **61**, 192–197.

74 Houston, A.B., Pollock, J.C.S., Doig, W.B., *et al.* (1990) Anomalous origin of the left coronary artery from the pulmonary trunk: elucidation with colour Doppler flow mapping. *British Heart Journal* **63**, 50–54.

75 Rodgers, D.M., Wolf, N.M., Barrett, M.J., *et al.* (1982) Two-dimensional echocardiographic features of coronary arteriovenous fistula. *American Heart Journal* **104**, 872–874.

76 Ke, W.L., Wang, N.K., Lin, Y.M., *et al.* (1988) Right coronary artery fistula into right atrium: diagnosis by color Doppler echocardiography. *American Heart Journal* **116**, 886–889.

77 Currie, P.J., Seward J.B., Chan, K.J., *et al.* (1985) Continuous wave Doppler determination of right ventricular pressure: a simultaneous Doppler-catheterisation study in 127 patients. *Journal of the American College of Cardiology* **6**, 750–756.

Chapter 9: Valvular heart disease

J.C. Rodger

Valvular disease can be assessed comprehensively using the combination of imaging and Doppler echocardiography. Patients in whom the likelihood of coexisting coronary heart disease is low, and who thus do not require coronary angiography, can proceed to valve surgery on the evidence of the echocardiographic findings alone. Transoesophageal echocardiography has a limited but specific role in the assessment of valve lesions, and is dealt with elsewhere (Chapters 12 and 14). This account is confined to echocardiography from the transthoracic approach. In line with current clinical practice, it concentrates on cross-sectional and Doppler echocardiography and places less emphasis on the M-mode.

Mitral valve

Assessment of the mitral valve requires imaging in three views. Diastolic motion of the leaflets and the anatomy of the subvalvar apparatus are optimally displayed in the parasternal long axis view. Systolic coaptation of the leaflets is often best seen in the apical four-chamber view. The size and shape of the mitral orifice should be examined on parasternal short axis images.

Normal mitral valve

Echoes from the leaflets are thin (Fig. 9.1). In diastole the leaflets separate widely; the anterior leaflet is always clearly visible but on parasternal long axis images, it can be difficult to differentiate the posterior leaflet from the underlying left ventricular posterior wall. In systole, coaptation of the leaflets is extensive (it is not confined to their tips) and the closed valve domes towards the left atrium. Prolapse of the closed valve behind the plane of the mitral ring in the apical four-chamber view (see Fig. 9.9a) is normal but prolapse in the parasternal long axis view is not [1]. The apparent discrepancy has been explained by a study which showed that the normal mitral ring is saddle shaped with its anterior and posterior portions turning upwards and its sides downwards [2]. On the M-mode (Fig. 9.2), the echograms from the anterior and posterior leaflets are M and W shaped, respectively, in diastole and both are anteriorly directed throughout systole.

'Physiological' mitral regurgitation occurs in up to 60% of normal young adults [3]. It is recognized using colour flow imaging or pulsed Doppler as a regurgitant jet appearing briefly in systole and confined to the immediate vicinity of the point of leaflet coaptation.

Mitral stenosis

Congenital mitral stenosis is rare; the echocardiographic features are essentially as in acquired stenosis. Acquired stenosis is invariably the result of rheumatic involvement. The rheumatic process causes thickening, calcification, shortening and fusion of the mitral leaflets and of their chordae tendineae.

Echoes from the leaflets are thickened (Fig. 9.3). Particularly thick and bright echoes reflect calcification. In mild stenosis, long axis images may show that restriction of anterior leaflet mobility is confined to its tip. Posterior leaflet mobility is always grossly restricted. This feature, useful in the diagnosis of mild rheumatic involvement, is often best appreciated on the M-mode which shows the posterior leaflet moving forward with the anterior leaflet during diastole (Fig. 9.4). The extent of commisural fusion can be determined from short axis images of the mitral orifice (Fig. 9.5) and the extent of subvalvar disorganization can be determined from long axis views. Thrombus within the body of the left atrium but not within the atrial appendage can be identified from the transthoracic approach. A degree of left atrial enlargement is inevitable; atrial size is conventionally measured as its transverse dimension, behind the aortic root, in the parasternal long axis view (normally <4 cm).

Valve area and thus the severity of stenosis, can be estimated by planimetry of the mitral orifice in the parasternal short axis view. Provided that the orifice, which is funnel shaped, is measured where it is narrowest, the accuracy is good [4].

(a)

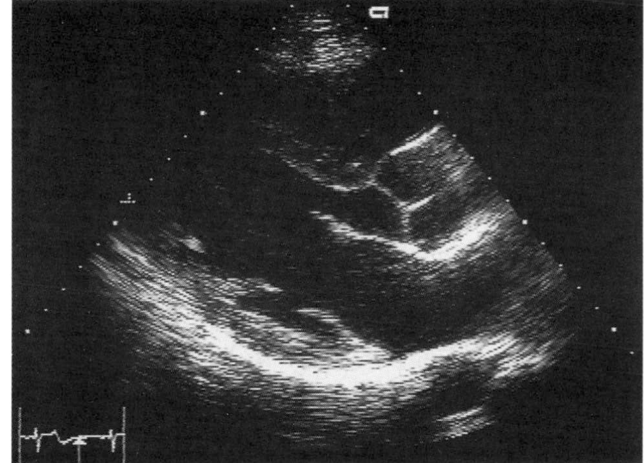

(b)

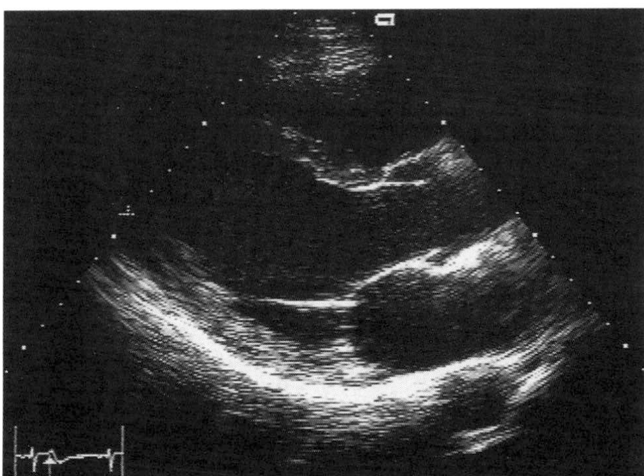

Fig. 9.1 Normal heart. Parasternal long axis images in (a) diastole and (b) systole.

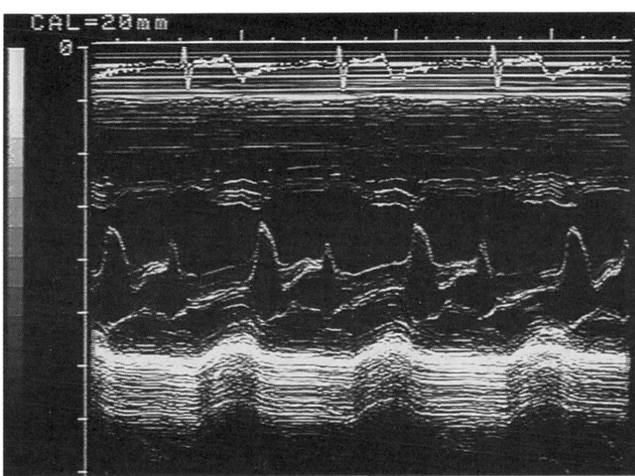

Fig. 9.2 M-mode record from normal mitral valve. The valve opens in early diastole, then partially closes and reopens with atrial systole. The two leaflets move in opposite directions during diastole; both are anteriorly directed throughout systole.

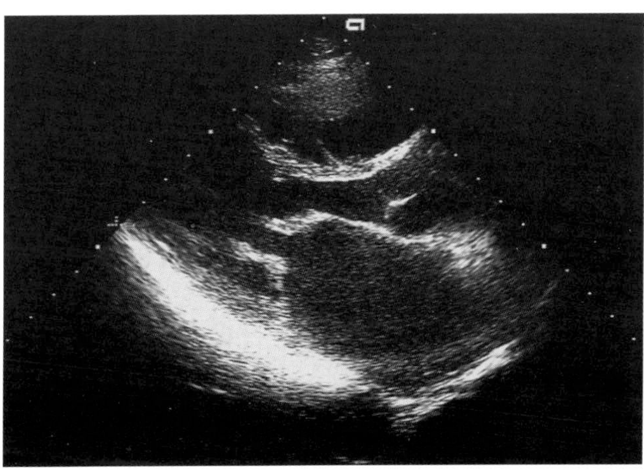

Fig. 9.3 Parasternal long axis diastolic image of rheumatic mitral valve. The leaflets are thick, their motion is restricted with the anterior leaflet doming towards the left ventricle. The chordae tendineae are thick, possibly calcified and short; there is subvalvar stenosis. The left atrium is enlarged.

DOPPLER ASSESSMENT

Continuous wave (CW) Doppler quantification of mitral stenosis (Fig. 9.6) is accurate; recordings are made from an apical probe position. The mitral pressure gradient can be measured at any point on the flow velocity profile [5] by substituting the measured velocity for v in the modified Bernoulli equation, $P = 4v^2$. However, instantaneous and mean gradients measured in this way are altered by a number of variables including heart rate and the volume of transmitral flow. The pressure half-time, which is the time taken for the mitral pressure gradient to fall to half of its initial level, is less dependent on these factors and is the preferred index of stenosis [6]. The normal mitral pressure half-time is less than 60 ms; values in mitral stenosis range from 100 to 400 ms. Except in the presence of severe aortic regurgitation or reduced left ventricular compliance [7] (e.g. as a result of associated aortic stenosis), the pressure half-time, and the estimate of valve area that can be derived from it, agree well with measurements made at cardiac catheterization [6].

With colour flow Doppler, the acceleration of blood flow as it approaches the stenotic orifice is seen (Fig. 9.7) as a series of hemispheric bands of alternating red and blue (due to aliasing). Flow through the stenotic orifice is displayed as a jet of high velocity laminar flow; jet direction is often eccentric [8]. Colour flow provides insight into the mechanics of blood flow but adds nothing to the quantification of mitral stenosis.

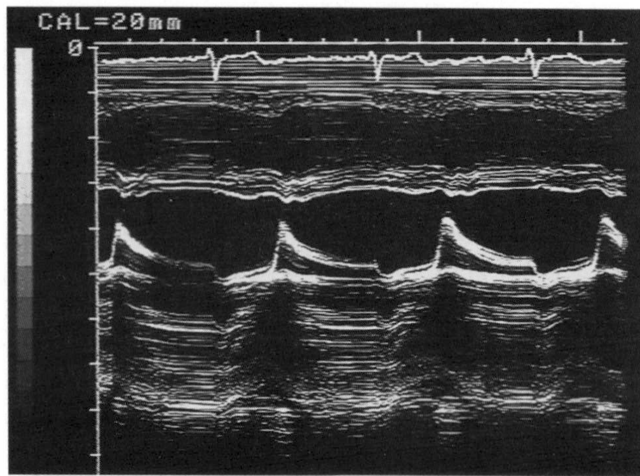

Fig. 9.4 M-mode record from mildly stenotic rheumatic mitral valve. Echoes from both leaflets are thick. The posterior leaflet is immobile. Rhythm is atrial fibrillation, late diastolic reopening of the valve is thus absent.

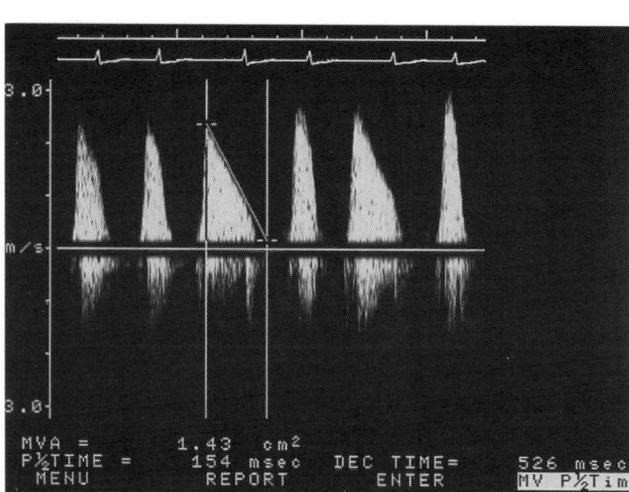

Fig. 9.6 Continuous wave Doppler record from mildly stenotic rheumatic mitral valve showing measurement of pressure half-time.

(a)

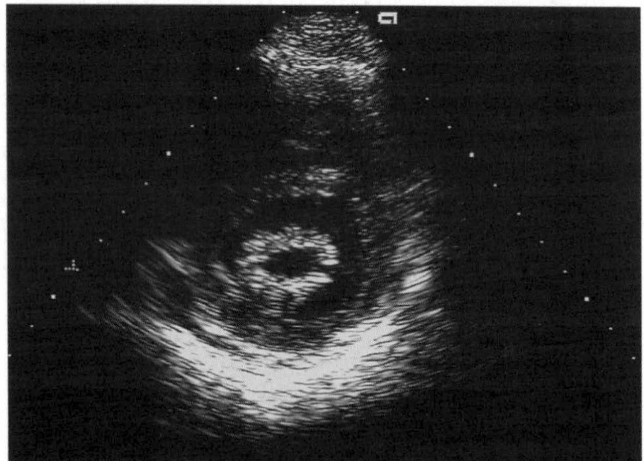

(b)

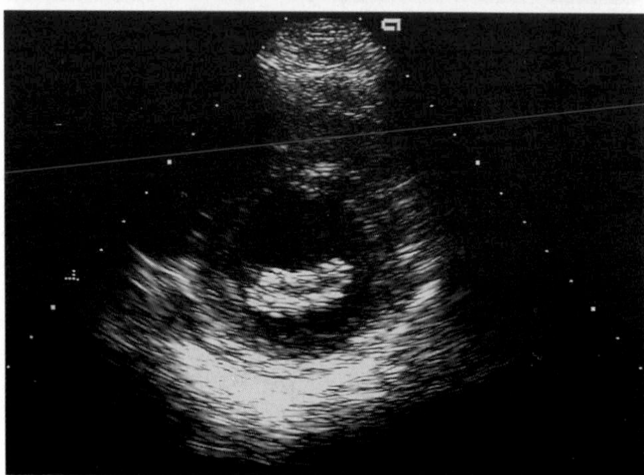

Fig. 9.5 Parasternal short axis images of rheumatic mitral valve in (a) diastole and (b) systole. Some anterior leaflet mobility is retained; there is commisural fusion medially. Orifice size is moderately reduced; mitral valve area by planimetry was 1.1 cm².

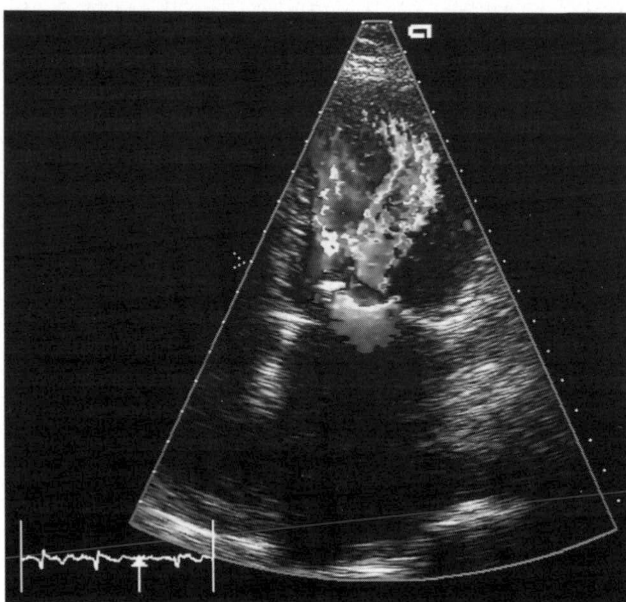

Fig. 9.7 Colour flow Doppler record from stenotic rheumatic mitral valve in diastole (see text). For colour, see Plate 9.7 (between pp. 308 and 309).

CLINICAL DECISION

Assessment of the patient with mitral stenosis does not only involve a look at the valve, a search for atrial thrombus and measurement of the pressure half-time. The examination should also include Doppler assessment of the pulmonary artery systolic pressure (see Fig. 9.25), a brief evaluation of left ventricular function (see Chapter

10), and a search for coexisting valve lesions. All of this can be done from the transthoracic approach.

The valve's suitability for balloon valvuloplasty can be reliably assessed using a 'splittability score' which takes account of mobility, thickening and calcification of the leaflets and disorganization of the subvalvar apparatus [9]. This too can be achieved from the transthoracic approach and it is only because of its ability to demonstrate thrombus within the atrial appendage (a relative contraindication to valvuloplasty) that the transoesophageal approach is often preferred.

Mitral regurgitation

The three basic causes of mitral regurgitation are an abnormality of the leaflets (floppy valve or associated with rheumatic mitral stenosis), calcification of the mitral ring and dilatation of the ring (producing functional regurgitation).

FLOPPY MITRAL VALVE

The floppy valve is the result of myxomatous degeneration of the leaflets and their chordae. Myxomatous degeneration may be confined to the mitral but may also involve the aortic valve and, less commonly, all four valves may be affected. The floppy mitral predisposes the patient to malign arrhythmias, it is prone to infection, small thrombi (not detectable echocardiographically) can form in its interstices and it can become acutely regurgitant due to chordal rupture. The diagnosis is thus an important one and, though there are characteristic auscultatory features, it can easily be missed clinically.

The floppy mitral valve (Figs 9.8, 9.9) is recognized by its billowing motion, the apparent thickening (due to folding) of its voluminous cusps and by the laxity of its subvalvar apparatus. Significant systolic prolapse (i.e. prolapse seen in both the apical four-chamber and parasternal long axis views) of one or both leaflets is characteristic. Anterior leaflet prolapse is typically gross, with the cusp arching backwards and upwards within the left atrium; displacement of the prolapsed posteror leaflet is usually less dramatic [10,11].

The M-mode features (Fig. 9.10) are increased diastolic excursion, additional echoes due to folding of the leaflets and holosystolic sagging or late systolic posterior motion of the leaflets [12]. M-mode echocardiography should not be neglected in the diagnosis and assessment of the floppy mitral. It will identify prolapse which is confined to late systole and the chaotic motion of a cusp which has become flail (Fig. 9.11) as the result of chordal rupture: neither of these is readily appreciated on cross-sectional imaging. Valves with apparently myxomatous leaflets but which move and function normally are sometimes seen. The diagnosis of floppy mitral should be reserved for valves with the combination of myxomatous degeneration and significant systolic prolapse. The term mitral valve prolapse has caused confusion. On the one hand, some clinicians regard it as synonymous with floppy mitral valve. On the other hand, it has been used as a diagnostic label (with implications for the patient's management) when all that has been observed is trivial prolapse of an otherwise normal valve. The recognition that minor prolapse confined to the four-chamber view [1] and trivial regurgitation [3] are normal findings should do much to end the confusion [13].

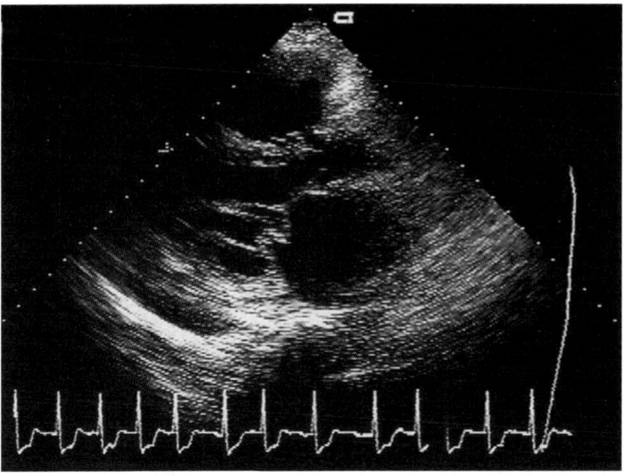
(a)

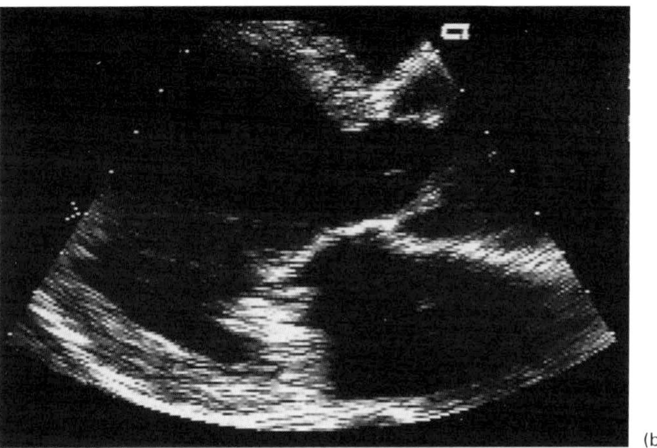
(b)

Fig. 9.8 Parasternal long axis systolic images of floppy mitral valves. Anterior leaflet prolapse is shown in (a) and posterior leaflet prolapse which is unusually gross in (b).

CALCIFICATION OF THE MITRAL RING

Calcification of the mitral ring is common in elderly subjects. It is a component of the degenerative calcification

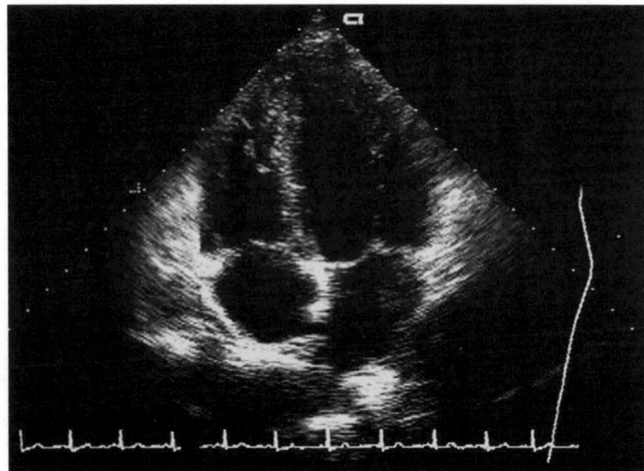
(a)

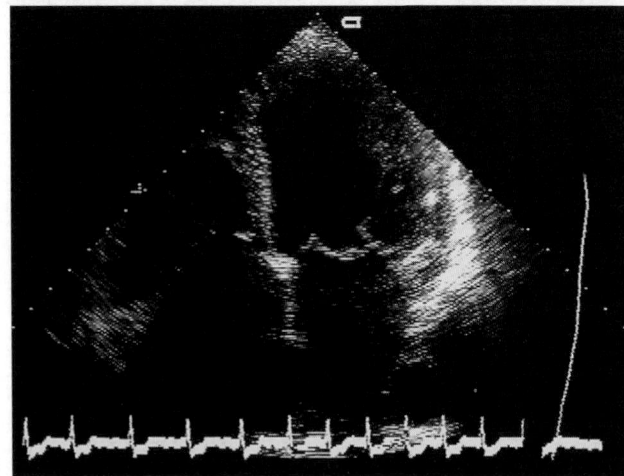
(b)

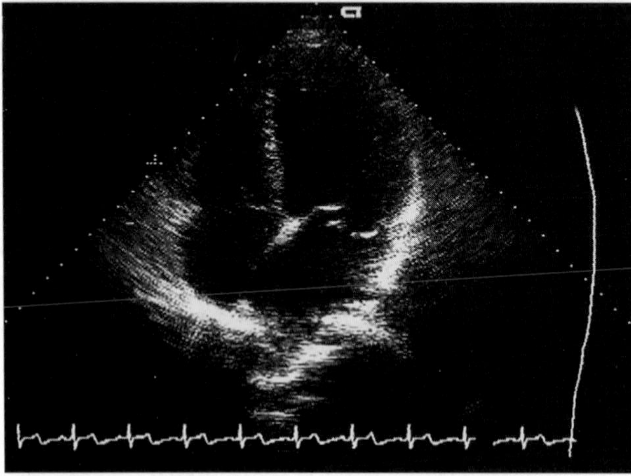
(c)

Fig. 9.9 Apical four-chamber systolic images. (a) Doming of the closed leaflets of a normal mitral valve; a normal finding. In (b) anterior mitral leaflet prolapse and in (c) posterior leaflet prolapse; both valves are floppy.

which affects the fibrous skeleton of the heart and is thus often associated with calcification of the base of the aortic leaflets and occasionally of the interventricular septum. It causes mitral regurgitation and very occasionally, trivial stenosis.

Typically, blocks of calcium are seen in the angle between the leaflets and the myocardium of the left ventricle in both parasternal long axis and apical four-chamber images (Fig. 9.12; see also Fig. 9.17). Though the calcification often encroaches on the base of the leaflets, the mobility of the remainder of the cusps is unimpaired; their normal motion is often best appreciated on the M-mode (Fig. 9.13). The calcified ring appears on the M-mode as a band of dense echoes closely related to the left ventricular posterior wall and moving with it [14].

The regurgitant jet can always be recorded with CW Doppler. However, as the calcification impedes the transmission of the Doppler signal, colour flow from the precordium may fail to identify the point of origin of the regurgitant jet.

FUNCTIONAL MITRAL REGURGITATION

Functional regurgitation is mild. It is the result of left ventricular dilatation which produces displacement of the papillary muscles and dilatation of the mitral ring. It is thus seen in coronary heart disease, dilated cardiomyopathy, aortic regurgitation, etc. Echoes from the mitral leaflets are normal; their amplitude of motion is usually small, coaptation is not obviously abnormal and there is no prolapse. On colour flow the regurgitant jet is small and does not extend far beyond the point of leaflet coaptation.

ISCHAEMIC MITRAL REGURGITATION

In patients with coronary heart disease, mitral regurgitation is usually functional. Severe regurgitation occasionally develops in the context of acute myocardial infarction, as a result of papillary muscle necrosis. This either causes rupture of the muscle (the detached part will be seen lying free within the left ventricle) or tearing of the chordae (these will be seen as highly mobile linear echoes) from their point of insertion on it. In both cases a portion of the cusp tissue will become flail; its motion will be chaotic and independent of the rest of the valve.

DOPPLER ASSESSMENT OF MITRAL REGURGITATION

Doppler echocardiography is a sensitive method for detecting mitral regurgitation. With colour flow, the point or points of origin of the regurgitation can be defined.

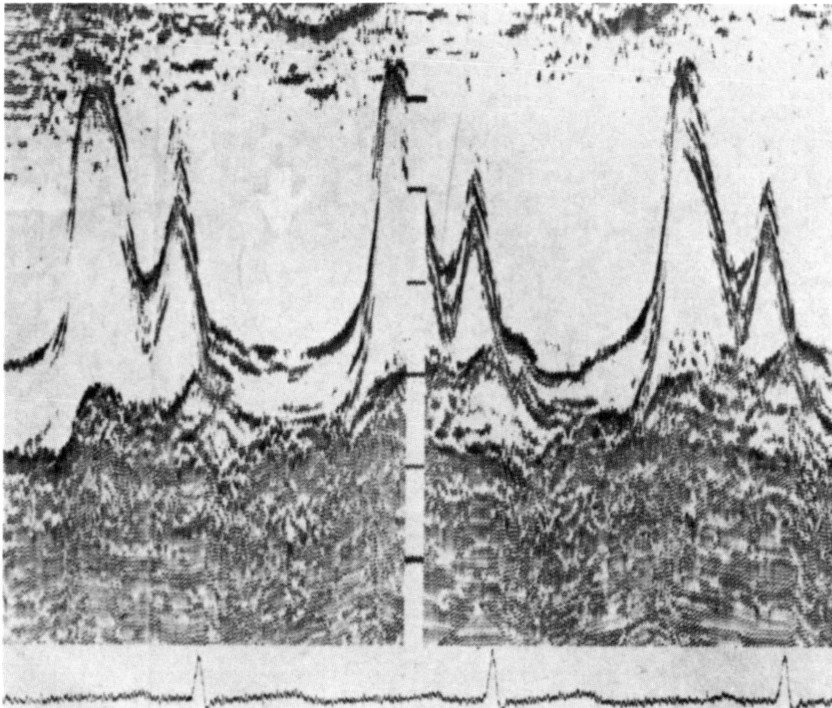

Fig. 9.10 M-mode record from a floppy mitral valve. Leaflet echoes are multiple giving the appearance of thickening. They sag posteriorly throughout systole (Courtesy of the *British Medical Bulletin*, **36**, 261.)

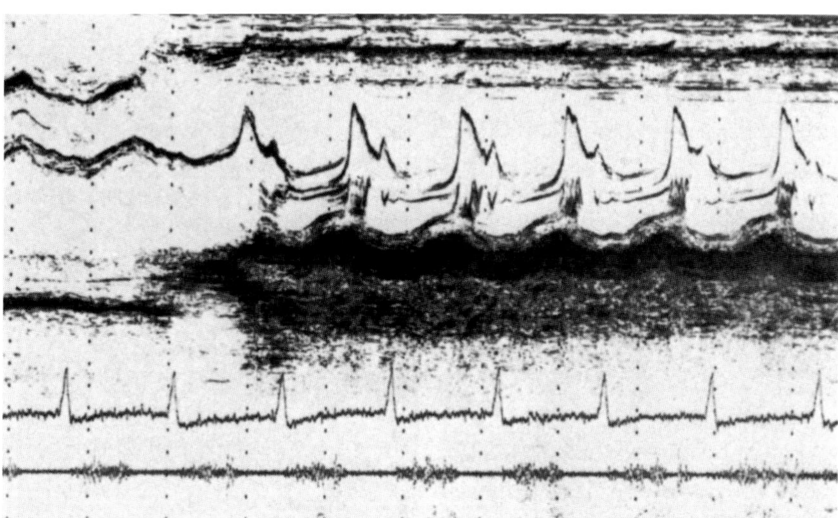

Fig. 9.11 M-mode record showing flail mitral posterior leaflet. Its motion at the onset of diastole is paradoxical and it flutters in early diastole.

Colour flow also displays the direction of the regurgitant jet and this can be of some diagnostic value. For example, in anterior leaflet prolapse the jet is directed upwards and towards the lateral wall of the left atrium whereas in posterior leaflet prolapse the jet is directed medially towards the interatrial septum [15] (Fig. 9.14).

Doppler assessment of the severity of mitral regurgitation is at best semi-quantitative. It can be concluded that severe regurgitation is likely if CW recordings (Fig. 9.15) show increased intensity of the regurgitant jet (compared with that of the forward flow signal) or decreased velocity of the regurgitant jet in late systole [16]. Though it is more accessible from the transoesophageal approach, pulmonary venous flow can frequently be recorded from the precordium [17]; it is accepted that reversal of systolic flow (normally directed towards the atrium) is good evidence of severe regurgitation [18].

Colour flow can provide information about the severity

of regurgitation. However, contrary to initial expectations, the presence of turbulent as opposed to laminar flow has been shown not to be a good indicator of severity. Also, the area of the regurgitant jet correlates poorly with angiographic grading of severity [19] and has been found to depend not just on the regurgitant volume but also on a number of variables including the pressure gradient driving the regurgitation and machine settings [20]. Recently, interest has centred on examination of the velocity of flow entering the regurgitant orifice on its ventricular side and on measurement of the proximal isovelocity surface area (PISA). As for a stenotic orifice, flow accelerates as it converges on the regurgitant orifice and is seen (because of aliasing) as alternating hemispheric bands of red and blue (Fig. 9.14b). The velocity of flow is highest near to the orifice and, assuming that flow can be represented as a series of hemispheric shells of equal and increasing velocity, flow rate can be calculated from the surface area of the hemisphere nearest the orifice and the velocity within it [21]. The method is largely independent of colour system gain and other equipment factors [22]. In the absence of a PISA signal, significant regurgitation is highly unlikely; it is not yet clear whether the size of the PISA signal is a reliable guide to severity.

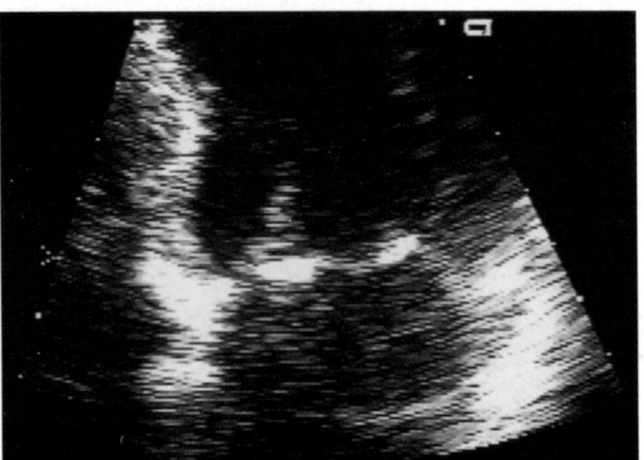

Fig. 9.12 Apical four-chamber diastolic image from a patient with calcification of the mitral ring and normal mitral leaflets (only the anterior leaflet is seen here).

CLINICAL DECISION

For many clinical purposes mitral regurgitation does not need to be measured with a high level of precision. The mitral Doppler data should be considered in the context of the clinical picture, the pulmonary artery pressure and the findings on imaging of the valve and the remainder of the left heart. Taken together these provide a useful and valid assessment of severity.

The transoesophageal approach is unnecessary for the routine evaluation of the regurgitant mitral valve. However, the clarity of the information it provides on valve morphology and jet origin makes it useful to the surgeon contemplating valve repair. The transoesophageal approach is thus usually preferred for preoperative and intraoperative studies (see Chapter 14).

Aortic valve

Assessment of the structure of the aortic valve requires imaging in the parasternal short and long axis views. The

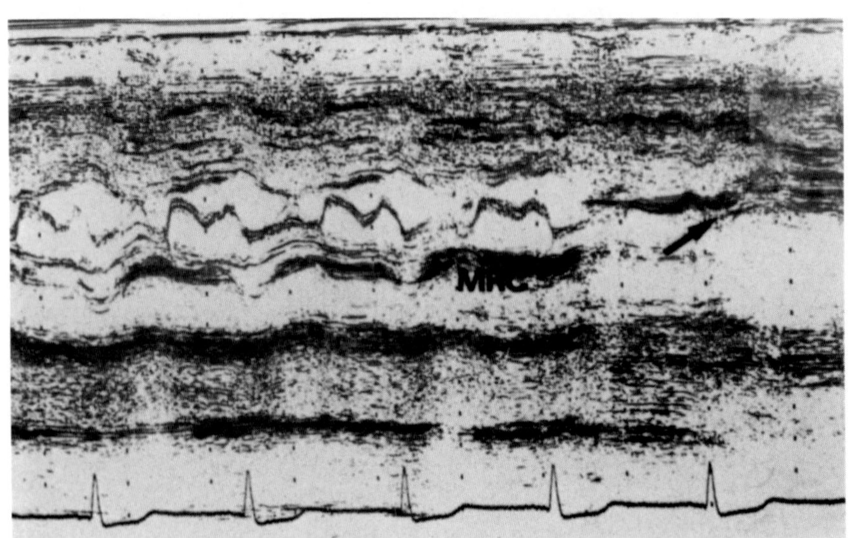

Fig. 9.13 M-mode showing calcification of the mitral ring (MRC). Calcification extends to the aortic root (arrow). The aortic valve is calcified and the left ventricle is hypertrophied; the patient had severe aortic stenosis.

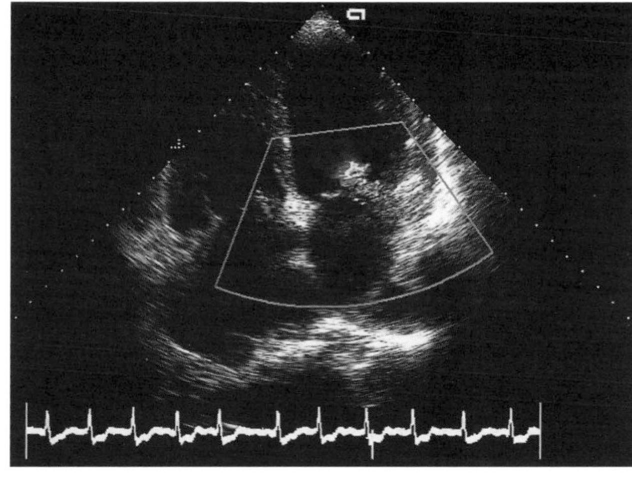
(a)

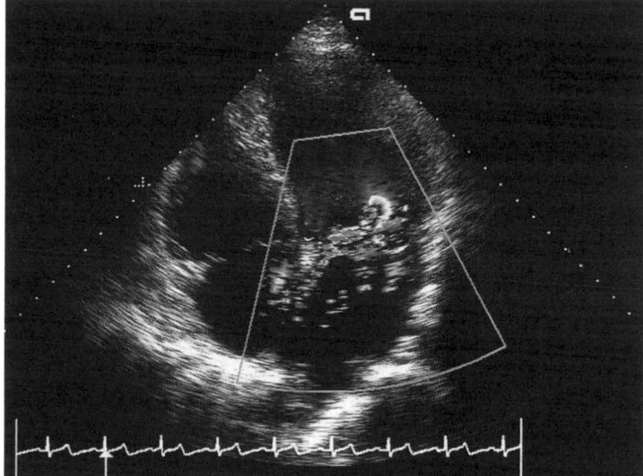
(b)

Fig. 9.14 Colour flow Doppler records (apical four chamber, systole) from floppy mitral valves with (a) mitral anterior leaflet prolapse, and (b) mitral posterior leaflet prolapse. In (a) the regurgitant jet is directed laterally and in (b) medially towards the interarterial septum. Acceleration of flow as it approaches the mitral on its ventricular side, more obvious in (b), is in keeping with severe regurgitation. For colour, see Plate 9.14 (between pp. 308 and 309).

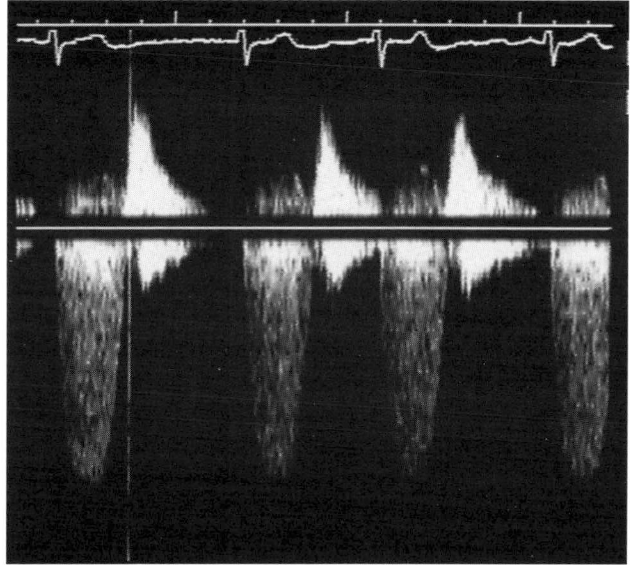
(a)

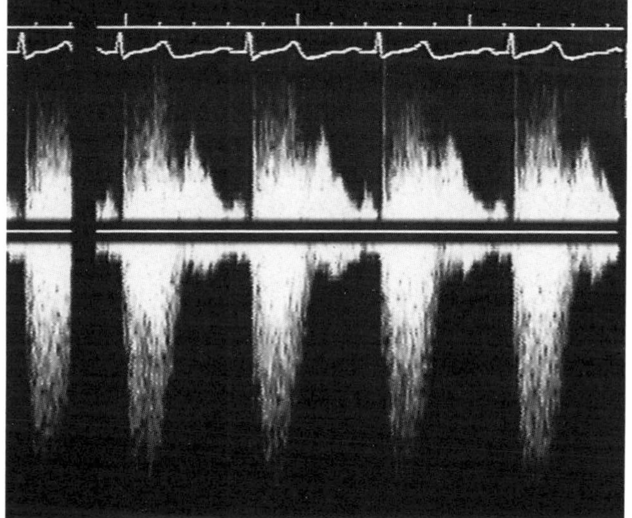
(b)

Fig. 9.15 Continuous wave Doppler records of mitral flow regurgitant rheumatic (a) and floppy (b) valves (same valve as Fig. 9.14). In (b) despite the absence of mitral stenosis, the velocity of forward flow is increased and the intensity of the regurgitant jet is comparable to that of the forward flow; both features in keeping with severe regurgitation. Regurgitant flow was directed across the plane of the interrogating beam and is thus recorded above and below the baseline.

orifice and all three cusps are seen in the short axis view; only the right and non-coronary cusps are usually seen in the long axis view. Except in the context of infective endocarditis, transoesophageal echocardiography adds nothing to the information obtained from the transthoracic approach.

Normal aortic valve

The valve lies within the aortic root. The aortic root is bounded above by the supra-aortic ridge and below by the aortic annulus, the interventricular septum and the base of the mitral anterior leaflet [23].

The three cusps are approximately the same size; echoes from them are thin. When the valve opens, they fold against the aortic root to which they are attached at the supra-aortic ridge. In diastole, their line of coaptation is Y shaped on short axis images and can be seen on long axis images to extend for a short distance below their edges (Fig. 9.16; see also Fig. 9.1).

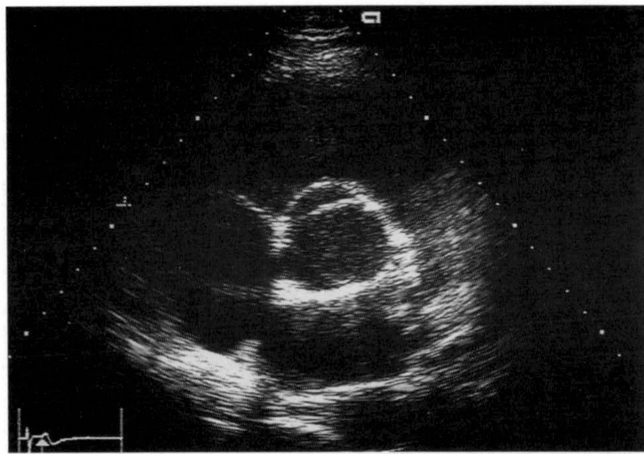
(a)

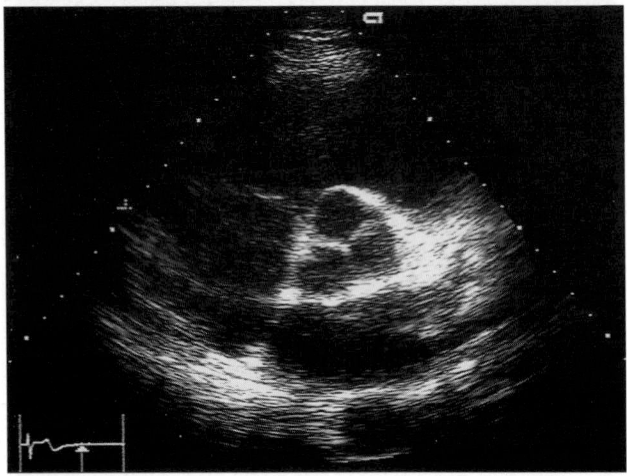
(b)

Fig. 9.16 Short axis images of normal aortic valve in (a) systole and (b) diastole.

Trivial regurgitation is a normal finding but is less common than 'physiological' regurgitation of the other valves [3].

Aortic stenosis

Congenital stenosis is dealt with elsewhere (see Chapter 8); systolic doming seen in the parasternal long axis view is characteristic. The commonest cause of acquired aortic stenosis is degenerative (senile) calcification of a normal valve; there is usually associated calcification of the mitral ring (Fig. 9.17). Other recognized causes are rheumatic heart disease and calcification of a congenitally bicuspid valve. In degenerative disease, calcification begins at the base of the cusps. In rheumatic disease (Fig. 9.18), thickening and calcification start at the edge of the cusps and commissural fusion occurs early. Both processes lead to extensive calcification which eventually obscures valve morphology.

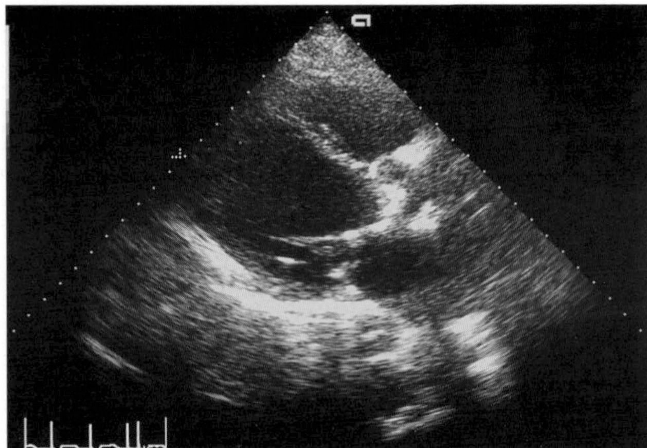

Fig. 9.17 Parasternal long axis image showing degenerative calcification of the aortic valve. There is also calcification of the mitral ring (the leaflets are normal) and of the tip of the posterior papillary muscle.

Parasternal short axis images provide the best information on leaflet mobility and orifice size but parasternal long axis imaging is necessary for a complete assessment of the extent of calcification.

Though planimetry of the aortic valve area is of no value in the quantification of stenosis, imaging does provide a useful guide to its severity. Thus, trivial stenosis with mild impairment of cusp mobility (often best demonstrated on the M-mode) and normal left ventricular wall thickness can be confidently differentiated from moderate to severe stenosis.

DOPPLER ASSESSMENT

Continuous wave Doppler is used for the quantification of aortic stenosis (Fig. 9.19). Provided that care is taken to obtain the maximum velocity of systolic flow (by recording from apical, right parasternal and suprasternal probe positions), Doppler gradients derived from the modified Bernoulli equation (see mitral stenosis) agree well with instantaneous gradients measured at cardiac catheterization [24]. However, it is not the instantaneous but the peak-to-peak gradient that is usually measured at catheterization and this is always lower than the Doppler gradient.

The Doppler gradient, like the catheter gradient is dependent not just on orifice size but also on the volume of flow. It will be underestimated when left ventricular function is compromised and will be overestimated when stroke volume is increased, e.g. by anaemia or significant aortic regurgitation. In practice it may be sufficient to recognize that the gradient may have been over- or underestimated. However, the effect of flow can be discounted if

(a)

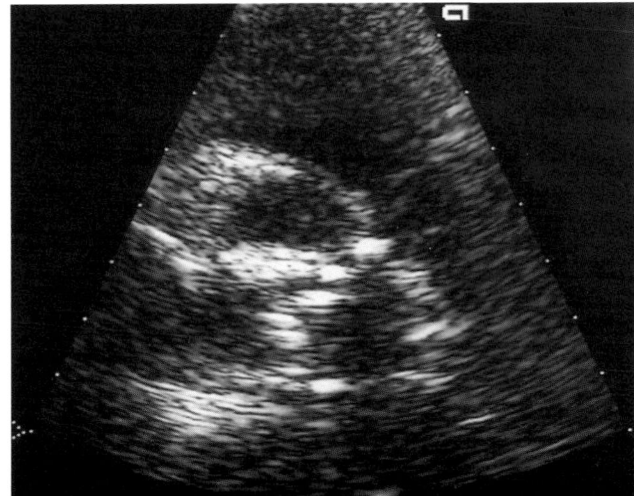

(b)

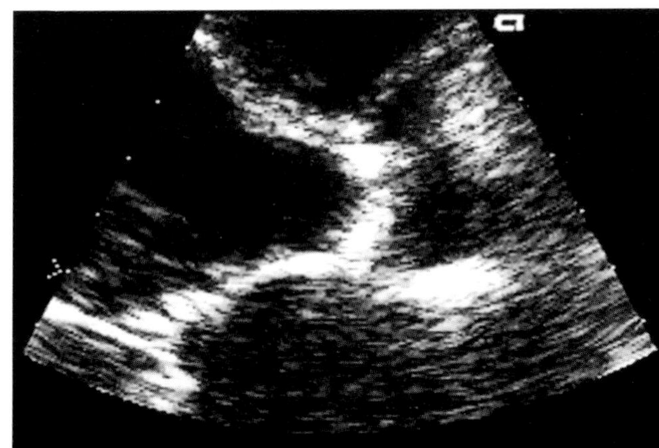

(c)

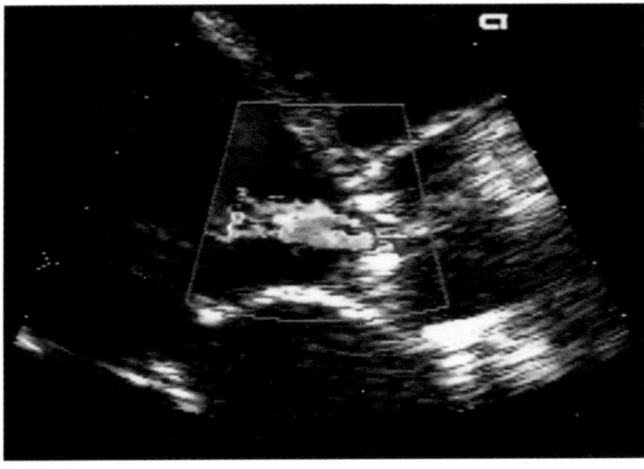

Fig. 9.18 Rheumatic aortic valve. (a) Parasternal short axis showing thickening and calcification of the edge of the leaflets. The long axis images in (b) systole and (c) diastole demonstrate the rigidity of the leaflets, the stenotic orifice and, with colour flow, a central regurgitant jet. For colour, see Plate 9.18 (between pp. 308 and 309).

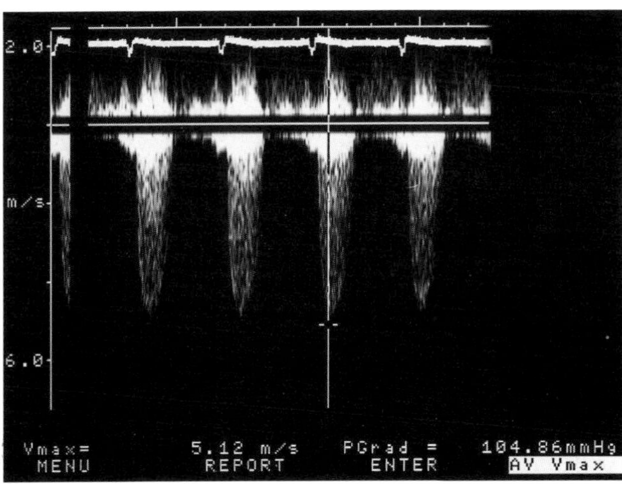

Fig. 9.19 Continuous wave Doppler record from apical probe position of flow velocity across a severely stenotic aortic valve; measurement of the gradient is shown.

valve area is calculated using the continuity equation [25,26]. The method involves measurement of the aortic dimension below the valve and the peak velocity of flow below (using pulsed Doppler) and above the valve; details are beyond the scope of this chapter.

CLINICAL DECISION

With Doppler, it is now possible to make serial measurements of the gradient or, for better reproducibility, of the valve area. This is clinically important but should also provide new information about the natural history of aortic stenosis. Serial data obtained so far show that in asymptomatic stenosis, the rate of progression (judged from the Doppler gradient) is linear rather than exponential, highly variable from patient to patient and cannot be predicted from the initial severity of the lesion [27].

Aortic regurgitation

The fundamental causes of aortic regurgitation are dilatation of the aortic root or an abnormality of the valve itself. Regurgitation may accompany stenosis and is then usually mild. Pure aortic regurgitation is a feature of the floppy aortic valve and can develop in a bicuspid valve, particularly if there is associated aortic root dilatation [28]. Provided that it extends far enough into the left ventricular cavity, turbulent aortic regurgitant flow (Fig. 9.20a) produces fluttering of the mitral anterior leaflet. This feature is best appreciated on M-mode records (Fig. 9.20b): its absence does not exclude aortic regurgitation.

(a)

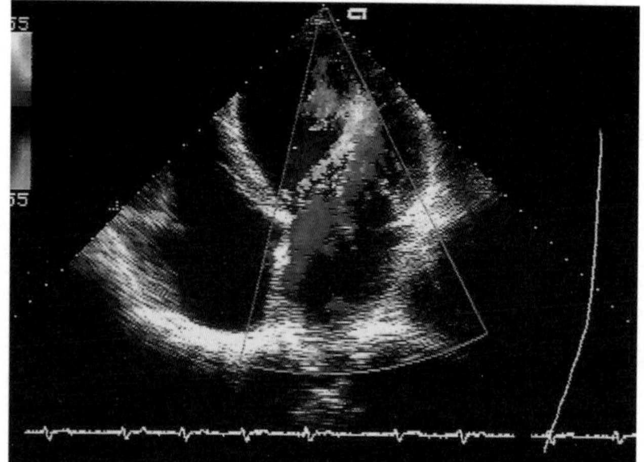

(b)

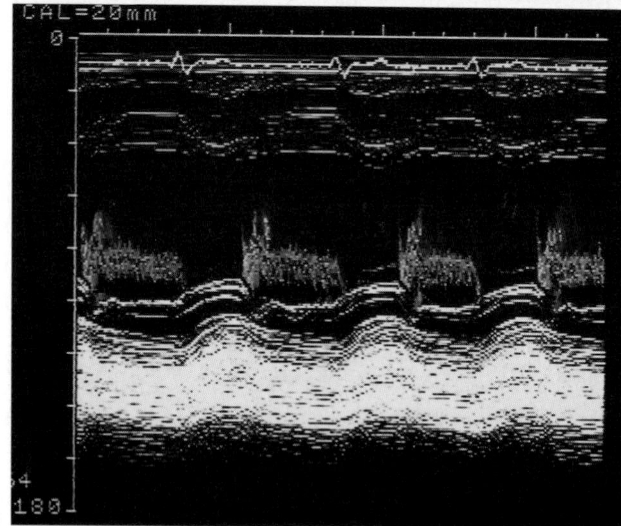

Fig. 9.20 (a)Apical four-chamber diastolic image. Turbulent aortic regurgitant flow extends across the front of normal mitral anterior leaflet to mix with mitral forward flow. (b) Colour M-mode shows the aortic regurgitant flow producing diastolic oscillation of the mitral anterior leaflet. For colour, see Plate 9.20 (between pp. 308 and 309).

FLOPPY AORTIC VALVE

As with the floppy mitral valve there is myxomatous degeneration of the leaflets and leaflet prolapse. Regurgitation is typically mild but the leaflets can tear and regurgitation is then acute and severe. A floppy aortic valve rarely occurs in isolation. The mitral valve is usually also floppy and, less often, all four valves are floppy [10,29]. The voluminous cusps fold and on cross-sectional images look thickened and, when they move, heavy. Their amplitude of motion is not impaired. Cusp prolapse into the left ventricular outflow tract can be identified on parasternal long axis images (Fig. 9.21; see also Fig. 9.27).

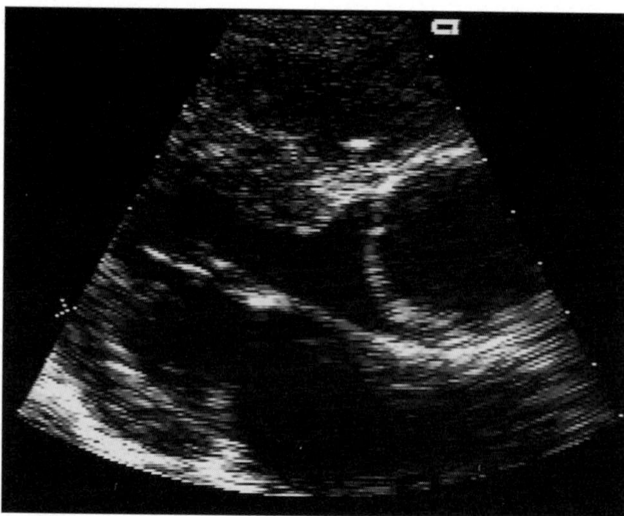

Fig. 9.21 Parasternal long axis diastolic image showing floppy aortic valve prolapsing into the left ventricular outflow tract.

The M-mode features (Fig. 9.22) are apparent thickening of the cusps which open wide and often oscillate in systole and come together in diastole to produce multiple centrally positioned echoes [10,30].

BICUSPID AORTIC VALVE

The congenitally bicuspid valve may be functionally normal, regurgitant or, particularly in later life, stenotic. Whatever the functional status of the valve, dilatation of the aortic root is a frequent association and the two abnormalities may reflect a common developmental defect [28,31].

Provided that the valve is not heavily calcified, the diagnosis is easily made on parasternal short axis images. The two cusps are of unequal size, and a ridge on one of them marks the site of leaflet fusion; the orifice is oval (Fig. 9.23).

DILATATION OF THE AORTIC ROOT

The aortic cusps are attached to the aortic root. Root dilatation (normal dimension <3.5 cm) thus produces failure of cusp coaptation. Its causes are idiopathic (there is a recognized association with bicuspid aortic valve), inflammatory, Marfan's syndrome and ageing. Precordial imaging in the parasternal long axis view usually provides adequate information but the transoesophageal approach may be necessary if dissection of the aortic root is suspected.

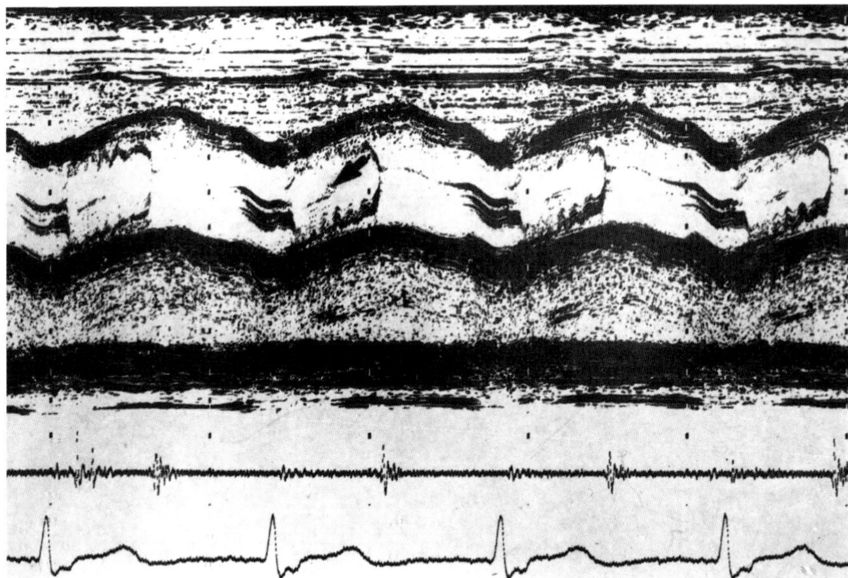

Fig. 9.22 M-mode record from floppy aortic valve. See text. There is gross systolic oscillation of the cusps. The structure arrowed is the left coronary cusp. (Courtesy of the *British Heart Journal* (1982), **47**, 337.)

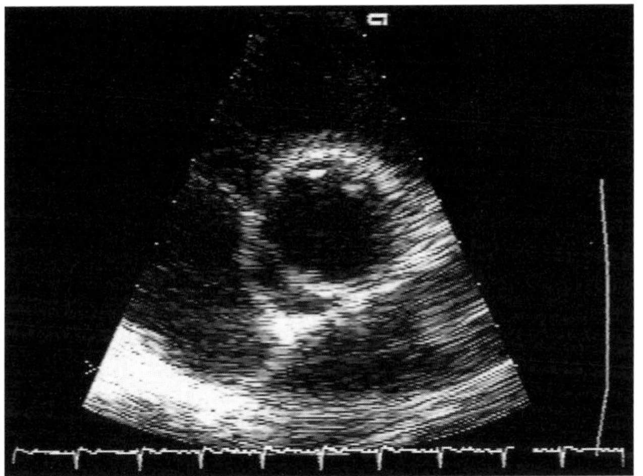

(a)

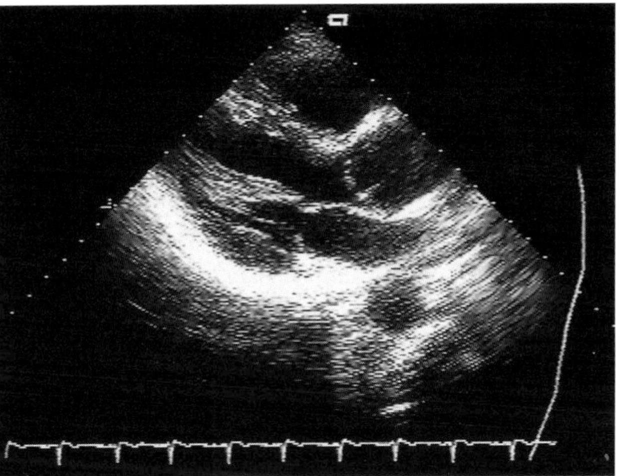

(b)

Fig. 9.23 Bicuspid aortic valve. (a) Parasternal short axis image of the open valve. There are lateral and medial commisures. The ridge on the anterior leaflet marks the site of leaflet fusion. (b) Parasternal long axis image of the closed valve. The anterior is the larger leaflet; it is prolapsing. Aortic root dimension is normal.

DOPPLER ASSESSMENT OF AORTIC REGURGITATION

Doppler is much more sensitive than auscultation and at least as sensitive as angiography for the detection of aortic regurgitation. It is accepted that quantification of aortic regurgitation by CW Doppler is accurate. Severe regurgitation is associated with a high velocity, high intensity (compared with the systolic signal) regurgitant jet. Measurement of the pressure half-time (see mitral stenosis) of the aortic diastolic flow velocity profile (Fig. 9.24) gives a useful estimate of severity; with values of less than 400 ms indicating at least moderately severe regurgitation. The method which is independent of heart rate, agrees well with angiographic estimates of severity [32]. However, like them, it will overestimate the severity if left ventricular end-diastolic pressure is raised as a result of ventricular dysfunction. Colour flow is a sensitive method for detecting regurgitation and will identify its point of origin. The regurgitant jet appears as an area of turbulent

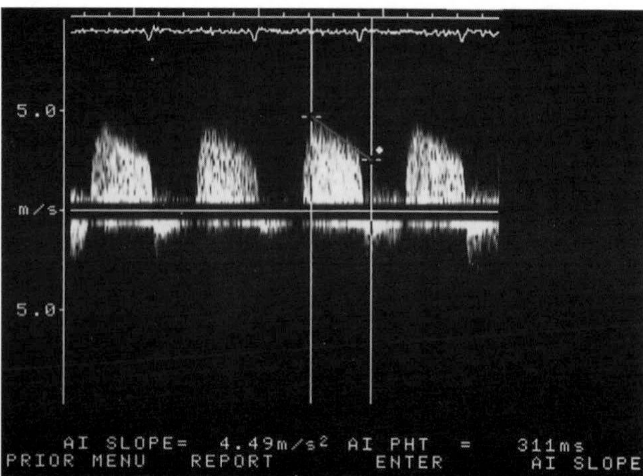

Fig. 9.24 Continuous wave Doppler record from apical probe position of flow velocity across a regurgitant aortic valve. The measured pressure half-time indicates moderately severe regurgitation.

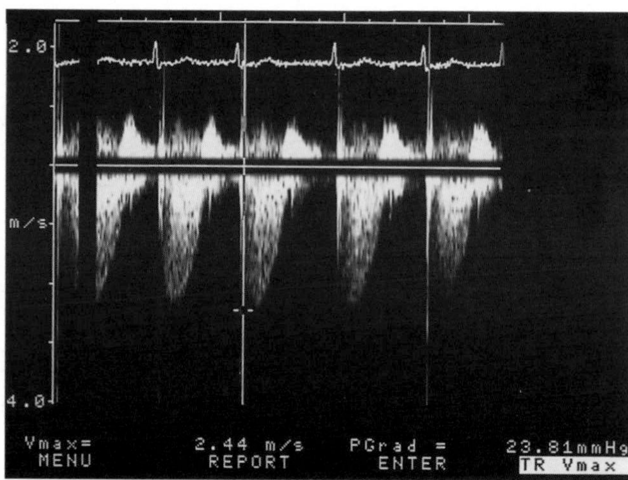

Fig. 9.25 Continuous wave Doppler record of tricuspid flow. Estimated pulmonary artery systolic pressure is 34 mmHg. See text.

flow extending a variable distance into the left ventricular cavity in diastole (see Fig. 9.20a). Maximum jet area which probably depends more on jet velocity than volume, provides no reliable information on the severity of regurgitation. However, jet width just below the valve (see Fig. 9.18c) in the parasternal long axis view (expressed as a pecentage of the width of the outflow tract) has been shown to correlate closely with angiographic grading of severity [33]. In routine practice, the results should be interpreted with some caution as the method can be influenced by instrumentation and operator factors.

CLINICAL DECISION

Assessment of the severity of aortic regurgitation should not rely on Doppler alone. The size of the left ventricular cavity is a guide to severity and M-mode measurements of the left ventricular dimension are useful in the serial assessment of patients. Also, the M-mode, by demonstrating premature closure of the mitral valve (see Fig. 9.31), can be of key importance in the diagnosis of acute severe regurgitation.

Tricuspid valve

Normal tricuspid valve

The anterior and septal leaflets are seen in the apical four-chamber (see Fig. 9.9a) and parasternal short axis views. The posterior leaflet is seen in the parasternal right ventricular inflow long axis view. No view provides a satisfactory short axis view of the orifice. 'Physiological' tricuspid regurgitation is a normal finding. It has been detected in up to 100% of normal young adults [3].

Pulmonary artery systolic pressure can be calculated (Fig. 9.25) from the tricuspid regurgitant jet [34]. The peak velocity of regurgitant flow is used to calculate the systolic gradient between the right ventricle and right atrium. Addition of the right atrial pressure (estimated from the jugular venous pulse or assumed to be, say, 10 mmHg) to this gradient provides an estimate of right ventricular systolic pressure. Provided that there is no obstruction to right ventricular outflow, this in turn reflects pulmonary artery systolic pressure. The accuracy of the method is acceptable. When the Doppler signal from the regurgitant jet is too weak to measure, it can be amplified by intravenous injection of fluid containing microbubbles. The velocity of the jet is unaltered by the process of contrast enhancement [35].

Tricuspid stenosis

Tricuspid stenosis is the result of rheumatic or carcinoid (see below) heart disease. Rheumatic disease of the tricuspid valve is unusual. It typically results in combined stenosis and regurgitation with the latter predominating; isolated stenosis is rare. There is always associated rheumatic involvement of the mitral and often also of the aortic valve. On cross-sectional images (Fig. 9.26) the leaflets appear thickened (calcification is rare). Their mobility is reduced and in diastole they dome towards the right ventricle. The subvalvar apparatus is thickened and shortened [36]. As planimetry of the orifice is not feasible, the stenosis cannot be quantified. However, when right

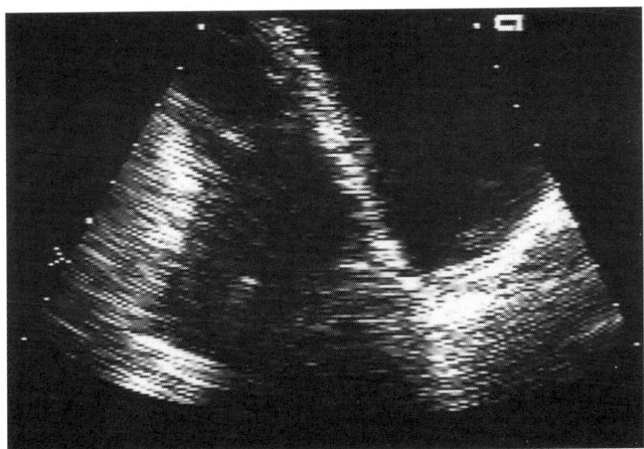

Fig. 9.26 Apical four-chamber diastolic image of rheumatic tricuspid valve. The leaflets are thick and rigid. They dome towards the right ventricle.

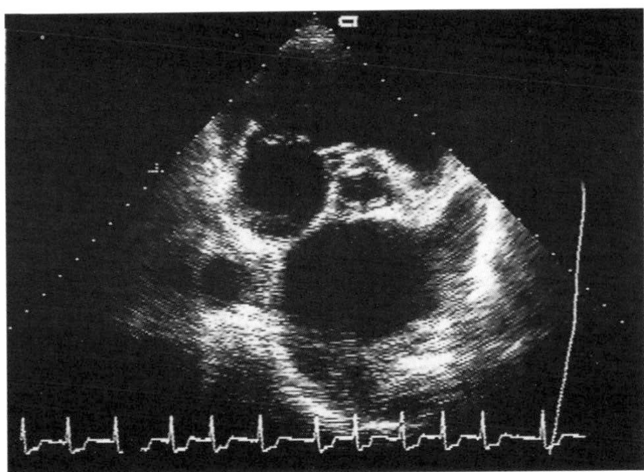

Fig. 9.27 Parasternal systolic short axis image. The tricuspid valve is floppy; the anterior leaflet is voluminous, the septal leaflet is prolapsing. The aortic valve is also floppy; the leaflets appear thick but open normally.

atrial enlargement is disproportionate to any right ventricular enlargement, it can be concluded that stenosis is likely to be significant.

Quantification of tricuspid stenosis is possible with CW Doppler. Estimates of valve area derived from measurement of the pressure half-time (see mitral stenosis) of the diastolic flow velocity profile agree well with invasive estimates [16].

Tricuspid regurgitation

Tricuspid regurgitation may be functional or the result of intrinsic disease of the valve as in rheumatic heart disease, carcinoid heart disease and floppy valve. Regurgitation is usually the dominant lesion in rheumatic involvement of the tricuspid valve (see tricuspid stenosis).

FUNCTIONAL TRICUSPID REGURGITATION

This is the usual cause of tricuspid regurgitation. It is the result of raised right ventricular systolic pressure and the associated dilatation of the right ventricle and tricuspid valve ring. Cross-sectional imaging shows normal leaflets, the dilated ventricle and, if the regurgitation is other than mild, right atrial enlargement. The size of the tricuspid ring can be assessed on cross-sectional images and when combined with the colour flow estimate of the severity of regurgitation, provides an accurate guide to the need for annuloplasty [37].

FLOPPY TRICUSPID VALVE

This does not occur in isolation (see floppy mitral) [10]. Cross-sectional imaging (Fig. 9.27) shows voluminous leaflets, a lax subvalvar apparatus and prolapse of one or more of the leaflets above the plane of the tricuspid annulus. Prolapse is usually best seen in the apical four-chamber view. Typically the regurgitation is not severe and there is thus no enlargement of the right heart chambers.

CARCINOID HEART DISEASE

About 50% of patients with carcinoid tumours have cardiac involvement. Fibrous plaques form on the endocardium of the right atrium, right ventricle and right heart valves. The tricuspid valve becomes predominantly regurgitant; accompanying stenosis is mild. On cross-sectional images (Fig. 9.28), the leaflets appear thickened, rigid and tethered and the valve may be fixed in a half-open position. Typically, there is enlargement of both the right atrium and the right ventricle [38].

DOPPLER ASSESSMENT OF TRICUSPID REGURGITATION

With colour flow Doppler, the presence of turbulent as opposed to laminar flow is not a guide to the severity of the regurgitation. The area of the regurgitant jet provides only a rough estimate of severity; the limitations of the method are as for mitral and aortic regurgitation. Reversal of systolic flow on pulsed Doppler recordings from the hepatic veins is good evidence of severe regurgitation [39].

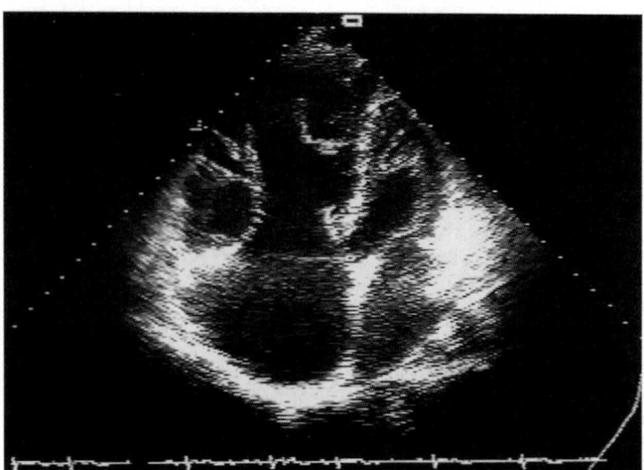

Fig. 9.28 Carcinoid heart disease. Apical four-chamber end-diastolic image. The tricuspid leaflets and their chordae tendineae are thick and rigid. The valve was fixed in this open position. Fibrous endocardial plaques are seen as bright echoes.

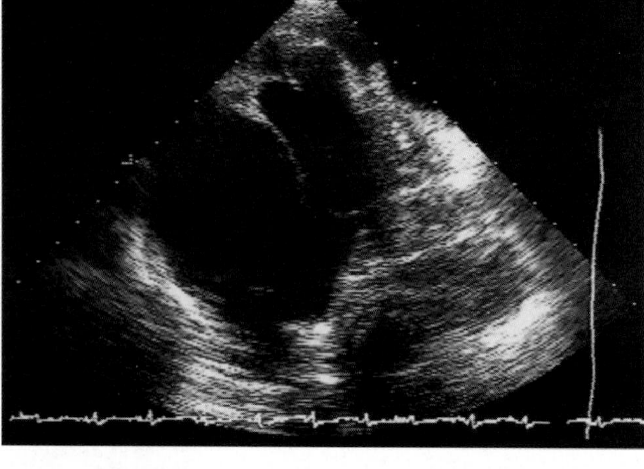

Fig. 9.29 Modified parasternal short axis image displaying the main pulmonary artery, its bifurcation and the pulmonary valve. The aorta is dilated.

Pulmonary valve

The pulmonary valve is best seen in the parasternal short axis view or in a modification of that view designed to display the main pulmonary artery and its bifurcation (Fig. 9.29). The right and left cusps are seen; the anterior is not. Ordinarily, the orifice cannot be imaged in its short axis.

In up to 100% of normal young adults, Doppler will demonstrate 'physiological' regurgitation, confined to the immediate vicinity of the valve [3]. Pulmonary stenosis is usually congenital (see Chapter 8). Rheumatic involvement with combined stenosis and regurgitation has been described but is excessively rare, invariably mild and never occurs as an isolated lesion. Carcinoid heart disease (Fig. 9.30) is the best example of an acquired lesion. It results in stenosis with lesser regurgitation. The valve is thickened and rigid and is often fixed in a half-open position. There is always associated involvement of the tricuspid valve and enlargement of both right heart chambers is usual [38].

CW Doppler gradients agree well with pulmonary systolic gradients obtained invasively. They are best made with reference to the image in the modified short axis view [40]. When pulmonary regurgitation is significant, colour flow will demonstrate a wide jet extending through the outflow tract into the right ventricle.

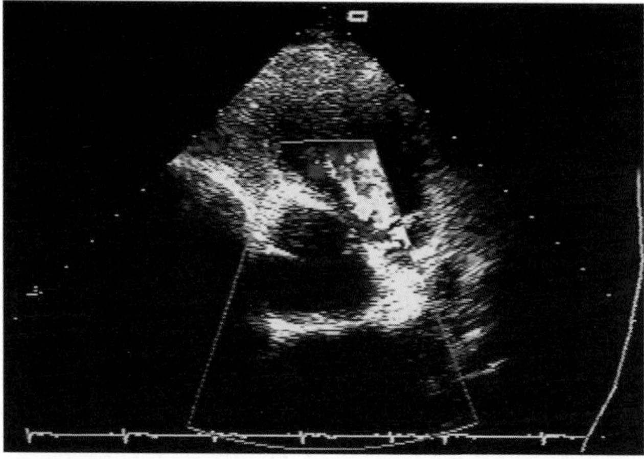

Fig. 9.30 Colour flow Doppler showing wide regurgitant jet in patient with carcinoid disease and significant pulmonary regurgitation. The valve is thick. For colour, see Plate 9.30 (between pp. 308 and 309).

Infective endocarditis

The clinical features of right and left heart infective endocarditis are different [41]. Right-sided endocarditis develops on a previously normal valve. Infection is typically introduced by intravenous drug abuse or by an indwelling intravenous line. Valve disruption is unusual and haemodynamic upset and heart failure are rare. Left-sided infective endocarditis usually develops on a congenitally abnormal valve, typically a bicuspid aortic valve but floppy valves are also susceptible. Valve disruption and thus haemodynamic upset and heart failure are common (Fig. 9.31). Echocardiography can demonstrate vegetations and can thus clinch the diagnosis of infective endocarditis. Vegetations are seen at their most gross as clusters of bright mobile echoes (Fig. 9.32). They are usually related to a valve leaflet but are occasionally seen

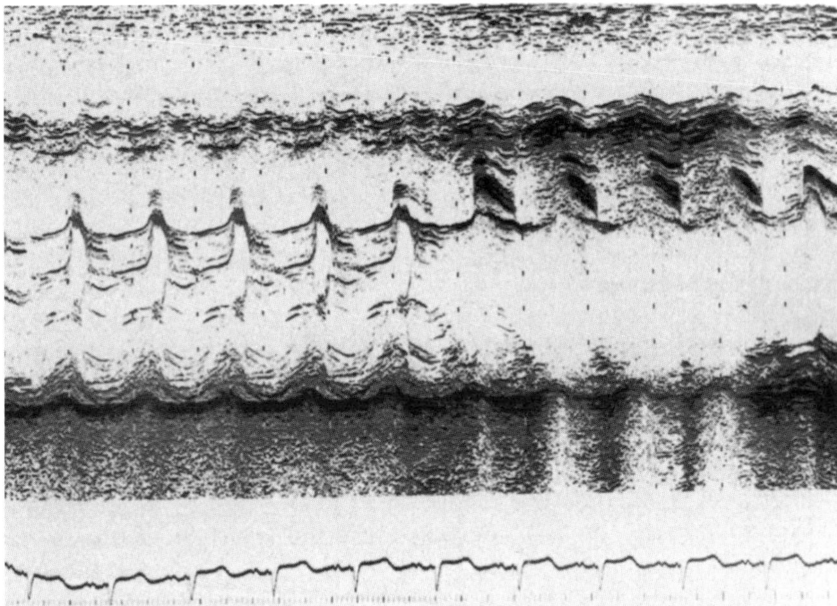

Fig. 9.31 M-mode record from patient with infective endocarditis on a calcified bicuspid aortic valve. Diastolic echoes in the left ventricular outflow tract are prolapsing vegetations. The left ventricle is dilated. The mitral valve closes prematurely (before the P wave of the electrocardiogram), indicating that regurgitation is severe and acute.

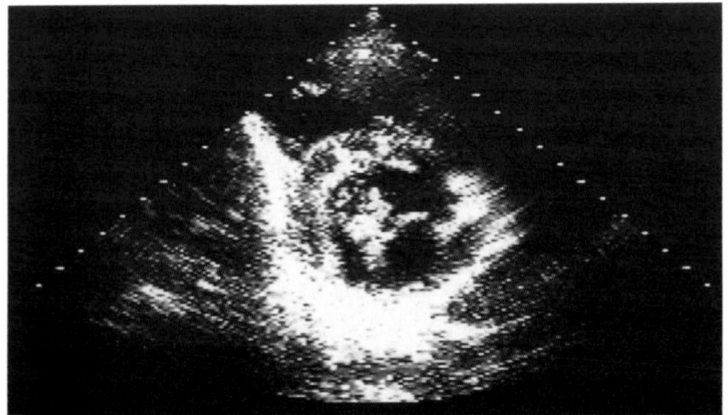

Fig. 9.32 Parasternal short axis image from a patient with infective endocarditis. There are vegetations on the mitral valve.

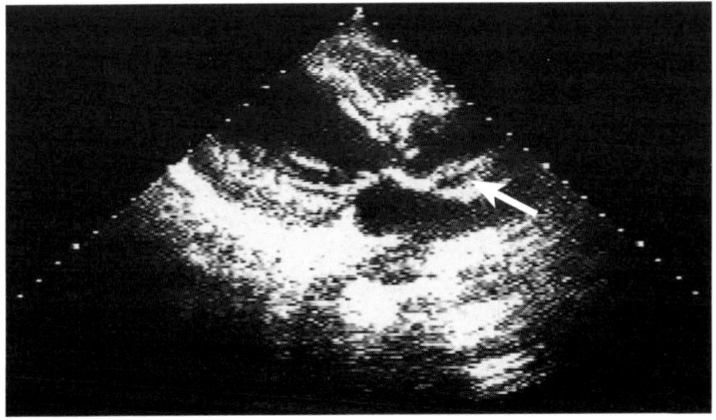

Fig. 9.33 Parasternal long axis image from a patient with infective endocarditis. There are vegetations on the aortic valve and an abscess of the aortic root (arrow).

on the myocardium adjacent to an infected tricuspid valve. Vegetations or sterile thrombi can form on the interventricular septum when infection has been caused by a Swan–Ganz catheter. For the detection of left heart vegetations, and particularly in the presence of a prosthetic valve, the transoesophageal is clearly superior to the transthoracic approach [42]. Neither can identify vegetations of less than 3 mm. Also, current technology cannot distinguish between active and healed vegetations.

Extension of infection produces periannular (ring) abscesses (Fig. 9.33), mycotic aneurysms, chordal rupture and valve dehiscence. For left heart infections, these are more readily detected from the transoesophageal approach [43].

Assessment of the patient with infective endocarditis must include colour flow Doppler (looking for leaks and fistulae), Doppler quantification of any regurgitant lesions and an evaluation of chamber size and function.

Acknowledgements

The technical assistance of John Jarvie, Mary Kerr and Rhona Shanks is gratefully acknowledged.

References

1 Levine, R.A., Stathogiannis, E., Newell, J.B., Harrigan, P., Weyman, A.E. (1988) Reconsideration of echocardiographic

standards for mitral valve prolapse: lack of association between leaflet displacement isolated to the apical four chamber view and independent echocardiographic evidence of abnormality. *Journal of the American College of Cardiology* **11**, 1010–1019.

2 Levine, R.A., Handschumacher, M.D., Sanfilippo, A.J., *et al.* (1989) Three-dimensional echocardiographic reconstruction of the mitral valve, with implications for the diagnosis of mitral valve prolapse. *Circulation* **80**, 589–598.

3 Jobic, Y., Slama, M., Tribouilloy, C., *et al.* (1993) Doppler echocardiographic evaluation of valve regurgitation in healthy volunteers. *British Heart Journal* **69**, 109–113.

4 Glover, M.U., Warren, S.E., Vieweg, W.V.R., *et al.* (1983) M-mode and two-dimensional echocardiographic correlation with findings at catheterization and surgery in patients with mitral stenosis. *American Heart Journal* **105**, 98–102.

5 Hatle, L., Brubakk, A., Tromsdal, A., Angelsen, B. (1978) Noninvasive assessment of pressure drop in mitral stenosis by Doppler ultrasound. *British Heart Journal* **40**, 131–140.

6 Hatle, L., Angelsen, B., Tromsdal, A. (1979) Noninvasive assessment of atrio-ventricular pressure half-time by Doppler ultrasound. *Circulation* **60**, 1096–1104.

7 Karp, K., Teien, D., Bjerle, P., Eriksson, P. (1989) Reassessment of valve area determination by the pressure half-time method. Impact of left ventricular stiffness and peak diastolic pressure difference. *Journal of the American College of Cardiology* **13**, 594–599.

8 Khandheria, B.K., Tajik, A.J., Reeder, G.S., *et al.* (1986) Doppler color flow imaging: a new technique for visualization of the blood flow jet in mitral stenosis. *Mayo Clinic Proceedings* **61**, 623–630.

9 Wilkins, G.T., Weyman, A.E., Abascal, V.M., *et al.* (1988) Percutaneous balloon dilatation of the mitral valve. An analysis of echocardiographic variables related to outcome and the mechanism of dilatation. *British Heart Journal* **60**, 299–308.

10 Morganroth, J., Jones, R.H., Chen, C.C., Naito, M. (1980) Two-dimensional echocardiography in mitral, aortic and tricuspid valve prolapse. *American Journal of Cardiology* **46**, 1164–1177.

11 Marcus, R.H., Sareli, P., Pocock, W.A., *et al.* (1989) Functional anatomy of severe mitral regurgitation in active rheumatic carditis. *American Journal of Cardiology* **63**, 577–584.

12 de Maria, A.N., King, J.F., Bogren, H.G., Lies, J.E., Mason, D.T. (1974) The variable spectrum of echocardiographic manifestations of the mitral valve prolapse syndrome. *Circulation* **50**, 33–41.

13 Devereux, R.B., Kramer-Fox, R., Brown, W.T., *et al.* (1989) Mitral valve prolapse: causes, clinical manifestations, and management. *Annals of Internal Medicine* **111**, 305–317.

14 D'Cruz, I.A., Cohen, H.C., Prabhu, R., Bisla, V., Glick, G. (1977) Clinical manifestations of mitral annulus calcification, with emphasis on its echocardiographic features. *American Heart Journal* **94**, 367–377.

15 Yoshida, K., Yoshikawa, J., Hozumi, T., *et al.* (1990) Value of acceleration flows and regurgitant jet direction by colour Doppler flow mapping in the evaluation of mitral valve prolapse. *Circulation* **81**, 879–885.

16 Hatle, L., Angelsen, B. (1982) *Doppler Ultrasound in Cardiology. Physical Principles and Clinical Applications.* Lea & Febiger, Philadelphia.

17 Rossvoll, O., Hatle, L.K. (1993) Pulmonary venous flow velocities recorded by transthoracic Doppler ultrasound: relation to left ventricular diastolic pressures. *Journal of the American College of Cardiology* **21**, 1687–1696.

18 Kamp, O., Huitink, H., van Eenige, M.J., Visser, C.A., Roos, J.P. (1992) Value of pulmonary venous flow characteristics in the assessment of severity of native mitral valve regurgitation: an angiographic correlated study. *Journal of the American Society of Echocardiography* **5**, 239–246.

19 Spain, M.G., Smith, M.D., Grayburn, P.A., *et al.* (1989) Quantitative assessment of mitral regurgitation by Doppler color flow imaging. Angiographic and hemodynamic correlations. *Journal of the American College of Cardiology* **13**, 585–590.

20 Simpson, I., Valdes-Cruz, L., Sahn, D., *et al.* (1989) Doppler color flow mapping of simulated *in vitro* regurgitant jets. Evaluation of the effects of orifice size and hemodynamic variables. *Journal of the American College of Cardiology* **13**, 1195–1207.

21 Recusani, F., Bargiggia, G.S., Yoganathan, A.P., *et al.* (1991) A new method for quantification of regurgitant flow rate using color Doppler flow imaging of the flow convergence region proximal to a discrete orifice, an *in vitro* study. *Circulation* **83**, 594–604.

22 Utsunomiya, T., Ogawa, T., Doshi, R., *et al.* (1991) Doppler color flow 'proximal isovelocity surface area' method for estimating volume flow rate: effects of orifice shape and machine factors. *Journal of the American College of Cardiology* **17**, 1103–1111.

23 Guiney, T.E., Davies, M.J., Parker, D.J., Leech, G.J., Leatham, A. (1987) The aetiology and course of isolated severe aortic regurgitation: a clinical, pathological, and echocardiographic study. *British Heart Journal* **58**, 358–368.

24 Hatle, L., Angelsen, B.A., Tromsdal, A. (1980) Non-invasive assessment of aortic stenosis by Doppler ultrasound. *British Heart Journal* **43**, 284–292.

25 Hegranaes, L., Hatle, L. (1985) Aortic stenosis in adults. Non-invasive estimation of pressure differences by continuous wave Doppler echocardiography. *British Heart Journal* **54**, 396–404.

26 Richards, K.L., Cannon, S.R., Miller, J.F., *et al.* (1986) Calculation of aortic valve area by Doppler echocardiography. A direct application of the continuity equation. *Circulation* **73**, 964–969.

27 Roger, V.L., Tajik, A.J., Bailey, K.R., Oh, J.K., Taylor, C.L., Seward, J.B. (1990) Progression of aortic stenosis in adults: new appraisal using Doppler echocardiography. *American Heart Journal* **119**, 331–338.

28 Sadee, A.S., Becker, A.E., Verheul, H.A., Bouma, B., Hoedemaker, G. (1992) Aortic valve regurgitation and the congenitally bicuspid aortic valve: a clinico-pathological correlation. *British Heart Journal* **67**, 439–441.

29 Rippe, J.M., Angoff, G., Sloss, L.J., Wynne, J., Alpert, J.S. (1979) Multiple floppy valves: an echocardiographic syndrome. *American Journal of Medicine* **66**, 817–824.

30 Rodger, J.C., Morley, P. (1982) Abnormal aortic valve echoes in mitral prolapse. *British Heart Journal* **47**, 337–343.

31 Hahn, T.R., Roman, M.J., Mogtader, A.H., Devereux, R.B. (1992) Association of aortic dilatation with regurgitant, stenotic and functionally normal bicuspid aortic valves. *Journal of the American College of Cardiology* **19**, 283–288.

32 Teague, S.M., Heinsimer, J.A., Anderson, J.L., *et al.* (1986) Quantification of aortic regurgitation utilizing continuous wave Doppler ultrasound. *Journal of the American College of Cardiology* **8**, 592–599.

33 Perry, G.J., Helmcke, F., Nanda, N.C., *et al.* (1987) Evaluation of aortic insufficiency by Doppler color flow mapping. *Journal of the American College of Cardiology* **9**, 952–959.

34 Hatle, L., Rosketh, R. (1981) Noninvasive estimation of pulmonary artery systolic pressure with Doppler ultrasound. *British Heart Journal* **45**, 157–165.

35 Waggoner, A.D., Barzilai, B., Perez, J.E. (1990) Saline contrast enhancement of tricuspid regurgitant jets detected by Doppler colour flow imaging. *American Journal of Cardiology* **65**, 1368–1371.

36 Daniels, S.J., Mintz, G.S., Kotler, M.N. (1983) Rheumatic tricuspid valve disease. Two-dimensional echocardiographic, hemodynamic, and angiographic correlations. *American Journal of Cardiology* **51**, 492–496.

37 Chopra, H.K., Nanda, N.C., Fan, P., *et al.* (1989) Can two-dimensional echocardiography and Doppler color flow mapping identify the need for tricuspid valve repair? *Journal of the American College of Cardiology* **14**, 1266–1274.

38 Callahan, J., Wroblewski, E.M., Reeder, G.S., *et al.* (1982) Echocardiographic features of carcinoid heart disease. *American Journal of Cardiology* **50**, 762–768.

39 Pennestri, F., Loperfido, F., Salvatori, M.P., *et al.* (1984) Assessment of tricuspid regurgitation by pulsed Doppler ultrasonography of the hepatic veins. *American Journal of Cardiology* **54**, 363–368.

40 Lima, C.O., Sahn, D.J., Valdes-Cruz, L.M., *et al.* (1983) Noninvasive prediction of transvalvular pressure gradient in patients with pulmonary stenosis by quantitative two-dimensional echocardiography Doppler studies. *Circulation* **67**, 866–871.

41 Chan, P., Ogilby, J.D., Segal, B. (1989) Tricuspid valve endocarditis. *American Heart Journal* **117**, 1140–1146.

42 Mugge, A., Daniel, W.G., Frank, G., Lichtlen, P.R. (1989) Echocardiography in infective endocarditis: reassessment of prognostic implications of vegetation size determined by the transthoracic and the transesophageal approach. *Journal of the American College of Cardiology* **14**, 631–638.

43 Daniel, W.G., Mugge, A., Martin, R.P., *et al.* (1991) Improvement in the diagnosis of abscesses associated with endocarditis by transesophageal echocardiography. *New England Journal of Medicine* **324**, 795–800.

Chapter 10: Left ventricular function

T. McDonagh

Echocardiography has become an invaluable tool in the non-invasive assessment of left ventricular function. This has coincided with an increase in the prevalence, incidence and the emergence of therapeutic advances for the syndrome of chronic heart failure [1,2].

Chronic heart failure (CHF) is not a diagnosis *per se* but a clinical syndrome whose symptoms and signs are ultimately due to cardiac dysfunction. In Western industrialized societies, CHF is most commonly attributable to left ventricular dysfunction, in particular to left ventricular systolic dysfunction, mainly arising as the result of ischaemic heart disease, usually due to a myocardial infarction. Moreover, we are now increasingly aware that CHF lies at the endstage of a continuum which is often preceded by a long latent phase of asymptomatic left ventricular systolic dysfunction, where the disease is clinically silent but left ventricular damage is present. A smaller proportion of CHF is due to diastolic dysfunction of the left ventricle [3]. This is thought to be associated with a better prognosis than systolic dysfunction [4].

Recent therapeutic advances have shown that patients with both symptomatic and asymptomatic left ventricular systolic dysfunction benefit, in terms of mortality and morbidity, from treatment with angiotensin-converting enzyme inhibitors [5,6]. Unfortunately, the diagnosis of CHF is often inaccurate because its symptoms and signs lack sensitivity and specificity [7]. Echocardiography has a pivotal role initially in the establishment of the diagnosis of left ventricular dysfunction, and then in the characterization of the nature of that dysfunction, i.e systolic or diastolic. The latter role is useful in risk stratification, as the presence of systolic dysfunction confers a poorer prognosis [8], as well as being invaluable in guiding further management.

Other imaging modalities are useful in assessing left ventricular function. Contrast angiography remains the gold standard for systolic function but is invasive and therefore has limited application. Radionuclide ventriculography provides accurate and reproducible measures of left ventricular systolic function. It is, however, more limited in its ability to give other information, is less widely available than echocardiography and involves the use of radioactive isotopes. While magnetic resonance imaging is having an emerging role in assessing left ventricular function, its position remains to be established. Echocardiography provides the nearest we have to an ideal test for left ventricular function, being widely available, non-invasive and by its power in providing other important information about the heart such as valve function, structural abnormalities and its ability to aid in the diagnosis of cardiomyopathies (all of which may manifest as heart failure).

In this chapter the assessment of left ventricular function is considered under four main headings: global systolic function, regional systolic function, associated abnormalities and diastolic function.

Global systolic function

There are numerous parameters to describe the overall contractile function of the left ventricle. The most commonly quoted is the left ventricular ejection fraction (LVEF). This is chiefly because it is a measure of left ventricular function which has both clinical and prognostic significance [9,10]. Quantifying left ventricular performance has become important since the major heart failure and postmyocardial dysfunction treatment trials used ejection fraction cut-offs as entry criteria. In the studies of left ventricular dysfunction (SOLVD) trials, patients with an LVEF of less than or equal to 35% benefited from angiotensin-converting enzyme inhibitor therapy [5,6], while it was an LVEF of less than or equal to 40% in the survival and ventricular enlargement (SAVE) study [11]. LVEF can be obtained from different echocardiographic modes. LVEF and various other parameters used to describe systolic function are considered in greater detail below.

Single plane measurements

M-MODE

Perhaps the simplest and most frequently used method for assessing left ventricular function is that obtained by two-dimensional (2D) guided M-mode echocardiography. This is usually carried out in the parasternal long axis view, but can also be obtained from the parasternal short axis view at the mitral valve level. Measurements should be made at the level of the tips of the mitral valve leaflets with the M-mode beam perpendicular to the interventricular septum and the left ventricular posterior wall (Fig. 10.1). This is in accordance with the American Society of Echocardiography leading edge to leading edge methodology, and employing the criteria of Schieken *et al.* to determine acceptable image quality for M-mode recordings [12]. For accurate measurements, the mean of three cardiac cycles should be taken.

The simplest measurements obtained by this method are the left ventricular end-diastolic (LVEDD) and systolic (LVESD) dimensions. The normal range of these vary with sex and height, but an LVEDD over or equal to 5.6 cm is usually considered dilated. Various derived measurements using these two basic parameters are often used in clinical practice.

Fractional shortening (FS) is the degree of change of the M-mode dimension of the left ventricle from diastole to systole. It is directly related to the ejection fraction [13] and is calculated from the formula:

$$\text{FS}\ (\%) = 100 \times \frac{(\text{LVEDD} - \text{LVESD})}{\text{LVEDD}}.$$

LVEF is the left ventricular volume in diastole minus that in systole, divided by the diastolic volume and expressed as a percentage. The lengths outlined above are converted to volumes by the Teicholz formula [3]:

$$\text{Volume} = \left(7/24 + \text{the dimension}\right)/\text{dimension}.$$

While these measurements can be useful and convenient, they can only be used to describe left ventricular function meaningfully in the absence of a regional wall motion abnormality.

Other single plane measurements which try to take some account of asymmetric contraction are left ventricular areas, volumes or ejection fractions derived from tracing around the endocardium of the left ventricle (in systole and diastole) in one of either the long axis, short axis, apical four- or two-chamber views. These methods rely on converting the subsequent lengths and areas obtained to volumes by making assumptions about the geometry of the heart, e.g. the area length method from the apical two-chamber view. These methods have been shown to correlate well with cavity volumes derived angiographically or from radionuclide ventriculography [14]. However, they share the limitations of M-mode measures in that they are not accurate in the presence of regional wall motion abnormalities [15]. This is hardly surprising as the assumptions made about the geometry

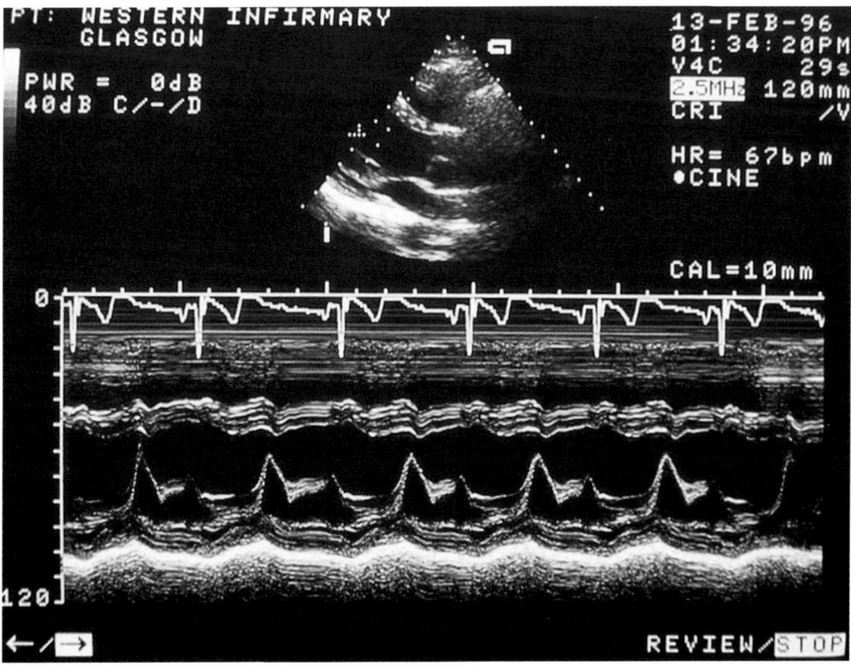

Fig. 10.1 M-mode slide.

of the healthy heart are unlikely to be maintained in the diseased and poorly contractile one.

A number of other M-mode variables relate to survival in subjects with reduced left ventricular function. These include the left ventricular end-diastolic size indexed to body surface area, the systolic diameter/wall thickness ratio and the mitral E point septal separation (the distance between the E point of the mitral valve and the interventricular septum) [16,17].

BIPLANE METHODS

Measurements utilizing more than one echocardiographic plane produce more accurate measures of left ventricular function. Of these, the modified biplane Simpson's rule for the determination of left ventricular volumes provides the most accurate measure of ejection fraction obtainable by echocardiography [18]. Its correlation with radionuclide and angiographic measures of LVEF is superior to other echocardiographic calculations [19]. It is also the most valid measurement in the presence of a regional wall motion abnormality [20]. It is obtained by tracing around the endocardium in systole and diastole, in triplicate, in the apical four- and two-chamber views (Fig. 10.2). It is unfortunately time-consuming and labour intensive. It also depends on having at least 80% of the endocardium available for analysis. As such its use is mainly restricted to research settings. Automated border detection has allowed on-line analysis and this may become available in the future. At the moment there are problems with obtaining adequate images for automatic detection in 25–50% of cases and, despite earlier promising correlations with left ventricular volumes, adaptation of the method to subjects with diseased hearts resulted in much poorer agreement with radionuclide and angiographic methods [21].

Due to the laborious nature of the manual biplane methods for assessing left ventricular function, the most commonly used parameter in clinical practice is the so-called 'eyeball' technique, whereby the ventricle is described as having either normal function or function that is mildly, moderately or severely impaired. In skilled hands the eyeball technique correlates well with angiographic and radionuclide measures of left ventricular function [19].

A word of caution is required regarding the quantification of left ventricular function by echocardiography. All measures of left ventricular function are subject to variability and error. There is appreciable intra- and interobserver variation in the conversion of the 2D image to figures as well as the error introduced by different sonographers acquiring the images, the different hardware used to obtain the images and the variation in software and the geometric formulas which are used to derive the left ventricular areas, volumes and, ultimately, ejection fraction. For these reasons, normal ranges for left ventricular function should be interpreted in the light of the normal range for the centre using particular equipment and personnel [22]. Normal ranges in textbooks for LVEF must be treated with some caution as they are based on small numbers of healthy young adults; there are very few population-based studies. The lower end of the normal range for echocardiographic ejection fraction varies from 40 to 50%.

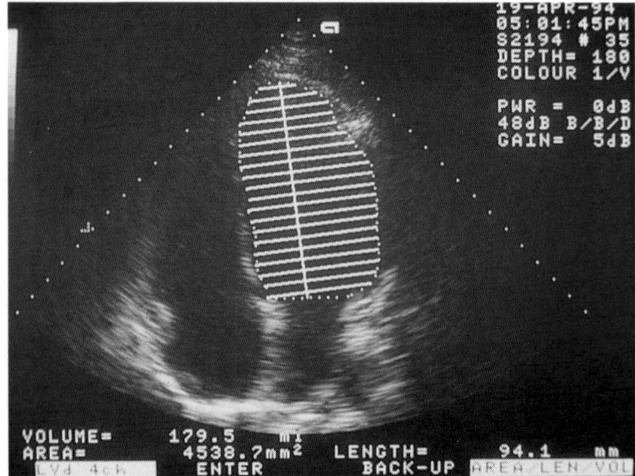

(a)

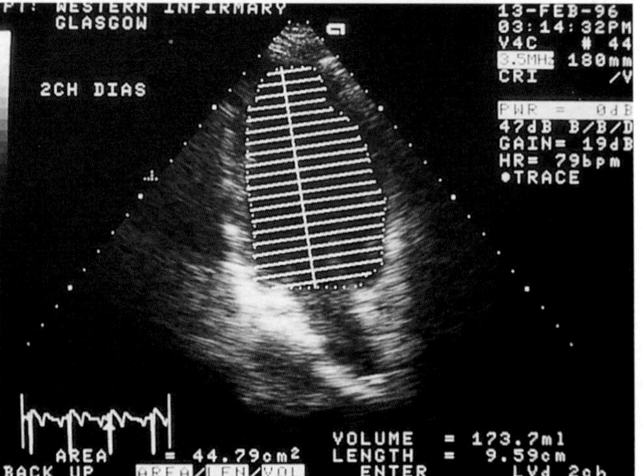

(b)

Fig. 10.2 Apical (a) four- and (b) two-chamber views with Simpson's rule.

DOPPLER ECHOCARDIOGRAPHY

The change in left ventricular pressure over time ($\Delta P/\Delta t$) and the maximum rate of the pressure change ($\Delta P/\Delta t_{max}$), usually measured during cardiac catheterization are good indicators of the contractile state of the myocardium. They can be derived in left ventricular systolic dysfunction by Doppler echocardiography of the (frequently present) mitral regurgitant jet. Using continuous wave Doppler

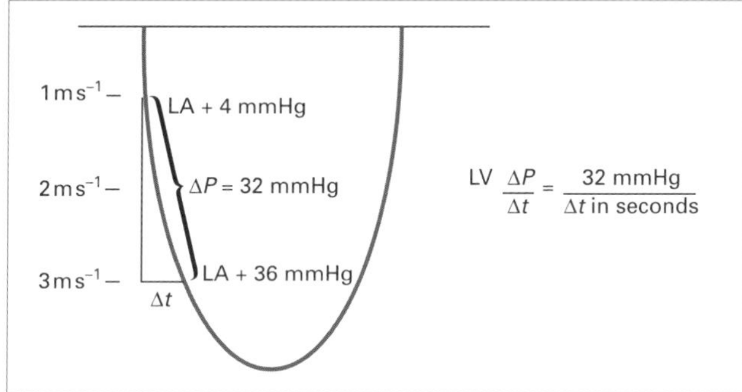

Fig. 10.3 The mitral regurgitant jet is converted to pressures using the modified Bernoulli equation. The time taken to measure the signal rise from 1 to 3 $m\,s^{-1}$ is measured. This equates to a change in left ventricular (LV) pressure from left atrial (LA) pressure + 4 mmHg to LA pressure + 32 mmHg.

echocardiography of the mitral regurgitant jet in the apical four-chamber view and applying the modified Bernoulli equation, allows a plot of the left ventricular $\Delta P/\Delta t$ from the first derivative of the pressure gradient plot [23,24] (Fig. 10.3).

Regional wall motion

Echocardiography is a powerful tool for evaluating regional wall motion abnormalities. This is one of its main advantages over radionuclide ventriculography [25]. As ischaemic heart disease (IHD) is the commonest cause of left ventricular systolic dysfunction, regional wall motion abnormalities are very prevalent in the condition. However, the absence of a regional wall motion problem does not rule out IHD as the aetiology of the left ventricular systolic dysfunction, as a globally hypokinetic left ventricle can occur in coronary heart disease and, similarly, regional wall motion abnormalities are not infrequent in dilated cardiomyopathies, both idiopathic, and from other causes.

The assessment of regional wall motion offers some advantages over global measures such as ejection fraction, which gives a rough guide to prognosis especially after myocardial infarction, as non-infarcted areas can compensate by contracting more vigorously. In this instance regional wall motion scoring is more accurate in risk stratification for prognostic purposes [26]. Wall motion scoring can be used to describe qualitatively the site and extent of, for example, an infarct, or it can be used to indirectly measure global left ventricular function by the calculation of a wall motion score index.

There are several schemes for analysing regional wall motion. Wall motion is quantified as a wall motion score index by adding the segment scores and dividing by the numbers of segments. The most widely used quantitative method is the ASE (American Society of Echocardiography) 16 segment method (Fig. 10.4). This has the advantage of allowing assessment of the segments from the three short axis views (at the level of the mitral valve, mid papillary muscles and apex) or by visualizing the segments in the parasternal long axis and apical four- and two-chamber views. These segments correspond to coronary artery distributions. The scoring system normally applied with this system qualitatively assesses each segment on a scale of 1–4, with 1 corresponding to normokinesia, 2 hypokinesia, 3 akinesia and 4 dyskinesia. High scores are associated with a poor prognosis.

Recently, a simpler wall motion score index using the nine segment method has become widely used [27]. It is simpler to obtain; segments can be substituted from all the standard 2D views. A decremental scoring system is used whereby, 0 = akinesia, 1 = hypokinesia, 2 = normokinesia and −1 = dyskinesia. The wall motion score index, derived by summing the scores and dividing by the number of segments, correlates well with the LVEF. Such a method was used to recruit patients in the TRACE study, where the use of an angiotensin-converting enzyme inhibitor was found significantly to reduce mortality in subjects with postmyocardial infarction, whose wall motion score index was less than or equal to 1.2, corresponding to a LVEF of less than or equal to 35% [28]. This measurement is obtainable much more easily than the Simpson's biplane ejection fraction.

Associated abnormalities

Echocardiography is also very useful in the detection of structural abnormalities frequently associated with or caused by systolic dysfunction. These include left ventricular aneurysms, thrombi, mitral incompetence, ventricular septal defects and pericardial effusions.

The presence of pulmonary hypertension is also associated with a poor prognosis in left ventricular systolic dysfunction [29]. It can be assessed by Doppler echocardiography indirectly by measuring the peak velocity of the tricuspid regurgitant jet. Using the Bernoulli equation and adding a correction for the right atrial pressure, i.e. $4 \times V^2_{max} + 6$ mmHg allows estimation of the pulmonary artery systolic pressure in millimetres of mercury.

An ever-increasing application of transthoracic echocardiography in the assessment of left ventricular function is the use of stress echocardiography. An increasing body of evidence suggests that hibernating myocardium (i.e. cardiac muscle that is hypoperfused but viable) may occur in up to 45% of patients with coronary artery disease [30]. Hibernating myocardium is hypocontractile. This is reversible by revascularization. Low dose dobutamine echocardiography has a similar sensitivity to

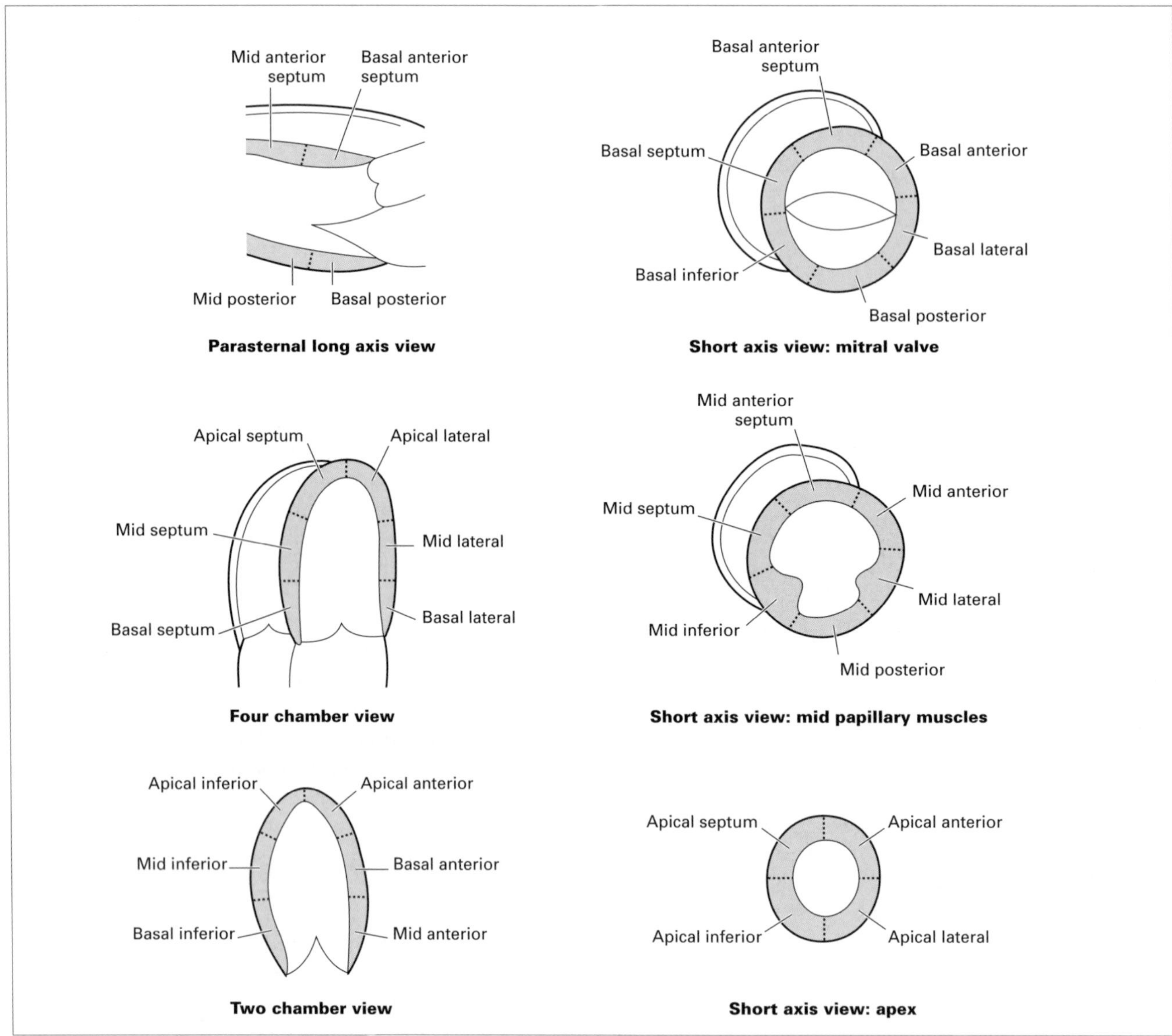

Fig. 10.4 ASE 16 segment method.

redistribution thallium scintigraphy in detecting hibernation [31]. Classically, wall segments change from akinetic to kinetic on the low dose dobutamine but deteriorate at high dose dobutamine. This so-called biphasic response has the best predictive value for the presence of hibernating myocardium [32].

Diastolic function

The definition of diastolic dysfunction, where there is abnormal relaxation of the left ventricle is much more confused than that of systolic dysfunction. Diastole itself is a complex mixture of active and passive relaxation (compliance). Numerous measurements have been advocated but none has achieved widespread application.

Diastolic dysfunction occurs in a number of pathological processes affecting the heart. It is often seen in left ventricular hypertrophy, hypertrophic cardiomyopathy and in infiltrative states such as amyloid. It can also coexist with systolic dysfunction due to IHD.

Diastolic function is most often assessed by examination of the mitral valve inflow pattern using pulsed wave (PW) Doppler echocardiography [33]. The PW sampling callipers should be placed between the tips of the mitral valve leaflets in the apical four-chamber view. The

Doppler beam should be parallel to the direction of flow. Measurements should not be made if the angle between the Doppler beam and the inflow jet is over 30° or if the heart rate is over 100 beats min^{-1}. The Doppler measurements made should be from a minimum of five readings to minimize the influence of respiration on the envelopes [34].

The resultant tracing is shown in Fig. 10.5. The E wave is caused by early, passive ventricular filling and the smaller A wave is due to atrial contraction. The E wave is normally greater than the A wave. The relationship between these two parameters is normally expressed as the E/A ratio and should be greater than 1. However, the situation is complicated by the fact that the E/A ratio reduces with age (presumably as the myocardium becomes stiffer due to replacement by fibrous tissue, with a reduction in its compliance) [35]. E/A ratios should therefore be age-corrected.

Due to the complexity of diastolic filling, a single variable such as the peak E or A velocity or their ratio cannot reliably describe abnormality. Therefore, other parameters are normally combined. These include the deceleration time of the peak velocity of the E wave and the isovolumic relaxation time (IVRT) [36].

The IVRT represents the period of time from aortic valve closure to mitral valve opening. Accurate measurement requires concurrent phonocardiography on the mitral valve inflow signal or placement of the PW sampler so that it simultaneously samples mitral inflow and aortic outflow. The IVRT reflects the rate of myocardial relaxation and is probably the most sensitive indicator of impaired relaxation [36]. The normal range varies from 60 to 90 ms.

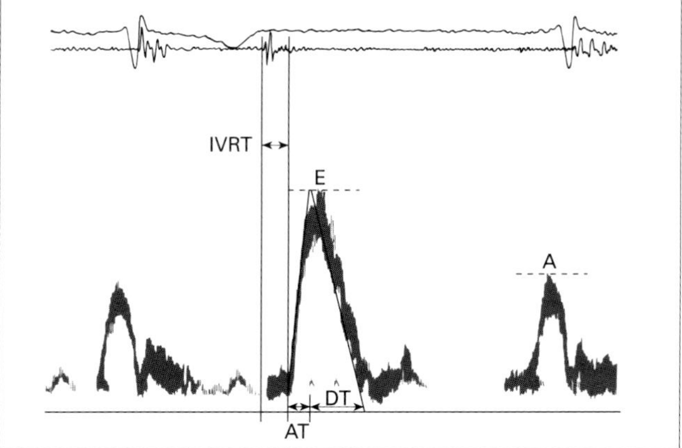

Fig. 10.5 Mitral valve inflow pattern using pulsed wave Doppler echocardiography. AT, acceleration time; DT, deceleration time; IVRT, isovolumic relaxation time.

The deceleration time (DT) is measured as the interval of time from the peak of the E wave to the intersection of the flow velocity envelope with the baseline. The mean value is 193 ± 23 ms. Heart rate has little effect on the DT. A prolonged DT is a more sensitive index than E/A ratio in detecting abnormal myocardial relaxation [37].

Two general patterns of diastolic dysfunction are recognized by mitral inflow Doppler parameters. The first is the abnormal relaxation pattern [36], characterized by a prolonged IVRT, prolonged DT (>250 ms) with an E/A ratio of less than 1. This is found in IHD, hypertension, advanced age and dilated, infiltrative and hypertrophic cardiomyopathies. The second type is the restrictive pattern, characterized by a decreased IVRT, short DT (<150 ms) and an increase in the E/A ratio. This pattern is reported in the advanced stages of cardiac amyloid, hypertrophic obstructive cardiomyopathy with mitral incompetence and end-stage dilated cardiomyopathy, constrictive pericarditis and when the pulmonary capillary wedge pressure is over or equal to 16 mmHg [33]. The picture is further complicated by the fact that an E/A ratio and DT which fall within the normal range does not rule out diastolic dysfunction as there can be an evolving continuum from the relaxation deficit to the restrictive pattern meaning that some patients have normal patterns; so-called 'pseudo-normalization' [38].

Diastolic function can also be assessed by examining the pattern of pulmonary venous flow. While this is more usually attempted at transoesophageal studies, it is also possible by transthoracic echocardiography. Normally a triphasic pattern is seen, with forward flow occurring during both ventricular systole and atrial diastole with flow reversal during atrial contraction [36]. Impaired ventricular relaxation results in a reduction in pulmonary venous flow during ventricular diastole. The restrictive defect increases the atrial reversal.

Conclusion

Echocardiography plays a pivotal role in the assessment of left ventricular function. Its only real weakness has been in the reliable quantification of left ventricular function which has inevitably followed on from the results of the angiotensin-converting enzyme inhibitor clinical trials. Echocardiography is set to become more important as advances in ultrasound technology and the availability of contrast agents allow quantification of left ventricular function to become more accurate.

References

1 Gillum, R.F. (1987) Heart failure in the United States 1970–1985. *American Heart Journal* **113**, 1043–1045.

2 Swedberg, K., Idanpaan Heikkila, U., Remes, J., *et al.* (1987) Effects of enalapril on mortality in severe congestive heart failure. Results of the Cooperative North Scandinavian Enalapril Survival Study (CONSENSUS). *New England Journal of Medicine* **316**, 1429–1435.

3 Soufer, R., Wohlgelertner, D., Vita, N.A., Amuchestegui, M., Sostman, H.D., Berger, H.J. (1985) Intact systolic left ventricular function in congestive heart failure. *American Journal of Cardiology* **55**, 1032–1036.

4 Dougherty, A.H., Nacarelli, G.V., Gray, E.L., Hicks, C.H., Goldstein, R.A. (1984) Congestive heart failure with normal systolic function. *American Journal of Cardiology* **54**, 778–782.

5 The SOLVD Investigators (1991) Effect of enalapril on survival in patients with reduced left ventricular ejection fractions and congestive heart failure. *New England Journal of Medicine* **325**, 293–302.

6 The SOLVD Investigators (1992) Effect of enalapril on mortality and the development of heart failure in asymptomatic patients with reduced left ventricular ejection fractions. *New England Journal of Medicine* **327**, 685–691. [published erratum appears in *New England Journal of Medicine*, 1992, **327**, 1768.]

7 Wheeldon, N.M., MacDonald, T.M., Flucker, C.J., McKendrick, A.D., McDevitt, D.G., Struthers, A.D. (1993) Echocardiography in chronic heart failure in the community [see comments]. *Quarterly Journal of Medicine* **86**, 17–23.

8 McKee, P.A., Castelli, W.P., McNamara, P.M., Kannel, W.B. (1971) The natural history of congestive heart failure: the Framingham study. *New England Journal of Medicine* **285**, 1441–1446.

9 Murray, J.A., Chinn, N., Peterson, D.R. (1974) Influence of left ventricular function on early prognosis in atherosclerotic heart disease. *American Journal of Cardiology* **33**, 159.

10 Nelson, N.B., Cohn, P.F., Garlin, R. (1975) Prognosis in medically treated coronary artery disease. Influence of ejection fraction compared to other parameters. *Circulation* **52**, 408.

11 Pfeffer, M.A., Braunwald, E., Moye, L.A., *et al.* (1992) Effect of captopril on mortality and morbidity in patients with left ventricular dysfunction after myocardial infarction. Results of the survival and ventricular enlargement trial. The SAVE Investigators. *New England Journal of Medicine* **327**, 669–677.

12 Schieken, R., Clarke, W., Mahoney, L., Lauer, R. (1979) Measurement criteria for group echocardiographic studies. *American Journal of Epidemiology* **110**, 504–514.

13 Fortun, N., Hood, W.J., Sherman, M., Craige, E. (1971) Determination of left ventricular volumes by ultrasound. *Circulation* **44**, 575.

14 Folland, E.D., Parisi, A.F., Moynihan, P.F., Jones, D.R., Feldman, C.L., Tow, D.E. (1979) Assessment of left ventricular ejection fraction and volumes by real-time, two-dimensional echocardiography. *Circulation* **60**, 760–766.

15 Gueret, P., Meerbaum, S., Wyatt, H., *et al.* (1980) Two-dimensional echocardiographic quantitation of left ventricular volumes and ejection fraction. Importance of accounting for dyssynergy in short-axis reconstruction models. *Circulation* **62**, 1308–1318.

16 Lee, T.H., Hamilton, M.A., Stevenson, L.W., *et al.* (1993) Impact of left ventricular cavity size on survival in advanced heart failure. *American Journal of Cardiology* **72**, 672–676.

17 Wong, M., Johnson, G., Shabetai, R., *et al.* (1993) Echocardiographic variables as prognostic indicators and therapeutic monitors in chronic congestive heart failure. Veterans Affairs cooperative studies V-HeFT I and II. V-HeFT VA Cooperative Studies Group. *Circulation* **87**, V165–V170.

18 Schiller, N.B., Acquatella, H., Ports, T.A., *et al.* (1979) Left ventricular volume from paired biplane two-dimensional echocardiography. *Circulation* **60**, 547–555.

19 Stamm, R.B., Carabello, B.A., Mayers, D.L., Martin, R.P. (1992) Two-dimensional echocardiographic measurement of left ventricular ejection fraction: prospective analysis of what constitutes an adequate determination. *American Heart Journal* **104**, 136–144.

20 Albin, G., Rahko, P.S. (1990) Comparison of echocardiographic quantitation of left ventricular ejection fraction to radionuclide angiography in patients with regional wall motion abnormalities. *American Journal of Cardiology* **65**, 1031–1032.

21 Herregods, M.C., Vermylen, J., Bynens, B., De Geest, H., Van de Werf, F. (1993) On -line quantification of left ventricular function by automatic boundary detection system and comparison with radionuclide ventriculography and ultrasonic backscatter imaging. *American Journal of Cardiology* **72**, 195–199.

22 Ray, S.G., Metcalfe, M.J., Oldroyd, K.G., *et al.* (1995) Do radionuclide and echocardiographic techniques give a universal cut-off value for left ventricular ejection fraction that can be used to select patients for treatment with ACE inhibitors after myocardial infarction? *British Heart Journal* **73**, 466–469.

23 Recusani, F. (1991) Noninvasive assessment of left ventricular function with continuous wave Doppler echocardiography. *Circulation* **83**, 2141–2143.

24 Chen, C., Rodriguez, L., Lethor, J.P. (1994) Continuous wave Doppler echocardiography for noninvasive assessment of left ventricular dP/dt and relaxation time constant from mitral regurgitation spectra in patients. *Journal of the American College of Cardiology* **23**, 970–976.

25 Van Reet, R.E., Quinones, M.A., Poliner, L.R., *et al.* (1984) Comparison of two-dimensional echocardiography with gated radionuclide ventriculography in the evaluation of global and regional left ventricular function in acute myocardial infarction. *Journal of the American College of Cardiology* **3**, 243–252.

26 Kan, G., Visser, C.A., Koolen, J.J., Dunning, A.J. (1986) Short and long term predictive value of admission wall motion score in acute myocardial infarction. A cross sectional echocardiographic study of 345 patients. *British Heart Journal* **56**, 422–427.

27 Kober, L., Torp-Pedersen, C., Carlsen, J., Videbaek, R., Egeblad, H. (1994) An echocardiographic method for selecting high risk patients shortly after acute myocardial infarction, for inclusion in multi-centre studies (as used in the TRACE study). *European Heart Journal* **15**, 1616–1620.

28 Kober, L., Torp-Pedersen, C., Carlsen, J.E., *et al.* (1995) A clinical trial of the angiotensin-converting enzyme trandolapril in patients with left ventricular dysfunction after myocardial infarction. *New England Journal of Medicine* **327**, 1670–1676.

29 Abramson, S., Burke, J., Kelly, J.L., *et al.* (1992) Pulmonary hypertension predicts mortality and morbidity in patients with dilated cardiomyopathy. *Annals of Internal Medicine* **116**, 888–895.

30 Lewis, S.J., Sawada, S.G., Ryan, T., *et al.* (1991) Segmental wall motion abnormalities in the absence of clinically documented myocardial infarction. Clinical significance of hibernating myocardium. *American Heart Journal* **121**, 1088.

31 Cigarroa, C.G., de Filippi, C.R., Brickner, M.E. (1993) Dobutamine stress echocardiography identifies hibernating myocardium and predicts recovery of left ventricular function after coronary revascularisation. *Circulation* **38**, 430.

32 Alfridi, I., Kleidman, N.S., Raizner, A.E., Zoghbi, W.A. (1995) Dobutamine echocardiography in myocardial hibernation.

Optimal dose and accuracy in predicting recovery of left ventricular function after coronary angioplasty. *Circulation* **91**, 663.

33 Thomas, J.D., Weyman, A.E. (1991) Echocardiographic Doppler evaluation of left ventricular diastolic function—physics and physiology. *Circulation* **84**, 977–990.

34 Benjamin, E.J., Levy, D., Anderson, K.M., *et al.* (1992) Determinants of Doppler indexes of left ventricular diastolic function in normal subjects (the Framingham Heart Study). *American Journal of Cardiology* **70**, 515.

35 Pearson, A.C., Gudipati, C.V., Labovitz, A.J. (1991) Effects of aging on left ventricular structure and function. *American Heart Journal* **121**, 622–627.

36 Nishimura, R.A., Abel, M.D., Hatle, L.K., Tajik, A.J. (1989) Assessment of diastolic function of the heart: background and current applications of Doppler echocardiography. *Mayo Clinics Proceedings* **64**, 181–204.

37 Himura, Y., Toshiaki, K., Kambayashi, M. (1991) Importance of left ventricular systolic function in the assessment of left ventricular diastolic function with Doppler transmitral flow velocity recording. *Journal of the American College of Cardiology* **18**, 753–760.

38 Taylor, R., Waggoner, A.D. (1992) Doppler assessment of left ventricular diastolic dysfunction: a review. *Journal of the American Society of Echocardiography* **5**, 603–612.

Chapter 11: Cardiomyopathies and pericardial disease

C.A. Roobottom & P. Wilde

Pericardial disease

Many diseases affect the pericardium but the response of the pericardial tissues is limited and manifests itself in only three ways as pericardial effusion, pericardial thickening or pericardial masses. While other imaging techniques, particularly magnetic resonance imaging (MRI), may be more sensitive than echocardiography in certain aspects of pericardial disease [1] it remains an excellent method of demonstrating the majority of pericardial diseases and, because of its simplicity and wide availability, should be considered the primary imaging investigation in all patients suspected of pericardial disease.

Normal appearances of the pericardium

The normal pericardium consists of two layers, fibrous and visceral. The fibrous layer is conical in shape and is continuous with the diaphragm below and fuses with the origin of the great vessels above. It is usually not identifiable in normal patients. The visceral pericardium is occasionally visualized as a thin echogenic line that should be less than 3 mm thick. It lines the fibrous pericardium and covers the majority of the heart with reflections at the base of the great vessels and the pulmonary veins. There is therefore no space behind the left atrium. Whilst the two layers are separated in healthy subjects by up to 20 ml of fluid this is not usually discernible at echocardiography and demonstration of more than 1–2 ml of fluid should be considered abnormal.

Diagnosis of a pericardial effusion

Collection of abnormal amounts of fluid usually produces an echo-free space surrounding the heart. In order to detect effusions accurately it is important to set the gain controls carefully to allow epicardial fat to be differentiated from fluid, the former containing multiple low level echoes. It is also important to set the depth significantly deeper than the posterior heart wall to avoid missing a posterior effusion.

Effusions can be demonstrated both on two-dimensional (2D) and M-mode echocardiography. On M-mode examination pericardial fluid is demonstrable as an echo-free space between the layers of pericardium, mostly posterior to the left ventricle (Fig. 11.1), but not behind the left atrium. However, 2D echocardiography gives greater appreciation of the distribution of fluid than M-mode studies (Fig. 11.2) and is more sensitive as effusions, particularly if small, chronic or of an inflammatory aetiology may be localized and missed if M-mode examination is used in isolation [2]. A number of conditions and normal variants can produce echo-free areas and must be differentiated before a diagnosis of pericardial effusion is made (Table 11.1). These can be differentiated by knowledge of their typical site and the search for fluid in extrapericardial locations. Care must be taken to ensure that isoechoic effusions are not overlooked. These occur in effusions of an infective or traumatic aetiology and appear as a rind of echoes that obliterate or reduce the typical echo-free space [3].

Once diagnosed a pericardial effusion should be assessed in terms of size and appearance, and a search for an underlying cause begun. The heart should be examined in detail to look for evidence of abnormal cardiac function and any evidence to suggest that the effusion is causing cardiac tamponade. Quantification of the size of the effusion is best made by experience and should be described as small, moderate or large. More complex methods of quantification by subtraction of estimated cardiac volume from pericardial sac volume can be used but are only an approximation and can be unreliable.

Several features are useful in indicating the aetiology of the pericardial effusion. Thickening (predominantly of the serous) pericardium with fibrous strands projecting into the fluid is often seen in infective and inflammatory effusions. Masses within the effusion commonly occur with malignancy and haemorrhagic effusions. Mobile masses are usually fibrous in nature whilst neoplastic masses are more often adherent to the pericardium.

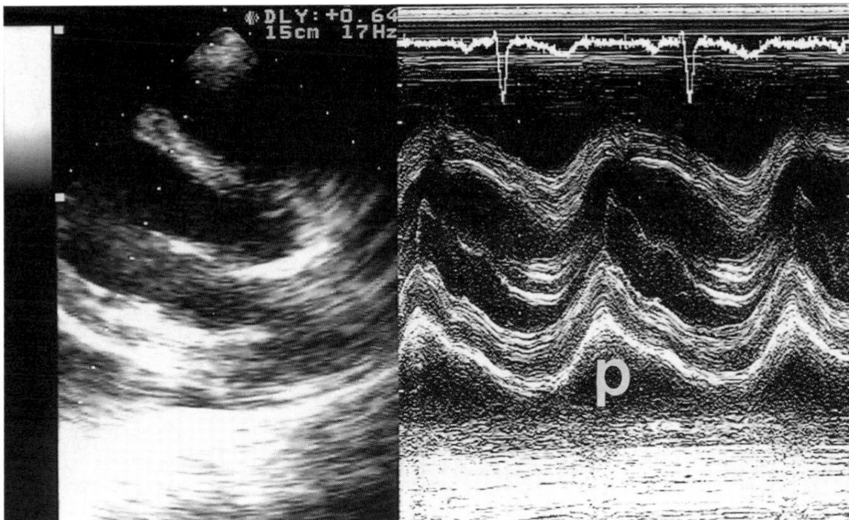

Fig. 11.1 Long axis parasternal view with the accompanying M-mode trace showing a simple pericardial effusion demonstrating an echo-free space and posteriorly (p) to the left ventricle.

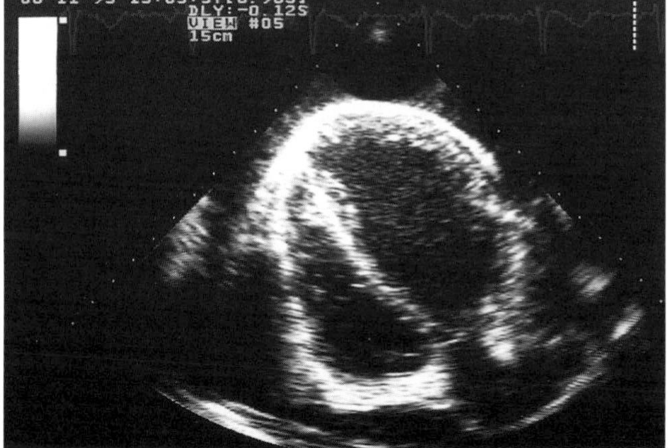

(a)

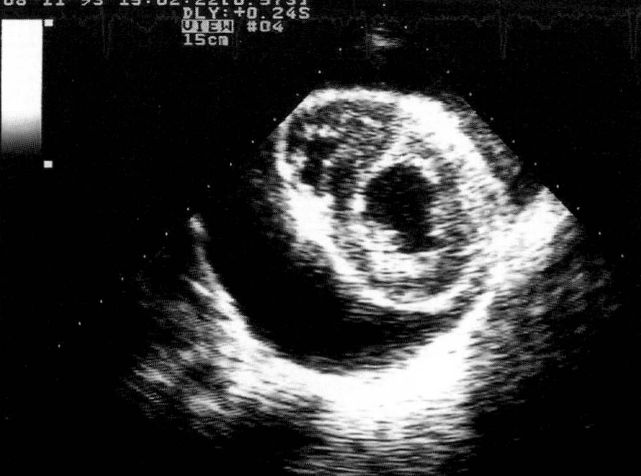

(b)

Fig. 11.2 Two-dimensional echocardiography of a large pericardial effusion both in apical four-chamber (a) and short axis (b) views.

Table 11.1 Echo-poor structures that may mimic pericardial effusions

Normal structures or variants	Pericardial fat pads Subepicardial fat Descending aorta Enlarged left atrium Pericardial cyst
Fluid collections	Pleural effusion Ascites
Abnormal masses	Pericardial tumours Morgagni hernias

Simple effusions are the most common and may occur with any of the possible causes of effusion (see Table 11.2). Features suggesting cardiac tamponade are discussed below.

Specific types of pericardial effusion

INFECTIVE PERICARDITIS

Viral pericarditis is the most common cause of pericardial effusion and presents as a simple effusion. This may be accompanied by impairment of ventricular contractility if there is associated myocarditis.

Pyopericardium secondary to bacterial infection is uncommon. Spread is either direct or haematogenous in nature. The effusion is often echogenic (Fig. 11.3) and can be difficult to appreciate. Occasionally a pericardial 'peel' may be seen lying within the pericardial effusion [3]. Pericardial tamponade may develop rapidly in bacterial

Table 11.2 Causes of pericardial effusion

Infective	Viral Bacterial Tuberculous
Autoimmune	Dressler's syndrome Rheumatoid arthritis Systemic lupus erythematosus Rheumatic fever
Secondary to myocardial disease	Heart failure (whatever cause) Myocarditis Myocardial infarction Myocardial trauma Aortic dissection
Malignancy	Metastastic Direct involvement Lymphomatous Primary myocardial and pericardial
Systemic disease	Uraemia Myxoedema

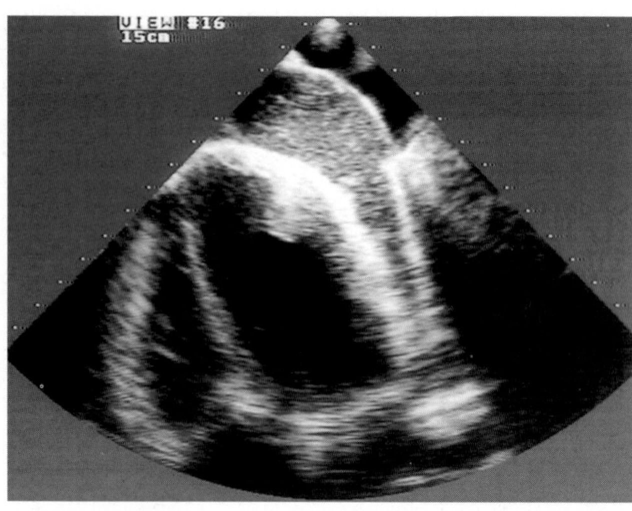

Fig. 11.3 An example of a complicated pericardial effusion in a patient with a pyopericardium. Note the high level of echoes seen in the effusion.

pyocardium and drainage should be performed in all cases. Despite appropriate drainage and medical treatment there is a tendency to reoccurrence and loculation. Pericardial constriction is an unpredictable but not infrequent occurrence that can occur rapidly and require surgical intervention in the acute stage [4] or more commonly several months to years after the acute event. For this reason regular follow-up scans for several years are recommended.

Tuberculous pericarditis may present with pericardial effusion, pericarditis or pericardial constriction. It is always secondary to infection elsewhere but may be the presenting feature. Features include irregular thickening of the pericardium and strands crossing the pericardial space [5] but these are not specific. Effusions are often large at presentation and may produce tamponade, but the rate of its progression is often slower than that of other aetiologies. Antituberculous therapy brings about a reduction in the size of the effusion but is associated with an increased incidence of pericardial thickening and, eventually, pericardial constriction.

Pericardial effusions may also be caused by infradiaphragmatic infections including bacterial subphrenic abscesses and hydatid and amoebic liver abscesses. These tend to be simple in nature unless they have directly breached the diaphragm.

UNDERLYING MYOCARDIAL DISEASE

Pericardial effusions are commonly seen in patients with heart failure and although they may reach considerable size they are unlikely to cause tamponade. The main role of echocardiography is in assessment of myocardial and valvular function.

Small or moderately sized pericardial effusions are seen in approximately one third of patients with myocardial infarction [6]. Because of their higher incidence in large infarcts they are associated with a worse prognosis. Haemopericardium is occasionally seen in patients' postinfarct who experience a sudden deterioration in their condition. This is usually rapidly fatal but when seen the effusion has a low echo pattern compared to other 'complex' effusions as the clot is usually acute. Pericardial effusions are seen weeks to months postinfarct and form part of the spectrum of Dressler's syndrome. The latter only require observation as they very rarely cause either tamponade or pericardial constriction.

Aortic disease is rarely associated with pericardial effusion but when seen is an important sign with sinister implications. Haemopericardium may complicate aortic dissection or rupture, particularly in patients with annuloaortic ectasia. As with myocardial rupture, acute clot appears as low level echoes within the pericardial space and there is often rapid progression to tamponade.

SECONDARY TO MALIGNANCY

Malignant pericardial effusions are common and usually metastatic, (especially from bronchus or breast) or secondary to local invasion from adjacent malignancy, including lymphoma [7]. The effusions usually appear complicated on echocardiography (Fig. 11.4). There may

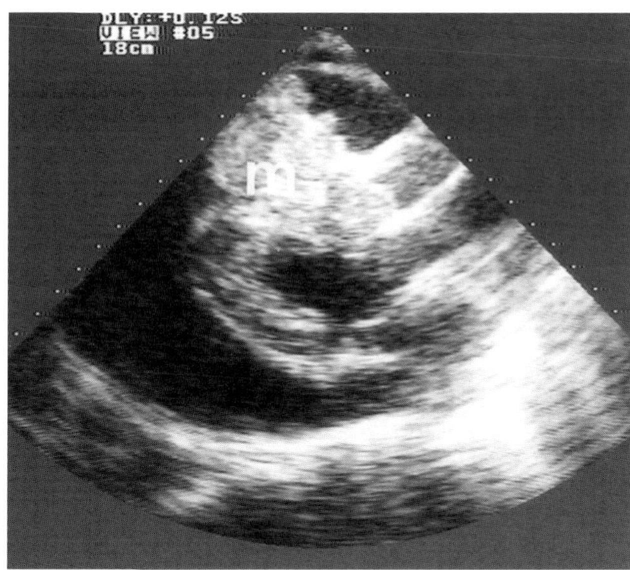

Fig. 11.4 A long axis parasternal view demonstrating a malignant pericardial effusion. The pericardium can be seen to be thickened anteriorly and there is a large echogenic mass (m) which is directly involving the myocardium. Histology showed this to be a sarcoma.

be pericardial thickening, pericardial fibrinous strands or echogenic fluid due to either malignant cells or haemopericardium. There is a high incidence of progression to tamponade and therefore a careful search for features suggesting it should be made.

The commonest primary malignant tumour of the pericardium is mesothelioma, but local invasion from an adjacent pleurally based primary tumour is more common. Either may present as an asymptomatic effusion, pericarditis or constrictive pericarditis [8]. Echocardiography reveals pericardial thickening that may be in the form of local plaques or generalized pericardial thickening with or without effusion. Prognosis is very poor with most patients dying within 6 months of presentation.

Benign pericardial tumours are rare, usually of mesenchymal origin (i.e. fibroma, lipoma, angioma and neurofibroma), and are associated with a good prognosis unless they are large or complicated by pericardial effusion (both of which are common with teratoma).

TRAUMA AND SURGERY

Pericardial effusion is not uncommon postsurgery. It is usually secondary to haemopericardium and is echogenic in nature. This may be compounded or initiated by the anticoagulation regime associated with some valve prostheses. Effusions may be simple or loculated in nature and are associated with a high incidence of tamponade—which may take up to 3 months to develop [9]. There is a tendency for postsurgical pericardial effusions to loculate and thus tamponade may only involve a single cardiac chamber or even the superior vena cava [10].

Haemopericardium may complicate penetrating and blunt trauma and, because of its rapid accumulation often leads to severe tamponade. It can occasionally complicate intracardiac catheterization or interventional techniques. Echocardiographic assessment should include a search for impairment of ventricular function (either due to direct myocardial trauma or coronary artery damage) as well as mitral valve, ventricular septal and aortic rupture (which commonly occurs at the isthmus or aortic root).

Pericardial thickening and constriction

Pericardial thickening occurs following haemopericardium, malignant infiltration (particularly post-treatment) and following pericarditis of whatever cause, but particularly after tuberculous infection. With constrictive pericarditis there is fusion of the two layers of pericardium which become thickened and non-distensible. This results in a restriction of cardiac filling and subsequent increase in systemic and pulmonary venous pressure and reduced cardiac output. Onset of constriction varies between several weeks to several years.

Echocardiography is insensitive in differentiating normal from thickened pericardium [11] and in demonstration of pericardial thickening proven on computed tomography (only detecting 29% in one comparative study [12]). However, it is of use in the diagnosis of pericardial constriction. Whilst there is no single sign that will reliably diagnose it, there are a number of features that are suggestive of haemodynamically important restriction of cardiac filling which occurs in constriction. In this regard M-mode echocardiography is superior to 2D echocardiography. The latter may show a normal-sized heart (possibly with an enlarged left atrium, as this is not completely surrounded by pericardium) with evidence of a sudden stop in ventricular diastolic filling and associated reduced wall motion, but these features are subjective and unreliable.

M-mode features of constriction within the ventricles include exaggerated movement of the septum compared to the left ventricular free wall (sensitive but non-specific), flattening of posterior wall movement in diastole with an abrupt and premature end to ventricular filling and early opening of the pulmonary valve. In the atria the features are early diastolic septal kick or septal notch, an atrial systolic notch and enlargement of the left atria, inferior vena cava and hepatic veins [11–13]. The presence of several of these signs in the appropriate clinical situation is highly suggestive of constrictive pericarditis.

It is important to appreciate that all of the above features are also seen in restrictive cardiomyopathy. As the treatment for constrictive pericarditis is surgical, and for restrictive cardiomyopathy is conservative, it is important to differentiate the two. This problem is not unique to echocardiography and is just as problematic with cardiac catheter. The demonstration of pericardial thickening is helpful in differentiating the two, and computed tomography or MRI should be considered if thickening is not seen on echocardiography. Following surgical treatment rescanning is recommended to ensure normalization of the echocardiographic abnormalities. If this does not occur the diagnosis of restrictive cardiomyopathy should be considered.

Cardiac tamponade

The haemodynamic effects of an effusion are dependent on a number of factors, namely the speed of accumulation, the elasticity of the pericardium and the presence of coexisting cardiac impairment. The size of effusion is generally not important and the rapid development of a small effusion is more significant than the slow accumulation of a large one. Consideration for drainage should therefore be decided upon the clinical condition of the patient. There are, however, a number of echocardiographic signs which although not absolute may be helpful in the differentiation of cardiac tamponade from a simple effusion. Although isolated left ventricular tamponade has been described [14], the majority of signs that correlate well with tamponade are secondary to pressure effects of the tamponade on the compliant right-sided chambers. Diastolic right atrial [15] and right ventricular [16] compression are seen both on M-mode and 2D echocardiography. Right atrial inversion represents part of this spectrum and has a reported sensitivity of 100% and specificity of 82% [17]. Diastolic right ventricular compression and collapse [18] are also sensitive for tamponade. They are, however, not specific as any cause of abnormal wall motion can mimic these appearances. The presence of normal atrial and ventricular wall motion does, however, essentially exclude tamponade.

Abnormalities in cardiac filling bring about secondary changes in transvalvular flow that can be detected on Doppler examination. Intrapericardial pressures are raised in inspiration which bring about a reduction in early mitral flow velocity both at the beginning of diastole and during atrial systole [19,20] and a corresponding increase in early tricuspid flow both in early diastole and early atrial contraction. These result in increased pulmonary artery flow velocity and reduced aortic flow velocity.

Flow changes are also seen in the superior and inferior vena cava and hepatic veins [19,21]. Of these the respiratory changes seen in the inferior vena cava are the most specific [22]. Because of impaired right ventricular filling there is raised central venous pressure. This results in a reduction in the variation of the diameter of the inferior vena cava with respiration that is normally seen. The percentage decrease in the inferior vena caval diameter after inspiration (the 'caval respiratory index') closely correlates with central venous pressure [22]. These changes, however, reflect raised central venous pressure and are not specific to tamponade [21]. However, because of their high sensitivity, they are a useful sign in the appropriate clinical context.

Pericardial aspiration

Pericardial aspiration is required both to obtain diagnostic samples and for the treatment of pericardial tamponade. Echocardiography allows the examiner to choose an appropriate site for insertion of the needle avoiding both lung and liver and to make an assessment as to the depth of puncture required. It is relatively simple and associated with a low incidence of complications [23]. In many cases ultrasound imaging can be used to select a site for puncture and the procedure can then follow without further imaging. The conventional subxiphoid site is not always the most suitable for aspiration and more lateral positions are often much nearer to the pericardial fluid collection. In difficult or loculated effusions echocardiography can be used to visualize directly the insertion of drainage needles or drainage catheters. The scan plane chosen should allow visualization of the whole needle and especially the tip. Once the pericardium has been punctured confirmation of the position of the needle tip can be made by injecting saline through it. In certain cases percutaneous balloon pericardotomy is appropriate and may avoid surgery [24].

Cardiomyopathies

Classification

Cardiomyopathies are generalized diseases of heart muscle commonly of unknown aetiology; however, specific heart muscle diseases of known aetiology can also be classified as cardiomyopathies. Both result in changes in cardiac function and structure. Cardiomyopathies are broadly separated into three groups identified by both haemodynamic and pathological characteristics, namely (a) dilated; (b) hypertrophic; and (c) restrictive [25]. These provide a useful framework for describing the haemodynamics and pathophysiological changes seen. However, the boundaries between the three groups are indistinct and may not always be respected by any given pathological process.

The essential feature of dilated cardiomyopathy is dilatation of the left or right ventricle or both in response to impaired systolic function and hypokinesis with subsequent diminished ventricular emptying. Signs of congestive cardiac failure may develop but are not required for diagnosis.

Hypertrophic cardiomyopathy is characterized by unexplained hypertrophy of the left ventricle, often only involving the septum. The left ventricular volume is normal or reduced and the myocardial contractility is increased. The primary haemodynamic abnormality is usually impaired left ventricular filling associated with raised diastolic pressure.

In restrictive cardiomyopathy there is reduced ventricular compliance that results in impaired ventricular filling. This is often associated with reduced ventricular contractility and thus brings about effects haemodynamically which are a hybrid of the other forms of cardiomyopathy.

Using simple measurements—ventricular internal dimensions, wall thickness and contractility (shortening fraction) and ejection fraction estimation—echocardiography can differentiate the three forms of cardiomyopathy in the majority of cases. It also allows assessment of the severity of the disease as well as recognizing a number of their complications. For these reasons echocardiography is central in the diagnosis and management of patients with cardiomyopathy.

Dilated cardiomyopathy

Dilated cardiomyopathy (DCM) is characterized by a reduction in cardiac contractility and dilatation of both ventricles. Clinically this presents with congestive cardiac failure and differentiation has to be made between DCM and other causes of cardiac enlargement, primarily ischaemic heart disease. The diagnosis of DCM is essentially one of exclusion.

ECHOCARDIOGRAPHIC FEATURES

The primary echocardiographic feature of DCM is of dilated poorly contracting ventricles with increased end-systolic and end-diastolic dimensions (Fig. 11.5). 2D echocardiography shows this reduction in contractility is diffuse (an important differentiating feature from ischaemic disease, see below). Although left ventricular mass is markedly increased [26] because of ventricular dilatation, ventricular wall thickness is normal or slightly reduced. Atrial and venous dilatation frequently accompany ventricular dilatation and are subsequent on elevated ventricular filling pressures. M-mode echocardiography confirms 2D findings and often also demonstrates premature closure of the aortic valve that is secondary to the reduced stroke volume seen in these patients. DCM is often associated with mitral regurgitation. This is secondary to stretching of the atrioventricular annular ring and subvalvular apparatus as well as myocardial impairment of the papillary muscles. A frequently encountered problem is the differentiation of mitral regurgitation secondary to DCM from ventricular dilatation due to volume overload secondary to a 'primary' valvular lesion. Indications that are useful in differentiating the two are that the valve appears entirely normal in DCM but is frequently distorted in primary

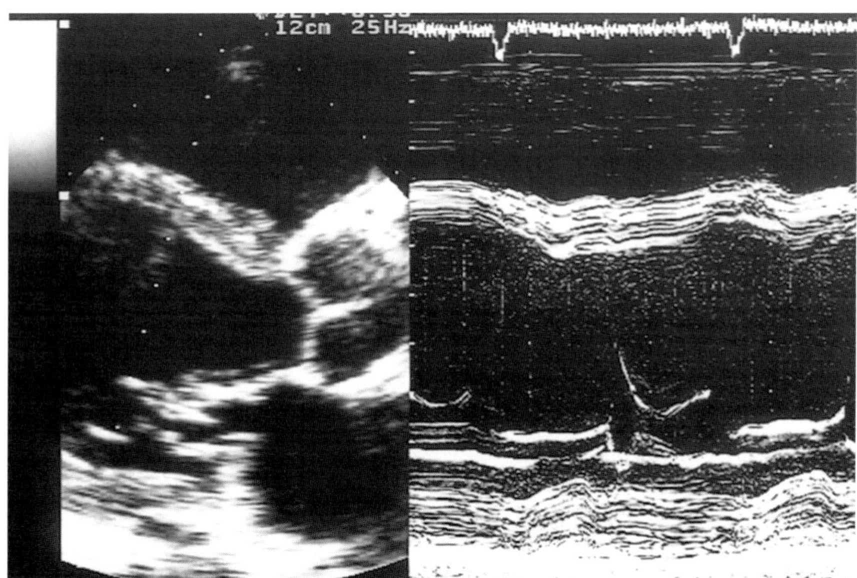

Fig. 11.5 Parasternal long axis view of the left ventricle in a patient with a dilated cardiomyopathy. The accompanying M-mode trace shows considerable increase in distance of the anterior leaflet of the mitral valve from the septum, a good sign of ventricular dilatation.

mitral regurgitation. The size of the jet as seen with colour Doppler is usually larger in primary valve disease than DCM and the left atrium is usually larger with the latter. However, even using these indicators, the primary aetiology is frequently uncertain.

It has been suggested that echocardiography has some role in assessing prognosis in patients with DCM. Patients with left ventricular hypertrophy or atrial fibrillation are said to have a better prognosis while those with thin ventricular walls, high end-diastolic pressures and ventricular arrhythmias are said to be worse. The severity of ventricular dilatation, interestingly, does not appear to be a reliable indicator of mortality. Unfortunately, these prognostic features are not reliable enough to be of any use in selecting patients for consideration for cardiac transplantation.

One important subgroup of DCM are those patients with isolated right ventricular dilatation for which no other cause—such as pulmonary hypertension, valvular or congenital heart disease—can be found. These patients appear to be at risk of life-threatening arrhythmias and a high risk of sudden death [27] and are therefore an important group to identify. In this subgroup the left ventricle is characteristically normal.

Another possible role of echocardiography is its use in the identification of a subgroup of patients requiring anticoagulation. Ventricular dilatation and hypokinesis lead to low intraventricular velocities that can be seen on 2D echocardiography as swirling areas of echogenicity. This relative stasis predisposes to cellular aggregation and thrombus formation. The thrombus seen in DCM is felt to have a higher incidence for embolization than postmyocardial infarct and recognition of the above features is frequently an indication for anticoagulation.

DIFFERENTIAL DIAGNOSIS

Generalized ventricular dilatation and hypokinesis with relatively normal wall thickness in the absence of significant valvular or congenital heart disease is suggestive of DCM. However, echocardiographic differentiation 1from secondary heart muscle disorders such as alcoholic cardiomyopathy is impossible and a search for a definitive aetiology must always be sought. Echocardiography is a useful tool as it can help exclude a number of conditions, such as congenital and significant valvular heart disease. However, the differentiation of DCM from left ventricular failure of an ischaemic aetiology is more difficult and often impossible. Differentiation from a single transmural infarct is usually possible because this produces focal rather than diffuse hypokinesis. Multiple infarcts, however, can produce generalized hypokinesis identical to DCM. The identification of myocardial scarring is sometimes possible as focal myocardial thinning or an area of increased echogenicity (Fig. 11.6). Often the two conditions are identical in appearance on echocardiography. Differentiation may also be difficult on left ventriculography, the presence or absence of coronary artery disease being the only helpful distinguishing feature.

Hypertrophic cardiomyopathy

Hypertrophic cardiomyopathy (HCM) is inherited as an autosomal dominant trait with variable inheritance.

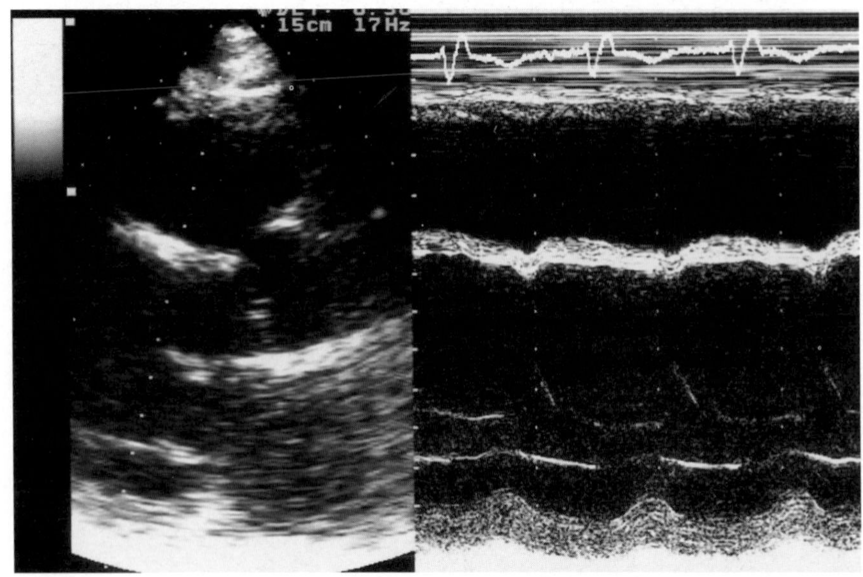

Fig. 11.6 Parasternal long axis view and accompanying M-mode trace of a dilated and poorly contracting left ventricle. Whilst the general appearances are similar to those of a dilated cardiomyopathy, the thin and echogenic septum suggests previous ischaemic damage.

Associations also exist with Noonan's syndrome and Friedreich's ataxia. The condition is characterized by increased ventricular contraction with ejection fractions of 80% or over, and ventricular thickening of varying distribution (see below). The powerful contractions and ventricular thickening are associated with labile, often variable pressure gradients within the left ventricular cavity and mitral valve dysfunction including mitral regurgitation.

Echocardiographic criteria are central in the diagnosis of HCM and M-mode features have been used extensively in the past [28]. These are: (a) the presence of asymmetrical hypertrophy of the intraventricular septum (ASH), defined as a ratio of septal to posterior left ventricular end-diastolic thickness of equal to or greater than 1.3:1 [29]; (b) premature mid-systolic closure of the aortic valve [30,31]; and (c) systolic anterior motion of the mitral valve (SAM) [32].

These echocardiographic features are, however, not either all obligatory or unique to HCM, as was originally believed. They can be seen in a variety of other cardiac anomalies with no common pathophysiological mechanism [32,33]. 2D echocardiography and the various forms of Doppler echocardiography are more recent developments that have enhanced our understanding of HCM as well as improving the overall sensitivity and specificity of the examination. For example 2D echocardiography has allowed the realization that oblique sectioning of the ventricle causing overestimation of ventricular size and wall thickness was a frequent occurrence with M-mode used in isolation, thus causing many false positive diagnoses.

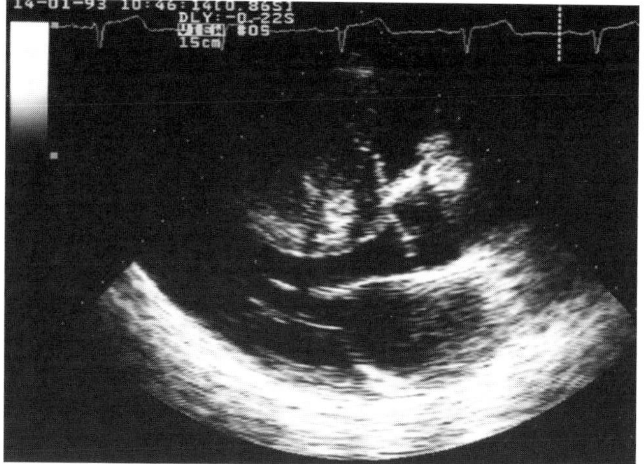

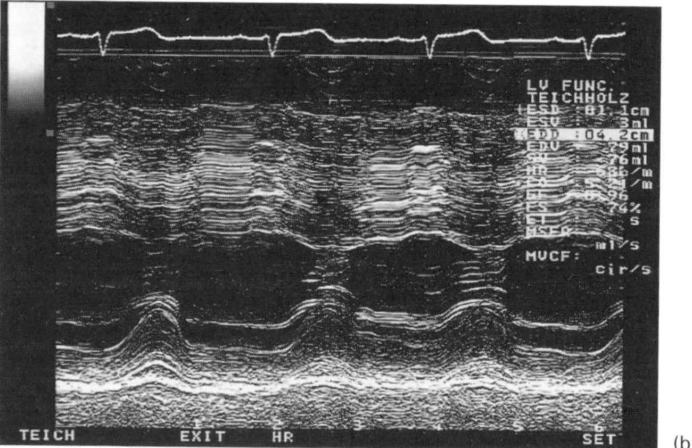

Fig. 11.7 (a) Parasternal long axis and (b) subsequent M-mode tracing showing markedly asymmetrical hypertrophy of the interventricular septum with a normal left ventricular free wall in a patient with HCM.

ECHOCARDIOGRAPHIC FEATURES

Ventricular hypertrophy

The use of 2D echocardiography has allowed appreciation of the inhomogeneity of ventricular hypertrophy seen in HCM. Hypertrophy is most frequently seen as ASH (Fig. 11.7). Although this hypertrophy usually involves the anterior septum to various extents and severities it may only involve the left ventricular apex, mid or posterior septum or lateral wall [34]. Frequently, the wall thickening is markedly heterogeneous even over short distances.

Other forms of hypertrophy are also described. Shapiro and McKenna [35] defined three patterns of left ventricular hypertrophy: asymmetrical left ventricular in 55%, symmetrical in 31% and distal/apical in 14% (Fig. 11.8). Differentiation between the subgroups is a worthwhile exercise as it has been suggested that the predominantly apical pattern is associated with mild symptoms and few adverse prognostic features [36] as well as typical giant negative T waves on the electrocardiogram (ECG). Differentiation of the subtypes requires multiple short axis views with 2D echocardiography. Care is required to

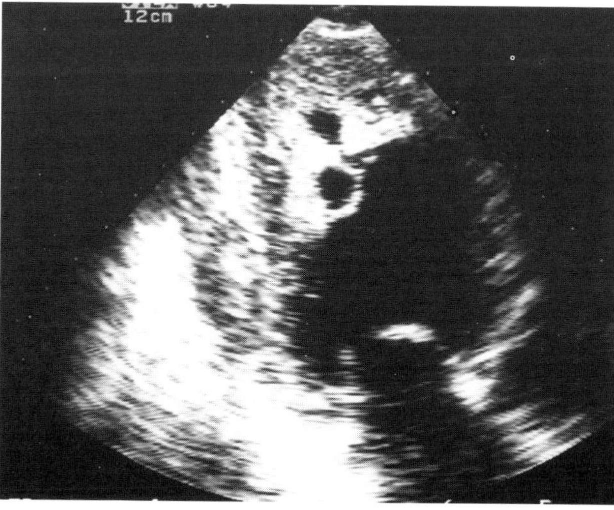

Fig. 11.8 An example of one of the variants of HCM, in this case there is myocardial thickening at the apex with relatively normal free wall and septum. This represents the localized apical variant of HCM.

ensure oblique cuts are avoided as these will cause false positive results, particularly of the apical subtype. Differentiation of symmetrical left ventricular HCM from secondary causes is particularly difficult and is often a diagnosis of exclusion or reliant on a good family history. Hypertrophy is seen within the right ventricle frequently (44% in one study [37]) and is usually associated with severe disease and arrhythmias.

Ventricular septal wall thickening is frequently associated with left ventricular outflow tract obstruction but its severity appears to be independent of wall thickness. Another association includes thickening of the proximal endocardial surface immediately opposite the mitral valve and is secondary to repeated contact between the valvular and mural endocardium secondary to SAM.

Mitral valve effects

HCM produces signs within the mitral valve and these are best assessed with apical four-chamber and parasternal long axis views utilizing both M-mode, 2D and Doppler echocardiography. The most well-known sign is that of SAM (Fig. 11.9), yet its aetiology remains unclear. It is either secondary to abnormal displacement of the papillary muscles in systole [38], a venturi effect (the cusps being drawn into the low pressure created by high blood flow in the left ventricular outflow tract) [39] or secondary to abnormal mitral cusp coaptation at the onset of systole in association with the small left ventricular cavity [40]. There does appear to be a direct relationship between the presence and duration of SAM and the presence of left ventricular outflow gradient measured at cardiac catheterization [41]; but whether it is a reliable indicator of left ventricular obstruction is debatable.

Mitral regurgitation is a well-recognized association of HCM and is a frequent association of both SAM and intraventricular gradients [42]. This is usually easy to visualize using colour flow imaging that shows a jet of 'mosaic' colour directed anteriorly within the left atrium that may sometimes be difficult to differentiate from the turbulent jet seen in the outflow tract. The severity of the regurgitation appears to be related to the presence of SAM and the severity of the outflow tract gradient. Its aetiology remains unclear but is probably secondary to distortion of the mitral apparatus [42].

Pressure abnormalities

In HCM there are abnormalities both of diastolic filling and ventricular ejection. In diastole there is impaired relaxation, compliance and therefore filling of the left ventricle. Abnormal filling brings about changes in flow velocities and times that can be detected with pulsed wave Doppler examination. These are detected by positioning the sample volume in the inflow region of the left ventricle and are as follows: (a) the early diastolic peak (E wave) is reduced and prolonged; (b) the late diastolic peak (A wave) is increased; and (c) the ratio of the two E/A is reduced. While these indices are sensitive for HCM they are non-specific and seen with any cause of reduced compliance [43].

The reduced filling, thickened ventricular walls and overactive ventricular contractions all predispose to the systolic abnormality seen in HCM, that is intraventricular

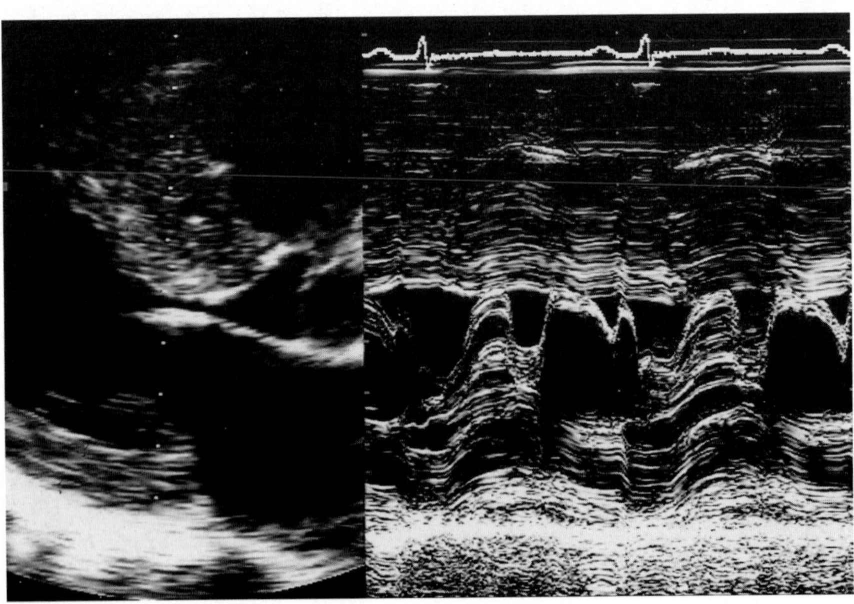

Fig. 11.9 Parasternal long axis view and M-mode trace demonstrating asymmetrical hypertrophy of the left ventricle and anterior systolic motion of the anterior leaflet of the mitral valve. There is also anterior motion of the mitral apparatus seen in this patient with HCM.

pressure gradients and outflow tract obstruction. These pressure gradients can be estimated using Doppler echocardiography and the modified Bernoulli equation: $\Delta P = 4v^2$ (where p = pressure gradient, v = peak velocity in $m\,s^{-1}$ [44]. In contrast to fixed obstruction the flow velocity seen with left ventricular outflow obstruction in HCM shows a slow and gradual increase that only reaches a peak in late systole and is therefore different in shape to aortic stenosis (Fig. 11.10). Obstruction varies in severity and may be absent in the resting state. Because of this obstruction there is secondary premature closure of the aortic valve (Fig. 11.11).

Intracavity gradients can be demonstrated elsewhere within the left ventricle and colour flow imaging is particularly useful in this regard. In the normal apical four-chamber view homogeneous 'blue' colour coding is seen at the apex of the left ventricle that becomes brighter as it moves towards the ventricular outflow with aliasing commonly seen immediately below the aortic valve. In HCM there is a generalized increase in intracavity blood velocity in systole which results in a generalized lighter hue of blue and aliasing with a mosaic pattern occurring closer to the apex, at mid ventricular level. If SAM is present there is usually a mosaic pattern adjacent to it due

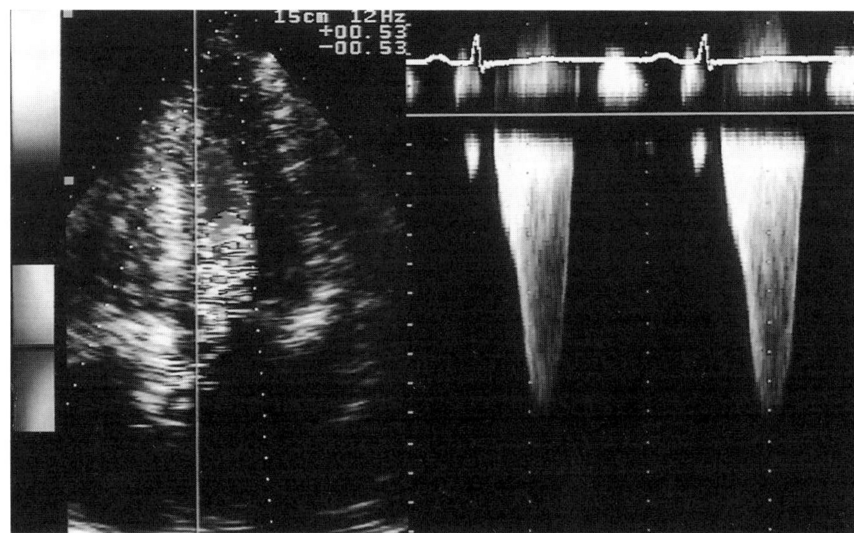

Fig. 11.10 Apical four-chamber view with colour flow imaging of the left ventricle showing aliasing in mid left ventricle indicating a ventricular gradient. Doppler analysis at the same level shows a slow and later peak of flow compared to what is seen in aortic stenosis. For colour, see Plate 11.10 (between pp. 308 and 309).

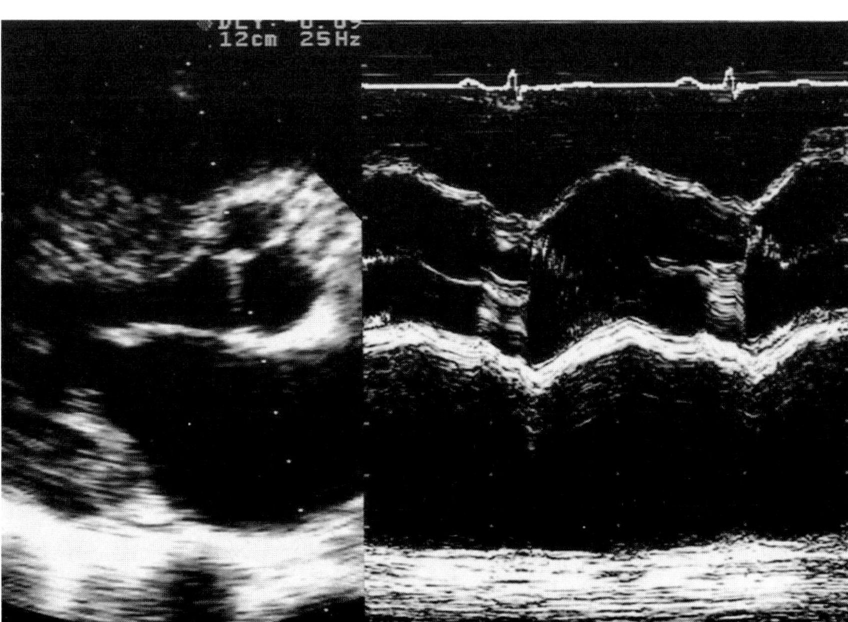

Fig. 11.11 M-mode echocardiography through the aortic valve showing premature closure due to outflow tract obstruction in this patient with HCM.

to the turbulence caused by the anteriorly displaced mitral apparatus. Occasionally turbulent flow is seen at the apex and is a fairly specific sign of HCM [38]. The increased intracardiac velocities can be confirmed by using pulsed wave Doppler examination.

Differential diagnosis

A number of normal variants and disease can simulate HCM. Of the normal variants the commonest is bending of the ventricular septum simulating ASH, particularly in the elderly. Another major diagnostic difficulty occurs in some athletes with either symmetrical or asymmetrical ventricular wall thickening. Differentiation can usually be made by the fact that athletes are bradycardic and have intracavity dimensions which are the upper limit of normal. In HCM patients dimensions are at the low end of normal particularly at end-systole.

Asymmetrical hypertrophy may occur in conditions which either cause thinning of the free wall (e.g. transmural myocardial infarct) or hypertrophy of the septum (often due to pulmonary hypertension). Conditions which usually cause generalized left ventricular hypertrophy such as hypertension can be asymmetric and can present diagnostic problems. Infiltrative conditions such as amyloidosis can also be focal but the reduced ventricular contractility usually differentiates them from HCM.

Of particular difficulty is the differentiation of the subgroup of HCM patients with the generalized ventricular hypertrophy from other causes of hypertrophy. This often is a diagnosis of exclusion.

Restrictive cardiomyopathy

Restrictive cardiomyopathy is the rarest form of cardiomyopathy in which the primary abnormality is reduced ventricular compliance and consequently a restriction of ventricular filling. Its cause, as with most other cardiomyopathies is unknown. There are, however, a number of infiltrative disorders of the myocardium that have similar physiological effects on the ventricle and are described under the same generic term [45].

ECHOCARDIOGRAPHIC FEATURES

The cardinal echocardiographic features of restrictive cardiomyopathy are of small normally contracting ventricles with a bilateral atrial enlargement (Fig. 11.12). Early ventricular filling is normal and this is followed by an abrupt halt to filling as the non-compliant chambers fail to expand any further. This halt to filling may be visible on 2D echocardiography but is best appreciated on the M-mode trace. In the normal left ventricle there is a smooth progressive increase in diastolic dimensions from early to late diastole. In restrictive cardiomyopathy the increase in ventricular dimensions is confined to early diastole with the remaining wall movement in diastole remaining constant and therefore showing as a horizontal line. Other features seen include early diastolic septal kick or an atrial systolic notch and enlargement of the inferior vena cava and hepatic veins.

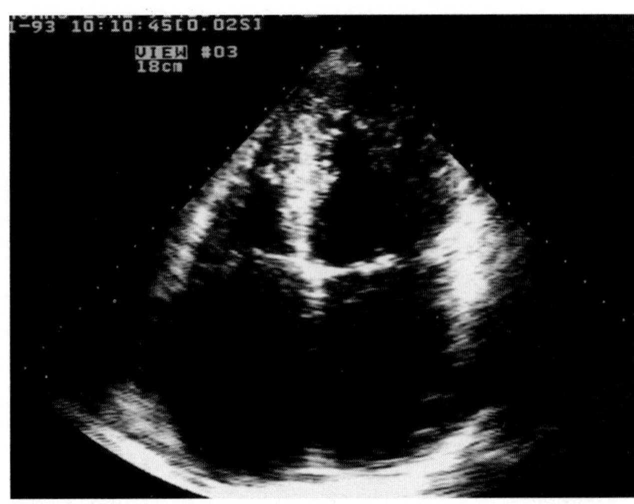

Fig. 11.12 Apical four-chamber view in a patient with restrictive cardiomyopathy demonstrating dilatation of both atria with normal-sized ventricles suggesting reduced compliance at the ventricular level.

Doppler studies may reveal increased flow reversal on respiration and shortened mitral and tricuspid deceleration times with a further shortening with inspiration [46] but these also occur with pericardial constriction.

Certain features may be specific of certain types of restrictive cardiomyopathy. Cardiac amyloid is the most frequent infiltrative disorder of the myocardium and is most commonly secondary to myeloma or of primary aetiology. Infiltration begins subendocardially and therefore may present on echocardiography as thickening of the ventricular walls, which are hyperechoic, with a normal or reduced cavity size. Infiltration also occurs in the endocardium and coronary arteries and results in thrombus formation and arrhythmias, respectively.

Endomyocardial fibrosis is another cardiac disease which presents with features of a restrictive cardiomyopathy with additional suggestive features. Pathologically, the condition is characterized by endocardial infiltration of eosinophils followed by granulation tissue and endarteritis. This results in endocardial fibrosis and thrombus formation which can be visualized on echocardiography as thickening of the inner ventricular wall, particularly at the apex often with adjacent thrombus. The fibrotic process also affects the valvular chordae and results in tethering of the mitral valve leaflets with associated valvular incompetence.

References

1 Hartnell, G.G., Rosevec, A., Waring, J., Vann Jones, J., Wilde, R.P.H., Goddard P.R. (1988) Magnetic resonance in the assessment of pericardial disease. *British Journal of Radiology* **61**, 779–780.
2 Windle, J.R., Felix, G., Pinsky, W.W., Kugler, J.D. (1983) False negative findings in pericardial effusion using M-mode echocardiography. *Pediatric Cardiology* **4**, 225–228.
3 Wolf, W.J. (1986) Echocardiographic features of a purulent pericardial peel. *American Journal of the Heart* **111**, 990–992.
4 Bjorkhem, G., Lunderstrom, N.R., Vitarelli, A. (1984) Sequential study of echocardiographic changes in purulent pericarditis. *Pediatric Cardiology* **5**, 317–332.
5 Chia, B.L., Choo, M., Tan, A., Ee, B. (1984) Echocardiographic abnormalities in tuberculous pericardial effusion. *American Heart Journal* **107**, 1034–1036.
6 Kaplan, K., Davison, R., Parker, M., *et al.* (1985) Frequency of pericardial effusion as determined by M-mode echocardiography in acute myocardial infarction. *American Journal of Cardiology* **55**, 335–337.
7 Armstrong, W.F., Buck, J.D., Hoffman, R., Waller, B.F. (1986) Cardiac involvement by lymphoma: detection and follow-up by two-dimensional echocardiography. *American Heart Journal* **112**, 627–631.
8 Coplan, N.L., Kennish, A.J., Burgess, N.L., Deligish, L., Goldman, M.E. (1984) Pericardial mesothelioma masquerading as a benign pericardial effusion. *Journal of the American College of Cardiology* **4**, 1307–1310.
9 D'Cruz, I.A., Kensey, K., Campbell, C., Replogle, R., Jain, M. (1985) Two-dimensional echocardiography in cardiac tamponade occurring after cardiac surgery. *Journal of the American College of Cardiology* **5**, 1250–1252.
10 Fyke, F.E., Tancredi, R.G., Shub, C., Julsrud, P.R., Sheedy, P.F. (1985) Detection of intrapericardial hematoma after open heart surgery: the roles of echocardiography and computed tomography. *Journal of the American College of Cardiology* **5**, 1496–1499.
11 Voelkel, A.G., Pietro, D.A., Folland, E.D., Fisher, M.I., Parisi, A.F. (1978) Echocardiographic features of constrictive pericarditis. *Circulation* **58**, 871–875.
12 Sutton, F.J., Whitley, N.O., Applefield, M.M. (1985) The role of echocardiography and computed tomography in the evaluation of constrictive pericarditis. *American Heart Journal* **109**, 350–355.
13 Candel-Riera, J., Gutierrez-Palau, L., Garcia-Del-Castillo, H., Permanyer-Milralada, G., Soler-Soler, J. (1985) Atrial systolic notch and early diastolic notch on the interventricular septal echocardiogram in constrictive pericarditis. *Journal of the American College of Cardiology* **5**, 1020–1021.
14 Davies, S.W., Youhanna, A., Copp, M. (1992) Severe rheumatic mitral stenosis with pericardial effusion causing left ventricular tamponade. *British Heart Journal* **67**, 269–270.
15 Kronzon, I., Cohen, M.L., Winer, H.E. (1983) Diastolic atrial compression; a sensitive echocardiographic sign of cardiac tamponade. *Journal of the American College of Cardiology* **2**, 770–775.
16 Singh, S., Wann, S., Schuchard, G.H., *et al.* (1984) Right ventricular and right atrial collapse in patients with cardiac tamponade—a combined echocardiographic and hemodynamic study. *Circulation* **70**, 966–971.
17 Gillam, L.D., Guyer, D.E., Gibson, T.C., King, M.E., Marshall, J.E., Werman, A.E. (1983) Hydrodynamic compression of the right atrium: a new echocardiographic sign of cardiac tamponade. *Circulation* **68**, 294–301.
18 Armstrong, W.F., Schilt, B.F., Helper, D.J., Dillon, J.C., Feigenbaum, H. (1982) Diastolic collapse of the right ventricle with cardiac tamponade: an echocardiographic study. *Circulation* **65**, 1491–1496.
19 Spodick, D.H., Paldino, D., Flessas, A.P. (1983) Respiratory effects on systolic time intervals during pericardial effusion. *American Journal of Cardiology* **51**, 1033–1035.
20 Appleton, C.P., Hattle, L.K., Popp, R.L. (1988) Cardiac tamponade and pericardial effusion: respiratory variation in transvalvular flow velocities studied by Doppler echocardiography. *Journal of the American College of Cardiology* **11**, 1020–1030.
21 Fowler, N.O. (1988) The significance of echocardiographic Doppler studies in cardiac tamponade. *Journal of the American College of Cardiology* **11**, 1031–1035.
22 Himelman, R.B., Kircher, B., Rockey, D.C., Schiller, N.B. (1988) Inferior vena cava plethora with blunted respiratory response: a sensitive echocardiographic sign of tamponade. *Journal of the American College of Cardiology* **12**, 1470–1477.
23 Callahan, J.A., Seward, J.B., Nishimura, R.A., *et al.* (1985) Two dimensional echocardiographically guided pericardiocentesis: experience in 117 consecutive patients. *American Journal of Cardiology* **55**, 476–479.
24 Jackson, G., Keane, D., Mishra, M. (1992) Percutaneous balloon pericardotomy in the management of recurrent malignant pericardial effusions. *British Heart Journal* **68**, 613–615.
25 Goodwin, J.F. (1982) The frontiers of cardiomyopathy. *British Heart Journal* **48**, 1–18.
26 Nihoyannopolous, P., Yonezawa, Y., Dickie, C., McKenna, W.J., Oakly, C.M. (1988) Accelerated intraventricular systolic flow differentiates patients with hypertrophic cardiomyopathy from those with secondary causes of hypertrophy. *British Heart Journal* **59**, 127 (abstract).
27 Foale, R.A., Nihoyannopolous, P., Ribero, P. *et al.* (1986) Right ventricular abnormalities in ventricular tachycardia of right ventricular origin: relation to electrophysiological features. *British Heart Journal* **56**, 45–54.
28 Rosen, R.M., Goodman, D.J., Ingham, R.E., Popp, R.L. (1974) Echocardiographic criteria in the diagnosis of idiopathic hypertrophic subaortic stenosis. *Circulation* **50**, 747–749.
29 Henry, W.L., Clark, C.E., Epstein, S.E. (1973) Asymmetric septal hypertrophy: echocardiographic identification of the pathognomonic anatomic abnormality of IHSS. *Circulation* **47**, 225–233.
30 Feignbaum, H. (1976) Clinical applications of echocardiography. *Progress in Cardiovascular Disease* **53**, 258–268.
31 Shah, P.M., Gramiak, R., Kramer, D.H. (1969) Ultrasound localisation of left ventricular outflow obstruction in hypertrophic obstructive cardiomyopathy. *Circulation* **40**, 3–11.

32 Maron, B.J., Gottdiener, J.S., Perry, L.W. (1981) Specificity of systolic anterior motion of the anterior mitral leaflet for hypertrophic cardiomyopathy: prevalence in a large population of patients with other cardiac disease. *British Heart Journal* **45**, 206–212.

33 Larter, W.E., Allen, H.D., Sahn, D.J., Goldberg, S.J. (1976) The asymmetrical hypertrophied septum: further differentiation of its causes. *Cirulation* **53**, 19–27.

34 Maron, D.J., Gottdiener, J.S., Epstein, S.E. (1981) Patterns and significance of distribution of left ventricular hypertrophy in hypertrophic cardiomyopathy. A wide angle two-dimensional echocardiographic study of 125 patients. *American Journal of Cardiology* **49**, 418–428.

35 Shapiro, L.M., McKenna, L. (1983) Distribution of left ventricular hypertrophy in hypertrophic cardiomyopathy: a two-dimensional echocardiographic study. *American College of Cardiology* **2**, 437.

36 Yamaguchi, H., Ishimura, T., Nishiyama, S. (1979) Hypertrophic non-obstructive cardiomyopathy with giant negative T waves (apical hypertrophy); ventricular and echocardiographic features in 30 patients. *American Journal of Cardiology* **44**, 401–412.

37 McKenna, W.J., Klienebenne, A., Nihoyannopolous, P., Foale, R. (1988) Echocardiographic measurement of right ventricular wall thickness in hypertrophic cardiomyopathy: relation to clinical and prognostic features. *Journal of the American College of Cardiology* **11**, 351–358.

38 Levine, R., Vlachakes, G.J., Giesking, E. *et al.* (1989) New insights into the mechanism of obstruction in hypertrophic cardiomyopathy: experimental models. *Circulation* **80**, 662.

39 Henry, W.L., Clark, C.E., Griffiths, J.M., Epsein, S.E. (1975) Mechanism of left ventricular obstruction in patients with asymmetric septal hypertrophy (idiopathic subaortic stenosis). *American Journal of Cardiology* **35**, 337–345.

40 Shah, P.M., Taylor, R.D., Wong, M. (1981) Abnormal mitral valve coaptation in hypertrophic obstructive cardiomyopathy: proposed role in systolic anterior motion of the mitral valve. *American Journal of Cardiology* **48**, 258–263.

41 Pollick, C., Rakowski, H., Wigle, E.D. (1984) Muscular subaortic stenosis: the quantitative relationship between systolic anterior motion and the pressure gradient. *Circulation* **69**, 43–47.

42 Yonezawa, Y., Nihoyannopoulos, P., McKenna, W.J., Doi, J.L., Ozawa, T. (1988) Mitral regurgitation in hypertrophic cardiomyopathy. A colour Doppler echocardiographic study. *American Journal of Noninvasive Cardiology* **2**, 195–198.

43 Grossman, W., McLaurin, L.P. (1976) Diastolic properties of the left ventricle. *Annals of Internal Medicine* **84**, 316–326.

44 Sasson, Z., Yock, P.G., Hatle, L.K., Alderman, E.L., Popp, R.L. (1988) Doppler echocardiographic determination of the pressure gradient in hypertrophic cardiomyopathy. *Journal of the American College of Cardiology* **11**, 752–756.

45 Goodwin, J.F. (1982) The frontiers of cardiomyopathy. *British Heart Journal* **48**, 1–18.

46 Appleton, C.P., Hatle, L.K., Popp, R.L. (1988) Demonstration of restrictive ventricular physiology by Doppler echocardiography. *Journal of the American College of Cardiology* **11**, 757–768.

Chapter 12: Prosthetic valve function

T.J. Edwards & I.A. Simpson

The first successful heart valve replacements were performed in the early 1960s with the use of mechanical valve prostheses [1,2]. Since then prosthetic valve replacement has evolved as the standard treatment for haemodynamically significant valve lesions. Despite advances in design, prosthetic valve dysfunction remains a significant problem. Certain mechanisms of dysfunction are common to all valve types and others more specific for particular prosthetic designs. Echocardiography is now the non-invasive method of choice for the assessment of prosthetic valve function. It has many advantages, particularly the fact that it can be repeated frequently and used for serial evaluation without the attendant risks of cardiac catheterization. M-mode and two-dimensional (2D) imaging, pulsed and continuous wave Doppler, and Doppler colour flow mapping each have values and limitations in the assessment of prosthetic valve function but when used together they provide a comprehensive assessment of valve integrity. The main limitation of transthoracic echocardiography is the suboptimal imaging due to acoustic reverberations from the non-biological material used in prosthetic valves and occasionally due to poor acoustic windows in non-echogenic subjects. Transoesophageal echocardiography can overcome these problems and can be used perioperatively and in the intensive care setting when transthoracic imaging is often impractical or inadequate. Currently available transducers allow for high frequency multiplane transoesophageal imaging utilizing all of the above ultrasound modes. This chapter provides a background to prosthetic valve function and the role of modern echocardiographic techniques in its assessment.

Types of prosthetic valve

Prostheses in current use fall into two broad groups, mechanical and biological. Since there are considerable differences in the structural design and functional characteristics of these valves, the echocardiographic appearances can be quite diverse even when the prosthesis is functioning normally. A sound understanding of the design of prosthetic valves from an echocardiographic perspective is therefore quite valuable.

Biological valves

Biological valves include aortic homografts, porcine xenografts and bovine pericardial prostheses.

Aortic homografts have been used clinically since 1962 [3]. Chemical sterilization of valves was abandoned in 1968 due to a high incidence of valve failure and was replaced with the antibiotic sterilized aortic homograft. These are usually stored at 4°C although cryopreservation of the homograft may further improve the long-term durability of the valve [4]. A freehand insertion technique is used to implant homografts, therefore the valves have no stent or sewing ring. The absence of significant echocardiographic artefacts is an advantage for follow-up of valve function although not in itself an indication for choosing this type of valve.

Porcine bioprostheses have been used clinically since 1965 [5]. The largest experience has been with the glutaraldehyde preserved, frame-mounted Hancock and Carpentier–Edwards porcine valves. These valves have significant differences in stent design. The effective orifice of the porcine aortic valve is limited by a shelf of myocardium in the base of the right coronary cusp. In the Carpentier–Edwards prosthesis the valve is attached to an asymmetric stent to minimize the prominence of the muscular shelf. The original Hancock valve was perfectly round with no attempt to modify the restriction of the septal shelf. In 1976 the Hancock modified orifice valve was developed to improve haemodynamics by replacing the muscular-based septal leaflet with a larger non-coronary leaflet. In the early 1980s the Carpentier–Edwards supra-annular prosthesis was developed, also to improve the haemodynamic properties. Neither of these developments, however, improved valve durability [6,7]. More recent advances in bioprosthetic valve design should improve durability and further improve haemodynamic function [8]. Zero pressure fixation techniques preserve collagen architecture and improve the elastic properties of the valve and antimineralization treatment mitigates (although does not prevent) dystrophic calcification of bioprostheses [9–11]. The Medtronic Intact valve (Fig. 12.1) is a new generation bioprosthesis employing zero pressure fixation and an anticalcific agent (toluidine blue) [12]. The St Jude Medical Toronto stentless porcine valve (Fig. 12.2) [13] should provide superior haemodynamic results to stented porcine valves because the obstruction caused by the stent and the sewing cuff is eliminated. Additionally the durability of the valve should be enhanced as the aortic sinuses of the host may allow for better dissipation of the mechanical stress to which the leaflets are subjected during diastole.

Pericardial bioprostheses were initially promising especially with regard to their haemodynamic profile. The long-term durability of these valves, however, proved to be poor compared with porcine valves [14] and they are no longer available for implantation.

Mechanical valves

Mechanical valves include caged ball, tilting disc and hinged bileaflet valves [15]. Ball valves have been used since 1960 [1,2], disc valves since 1969 [16] and bileaflet valves since 1977 [17].

The Starr–Edwards caged ball valve prosthesis (Fig. 12.3) consists of a barium impregnated silastic ball inside a stellite cage with a seamless cloth sewing ring. Since its introduction in 1960 several modifications have led to the model 6120 mitral valve in 1965 and the model 1260 aortic valve in 1968 which have been in continuous use since. Totally cloth-covered prostheses were introduced in 1967 but were discontinued in 1982 when they did not demonstrate any advantage with respect to thromboembolic risk. The main disadvantage of caged ball prostheses is the relatively large space occupied by the prosthesis which is a potential problem in patients with small left ventricles or narrow aortas.

Single disc and bileaflet valves comprise pyrolytic carbon discs within titanium or pyrolytic carbon housing attached to Teflon or Dacron sewing rings. Single disc valves include the Medtronic Hall, Omniscience and Bjork Shiley. The Bjork Shiley valve (Fig. 12.4) first introduced in 1969 had a free-floating central tilting disc retained by a pair of struts. In 1976 the convexoconcave disc was introduced to improve haemodynamic function and decrease the incidence of thromboembolism. This design suffered serious durability problems with cases of strut fracture and disc escape. Strut fracture was more common in a group of large sized 70° valves manufactured in 1981 and 1982 with an incidence of 0.29% per year. These were withdrawn in 1983. For the 60° convexoconcave valve the estimated incidence of strut fracture is 0.02% for the 19–27 mm valves and 0.08% for the 29–33 mm valves [15]. Prophylactic replacement of these 60° convexoconcave valves is not recommended as the risk of reoperation is likely to be higher than the risk of strut fracture [18]. All convexoconcave valves were withdrawn by the manufacturer in 1986. The Bjork Shiley monostrut valve was developed to eliminate the possibility of strut fracture. This valve has an opening angle of 70°. This model has been used extensively in European centres since 1982 with no cases of strut fracture.

The Medtronic Hall prosthesis was first implanted in 1977. The open disc angle of the aortic valve is 75° and the mitral 70° with a closed disc angle of 0° for both. The Omniscience valve has an open disc angle of 80° and closed disc angle of 12°.

The St Jude Medical and Carbomedics valves are bileaflet valves (Fig. 12.5). The St Jude valve was first

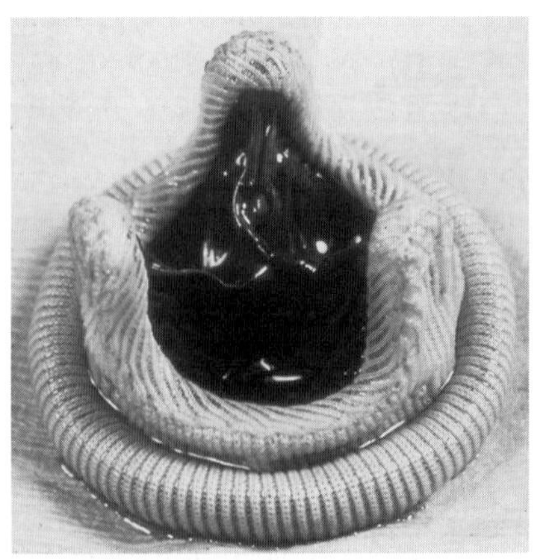

Fig. 12.1 A Medtronic Intact porcine bioprosthesis.

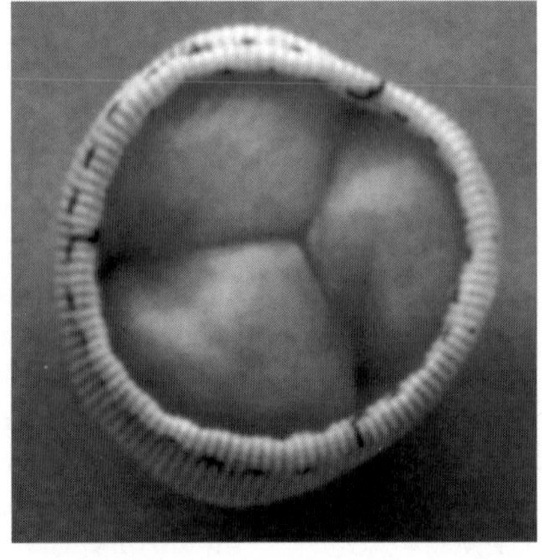

Fig. 12.2 A St Jude Medical Toronto stentless porcine valve.

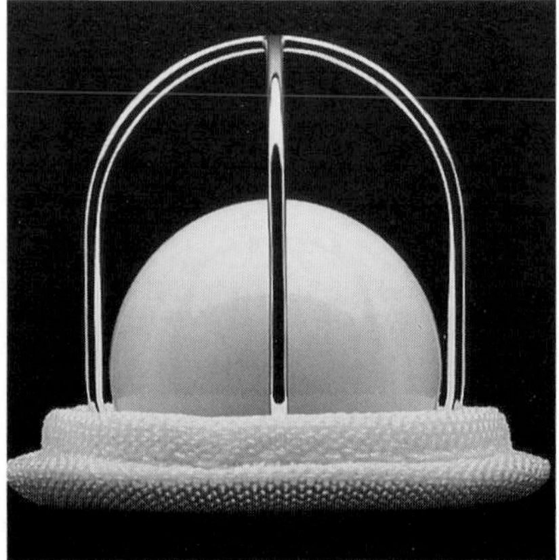

Fig. 12.3 A Starr–Edwards caged ball prosthesis.

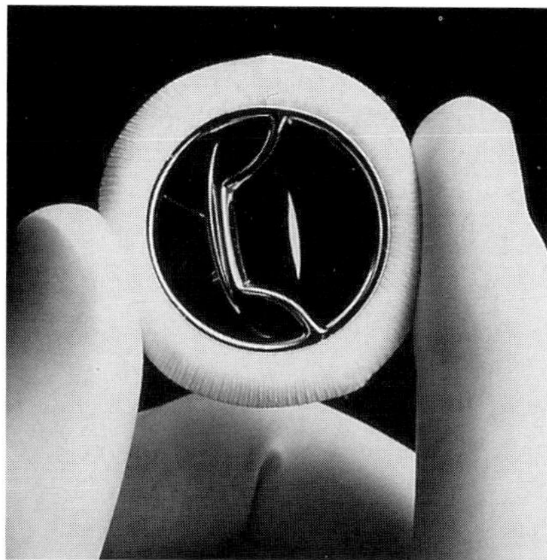

Fig. 12.4 A Bjork Shiley tilting disc prosthesis.

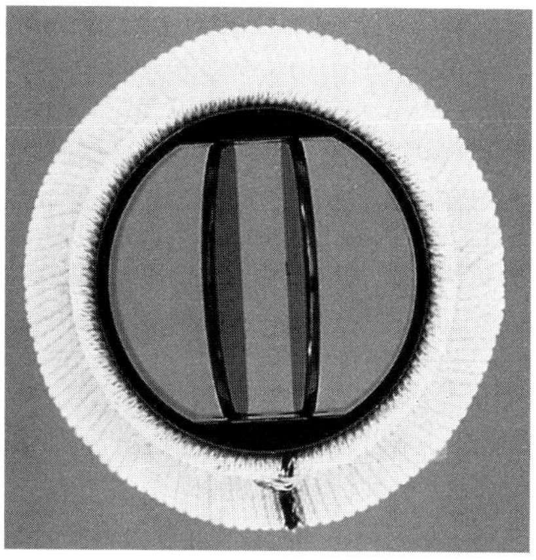

Fig. 12.5 A Carbomedics bileaflet prosthesis.

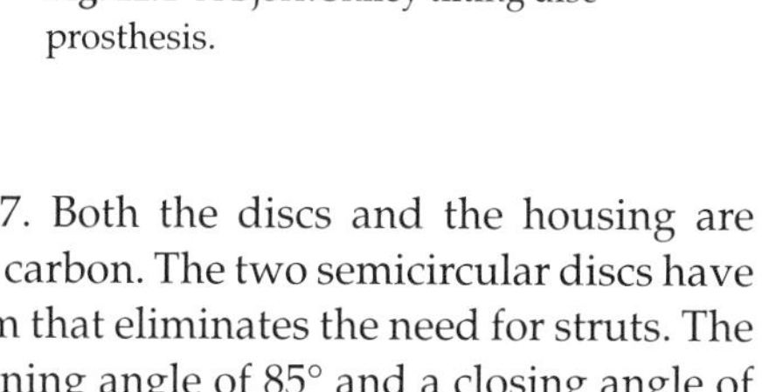

implanted in 1977. Both the discs and the housing are made of pyrolytic carbon. The two semicircular discs have a pivot mechanism that eliminates the need for struts. The discs have an opening angle of 85° and a closing angle of 30–35°. The flow across the valve is nearly laminar and can be measured at any point in the open position.

Atrioventricular valve rings may be used in more conservative tricuspid and mitral valve surgery. Mitral valve repair is an increasingly accepted alternative to valve replacement especially in cases of mitral regurgitation. Annuloplasty techniques for this operation include the use of flexible and rigid rings and a suture only technique. The most extensively used ring is the Carpentier–Edwards which consists of a rigid ring of titanium alloy. This remodels the annulus to the size and shape of the ring. The Duran ring is flexible and simply reduces the annulus to the size of the ring allowing changes in shape during the cardiac cycle. The mitral valve plays an important role in the geometry and mechanics of the left ventricle and annuloplasty techniques which maintain the structural and functional integrity of the mitral valve are likely to improve postoperative left ventricular function [19]. Table 12.1 lists the more common valve types.

Table 12.1 Types of prosthetic valve

Biological valves	
Homograft	
Porcine	Hancock (standard and modified orifice)
	Carpentier–Edwards (standard and supra-annular)
	Medtronic Intact
	St Jude Medical Toronto Stentless
Mechanical valves	
Caged ball	Starr–Edwards
Disc	Medtronic Hall
	Bjork Shiley
	Omniscience
Bileaflet	St Jude
	Carbomedics
Annular ring	Carpentier–Edwards
	Duran

Normal prosthetic valve function and potential complications

Prosthetic valve replacement of diseased native valves will provide improved haemodynamic function giving symptomatic and often prognostic benefit for the patient. The haemodynamic function of prosthetic valves will not equal that of normal native valves and prosthetic valve replacement brings with it the potential for complications which may themselves be life-threatening. An appreciation of the normal function and flow characteristics of prosthetic valves as well as a knowledge of the possible complications is essential in interpreting the echocardiographic findings.

All prosthetic valves are at least mildly stenotic and relatively high pressure gradients can occur with normal prosthetic function [20]. Generally gradients are higher for ball and cage valves and lowest for tissue valves. Bileaflet valves tend to have larger effective orifice areas than the tilting disc design especially in the larger sizes due to the larger opening angles and lack of obstructive struts [21]. The smaller the valve the higher the gradient. All normally functioning mechanical valves have an inherent regurgitant volume. The regurgitant volume is the sum of the closure flow and the leakage flow for a valve. The closure flow is the volume of backflow required to close the valve. Leakage flow is the volume passing through the valve after the valve has returned to the closed position [22]. For mechanical valves the regurgitant fraction ranges from 8% for smaller valves to 13% for larger valves [20], the difference due largely to an increase in leakage volume. The tilting disc valves generally have better regurgitant characteristics than bileaflet valves due to the lower leakage volumes and the smaller opening angle giving a more rapid closure of the valve. Doppler colour flow mapping is sensitive enough to detect this normal regurgitant flow particularly with transoesophageal imaging and an appreciation of the normal regurgitant flow characteristics will allow the echocardiographer to distinguish normal from pathological regurgitation.

Leakage flow is generally negligible for bioprosthetic valves. Mild valvar regurgitation, however, is not uncommon for homograft valves (Fig. 12.6). Homograft insertion is a technically demanding procedure and aortic regurgitation has been reported in up to 23% of patients postoperatively although in this series the regurgitation was severe in only 4% [23]. Valvar regurgitation through a homograft valve therefore does not necessarily represent structural valve degeneration if it was present postoperatively, is not progressive on serial evaluation and the valve has an otherwise normal echocardiographic appearance. The regurgitation detected echocardiographically may not be apparent clinically.

Unlike the 'physiological' valvar regurgitation through a prosthetic valve a paravalvar leak is always pathological. It is a result of partial valve dehiscence either from stitch rupture or as a consequence of infective endocarditis. Differentiating valvar from paravalvar regurgitation

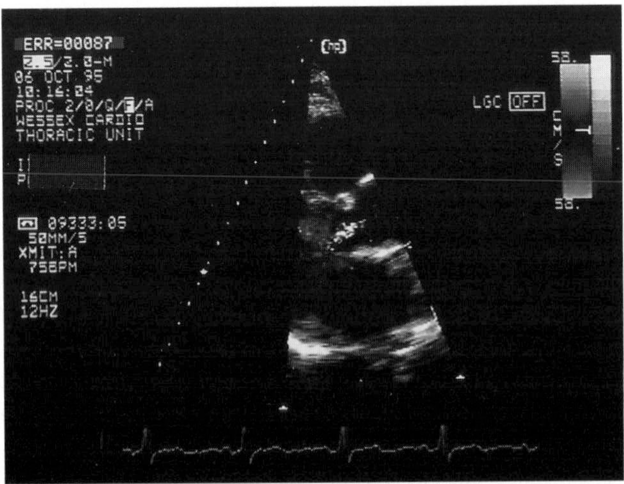

Fig. 12.6 Regurgitation through an otherwise normal aortic homograft. This was present postoperatively and did not represent structural valve degeneration. For colour, see Plate 12.6 (between pp. 308 and 309).

by ultrasound techniques is of considerable clinical importance although it can be difficult on occasions even with transoesophageal echocardiography.

Inteference with valve function from intracardiac structures is a potential problem requiring special care at implant especially with the lower profile mechanical valves. Fibrous ingrowth or pannus formation may cause similar problems at a later date.

Prosthetic–ventricular mismatch for valves in the mitral position is a problem with high profile valves such as stented biological valves and caged ball prostheses. The stent or cage may overprotrude into the left ventricular cavity particularly in cases of valve replacement for rheumatic mitral stenosis with a small left ventricular cavity. This can cause left ventricular outflow tract obstruction and rarely erosion (or even rupture) of the posterolateral left ventricular wall [24,25].

Left ventricular outflow tract obstruction has also been described following mitral valve repair using annular ring devices [26]. This is caused by systolic anterior motion of the mitral valve and is usually a dynamic phenomenon open to pharmacological manipulation. Residual mitral regurgitation is the other main complication of conservative mitral valve surgery and is the commonest cause of early reoperation [27–29].

All prosthetic valves carry the risk of endocarditis. The risk is as great for biological valves as for mechanical valves [30,31] although it has been reported to be lower for homografts in the perioperative period [23,32]. Endocarditis may affect the valve leaflets or the sewing ring. Due to the involvement of the sewing ring perivalvular extension of infection leading to paraprosthetic regurgitation, paravalvar abscess and spread to adjacent structures can affect 54–60% of cases of prosthetic valve endocarditis [33]. Involvement of the valve leaflets of biological valves may cause progressive and often acute valve degeneration. Involvement of the occluding device of mechanical valves can cause valve stenosis by interfering with valve opening and also regurgitation by preventing complete valve closure. Vegetations in any position have the potential to embolize. The likelihood of embolization is difficult to predict from the echocardiographic appearance although there is some evidence that vegetations greater than 1 cm diameter are more likely to embolize.

The major differences in the complications of biological and mechanical valves arise from the greater thrombogenicity of mechanical valves (and the consequent need for lifelong anticoagulation) and the incidence of structural valve degeneration affecting tissue valves. Perhaps surprisingly, the incidence of thromboembolic complications does not differ significantly between the two valve types [30] suggesting that factors other than valve type play a significant role. Valve thrombosis, however, is more common for mechanical valves and in a similar way to valvar vegetations may lead to both stenosis and regurgitation. The low thrombogenicity and excellent haemodynamic profiles made tissue valves the valve of choice in most centres in the 1970s and early 1980s. It became apparent, however, that biological valves had a significant incidence of structural valve degeneration requiring reoperation [34–40]. The incidence of structural valve degeneration for tissue valves is approximately 10–30% at 10 years and 42–70% at 15 years. The incidence of degeneration is higher in younger patients and for valves in the mitral position. The failure rates are similar for homografts and porcine valves although the mode of failure differs. Calcific degeneration of porcine valves may cause stenosis or regurgitation. Calcification is less common in homografts and when it does occur is more likely to have a minor effect on leaflet mobility but predisposes to leaflet rupture making regurgitation the commonest mode of failure [41]. In contrast the currently available mechanical prostheses have proven long-term durability. There have been no cases of structural failure of the Starr–Edwards, Medtronic Hall or Omniscience valves and only 10 cases of fracture in St Jude valves [42].

The morbidity associated with tissue valves from structural valve degeneration and the need for reoperation outweighs the risks of bleeding complications associated with anticoagulation for mechanical valves at approx. 12 years [31]. Tissue valves are now only the valve of choice when anticoagulation is contraindicated or for elderly patients in the aortic position. However, the long-term durability of current generation bioprostheses is yet to be determined and may influence this policy in the future.

The broad spectrum of normality for prosthetic valve function and the wide range of pathological conditions affecting these prostheses make a comprehensive assessment of their function a significant challenge for modern ultrasound techniques and requires an appreciation of the values of each of the echocardiographic modes from both transthoracic and transoesophageal windows.

Echocardiographic assessment of prosthetic valves

M-mode

The use of M-mode echocardiography for direct visualization of valve prostheses is largely of historical interest but it still plays a role in assessing the effects of valve dysfunction on the cardiac chamber size and function. Nevertheless a brief description of the common findings is worthwhile. The basis of M-mode echocardiography is that reflected ultrasound can be used to identify the position of the reflected structure by the time from ultrasound transmission to reception. This assumes that the speed of ultrasound in the biological tissue is constant, a situation that is not true when a mechanical valve is *in situ*, particularly a ball and cage prosthesis. The speed of ultrasound through a sialastic ball is slower than through biological tissue and this has the artefactual effect of increasing the apparent depth of the ball. This will give the impression that the posterior aspect of the ball in an aortic valve replacement lies within the cavity of the left atrium when viewed from the parasternal view.

M-mode can be used for tracing the time course of motion of prosthetic valve opening and closing. The opening and closing of mechanical valve occluders and tissue valve leaflets should be vertical and of large amplitude. Atrioventricular valves should remain open during diastole and ventriculoarterial valves during systole. Simultaneous phonocardiography is useful in the timing of prosthetic valve opening and closing relative to the corresponding native valve (although this is now rarely used). Values of maximum excursion of occluder devices on M-mode are available from the manufacturer and the range of time delay in opening and closing from the literature [43]. Reduction in the excursion of the occluding device or the opening angle, or a delay in the valve opening suggest prosthetic valve obstruction. This may be intermittent and several cycles need to be recorded [44]. For biological valves thickening of valve cusps may be seen in addition to reduction in opening angle and leaflet excursion indicating valve stenosis or obstruction.

There are several limitations of M-mode for assessing valve function. The ultrasound beam must be aligned parallel to valve opening for any measurements to be reliable. This is aided by using 2D imaging to guide the position of the M-mode cursor. A reduced cardiac output from impaired left ventricular function may give reduced opening angle and leaflet/occluder excursion in the case of a normally functioning prosthesis. There is also a wide variation in the opening times of valves dependent upon factors such as heart rate, rhythm and preload. M-mode is generally of little use in assessing valve dysfunction when regurgitation is the main problem although the presence of fluttering of tissue valve leaflets suggests the presence of valvar regurgitation.

2D imaging

The spatial orientation inherent in 2D imaging facilitates greater visualization of prosthetic valves and surrounding structures than M-mode alone. The 2D examination remains the keystone of ultrasound assessment of prosthetic valves.

Due to the acoustic reverberations from the non-biological material of prosthetic valves it is important to use all the available acoustic windows and transducer positions and manoeuvres to optimize the imaging of all the prosthetic valve elements. Alignment of the transducer beam parallel to the opening of the valve will minimize the interference from the sewing ring in visualizing the valve occluder or leaflets. From the transthoracic approach this is often best achieved from the apical view for both aortic and mitral prostheses. The apical view will only allow imaging of the ventricular aspect of the valves. The parasternal window allows imaging of the ascending aorta and may provide satisfactory views of the left atrium and atrial aspect of the mitral valve. The transoesophageal approach, however, is usually required to provide adequate diagnostic information for valves in the mitral position. Finding a suitable imaging window can be particularly difficult in patients with two prosthetic valves. In patients with an aortic and mitral prosthesis it may not be possible to obtain satisfactory images of the mitral valve from the transthoracic approach and from the transoesophageal approach it can be very difficult to image the aortic prosthesis. In such patients multiple imaging planes from both the transthoracic and transoesophageal windows will be required to provide a comprehensive assessment of both valves.

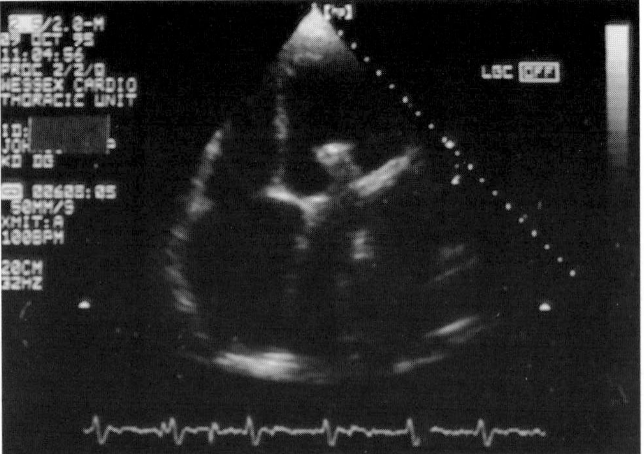

(a)

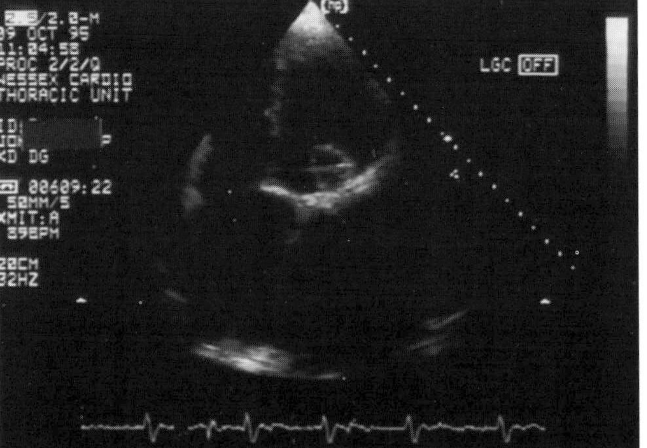

(b)

Fig. 12.7 Transthoracic 2D imaging of a Starr–Edwards mitral valve prosthesis (a) open and (b) closed.

MECHANICAL VALVES

Artefactual acoustic reverberations are greater with mechanical valves as both the valve occluding device and the sewing ring comprise non-biological material. Nevertheless 2D imaging of all the valve elements is possible and should distinguish normal from abnormal function.

In a caged ball prosthesis both the cage and ball can be seen. The ball should move smoothly to the cage apex. A reduction in the excursion of the ball implies the presence of obstructing tissue such as thrombus or vegetation. The orientation of the valve cage can be determined. In the mitral position this should be towards the left ventricular apex and the left ventricular outflow tract adjacent to the valve should not be narrowed (Fig. 12.7).

For tilting disc valves the maximal motion of the disc can be determined. For valves in the mitral position the larger portion of the disc will tilt into the ventricle and the smaller portion into the atrium. Usually only the movement of the larger portion can be seen, the movement of the smaller portion being obscured by the sewing ring. Likewise for valves in the aortic position the larger portion of the disc will tilt into the ascending aorta. The larger valve orifice can be determined from the disc movement and for valves in the mitral position the larger orifice should be directed towards the left ventricular apex to minimize turbulence in the outflow tract. Obstructing tissue can restrict the opening angle of the disc implying stenosis of the valve and can also prevent the closure of the disc which will cause significant regurgitation.

The individual discs of a bileaflet valve can be seen. When the valve is open the discs are parallel and when closed they appear to form two sides of a triangle depending on the closure angle (Fig. 12.8). Because the flow across bileaflet valves should be relatively uniform the orientation of the valve is of less importance. As in tilting disc valves any reduction in the normal opening and closing motion of the discs can be seen and both leaflets can be evaluated separately. This is important as obstructing tissue may affect one disc and not the other. Care should be taken to observe the valve in a plane where the movement of both leaflets can be seen to prevent the incorrect conclusion that one disc is not working normally.

BIOLOGICAL VALVES

Acoustic shadowing is less of a problem with biological valves. Porcine xenografts have non-biological material in

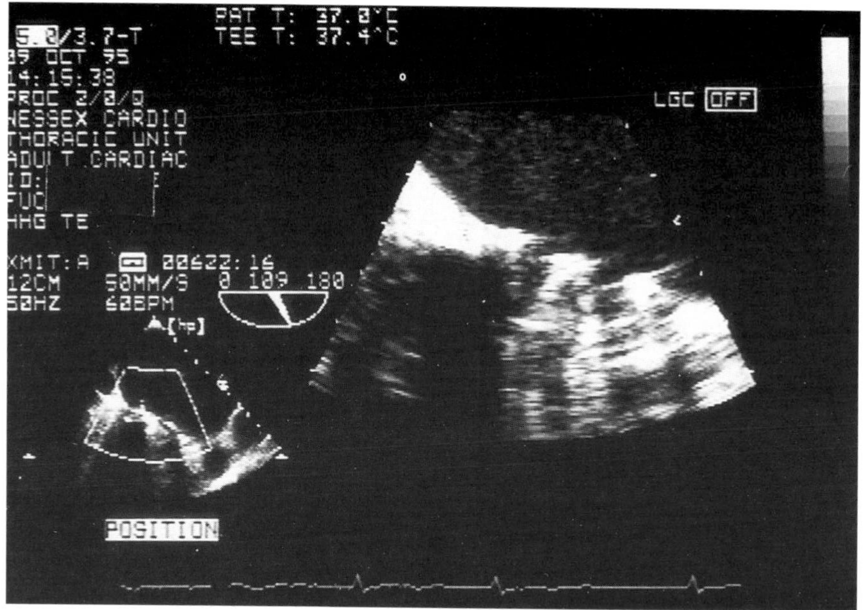

(a)

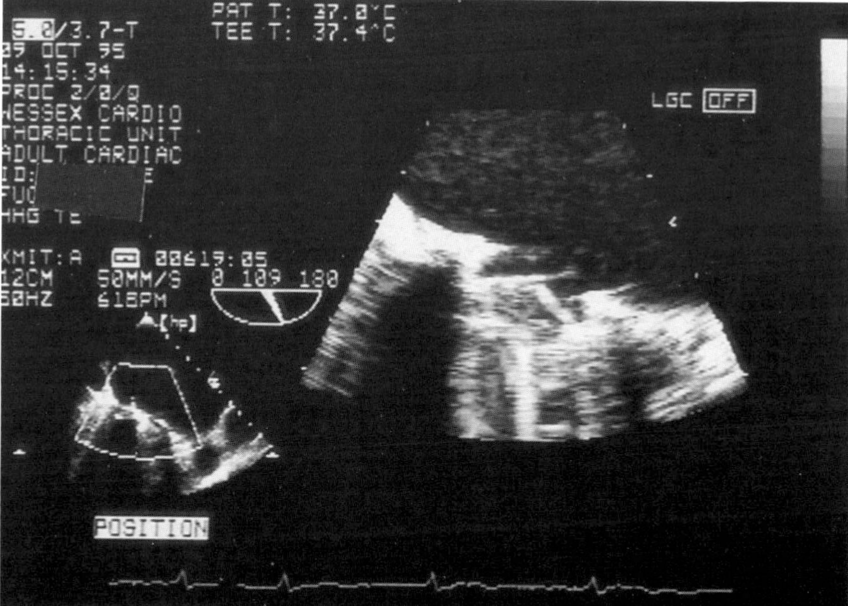

(b)

Fig. 12.8 Transoesophageal imaging of a Carbomedics bileaflet valve (a) open and (b) closed.

the valve stents (Fig. 12.9) and sewing ring and homografts have no non-biological material. This makes adequate imaging easier and more likely from the transthoracic approach (Fig. 12.10). In a longitudinal plane two valve stents can be seen and all three imaged if the valve is viewed in cross-section. It should be possible to visualize all three leaflets of a biological valve. The valve leaflets should be thin and mobile similar to normal native aortic valve leaflets. Degenerative changes will appear as thickening and calcification of the leaflets. The movement of the valve leaflets will be restricted if the valve becomes stenotic. Degeneration of the valve can result in a cusp tear. This is occasionally an acute event resulting in severe acute regurgitation. Prolapse of all or part of the valve cusp into the dependent chamber can be seen on 2D imaging. Occasionally fibrin deposited on stitch material can mimic the appearance of a flail cusp. Doppler colour flow mapping should clarify the situation by identifying significant regurgitation in the case of a flail cusp.

MECHANICAL AND BIOLOGICAL VALVES

For all prosthetic valves the contours of the valve and

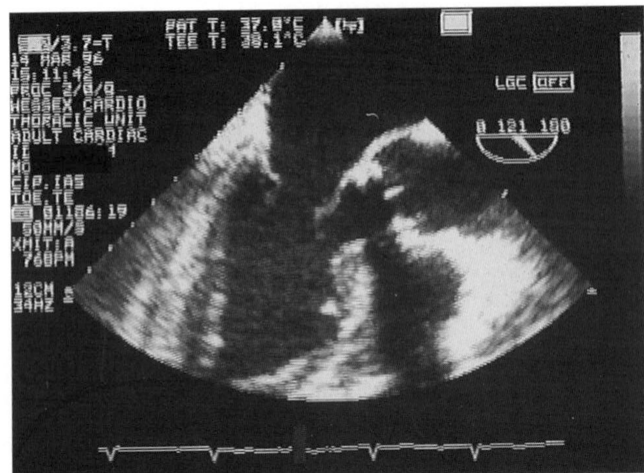

(a)

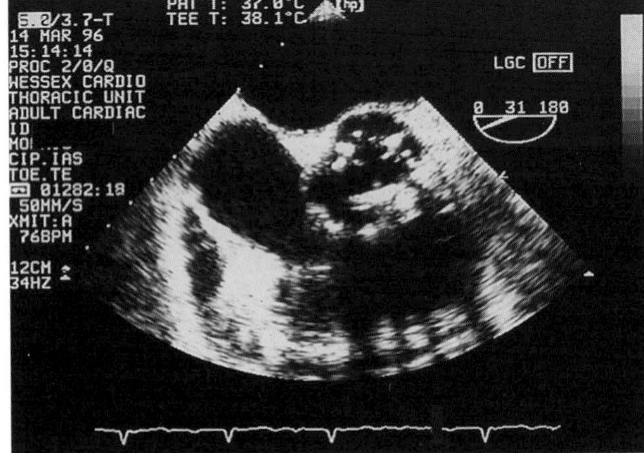

(b)

Fig. 12.9 Transoesophageal imaging of a Medtronic Intact porcine aortic prosthesis in (a) the longitudinal axis and (b) the cross-sectional short axis.

sewing ring should be smooth and regular without unusual protrusions or echo densities. Thombi and vegetations will appear as echodense masses attached to the valve or sewing ring usually with movement independent of the valve. Due to the non-biological material it is often difficult to distinguish true echo-dense masses and those produced by artefact unless they are large and protrude from the valve plane into the cardiac chambers. Transoesophageal echocardiography is more sensitive than transthoracic for the detection of smaller thrombi or vegetations. Paravalvar abscesses in endocarditis can be seen as echo-free spaces surrounding the valve sewing ring. Further complications of endocarditis such as fistulous connections or perforation of the anterior mitral valve leaflet can be diagnosed by loss of continuity of the particular structure although demonstration of blood flow through such fistulae by Doppler techniques is usually required to confirm the diagnosis. Again transoesophageal echocardiography is more sensitive in the diagnosis of the complications of endocarditis and this will be discussed in more detail below.

The motion of the sewing ring should be assessed for all prosthetic valves. The sewing ring should move with the native valve annulus. Abnormal rocking motion of the valve is seen with partial dehiscence of the valve from the annulus [45].

Assessment of left ventricular function from the 2D study is important in the interpretation of prosthetic valve function in several ways. In cases of significant valve regurgitation and normal left ventricular systolic function the left ventricle will appear dynamic on imaging with an increased end-diastolic volume and a normal or exaggerated ejection fraction. In addition, septal motion postcar-

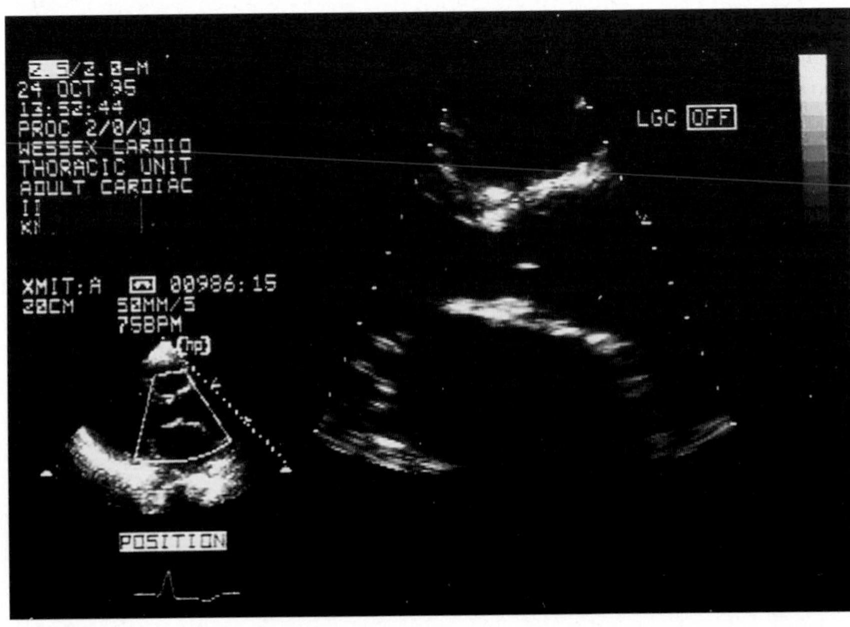

Fig. 12.10 Transthoracic imaging of a St Jude Toronto stentless porcine aortic prosthesis. The absence of stents improves the imaging of the valve leaflets.

diac surgery is normally paradoxical. The mechanism for this is poorly understood and septal motion often returns to normal with time. In the case of significant volume overload the septal motion can be normal or exaggerated. The absence of paradoxical septal motion in the early stages postvalve replacement may imply volume overload from a significant regurgitant lesion. The left ventricular systolic function should always be considered when interpreting the Doppler-derived aortic valve gradients. In the presence of a poorly functioning left ventricle the valve gradient may be within normal limits despite significant valve dysfunction whereas a hypertrophied ventricle with normal systolic function may give high pressure gradients across normally functioning prostheses especially with the smaller sized valves.

As with M-mode, 2D echo is of limited use in the quantitation of stenosis or regurgitation. Restricted movement of valve occluders or leaflets implies that the valve is stenotic. Prolapse of bioprosthetic leaflets or sticking of mechanical valve discs will imply a significant valvar leak and rocking of the sewing ring implies a significant paravalvar leak. Increase in the dependent chamber size is a less sensitive and less specific indicator of regurgitation. Quantitation of the degree of stenosis or regurgitation relies largely on Doppler techniques.

Conventional pulsed and continuous wave Doppler

Pulsed wave Doppler samples the velocity at a particular point along the line of interest. This is used for low velocity flow such as mitral forward flow or when the velocity sampled is likely to be less than the maximum flow along the line of interest such as in the left ventricular outflow tract. Continuous wave Doppler will display the maximum velocity along the line of interest and can be used for high velocity flow. Continuous wave Doppler is usually required to measure the peak velocities of aortic prosthetic valve forward and regurgitant flow and mitral regurgitation. In the case of aortic and mitral regurgitation pulsed wave Doppler is unlikely to be able to measure the peak flow but can be used to map the area in which regurgitation is detected within the dependent chamber.

Alignment of the Doppler signal with the direction of blood flow is important to avoid underestimation of the blood flow velocity. Use of 2D imaging with superimposed Doppler colour flow mapping aids the correct alignment of the Doppler signal.

As with native valves the pressure gradient across prosthetic valves can be estimated from the modified Bernoulli equation $P = 4v^2$. This equation has theoretical limitations when applied to prosthetic valves. The modified equation assumes that the velocity distal to the stenosis (v_1) is significantly larger than the velocity proximal to the stenosis (v_0) making v_0^2 negligible relative to v_1^2. In the measurement of prosthetic valve gradients the proximal and distal velocities may not be greatly different and the equation

$$P = 4(v_1^2 - v_0^2)$$

may be more accurate. The other assumption of both of these equations is that viscous forces within normal cardiac structures are negligible. This assumption does not necessarily apply to prosthetic heart valves. Despite these theoretical limitations pressure gradients derived from continuous wave Doppler using the modified Bernoulli equation have been validated against catheter-derived gradients for biological and mechanical prostheses in the aortic, mitral and tricuspid positions [46,47].

PROSTHETIC VALVE FORWARD FLOW

Aortic valves

Aortic flow may be adequately assessed apically although often the right parasternal or the suprasternal window will provide a better signal. The transoesophageal window seldom adds to the continuous wave Doppler assessment of aortic flow due to the difficulty aligning the signal with transaortic flow from this approach. As with native valves the peak Doppler-derived aortic valve gradient correlates with the peak instantaneous catheter-derived gradient and will appear to overestimate the more commonly measured peak-to-peak catheter gradient.

Prosthetic valves are inherently mildly stenotic and consequently the calculated pressure gradients across normally functionally aortic prostheses will exceed those of normal native valves. Valve gradients are usually highest for ball and cage valves and lowest for bioprostheses. Aortic homografts and the stentless porcine valves may have gradients similar to normal native valves due to the absence of obstructing valve stents. Normal ranges of pressure gradients are available for the various types of prostheses. Table 12.2 demonstrates the normal values for four different types of aortic prosthesis.

The most reliable reference value for a particular patient is provided by a baseline postoperative Doppler assessment. Pressure gradients across normally functioning prostheses vary greatly between individual patients and comparison of the follow-up haemodynamic data with the baseline data for that particular patient is far more valuable than reference to the quoted normal range for the valve type. With reference to the normal valve gradient for a particular patient valve stenosis can be reliably diagnosed and quantitated by elevated transvalvar gradients.

There are, however, limitations to relying on pressure gradients to diagnose obstruction/stenosis. The valve

Table 12.2 Values for normally functioning aortic valve prostheses (with permission from Heldman and Gardin [48])

Valve type	Peak velocity ($m s^{-1}$)	Peak gradient (mmHg)	Mean gradient (mmHg)
St Jude	2.3 ± 0.6	22 ± 12	12 ± 7
Bjork Shiley	2.6 ± 0.5	27 ± 9	14 ± 6
Starr–Edwards	3.2 ± 0.2	40 ± 3	24 ± 4
Tissue	2.1 ± 0.5	19 ± 9	11 ± 5

gradient depends not only on valve function but upon haemodynamic factors such as cardiac output and heart rate. Relatively high transvalvar gradients may be recorded across normally functioning valves and valve gradients have been shown to nearly double on maximal exertion [49,50]. Conversely, a patient with a failing left ventricle due to valve obstruction or stenosis may have a maximum pressure gradient within the normal range for that particular valve despite the valvar dysfunction.

In such cases calculation of the valve area may give a more reliable index of valve integrity. For aortic valves the continuity principle is used to calculate area according to the equation

$$AVA = LVOT_{area} \times LVOT_{VTI}/AV_{VTI}$$

where AVA = aortic valve area, LVOT = left ventricular outflow tract, AV = aortic valve and VTI = velocity time integral. The left ventricular outflow tract area is calculated by measurement of the inner diameter of the left ventricular outflow tract just below the aortic valve. The left ventricular outflow tract velocity time integral is calculated from the pulsed wave Doppler signal sampled in the left ventricular outflow tract at the same point as the diameter measurement. The velocity time integral is the area under the velocity : time curve and allows calculation of blood flow if the cross-sectional area is known. The simplified continuity equation uses velocity measurements if calculation of the velocity time integral is not available:

$$AVA = LVOT_{area} \times LVOT\,.\,V_{max}/AV\,.\,V_{max}$$

where V_{max} = maximal blood flow velocity. The calculation of prosthetic aortic valve area using this principle has been validated against *in vitro* measurements [51]. It has also been shown that effective valve areas of <1.0 cm^2 tended to be associated with obstruction documented at surgery [52] although prosthetic valve areas of <1 cm^2 can be found with the smaller sizes of normally functioning aortic prostheses.

Mitral valves

Transmitral flow is best assessed from the apical window in a transthoracic study. The transoesophageal approach allows more accurate alignment of the Doppler signal and overcomes the problem of flow masking of regurgitation from the prosthesis. As with aortic prostheses transprosthetic gradients in the mitral position will be higher than normal native valves and reference to the baseline values for the individual patient will be of greater value than the quoted normal range for a particular valve. Table 12.3 demonstrates the normal values for four different prostheses.

Mitral valve area can be calculated from the continuity equation or the pressure half-time method:

$$MVA = LVOT_{area} \times LVOT_{VTI}/MV_{VTI}$$

$$MVA = 220/\text{pressure half-time}$$

where MVA = mitral valve area and MV = mitral valve. The estimated prosthetic mitral valve area by pressure half-time has been shown to correlate with catheter-derived valve area [53,54]. Kapur *et al.* found that valve areas of <1.1 cm^2 calculated from the pressure half-time were associated with obstruction confirmed at surgery [52]. Dumensil *et al.* [55] found that the continuity equation is a more accurate method of calculating prosthetic mitral valve area when validated against an *in vitro* model. The pressure half-time method in this study overestimated the valve area. This may be due to the inertia of the valve giving a higher early diastolic pressure and a steeper deceleration slope (from which the pressure half-time is calculated). The continuity equation, however, will be inaccurate in the presence of significant mitral or aortic regurgitation and in such cases the pressure half-time is likely to be more accurate.

PROSTHETIC VALVE REGURGITANT FLOW

Pulsed and continuous wave Doppler are highly sensitive in the detection of valve regurgitation although masking of the signal by prosthetic material is a problem for mitral valves. These Doppler modes are of less value in the quantitation of regurgitation although they can be used as an index of severity in several ways. Mapping of the regurgitant jet area within the dependent chamber by pulsed wave Doppler allows semiquantitation of regurgitation but is time-consuming and has been superseded by Doppler colour flow mapping.

Calculation of the volume of blood flow across the mitral valve and aortic valve or left ventricular outflow tract using the velocity time integral and orifice area allows a regurgitant fraction to be calculated for aortic or mitral regurgitation from the continuity principle. Small

Table 12.3 Values for normally functioning mitral valve prostheses (with permission from Heldman and Gardin [48])

Valve type	Peak velocity ($m s^{-1}$)	Peak gradient (mmHg)	Mean gradient (mmHg)	Orifice size (cm^2)
St Jude	1.6 ± 0.3	11 ± 4.0	5 ± 2.0	3.0 ± 0.6
Bjork Shiley	1.6 ± 0.3	10 ± 3.0	5 ± 2.0	2.2 ± 0.4
Starr–Edwards	1.8 ± 0.4	13 ± 5	5 ± 2.0	2.1 ± 0.5
Tissue	1.5 ± 0.3	9.9 ± 3.4	4.8 ± 1.7	2.0 ± 0.5

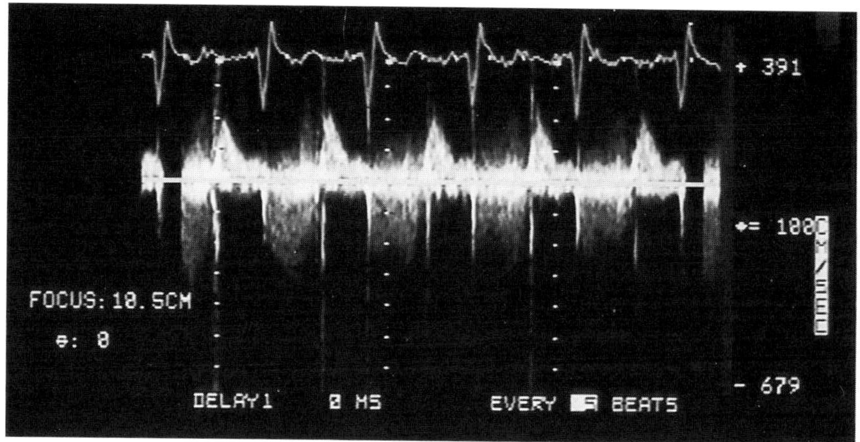

Fig. 12.11 Continuous wave Doppler of mitral forward flow in a case of severe regurgitation demonstrating a high peak forward flow and normal deceleration slope.

inaccuracies in measurement, however, may give a large inaccuracy in the regurgitant fraction.

Severe mitral regurgitation will give a high peak forward velocity across the mitral valve. If the valve opening is normal the pressure half-time will be normal. This principle is particularly important for transthoracic studies of mitral prostheses as the regurgitation may be masked by the prosthesis. The combination of a high forward velocity in the presence of a normal valve area by pressure half-time method suggests severe regurgitation and will be an indication for further imaging from the transoesophageal approach (Fig. 12.11).

The pressure half-time of aortic regurgitation has been used to assess its severity. The more severe the regurgitation the more rapid the equalization of aortic and left ventricular diastolic pressure and the steeper the descent of the continuous wave Doppler velocity trace. A pressure half-time measured from the deceleration slope of <300 ms suggests severe aortic regurgitation.

Doppler colour flow mapping

PROSTHETIC VALVE FORWARD FLOW

Colour flow mapping of transprosthetic flow enables the echocardiographer to align the continuous wave Doppler with the direction of flow allowing a more accurate assessment of transvalvar gradients. This is more important for prosthetic than native valves as prosthetic valves may have eccentric and multiple jets.

Caged ball valves will appear to have two jets of flow around the ball (as imaging is 2D) (Fig. 12.12). Tilting disc valves will have one major and one minor jet corresponding to the major and minor orifices. Correct orientation of the major orifice towards the left ventricular apex is important at implant as this causes less turbulence on the ventricular side of the valve. Bileaflet valves may be seen to have three jets of flow. Failure to identify separately each of the jets of flow across mechanical valves may indicate obstruction to flow but from the transthoracic approach is as likely to represent inadequate imaging.

Biological valves should only have one jet of colour flow. Measurement of the maximal jet width at its origin for biological valves in the mitral position correlates with the effective valve area calculated at catheter and a jet width of ≤0.8 cm has been shown to be associated with obstruction confirmed at surgery [52].

PROSTHETIC VALVE REGURGITANT FLOW

Doppler colour flow mapping has proved to be most useful for evaluation of prosthetic valve regurgitation. The regurgitant flow is seen as a reversed, mosaic coloured pattern in the dependent chamber upon closure of the valve. The site of the regurgitation, the width of the jet at the regurgitant orifice, and the area occupied by the jet in the dependent chamber are readily visualized allowing a quicker and more accurate assessment of the severity of the regurgitation than methods using pulsed wave and continuous wave Doppler modes.

Doppler colour flow mapping is sensitive enough to detect the normal closing and leakage volume from a mechanical valve. From the transthoracic view (Fig. 12.13) this is often masked by artefact from the valve and the normal regurgitant flow of mechanical valves is best visualized from transoesophageal imaging. Transoesophageal echocardiography (Fig. 12.14) will also readily distinguish this normal flow from pathological regurgitation. Normal regurgitation is seen within the valve ring, is of low velocity and occupies only a small area within the dependent chamber. Caged ball prostheses exhibit two regurgitant jets just within the valve ring. The flow is mostly early systolic representing closure rather than leakage flow. Tilting disc and bileaflet valves exhibit holosystolic regurgitant flow. Tilting disc valves may produce two peripheral jets although they may appear to have only one central regurgitant jet. Bileaflet valves produce two peripheral jets and often a third central jet.

Pathological regurgitation is of higher velocity, occupying a significant area within the dependent chamber. Visualization of the regurgitant colour flow jet and the flow convergence region (see below) helps to distinguish valvar from paraprosthetic regurgitation. Correct categorization is possible in approximately 90% of mitral and 80% of aortic prostheses from the transthoracic approach in relation to the findings at surgery [52]. This sensitivity is increased with transoesophageal echocardiography. As well as aiding the diagnosis of the causative pathology the differentiation of valvar from paravalvar regurgitation has implications for the surgical management as a paravalvar leak may be amenable to repair rather than replacement.

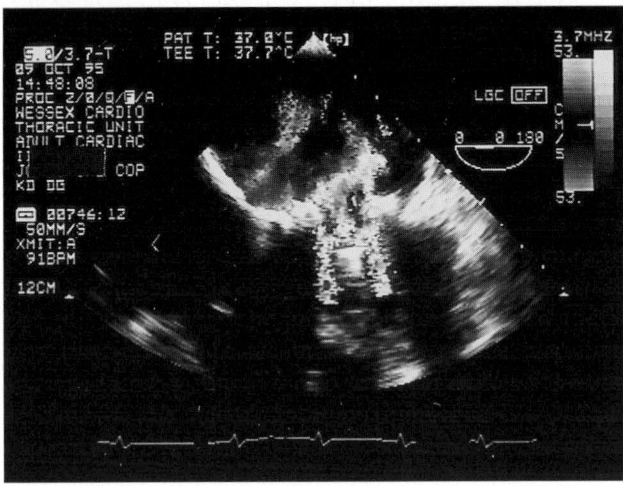

Fig. 12.12 Doppler colour flow mapping of normal forward flow through a caged ball prosthesis. For colour, see Plate 12.12 (between pp. 308 and 309).

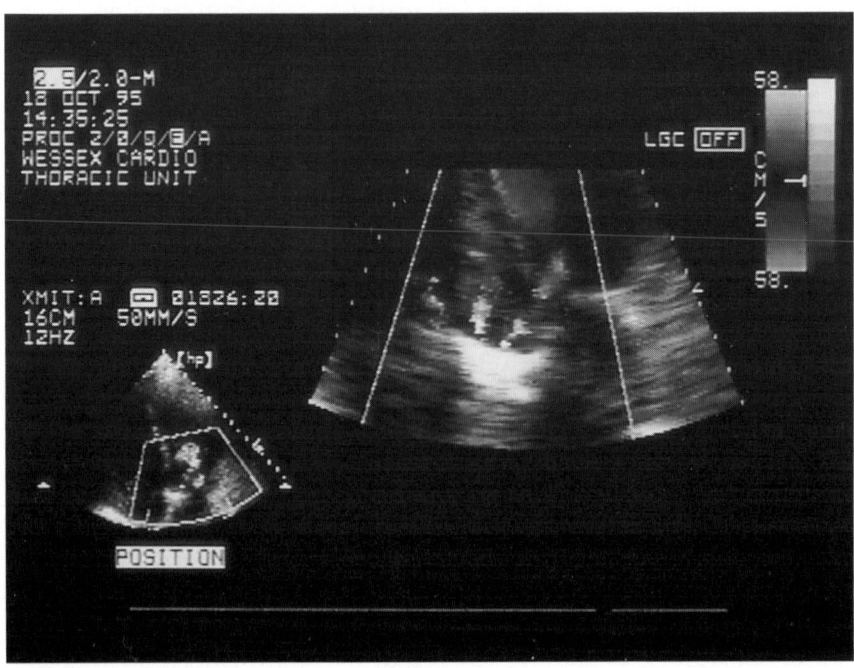

Fig. 12.13 Transthoracic imaging of normal regurgitant flow through an aortic bileaflet prosthesis. For colour, see Plate 12.13 (between pp. 308 and 309).

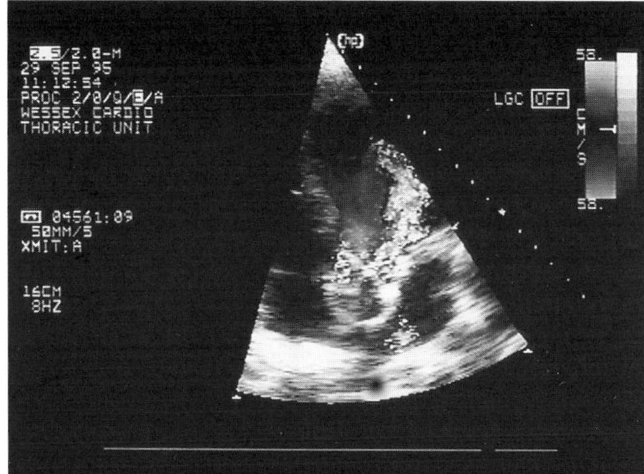

(a)

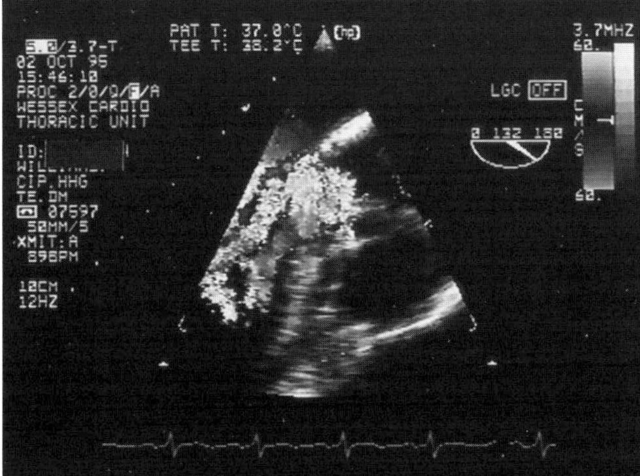

(b)

Fig. 12.14 Significant regurgitation due to structural valve degeneration of an aortic homograft from (a) transthoracic and (b) transoesophageal windows. For colour, see Plate 12.14 (between pp. 308 and 309).

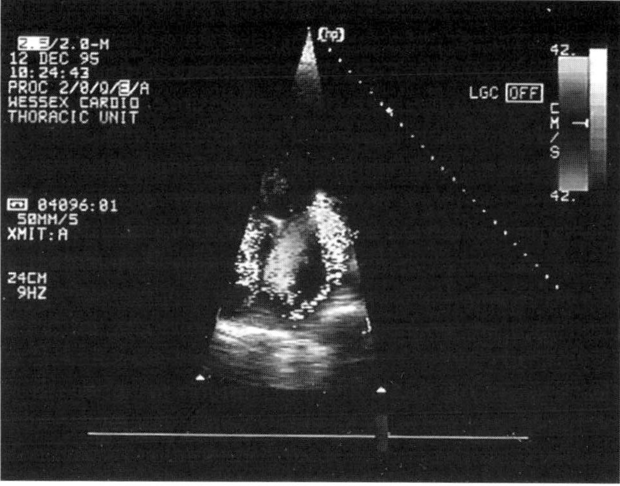

Fig. 12.15 Eccentric wall jet of severe paraprosthetic mitral regurgitation. For colour, see Plate 12.15 (between pp. 308 and 309).

Quantitation of regurgitation involves assessment of regurgitant jet width at its origin and the maximal jet area within the dependent chamber [52]. The maximal area of prosthetic mitral regurgitation assessed by planimetry and expressed as a ratio of the left atrial area has been shown to correlate with angiographic assessment of mitral regurgitation. Areas of <20%, 20–40% and >40% represent mild, moderate and severe regurgitation, respectively. The use of jet areas alone may be an unreliable indicator of the severity of the regurgitation when the jet is eccentric and hugs the wall of the left atrium (Fig. 12.15). In such cases the apparent size of the jets is reduced and the jet may not be imaged in certain views. The presence of a wall jet implies that the regurgitation is likely to be severe and care should be taken to image the regurgitation in several planes to determine the width of the regurgitant orifice and the limits of the regurgitant jet within the atrium. In severe regurgitation wall jets will often cause colour flow reversal or aliasing of the colour flow Doppler signal within the atrial appendage and one or more pulmonary veins and the jet can circle the entire left atrium in very severe regurgitation. Adequate assessment of prosthetic mitral regurgitation usually requires transoesophageal imaging. The severity of aortic regurgitation can be assessed by the maximal diameter of the regurgitant jet at its origin expressed as a ratio of the left ventricular outflow tract inner diameter taken at the same point. Ratios of <24%, 25–46%, 47–64% and ≥65% represent grades I–IV, respectively.

As with most attempts to quantitate regurgitation there are limitations to these methods. Regurgitant jet areas are dependent upon fluid dynamic factors other than regurgitant volume and the appearance of the jet area will also depend on instrumentation factors. Doppler colour flow mapping can add further to the assessment of regurgitation by identifying a flow convergence region (Fig. 12.16). Within this region the regurgitant stream narrows and accelerates proximal to the regurgitant orifice. The presence of colour flow convergence suggests significant regurgitation and this flow convergence region has been used to quantitate mitral regurgitation in native valves. The flow rate within the flow convergence region is given by the value $2\pi r^2 vr$ where $2\pi r^2$ is the hemispheric area and vr the velocity at a distance r from the regurgitant orifice. (This calculation is based on the principle that the flow convergence region comprises isovelocity hemispheric surfaces when the size of the regurgitant orifice is small enough for its shape to be considered insignificant.) According to the continuity principle this flow rate equals that through the regurgitant orifice [56].

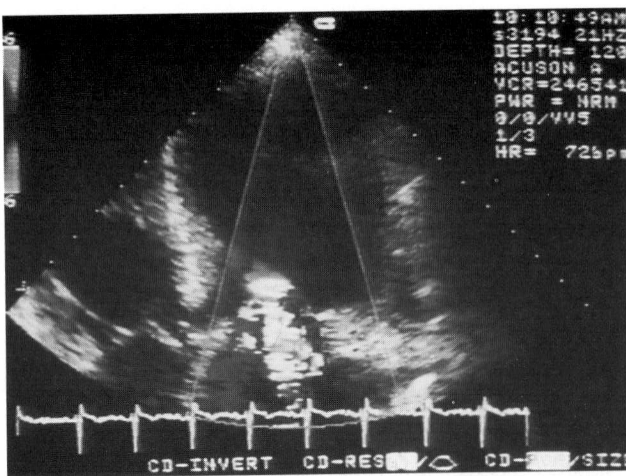

Fig. 12.16 Region of colour flow convergence on the ventricular aspect of a severely regurgitant mitral valve. For colour, see Plate 12.16 (between pp. 308 and 309).

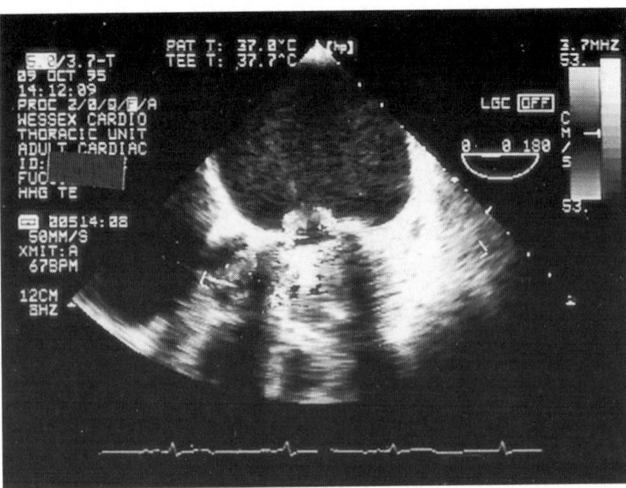

Fig. 12.17 Normal regurgitant flow through a mitral bileaflet prosthesis. For colour, see Plate 12.17 (between pp. 308 and 309).

Transoesophageal echocardiography

Transoesophageal echocardiography overcomes many of the limitations of transthoracic echocardiography. The close proximity of the oesophagus to the heart, the lack of intervening surfaces, and the use of higher frequency transducers provides superior quality imaging of the heart and valvar structures. Transoesophageal echocardiography provides an unobstructed view of the left atrium, left atrial appendage, mitral valve, right atrium and appendage, aortic root and ascending aorta, overcoming the limitations encountered as a result of attenuation and accoustic shadowing from prosthetic valves. Transoesophageal echocardiography can be performed perioperatively and in the intensive care setting when transthoracic echocardiography is often of little help.

Initially single plane 2D imaging was the only mode available. Currently available transducers allow multiplane imaging with all of the echocardiographic modes discussed above.

Transoesophageal echocardiography can be performed safely in the conscious patient with a very low risk of complication [57]. Perhaps the major concern is the incidence of bacteraemia and the risk of endocarditis. The incidence of bacteraemia has been reported as similar to gastroscopy, 7–16% [58]. There has, however, been only one case of streptococcal endocarditis temporally related to transoesophageal echocardiography and no cases with a proven causal relationship. Suspected endocarditis is often the indication for a transoesophageal study in patients with prosthetic valves and prophylactic antibiotic treatment would be likely to mask the bacteriological diagnosis in such cases. It is not routine practice at the authors' unit to give prophylactic antibiotics prior to transoesophageal echocardiography in patients with prosthetic valves.

MITRAL PROSTHESES

One of the major values of transoesophageal echocardiography is the assessment of prosthetic mitral valve function particularly regurgitation [59,60] (Fig. 12.17). Transoesophageal echocardiography allows high quality images of the left atrium and atrial surface of the valve which are frequently not possible from the transthoracic views. From the transthoracic approach mitral regurgitation is often masked by acoustic shadowing from the prosthesis. This can be partly overcome by the parasternal views. However, if the patient also has an aortic valve prosthesis adequate imaging of the left atrium and any mitral regurgitation may not be possible from any of the transthoracic windows. From the transoesophageal window the mitral valve is best imaged from both the transverse and longitudinal planes. The transgastric short axis view is also particularly useful to delineate a region of partial valve dehiscence and regurgitation (Fig. 12.18). When imaging mitral prostheses it is important to anteflex and retroflex the transducer and to scan the entire sewing ring anteriorly and posteriorly as well as from medial to lateral.

Transoesophageal echocardiography has been shown to have greater sensitivity and accuracy than transthoracic echocardiography in detecting and localizing regurgitation from mechanical and biological mitral valve prostheses [61–64]. As discussed earlier transoesophageal

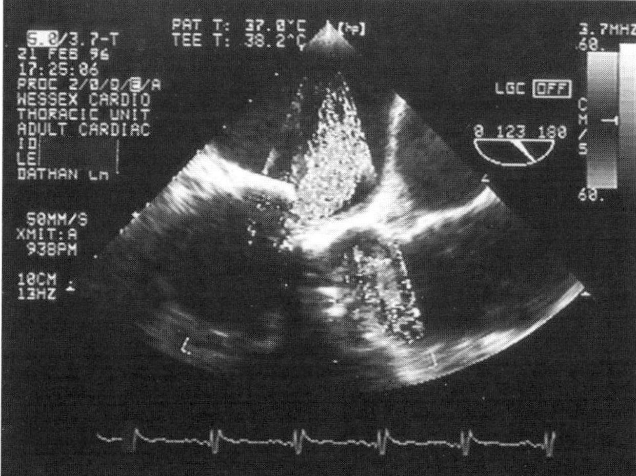

Fig. 12.18 Paraprosthetic mitral regurgitation: (a) a region of partial valve dehiscence, and (b) a broad regurgitant jet. For colour, see Plate 12.18 (between pp. 308 and 309).

Doppler colour flow mapping is far more sensitive than transthoracic in detecting the normal leakage volume from a prosthetic valve and in distinguishing paraprosthetic from valvar regurgitation. The sensitivity is such that occasionally in the early postoperative period small and insignificant paraprosthetic regurgitant jets can be seen through the sutures which disappear with time due to endothelialization of the suture ring. With significant paraprosthetic regurgitation abnormal rocking of the valve and a region of partial valve dehiscence are often seen. Semi-quantitation of mitral regurgitation by Doppler colour flow mapping of regurgitant jet areas and measurement of the width of the jet at its origin are more accurate from transoesophageal imaging [59,65,66]. Assessment of the severity of mitral regurgitation is further enhanced by imaging of the pulmonary veins and pulsed wave Doppler interrogation of pulmonary venous flow [67,68]. This is rarely possible from the transthoracic view. Normal pulmonary venous flow is quadriphasic with flow reversal seen only in late diastole (due to atrial contraction). Blunting of systolic forward flow or systolic flow reversal suggest severe regurgitation (Fig. 12.19). It is important to interrogate right and left pulmonary veins as the mitral regurgitant jet may be eccentric and flow reversal may be seen in the right-sided pulmonary veins and not the left and vice versa.

Transoesophageal imaging allows clear views of the left (and right) atrial appendage which is the commonest site of thrombus formation within the left atrium (Fig. 12.20) and rarely seen from transthoracic views even in the most echogenic patients with normal native valves. Patients with an enlarged left atrium or a stenotic mitral valve may also show spontaneous echo contrast within the atrium or atrial appendage. Spontaneous contrast is rarely seen with significant mitral regurgitation.

Clear views of the interatrial septum can be obtained with transoesophageal imaging. Bulging of the septum in the direction of the right atrium will occur with a high left atrial pressure from significant mitral regurgitation although this is a far less sensitive and specific measure of severity than other indices.

Pulsed and continuous wave Doppler measurements provide haemodynamic assessment of mitral forward flow and calculation of mitral valve area. These measurements are more easily performed from transoesophageal imaging although are usually adequate from the transthoracic views.

The aetiology of mitral valve dysfunction is also more accurately assessed from the transoesophageal view. The opening and closing of mechanical device occluders and the leaflets of biological valves are better visualized especially with multiplane transducers. Calcification, immobility or prolapse of tissue valve leaflets and restricted movements of mechanical valve occluders can be determined with greater accuracy. Vegetations or thrombi that may be masked by artefact or too small to be seen from transthoracic views can be diagnosed accurately.

AORTIC PROSTHESES

The aortic valve is best imaged from the longitudinal and basal short axis views. Transoesophageal echocardiography of prosthetic aortic valves provides superior imaging to transthoracic echocardiography although haemodynamic evaluation of aortic prosthetic function may be better performed from the transthoracic view. Due to the direction of blood flow across the aortic valve alignment of the continuous wave Doppler is usually easier from the transthoracic windows. The transgastric view may provide the best alignment when performing a transoeso-

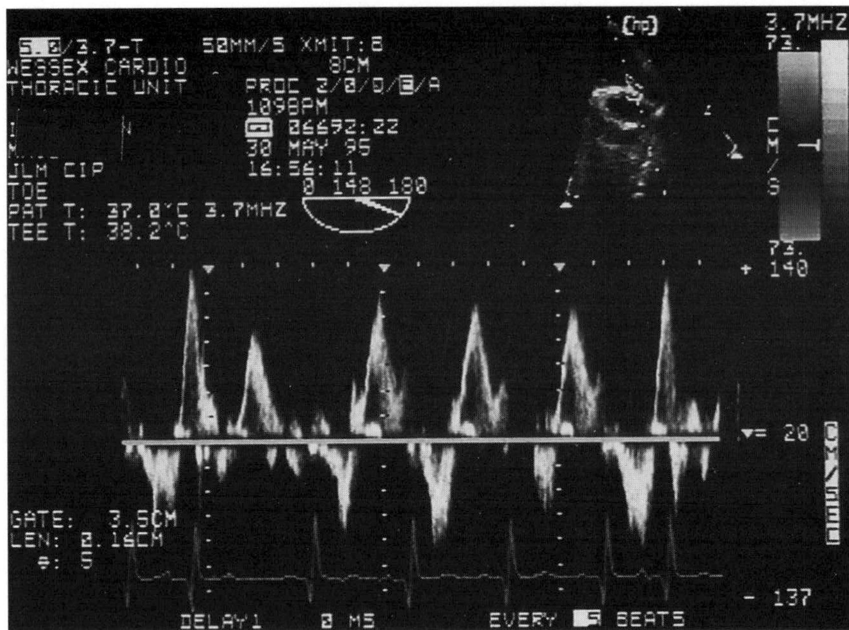

Fig. 12.19 Pulmonary venous flow showing systolic flow reversal in a case of severe mitral regurgitation.

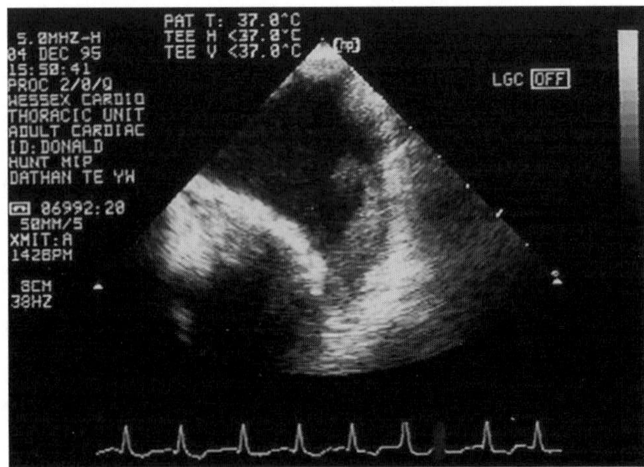

Fig. 12.20 Thrombus in the left atrial appendage of a patient with a mitral valve replacement.

phageal echo. Assessment of aortic regurgitation by transoesophageal echocardiography is similar to that by transthoracic echocardiography and transoesophageal echocardiography may add little to a good transthoracic study in the quantitation of aortic regurgitation. The better imaging provided of the ascending aorta, however, can reveal diastolic flow reversal on colour flow mapping in cases of severe aortic regurgitation. This may not be seen from a transthoracic study.

Transoesophageal echocardiography is important in demonstrating the underlying pathology of prosthetic aortic valve dysfunction and in distinguishing valvar from paravalvar regurgitation [69]. As with prosthetic mitral valves transoesophageal imaging is both more sensitive and specific in diagnosing the cause of aortic prosthetic dysfunction (Fig. 12.21). Superior imaging of the ascending aorta provides diagnostic information in cases of aortic pathology such as aneurysmal dilatation or aortic dissection.

A major limitation to transoesophageal imaging of aortic prostheses occurs with cases of aortic and mitral valve replacement when the aortic prosthesis and the left ventricular outflow tract may be masked by acoustic reverberations from the mitral prosthesis despite imaging in several planes. In such cases transthoracic echocardiography may provide the only adequate imaging.

TRICUSPID AND PULMONARY VALVES

Less information exists on transoesophageal echocardiography of tricuspid and pulmonary valves. Both are often adequately visualized from transthoracic echocardiography but transoesophageal imaging will provide additional information on the degree and cause of any valve dysfunction.

ENDOCARDITIS

Transoesophageal echocardiography should be considered an essential investigation in the assessment of suspected or proven prosthetic valve endocarditis.

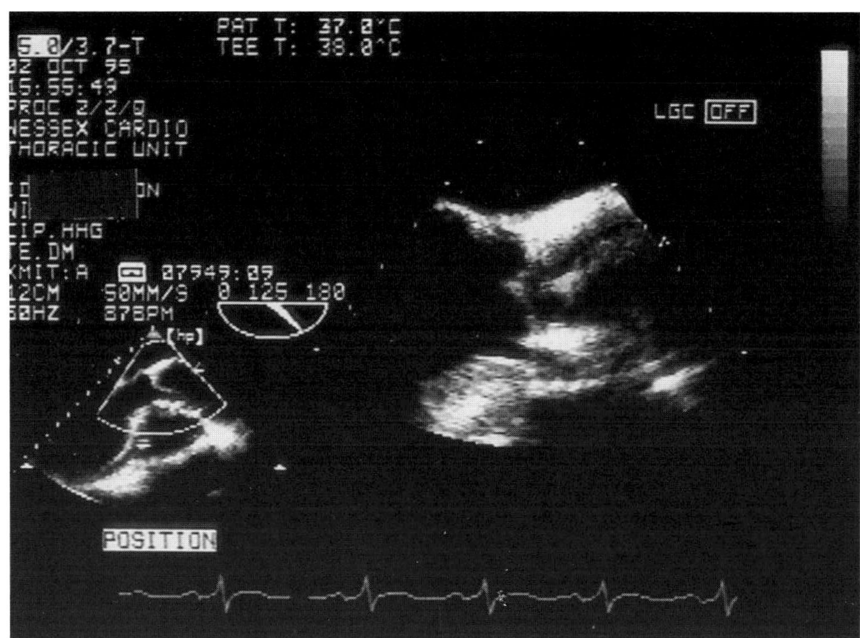

Fig. 12.21 Severe degenerative change in an aortic homograft. A partial flail cusp is responsible for the regurgitation and a vegetation is excluded (same patient as Fig. 12.6).

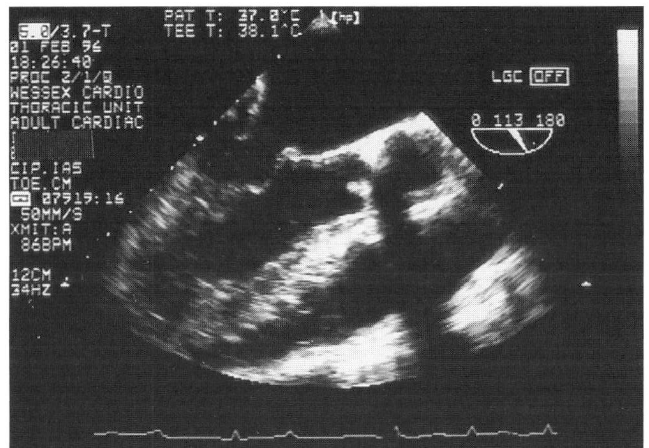

Fig. 12.22 A vegetation on a prosthetic valve.

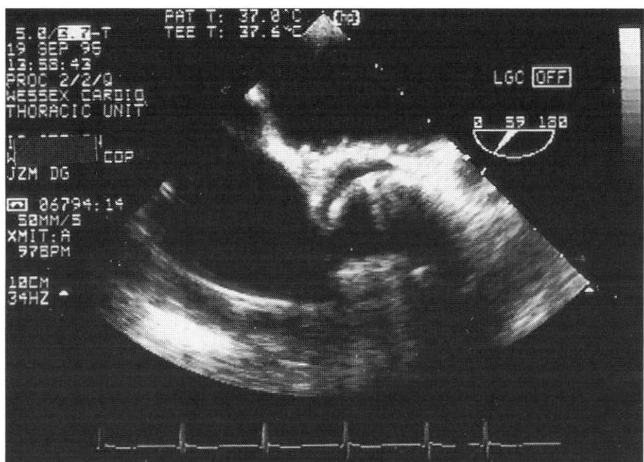

Fig. 12.23 An abscess cavity surrounding a prosthetic aortic valve.

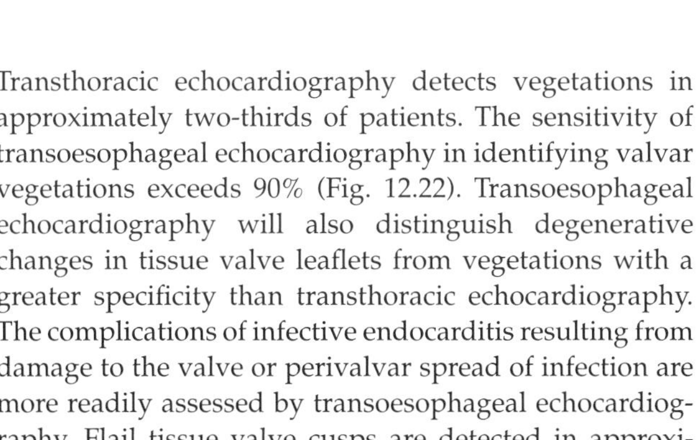

Transthoracic echocardiography detects vegetations in approximately two-thirds of patients. The sensitivity of transoesophageal echocardiography in identifying valvar vegetations exceeds 90% (Fig. 12.22). Transoesophageal echocardiography will also distinguish degenerative changes in tissue valve leaflets from vegetations with a greater specificity than transthoracic echocardiography. The complications of infective endocarditis resulting from damage to the valve or perivalvar spread of infection are more readily assessed by transoesophageal echocardiography. Flail tissue valve cusps are detected in approximately 90% of surgically confirmed cases compared to 40% by transthoracic echocardiography. The sensitivity for detection of abscesses (Fig. 12.23) complicating endocarditis in native and prosthetic valves has been reported as 28.3 and 87%, respectively, for transthoracic and transoesophageal echocardiography [70]. (A possible source of confusion can arise from imaging the transverse sinus in the horizontal axis from the transoesophageal window; this can occasionally be mistaken for an aortic root abscess cavity if the anatomy of this structure is not appreciated.) Subaortic complications in prosthetic aortic valve endocarditis are more readily detected by transoesophageal echocardiography. Involvement of the mitral aortic intervalvular fibrosa and the anterior mitral valve leaflet can lead to abscess and aneurysm formation. This can then rupture leading to communication between the left ventricle and left atrium. This region is best imaged in the longitudinal axis from the transoesophageal view and close attention should be paid to this region in all cases of prosthetic aortic valve endocarditis [71].

INTRAOPERATIVE TRANSOESOPHAGEAL ECHOCARDIOGRAPHY

The introduction of transoesophageal echocardiography has facilitated continuous echocardiographic monitoring during surgical procedures without obstructing the surgeon. The two main uses of intraoperative transoesophageal echocardiography are monitoring left ventricular function and assessing the efficacy of surgical intervention before discontinuing bypass.

Global and regional left ventricular function can be accurately assessed, most often using the transgastric short axis view at the mid papillary muscle level. The left ventricular fractional area change is the short axis equivalent of the ejection fraction and accurately reflects global left ventricular function. Recently introduced automated border detection systems allow the on-line calculation of cross-sectional areas and fractional area change. (The latest software will also allow on-line volume calculations and ejection fraction utilizing the left ventricular long axis views.) The end-diastolic area or volume may also provide a more useful measure of preload than measurement of the pulmonary capillary wedge pressure especially in the presence of altered left ventricular diastolic function or mitral valve disease. As the myocardium supplied by all three major coronary arteries is represented in the short axis view this is also useful for monitoring segmental wall motion abnormalities. Within seconds after the interruption of myocardial blood flow normal inward motion and thickening of the affected myocardium ceases. This systolic wall motion abnormality has been shown to be a more sensitive index of perioperative ischaemia than ST segment changes or a rise in pulmonary capillary wedge pressure.

Despite its value in monitoring perioperative left ventricular function transoesophageal echocardiography is not used routinely for this purpose mainly because of its demands upon operator time and use of equipment. The field in which intraoperative transoesophageal echocardiography has been shown to be an efficient use of resources is mitral valve reconstructive surgery. Mitral valve repair has become an increasingly accepted alternative to valve replacement mainly for cases of mitral regurgitation. It is now widely accepted that mitral valve repair provides a lower operative mortality, lower thromboembolic risk, improved postoperative left ventricular function and improved survival compared with mitral valve replacement. Preoperative transoesophageal echocardiography allows accurate assessment of mitral valve morphology and the cause of the regurgitation such as prolapsing leaflet or ruptured chordae (Fig. 12.24). This helps determine the suitability for repair and the type of repair necessary. Intraoperative transoesophageal echocardiography provides an immediate assessment of the results of the repair (Fig. 12.25) and is a more sensitive indicator of residual mitral regurgitation than either saline insufflation of the flaccid left ventricle or evaluation of the v wave of the pulmonary capillary wedge pressure [72]. Identification of significant residual regurgitation or stenosis of the valve will allow the surgeon immediately to revise the repair or replace the valve. Systolic anterior motion of the mitral valve has been described after mitral valve repair particularly with the insertion of a rigid annular ring. This may be associated with significant mitral regurgitation. This is often a dynamic phenomenon which will respond to volume expansion and manipulation of inotropes. Intraoperative transoesophageal echocardiography will identify systolic anterior motion and its response to conservative measures and determine whether or not the repair needs to be revised.

Table 12.4 Indications for transoesophageal echocardiography

Inadequate transthoracic imaging due to poorly echogenic subject or flow masking from prosthetic material
All cases of suspected or proven prosthetic valve endocarditis
Any thromboembolic event in a patient with a prosthetic valve
Prosthetic mitral regurgitation

INDICATIONS FOR TRANSOESOPHAGEAL ECHOCARDIOGRAPHY

Table 12.4 outlines the indications for performing a transoesophageal echocardiogram in patients with prosthetic valves.

Conclusion

All patients with prosthetic valves should have a postoperative transthoracic echocardiogram to provide baseline haemodynamic data for future reference. At follow-up and for all cases of suspected prosthetic valve dysfunction

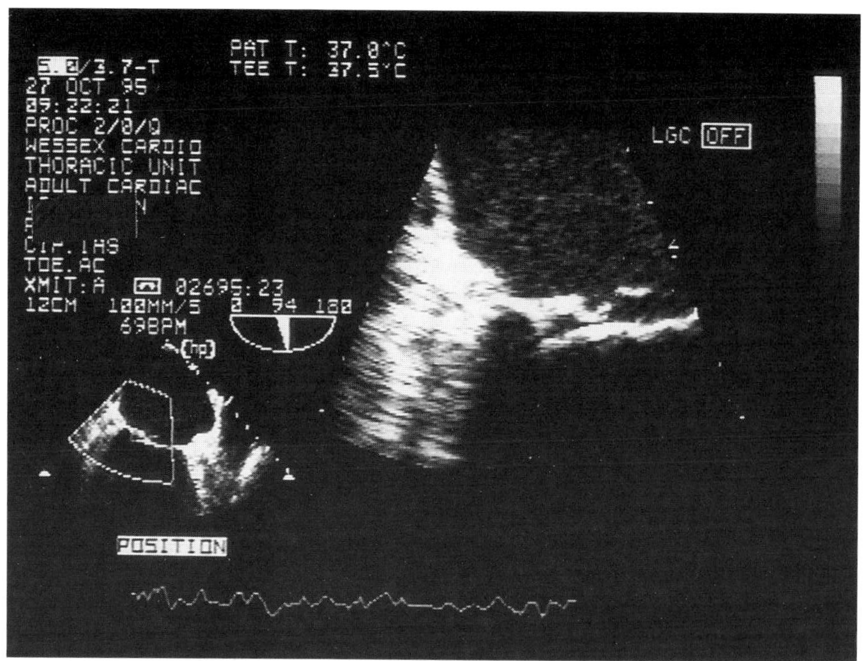

(a)

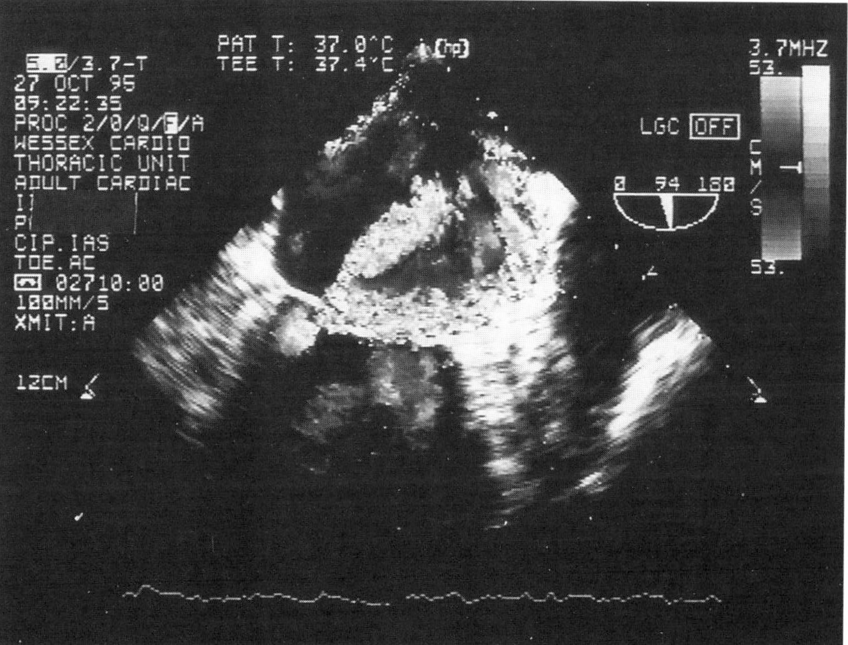

(b)

Fig. 12.24 A flail posterior mitral valve leaflet due to ruptured chordae (a), with a broad jet of regurgitation (b). For colour, see Plate 12.24 (between pp. 308 and 309).

a transthoracic study employing all echocardiographic modes should be performed after the clinical assessment of the patient. Transoesophageal echocardiography will be necessary in cases where transthoracic imaging is inadequate. In addition transoesophageal echocardiography should be considered an essential investigation in all cases of suspected or proven prosthetic valve endocarditis, in patients with a prosthetic valve presenting with a thromboembolic event, and in patients in whom there is evidence of prosthetic valve dysfunction from transthoracic echocardiography.

The combination of transthoracic and transoesophageal echocardiography should provide a comprehensive assessment of prosthetic valve function obviating the need for invasive investigations in the majority of patients.

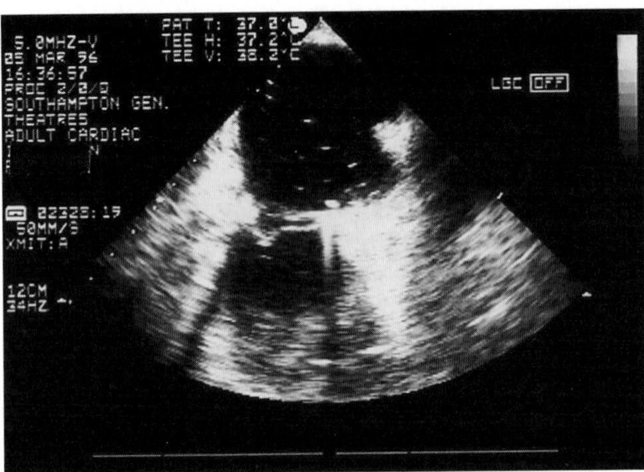

Fig. 12.25 The same valve post repair as in Fig. 12.24.

References

1 Harken, D.E., Soroff, H.S., Taylor, W.J., Lefemine, A.A., Gupta, S.K., Lunzer, S. (1960) Partial and complete prostheses in aortic insufficiency. *Journal of Thoracic Cardiovascular Surgery* **40**, 744–762.

2 Starr, A., Edwards, M.L. (1961) Mitral valve replacement: clinical experience with a ball–valve prosthesis. *Annals of Surgery* **154**, 726–740.

3 Ross, D.N. (1962) Homograft replacement of the aortic valve. *Lancet* **ii**, 487.

4 McGiffin, D.C., O'Brien, M.F., Stafford, E.G., Gardner, M.A., Polner, P.G. (1988) Long-term results of the viable cryopreserved allograft aortic valve: continuing evidence for superior valve durability. *Journal of Cardiac Surgery* suppl. **3**(3), 289–296.

5 Binet, J.P., Duran, C.G., Carpentier, A., Langlois, J. (1965) Heterologous aortic valve transplantation. *Lancet* **ii**, 1275.

6 Cohn, L.H., Disera, V.J., Collins, J.J. (1989) The Hancock modified-orifice porcine bioprosthetic valve 1976–1988. *Annals of Thoracic Surgery* **48**, 581–582.

7 Jamieson, W.R.E., Tyers, G.F.O., Miyagishima, R.T., Germann, E., Janusz, M.T., Ling, H. (1991) Carpentier–Edwards porcine bioprostheses: comparison of standard and supra annular prostheses at 7 years. *Circulation* **84**(suppl. III), III-145 to III-152.

8 Valente, M., Minarini, M., Maizza, A.F., Bortolotti, U., Thiene, G. (1992) Heart valve bioprosthesis durability: a challenge to the new generation of porcine valves. *European Journal of Cardiothoracic Surgery* **6**(suppl.), S82–S90.

9 Vesely, I., Lozan, A. (1993) Natural preload of aortic valve leaflet components during glutaraldehyde fixation: effects on tissue mechanics. *Journal of Biochemistry (USA)* **26**(2), 121–131.

10 Flomenbaum, M.A., Schoen, F.J. (1993) Effects of fixation backpressure and antimineralisation treatment on the morphology of porcine aortic bioprosthetic valves. *Journal of Thoracic Cardiovascular Surgery* **105**(1), 154–164.

11 Vesely, I. (1991) Analysis of the Medtronic Intact bioprosthetic valve. Effects of zero pressure fixation. *Journal of Thoracic Cardiovascular Surgery* **101**(1), 90–99.

12 Jaffe, W.M., Barratt-Boyes, B.G., Sadri, A., Gavin, J.B., Coverdale, H.A., Neutze, J.M. (1989) Early follow up of patients with the Medtronic Intact porcine valve. *Journal of Thoracic Cardiovascular Surgery* **98**, 181–192.

13 David, T.E., Pollick, C., Bos, J. (1990) Aortic valve replacement with stentless porcine aortic bioprosthesis. *Journal of Thoracic Cardiovascular Surgery* **99**, 113–118.

14 Teoh, K.H., Ivanov, J., Weisel, R.D., Darcel, I.C., Ralowski, H. (1989) Survival and bioprosthetic valve failure; ten year follow up. *Circulation* **80**(suppl. I), I-8 to I-15.

15 Wernly, J.A., Crawford, M.H. (1991) Choosing a prosthetic heart valve. *Cardiology Clinics* **9**, 329–338.

16 Bjork, V.O. (1969) A new tilting disc valve prosthesis. *Scandinavian Journal of Thoracic and Cardiovascular Surgery* **3**, 1–10.

17 Emery, R.W., Mettler, E., Nicoloff, D.M. (1979) A new cardiac prosthesis: the St Jude Medical cardiac valve: *in vivo* results. *Circulation* **60**(suppl.), 1148–1154.

18 Hiratzka, L.F., Kouchoukos, N.T., Grunkemeier, G.L., *et al.* (1988) Outlet strut fracture of the Bjork–Shiley 60° convexo-concave valve: current information and recommendations for patient care. *Journal of the American College of Cardiology* **2**, 1130.

19 David, T.E., Komeda, M., Pollick, C., Burns, R.J. (1989) Mitral valve annuloplasty: the effect of the type on left ventricular function. *Annals of Thoracic Surgery* **47**, 524–528.

20 Demensil, J.G., Yoganathan, A.P. (1992) Valve prosthesis haemodynamics and the problem of high transprosthetic pressure gradients. *European Journal of Cardiothoracic Surgery* **6**(suppl. I), S34–37.

21 Walker, P.G., Yoganathan, A.P. (1992) *In vitro* pulsatile flow haemodynamics of five mechanical aortic heart valve prostheses. *European Journal of Cardiothoracic Surgery* **6**(suppl. I), S113–123.

22 Rashtian, M.Y., Stevenson, D.M., Allen, D.T., *et al.* (1990) Flow characteristics of bioprosthetic heart valves. *Chest* **98**(2), 365–375.

23 Virdi, I.S., Monro, J.L., Ross, J.K. (1986) 11-year experience of aortic valve replacements with antibiotic sterilised homograft valves in Southampton. *Thoracic and Cardiovascular Surgeon* **34**, 277–282.

24 Bortolotti, U., Thiene, G., Casarotto, D., Mazzucco, A., Gallucci, V. (1980) Left ventricular rupture following mitral valve replacement with a Hancock bioprosthesis. *Chest* **77**, 235–237.

25 Thiene, G., Bortolotti, U., Casarotto, D., Valfre, C., Gallucci, V. Prosthesis left ventricle disproportion in mitral valve replacement with the Hancock bioprosthesis: pathologic observations. In: Sebening, F., Klovekorn, W.P., Meisner, H., Struck, E. (eds) *Bioprosthetic Cardiac Valves*. Deutsches Herzzentrum, Munich, pp. 357–365.

26 Mihaileanu, S., Marino, J.P., Chauvaud, S., *et al.* (1988) Left ventricular outflow obstruction after mitral valve repair (Carpentier's technique)—proposed mechanisms of disease. *Circulation* **78**(suppl. I), 78–84.

27 Deloche, A., Jebara, V.A., Relland, J.Y.M., *et al.* (1990) Valve repair with Carpentier techniques. The second decade. *Journal of Thoracic Cardiovascular Surgery* **99**, 990–1002.

28 Chauvaud, S.M., Deleuze, P., Perier, P.M., *et al.* (1986) Failures in reconstructive mitral valve surgery. *Circulation* **74**, 393.

29 Stewart, W.J., Currie, P.J., Salcedo, E.E., *et al.* (1990) Intraoperative Doppler colour flow mapping for decision making in valve repair for mitral regurgitation. *Circulation* **81**, 556–566.

30 Grunkemeier, G.L., Rashimtoola, S.H. (1990) Artificial heart valves. *Annual Review of Medicine* **41**, 251–263.

31 Bloomfield, P., Wheatley, D.J., Prescott, R.J., Miller, H.C. (1991) Twelve year comparison of a Bjork Shiley mechanical heart valve

with a porcine bioprosthesis. *New England Journal of Medicine* **324**, 573–579.

32 Barrett-Boyes, B.G., Roche, A.H.G., Subramanyan, R., *et al.* (1987) Long-term follow-up of patients with antibiotic sterilized aortic homograft valve inserted freehand in the aortic position. *Circulation* **75**, 768–777.

33 Carpenter, J.L. (1991) Perivalvular extension of infection in patients with infectious endocarditis. *Review of Infectious Diseases* **13**, 127–138.

34 Gallo, J., Nistal, F., Blasquez, R., Arbe, E., Artinano, E. (1988) Incidence of primary tissue valve failure in porcine bioprosthetic heart valves. *Annals of Thoracic Surgery* **45**, 66–70.

35 Cohn, L.H., Collins, J.J., Disesa, V.J., *et al.* (1989) Fifteen-year experience with 1678 Hancock porcine bioprosthetic heart valve replacements. *Annals of Surgery* **210**, 435–442.

36 Magilligan, D.J., Lewis, J.W., Stein, P., Alam, M. (1989) The porcine bioprosthetic heart valve: experience at 15 years. *Annals of Thoracic Surgery* **48**, 324–330.

37 Jones, E.L., Weintraub, W.S., Craver, J.M., *et al.* (1990) Ten-year experience with the porcine bioprosthetic valve: interrelationship of valve survival and patient survival in 1050 valve replacements. *Annals of Thoracic Surgery* **49**, 370–384.

38 Akins, C.W., Carroll, D.L., Buckley, M.J., Daggett, W.M., Hilgenberg, A.D., Austen, W.G. (1990) Late results with Carpentier–Edwards porcine bioprosthesis. *Circulation* **82**(suppl. IV), IV-65 to IV-74.

39 Jamieson, W.R.E., Allen, P., Miyagishima, R.J., *et al.* (1990) The Carpentier–Edwards standard porcine bioprosthesis. *Journal of Thoracic Cardiovascular Surgery* **99**, 543–561.

40 Gallucci, V., Mazzucco, A., Bartollotti, U., *et al.* (1988) The standard Hancock porcine bioprosthesis: overall experience at the University of Padova. *Journal of Cardiac Surgery* suppl. **3**, 337–345.

41 Jamieson, W.R.E., Rosado, L.J., Munro, A.I., *et al.* (1988) Carpentier–Edwards standard porcine bioprosthesis: primary tissue failure (structural valve deterioration) by age groups. *Annals of Thoracic Surgery* **46**, 155–162.

42 Arom, K.V., Nicoloff, D.M., Kersten, T.E., *et al.* (1987) St Jude Medical prosthesis: valve related deaths and complications. *Annals of Thoracic Surgery* **43**, 591–598.

43 Lewis, R., Rittgers, S.E., Boudulas, H. (1980) A critical review of the systolic time intervals. *American Heart Association Monograph* **66**, 73.

44 Veenendoal, M., Nanda, N.C. (1980) Noninvasive diagnosis of mitral prosthesis malfunction. *American Journal of Medicine* **69**, 458–462.

45 Mehta, A., Kessler, K.M., Tamer, D., *et al.* (1981) Two dimensional echocardiographic observations in major detachment of a prosthetic valve. *American Heart Journal* **101**, 231–233.

46 Burstow, D.J., Nishimura, R.J., Bailey, K.R., *et al.* (1989) Continuous wave Doppler echocardiographic measurement of prosthetic valve gradients: a simultaneous Doppler–catheter correlative study. *Circulation* **80**, 504–514.

47 Wilkins, G.T., Gilliam, L.D., Kritzer, G.L., Levine, R.A., Palacios, I.F., Weyman, A.E. (1986) Validation of continuous wave Doppler echocardiographic measurements of mitral and tricuspid prosthetic valve gradients: a simultaneous Doppler–catheter study. *Circulation* **74**, 786–795.

48 Heldman, D., Gardin, J.M. (1989) Evaluation of prosthetic valves by Doppler echocardiography. *Echocardiography* **6**, 63–77.

49 Williams, G.A., Labovitz, A.J. (1985) Doppler haemodynamic evaluation of prosthetic (Starr–Edwards and Bjork Shiley) and bioprosthetic (Hancock and Carpentier–Edwards) cardiac valves. *American Journal of Cardiology* **56**, 325–332.

50 Tatenini, S., Barnes, H.B., Pearson, A.C., Halbe, D., Woodruff, R., Labovitz, A.J. (1989) Rest and exercise evaluation of St Jude Medical and Medtronic Hall prostheses. *Circulation* **80**(suppl. I), 116–123.

51 Dumensil, J.G., Honos, G.N., Lemieux, M., Beauchemin, J. (1990) Validation and applications of indexed aortic prosthetic valve areas calculated by Doppler echocardiography. *Journal of the American College of Cardiology* **16**, 637–643.

52 Kapur, K.K., Fan, P., Nauda, N.C., Yoganathan, A.P., Goyal, R. (1989) Doppler colour flow mapping in the evaluation of prosthetic mitral and aortic valve function. *Journal of the American College of Cardiology* **13**, 1561–1571.

53 Alam, M., Rosman, H.S., Lakier, J.B., *et al.* (1987) Doppler and echocardiographic features of normal and dysfunctioning bioprosthetic valves. *Journal of the American College of Cardiology* **10**, 851–858.

54 Sagar, K.B., Wann, L.S., Paulsen, W.H.J., *et al.* (1986) Doppler echocardiographic evaluation of Hancock and Bjork Shiley prosthetic valves. *Journal of the American College of Cardiology* **7**, 681–687.

55 Dumensil, J.G., Honos, G.N., Lemieux, M., Beauchemin, J. (1990) Validation and applications of mitral prosthetic valvar areas calculated by Doppler echocardiography. *American Journal of Cardiology* **65**, 1443–1448.

56 Bargiggia, G.S., Tronconi, L., Sahn, D.J., *et al.* (1991) A new method for quantitation of mitral regurgitation based on colour flow Doppler imaging of flow convergence proximal to regurgitant orifice. *Circulation* **84**(4), 1481–1489.

57 Daniel, W.G., Erbel, R., Kasper, W., *et al.* (1991) Safety of transoesophageal echocardiography: a multicentre survey of 10 419 examinations. *Circulation* **83**, 817–821.

58 Ansari, A. (1993) Transoesophageal two dimensonal echocardiography. Current perspectives. *Progress in Cardiovascular Disease* **35**(5), 349–397.

59 Khandheria, B.K., Seward, J.B., Oh, J.K., *et al.* (1991) Value and limitations of transoesophageal echocardiography in assessment of mitral valve prostheses. *Circulation* **83**, 1956–1968.

60 Yoshida, K., Yoshikawa, J., Yamaura, Y., *et al.* (1990) Assessment of mitral regurgitation by biplane transoesophageal colour Doppler flow mapping. *Circulation* **82**, 1121–1126.

61 Alam, M., Serwin, J.B., Rosman, H.S., *et al.* (1990) Transoesophageal colour flow Doppler and echocardiographic features of normal and regurgitant St Jude Medical prostheses in the aortic position. *American Journal of Cardiology* **66**, 873–875.

62 Hixson, C.S., Smith, M.D., Mattson, M.D., *et al.* (1992) Comparison of transoesophageal colour flow Doppler imaging of normal mitral regurgitation jets in St Jude Medical and Medtronic Hall cardiac prostheses. *Journal of the American Society of Echocardiography* **5**, 57–62.

63 Lange, H.W., Olson, J.D., Pederson, W.R., *et al.* (1991) Transoesophageal colour Doppler echocardiography of the normal St Jude Medical mitral valve prosthesis. *American Heart Journal* **122**, 489–494.

64 Mohr, K.S., Kupferwaser, I., Erbel, R., *et al.* (1990) Regurgitant flow in apparently normal valve prostheses: improved detection

and semiquantitative analysis by transoesophageal two-dimensonal colour-coded Doppler echocardiography. *Journal of the American Society of Echocardiography* **3**, 187–195.

65 Alam, M., Serwin, J.B., Rosman, H.S., *et al.* (1991) Transoesophageal echocardiographic features of normal and dysfunctioning bioprosthetic valves. *American Heart Journal* **121**, 1149.

66 Van den Brink, R.B.A., Visser, C.A., Basart, D.C.G., *et al.* (1989) Comparison of transthoracic and transoesophageal colour Doppler flow imaging in patients with mechanical prostheses in the mitral valve position. *American Journal of Cardiology* **63**, 1471.

67 Klein, A.L., Cohen, G.I., Davison, M.B., *et al.* (1991) Importance of sampling both pulmonary veins in the transoesophageal assessment of severity of mitral regurgitation. *Journal of the American College of Cardiology* **17**, 199A.

68 Klein, L.A., Obarski, T.P., Stewart, W.J., *et al.* (1991) Transoesophageal Doppler echocardiography of pulmonary venous flow: a new marker of mitral regurgitation severity. *Journal of the American College of Cardiology* **188**, 518–526.

69 Dittrich, H.C., McCann, H.A., Walsh, T.P., *et al.* (1990) Transoesophageal echocardiography in the evaluation of prosthetic and native aortic valves. *American Journal of Cardiology* **66**, 758.

70 Daniel, W.G., Mugge, A., Martin, R.P., *et al.* (1991) Improvement in the diagnosis of abscesses associated with endocarditis by transoesophageal echocardiography. *New England Journal of Medicine* **324**, 795–800.

71 Karalis, D.G., Bansal, R.C., Hauck, A.J., *et al.* (1992) Transoesophageal echocardiographic recognition of subaortic complications in aortic valve endocarditis. *Circulation* **86**(2), 353–362.

72 Kalman, J.M., Jones, E.F., Lubicz, S., Buxton, B.B., Tonkin, A.M., Calafiore, P. (1993) Evaluation of mitral valve repair by intraoperative transoesophageal echocardiography. *Australia and New Zealand Journal of Medicine* **23**, 463–469.

Chapter 13: Cardiac masses

J. Weir

Mass lesions in the heart are readily detectable by cross-sectional echocardiography and especially by the transoesophageal techniques [1]. Often these lesions are discovered by accident while the patient is being investigated either for symptoms of heart failure, arrhythmias or valvular obstruction or because there is a history of pulmonary or systemic emboli or occasionally because of a systemic illness with known cardiac complications.

Lesions in the mediastinum and/or pericardium cause their effects by compression and, if malignant, often by accompanying invasion and associated pericardial fluid. Mass lesions developing in the myocardium or endocardium cause their effects depending on their size, position and nature.

For the purposes of description, two varieties of 'mass' lesions are described, those associated with or caused by foreign bodies and those due to cardiac tumours.

Foreign bodies

Considered within this broad category are pacemakers, other intravenous lines, prosthetic valves, vegetations, thrombi and true foreign bodies such as bullets and displaced venous filters.

Pacemaker implants

Pacemaker wires are frequently seen on echocardiography, crossing the tricuspid valve and embedding themselves into the apex of the right ventricle. The majority cause no problems but both thrombus and infection may occur on the wire and produce an echogenic mass on ultrasound either in the atrium, the ventricle or at the level of the tricuspid valve. Platelet thrombi due to pacemaker wires are relatively rare occurrences and may be dissolved by appropriate anticoagulant therapy [2,3]. The thrombus may be sessile or pedunculated and may occur anywhere on the pacemaker wire, not necessarily at the catheter tip. Figure 13.1 shows an echogenic mass attached to a pacemaker wire at the level of the tricuspid valve in a patient who had repeated pulmonary emboli unresponsive to anticoagulation. Percutaneous removal of the pacemaker can be associated with stripping of the thrombus and a significant risk of major fatal pulmonary embolism. Open heart surgery on bypass may occasionally be warranted if repeated emboli are caused by a persistent thrombus.

Intravenous catheters

Central venous lines and other right heart catheters in patients with prolonged intravenous feeding, long-term antibiotics or chemotherapy, are all potential sources for thrombus formation and infection [4]. The risks are considerably increased in patients who are also immunocompromised, where opportunistic infections (e.g. *Candida*) may occur [5,6]. Catheters in the venous system may also disintegrate and migrate, resulting in partial obstruction often to a pulmonary artery and act as a source for thrombus formation. Retrieval may be complicated but is often resolved by snare procedures under interventional radiology control [7].

Prosthetic valves

Although prosthetic valves are covered elsewhere in this text (see Chapter 12), disintegration of such a valve may cause a mass effect on echocardiography. Figure 13.2 demonstrates an apparent 'floating body' in the left ventricle in a patient with a Starr–Edwards mitral prosthesis. A strut of the valve cage had partially separated and although attached to the prosthetic valve, was able to move freely during the cardiac cycle, within the body of the left ventricle. The valve was subsequently replaced after X-ray screening confirmed the echocardiographic findings. Discs can also become separated from their attachments and may migrate out of the heart to lodge in the aorta or one of its branches, resulting in embolic phenomena combined with torrential valvular regurgitation.

Vegetations

If vegetations are greater than 2 mm in size, they are

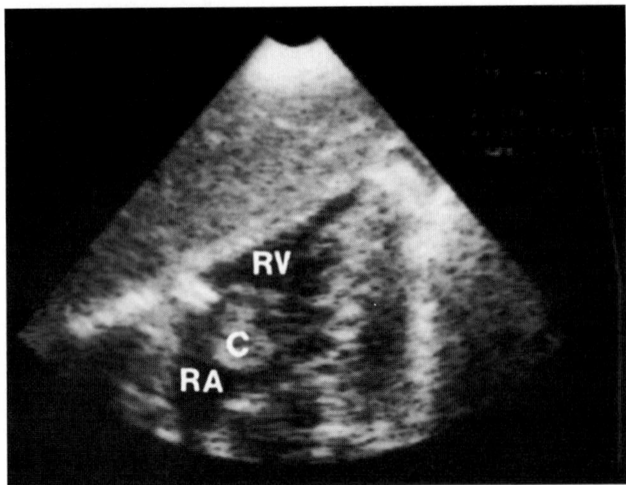

Fig. 13.1 Subcostal view of the right ventricle (RV) and right atrium (RA) with an echogenic mass (C) at the level of the tricuspid valve attached to a pacemaker wire.

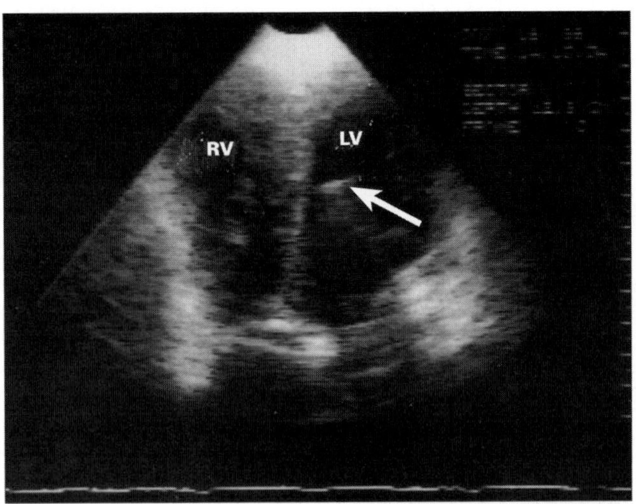

(a)

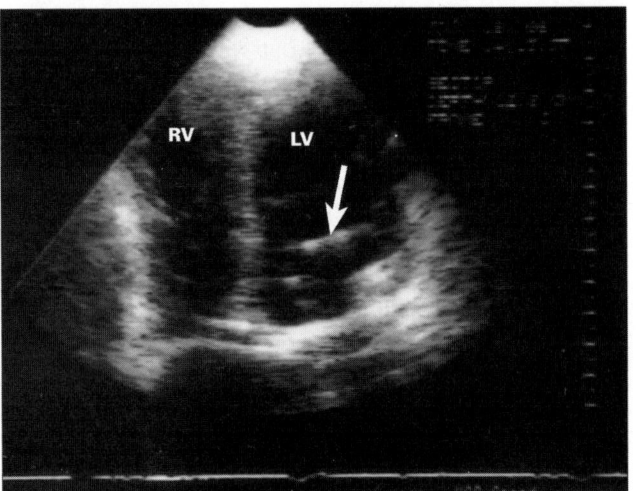

(b)

Fig. 13.2 (a,b) Apical four-chamber views of a prosthetic mitral valve with a floating 'foreign body' (arrow) in the body of the left ventricle (LV). RV, right ventricle.

usually detected by transthoracic echocardiography. However, smaller lesions, lesions in odd places (e.g. on the edges of a ventricular septal defect), and better visualization and characterization of known lesions all require the use of transoesophageal echocardiography [8]. The full spectrum of vegetations is discussed in Chapters 9 and 12, however, inclusion here is necessary because they produce echogenic 'mass' effects. Vegetations may be infective or non-infective [9], active or inactive, and all have the capability of producing emboli. The characteristic transoesophageal echocardiographic appearances of vegetations on the atrial side of an infective prosthetic mitral valve are shown in Fig. 13.3.

Thrombus formation

Thrombi may develop in any of the cardiac chambers and cause a variety of different clinical effects depending on their size, position, aetiology and embolic potential.

RIGHT ATRIUM

A right atrial thrombus usually results from a pacemaker wire or other long-term intravenous catheter as described above. Infection may coexist, there being no specific echocardiographic features to distinguish between sterile and septic thrombi. Occasionally, congestive cardiac failure with stasis may cause a pure right atrial thrombus [10].

LEFT ATRIUM

Thrombi are much more common in the left atrium than in the right atrium. They vary in size from small mural plaques to giant 'ball' thrombi causing functional mitral stenosis. Transthoracic echocardiography is relatively poor in detecting left atrial thrombi particularly as the atrial appendage, where a considerable number of thrombi form, is not routinely visible. One considerable advantage of transoesophageal echocardiography is that the left atrium is fully visualized, especially the appendage, and small thrombi (Fig. 13.4) as well as large thrombi are readily detectable [11–14]. It is now accepted that transoesophageal echocardiography is necessary in all cases where the diagnosis of the presence of a left atrial

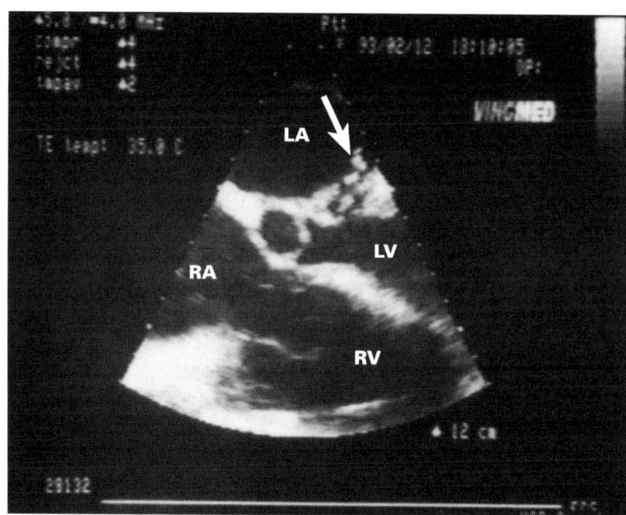

Fig. 13.3 Transoesophageal echocardiographic view of vegetations (arrow) on the atrial side of a prosthetic mitral valve. LA, left atrium; LV, left ventricle; RA, right atrium; RV, right ventricle.

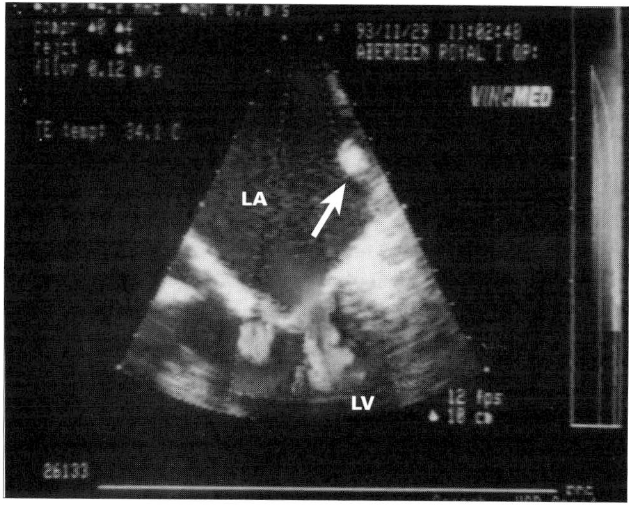

Fig. 13.4 Transoesophageal echocardiographic view of a thrombus in the left atrial appendage (arrow) in a patient with mitral stenosis as shown by the colour jet into the left ventricle (LV). LA, dilated left atrium. For colour, see Plate 13.4 (between pp. 308 and 309).

thrombus may alter patient management. Most thrombi will resolve on appropriate anticoagulant therapy and transoesophageal echocardiography is used to monitor the response [15]. Left atrial 'ball' thrombus is relatively rare, usually occurring in a dilated atrium secondary to postrheumatic mitral valve disease and may be fatal. Figure 13.5 demonstrates a free-floating ball thrombus in the left atrium in a patient with postrheumatic mitral stenosis. Echocardiographic differentiation from an atrial

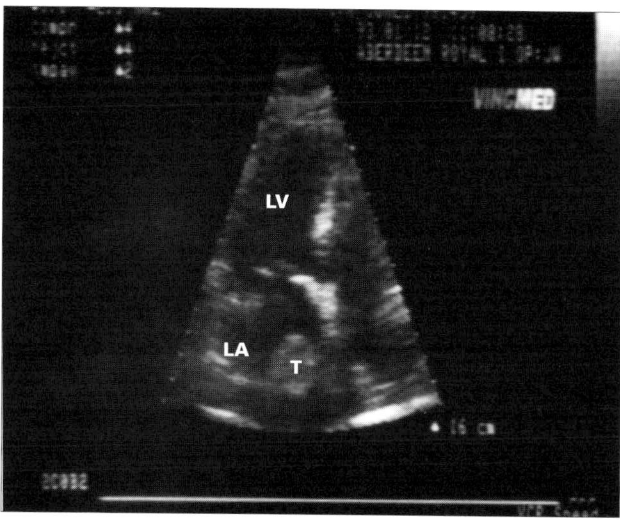

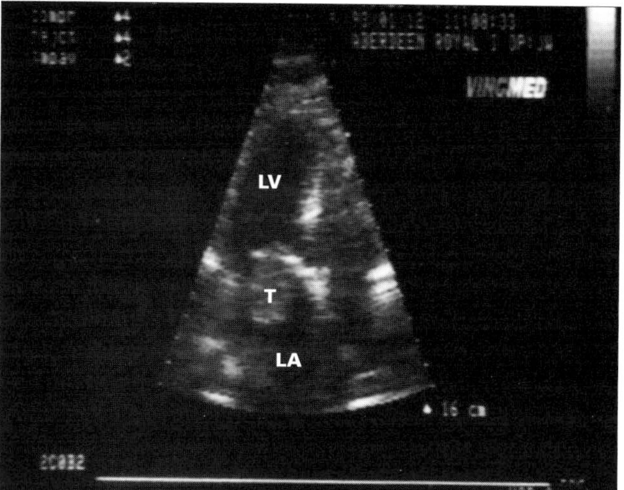

Fig. 13.5 (a,b) Apical four-chamber views of a free-floating ball thrombus (T) within the left atrium (LA). LV, left ventricle.

myxoma may be difficult if the thrombus is attached to an atrial wall. Ball thrombi have a poor prognosis, may embolize or obstruct, do not respond well to anticoagulation and where possible should be removed at cardiac surgery [16].

RIGHT VENTRICLE

Thrombi in the right ventricle are rare, again associated with pacemakers or other catheters, but are also seen in patients with a dilated cardiomyopathy or following right ventricular infarction [17]. Pedunculated right ventricular thrombus has also been described due to the repeated blunt anterior chest wall trauma of boxing, the patient initially diagnosed as having a possible myxoma [18].

LEFT VENTRICLE

This chamber is the commonest site for intracardiac thrombi, most occurring either after a myocardial infarction and wall damage or associated with a dilated cardiomyopathy. Patients with acute anterior myocardial infarctions may develop both early and late left ventricular thrombi, with significant embolic complications and echocardiography can be used to diagnose and follow these thrombi [19,20]. The echocardiographic appearances of thrombi depend on their structure, longevity and position. Early thrombus may be relatively echolucent, but its echogenicity increases with age. If the thrombus is large, it may liquefy in the centre and become echolucent. Thrombi may be large or small, sessile or pedunculated, mobile or static. Thrombi that are visualized floating with a frond-like appearance (Fig. 13.6) are more likely to embolize than the fixed, consolidated type (Fig. 13.7). One author suggests that cross-sectional echocardiography may be able to assess high risk thrombi by texture analysis [21]. The surface of a thrombus also varies with time, changing as it becomes incorporated into the ventricular wall and endothelialized, resulting in an increase in echogenicity. Examples of the variability of left ventricular thrombi are shown in Figs 13.8–13.10. As in the right ventricle, repeated blunt anterior chest wall trauma may also cause left ventricular thrombi but both are rare [22].

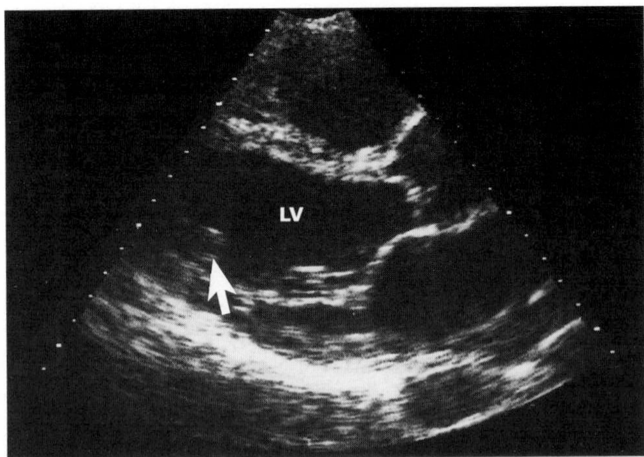

(a)

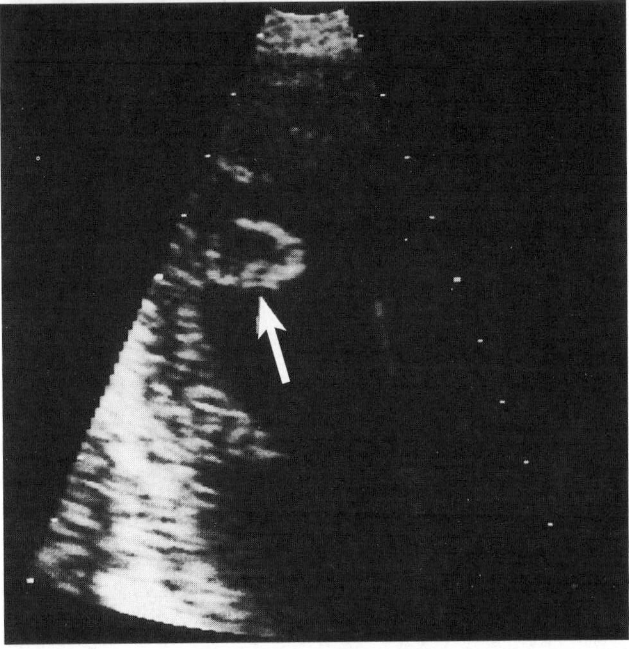
(b)

Fig. 13.6 (a) Long axis view of the left ventricle (LV) showing the ring appearance of a friable thrombus (arrowhead). (b) Apical two-chamber view of the same patient as (a) showing the mobile frond-like appearance of a recent thrombus formation (arrow). LV, left ventricle.

Miscellaneous

The migration of inferior vena cava filters to the right heart has been described, producing echocardiographic masses of bizarre appearance [23,24]. Echocardiography has also gained a place in the investigation of patients with penetrating cardiac trauma due to bullet wounds [25], and intraoperative ultrasound has been used to detect small intracardiac foreign bodies at surgery [26]. Rarely, other pieces of metal may be seen in the heart as in the case described by Jagmeet *et al.* [27] of a schizophrenic with a needle found lying across the interventricular septum!

MISCELLANEOUS LESIONS

1 Dissecting intramyocardial haematomas may occur as a result of trauma, myocardial infarction, postsurgery or rarely spontaneously. The condition may present as a pseudotumour of either the left or right ventricle [28] and is virtually indistinguishable echocardiographically from a true tumour.

2 The left ventricular outflow tract may be the site for a prolapsing intimal tear resulting from a dissecting aortic aneurysm (Fig. 13.11), the intima moving to and fro across the aortic valve during cardiac contraction. This is associated with torrential aortic regurgitation.

3 Figure 13.12 demonstrates a large echolucent space within the myocardium in a patient with an intramyocardial hydatid cyst that was partially compressing the left ventricle. Hydatid cysts may occur within the pericardium or rarely within the myocardium itself, with rupture and secondary infection as possible complications.

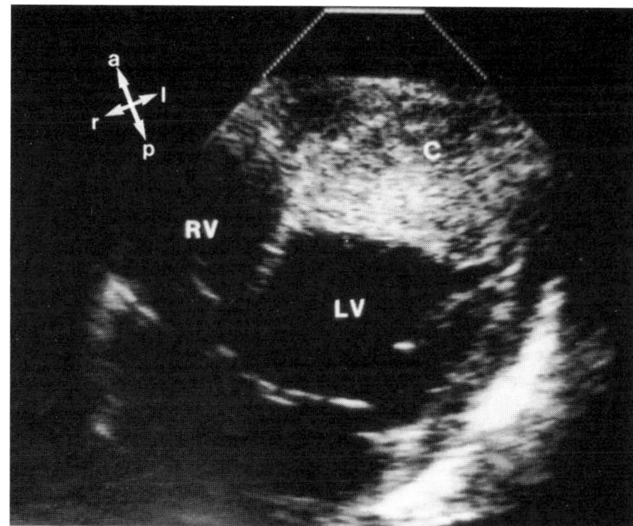

Fig. 13.7 Echogenic clot (c) in an apical aneurysm. LV, left ventricle; RV, right ventricle.

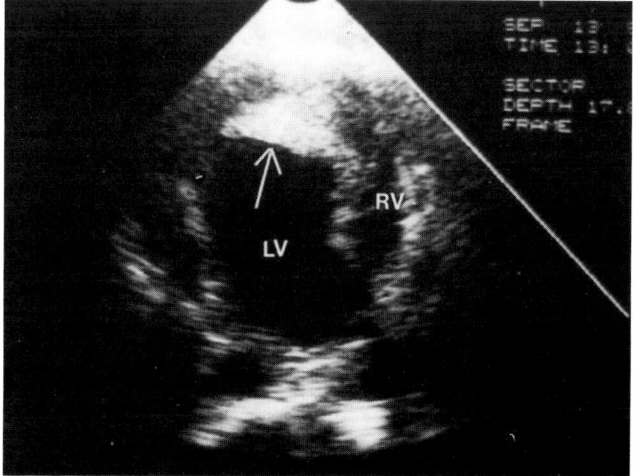

Fig. 13.8 Highly echogenic thrombus (arrow) at the apex of the left ventricle (LV). RV, right ventricle.

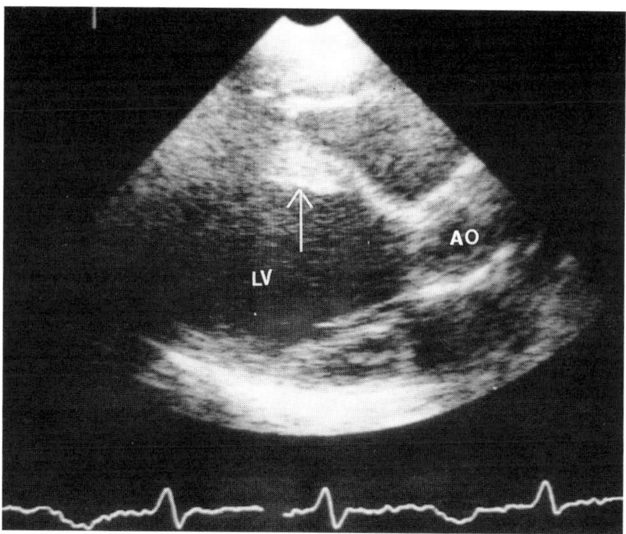

Fig. 13.9 Long axis view of thrombus (arrow) attached to an infarcted septum. Note the increased echogenicity of the clot surface that is covered by endothelium. AO, aorta; LV, left ventricle.

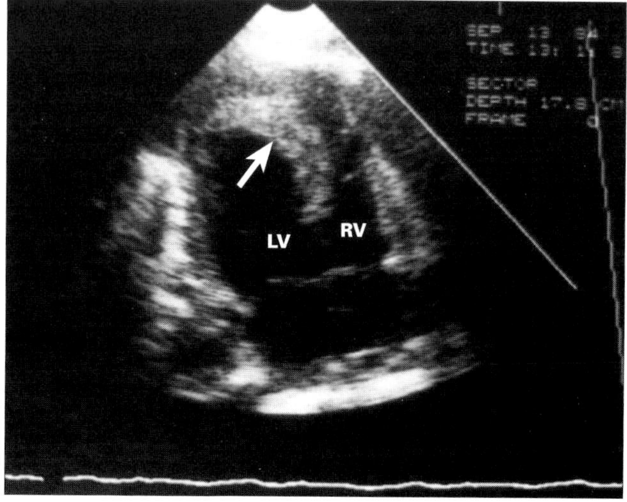

Fig. 13.10 Apical four-chamber view showing echogenic curvilinear thrombus (arrow) attached to the left ventricular (LV) apex. RV, right ventricle.

Tumours

The commonest tumours of the heart and pericardium are secondary deposits from frequently occurring primary carcinomas such as those from the breast and bronchus. Pericardial deposits usually present with pericardial fluid with or without tamponade. Myocardial deposits are rarely diagnosed during life but are present at post-mortem in a significant proportion (10%) of patients who die from carcinomatosis. Secondary tumours occurring within the heart cavities are described in more detail below.

Primary cardiac tumours are rare, and may be benign or malignant. They occur at any age, Groves *et al.* [29] describing 11 cases of cardiac tumours in the fetus, the majority being rhabdomyomas, some of which were associated with tuberous sclerosis. There are also recent reports in the literature of preoperative diagnosis of cardiac tumours by transvenous biopsy under transoesophageal guidance [30], a useful addition to the current techniques as cardiac masses have a wide spectrum of possible pathology.

Extrinsic lesions

Figure 13.13 demonstrates a large tumour anterior to the heart, invading the pericardium, the anterior wall of the right ventricle and extending into the body of the right ventricle and outflow tract. The tumour also encircles the great vessels. Percutaneous biopsy showed undifferentiated carcinoma from an unknown primary. Malignant thymomas may also invade the right heart [31] with intracavitary extension.

Very rarely a phaeochromocytoma may be detected in an intrapericardial site, initially described by Besterman *et al.* [32] where the left atrium was shown to be compressed on angiography and more recently by Rosamond *et al.* [33] who described on echocardiography, a compressive lesion in the atrioventricular groove close to the tricuspid valve.

Another very rare entity is intracardiac thyroid heterotopia that may cause a mass effect [34]. Ectopic thyroid tissue may be distributed in the myocardium, pericardium, aortic arch, mediastinum and diaphragm, due to aberrant migration early in fetal life. Most of the documented cases, however, do not present until middle-age indicating the very slow growth of the cells over time. If the tissue occurs in the myocardium, it tends to appear on the right side of the interventricular septum and cause right-sided obstruction. It has to be differentiated from the more commonly occurring (but also rare) metastatic thyroid carcinoma, which also has a right heart predominance.

Secondary malignant tumours

Intracavitary secondary malignant tumours of the heart while rare, are important because of the possible surgical treatment that may be indicated. They are usually right sided but may occasionally be seen in the left heart. There are two mechanisms that produce this type of tumour. Firstly, a primary tumour directly extends into the venous system, e.g. from the kidney, and may extend intravascularly to reach the heart. The second method of spread is by true metastatic dissemination to the endocardium. Both present with intracavitary masses but differentiation

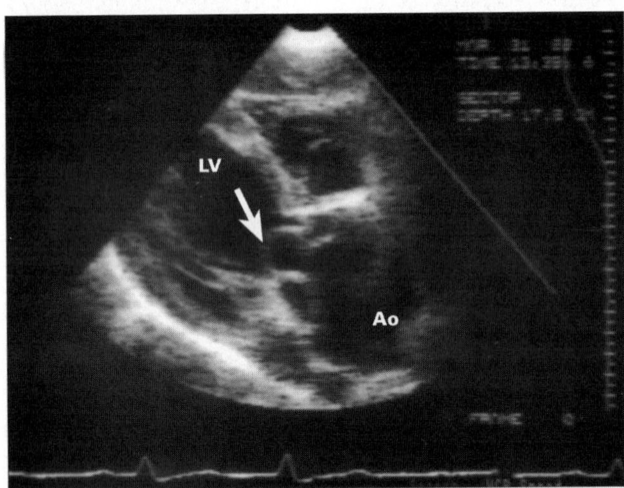

Fig. 13.11 Subcostal view showing prolapsed intima (arrow) through an incompetent aortic valve. Note the gross aortic aneurysmal dilatation (Ao). LV, left ventricle.

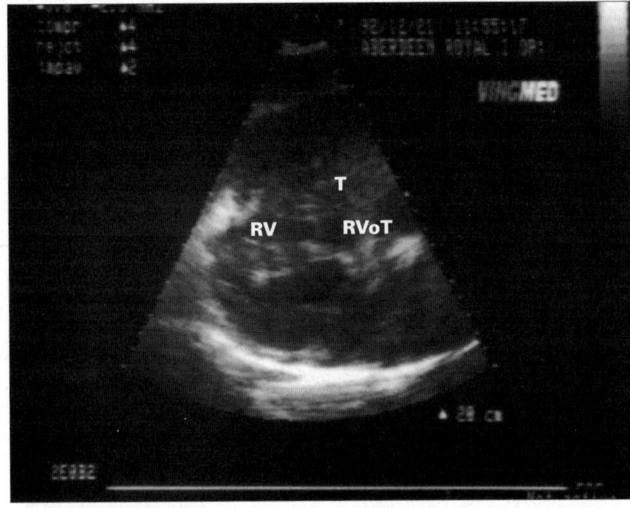

Fig. 13.13 Large tumour (T) invading pericardium, right ventricle (RV) and right ventricular outflow tract (RVoT). Pathology—undifferentiated carcinoma.

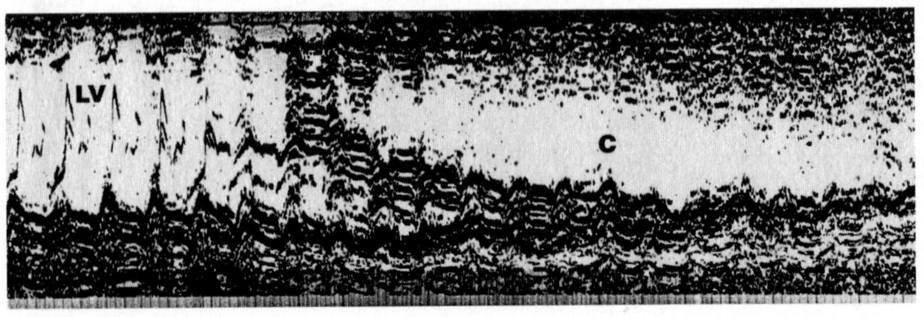

Fig. 13.12 M-mode echocardiogram of the left ventricle (LV) in a patient with a large echolucent myocardial hydatid cyst (C), that was excised intact at surgery.

is important as it may considerably alter patient management.

DIRECT EXTENSION TUMOURS

Right-sided tumours arise from one of two main sources, the kidney or liver. Kidney tumours commonly invade the renal vein with occasional tumour extension into the inferior vena cava. The tumour may grow proximally up the inferior vena cava and into the right atrium and even into the right ventricle and outflow tract. Figure 13.14 demonstrates a large mass in the right atrium which could be traced back to the right kidney, the patient presenting with lower limb oedema without any urinary symptoms. Shahian *et al.* [35] describe 10 patients with intracaval extension of a renal tumour to the right atrium, seven of whom had complete tumour removal under hypothermic circulatory arrest with a reasonable long-term survival in several cases. A patient with a left ventricular renal metastasis has also been described, who had previously been successfully treated for inferior vena cava and right atrial extension of the original tumour [36]. Wilms' tumour may also directly extend to the right heart [37].

Hepatocellular carcinoma with direct invasion of the hepatic veins, inferior vena cava and right atrium has also been described [38]. There is another rare entity, intravenous leiomyomatosis, which originates in the uterus, spreading by direct extension into the inferior vena cava and right atrium, and although 'benign' carries a poor prognosis if not recognized [39].

Direct intracavitary involvement of the left heart by tumour is occasionally caused by lung carcinoma invading the pulmonary veins and extending into the left atrium [40]. This happens more frequently than is currently recognized, although it is rarely demonstrated on echocardiography, magnetic resonance imaging (MRI) or computed tomography (CT) being preferable in the staging of mediastinal spread of lung carcinoma. The use of transoesophageal echocardiography in the staging of lung tumours will undoubtedly increase the diagnosis of left atrial tumour extension as at postmortem, up to 5% of these tumours directly involve the heart.

METASTATIC SECONDARY TUMOURS

Figure 13.15 demonstrates a large mobile mass in the right atrium in a 22-year-old male with known metastatic testicular seminoma. The atrial mass was diagnosed on echocardiography performed for his new systolic murmur. The mass regressed considerably on chemotherapy as did his multiple intrapulmonary deposits but unfortunately all returned in the final stages of his disease. Germ cell tumours may also involve the right ventricle [41], and spread to the right heart in these tumours should always be considered if the patient develops a new murmur.

Other tumours metastasizing to the heart include melanoma [42], chorion carcinoma [43] and liposarcoma [44]. The finding of an intracavitary mass in any of the cardiac chambers may be due to a metastasis even if there is no known primary. However, it is rarely possible to definitely diagnose the type of lesion as echocardio-

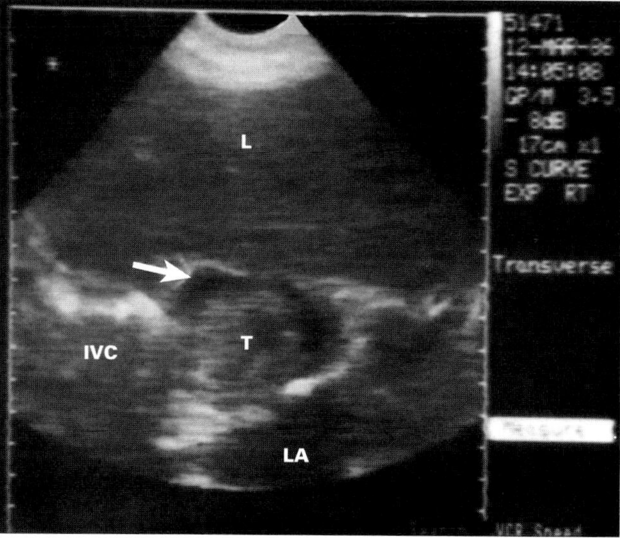

Fig. 13.14 Subcostal view through left lobe of liver (L) in a patient with a large tumour (T) in the right atrium (arrow) arising from the right kidney via the inferior vena cava (IVC). LA, left atrium.

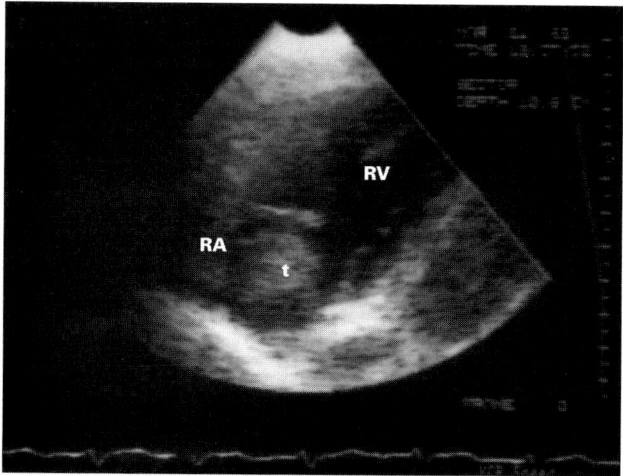

Fig. 13.15 Long axis view through the right ventricle (RV) and right atrium (RA) in a patient with a right atrial tumour metastasis (t) from a testicular seminoma.

graphically, there is little difference in the appearances between primary or secondary, malignant or benign masses.

Primary cardiac tumours

Benign

MYXOMA

The commonest primary benign tumour of the heart is a myxoma, most frequently arising from the left side of the intra-atrial septum [45]. The tumour may also be found in the right atrium [46,47], the right ventricle [48], on the eustachian valve [49], the mitral valve [50] and very rarely in the left ventricle [51].

Examples of left atrial myxoma in three patients are shown in Figures 13.16–13.18. There is a variability of echocardiography appearances in these tumours. Some are relatively echolucent and difficult to see because of their jelly-like consistency, while others contain flecks of calcification (as in Fig. 13.18b) and are more echogenic. A few have cystic spaces within the tumour itself. Clinical symptoms of cardiac myxomas can be separated into three groups: those due to obstruction at the atrial or valve level; secondary systemic manifestations such as fever, weight loss, high erythrocyte sedimentation rate and anaemia; and cases presenting with embolic phenomena [45]. It is important to echocardiographically screen patients with systemic emboli as left atrial myxomas may be clinically silent yet because of their consistency have a tendency to embolize.

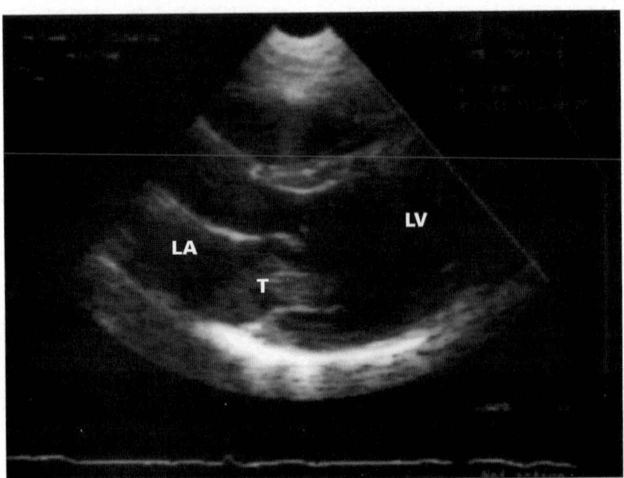

Fig. 13.16 Long axis view of a patient with a small left atrial myxoma (T) prolapsing through the mitral valve, who presented with a systemic embolus to her leg. LA, left atrium; LV, left ventricle.

Multiple myxomas may be sporadic or associated with 'syndrome myxoma' [52]. Syndrome myxoma is a familial entity associated with multiple, recurrent myxomas, peripheral and endocrine neoplasms, and cutaneous abnormalities including blue naevi and freckles. These patients form a younger subset than the sporadic, single or multiple non-familial cases. Myxoma is the third commonest cardiac tumour in childhood. The other benign cardiac tumours associated with hereditary syndromes are rhabdomyomas and fibromas.

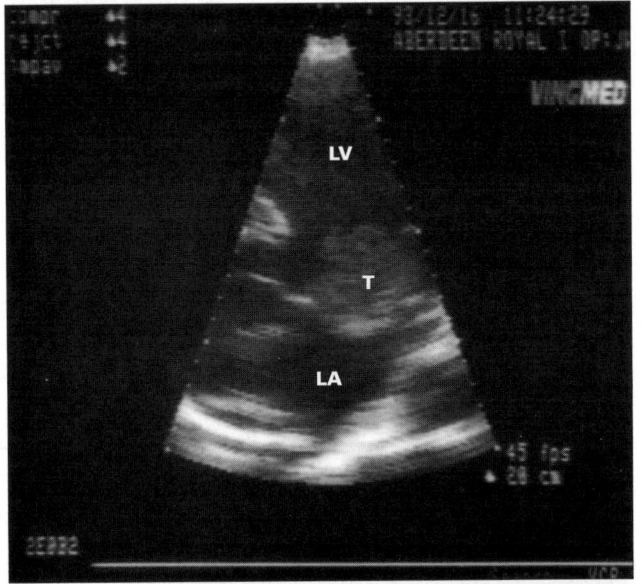

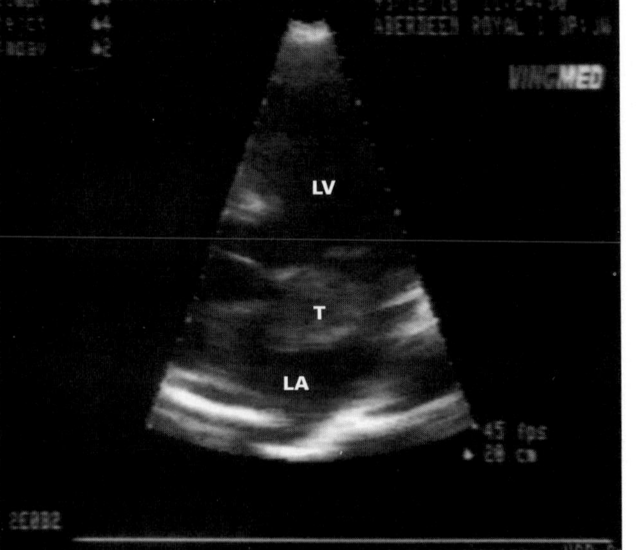

Fig. 13.17 (a,b) Apical two-chamber views of a larger, more echogenic left atrial myxoma (T) than seen in Fig. 13.6. LA, left atrium; LV, left ventricle.

(a)

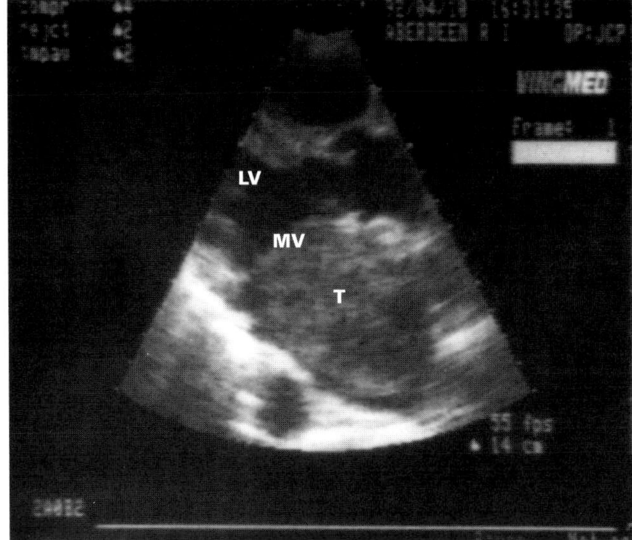

(b)

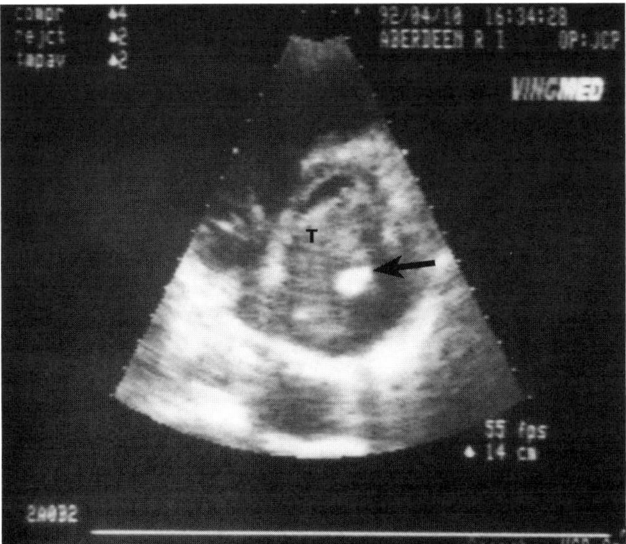

Fig. 13.18 (a) Long and (b) short axis views of a large, highly echogenic left atrial myxoma (T) almost obliterating the atrial cavity, and containing flecks of calcification (arrow) with the typical acoustic shadow deep to the calcium. LV, left ventricle; MV, mitral valve.

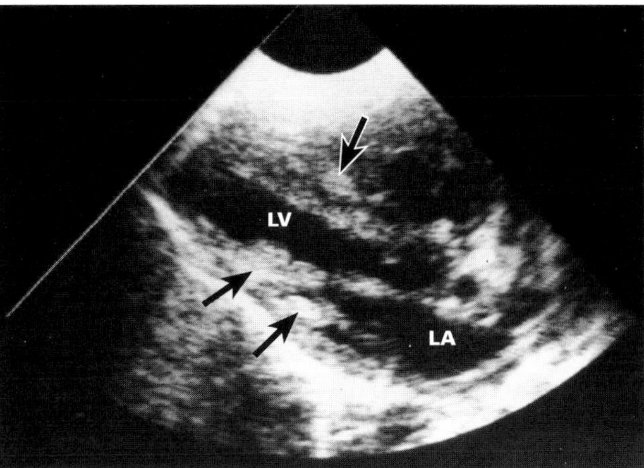

Fig. 13.19 Multiple circular areas of increased echogenicity due to multiple rhabdomyomas, in the interventricular septum, the posterior left ventricular wall and the papillary muscles (arrows) in a neonate with tuberous sclerosis. LA, left atrium; LV, left ventricle.

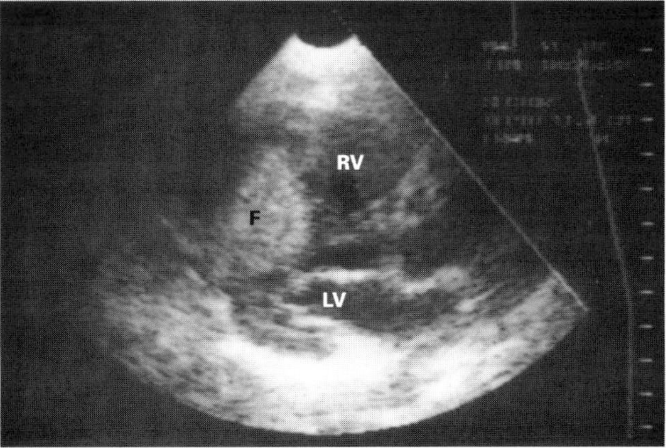

Fig. 13.20 Long axis views of a 10-year-old boy with a large echogenic fibroma (F) of the muscular interventricular septum causing distortion of both ventricular cavities. LV, left ventricle; RV, right ventricle.

RHABDOMYOMA

Cardiac rhabdomyomas are the commonest cardiac tumours in children, and occur in approximately 30% of patients with tuberous sclerosis [53,54]. The tumours are usually buried within the myocardium in cases associated with tuberous sclerosis, whereas in the sporadic cases, the tumour is more likely to be intracavitary. Multiple rhabdomyomas are shown in Fig. 13.19 in a neonate with other clinical features of tuberous sclerosis. This patient was followed by serial echocardiography for several years, the tumours gradually decreasing in size, to be virtually undetectable at 5 years of age, similar to other reported cases [55].

FIBROMA

Cardiac fibromas are the second commonest childhood cardiac tumour, a few being associated with the naevoid basal cell carcinoma syndrome. The tumour is usually solitary and sited in the interventricular septum (Fig. 13.20). It may cause disturbance to the conducting mechanism of the heart, obstruction to either ventricle or be asymptomatic [56,57].

OTHER BENIGN TUMOURS

A variety of intracardiac benign masses have been described including aortic and mitral fibroelastomas [58–60], known also as giant Lambl's excrescences, which are thought to arise on or near valves as a result of fibrin deposition at sites of minor endothelial damage; valvular hamartomas [61], rare cystic structures of either the mitral or tricuspid valves; cavernous haemangiomas of the right heart [62,63]; and lipomas [64] which may lie within the atrial septum, the ventricular septum or in the bodies of the left or right ventricles.

CARCINOID DISEASE OF THE HEART

Malignant gastrointestinal carcinoid tumours are associated with endocardial deposition of myofibromatous tissue, principally in the right heart, resulting in thickened tricuspid and pulmonary valves and reduced atrial and ventricular function [65].

Malignant

Angiosarcomas and rhabdomyosarcomas account for the majority of malignant primary cardiac tumours, forming approximately 20% of all primary tumours of the heart, the rest being in the benign group described above.

Angiosarcoma is the commonest malignant primary tumour, almost always occurring in the right atrium or in the nearby pericardium and being invasive with a poor prognosis. About half the reported cases also have metastases [66,67]. Primary rhabdomyosarcoma [68], leiomyosarcoma [69], fibrosarcoma [70] and malignant mesenchymomas [71,72] have all been described, are rare and may be echocardiographically indistinguishable from their benign counterparts.

Most of these malignant tumours were previously only diagnosed at postmortem but with the increasing use of wider investigative procedures such as transoesophageal ultrasound and MRI, these patients are now presenting to the surgeon and echocardiographers should be aware of the wide pathological basis that exists in benign and malignant, primary and secondary cardiac tumours.

References

1 Mugge, A., Daniel, W.G., Haverich, A., Lichtlen, P.R. (1991) Diagnosis of noninfective cardiac mass lesions by two-dimensional echocardiography. Comparison of the transthoracic and transesophageal approaches. *Circulation* **83**, 70–78.

2 Porath, A., Avnun, L., Hirsch, M., Ovsyshcher, I. (1987) Right atrial thrombus and recurrent pulmonary emboli secondary to permanent cardiac pacing—a case report and short review of literature. *Angiology* **38**, 627–630.

3 Mugge, A., Gulba, D.C., Jost, S., Daniel, W.G. (1990) Dissolution of a right atrial thrombus attached to pacemaker electrodes: usefulness of recombinant tissue-type plasminogen activator. *American Heart Journal* **119**, 1437–1439.

4 Dick, A.E., Gross, C.M., Rubin, J.W. (1989) Echocardiographic detection of an infected superior vena caval thrombus presenting as a right atrial mass. *Chest* **96**, 212–214.

5 Paut, O., Kreitmann, B., Silicani, M.A., *et al.* (1992) Successful treatment of fungal right atrial thrombosis complicating central venous catheterization in a critically ill child. *Intensive Care Medicine* **18**, 375–376 (review).

6 Leung, W.H., Lau, C.P., Tai, Y.T., Wong, C.K., Cheng, C.H. (1990) *Candida* right ventricular mural endocarditis complicating indwelling right atrial catheter. *Chest* **97**, 1492–1493.

7 Oto, A., Tokgozoglu, S.L., Oram, A., *et al.* (1993) Late percutaneous extraction of an intracardiac catheter fragment. *Japanese Heart Journal* **34**, 117–119.

8 Taams, M.A., Gussenhoven, E.J., Bos, E., *et al.* (1990) Enhanced morphological diagnosis in infective endocarditis by transoesophageal echocardiography. *British Heart Journal* **63**, 109–113.

9 Ozkutlu, S., Saraclar, M., Atalay, S., Demircin, M., Ruacan, S. (1991) Two-dimensional echocardiographic diagnosis of tricuspid valve noninfective endocarditis due to protein C deficiency (lesion mimicking tricuspid valve myxoma). *Japanese Heart Journal* **32**, 139–145.

10 Tatsukawa, H., Okajima, Y., Furukawa, K., Katsume, H., Miyao, K., Nakagawa, M. (1989) Giant right atrial thrombus in Noonan syndrome combined with Eisenmenger's complex. *Chest* **95**, 930–932.

11 Chow, W.H., Chow, L.T., Ng, W. (1993) Free-floating but immobile ball thrombus in left atrium: diagnosis aided by transoesophageal echocardiography. *International Journal of Cardiology* **39**, 213–215.

12 Olson, J.D., Goldenberg, I.F., Pedersen, W., *et al.* (1992) Exclusion of atrial thrombus by transesophageal echocardiography. *Journal of the American Society of Echocardiography* **5**, 52–56.

13 Alam, M., Jafri, S.M. (1993) Ball-valve thrombus obstructing a bioprosthetic mitral valve. *Chest* **103**, 1599–1600.

14 Delphin, E., Smith, C. Jr, Weissman, C. (1993) Transesophageal echocardiographic diagnosis of a free-floating atrial thrombus. *Journal of Cardiothoracic and Vascular Anesthesia* **7**, 326–328.

15 Hwang, J.J., Kuan, P., Tzou, S.S., Fuh, M.C., Cheng, J.J., Lien, W.P. (1993) Resolution of left atrial thrombi after anticoagulant therapy in patients with rheumatic mitral stenosis: report of four cases. *Journal of the Formosan Medical Association* **92**, 72–77.

16 Wrisley, D., Giambartolomei, A., Lee, I., Brownlee, W. (1991) Left atrial ball thrombus: review of clinical and echocardiographic manifestations with suggestions for management. *American Heart Journal* **121**(6 Pt 1), 1784–1790 (review).

17 Isner, J.M., Roberts, W.C. (1978) Right ventricular infarction complicating left ventricular infarction secondary to coronary heart disease. *American Journal of Cardiology* **42**, 885–894.

18 Kessler, K.M., Mallon, S.M., Bolooki, H., Myerburg, R.J. (1981) Pedunculated right ventricular thrombus due to repeated blunt chest trauma. *American Heart Journal* **102**, 1064–1069.

19 Domenicucci, S., Chiarella, F., Bellotti, P., Lupi, G., Scarsi, G., Vecchio, C. (1990) Early appearance of left ventricular thrombi after anterior myocardial infarction: a marker of higher in-hospital mortality in patients not treated with antithrombotic drugs. *European Heart Journal* **11**, 51–58.

20 Kontny, F., Dale, J., Nesvold, A., Lem, P., Soberg, T. (1993) Left ventricular thrombosis and arterial embolism in acute anterior myocardial infarction. *Journal of Internal Medicine* **233**, 139–143.

21 Lloret, R.L., Cortada, X., Bradford, J., Metz, M., Kinney, E.L. (1985) Classification of left ventricular thrombi by their history of systemic embolisation using pattern recognition of two dimensional echocardiograms. *American Heart Journal* **110**, 761–765.

22 Rechavia, E., Imbar, S., Birnbaum, Y., Strasberg, B., Sclarovsky, S. (1993) Protruding left ventricular thrombus formation following blunt chest trauma. *American Heart Journal* **125**, 893–896.

23 Alam, M., Levine, T.B. (1993) Echocardiographic features of embolized inferior venacaval filter to the right ventricle—a case report. *Angiology* **44**, 338–340.

24 Dorsa, F.B., Gindea, A.J., Kralik, M., Tice, D.A. (1992) Misplaced Greenfield filter: diagnosis by transesophageal echocardiography. *Journal of the American Society of Echocardiography* **5**, 437–438.

25 Xie, S.W., Picard, M.H. (1992) Two-dimensional and color Doppler echocardiographic diagnosis of penetrating missile wounds of the heart: chronic complications from intracardiac course of a bullet. *Journal of the American Society of Echocardiography* **5**, 81–84.

26 Shaikh, K., Cilley, J., O'Connor, W., DelRossi, A.J. (1989) Intraoperative echocardiography: a useful tool in the localization of small intracardiac foreign bodies. *Journal of Cardiovascular Surgery* **30**, 42–43.

27 Jagmeet, P.S., D'Silva, S., Lokhandwala, Y.Y., Dalvi, B.V. (1992) Intracardiac needle in a man with self-injurious behaviour presenting with only a heart murmur. *Thoracic and Cardiovascular Surgeon* **40**, 231–233.

28 Mohan, J.C., Agarwala, R., Khanna, S.K. (1992) Dissecting intramyocardial hematoma presenting as a massive pseudotumor of the right ventricle. *American Heart Journal* **124**, 1641–1642.

29 Groves, A.M., Fagg, N.L., Cook, A.C., Allan, L.D. (1992) Cardiac tumours in intrauterine life. *Archives of Disease in Childhood* **67**(10 special no.), 1189–1192.

30 Salka, S., Siegel, R., Sagar, K.B. (1993) Transvenous biopsy of intracardiac tumor under transesophageal echocardiographic guidance. *American Heart Journal* **125**, 1782–1784.

31 Missault, L., Duprez, D., De Buyzere, M., Cambier, B., Adang, L., Clement, D. (1992) Right atrial invasive thymoma with protrusion through the tricuspid valve. *European Heart Journal* **13**, 1726–1727.

32 Besterman, E., Bromley, L.L., Peart, W.S. (1974) An intrapericardial phaeochromocytoma. *British Heart Journal* **36**, 318–320.

33 Rosamond, T.L., Hamburg, M.S., Vacek, J.L., Borkon, A.M. (1992) Intrapericardial pheochromocytoma. *American Journal of Cardiology* **70**, 700–702.

34 Ansani, L., Percoco, G., Zanardi, F., Peranzoni, P., Gamba, G., Antonioli, G. (1993) Intracardiac thyroid heterotopia. *American Heart Journal* **125**, 1797–1801.

35 Shahian, D.M., Libertino, J.A., Zinman, L.N., Leonardi, H.K., Eyre, R.C. (1990) Resection of cavoatrial renal cell carcinoma employing total circulatory arrest. *Archives of Surgery* **125**, 727–731.

36 Sobue, T., Iwase, M., Iwase, M., *et al.* (1993) Solitary left ventricular metastasis of renal cell carcinoma. *American Heart Journal* **125**, 1801–1802.

37 Farooki, Z.Q., Henry, J.G., Green, E.W. (1975) Echocardiographic diagnosis of right atrial extension of Wilms' tumor. *American Journal of Cardiology* **36**, 363–367.

38 Pellicelli, A.M., Barba, J., Gomez, A.J., Borgia, M.C. (1992) Echocardiographic follow-up of right atrial tumoral invasion by hepatocarcinoma: a case report. *Cardiologia* **37**, 151–153.

39 Podolsky, L.A., Jacobs, L.E., Ioli, A., Kotler, M.N. (1993) TEE in the diagnosis of intravenous leiomyomatosis extending into the right atrium. *American Heart Journal* **125**(5 Pt 1), 1462–1464.

40 Popovic, A.D., Harrigan, P., Sanfilippo, A.J., Weyman, A.E. (1989) Echocardiographic detection of left atrial extension of bronchial carcinoma. *Journal of the American Medical Association* **261**, 1478–1480.

41 Pickuth, D., Eeles, R., Mason, M., Pumphrey, C., Goldstraw, P., Horwich, A. (1992) Intracardiac metastases from germ cell tumours—an unusual but important site of metastasis. *British Journal of Radiology* **65**, 672–673.

42 Sheldon, R., Isaac, D. (1991) Metastatic melanoma to the heart presenting with ventricular tachycardia. *Chest* **99**, 1296–1298.

43 Kishore, A.G., Desai, N., Nayak, G. (1992) Choriocarcinoma presenting as intracavitary tumor in the left atrium. *International Journal of Cardiology* **35**, 405–407.

44 Schrem, S.S., Colvin, S.B., Weinreb, J.C., Glassman, E., Kronzon, I. (1990) Metastatic cardiac liposarcoma: diagnosis by transesophageal echocardiography and magnetic resonance imaging. *Journal of the American Society of Echocardiography* **3**, 149–153 (review).

45 Larsson, S., Lepore, V., Kennergren, C. (1989) Atrial myxomas: results of 25 years' experience and review of the literature. *Surgery* **105**, 695–698 (review).

46 Sommariva, L., Auricchio, A., Polisca, P., Penta de Peppo, A., Chiariello, L. (1993) Right atrial myxoma with atypical features of syndrome myxoma. *American Heart Journal* **126**, 256–258.

47 Ohshima, H., Kawashima, E., Ogawa, Y., Tobise, K., Onodera, S. (1993) Demonstration of the inner structure of a right atrial myxoma by transoesophageal echocardiography. *European Heart Journal* **14**, 132–134.

48 Lebovic, S., Koorn, R., Reich, D.L. (1991) Role of two-dimensional transoesophageal echocardiography in the management of a right ventricular tumour. *Canadian Journal of Anaesthesia* **38**, 1050–1054.

49 Teoh, K.H., Mulji, A., Tomlinson, C.W., Lobo, F.V. (1993) Right atrial myxoma originating from the eustachian valve. *Canadian Journal of Cardiology*, **9**, 441–443 (review).

50 Zamorano, J., Vilacosta, I., Almeria, C., San Roman, A., Alfonso, F., Sanchez-Harguindey, L. (1993) Diagnosis of mitral valve myxoma by transesophageal echocardiography. *European Heart Journal* **14**, 862–863.

51 Soma, Y., Ogawa, S., Iwanaga, S., *et al.* (1992) Multiple primary left ventricular myxomas with multiple intraventricular recurrences. *Journal of Cardiovascular Surgery* **33**, 765–767.

52 Vidaillet, U.J. Jr, Seward, J.B., Fyke, III F.E., Su, W.P.D., Tajik, A.J. (1987) Syndrome myxoma: a subset of patients with cardiac myxoma associated with pigmented skin lesions and peripheral and endocrine neoplasms. *British Heart Journal* **57**, 247–255.

53 Webb, D.W., Thomas, R.D., Osborne, J.P. (1993) Cardiac rhabdomyomas and their association with tuberous sclerosis. *Archives of Disease in Childhood* **68**, 367–370.

54 Giacoia, G.P. (1992) Fetal rhabdomyoma: a prenatal echocardiographic marker of tuberous sclerosis. *American Journal of Perinatology* **9**, 111–114 (review).

55 Matsuoka, Y., Nakati, T., Kawaguchi, K., Hayakawa, K. (1990) Disappearance of a cardiac rhabdomyoma complicating congenital mitral regurgitation as observed by serial two-dimensional echocardiography. *Pediatric Cardiology* **11**, 98–101.
56 Ceithaml, E.L., Midgley, F.M., Perry, L.W., Dullum, M.K. (1990) Intramural ventricular fibroma in infancy: survival after partial excision in two patients. *Annals of Thoracic Surgery* **50**, 471–472.
57 Tahernia, A.C., Bricker, J.T., Ott, D.A. (1990) Intracardiac fibroma in an asymptomatic infant. *Clinical Cardiology* **13**, 506–512.
58 Lewis, N.P., Williams, G.T., Fraser, A.G. (1989) Unusual and intraoperative epicardial echocardiographic features of a papillary tumour of the aortic valve. *British Heart Journal* **62**, 470–474.
59 Uchida, S., Obayashi, N., Yamanari, H., Matsubara, K., Saito, D., Haraoka, S. (1992) Papillary fibroelastoma in the left ventricular outflow tract. *Heart and Vessels* **7**, 164–167.
60 Thomas, M.R., Jayakrishnan A.G., Desai, J., Monaghan, M.J., Jewitt, D.E. (1993) Transesophageal echocardiography in the detection and surgical management of a papillary fibroelastoma of the mitral valve causing partial mitral valve obstruction. *Journal of the American Society of Echocardiography* **6**, 83–86.
61 Crotty, T.B., Edwards, W.D., Oh, J.K., Rodeheffer, R.J. (1991) Lipomatous hamartoma of the tricuspid valve: echocardiographic–pathologic correlations. *Clinical Cardiology* **14**, 262–266 (review).
62 Cunningham, T., Lawrie, G.M., Stavinoha, J. Jr, Quinones, M.A., Zoghbi, W.A. (1993) Cavernous hemangioma of the right ventricle: echocardiographic–pathologic correlates. *Journal of the American Society of Echocardiography* **6**(3 Pt 1), 335–340.
63 Palanivandi, R. Yang, S.S., Eldredge, W.J., *et al.* (1989) Cavernous lymphohemangioendothelioma of the right atrium—a case report. *Angiology* **40**, 768–771.
64 Alam, M., Silverman, N. (1993) Apical left ventricular lipoma presenting as syncope. *American Heart Journal* **125**, 1788–1790.
65 Lundin, L., Landelius, J., Andren, B., Oberg, K. (1990) Transoesophageal echocardiography improves the diagnostic value of cardiac ultrasound in patients with carcinoid heart disease. *British Heart Journal* **64**, 190–194.
66 Glancy, D.L., Morales, J.B. Jr, Roberts, W.C. (1968) Angiosarcoma of the heart. *American Journal of Cardiology* **21**, 413–419.
67 Sherman, D., Smith, C., Marboe, C., *et al.* (1993) Right atrial angiosarcoma causing a coronary artery fistula: diagnosis by transesophageal echocardiography. *American Heart Journal* **126**, 254–256.
68 Awad, M., Dunn, B., al Halees, Z., *et al.* (1992) Intracardiac rhabdomyosarcoma: transesophageal echocardiographic findings and diagnosis. *Journal of the American Society of Echocardiography* **5**, 199–202.
69 Fox, J.P., Freitas, E., McGiffin, D.C., Firouz-Abadi, A.A., West, M.J. (1991) Primary leiomyosarcoma of the heart: a rare cause of obstruction of the left ventricular outflow tract. *Australian and New Zealand Journal of Medicine* **21**, 881–883.
70 Sethi, K.K., Nair, M., Khanna, S.K. (1989) Primary fibrosarcoma of the heart presenting as obstruction at the tricuspid valve: diagnosis by cross-sectional echocardiography. *International Journal of Cardiology* **24**, 228–230.
71 Peters, P., Flachskampf, F.A., Hauptmann, S., Lo, H.B., Schuster, C.J. (1992) Bilocular atrial malignant mesenchymoma causing mitral and localized pulmonary vein flow obstruction: diagnosis by transoesophageal echocardiography. *European Heart Journal* **13**, 1585–1588.
72 McKenney, P.A., Moroz, K., Haudenschild, C.C., Shemin, R.J., Davidoff, R. (1992) Malignant mesenchymoma as a primary cardiac tumor. *American Heart Journal* **123**, 1071–1075 (review).

Chapter 14: Transoesophageal echocardiography

A. Deaner

To get the best ultrasound images the ultrasound transducer needs to lie as close to the tissue under interrogation as possible. Higher ultrasound frequencies can then be used and the interference produced by intervening structures avoided. This has lead to a proliferation of more invasive methods of ultrasound such as transrectal and transvaginal scanning. In cardiology the transoesophageal approach has found favour as it overcomes the most common limitations to optimum imaging, obesity and pulmonary disease.

Background

The first description of transoesophageal echo was by Frazin *et al.* in 1976 [1] and involved the positioning of an M-mode transducer behind the left atrium. In 1979 further descriptions of M-mode transoesophageal studies including the first descriptions of transoesophageal stress echocardiography came from Matsumoto *et al.* [2,3]. In 1980 Hisanaga *et al.* [4,5] described a simple rotating scanner that produced two-dimensional (2D) biplane images of cardiac structures. In 1982 Souquet *et al.* [6] described the first phased array transoesophageal instrument and in the same year Schluter [7] described the application of transoesophageal pulsed wave Doppler for assessing mitral regurgitation. Following these early reports the use of transoesophageal echo steadily increased. As well as cardiologists describing the appearances of various cardiac structures and pathology, anaesthetists used it to detect air emboli at the time of neurosurgical procedures [8] and for monitoring left ventricular function during major surgery.

Instrumentation

Transoesophageal probes are essentially converted gastroscopes. One or two ultrasound transducers are mounted distally and connected to a standard cardiac ultrasound unit by wires passing through the length of the scope. Three types of scopes are available, single (horizontal) plane, biplane and multiplane. Single plane probes have a single transducer at the tip of the scope, whereas biplane scopes have a horizontal plane transducer at the scope tip with a longitudinal plane transducer mounted 1–2 cm proximally. Multiplane probes have a single transducer mounted at the scope tip that can be turned through 180° by an internal mechanism either controlled manually or by a motor. The advantages of the latter two systems will be discussed below. A majority of scopes in present use have transducers of the multi-element phased array design (usually 64 elements) although single plane and multiplane scopes with mechanical transducers are available. As stated above, the proximity of the probe to the structures under examination enables transducers working at frequencies above those commonly used for precordial scanning to be used, most commonly 5 MHz. All commercially available systems have colour flow Doppler capability in addition to steerable pulsed wave Doppler and many now have steerable continuous wave Doppler. Adult scopes have a distal diameter of approximately 13–17 mm whilst miniaturized systems available for paediatric use have a distal diameter of 6–7 mm. Neonates weighing as little as 2.2 kg have been studied with the most recent scopes [9].

Examination

In our unit transoesophageal studies are carried out on ambulant patients in a room laid out specifically for this investigation. Facilities for administering sedation and full resuscitation equipment are required. The patient should be fasted for at least 4 h. We study a majority of our patients following sedation with midazolam and anaesthetize the pharynx with a lignocaine spray. Particular care to titrate the dose of midazolam according to patient need should be taken particularly in the elderly and those with pulmonary disease. The author routinely reverses sedation following the examination with the specific benzodiazipine antagonist, flumazenil and has this close at hand throughout the procedure in case of respiratory problems. A pulse oximeter is a useful method of detecting respiratory problems at an early stage. The patient is laid in the left lateral decubitus position and the scope passed by an experienced operator. A tooth guard is used if indicated and the scope lubricated with sterile gel. Many centres use a protective disposable sheath to protect against infection whilst others rely on chemical sterilization between cases. No consensus exists concerning the use of antibacterial prophylaxis against endocarditis; recent data suggests that significant bacteraemia during this investigation is extremely rare [10–12]. Once the scope has been passed into the oesophagus the various views of the heart are achieved by manipulating the tip of the instrument. The scope is passed up and down the oesophagus, rotated laterally in either direction and then the tip is anteverted or retroverted using the hand wheels at the control end of the probe. If a biplane scope is used then the tip is repositioned between horizontal and longitudinal views being taken. A multiplane scope allows the plane of imaging to be varied whilst viewing the image continuously.

Before undertaking the transoesophageal study a clinical history and examination should be taken and a full precordial examination carried out so that the operator has a clear idea of what he or she is likely to find. If the patient is only able to tolerate the scope for a short period the operator should initially view the areas of the heart most likely to produce useful information, followed by a more general scan.

A number of standard views of the heart are illustrated in Figs 14.1–14.4. Single plane transoesophageal echo is most impressive in its ability to view the atria, mitral valve and the proximal ascending and much of the descending thoracic aorta. The addition of the longitudinal plane improves views of the aortic valve, left ventricle, the distal ascending aorta and aortic arch. In addition, views of the right ventricular outflow tract and vena cava are improved. Multiplane probes have the great advantage of allowing each cardiac structure to be studied with varying planes of ultrasound without moving the transducer so that views can be optimized. This improves patient tolerance of the procedure and may shorten the length of a scan. Although little prospective work has been done to compare the diagnostic yield of the three modalities described, early experience suggests that multiplane scopes give the most comprehensive views of the left ventricular outflow tract, right ventricular outflow tract including the pulmonary artery and its two primary branches as well as allowing a more detailed assessment of native and prosthetic mitral and aortic leaks [13,14]. Additionally, multiplane scopes appear to improve the appreciation of complex congenital anatomy.

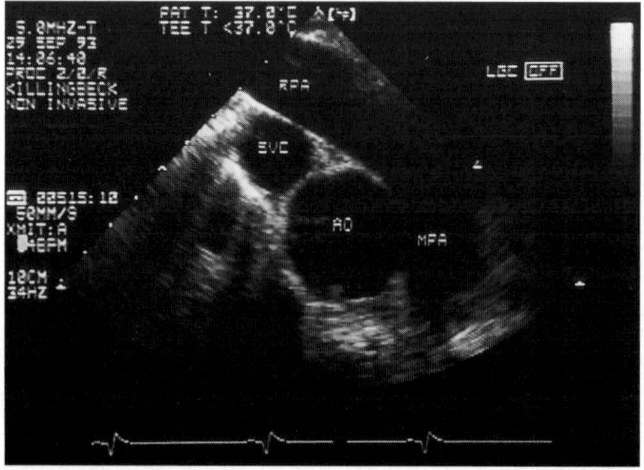

Fig. 14.1 View of normal main and right pulmonary artery (MPA + RPA), aorta (AO) and superior vena cava (SVC) taken with a multiplane probe.

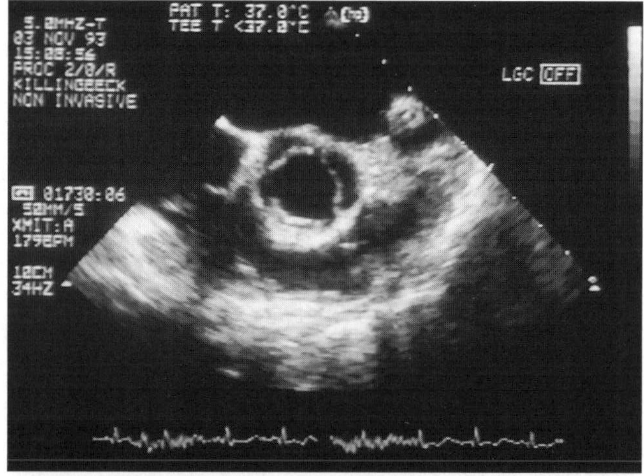

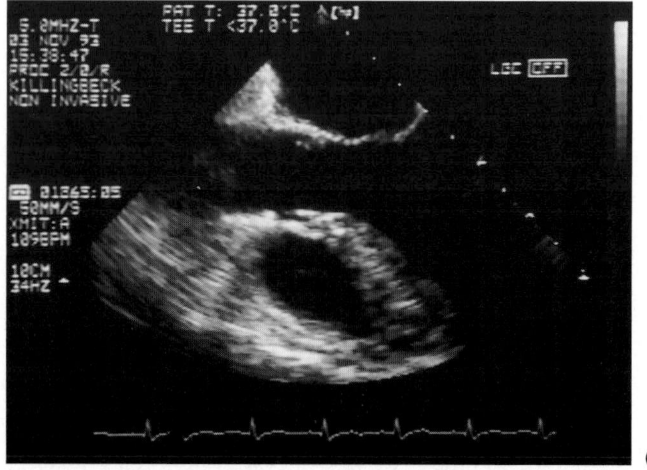

Fig. 14.2 Normal aortic valve seen in (a) short and (b) long axis, taken with multiplane probe.

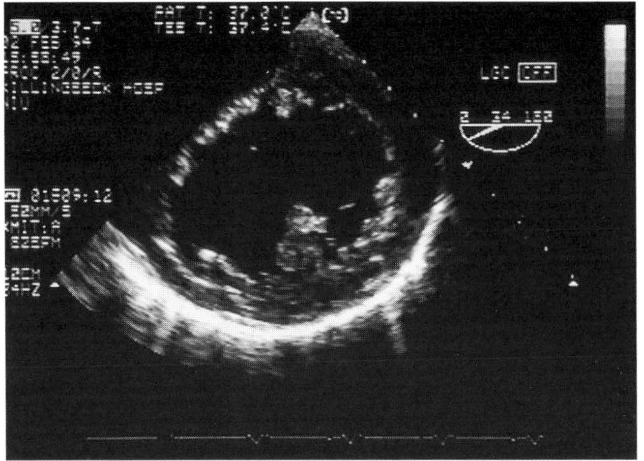

(a)

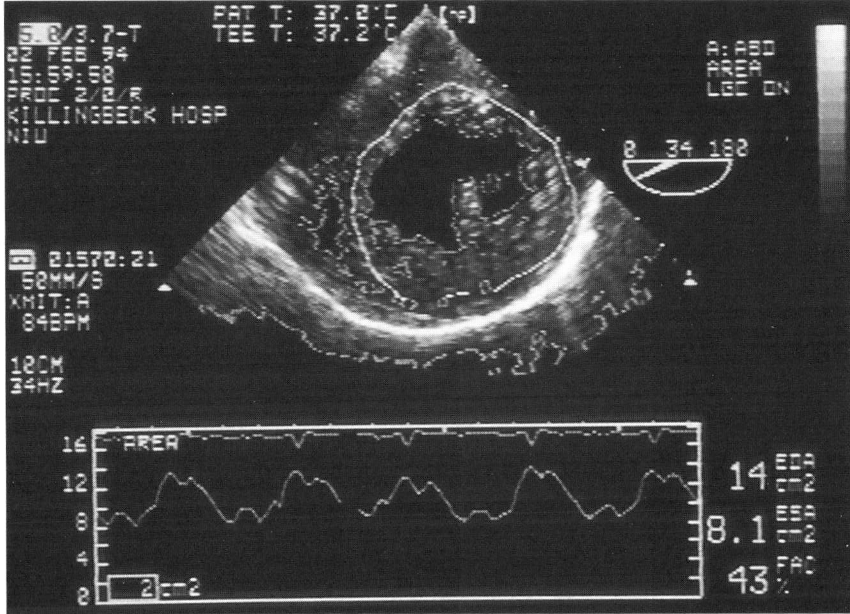

(b)

Fig. 14.3 (a) Cross-sectional view of the left ventricle taken from the gastric fundus and (b) illustrating the use of automated boundary location in the measurement of area changes between diastole and systole. For colour, see Plate 14.3 (between pp. 308 and 309).

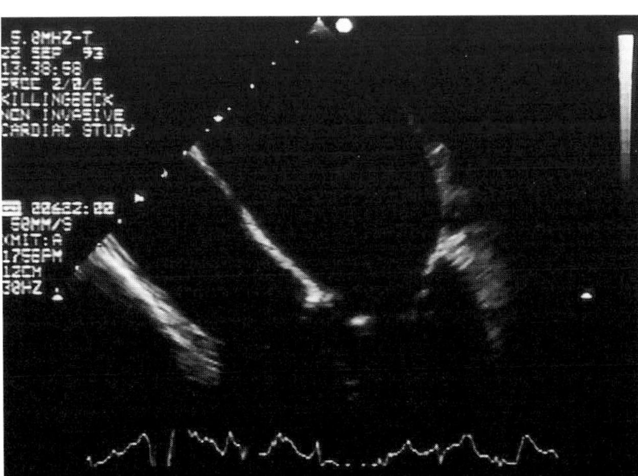

Fig. 14.4 Normal four-chamber view showing both atria and atrioventricular valves.

Indications

The principal indications for transoesophageal echo are shown in Table 14.1. The frequency of diagnoses found on transoesophageal scans carried out in the author's unit are shown in Table 14.2. This is fairly typical for a regional cardiothoracic unit with a large surgical work load, units in which surgery is not carried out will see fewer patients with prosthetic valves.

Transoesophageal scans may be carried out because of inadequate precordial images although in practice this is rather unusual. Others are done either because of a need to see structures in greater detail or because of technical difficulties in imaging specific anatomy from the chest wall such as the left atrial appendage or prosthetic heart valves. Many scans are requested for sick patients where the diagnosis is unclear. There is, however, little point in

Table 14.1 Common indications for transoesophageal echo

Clarify cause of valvar regurgitation
Assess prosthetic valve function
Exclude sources of systemic emboli
Find evidence of endocarditis or exclude complications of endocarditis
Clarify the nature of an intracardiac or pericardial mass
Assess congenital anomalies of the heart
Look for aortic dissection
Unable to get adequate precordial images (rarely sole indication)
Before percutaneous mitral valvuloplasty
Intraoperative assessment of valve repair or left ventricular function
Cardiac assessment of ventilated patients on the intensive care unit

Table 14.2 Distribution of diagnoses found on 307 consecutive adult patients undergoing transoesophageal scans in the author's unit. In a number of cases more than one diagnosis was made. (Excludes intraoperative scans.)

Diagnosis	Percentage of all transoesophageal echos
Mitral prosthesis	31
Aortic prosthesis	13
Mitral regurgitation	16
Aortic regurgitation	13
Intracardiac thrombus	10
Endocarditis	6
Congenital heart disease	6
Other diagnoses	9
Normal anatomy	13

carrying out an invasive procedure if it is unlikely to change the management of the patient. Having said this, transoesophageal echo has the great advantage of being tolerated even by very sick patients [15,16], and can be carried out on ventilated patients in the intensive care unit. In the operating theatre transoesophageal echo has two additional roles, monitoring left ventricular function and guiding surgical procedures such as mitral valve repair.

Transoesophageal echo has now become a routine procedure for the indications outlined in Table 14.2 and has been shown to be safe and well tolerated even when no sedation is used. In a survey of 15 centres carrying out over 10000 examinations only one fatality was described. In only 2.7% of cases did the operator fail to pass the probe or interrupt the examination (generally owing to intolerance of the probe in unsedated patients) [17]. The main contraindication to transoesophageal echo is any degree of dysphagia. In this situation the oesophagus should be fully investigated before it is blindly intubated. Significant respiratory compromise is a partial contraindication and certainly should limit the use of sedation. Other than a sore throat there are no common complications following this procedure. Potentially the most serious problem would be perforation of the oesophageal wall but fortunately this has never been reported. Respiratory depression, myocardial ischaemia and cardiac arrythmias may cause occasional problems but with careful monitoring and with the appropriate treatment at hand these should be limited in severity.

Mitral valve disease

Precordial transmitral Doppler using calculated pressure half-time remains the method of choice for estimating severity of mitral stenosis with echo but a transoesophageal echo will produce detailed views of the valve leaflets and apparatus (Fig. 14.5). An inspection of the left atrium will detect thrombus that may often be missed on precordial echo (Fig. 14.6) particularly in the left atrial appendage [18]. Transoesophageal echo is of particular use in assessing the suitability of a valve for balloon valvuloplasty and is now regarded as a prerequisite by many operators to exclude atrial thrombus [19–21]. Others have described its use in monitoring this procedure while it is in progress or even carrying it out under transoesophageal echo guidance only [22–24]. Following valvuloplasty transoesophageal echo will detect residual atrial septal shunts and changes in the severity of mitral regurgitation [25].

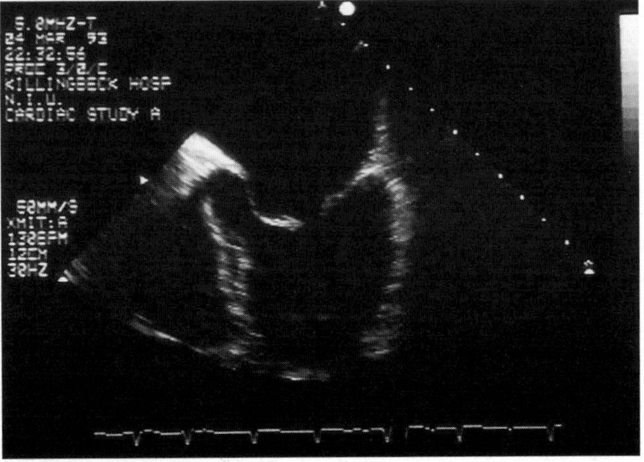

Fig. 14.5 View of stenotic mitral valve.

Transoesophageal echo has a greater role in the investigation of mitral regurgitation and in many instances will

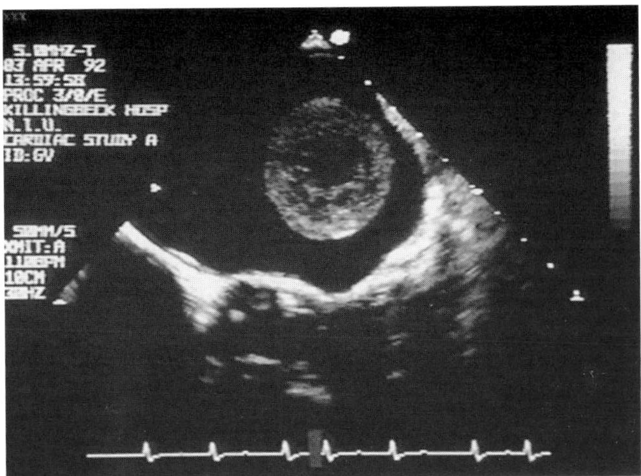

Fig. 14.6 Large ball thrombus seen in the left atrium of patient with severe mitral stenosis.

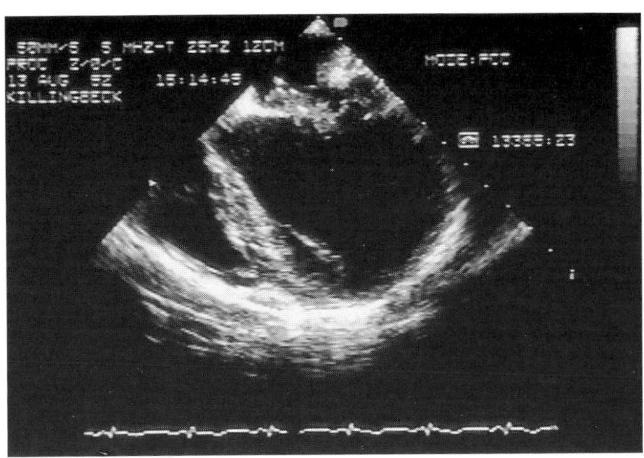

Fig. 14.7 Friable vegetations seen on both mitral leaflets.

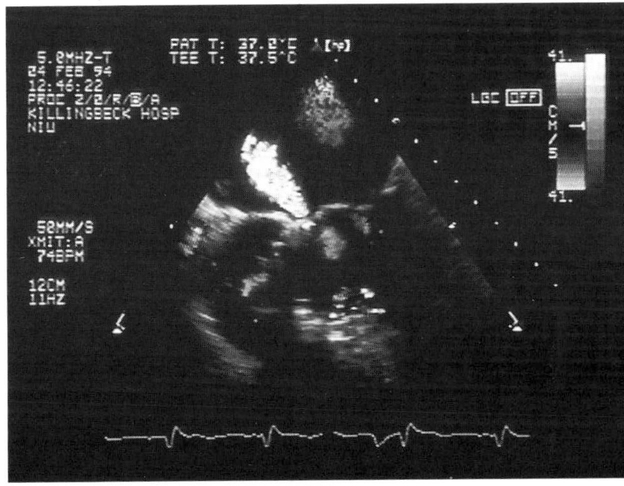

Fig. 14.8 View of a mechanical aortic prosthesis and a jet of mitral regurgitation through a hole at the base of the anterior mitral leaflet, a result of the aortic valve surgery. For colour, see Plate 14.8 (between pp. 308 and 309).

provide better information than transthoracic echo alone (Figs 14.7, 14.8) [26–29]. By producing detailed images of the valve the cause of significant mitral regurgitation can be clarified. Ruptured chordae, perforated leaflets and previously missed vegetations may be seen and advice on the possibility of valve repair can be offered to the surgeon [30–35]. The extent of the regurgitant jet shown on colour flow Doppler combined with the pattern of pulmonary venous flow measured by pulsed wave Doppler allows a semi-quantitative assessment of regurgitation. Severe mitral regurgitation is shown as a broad jet of colour flow with a mosaic of aliasing colours often filling much of the left atrium. The pulmonary venous flow pattern in severe mitral regurgitation includes significant reversed systolic flow as illustrated in Fig. 14.9 [36–38]. Methods of accurate quantitative assessment of the severity of mitral regurgitation have been keenly sought and include the use of flow convergence, measurements of colour flow jets in the left atrium and detailed analysis of the pulmonary venous flow trace; however, none has been widely adopted in clinical practice. Most cardiologists will make an overall assessment of regurgitation severity by reviewing clinical findings and then the precordial echo and other investigations in addition to the transoesophageal echo appearances.

Aortic valve disease

Aortic valve pathology may be better appreciated on transoesophageal study (Fig. 14.10) although views of this structure may not be as comprehensive as those of the mitral valve. Short axis views of the aortic valve are achieved in a proportion of patients with single plane probes but multiplane instruments mean that such views are possible in most cases. This may be of particular use when there is a significant doubt as to the presence of valvar aortic stenosis but will not allow a quantitative assessment of pressure drop to be made as even with a multiplane probe it is impossible to line up the Doppler sampling volume with flow through the left ventricular outflow tract. It has been suggested that transoesophageal echo allows accurate planimetry of aortic valve area in native valve stenosis [39,40] but this method is not routinely employed.

In suspected endocarditis the rate of detection of vegetations as well as the diagnosis of root abscesses will be improved. Transoesophageal echo may be useful when

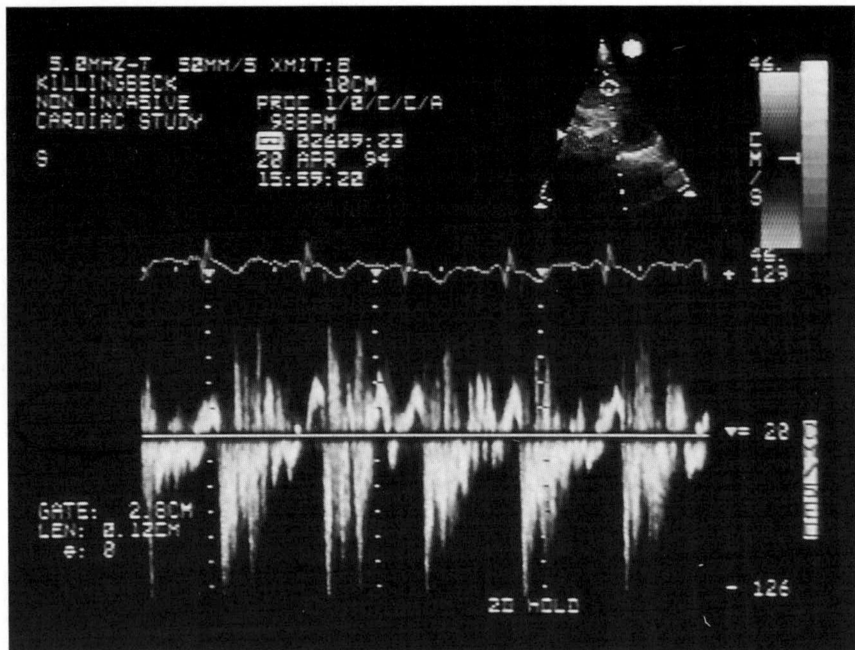

Fig. 14.9 Pulsed wave Doppler trace from the left lower pulmonary vein in a patient with severe mitral regurgitation. Note the reversed systolic flow. For colour, see Plate 14.9 (between pp. 308 and 309).

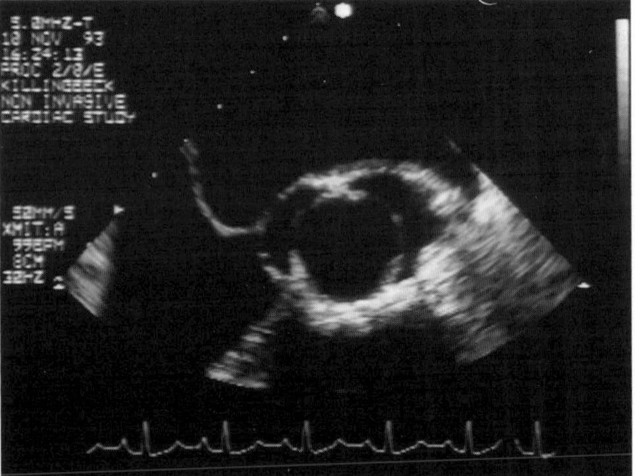

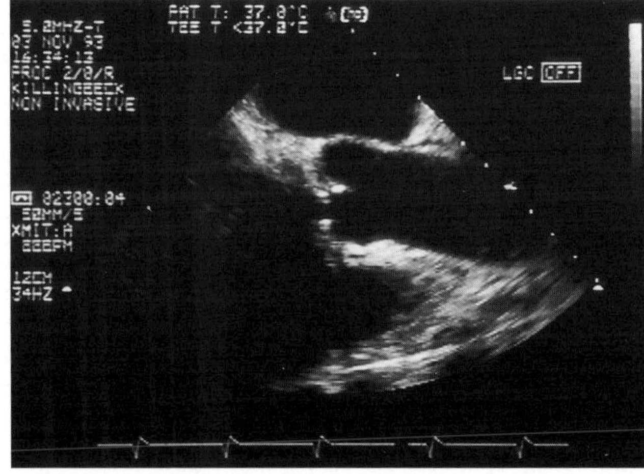

Fig. 14.10 (a) Bicuspid aortic valve seen in short axis with multiplane probe and (b) long axis view of aortic valve and root showing vegetation on aortic cusp.

non-valvar obstruction such as a subaortic membrane is suspected [41]. When there is a combination of valvar and dynamic left ventricular outflow tract obstruction transoesophageal echo will clarify the diagnosis particularly after aortic valve replacement [42,43].

Prosthetic valves

Most prosthetic valves are poorly imaged by precordial echo because of the echo reflective materials from which they are constructed. Precordial Doppler and 2D imaging may give important clues when prosthetic valve dysfunction is suspected but a transoesophageal study will frequently provide important additional information [44,45]. Best results are achieved when studying mitral prostheses as the atrial surface of the prosthesis is generally obscured by the ultrasonic shadow cast by the valve. Multiplane instruments have significantly improved the imaging of aortic prostheses but standard horizontal and longitudinal plane views are not as comprehensive as those of mitral prostheses [46]. The most frequent pathological processes affecting both biological and mechanical prostheses are thrombus formation (Fig. 14.11), endocarditis and paravalvular leaks (Fig. 14.12). Bioprosthetic valves

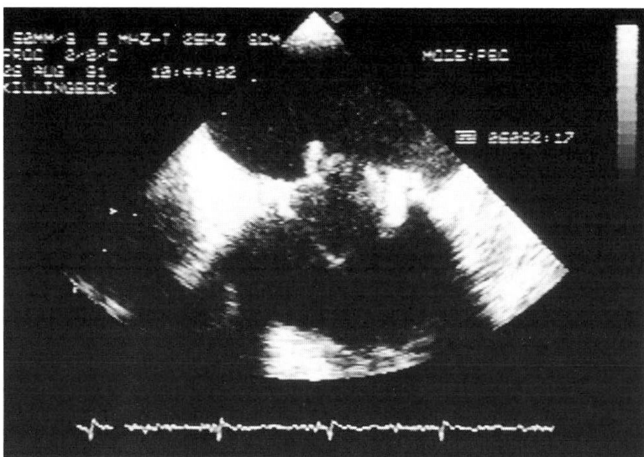

Fig. 14.11 Small thrombus shown attached to leaflet of bioprosthetic mitral valve.

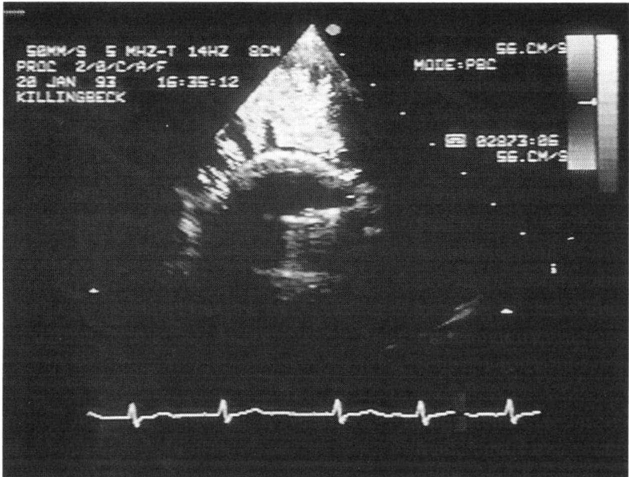

Fig. 14.12 Short axis view of a prosthetic mitral valve with an extensive paraprosthetic leak illustrated by colour flow Doppler. For colour, see Plate 14.12 (between pp. 308 and 309).

have the additional problem of degenerative changes leading to obstruction (Fig. 14.13) or regurgitation (Fig. 14.14). A number of studies have demonstrated the superiority of transoesophageal echo above precordial echo in detecting these abnormalities [44,45,47–51]. Cardiologists should, therefore, have a low threshold for requesting a transoesophageal scan when there is a clinical suspicion of prosthetic dysfunction even when the precordial study appears normal. Indications for transoesophageal echo to study aortic valve prostheses with a monoplane probe are limited to patients with restricted precordial views or to detect paravalvular leaks or other paravalvular pathology; however, as mentioned above multiplane probes

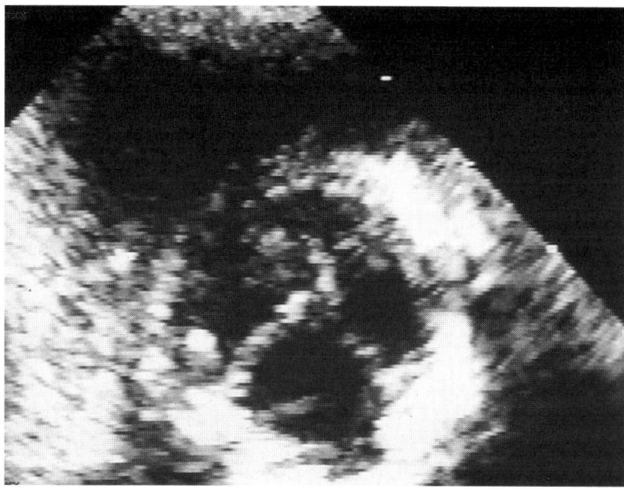

Fig. 14.13 Cross-sectional view of calcified and stenosed mitral bioprosthesis.

allow more comprehensive views of these valves and it is likely that the indications for transoesophageal echo examination of aortic valve prostheses will broaden to those of mitral valve prostheses.

Normal prosthetic valves are rarely totally competent. Transoesophageal studies of all types of mechanical prosthesis will detect a degree of regurgitation, each valve type having its own pattern of leak seen on colour flow mapping compatible with its 'normal' function [52,53]. An awareness of these patterns is necessary to avoid the inappropriate diagnosis of prosthetic valvular dysfunction.

Aortic pathology

As mentioned above, transoesophageal echo can image the aortic root, varying lengths of the ascending aorta, much of the arch and the descending aorta down to the level of the diaphragm. Not surprisingly it has been used in the diagnosis of a wide variety of acute and chronic aortic pathology.

Aortic dissection

Aortic dissection is a very dangerous condition so early diagnosis is essential. Until recently the standard method of diagnosis has been aortography. This is a highly invasive procedure as well as being expensive and time-consuming so a less invasive method of diagnosis was likely to be quickly adopted. Precordial echo is able to diagnose a number of patients with aortic dissection but has been shown to be insensitive. Transoesophageal echo is more sensitive than precordial echo in diagnosing dissection (Fig. 14.15) [54]. In addition to transoesophageal

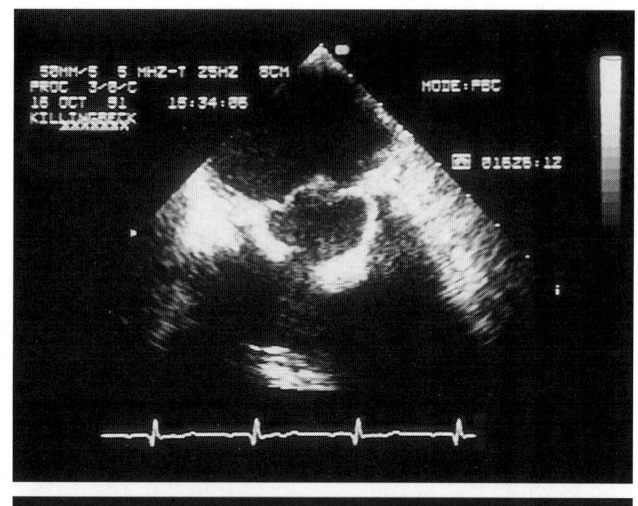
(a)

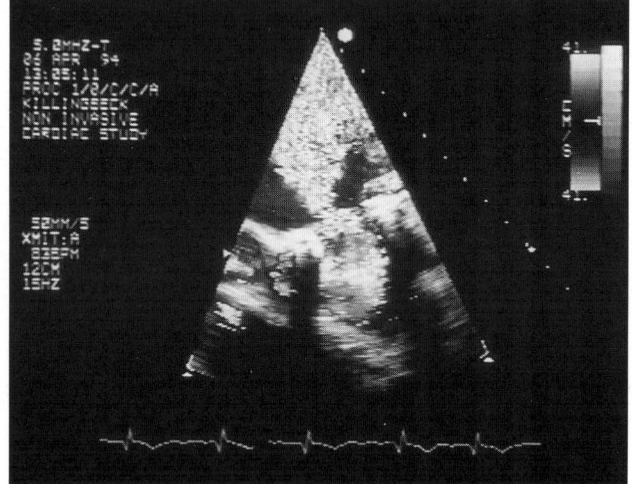
(b)

Fig. 14.14 (a) View of mitral bioprosthesis with prolapse of a torn leaflet back into the left atrium during systole and (b) the same valve with severe mitral regurgitation illustrated by a broad-based colour jet extending to the posterior atrial wall. For colour, see Plate 14.14 (between pp. 308 and 309).

(a)

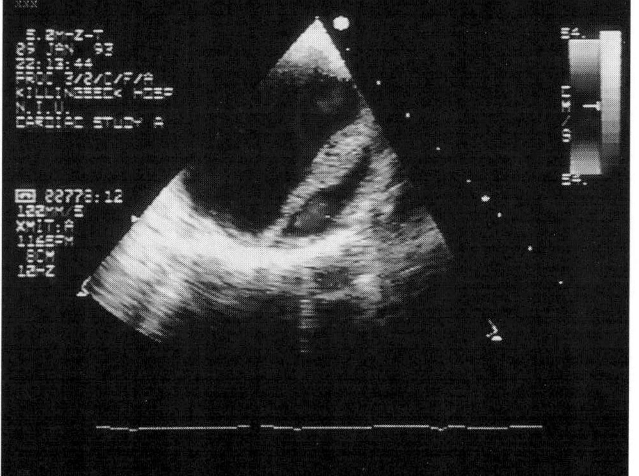
(b)

Fig. 14.15 (a) Type 1 aortic dissection with intimal flap easily identified in the aortic root and (b) seen extending into the descending aorta where colour flow Doppler helps to differentiate the true from the false lumen. For colour, see Plate 14.15 (between pp. 308 and 309).

echo, computed tomography (CT) scanning and latterly magnetic resonance imaging (MRI) have been shown to be useful in making this diagnosis [54–62]. Transoesophageal echo has the advantage over these two other modalities of portability and cost and gives additional information concerning left ventricular and valvar function. In DeBakey type I dissections transoesophageal echo can show the relation between a dissection flap and the aortic valve and coronary arteries and with the aid of colour flow Doppler can differentiate between the true and false lumen. The extent of a dissection can often be shown and entry and exit sites into and from the false lumen may be seen. The main limitation of transoesophageal echo is that a significant number of false positive diagnoses are sometimes made owing to echoes produced by reverberations in atheromatous aortic roots [63] but more often as a result of operator inexperience, resulting in decreased specificity. The study should be carried out only by experienced personnel and with great caution as there is a risk of extending the dissection during the procedure. Most cardiologists will only carry out a transoesophageal scan in a suspected dissection with the surgeon ready to operate. The patient should be heavily sedated or anaesthetized and ventilated and the blood pressure controlled by intravenous labetalol or a similar drug. Many cardiothoracic surgeons will now operate on the basis of a transoesophageal echo without recourse to cardiac catheterization.

Traumatic aortic rupture

Traumatic aortic rupture is an infrequent but extremely important diagnosis with few specific clinical signs apparent at initial presentation. A high suspicion for the diagnosis is thus necessary in significant blunt chest trauma so aortography is often carried out with a negative result. A number of recent reports suggest that transoesophageal echo can make this diagnosis with a high degree of sensitivity and a specificity as good or better than aortography [64–67]. Transoesophageal echo is certainly well suited to use in the accident and emergency unit or on the intensive care unit thus avoiding a prolonged visit to the catheter laboratory.

Transoesophageal echo is an accurate method of assessing thoracic aortic dilatation (Fig. 14.16) either secondary to atheromatous disease or cystic medial necrosis most commonly as part of Marfan's syndrome [68].

Transoesophageal echo can detect atheromatous plaques in the thoracic aorta (Fig. 14.17) [69,70] and recent studies have suggested that these may be a source of cerebral emboli [71–73]. Supporting the hypothesis that embolization of aortic plaque leads to cerebral events is the observation that 'protruding' plaques are found more frequently in those affected by such events [74,75].

Cardiac masses

Echocardiography has revolutionized the detection of intracardiac masses. These may be primary or secondary neoplasms, thrombus or vegetations. Many of these masses will be found most commonly in the atria and thus often will not be clearly visualized with transthoracic echo. Transoesophageal echo will help detect atrial masses that are missed on precordial scans and will provide better images of any mass that has been detected on a transthoracic scan enabling differentiation between different pathologies (Figs 14.18–14.20; see also Fig. 14.6), in addition it may help with the detection of extracardiac masses [76–78]. Transoesophageal echo will clarify the movement of masses in relation to other cardiac structures.

Transoesophageal echo has been shown to be more sensitive than precordial echo in the detection of atrial myxomas [79] and it has been shown to be a sensitive method for following up patients following excision of a myxoma and will detect rare cases of recurrence [80].

Other cardiac tumours are occasionally seen including benign tumours such as a papillary fibroelastoma (Fig. 14.21) or lipoma. The discovery of such benign masses may be coincidental and confusion may result particularly

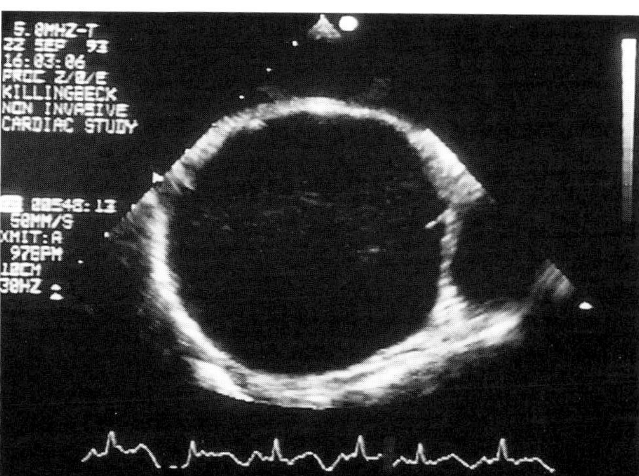

Fig. 14.16 Hugely dilated aortic root seen in cross-section (depth markers on the left are 1 cm apart).

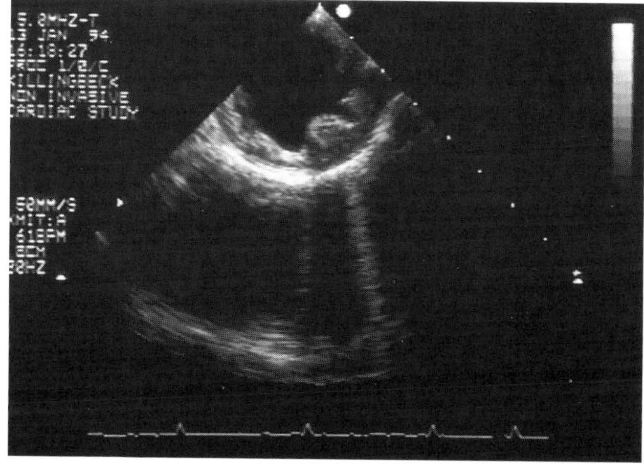

Fig. 14.17 Cross-sectional view of atheromatous descending aorta.

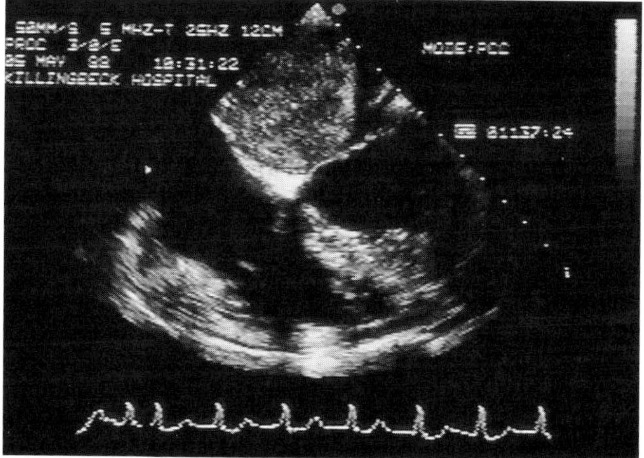

Fig. 14.18 Large left atrial mass confirmed to be a myxoma after excision.

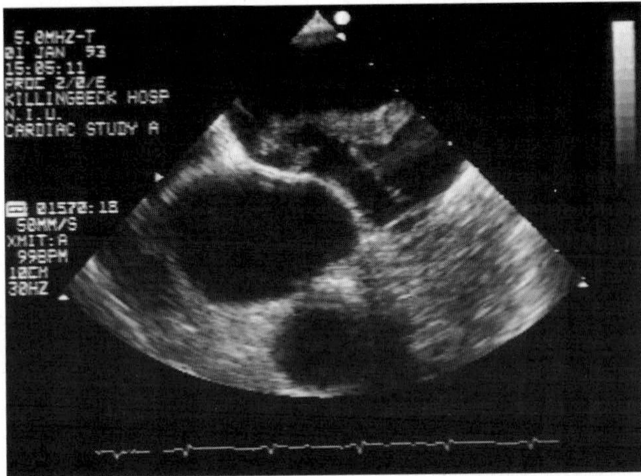

Fig. 14.19 Mass seen in left atrium attached to atrial septum, at surgery it was found to be venous thrombus passing through a large patent foramen ovale.

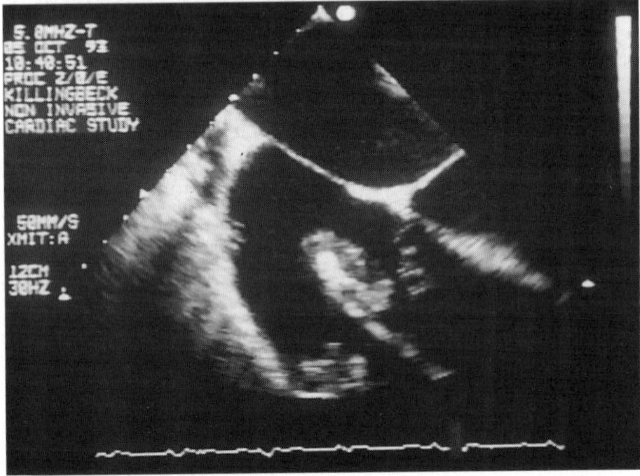

Fig. 14.20 Infected thrombus seen attached to ventricular pacing wire as it crosses the tricuspid valve.

if the transoesophageal echo has been carried out in order to exclude a source of embolus or to search for evidence of endocarditis. Secondary deposits or direct invasion from metastatic carcinomas are not uncommon and will be seen in more detail with transoesophageal echo.

Atrial thrombus

Clot in the left atrium is the commonest intracardiac source of embolism and is most frequently associated with an enlarged atrium and atrial fibrillation. Thrombus is very likely to be found when the mitral valve is stenosed or if there is inadequate anticoagulation when a prosthetic mitral valve is *in situ* (see Figs 14.6, 14.11). The left atrial

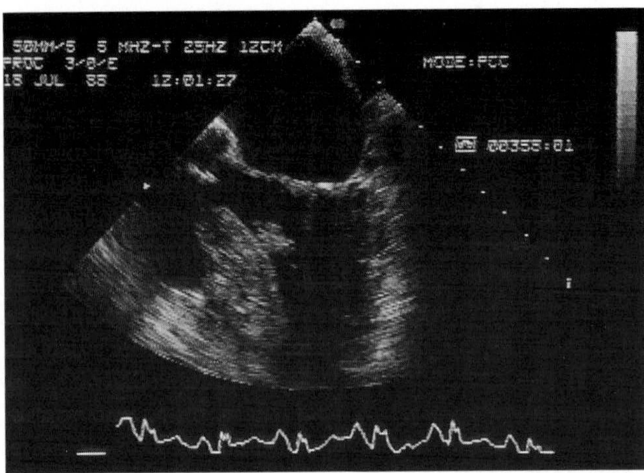

Fig. 14.21 Mass on ventricular septum later found to be a benign papillary fibroelastoma.

appendage is the commonest site for thrombus to be found and is rarely seen on precordial scan. Even extensive clot may be missed on precordial scan particularly if fresh. In all these situations transoesophageal echo is more sensitive than precordial echo and is certainly indicated following an embolic event in patients with such pathology [18,51].

A curious phenomenon known as spontaneous contrast is frequently seen on transoesophageal echo. It is recognized as a swirling cloudy appearance that may be ejected into the left ventricle during diastole. It is less frequently seen in the right atrium and may very occasionally be seen on precordial echo. The physical cause of this finding is the subject of much debate. It has been shown to be associated with increased atrial size, atrial fibrillation, mitral valve disease or prostheses and various haematological findings [81–85]. It is said to be less likely in the presence of significant mitral regurgitation [86]. An association with increased risk of thrombus formation has been shown in most studies but this has been disputed [87]. On balance most cardiologists now regard the presence of spontaneous contrast in the left atrium as an indication for anticoagulation certainly when found following an embolic event.

Other sources of systemic embolization

There is still debate regarding when a transoesophageal echo is indicated in the investigation of systemic embolization but certainly it is better than transthoracic echo at detecting possible sources of emboli [88–91]. Others have pointed out that although possible sources of emboli will frequently be detected there is often doubt regarding a definite causal relationship with an embolic event and therefore such findings may cause confusion [92,93]. As well as improving the detection of atrial thrombus, transoesophageal echo will detect left ventricular mural thrombus [94] although its sensitivity in this situation is less impressive. As mentioned above, transoesophageal echo detects areas of aortic atheroma which may be a source of embolism although other studies have shown that such atheroma is a marker of generalized arterial atherosclerosis [69,70] so it cannot be assumed that a particular aortic plaque has embolized. Cardiac tumours or vegetations may embolize and certainly transoesophageal echo will improve the detection of these abnormalities. It is well known that so-called 'paradoxical embolization' occurs across left-to-right shunts and a number of case reports describe the detection of clot found straddling the atrial septum with transoesophageal echo [95] (see Fig. 14.19). This may occur across an atrial septal defect but recent debate concerns the risk of such embolization across patent foramen ovale [96]. In support of patent foramen ovale as a conduit for paradoxical emboli has been the finding of an increased rate of asymptomatic deep venous thrombosis in patients with an embolic event and a patent foramen ovale [97]. One report has suggested that embolization only occurs if there is a significant right-to-left shunt shown with a contrast study [98]. Transoesophageal echo is a very sensitive method of detecting these defects which may be present in greater than 20% of the adult population. Recently, a high rate of systemic embolization has been described in patients with atrial septal aneurysms regardless of whether there is an associated shunt, such aneurysms being detected most frequently with transoesophageal echo which is able to see their structure in great detail (Fig. 14.22) [99,100].

It is likely that the debate regarding the role of transoesophageal echo will continue for some time and further research is required to clarify this difficult problem. A sensible approach is to reserve transoesophageal echo for young patients with embolic events with no obvious precipitant and for older patients with another predisposing cardiac abnormality such as a dilated atrium or mitral valve disease shown on precordial echo.

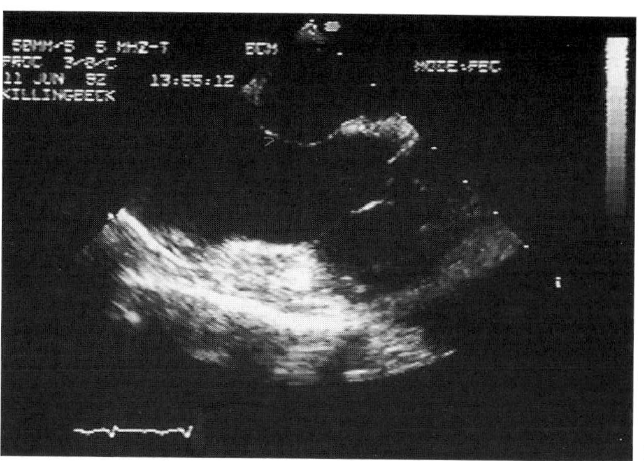

(a)

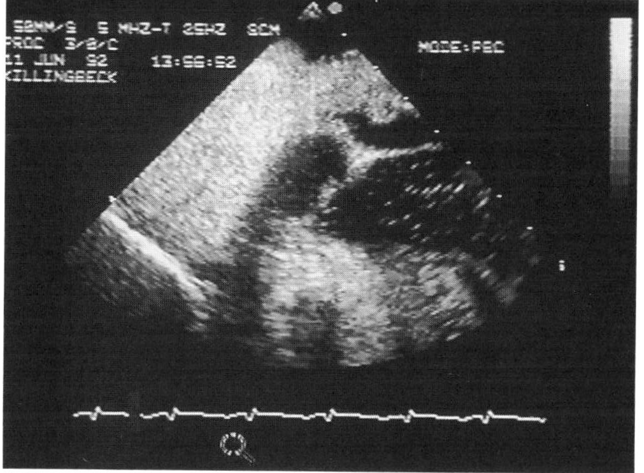

(b)

Fig. 14.22 (a) Atrial septum aneurysm with flow seen across it following a venous injection of echogenic contrast; (b) confirming an atrial septal defect (right-to-left flow can be demonstrated to some extent even when pulmonary artery pressure is normal).

Coronary arteries

Transoesophageal echo is able to produce images of the proximal coronary arteries. Although a number of reports have suggested that one can diagnose significant coronary stenoses with this method [101–104] and can sample coronary flow with pulsed wave Doppler [105], angiography remains the definitive investigation. Transoesophageal echo does, however, have an important role in clarifying congenital anomalies of the coronary arteries for instance when an aberrant coronary artery arises from the opposite coronary ostium and then passes between the aortic and pulmonary trunks [106–109]. In addition there have been numerous reports of transoesophageal echo imaging coronary artery fistulae allowing clarification of their site of drainage [110–114].

Pulmonary emboli

Precordial echo may indirectly suggest the diagnosis of massive pulmonary embolization by showing a dilated right heart and estimating raised pulmonary artery pressure. Transoesophageal echo has the additional benefit of imaging large central emboli (Fig. 14.23) and when available may quickly confirm this important diagnosis and replace more prolonged, risky and expensive investigations [115,116].

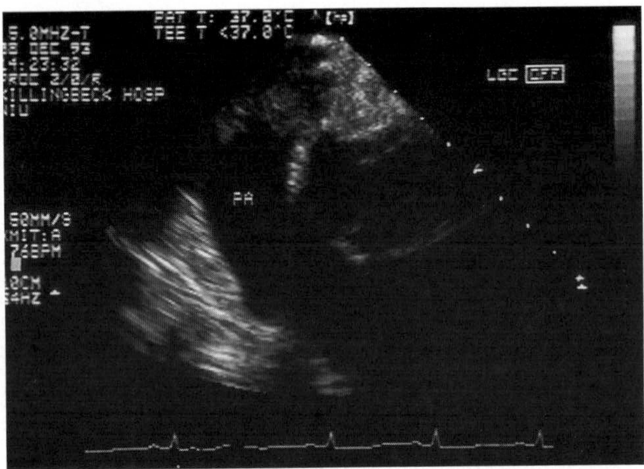

Fig. 14.23 Massive pulmonary embolus seen obstructing the right pulmonary artery.

Pericardial disease

Transoesophageal echo may be helpful when clarifying the nature of pericardial masses but this is only an occasional indication. Of more importance is its use in detecting localized thrombus adjacent to the right heart following cardiac surgery (Fig. 14.24). This may be a cause of cardiac tamponade that may be easily missed on transthoracic scans.

Congenital heart disease

Transoesophageal echo has been shown to have a useful role in the diagnosis and assessment of congenital heart disease in adults [117], adolescents [118], children and even neonates [9,119–121]. In most cases paediatric patients have an excellent echo window so the indications for transoesophageal echo are limited to specific complex anatomy and to monitor a child in the operating theatre and on the intensive care unit. In contrast adults and adolescents with congenital heart disease will often be difficult imaging subjects particularly following surgical interventions either corrective or palliative. In all these groups of patients transoesophageal echo has been shown to be of use in the diagnosis and assessment of congenital anomalies of systemic and pulmonary venous return [122], atrial morphology [123,124], atrioventricular valve anatomy [125], ventricular function, right and left ventricular outflow tracts, the atrial (Fig. 14.25) and ventricular septa [125–132], the pulmonary arteries, aorta [68] and ductus arteriosus [133]. In addition it is of use in the postoperative follow-up of patients with prosthetic valves, atrial baffles and those who have had a Fontan procedure [134]. Monitoring of interventions in the operating theatre and catheter laboratory with transoesophageal echo has been shown to be beneficial [135,136].

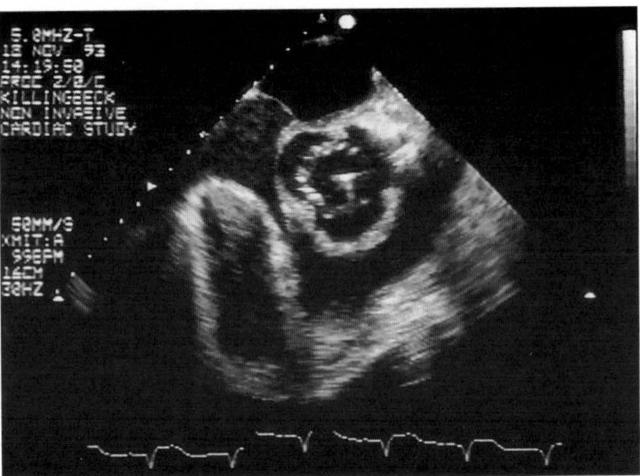

(a)

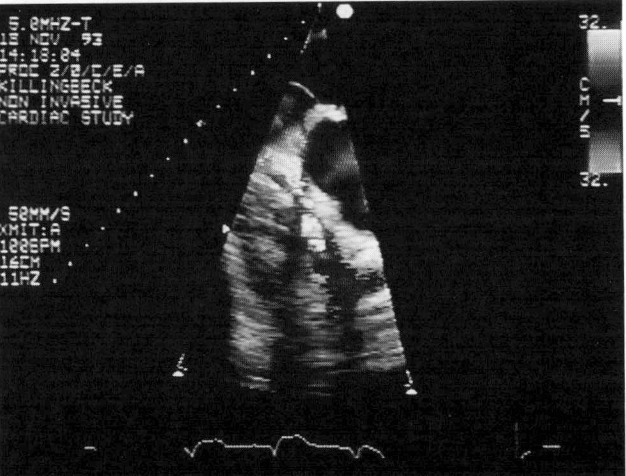

(b)

Fig. 14.24 (a) Aortic prosthetic valve in short axis with compression of the right heart by a localized postoperative pericardial collection in a patient with clinical signs of pericardial tamponade; (b) colour flow Doppler shows turbulent high velocity flow here confirming limitation of flow through the right heart. For colour, see Plate 14.24 (between pp. 308 and 309).

Intraoperative transoesophageal echocardiography

There are two broad indications for intraoperative transoesophageal echo, guidance of cardiac interventions and monitoring of left ventricular function. A less frequent indication is the detection of arterial air embolization during neurosurgery. Most often described is the utility of transoesophageal echo in guiding mitral valve repair [137]. A scan at the time of induction of anaesthesia will clarify the aetiology of regurgitation and suggest to the surgeon if a repair is possible. Once a repair has been attempted and the heart rewarmed then a further scan will show the degree of residual regurgitation (Fig. 14.26). It

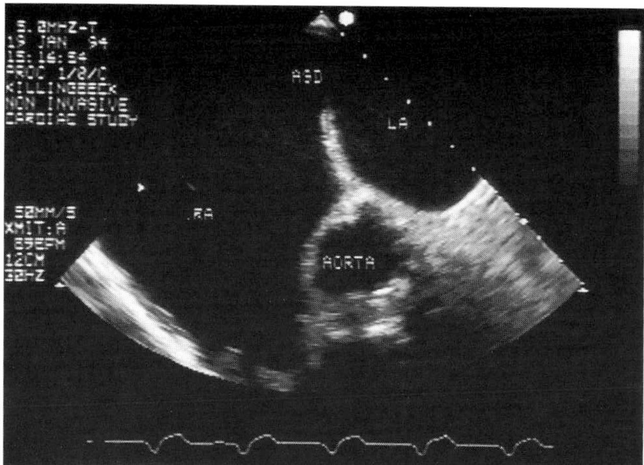

Fig. 14.25 Large secundum atrial secundum defect.

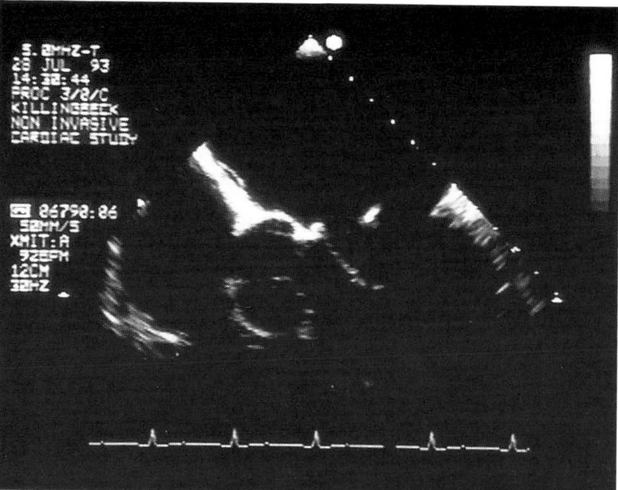
(a)

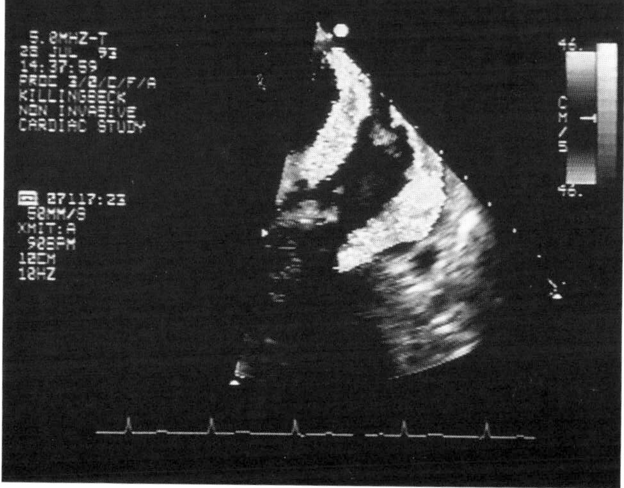
(b)

Fig. 14.26 (a) Following a mitral valve repair the flexible Duran ring has become separated from the mitral annulus at the base of the posterior mitral leaflet resulting in two significant regurgitant jets as seen with colour flow Doppler (b). For colour, see Plate 14.26 (between pp. 308 and 309).

has, however, been suggested that there are pitfalls in using transoesophageal echo in this situation. These include technical problems in imaging from the oesophagus during thoracotomy and variations in the apparent degree of residual regurgitation secondary to changes in left ventricular function in the postcardiac bypass period [138].

Transoesophageal echo has been used widely to monitor left ventricular function in a number of situations including during cardiac and non-cardiac surgery, during catheter laboratory interventions or during pharmacological stress or atrial pacing [139–145]. The method most frequently employed to estimate left ventricular function with transoesophageal echo has been to look at the short axis view from the transgastric position at papillary muscle level. Either areas of regional wall motion dysfunction can be searched for or percentage change in cross-sectional area between diastole and systole can be measured. If left atrial pressure (or pulmonary wedge pressure) is recorded simultaneously then pressure–area loops can be constructed thus giving a more meaningful estimate of ventricular function. The advent of automated boundary detection has simplified the process of measuring area changes during the cardiac cycle (see Fig. 14.3) [146] although this presently remains a research tool.

Three-dimensional reconstruction

Recently, several centres have described methods of producing three-dimensional (3D) images of cardiac structures using transoesophageal echo [147–149]. These images are produced by computer-generated reconstructions made from multiple views taken from set reference points. Two methods have been used. The first involves a rigid scope being pulled back along the oesophagus whilst serial horizontal plane images are taken. The second involves taking multiple views around a set axis using a multiplane probe with the transducer held in a set position. Echo images are then digitized and the reconstruction carried out at a computer work station. The 3D images can then be interrogated with the option to look at any chosen plane through the heart. The main limitation of these methods is the effect of movement of the heart and echo transducer during the cardiac and respiratory cycle although methods of compensating for this are used. The images produced using these techniques are impressive but currently lack the definition of standard transoesophageal echo. Its potential role in clinical practice is not yet clear.

Limitations of transoesophageal echo

Many of the limitations of transthoracic echo and Doppler, such as the semiquantitative nature of colour flow maps and other modes of Doppler in estimating the severity of valvular incompetence and the subsequent risk of significantly under- or overestimating the severity of leaks, apply to transoesophageal echo. An important additional concern derives from the ease with which an inexperienced operator can produce extremely clear images from the oesophagus. It is possible to be overly confident about one's ability to interpret such images with potentially serious consequences particularly when a surgeon is prepared to act on such evidence alone. Reporting of transoesophageal scans should be carried out by experienced operators only and interpretation of the report made in the context of the full clinical picture.

Conclusion

Transoesophageal echocardiography has been rapidly adopted as an indispensable diagnostic tool in cardiology. It is well tolerated and safe and in a number of situations has replaced more invasive and risky investigations. It has the advantages of portability and economy. It allows posterior cardiac anatomy to be studied in detail and will produce excellent images even in the obese and those with chest disease. To date most experience has been gained with monoplane scopes but latterly the advent of biplane and most recently multiplane scopes has promised an improvement in diagnostic yield particularly when studying the left and right ventricular outflow tracts and these probes are likely to become widely used.

References

1 Frazin, L., Talano, J.V., Stephanides, L., Loeb, H.S., Kopel, L., Gunnar, R.M. (1976) Esophageal echocardiography. *Circulation* **54**, 102–108.

2 Matsumoto, M., Oka, Y., Lin, Y.T., Strom, J., Sonnenblick, E.H., Frater, R.W. (1979) Transesophageal echocardiography; for assessing ventricular performance. *New York State Journal of Medicine* **79**, 19–21.

3 Matsumoto, M., Oka, Y., Strom, J., *et al.* (1980) Application of transesophageal echocardiography to continuous intraoperative monitoring of left ventricular performance. *American Journal of Cardiology* **46**, 95–105.

4 Hisanaga, K., Hisanaga, A., Hibi, N., Nishimura, K., Kambe, T. (1980) High speed rotating scanner for transesophageal cross-sectional echocardiography. *American Journal of Cardiology* **46**, 837–842.

5 Hisanaga, K., Hisanaga, A., Nagata, K., Ichie, Y. (1980) Transesophageal cross-sectional echocardiography. *American Heart Journal* **100**, 605–609.

6 Souquet, J., Hanrath, P., Zitelli, L., Kremer, P., Langenstein, B.A., Schluter M. (1982) Transesophageal phased array for imaging the heart. *Transactions on Biomedical Engineering* **29**, 707–712.

7 Schluter, M., Langenstein, B.A., Hanrath, P., Kremer, P., Bleifeld, W. (1982) Assessment of transesophageal pulsed Doppler echocardiography in the detection of mitral regurgitation. *Circulation* **66**, 784–789.

8 Furuya, H., Suzuki, T., Okumura, F., Kishi, Y., Uefuji, T. (1983) Detection of air embolism by transesophageal echocardiography. *Anesthesiology* **58**, 124–129.

9 Scott, P.J., Blackburn, M.E., Wharton, G.A., Wilson, N., Dickinson, D.F., Gibbs, J.L. (1992) Transoesophageal echocardiography in neonates, infants and children: applicability and diagnostic value in everyday practice of a cardiothoracic unit. *British Heart Journal* **68**, 488–492.

10 Pongratz, G., Henneke, K.H., von der Grun, M., Kunkel, B., Bachmann, K. (1993) Risk of endocarditis in transesophageal echocardiography. *American Heart Journal* **125**, 190–193.

11 Shyu, K.G., Hwang, J.J., Lin, S.C., *et al.* (1992) Prospective study of blood culture during transesophageal echocardiography. *American Heart Journal* **124**, 1541–1544.

12 Melendez, L.J., Chan, K.L., Cheung, P.K., Sochowski, R.A., Wong, S., Austin, T.W. (1991) Incidence of bacteremia in transesophageal echocardiography: a prospective study of 140 consecutive patients. *Journal of the American College of Cardiology* **18**, 1650–1654.

13 Daniel, W.G., Pearlman, A.S., Hausmann, D., *et al.* (1993) Initial experience and potential applications of multiplane transesophageal echocardiography. *American Journal of Cardiology* **71**, 358–361.

14 Seward, J.B., Khandheria, B.K., Freeman, W.K., *et al.* (1993) Multiplane transesophageal echocardiography: image orientation, examination technique, anatomic correlations, and clinical applications. *Mayo Clinic Proceedings* **68**, 523–551.

15 Foster, E., Schiller, N.B. (1992) The role of transesophageal echocardiography in critical care: UCSF experience. *Journal of the American Society of Echocardiography* **5**, 368–374.

16 Pearson, A.C., Castello, R., Labovitz, A.J. (1990) Safety and utility of transesophageal echocardiography in the critically ill patient. *American Heart Journal* **119**, 1083–1089.

17 Daniel, W.G., Erbel, R., Kasper, W., *et al.* (1991) Safety of transesophageal echocardiography. A multicenter survey of 10 419 examinations. *Circulation* **83**, 817–821.

18 Aschenberg, W., Schluter, M., Kremer, P., Schroder, E., Siglow, V., Bleifeld, W. (1986) Transesophageal two-dimensional echocardiography for the detection of left atrial appendage thrombus. *Journal of the American College of Cardiology* **7**, 163–166.

19 Thomas, M.R., Monaghan, M.J., Smyth, D.W., Metcalfe, J.M., Jewitt, D.E. (1992) Comparative value of transthoracic and transoesophageal echocardiography before balloon dilatation of the mitral valve. *British Heart Journal* **68**, 493–497.

20 Manning, W.J., Reis, G.J., Douglas, P.S. (1992) Use of transoesophageal echocardiography to detect left atrial thrombi before percutaneous balloon dilatation of the mitral valve: a prospective study. *British Heart Journal* **67**, 170–173.

21 Rittoo, D., Sutherland, G.R., Currie, P., Starkey, I.R., Shaw, T.R. (1993) The comparative value of transesophageal and transthoracic echocardiography before and after percutaneous mitral balloon valvotomy: a prospective study. *American Heart Journal* **125**, 1094–1105.

22 Vilacosta, I., Iturralde, E., San Roman, J.A., *et al.* (1992)

Transesophageal echocardiographic monitoring of percutaneous mitral balloon valvulotomy. *American Journal of Cardiology* **70**, 1040–1044.

23 Cormier, B., Vahanian, A., Michel, P.L., *et al.* (1991) Transoesophageal echocardiography in the assessment of percutaneous mitral commissurotomy. *European Heart Journal* **12**(suppl. B), 61–65.

24 Kultursay, H., Turkoglu, C., Akin, M., Payzin, S., Soydas, C., Akilli, A. (1992) Mitral balloon valvuloplasty with transesophageal echocardiography without using fluoroscopy. *Catheterization and Cardiovascular Diagnosis* **27**, 317–321.

25 Thomas, M.R., Monaghan, M.J., Metcalfe, J.M., Jewitt, D.E. (1992) Residual atrial septal defects following balloon mitral valvuloplasty using different techniques. A transthoracic and transoesophageal echocardiography study demonstrating an advantage of the Inoue balloon. *European Heart Journal* **13**, 496–502.

26 Castello, R., Fagan, L. Jr, Lenzen, P., Pearson, A.C., Labovitz, A.J. (1991) Comparison of transthoracic and transesophageal echocardiography for assessment of left-sided valvular regurgitation. *American Journal of Cardiology* **68**, 1677–1680.

27 Castello, R., Lenzen, P., Aguirre, F., Labovitz, A. (1992) Variability in the quantitation of mitral regurgitation by Doppler color flow mapping: comparison of transthoracic and transesophageal studies. *Journal of the American College of Cardiology* **20**, 433–438 (see comments).

28 Castello, R., Lenzen, P., Aguirre, F., Labovitz, A.J. (1992) Quantitation of mitral regurgitation by transesophageal echocardiography with Doppler color flow mapping: correlation with cardiac catheterization. *Journal of the American College of Cardiology* **19**, 1516–1521.

29 Kamp, O., Dijkstra, J.W., Huitink, H., *et al.* (1991) Transesophageal color flow Doppler mapping in the assessment of native mitral valvular regurgitation: comparison with left ventricular angiography. *Journal of the American Society of Echocardiography* **4**, 598–606.

30 Shyu, K.G., Lei, M.H., Hwang, J.J., Lin, S.C., Kuan, P., Lien, W.P. (1992) Morphologic characterization and quantitative assessment of mitral regurgitation with ruptured chordae tendineae by transesophageal echocardiography. *American Journal of Cardiology* **70**, 1152–1156.

31 Sochowski, R.A., Chan, K.L., Ascah, K.J., Bedard, P. (1991) Comparison of accuracy of transesophageal versus transthoracic echocardiography for the detection of mitral valve prolapse with ruptured chordae tendineae (flail mitral leaflet). *American Journal of Cardiology* **67**, 1251–1255.

32 Himelman, R.B., Kusumoto, F., Oken, K., *et al.* (1991) The flail mitral valve: echocardiographic findings by precordial and transesophageal imaging and Doppler color flow mapping. *Journal of the American College of Cardiology* **17**, 272–279.

33 Taams, M.A., Gussenhoven, E.J., Bos, E., *et al.* (1990) Enhanced morphological diagnosis in infective endocarditis by transoesophageal echocardiography. *British Heart Journal* **63**, 109–113.

34 Rohmann, S., Erbel, R., Gorge, G., *et al.* (1992) Clinical relevance of vegetation localization by transoesophageal echocardiography in infective endocarditis. *European Heart Journal* **13**, 446–452.

35 Erbel, R., Rohmann, S., Drexler, M., *et al.* (1988) Improved diagnostic value of echocardiography in patients with infective endocarditis by transoesophageal approach. A prospective study. *European Heart Journal* **9**, 43–53.

36 Klein, A.L., Obarski, T.P., Stewart, W.J., *et al.* (1991) Transesophageal Doppler echocardiography of pulmonary venous flow: a new marker of mitral regurgitation severity. *Journal of the American College of Cardiology* **18**, 518–526.

37 Kamp, O., Huitink, H., van Eenige, M.J., Visser, C.A., Roos, J.P. (1992) Value of pulmonary venous flow characteristics in the assessment of severity of native mitral valve regurgitation: an angiographic correlated study. *Journal of the American Society of Echocardiography* **5**, 239–246.

38 Klein, A.L., Stewart, W.J., Bartlett, J., *et al.* (1992) Effects of mitral regurgitation on pulmonary venous flow and left atrial pressure: an intraoperative transesophageal echocardiographic study. *Journal of the American College of Cardiology* **20**, 1345–1352.

39 Stoddard, M.F., Arce, J., Liddell, N.E., Peters, G., Dillon, S., Kupersmith, J. (1991) Two-dimensional transesophageal echocardiographic determination of aortic valve area in adults with aortic stenosis. *American Heart Journal* **122**, 1415–1422.

40 Hofmann, T., Kasper, W., Meinertz, T., Spillner, G., Schlosser, V., Just, H. (1987) Determination of aortic valve orifice area in aortic valve stenosis by two-dimensional transesophageal echocardiography. *American Journal of Cardiology* **59**, 330–335.

41 Poppele, G., Kruger, W., Langenstein, B., Hanrath, P. (1988) Membranous subvalvular aortic stenosis. Its detection by transthoracic and transesophageal 2D Doppler echocardiography. *Deutsche Medizinische Wochenschrift* **113**, 1224–1228 (in German).

42 Cutrone, F., Coyle, J.P., Novoa, R., Stewart, R., Currie, P.J. (1990) Severe dynamic left ventricular outflow tract obstruction following aortic valve replacement diagnosed by intraoperative echocardiography. *Anesthesiology* **72**, 563–566.

43 Laurent, M., Leborgne, O., Clement, C., *et al.* (1991) Systolic intra-cavitary gradients following aortic valve replacement: an echo-Doppler study. *European Heart Journal* **12**, 1098–1106.

44 Daniel, W.G., Mugge, A., Grote, J., *et al.* (1993) Comparison of transthoracic and transesophageal echocardiography for detection of abnormalities of prosthetic and bioprosthetic valves in the mitral and aortic positions. *American Journal of Cardiology* **71**, 210–215.

45 Herrera, C.J., Chaudhry, F.A., DeFrino, P.F., *et al.* (1992) Value and limitations of transesophageal echocardiography in evaluating prosthetic or bioprosthetic valve dysfunction. *American Journal of Cardiology* **69**, 697–699.

46 Karalis, D.G., Chandrasekaran, K., Ross, J.J. Jr, *et al.* (1992) Single-plane transesophageal echocardiography for assessing function of mechanical or bioprosthetic valves in the aortic valve position. *American Journal of Cardiology* **69**, 1310–1315.

47 Alam, M., Serwin, J.B., Rosman, H.S., Polanco, G.A., Sun, I., Silverman, N.A. (1991) Transesophageal echocardiographic features of normal and dysfunctioning bioprosthetic valves. *American Heart Journal* **121**, 1149–1155.

48 Khandheria, B.K., Seward, J.B., Oh, J.K., *et al.* (1991) Value and limitations of transesophageal echocardiography in assessment of mitral valve prostheses. *Circulation* **83**, 1956–1968.

49 Alam, M., Rosman, H.S., Polanco, G.A., Sheth, M., Garcia, R., Serwin, J.B. (1991) Transesophageal echocardiographic features of stenotic bioprosthetic valves in the mitral and tricuspid valve positions. *American Journal of Cardiology* **68**, 689–690.

50 Pedersen, W.R., Walker, M., Olson, J.D., *et al.* (1991) Value of transesophageal echocardiography as an adjunct to transthoracic echocardiography in evaluation of native and prosthetic valve endocarditis. *Chest* **100**, 351–356.

51 Scott, P.J., Essop, R., Wharton, G.A., Williams, G.J. (1991) Left atrial clot in patients with mitral prostheses: increased rate of detection after recent systemic embolism. *International Journal of Cardiology* **33**, 141–148.

52 Flachskampf, F.A., O'Shea, J.P., Griffin, B.P., Guerrero, L., Weyman, A.E., Thomas, J.D. (1991) Patterns of normal transvalvular regurgitation in mechanical valve prostheses. *Journal of the American College of Cardiology* **18**, 1493–1498.

53 Alam, M., Serwin, J.B., Rosman, H.S., *et al.* (1990) Transesophageal color flow Doppler and echocardiographic features of normal and regurgitant St Jude Medical prostheses in the mitral valve position. *American Journal of Cardiology* **66**, 871–873.

54 De Simone, R., Haberbosch, W., Iarussi, D., Iacono, A. (1990) Transesophageal echocardiography for the diagnosis of thoracic aorta aneurysms and dissections. *Cardiologia* **35**, 387–390.

55 Adachi, H., Kyo, S., Takamoto, S., Kimura, S., Yokote, Y., Omoto, R. (1990) Early diagnosis and surgical intervention of acute aortic dissection by transesophageal color flow mapping. *Circulation* **82**, IV19–IV23.

56 Roudaut, R.P., Marcaggi, X.L., Deville, C., *et al.* (1992) Value of transesophageal echocardiography combined with computed tomography for assessing repaired type A aortic dissection. *American Journal of Cardiology* **70**, 1468–1476.

57 Nienaber, C.A., Spielmann, R.P., von Kodolitsch, Y., *et al.* (1992) Diagnosis of thoracic aortic dissection. Magnetic resonance imaging versus transesophageal echocardiography. *Circulation* **85**, 434–447.

58 Tottle, A.J. Wilde, P., Hartnell, G.G., Wisheart, J.D. (1992) Diagnosis of acute thoracic aortic dissection using combined echocardiography and computed tomography. *Clinical Radiology* **45**, 104–108.

59 Erbel, R., Engberding, R., Daniel, W., Roelandt, J., Visser, C., Rennollet, H. (1989) Echocardiography in diagnosis of aortic dissection. *Lancet* **i**, 457–461.

60 Nienaber, C.A., von Kodolitsch, Y., Nicolas, V., *et al.* (1993) The diagnosis of thoracic aortic dissection by noninvasive imaging procedures. *New England Journal of Medicine* **328**, 1–9.

61 Nienaber, C.A., von Kodolitsch, Y., Siglow, V., *et al.* (1992) Detection of dissection of the thoracic aorta: improved specificity by magnetic resonance tomography in comparison with echocardiography techniques. *Zeitschrift für Kardiologie* **81**, 205–216 (in German).

62 Erbel, R., Borner, N., Steller, D., *et al.* (1987) Detection of aortic dissection by transoesophageal echocardiography. *British Heart Journal* **58**, 45–51.

63 Appelbe, A.F., Walker, P.G., Yeoh, J.K., Bonitatibus, A., Yoganathan, A.P., Martin, R.P. (1993) Clinical significance and origin of artifacts in transesophageal echocardiography of the thoracic aorta. *Journal of the American College of Cardiology* **21**, 754–760.

64 Galvin, I.F., Black, I.W., Lee, C.L., Horton, D.A. (1991) Transesophageal echocardiography in acute aortic transection. *Annals of Thoracic Surgery* **51**, 310–311.

65 Snow, C.C., Appelbe, A.F., Martin, T.D., Martin, R.P. (1992) Diagnosis of aortic transection by transesophageal echocardiography. *Journal of the American Society of Echocardiography* **5**, 100–102.

66 Sparks, M.B., Burchard, K.W., Marrin, C.A., Bean, C.H., Nugent, W.C. Jr, Plehn, J.F. (1991) Transesophageal echocardiography. Preliminary results in patients with traumatic aortic rupture. *Archives of Surgery* **126**, 711–713 (discussion).

67 Kearney, P.A., Smith, D.W., Johnson, S.B., Barker, D.E., Smith, M.D., Sapin, P.M. (1993) Use of transesophageal echocardiography in the evaluation of traumatic aortic injury. *Journal of Trauma* **34**, 696–701 (discussion).

68 Simpson, I.A., de Belder, M.A., Treasure, T., Camm, A.J., Pumphrey, C.W. (1993) Cardiovascular manifestations of Marfan's syndrome: improved evaluation by transoesophageal echocardiography. *British Heart Journal* **69**, 104–108.

69 Nihoyannopoulos, P., Joshi, J., Athanasopoulos, G., Oakley, C.M. (1993) Detection of atherosclerotic lesions in the aorta by transesophageal echocardiography. *American Journal of Cardiology* **71**, 1208–1212.

70 Fazio, G.P., Redberg, R.F., Winslow, T., Schiller, N.B. (1993) Transesophageal echocardiographically detected atherosclerotic aortic plaque is a marker for coronary artery disease. *Journal of the American College of Cardiology* **21**, 144–150.

71 Toyoda, K., Yasaka, M., Nagata, S., Yamaguchi, T. (1992) Aortogenic embolic stroke: a transesophageal echocardiographic approach. *Stroke* **23**, 1056–1061.

72 Horowitz, D.R., Tuhrim, S., Budd, J., Goldman, M.E. (1992) Aortic plaque in patients with brain ischemia: diagnosis by transesophageal echocardiography. *Neurology* **42**, 1602–1604.

73 Karalis, D.G., Chandrasekaran, K., Victor, M.F., Ross, J.J. Jr, Mintz, G.S. (1991) Recognition and embolic potential of intraaortic atherosclerotic debris. *Journal of the American College of Cardiology* **17**, 73–78.

74 Tunick, P.A., Perez, J.L., Kronzon, I. (1991) Protruding atheromas in the thoracic aorta and systemic embolization *Annals of Internal Medicine* **115**, 423–427 (see comments).

75 Katz, E.S., Tunick, P.A., Rusinek, H., Ribakove, G., Spencer, F.C., Kronzon, I. (1992) Protruding aortic atheromas predict stroke in elderly patients undergoing cardiopulmonary bypass: experience with intraoperative transesophageal echocardiography. *Journal of the American College of Cardiology* **20**, 70–77.

76 Reeder, G.S., Khandheria, B.K., Seward, J.B., Tajik, A.J. (1991) Transesophageal echocardiography and cardiac masses *Mayo Clinic Proceedings* **66**, 1101–1109 (see comments).

77 Mugge, A., Daniel, W.G., Haverich, A., Lichtlen, P.R. (1991) Diagnosis of noninfective cardiac mass lesions by two-dimensional echocardiography. Comparison of the transthoracic and transesophageal approaches. *Circulation* **83**, 70–78.

78 Alam, M., Sun, I. (1991) Transesophageal echocardiographic evaluation of left atrial mass lesions. *Journal of the American Society of Echocardiography* **4**, 323–330.

79 Obeid, A.I., Marvasti, M., Parker, F., Rosenberg, J. (1989) Comparison of transthoracic and transesophageal echocardiography in diagnosis of left atrial myxoma. *American Journal of Cardiology* **63**, 1006–1008.

80 Waller, D.A., Scott, P.J., Essop, R., Ettles, D.F., Saunders, N.R., Williams, G.J. (1992) The use of transoesophageal echocardiography for detecting early recurrence of atrial myxoma. *International Journal of Cardiology* **35**, 235–239.

81 Michalis, L.K., Thomas, M.R., Smyth, D.W., Why, H.J., Monaghan, M.J., Jewitt, D.E. (1993) Left atrial spontaneous echo contrast assessed by TEE in patients with either native mitral valve disease or mitral valve replacement. *Journal of the American Society of Echocardiography* **6**, 299–307.

82 de Belder, M.A., Lovat, L.B., Tourikis, L., Leech, G., Camm, A. (1993) Left atrial spontaneous contrast echoes—markers of thromboembolic risk in patients with atrial fibrillation. *European Heart Journal* **14**, 326–335.

83 Chen, Y.T., Kan, M.N., Chen, J.S., *et al.* (1990) Contributing factors to formation of left atrial spontaneous echo contrast in mitral valvular disease. *Journal of Ultrasound in Medicine* **9**, 151–155.

84 Black, I.W., Chesterman, C.N., Hopkins, A.P., Lee, L.C., Chong, B.H., Walsh, W.F. (1993) Hematologic correlates of left atrial spontaneous echo contrast and thromboembolism in nonvalvular atrial fibrillation. *Journal of the American College of Cardiology* **21**, 451–457.

85 Black, I.W., Hopkins, A.P., Lee, L.C., Walsh, W.F. (1991) Left atrial spontaneous echo contrast: a clinical and echocardiographic analysis. *Journal of the American College of Cardiology* **18**, 398–404.

86 Movsowitz, C., Movsowitz, H.D., Jacobs, L.E., Meyerowitz, C.B., Podolsky, L.A., Kotler, M.N. (1993) Significant mitral regurgitation is protective against left atrial spontaneous echo contrast and thrombus as assessed by transesophageal echocardiography. *Journal of the American Society of Echocardiography* **6**, 107–114.

87 Vigna, C., de Rito, V., Criconia, G.M., *et al.* (1993) Left atrial thrombus and spontaneous echo-contrast in nonanticoagulated mitral stenosis. A transesophageal echocardiographic study. *Chest* **103**, 348–352 (see comments).

88 Pearson, A.C., Labovitz, A.J., Tatineni, S., Gomez, C.R. (1991) Superiority of transesophageal echocardiography in detecting cardiac source of embolism in patients with cerebral ischemia of uncertain etiology. *Journal of the American College of Cardiology* **17**, 66–72.

89 Cujec, B., Polasek, P., Voll, C., Shuaib, A. (1991) Transesophageal echocardiography in the detection of potential cardiac source of embolism in stroke patients. *Stroke* **22**, 727–733.

90 Lee, R.J., Bartzokis, T., Yeoh, T.K., Grogin, H.R., Choi, D., Schnittger, I. (1991) Enhanced detection of intracardiac sources of cerebral emboli by transesophageal echocardiography. *Stroke* **22**, 734–739.

91 Black, I.W., Hopkins, A. P. Lee, L.C. Jacobson, B.M., Walsh, W.F. (1991) Role of transoesophageal echocardiography in evaluation of cardiogenic embolism. *British Heart Journal* **66**, 302–307.

92 de Belder, M.A., Lovat, L.B., Tourikis, L., Leech, G., Camm, A.J. (1992) Limitations of transoesophageal echocardiography in patients with focal cerebral ischaemic events. *British Heart Journal* **67**, 297–303 (see comments).

93 Pop, G., Sutherland, G.R., Koudstaal, P.J., Sit, T.W., de Jong, G., Roelandt, J.R. (1990) Transesophageal echocardiography in the detection of intracardiac embolic sources in patients with transient ischemic attacks. *Stroke* **21**, 560–565.

94 Chen, C., Koschyk, D., Hamm, C., Sievers, B., Kupper, W., Bleifeld, W. (1993) Usefulness of transesophageal echocardiography in identifying small left ventricular apical thrombus. *Journal of the American College of Cardiology* **21**, 208–215.

95 Nelson, C.W., Snow, F.R., Barnett, M., McRoy, L., Wechsler, A.S., Nixon, J.V. (1991) Impending paradoxical embolism: echocardiographic diagnosis of an intracardiac thrombus crossing a patent foramen ovale. *American Heart Journal* **122**, 859–862.

96 Hausmann, D., Mugge, A., Becht, I., Daniel, W.G. (1992) Diagnosis of patent foramen ovale by transesophageal echocardiography and association with cerebral and peripheral embolic events. *American Journal of Cardiology* **70**, 668–672.

97 Stollberger, C., Slany, J., Schuster, I., Leitner, H., Winkler, W.B., Karnik, R. (1993) The prevalence of deep venous thrombosis in patients with suspected paradoxical embolism. *Annals of Internal Medicine* **119**, 461–465.

98 Van camp, G., Schulze, D., Cosyns, B., Vandenbossche, JL. (1993) Relation between patent foramen ovale and unexplained stroke. *American Journal of Cardiology* **71**, 596–598.

99 Schneider, B., Hofmann, T., Meinertz, T., Hanrath, P. (1992) Diagnostic value of transesophageal echocardiography in atrial septal aneurysm. *International Journal of Cardiac Imaging* **8**, 143–152.

100 Schneider, B., Hanrath, P., Vogel, P., Meinertz, T. (1990) Improved morphologic characterization of atrial septal aneurysm by transesophageal echocardiography: relation to cerebrovascular events. *Journal of the American College of Cardiology* **16**, 1000–1009.

101 Memmola, C., Iliceto, S., Rizzon, P. (1993) Detection of proximal stenosis of left coronary artery by digital transesophageal echocardiography: feasibility, sensitivity, and specificity. *Journal of the American Society of Echocardiography* **6**, 149–157.

102 Yoshida, K., Yoshikawa, J., Hozumi, T., *et al.* (1990) Detection of left main coronary artery stenosis by transesophageal color Doppler and two-dimensional echocardiography. *Circulation* **81**, 1271–1276.

103 Taams, M.A., Gussenhoven, E.J., Cornel, J.H., *et al.* (1988) Detection of left coronary artery stenosis by transoesophageal echocardiography. *European Heart Journal* **9**, 1162–1166.

104 Reichert, S.L., Visser, C.A., Koolen, J.J., *et al.* (1990) Transesophageal examination of the left coronary artery with a 7.5 MHz annular array two-dimensional color flow Doppler transducer. *Journal of the American Society of Echocardiography* **3**, 118–124.

105 Iliceto, S., Marangelli, V., Memmola, C., Rizzon, P. (1991) Transesophageal Doppler echocardiography evaluation of coronary blood flow velocity in baseline conditions and during dipyridamole-induced coronary vasodilation *Circulation* **83**, 61–69 (see comments).

106 Alam, M., Brymer, J., Smith, S. (1993) Transesophageal echocardiographic diagnosis of anomalous left coronary artery from the right aortic sinus. *Chest* **103**, 1617–1618.

107 Salloum, J.A., Thomas, D., Evans, J. (1991) Transoesophageal echocardiography in diagnosis of aberrant coronary artery. *International Journal of Cardiology* **32**, 106–108.

108 Daliento, L., Fasoli, G., Mazzucco, A. (1993) Anomalous origin of the left coronary artery from the anterior aortic sinus: role of echocardiography. *International Journal of Cardiology* **38**, 89–91.

109 Henson, K.D., Geiser, E.A., Billett, J., Alexander, J.A., Akins, E.W., Bopitiya, C. (1992) Use of transesophageal

echocardiography to visualize an anomalous right coronary artery arising from the left main coronary artery (single coronary artery). *Clinical Cardiology* **15**, 462–465.

110 Sunaga, Y., Taniichi, Y., Okubo, N., *et al.* (1992) Biplane transesophageal echocardiographic study of left coronary artery to right atrium fistula. *American Heart Journal* **123**, 1058–1060.

111 Tsai, L.M., Chen, J.H., Teng, J.K., Fang, C.J., Lin, L.J., Kwan, C.M. (1992) Right coronary artery-to-left ventricle fistula identified by transesophageal echocardiography. *American Heart Journal* **124**, 1106–1109.

112 Samdarshi, T.E., Mahan, E.F., Nanda, N.C., Sanyal, R.S. (1991) Transesophageal echocardiographic assessment of congenital coronary artery to coronary sinus fistulas in adults. *American Journal of Cardiology* **68**, 263–266.

113 Arazoza, E.A., Bowser, M., Obeid, A.I. (1992) Coronary artery fistula: diagnosis by biplane transesophageal echocardiography. *Journal of the American Society of Echocardiography* **5**, 277–280.

114 Rubin, D.A., Zaki, A.M., Zaghlol, S., Abdala, S., Fahmy, A.R., Ziady, G. (1992) Visualization of coronary artery fistula with transesophageal echocardiography. *Journal of the American Society of Echocardiography* **5**, 173–175.

115 Rittoo, D., Sutherland, G.R. (1993) Acute pulmonary artery thromboembolism treated with thrombolysis: diagnostic and monitoring uses of transoesophageal echocardiography. *British Heart Journal* **69**, 457–459.

116 Wittlich, N., Erbel, R., Eichler, A., *et al.* (1992) Detection of central pulmonary artery thromboemboli by transesophageal echocardiography in patients with severe pulmonary embolism. *Journal of the American Society of Echocardiography* **5**, 515–524.

117 Ungerleider, R.M., Greeley, W.J., Kanter, R.J., Kisslo, J.A. (1992) The learning curve for intraoperative echocardiography during congenital heart surgery. *Annals of Thoracic Surgery* **54**, 691–696 (discussion).

118 Sreeram, N., Sutherland, G.R., Geuskens, R., *et al.* (1991) The role of transoesophageal echocardiography in adolescents and adults with congenital heart defects. *European Heart Journal* **12**, 231–240.

119 Lam J., Neirotti, R.A., Nijveld, A., Schuller, J.L., Blom-Muilwijk, C.M. Visser, C.A. (1991) Transesophageal echocardiography in pediatric patients: preliminary results. *Journal of the American Society of Echocardiography* **4**, 43–50.

120 Stumper, O., Kaulitz, R., Elzenga, N.J., *et al.* (1991) The value of transesophageal echocardiography in children with congenital heart disease. *Journal of the American Society of Echocardiography* **4**, 164–176.

121 Ritter, S.B. (1991) Transesophageal real-time echocardiography in infants and children with congenital heart disease. *Journal of the American College of Cardiology* **18**, 569–580.

122 Stumper, O., Vargas-Barron, J., Rijlaarsdam, M., *et al.* (1991) Assessment of anomalous systemic and pulmonary venous connections by transoesophageal echocardiography in infants and children. *British Heart Journal* **66**, 411–418.

123 Tuccillo, B., Stumper, O., Hess, J., *et al.* (1992) Transoesophageal echocardiographic evaluation of atrial morphology in children with congenital heart disease. *European Heart Journal* **13**, 223–231.

124 Stumper, O., Rijlaarsdam, M., Vargas-Barron, J., Romero, A., Hess, J., Sutherland, G.R. (1990) The assessment of juxtaposed atrial appendages by transoesophageal echocardiography. *International Journal of Cardiology* **29**, 365–371.

125 Sreeram, N., Stumper, O.F., Kaulitz, R., Hess, J., Roelandt, J.R., Sutherland, G.R. (1990) Comparative value of transthoracic and transesophageal echocardiography in the assessment of congenital abnormalities of the atrioventricular junction. *Journal of the American College of Cardiology* **16**, 1205–1214.

126 Schwinger, M.E., Gindea, A.J., Freedberg, R.S., Kronzon, I. (1990) The anatomy of the interatrial septum: a transesophageal echocardiographic study. *American Heart Journal* **119**, 1401–1405.

127 Gnanapragasam, J.P., Houston, A.B., Northridge, D.B., Jamieson, M.P., Pollock, J.C. (1991) Transoesophageal echocardiographic assessment of primum, secundum and sinus venosus atrial septal defects. *International Journal of Cardiology* **31**, 167–174.

128 Muhiudeen, I.A., Roberson, D.A., Silverman, N.H., Haas, G., Turley, K., Cahalan, M.K. (1990) Intraoperative echocardiography in infants and children with congenital cardiac shunt lesions: transesophageal versus epicardial echocardiography. *Journal of the American College of Cardiology* **16**, 1687–1695.

129 Roberson, D.A., Muhiudeen, I.A., Silverman, N.H., Turley, K., Haas, G.S., Cahalan, M.K. (1991) Intraoperative transesophageal echocardiography of atrioventricular septal defect. *Journal of the American College of Cardiology* **18**, 537–545.

130 Kronzon, I., Tunick, P.A., Freedberg, R.S., Trehan, N., Rosenzweig, B.P., Schwinger, M.E. (1991) Transesophageal echocardiography is superior to transthoracic echocardiography in the diagnosis of sinus venosus atrial septal defect. *Journal of the American College of Cardiology* **17**, 537–542.

131 Lin, S.L., Ting, C.T., Hsu, T.L., *et al.* (1992) Transesophageal echocardiographic detection of atrial septal defect in adults. *American Journal of Cardiology* **69**, 280–282.

132 Mehta, R.H., Helmcke, F., Nanda, N.C., Hsiung, M., Pacifico, A.D., Hsu, T.L. (1990) Transesophageal Doppler color flow mapping assessment of atrial septal defect. *Journal of the American College of Cardiology* **16**, 1010–1016.

133 Takenaka, K., Sakamoto, T., Shiota, T., Amano, W., Igarashi, T., Sugimoto, T. (1991) Diagnosis of patent ductus arteriosus in adults by biplane transesophageal color Doppler flow mapping. *American Journal of Cardiology* **68**, 691–693.

134 Fyfe, D.A., Kline, C.H., Sade, R.M., Greene, C.A., Gillette, P.C. (1991) The utility of transesophageal echocardiography during and after Fontan operations in small children. *American Heart Journal* **122**, 1403–1415.

135 Tumbarello, R., Sanna, A., Cardu, G., Bande, A., Napoleone, A., Bini, R.M. (1993) Usefulness of transesophageal echocardiography in the pediatric catheterization laboratory. *American Journal of Cardiology* **71**, 1321–1325.

136 Boutin, C., Musewe, N.N., Smallhorn, J.F., Dyck, J.D., Kobayashi, T., Benson, L.N. (1993) Echocardiographic follow-up of atrial septal defect after catheter closure by double-umbrella device. *Circulation* **88**, 621–627.

137 Freeman, W.K., Schaff, H.V., Khandheria, B.K., *et al.* (1992) Intraoperative evaluation of mitral valve regurgitation and repair by transesophageal echocardiography: incidence and significance of systolic anterior motion. *Journal of the American College of Cardiology* **20**, 599–609.

138 Mihaileanu, S., el Asmar, B., Acar, C., *et al.* (1991) Intra-operative transoesophageal echocardiography after mitral repair—specific conditions and pitfalls. *European Heart Journal* **12**(suppl. B), 26–29.

139 Smith, M.D., MacPhail, B., Harrison, M.R., Lenhoff, S.J., DeMaria, A.N. (1992) Value and limitations of transesophageal echocardiography in determination of left ventricular volumes and ejection fraction. *Journal of the American College of Cardiology* **19**, 1213–1222.

140 O'Kelly, B.F., Tubau, J.F., Knight, A.A., London, M.J., Verrier, E.D., Mangano, D.T. (1991) Measurement of left ventricular contractility using transesophageal echocardiography in patients undergoing coronary artery bypass grafting. The Study of Perioperative Ischemia (SPI) Research Group. *American Heart Journal* **122**, 1041–1049.

141 Pavlides, G.S., Hauser, A.M., Dudlets, P.I., Almany, S.L., Grines, C.L., O'Neill, W.W. (1991) Value of transesophageal echocardiography during complex or high-risk coronary interventions in the cardiac catheterization laboratory. *American Journal of Cardiology* **68**, 1452–1457.

142 Cunningham, A.J., Turner, J., Rosenbaum, S., Rafferty, T. (1993) Transoesophageal echocardiographic assessment of haemodynamic function during laparoscopic cholecystectomy. *British Journal of Anaesthesia* **70**, 621–625.

143 Kato, M., Nakashima, Y., Levine, J., Goldiner, P.L., Oka, Y. (1993) Does transesophageal echocardiography improve postoperative outcome in patients undergoing coronary artery bypass surgery? *Journal of Cardiothoracic and Vascular Anesthesia* **7**, 285–289.

144 Chapman, P.D., Doyle, T.P., Troup, P.J., Gross, C.M., Wann, L.S. (1984) Stress echocardiography with transesophageal atrial pacing: preliminary report of a new method for detection of ischemic wall motion abnormalities. *Circulation* **70**, 445–450.

145 Iliceto, S., Sorino, M., D'Ambrosio, G., *et al.* (1985) Detection of coronary artery disease by two-dimensional echocardiography and transesophageal atrial pacing. *Journal of the American College of Cardiology* **5**, 1188–1197.

146 Cahalan, M.K., Ionescu, P., Melton, H.E. Jr, Alder, S., Kee, L.L., Schiller, N.B. (1993) Automated real-time analysis of intraoperative transesophageal echocardiograms. *Anesthesiology* **78**, 477–485.

147 Martin, R.W., Bashein, G. (1989) Measurement of stroke volume with three-dimensional transesophageal ultrasonic scanning: comparison with thermodilution measurement. *Anesthesiology* **70**, 470–476 (see comments).

148 Martin, R.W., Bashein, G., Nessly, M.L., Sheehan, F.H. (1993) Methodology for three-dimensional reconstruction of the left ventricle from transesophageal echocardiograms. *Ultrasound in Medicine and Biology* **19**, 27–38.

149 Kuroda, T., Kinter, T.M., Seward, J.B., Yanagi, H., Greenleaf, J.F. (1991) Accuracy of three-dimensional volume measurement using biplane transesophageal echocardiographic probe: *in vitro* experiment. *Journal of the American Society of Echocardiography* **4**, 475–484.

Chapter 15: Intravascular echography

C. di Mario, N. Bom, W. Li & A.F.W. van der Steen*

Intravascular ultrasound has the unique advantage of allowing the study of vessel wall morphology and pathology beneath the endothelial surface [1,2]. Although earlier prototypes have been described and tested in the 1970s [3], the major impetus for the development of intracoronary ultrasound into a practical tool was a consequence of the introduction of catheter-based interventions for the treatment of atherosclerotic disease both in coronary and peripheral arteries. In the eagerness to introduce these various new techniques, a hypothetical mechanism was frequently assumed for the effects on atherosclerotic lesions.

An example of an erroneous interpretation of the results of such a procedure is provided by the original 'percutaneous transluminal angioplasty' described by Dotter and Judkins in 1964 [4]. Dotter theorized that the atheromatous plaque obstructing the lumen of an artery would be compressed by the coaxial catheter, much as fresh snow is compressed by footsteps. This theory was still held in 1978 when Grüntzig [5] introduced the balloon catheter that subsequently became accepted worldwide. The method certainly worked and a scientific explanation was not deemed necessary until it became evident that the positive initial results were often followed by restenosis months later [6]. As stated above intravascular ultrasound has the unique capability to characterize arterial wall structure in cross-sectional images [7]. When applied before and after catheter interventional procedures these images provide useful information, not only to the catheter procedure, but also on the pathophysiological changes occurring in the vessel wall as a result of intervention. These changes can be recorded and measured quantitatively by computer contour analysis as, for instance, described by Li *et al.* [8]. Qualitative information, such as exact localization and extent of plaque rupture and vessel wall dissection, may prove useful to better define criteria for the effectiveness and completeness of these catheter interventions [9].

Technique

Two approaches are currently applied to obtain cross-sectional images of the vessel wall. One approach is based on crystals mounted around the tip of a catheter and used in sequence, one by one or in subgroups, to scan around the circumference (multi-element electronic system) (Fig. 15.1a) while the other is based on mechanical rotation of a single crystal or a mirror (single element mechanical system) (Fig. 15.1b,c). Advantages and disadvantages can be summarized as follows.

Single element mechanical systems

Mechanical rotation of the ultrasound element permits a circumferential scan of the vessel wall perpendicular to the long axis of the catheter. Rotating an acoustic reflector in front of a fixed transducer is an alternative approach. In both cases the rotational force is provided by means of a long, flexible driving shaft through the catheter. The principle is simple but realizing a driving mechanism while keeping the catheter fully flexible and steerable as well as its miniaturization are challenging problems. Distortion of the image because of an unequal rotation of the element/mirror at the catheter tip is a limitation of these systems. The advantages of the mechanical probes are imaging with high resolution and absence of near-field artefact.

Multi-element electronic systems

Sixty-four transducer elements are mounted around the circumference of the tip of the catheter which is as thin as an angioplasty intracoronary catheter. The signal is processed and multiplexed via ultraminiaturized integrated circuits contained in the tip of the catheter. Each transducer element transmits and receives independently. Sensitivity of the individual elements is low, therefore

* In part presented in PhD thesis 'Intracoronary ultrasound' by Carlo di Mario, Rotterdam, October 1993, and in PhD thesis 'Image and signal processing in intravascular ultrasound' by Wenguang Li, June 1997.

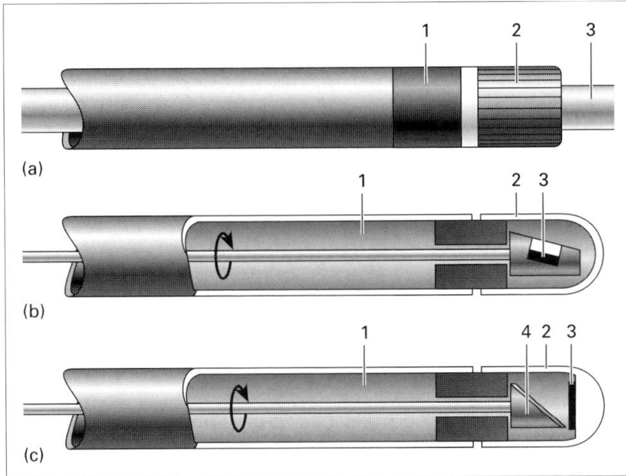

Fig. 15.1 (a) Contemporary array: (1) integrated electronic circuitry; (2) circumferential array with 64 elements; (3) central guide-wire. (b) Rotating element scanner: (1) flexible drive shaft with coaxial cable in catheter lumen connected to proximal motor unit; (2) ultrasonically transparent dome; (3) ultrasound transducer. (c) Rotating mirror scanner: (1) flexible drive shaft; (2) ultrasonically transparent dome; (3) fixed ultrasound transducer; (4) mirror body.

such elements have to be activated many times in order to average the summed signal above the noise level. Nevertheless frame rates are up to 30 frames s^{-1}. Systems that work with subgroups may yield a higher frame rate. An example of this approach was reported as early as in 1972 [10]. Advantages of these systems are: (a) the catheter shaft, containing conductive wires only, is very flexible; (b) a central lumen is available for guide-wire insertion; and (c) no distortion of the image due to inhomogeneous mechanical rotation is present.

Advantages of intravascular ultrasound

Intravascular ultrasound has three major advantages in comparison with angiography for the assessment of wall pathology.

Detection of wall pathology in apparently normal angiographic segments

Glagov *et al.* [11] have shown that coronary arteries undergo a progressive enlargement in relation to increases in plaque area, so that a reduction of lumen area is delayed until the atherosclerotic lesion occupies more than 40% of the area circumscribed by the internal elastic lamina. These findings explain why angiographically normal arterial segments may show an extensive atherosclerotic involvement at autopsy [12], by direct surgical inspection and on intraoperative epicardial high frequency echograms. Intravascular ultrasound has confirmed that significant and atherosclerotic changes may be present in angiographically normal arterial segments (Fig. 15.2) [12–14]. Furthermore, intravascular ultrasound can facilitate the assessment of the severity of intermediate lesions or of lesions not clearly visualized with angiography (ostial lesions, proximal lesions not clearly visualized in multiple projections with angiography). More recently, intravascular ultrasound has shown that negative remodelling of the artery may occur in peripheral and coronary atherosclerosis [15] and that arterial shrinkage is the main determinant of luminal narrowing in restenosis after angioplasty.

Detection of plaque eccentricity

An accurate assessment of lumen eccentricity with angiography requires an angiogram perpendicular to the maximal plaque thickness. Angiography determines the eccentricity of a stenosis comparing the proximal and distal segments of the vessel, assumed as 'normal' reference segments so that a misinterpretation is possible if the eccentric plaque also involves the reference segments. All the limitations here are caused by the fact that only the contrast-filled lumen is visualized in the image, and not the plaque itself. Conversely, intravascular ultrasound detects the eccentricity of the lesion from a direct measurement of the maximal and minimal thickness of the plaque so that the eccentricity index calculated with intravascular ultrasound is independent from the characteristics of the contiguous segments or the X-ray projection direction [16].

The advantage of the direct visualization of eccentric plaques is obvious in the guidance of percutaneous recanalization techniques which allow selective removal of atheromatous plaque, avoiding potentially dangerous procedures in areas of thin, normal wall [17].

Study of plaque composition in coronary arteries

Two types of atherosclerotic plaques can be distinguished (Fig. 15.3). 'Hard' plaques are seen as highly echogenic lesions and are likely to be composed of dense fibrous tissue. The additional presence of shadowing and duplicate echoes indicates the presence of calcific deposits. 'Soft' plaques are lesions with low echogenicity and may consist of thrombus, fibromuscular tissue or loose collagen. Occasionally, markedly hypoechoic areas can be identified within the plaque and are suggestive of lipid deposition or intraplaque necrotic degeneration.

Most atherosclerotic lesions are complex plaques with multiple components, thus explaining why most of the stenotic segments undergoing balloon dilation show areas

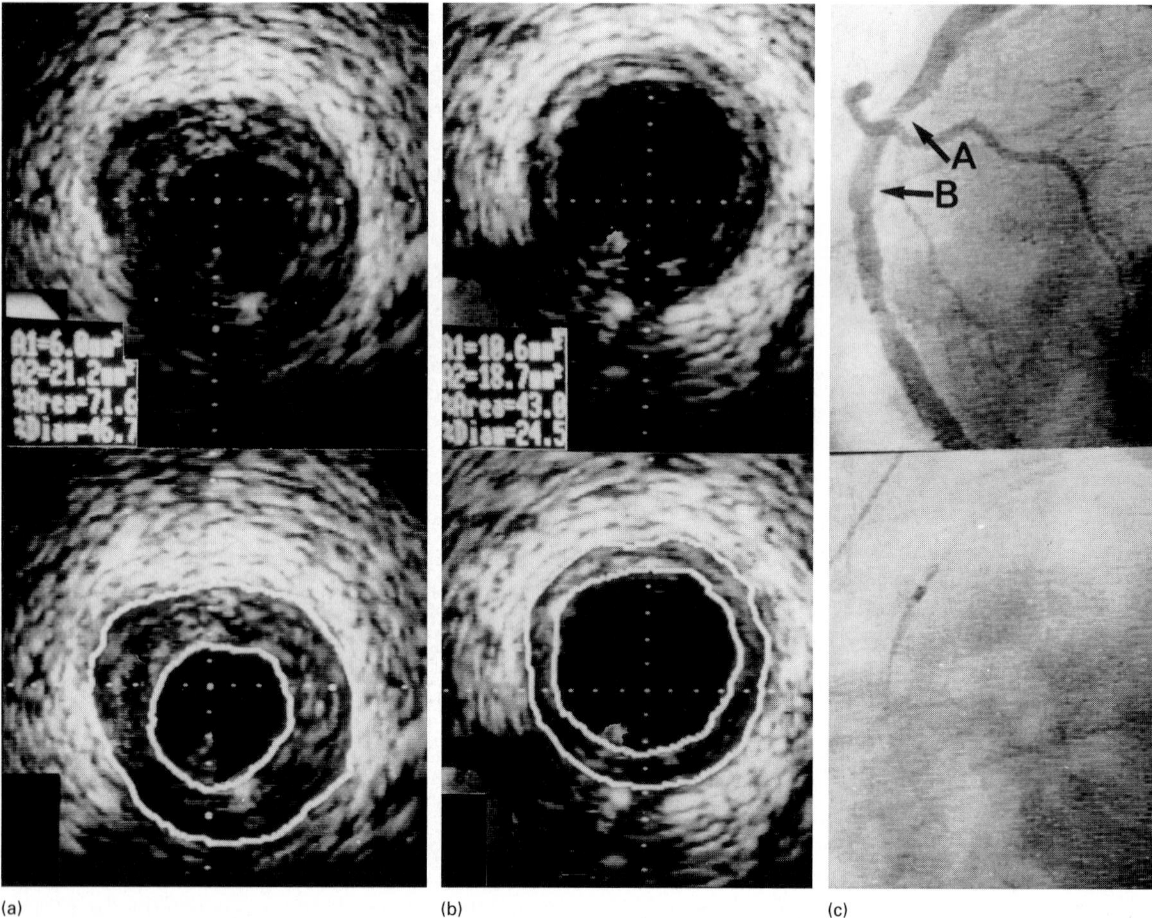

Fig. 15.2 (a) Ultrasonic image showing a large, concentric plaque at the site of a moderate stenosis in a proximal right coronary artery (position A), indicated by an arrow in the corresponding angiogram in (c). (b) Also in position B, apparently normal in the angiographic image, a diffuse intimal thickening induces a 43% cross-sectional area stenosis. (c) Corresponding angiogram (top) and angiographic documentation of the position of the ultrasound crystal (bottom). Calibration 0.5 mm.

of different echographic characteristics within the plaque ('mixed' plaques). Different echogenic characteristics of the culprit lesion have been reported in patients with stable and unstable syndromes. A prevalence of soft plaques with fewer intralesional calcium deposits has been reported by Hodgson *et al.* [18]. In the authors' experience, although echogenically 'soft' material was present in almost all of the 57 unstable lesions studied, the overall echographic characteristics of the plaque were similar in stable and unstable syndromes [19].

All this is offset to the earlier experiences obtained *in vitro* where, for instance, in peripheral arteries a more detailed classification into four echo descriptions seemed possible [20]. Based on the echogenicity of the atherosclerotic lesion, ultrasound could distinguish four basic types of plaque components:

1 hypoechoic—a reflection of a significant deposit of lipid;

2 soft echoes—reflective of fibromuscular tissue (intimal) proliferation as well as lesions that consist of fibromuscular tissue and diffusely dispersed lipid: the atherosclerotic lesion;

3 bright echoes—representative of collagen-rich fibrous tissues;

4 bright echoes with shadowing behind the lesion, representative of calcium.

Of the 54 arteries studied there was no histological evidence of atherosclerosis in four: this was confirmed with intravascular imaging. In seven specimens fibromuscular tissue was the only underlying disorder and on ultrasound it was recognized as soft echoes adjacent to the intimal surface. In the remaining 43 arteries, histology revealed the presence of an atherosclerotic lesion, either restricted to one particular area (in 19 cases) or involving the entire arterial vessel circumference (in 24 cases). Ultrasound examination had correctly assessed the presence

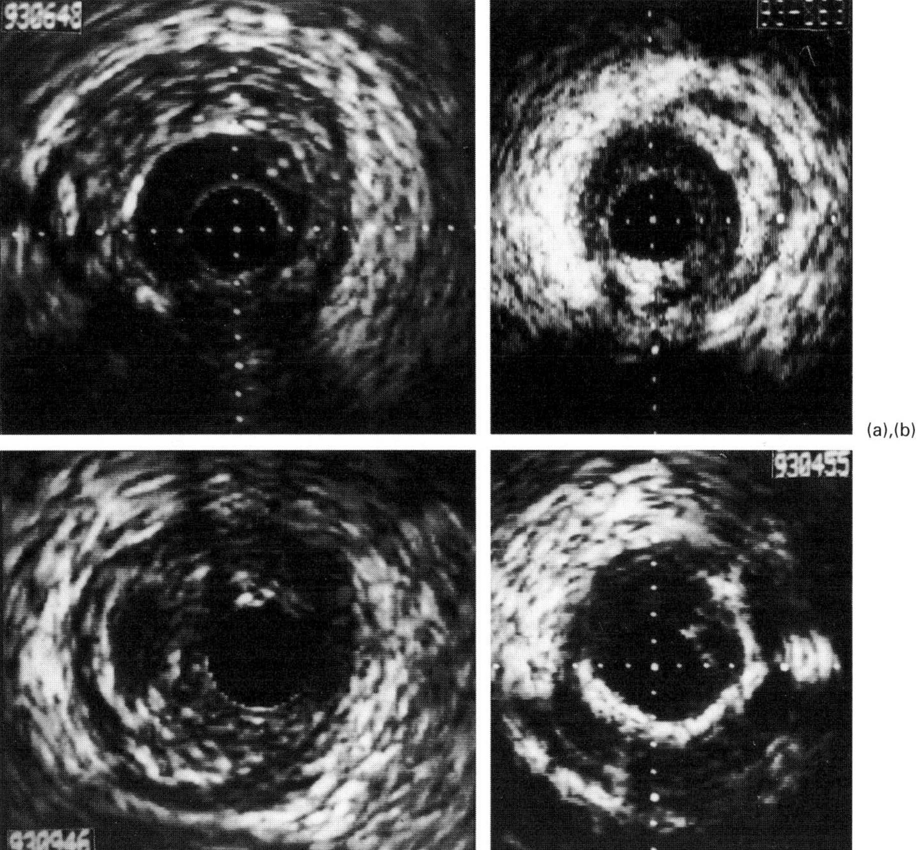

Fig. 15.3 Examples of different echographic characteristics of atherosclerotic plaques in four different patients. (a) Predominantly 'soft' plaque with a small calcification with shadowing at 9 o'clock. (b) Eccentric non-calcific 'hard' plaque. Note that the plaque echogenicity is similar to the echogenicity of the vascular adventitia. (c) Mixed plaque with an inner area of low echogenicity surrounded by a more echogenic structure. The image is suggestive of an area of lipid deposition enclosed in a fibrous cap. (d) Diffuse subendothelial calcification with shadowing and duplicate echoes (napkin ring).

and extent of the lesion involved. By systematically scanning the arteries with ultrasound from proximal to distal, at a 1 mm interval, it was noted that the location and composition of atherosclerotic plaques revealed marked variations.

Obviously also in peripheral vascular disease, knowledge of plaque composition may be helpful in deciding which lesions are more suitable for which specific treatment modality. 'Soft' plaques are more likely to be dilated by compression, stretching and superficial intimal tears. Alternatively, 'hard' or clearly calcific plaques have a higher risk of extensive dissection [21]. The presence of diffuse subendothelial calcification is associated with a lower success rate and higher risk of complications after directional coronary atherectomy, suggesting that alternative techniques such as rotational atherectomy should be used [22].

Most echo aspects so far described are also illustrated for the femoral artery in Fig. 15.4 [23]. Under fluoroscopy a radiopaque ruler is used to mark the position of the ultrasound catheter. Before intervention, a normal arterial segment is seen proximally (at level 24). From level 26 to 32.6 cm a long stenosis is observed. At level 26 the stenosis seen angiographically is 50–90%; with ultrasonography the stenosis is measured to be greater than 90%. At level 32 angiography and ultrasonography classify obstruction as 50–90% stenosis. An aneurysm is seen at level 33. At level 34 the obstruction is classified as less than 50% by both angiography and ultrasonography. Lesions seen at levels 26, 32 and 35 are classified as eccentric soft lesions. After balloon angioplasty, a normal cross-sectional site is seen at level 24 angiographically and on ultrasonography. At level 26 a dissection is seen with both techniques, but the degree of stenosis is discordant: less than 50% on angiography and 50–90% on ultrasonography. The obstruction is related to a large lesion dissected from the arterial wall. At level 32 a similar discordant analysis is found: on angiography less than 50% and on ultrasonography 50–90%. At level 34 an aneurysm is seen. Note the echogenicity of blood inside the aneurysm in the post-interventional photograph compared with other cross-sections in which saline is used to replace blood. At level 35 both angiography and ultrasonography reveal residual stenosis of less than 50%.

Mechanism of coronary interventions and restenosis

The possibility of measuring lumen area and area inside the external elastic lamina before and after coronary inter-

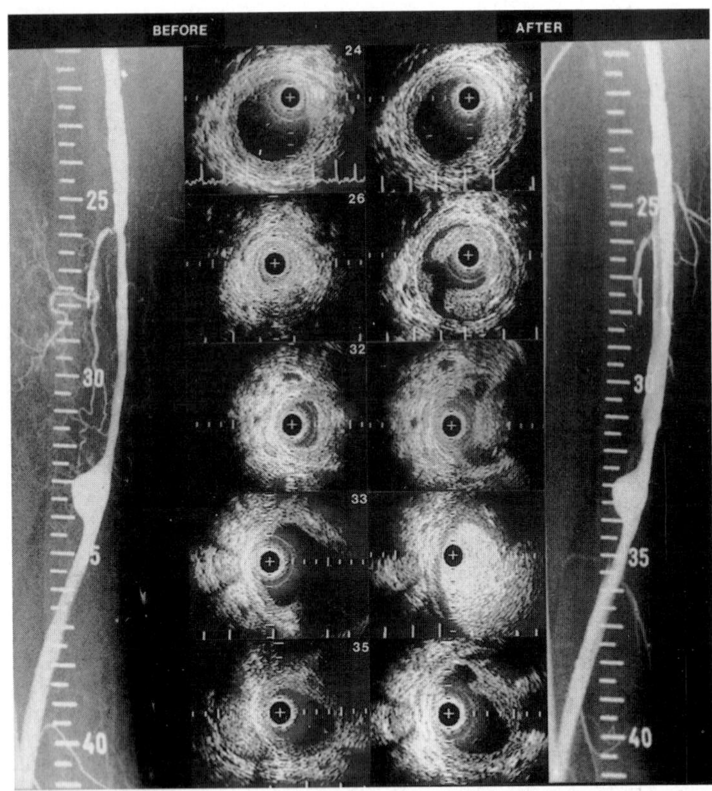

Fig. 15.4 Angiographic and intravascular ultrasonographic cross-sections obtained from superficial femoral artery before and after balloon angioplasty. Plus sign indicates centre of catheter position; calibration 1 mm. (Courtesy of E.J. Gussenhoven [23].)

ventions allows the study of the mechanism of balloon dilatation. Wall stretching with or without wall dissection has been reported as the main operative mechanism of balloon angioplasty in both coronary [24] and peripheral arteries [25]. A significant plaque compression (absolute reduction of plaque area) has been more recently reported [26,27]. The evaluation of a single cross-section, at the site of the minimal luminal cross-sectional area before and after angioplasty, may be insufficient for a complete assessment of the mechanism of balloon dilatation, thus explaining the differences in the results reported in the literature. In 18 coronary stenoses treated with balloon angioplasty and examined with three-dimensional (3D) intracoronary ultrasound, Mintz *et al.* [28] noted the presence of an axial redistribution of the plaque away from the narrowest cross-sectional area, without significant changes in the total plaque volume. Intracoronary ultrasound has shown that gain in luminal area is primarily achieved by plaque removal with directional coronary atherectomy [17,24]. However, the measurement of plaque area before and after directional coronary atherectomy allows the detection of individual cases with an unchanged or almost unchanged plaque area after treatment. These different mechanisms may have a prognostic value in the prediction of the long-term result after atherectomy.

Immediate complications and long-term results can be predicted based on the morphological findings after the interventional procedure [21]. Pathology studies have shown that intimal splits or cracks with localized medial dissection are normal operative mechanisms of balloon angioplasty. Extensive medial tears (>50% of the vessel circumference), however, are at risk of abrupt closure [29,30]. A 'smooth-walled' appearance is the most common angiographic pattern after balloon dilatation (41%), followed by intimal flaps (22%) and intraluminal haziness (17%) [31]. The presence of a dissection flap on angiography is a predictor of abrupt occlusion after angioplasty, resulting in a 6.5-fold increase of major complication in the following 24 h [32]. The identification of patients at high risk, requiring a prophylactic treatment such as the administration of abciximab or stent implantation, however, is not possible based on the angiographic findings. Furthermore, the presence of an angiographically visible dissection immediately after balloon angioplasty is not a predictor of late stenosis [33]. Intravascular ultrasound is more sensitive than angiography in detecting development of dissections following interventional procedures [34–38] and can identify circumferential and longitudinal extension of a dissection postangioplasty [39,40] (Fig. 15.5). An increased risk of abrupt occlusion requiring stent implantation or emergency coronary

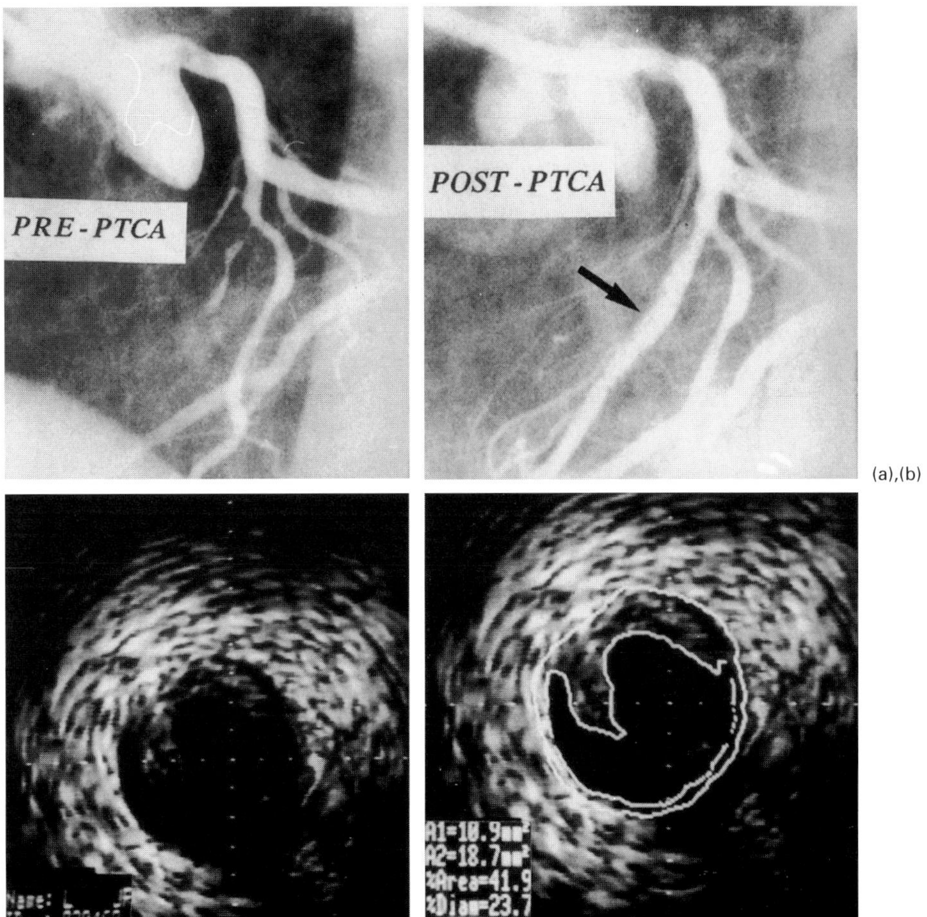

Fig. 15.5 (a) Prepercutaneous transluminal coronary angioplasty (PTCA) and (b) post-PTCA angiographic images with a post-PTCA ultrasonic observation (arrow) (c) showing a dissection of the mid segment of the left anterior descending coronary artery. The linear intraluminal defect visible on angiography is more clearly visualized as a large dissection and quantitatively assessed (d) in the ultrasound image.

bypass graft implantation was observed in the presence of circular dissections [24], major tears being observed four times more commonly in the adverse outcome group. These lesions also showed an increased risk of long-term restenosis (>50%) [41]. At the other extreme, a higher restenosis rate has been reported in the absence of intimal dissection, when only plaque stretching is the mechanism of lumen enlargement [37].

Intravascular ultrasound has confirmed previous observations from *in vitro* models showing that tears tend to occur at the junction between normal wall and plaque or between 'soft' tissue and calcific plates [42]. The qualitative and quantitative information provided by intravascular ultrasound may be used to reconstruct computerized models of the vessel and measure wall stress in order to predict risk and location of wall dissections [43].

Intravascular ultrasound gives a new insight into the causative mechanism of restenosis. Based on the results of serial intravascular ultrasound studies [44] the importance of neointimal hyperplasia in the process of restenosis has to be questioned. The increase in plaque area observed at the stenosis site from the measurements obtained immediately after angioplasty to the measurements obtained at 6 months follow-up, accounted for only 32% of the loss in luminal gain [44]. Furthermore, no significant changes of the echographic characteristics of the plaque were observed from the initial study to the follow-up study. Based on these findings, mechanisms which must be considered as an alternative to or in combination with neointimal hyperplasia are an overestimation of the initial luminal area gain by angiography because of undetected intraluminal flaps (pseudorestenosis), late thrombotic obliteration of dissection planes and a process of chronic recoil.

The metallic struts of current generation stents are poorly visible with fluoroscopy but are highly echogenic and show a clear and characteristic pattern with intravascular ultrasound [45]. An incomplete apposition of the struts to the vessel wall results in an increased risk of thrombosis and can be identified more easily with ultrasound than with angiography. A more frequent situation is the incomplete expansion of the stent due to the rigidity of the stenotic plaque. This suboptimal deployment, especially if the expansion of the stent is asymmetric, is not easily detected by angiography and prevents the normalization of luminal dimensions and restoration of a regular circular cross-sectional area. Ultrasound-guided inflations of short balloons within the stent can be used for the optimization of stent deployment. Intravascular ultrasound can also elucidate the mechanisms of restenosis within the stented segment and distinguish stent compression from neointimal proliferation [46].

Quantitative aspects

With computerized image processing techniques, quantitative information of the arterial cross-sectional dimensions can be obtained from intravascular ultrasound images. Generally, the computer analysis system is equipped with a frame-grabber to digitize the images from a videorecorder. The digital image data are then stored in the computer memory for off-line analysis. A mouse device is typically employed to perform manual contour tracing.

Quantification of lumen and lesion

The arterial lumen and lesion can be derived by tracing two boundaries. The boundary of the free lumen is defined as the leading edge of the blood–tissue interface. The boundary between the intimal plaque and the brighter external adventitia, often better detected because of the presence of an echolucent ring due to the sonolucent muscular media, identifies the area inside the external elastic membrane (EEMA) or original lumen. The areas of the lesion are simply calculated by subtracting the free lumen area from the EEMA. From the luminal contour, the maximum, minimum and mean diameters of the free lumen can be obtained. A photograph of the computer screen is shown in Fig. 15.6.

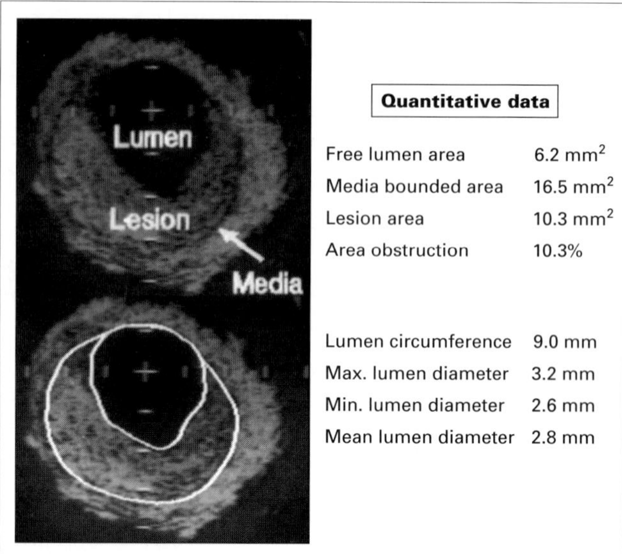

Lumen
Lesion
Media
Quantitative data
Free lumen area 6.2 mm²
Media bounded area 16.5 mm²
Lesion area 10.3 mm²
Area obstruction 10.3%
Lumen circumference 9.0 mm
Max. lumen diameter 3.2 mm
Min. lumen diameter 2.6 mm
Mean lumen diameter 2.8 mm

Fig. 15.6 Example of quantitative data being computed from a single cross-sectional image.

Dynamic analysis of wall contraction

The real-time intravascular ultrasound is capable of providing information about the dynamic contraction of the arterial wall during a cardiac cycle. Its potential clinical application is to study the wall compliance through a sequential measurement of the changes in the luminal dimensions in relation to blood pressure. The changes of the luminal dimensions can be obtained by tracking the wall motion dynamically with a semi-automatic contour detection algorithm. This technique is based on a template-matching method which is optimized using dynamic programming techniques. Figure 15.7 shows the curve of the luminal area as a function of time measured from two cardiac cycles.

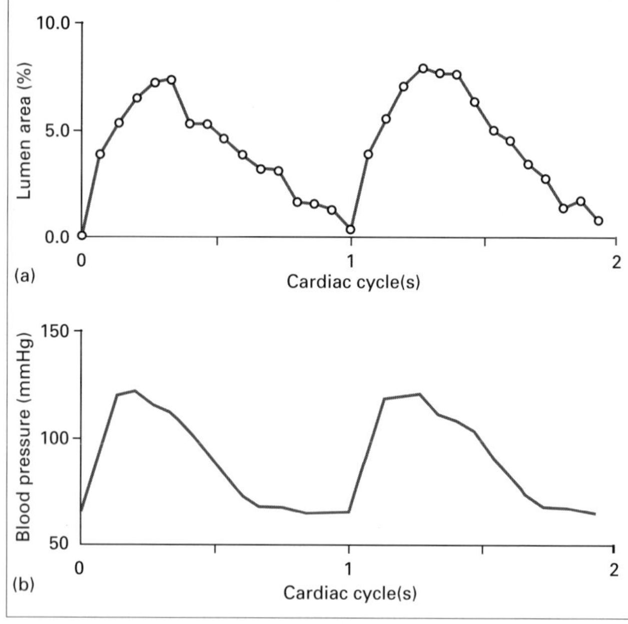

Fig. 15.7 Dimensional change of (a) lumen area and (b) corresponding pressure over two cardiac cycles.

3D reconstruction

By a steady withdrawal of the echo catheter, a sequence of the intravascular ultrasound images can be obtained to provide information along the long axis of the vessel. These longitudinally stacked ultrasonic scans can be used to reconstruct a 3D image of the vessel. Generally, 3D reconstruction from the ultrasound cross-sections comprises two steps, image segmentation and 3D modelling. In the segmentation procedure, the regions of the lumen and lesion are identified for each ultrasound image with semi- or fully automatic contour detection techniques. From the processed image data, the voxel modelling method can be applied to create the arterial objects in a 3D space. To visualize the 3D vessel image, processing is performed to project the arterial objects to the screen with a shading method. Figure 15.8 shows a 'cut-open' 3D display of the reconstructed vessel to visualize the details of the luminal surface and the distribution of the lesion.

Quantitative 3D intravascular ultrasound

Based on the 3D intravascular ultrasound reconstruction, it is possible to obtain plaque volume information in a semi-automatic way over the diseased arterial segment [47]. As indicated in Fig. 15.9, as a first step after the 3D reconstruction, two perpendicular longitudinal cross-sectional planes are selected. In these planes A and B, automatic contour analysis software based on minimum cost algorithm delineates the contours of plaque and media. As a second step (shown in the same figure) these contours correspond with starting points for a similar contour finding program in each transversal cross-sectional plane. In step 3, the contours are created through these points. Thus, for all planes, plaque or lumen area information is available. A practical example is illustrated in Fig. 15.10. From these data, the volumetric information is derived.

Volumetric blood flow measurement

With intravascular ultrasound, usually the video images are the obtained data. Using the radiofrequency (RF) ultrasonic echo signal, on which video information is based, further parameters can be derived. Looking at the temporal characteristics of these signals, the lumen boundary detection is significantly improved. It is well known that echoes from blood appear as varying speckles in the image, whereas wall echoes present a more stable echo appearance.

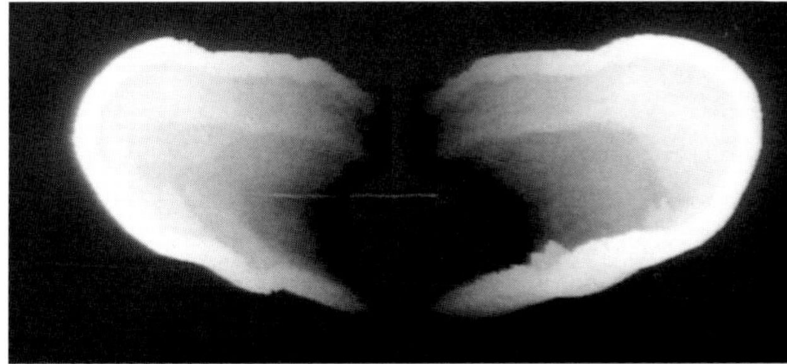

Fig. 15.8 Three-dimensional reconstruction of a vessel by the image segmentation procedure.

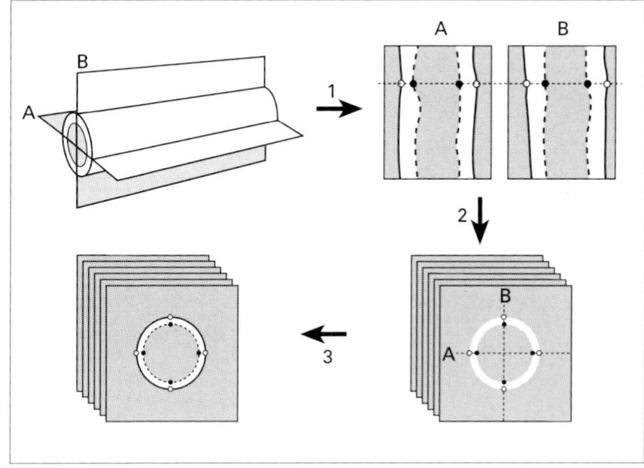

Fig. 15.9 Schematic illustration of the semi-automatic steps based on 3D reconstruction to derive volumetric information on lumen and plaque.

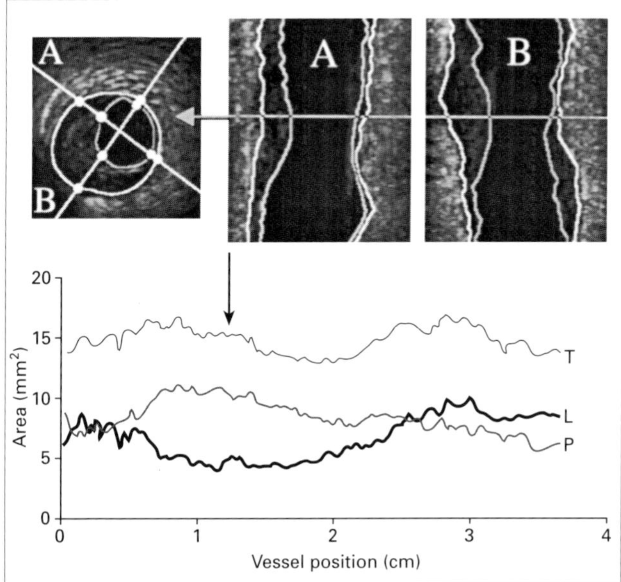

Fig. 15.10 Longitudinal and transverse cross-sectional planes with derived contours and resulting volumetric information. The arrow indicates the corresponding vessel position. Over the 4 cm long vessel segment the lumen (L) = 331 mm^3, the plaque (P) = 244 mm^3, and the total vessel (T) volume was 575 mm^3. The area–length diagram shows lumen, plaque and total vessel area measurements at each ultrasonic cross-section along the 4 cm assessed.

If the data acquisition is changed to the effect that ultrasonic pulses are transmitted twice or three times in the same direction before further rotation to compose of the entire image, it was shown that in the RF data blood could be well separated from wall echoes. With decorrelation techniques also blood velocity at any location in the cross-section could be derived. With non-Doppler techniques it has now become possible to derive blood volume flow from the regular intravascular echo image by integration of all velocity components [47,49]. To derive not only morphological information but also physiological data such as volume flow with the same echo imaging catheter is indeed a step forward. The alternative would have been a separate Doppler catheter or wire to derive velocity. Only with correct assumptions on profile and area measurements with quantitative angiography can a comparable flow be calculated with Doppler:

$$\text{Doppler flow} = V_{\text{mean}} \times \text{Angiographic lumen}_{\text{area}}.$$

Some results are shown in Fig. 15.11.

Limitations

The miniaturization of the currently available ultrasound catheter is still insufficient to allow the preinterventional study of a clinically significant stenosis of distal coronary arteries. Prototype catheter systems smaller than 3F are now under clinical evaluation.

The imaging wire tested in the Columbus Clinic, Milan, is a modification of the driving cable used in the mechanical 2.9F ultrasound catheters of Cvis/Scimed, USA (Micro View). It consists of metallic interwoven wires forming a flexible cable which is attached to a motor unit and rotated at 1800 rev min^{-1}. At the distal end of the cable, a 30 MHz piezoelectric crystal is mounted and connected by electrical cables to the central unit (Insight III, ClearView software, Cvis/Scimed). Although the imaging wire has the diameter of normal guide-wires (0.018 in) and is fairly flexible, its mechanical characteristics are still different from the characteristics of an angioplasty guide-wire. The absence of a floppy steerable distal end precludes its use as a rail to insert other devices inside the coronary arteries, and its insertion must be performed through a protective sheath which could be any catheter compatible with 0.018 in guide-wires.

Preliminary observations in 18 lesions confirmed the feasibility of the use of an ultrasound wire for monitoring of balloon expansion during stent implantation. After high pressure inflation, a moderate reduction of the stent lumen was observed during deflation, compatible with the recoil predicted for the stainless steel tubular stent used. Further improvements of the imaging wire mean it can examine the lesion before intervention to select type, size and length of the device to be used, guide accurate positioning of the device at the stenosis site and monitor the expansion of the balloon during inflation over its entire length.

All the elements of the catheter, including the distal end where the echo transducer is mounted, must be fully flexible in order to allow safe and successful passage through tortuous vessels, especially in intracoronary application. Furthermore, with currently available intravascular ultrasound systems, the image quality is not consistently adequate to allow a complete evaluation of vascular dimensions and morphological changes.

Limited steerability of the intravascular ultrasound

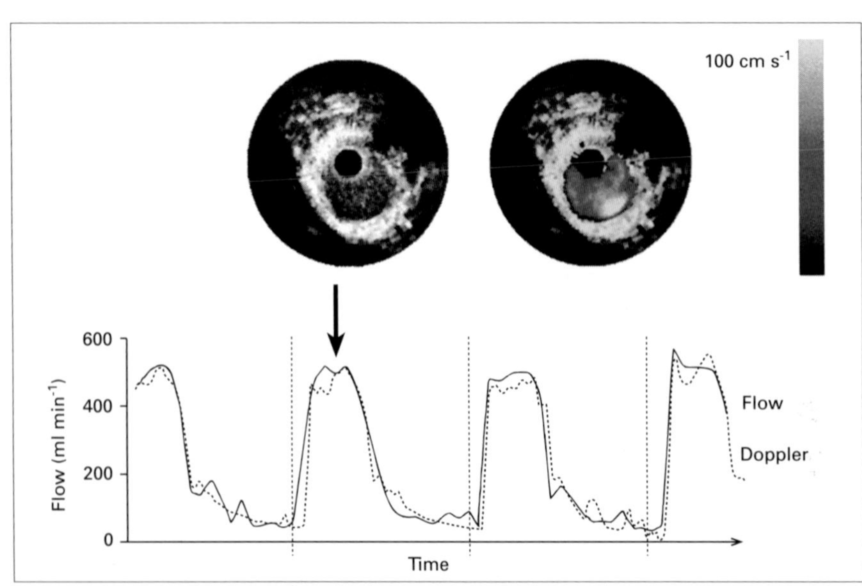

Fig. 15.11 Volume flow (—) in a renal artery obtained with the described RF method and compared to a Doppler measurement (---). The instantaneous velocity is colour-coded. For comparison the regular image is shown. For colour, see Plate 15.11 (between pp. 308 and 309).

catheters precludes correction for non-coaxial or eccentric intravascular position. The perpendicularity of the ultrasound beam to the vascular wall influences the intensity with which the structure is visualized and partial drop-outs occur above a critical angle of incidence [50].

Intravascular ultrasound is an expensive technology. The additional diagnostic and prognostic information during recanalization procedures must be confirmed in large studies to determine the optimal use of the technique.

Future developments

Efforts are being made to combine intravascular imaging with ablation techniques, so that the echographic cross-sectional image can be used for accurate application of the selected atherectomy technique aiming at maximal plaque removal without damage to the underlying vessel wall [51,52].

Forward imaging would make the assessment of vascular diseases more comprehensive and guide the crossing of chronic total occlusions. The implementation of software systems for on-line automatic quantification and 3D reconstruction [53], providing spatial orientation and safe application of ablation devices, is a research goal.

Analysis of the backscatter signals would allow a more accurate and quantitative characterization of plaque components. This could be achieved by spectral backscatter analysis [54–58] or by assessing the elastic properties of the vessel wall [59–63]. Much fundamental research has yet to be carried out in this area.

An improvement in image quality and a further miniaturization and increased flexibility of the ultrasound probes seem to be conflicting objectives with difficult technical solutions. The use of a miniaturized motor unit which can rotate the ultrasonic crystal at high speed avoiding the need for a long flexible drive shaft is an example of the many possible revolutionary technical solutions tested in this rapidly evolving field [64].

References

1 Roelandt, J.R.T.C., Di Mario, C., De Feyter, P.J., *et al.* (1992) Intravascular ultrasound: instrumentation, image interpretation, promises and pitfalls. In: Hanrath, P., Uebis, R., Krebs, W. (eds) *Cardiovascular Imaging by Ultrasound.* Kluwer Academic, Dordrecht, pp. 325–341.

2 Yock, P.G., Linker, D.T. (1990) Intravascular ultrasound. Looking below the surface of vascular disease. *Circulation* **81**, 1715–1718.

3 Bom, N., Lancée, C.T., Rijsterborgh, H., Ten Hoff, H., Roelandt, J.R.T.C. (1993) Intravascular ultrasound. From idea to clinical application. In: Roelandt, J., Gussenhoven, E.J., Bom, N. (eds) *Intravascular Ultrasound.* Kluwer Academic, Dordrecht, pp. 3–13.

4 Dotter, C.T., Judkins, M.P. (1964) Transluminal treatment of atherosclerotical obstruction: description of a new technique and a preliminary report of its application. *Circulation* **30**, 654–670.

5 Grüntzig, A.R. (1978) Transluminal dilatation of coronary artery stenosis. *Lancet* **i**, 263.

6 Castaneda-Zuniga, W.R., Formanek, A., Tadavarthy, M., *et al.* (1980) The mechanism of balloon angioplasty. *Radiology* **135**, 565–571.

7 Gussenhoven, E.J., Essed, C.E., Frietman, P., *et al.* (1989) Intravascular echographic assessment of vessel wall characteristics: a correlation with histology. *International Journal of Cardiac Imaging* **4**, 105–116.

8 Li, W., Gussenhoven, E.J., Zhong, Y., *et al.* (1991) Validation of quantitative analysis of intravascular ultrasound images. *International Journal of Cardiac Imaging* **6**, 247–253.

9 Borst, C., Rienks, R., Mali, W.P.T.M., Van Erven, L. (1989) Laser ablation and the need for intra-arterial imaging. *International Journal of Cardiac Imaging* **4**, 127–133.

10 Bom, N., Lancée, C.T., Van Egmond, F.C. (1972) An ultrasonic intracardiac scanner. *Ultrasonics* **10**, 72–76.

11 Glagov, S., Weisenberg, E., Zarins, C.K., *et al.* (1987) Compensatory enlargement of human atherosclerotic coronary arteries. *New England Journal of Medicine* **316**, 1371–1375.

12 Escaned, J., Haase, J., Di Mario, C., *et al.* (1993) Undetected coronary atheroma during qualitative angiographic analysis demonstrated by intravascular ultrasound and histological morphometry. *European Heart Journal* **14**, 426 (abstract).

13 Hermiller, J.B., Tenaglia, A.N., Kisslo, K.B., Stack, R.S., Davidson, C.J. (1993) *In vivo* validation of compensatory enlargement of atherosclerotic coronary arteries. *American Journal of Cardiology* **71**, 665–668.

14 Erbel, R., Ge, J., Schumann, D., *et al.* (1993) Differentiation of coronary syndromes with intracoronary ultrasound. In: Roelandt, J., Gussenhoven, E.J., Bom, N. (eds) *Intravascular Ultrasound.* Kluwer Academic, Dordrecht, pp. 33–39.

15 Pasterkamp, G. (1995) Diagnostic applications of intravascular ultrasound. PhD thesis, Utrecht.

16 Honye, J., Ashit, J., Tobis, J.M., *et al.* (1991) Atherosclerotic plaque eccentricity; a comparison of angiography and intravascular ultrasound imaging. *Circulation* **64**, II–701 (abstract).

17 Kimura, B.J., Fitzgerald, P.J., Amidon, T.M., Strunk, B.L., Yock, P.G. (1992) Guidance of directional coronary atherectomy by intracoronary ultrasound imaging. *American Heart Journal* **124**, 1385–1389.

18 Hodgson, M.J.B., Reddy, K.G., Suneja, R., Nair, R.N., Lesnefsky, E.J., Sheehan, H.M. (1993) Intracoronary ultrasound imaging: correlation of plaque morphology with angiography, clinical syndrome and procedural results in patients undergoing coronary angioplasty. *Journal of the American College of Cardiology* **21**, 35–44.

19 De Feyter, P.J., Escaned, J., Di Mario, C., *et al.* (1995) Combined intracoronary ultrasound and angioscopic imaging in patients with unstable angina. Target lesion characteristics. *Circulation* **92**, 1408–1413.

20 Gussenhoven, E.J., Essed, C.E., Frietman, P., *et al.* (1989) Intravascular echographic assessment of vessel wall characteristics: a correlation with histology. In: Bom, N., Roelandt, J. (eds) *Intravascular Ultrasound.* Kluwer Academic, Dordrecht, pp. 105–116.

21 Tenaglia, A.N., Buller, C.E., Kisslo, K.B., Phillips, H.R., Stack, R.S. (1992) Intracoronary ultrasound predictors of adverse outcomes

after coronary artery interventions. *Journal of the American College of Cardiology* **20**, 1385–1390.
22 Fitzgerald, P.J., Muhlberger, V.A., Moes, N.Y., *et al.* (1992) Calcium location within plaques as a predictor of atherectomy tissue retrieval: an intravascular ultrasound study. *Circulation* **86**, 516 (abstract).
23 Gerritsen, G.P., Gussenhoven, E.J., The, S.H.K., *et al.* (1993) Intravascular ultrasound before and after intervention: *in vivo* comparison with angiography. *Journal of Vascular Surgery* **18**, 31–40.
24 Tenaglia, A.N., Buller, C.E., Kisslo, K.B., Stack, R.S., Davidson, C.J. (1992) Mechanisms of balloon angioplasty and directional coronary atherectomy as assessed by intracoronary ultrasound. *Journal of the American College of Cardiology* **20**, 685–691.
25 The, S.H.K., Gussenhoven, W.J., Zhong, Y., *et al.* (1992) Effect of balloon angioplasty on femoral artery evaluated with intravascular ultrasound imaging. *Circulation* **86**, 483–493.
26 Losordo, D.W., Rosenfield, K., Pieczek, A., Baker, K., Harding, M., Isner, J.M. (1992) How does angioplasty work? Serial analysis of human iliac arteries using intravascular ultrasound. *Circulation* **86**, 1845–1858.
27 Baptista, J., Di Mario, C., Ozaki, Y., *et al.* (1994) Determinants of lumen and plaque changes after balloon angioplasty. A quantitative ultrasound study. *Journal of the American College of Cardiology* **23**, 414A (abstract).
28 Mintz, G.A., Kovach, J.A., Park, K.S. (1993) Conservation of plaque mass: a volumetric intravascular ultrasound analysis of patients before and after percutaneous transluminal coronary angioplasty. *Journal of the American College of Cardiology* **21**, 484A (abstract).
29 Mintz, G.A., Douek, P., Pichard, A.D., *et al.* (1993) Intravascular ultrasound comparison of *de novo* and restenotic coronary artery lesions. *Journal of the American College of Cardiology* **21**, 118 (abstract).
30 Waller, B.F. (1988) Morphologic correlates of coronary angiographic patterns at the site of percutaneous coronary angioplasty. *Clinical Cardiology* **11**, 817–822.
31 Waller, B.F., Orr, C.M., Pinkerton, C.A., Van Tassel, J., Peters, T., Slack, J.D. (1992) Coronary balloon angioplasty dissection 'the Good, the Bad and the Ugly'. *Journal of the American College of Cardiology* **20**, 701–706.
32 Holmes, D.R. Jr, Vliestra, R.E., Mock, M.B. (1983) Angiographic changes produced by percutaneous transluminal coronary angioplasty. *American Journal of Cardiology* **51**, 676–681.
33 Bredlau, C., Roubin, G.S., Leimgruber, P.P., Douglas, J.S., King, S.B., Gruentzig, A.R. (1985) In-hospital morbidity and mortality in patients undergoing elective coronary angioplasty. *Circulation* **72**, 1044–1052.
34 Hermans, W.R.M., Rensing, B.J., Foley, D.P., *et al.* (1992) Therapeutic dissection after successful coronary balloon angioplasty: no influence on restenosis or on clinical outcome in 693 patients. *Journal of the American College of Cardiology* **20**, 767–780.
35 Yock, P.G., Fitzgerald, P.J., Linker, D.T., *et al.* (1991) Intravascular ultrasound guidance for catheter based coronary interventions. *Journal of the American College of Cardiology* **6**, 39B–45B.
36 Yock, P.G., Fitzgerald, P.J., Sudhir, K. (1993) Intracoronary ultrasound scanning: clinical experience and new insights. In: Roelandt, J., Gussenhoven, E.J., Bom, N. (eds) *Intravascular Ultrasound*. Kluwer Academic, Dordrecht, pp. 17–28.
37 Werner, G.S., Sold, G., Buchwald, A., Wiegand, V. (1991) Intravascular ultrasound imaging of human coronary arteries after percutaneous transluminal angioplasty: morphologic and quantitative assessment. *American Heart Journal* **122**, 212–220.
38 Honye, J., Mahon, D.J., White, C.J., Ramee, S.R., Tobis, J.M. (1992) Morphological effects of coronary balloon angioplasty *in vivo* assessed by intravascular ultrasound imaging. *Circulation* **85**, 1012–1025.
39 Violaris, A.G., Linnemeier, T.J., Campbell, S., *et al.* (1992) Intravascular ultrasound imaging combined with coronary angioplasty. *Lancet* **339**, 1571–1572.
40 Kearney, P., Erbel, R., Ge, J., *et al.* (1993) Mechanisms of angioplasty analysed by coronary ultrasound before and after intervention. *European Heart Journal* **14**, 327.
41 Görge, G., Erbel, R., Gerber, T., *et al.* (1993) Intravascular ultrasound after PTCA and clinical outcome. A 6-month follow-up study. *Abstracts Xth Symposium on Echocardiology*. Erasmus University, Rotterdam, p. 65.
42 Fitzgerald, P.J., Pots, T.A., Yock, P.G. (1992) Contribution of localized calcium deposits to dissection after angioplasty. An observational study using intracoronary ultrasound. *Circulation* **86**, 64–70.
43 Lee, R.T., Loree, H.M., Cheng, G.C., Lieberman, E.H., Jaramillo, N., Schoen, F.J. (1993) Computational structural analysis based on intravascular ultrasound imaging before *in vitro* angioplasty: prediction of plaque fracture locations. *Journal of the American College of Cardiology* **21**, 777–782.
44 Coy, K.M., Park, J.C., Fishbein, M.C., *et al.* (1992) *In vitro* validation of three-dimensional intravascular ultrasound for the evaluation of arterial injury after balloon angioplasty. *Journal of the American College of Cardiology* **20**, 692–700.
45 Slepian, M.J. (1991) Application of intraluminal ultrasound imaging to vascular stenting. *International Journal of Cardiac Imaging* **6**, 285–311.
46 Lasky, W.K., Brady, S.T., Kussmaul, W.G., *et al.* (1993) Intravascular ultrasonic assessment of the results of coronary artery stenting. *American Heart Journal* **125**, 1576–1583.
47 Li, W. (1997) Image and signal processing in intravascular ultrasound. PhD thesis, Rotterdam.
48 Li, W., van der Steen, A.F.W., Lancée, C.T., Honkoop, J., Gussenhoven, E.J., Bom, N. (1996) Temporal correlation of blood scattering signals *in vivo* on radio frequency intravascular ultrasound. *Ultrasound in Medicine and Biology* **22**, 583–590.
49 Li, W., Van der Steen, A.F.W., Lancée, C.T., Céspedes, E.I., Bom, N. (1997) Estimation of local blood velocity and volume flow with intravascular ultrasound. *Ultrasound in Medicine and Biology* **23**, 430–441.
50 Di Mario, C., Madretsma, S., Linker, D., *et al.* (1992) The angle of incidence of the ultrasonic beam: a critical factor for image quality in intravascular ultrasonography. *American Heart Journal* **125**, 442–448.
51 Crowley, R.J., Hamm, M.A., Joshi, S.H., *et al.* (1991) Ultrasound guided therapeutic catheters: recent developments and clinical results. *International Journal of Cardiac Imaging* **6**, 145–156.
52 Aretz, H.T., Gregory, K.W., Martinelli, M.A., *et al.* (1991) Ultrasound guidance of laser atherectomy. *International Journal of Cardiac Imaging* **6**, 231–238.
53 Di Mario, C., Li, W., Linker, D.T., Gussenhoven, E.J., Serruys, P.W., Roelandt, J.R.T.C. (1993) Three-dimensional reconstruction

in intravascular ultrasound. Promises and practical problems. *International Journal of Cardiac Imaging* **18**, 63–67.

54 Wickline, S.A., Miller, J.G., Recchia, D., *et al*. (1994) Beyond intravascular imaging: quantitative ultrasonic tissue characterization of vascular pathology. *IEEE Ultrasonic Symposium* **3**, 1589–1597.

55 Bom, N., Li, W., Van der Steen, A.F.W., *et al*. (1995) Intravascular ultrasound: technical update 1995. In: De Feyter, P.J., Di Mario, C., Serruys, P.W. (eds) *Quantitative Coronary Imaging*. Barjesteh, Meeuwes & Co, Rotterdam, pp. 89–106.

56 Wilson, L.S., Neale, M.L., Talhami, H.E., Appleberg, M. (1994) Preliminary results from attenuation-slope mapping of plaque using intravascular ultrasound. *Ultrasound in Medicine and Biology* **20**, 529–542.

57 Bridal, S.L., Fornès, P., Bruneval, P., Berger, G. (1997) Parametric (integrated backscatter and attenuation) images constructed using backscattered radio frequency signals (25–56 MHz) from human aortae *in vitro*. *Ultrasound in Medicine and Biology* **23**, 215–229.

58 Spencer, T., Ramo, M.P., Salter, D.M., *et al*. (1997) Characterization of atherosclerotic plaque by spectral analysis of intravascular ultrasound: an *in vitro* methodology. *Ultrasound in Medicine and Biology* **23**, 191–203.

59 De Korte, C.L., Céspedes, E.I., Van der Steen, A.F.W., Lancée, C.T. (1997) Intravascular elasticity imaging using ultrasound: feasibility studies in phantoms. *Ultrasound in Medicine and Biology* **23**, 735–746.

60 Céspedes, E.I., de Korte, C.L., van der Steen, A.F.W., von Birgelen, C., Lancée, C.T. (1997) Intravascular elastography: principles and potentials. *Seminars in Interventional Cardiology* **2**, 55–62.

61 Ryan, L.K., Foster, F.S. (1997) Tissue equivalent vessel phantoms for intravascular ultrasound. *Ultrasound in Medicine and Biology* **23**, 261–273.

62 Talhami, H.E., Wilson, L.S., Neale, M.L. (1994) Spectral tissue strain: a new technique for imaging tissue strain using intravascular ultrasound. *Ultrasound in Medicine and Biology* **20**, 759–772.

63 Shapo, B.M., Crowe, J.R., Skovoroda, A.R., Eberle, M.J., Cohn, N.A., O'Donnell, M. (1996) Displacement and strain imaging of coronary arteries with intraluminal ultrasound. *IEEE Symposium on Ultrasonics, Ferroelements, Frequency Control* **43**, 234–246.

64 Lancée, C.T., Bom, N., Van Egmond, F.C., Honkoop, J., Roelandt, J.R.T.C. (1993) A micromotor system for intraluminal ultrasound scanning. *Thoraxcentre Journal* **5**, 8–12.

Part 3
Vascular System

Chapter 16: Carotid imaging and plaque morphology

P.S. Sidhu, J.P. Woodcock, S. Gorman & N. Pugh

Carotid imaging

P.S. SIDHU

History

Cerebrovascular disease, strokes and transient ischaemic attacks (TIAs), are a significant health problem. A completed stroke, rendering the patient permanently disabled, constitutes a major rehabilitation issue involving a wide spectrum of health-care and community workers which therefore implies a vast health-care expense. Prevention of cerebrovascular disease would logically reduce this morbidity and expense, and a reliable, non-invasive, low cost screening method for the assessment of risk factors for stroke, in particular the presence of atheromatous disease of the carotid bifurcation, would be useful.

The concept that transient strokes were due to 'vasospasm' was not discredited until 1948 [1]. In 1954 extracranial artery atheroma was first associated with ischaemic stroke and there was speculation that surgery might be effective in treating the signs and symptoms of extracranial carotid occlusion [2]. The first successful reconstruction of a stenosed carotid artery was later that same year, in a patient with TIAs, and this heralded the development of carotid endarterectomy for extracranial carotid artery disease [3]. By 1985, this operation had become one of the commonest surgical procedures in the USA, estimated at 107000 operations per year. Surgery on the carotid arteries is not without significant risk; serious perioperative complications are estimated at under 4% in units performing the procedure regularly to approximately 10% in other centres without regular experience [4,5]. Long-term results of carotid balloon dilatation and metallic stent insertion using endovascular techniques are as yet unavailable to compare with the results of endarterectomy [6].

Uncertainty about the appropriate management of TIAs and the efficacy of carotid endarterectomy [7,8], led to the institution of two large trials to assess the benefit of surgery and to determine the level of perioperative risk at which the procedure would become acceptable. In 1991 both the European Carotid Surgery Trial (ECST) [9] and North American Symptomatic Carotid Endarterectomy Trial (NASCET) [10] reported their preliminary findings, establishing carotid endarterectomy as a useful procedure which provided the best prophylaxis against stroke in patients with severe disease. Both ECST and NASCET reported the benefits of carotid endarterectomy in symptomatic patients with a greater than 70% diameter reduction of the internal carotid artery (ICA) ipsilateral to the symptomatic hemisphere and symptoms appropriate to that carotid supply territory.

In 1994 the Asymptomatic Carotid Atherosclerosis Study (ACAS) was terminated when interim results reported that over a 5-year follow-up period carotid endarterectomy reduced the risk for ipsilateral stroke by 5.8% in symptom-free patients with 60% or greater ICA diameter reduction when compared with medical treatment alone [11]. An accurate non-invasive assessment of the degree of stenosis therefore assumes great importance.

The first non-invasive studies (oculopneumoplethysmography) detected alterations in vascular beds in and around the orbit, distal to the carotid bifurcation, offering high specificity but no clue to the site of the abnormality [12]. Systems were than developed to use Doppler probes placed directly on the neck to detect obstructing lesions by identifying abnormal flow patterns. Doppler and B-mode ultrasound were first linked as duplex machines in 1974, they allowed the placement of the Doppler sample probe at a specific site in a specific vessel [13]. Colour Doppler now forms an integral part of the examination in most centres and enables flow in the vessel to be assessed rapidly and the spectral information to be obtained at the point of maximum stenosis [14]. These Doppler-derived velocity parameters can than be used to detect and quantify stenoses of the ICA.

Carotid angiography, long considered the 'gold standard' for evaluating a stenosis of the ICA, carries a complication rate of 0.2–4%, with symptomatic patients having a higher risk [15]. Angiography has limitations and is expensive. The most cost-effective method of evaluating

Table 16.1 Indications for a carotid Doppler ultrasound examination

Reversible neurological deficit, a TIA or amaurosis fugax
Permanent neurological deficit or a stroke of unknown aetiology
Known atherosclerotic peripheral vascular disease and coronary artery disease
Patients listed for coronary artery bypass grafting
Hypertension, diabetes mellitus, hyperlipidaemia
Asymptomatic carotid bruit
Postendarterectomy patients

patients with symptoms of carotid TIAs is Doppler ultrasound [16] which eliminates the risks associated with angiography [17].

Indications for carotid Doppler ultrasound

Every patient with risk factors for cerebrovascular disease should undergo a carotid Doppler ultrasound (Table 16.1). More importantly, in any patient suspected of having a TIA, a carotid ultrasound examination is mandatory. This is the primary aim of any non-invasive screening imaging modality, to identify a potentially treatable lesion. It is also wise to subject any patient undergoing coronary artery bypass grafting to a screening ultrasound examination prior to surgery, as the incidence of coexisting carotid atherosclerotic disease in these patients is high [18]. There is potential for a hypoperfusion injury during cardiac bypass in the presence of significant carotid stenosis, and arrangements can be made to do both the carotid endarterectomy and coronary bypass procedure at the same time. The presence of a bruit on clinical examination should warrant an ultrasound examination, as the presence of atheromatous disease at the carotid bifurcation is not insignificant in this group of patients [19].

Normal extracranial anatomy

The normal anatomical configuration of the great vessels of the head and neck, as they arise off the aorta, is for the right common carotid artery (CCA) to arise from the innominate artery and for the left CCA to arise directly from the aortic arch. The right vertebral artery (VA) arises from the proximal right subclavian artery, while the left VA arises from the proximal left subclavian artery (Fig. 16.1). There are numerous variations to the site of the origin of the right and left common carotid arteries, but this has little effect on the Doppler ultrasound examination of the extracranial carotid artery. The site of origin of the vertebral arteries is less varied.

In the majority of patients the CCA is medial to the jugular vein and can be distinguished from the compressible jugular vein, as the CCA is smaller, pulsatile and assumes a more circular configuration (Fig. 16.2). The jugular vein may be used as an acoustic window if only light pressure is applied with the probe during the examination. The CCA divides into the ICA and the external carotid artery (ECA) at the level of the fourth cervical vertebrae, although the level of this division may vary from T2 to C1 [20] (Fig. 16.3). The location of the carotid bulb is a matter of debate; most physicians (but not anatomists) regard the bulb as the area of dilatation proximal to the ICA, after the origin of the ECA [21]. In 80% of patients the ICA lies posterior and lateral to the ECA. The two vessels have a number of distinguishing features to aid in their differentiation, which becomes less of a problem with experience (Table 16.2, Fig. 16.4). The ECA supplies a high resistance area and this is reflected in the spectral waveform, in contrast to the ICA which supplies the brain as an end-organ and displays a low resistance spectral waveform (see Fig. 16.1). The 'temporal tap' may be used to distinguish between the ECA and the ICA, but is not always specific [22] (Fig. 16.5). Several centimetres of both the ICA and ECA may be examined when the bifurcation is at the normal level.

Scanning technique

Carotid artery

The examination is performed with the patient lying comfortably in a supine position, with the neck slightly extended, chin straight ahead, with the ability to turn the head during the course of the examination. It is important to be comfortable as the examination will normally take between 10 and 20 min or even longer with a difficult case. The examiner evaluates the carotid artery by sitting at the level of the patient's shoulders facing the patient, reaching across the patient's chest to examine the left side. An approach anterior to the sternocleidomastoid muscles, using the jugular vein as an acoustic window, is usually adequate, but sometimes an approach posterior to the sternocleidomastoid muscle is necessary. Scanning from above the patient is used by some sonographers, which may be disorientating and needs skill with the use of both hands. Needless to say the examiner must be as comfortable as the patient during the examination [20].

The examination is normally conducted in two parts. Initially, the examination is performed using grey-scale only, as this permits the evaluation of the arterial wall and detects the presence of any plaque disease which may be of very low reflectivity and so be obscured by colour images. The highest possible imaging frequency should

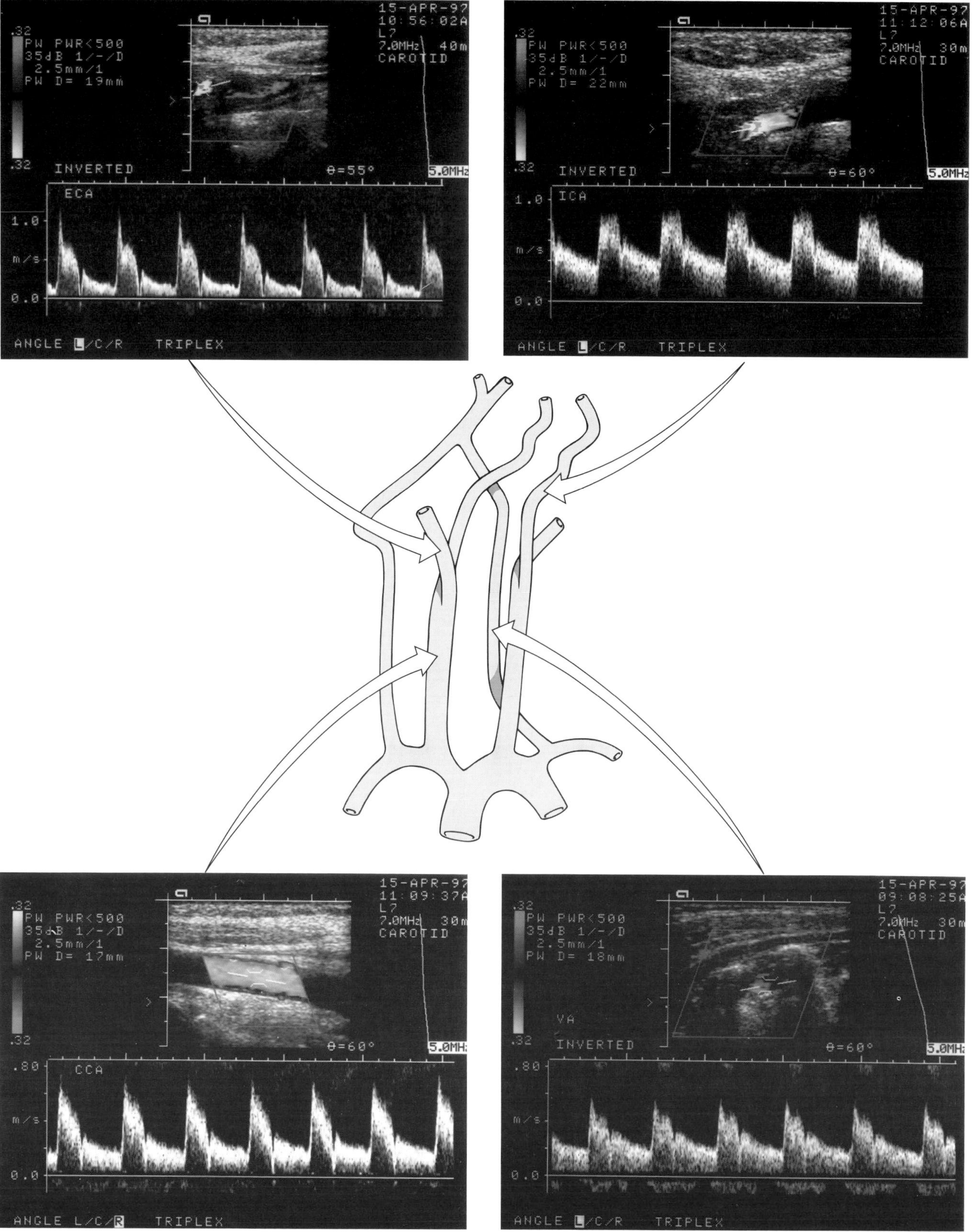

Fig. 16.1 Diagram of the normal anatomy of the extracranial carotid arterial system arising off the aortic arch. The normal spectral Doppler waveform patterns for each artery is indicated. CCA, common carotid artery; ECA, external carotid artery; ICA, internal carotid artery; VA, vertebral artery. For colour, see Plate 16.1 (between pp. 308 and 309).

Table 16.2 Differences between the ECA and the ICA on Doppler ultrasound examination

	ICA	ECA
Location	Posterior/lateral	Anterior/medial
Size	Larger	Smaller
Branches	None	Present
Waveform	Low resistance	High resistance
Temporal tap	Absent	Present

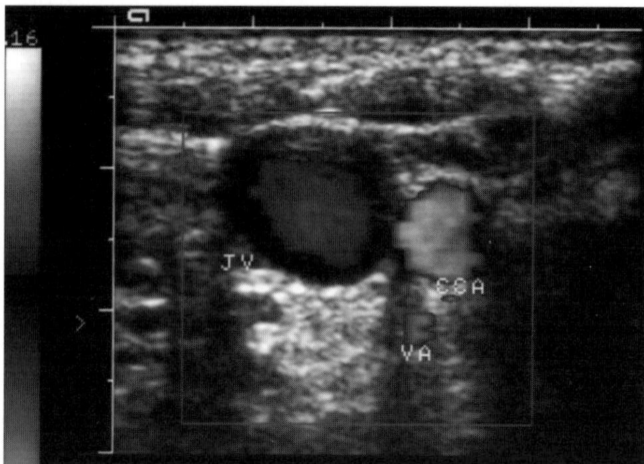

Fig. 16.2 Transverse section through the root of the neck, showing the common carotid artery (CCA), jugular vein (JV) and vertebral artery (VA). For colour, see Plate 16.2 (between pp. 308 and 309).

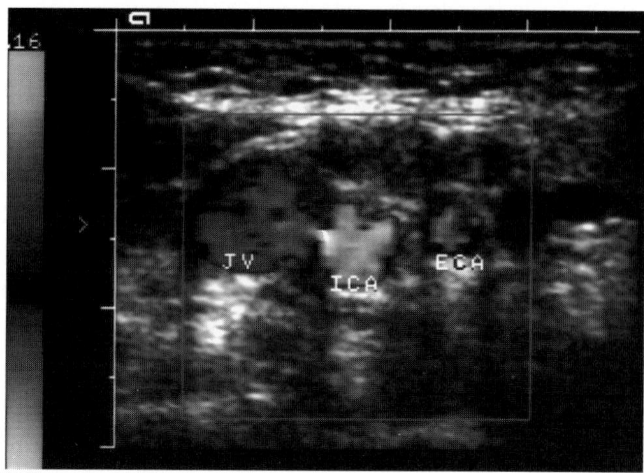

Fig. 16.3 Transverse section at the level of the bifurcation of the CCA into the internal carotid artery (ICA) laterally and the external carotid artery (ECA) medially. JV, jugular vein. For colour, see Plate 16.3 (between pp. 308 and 309).

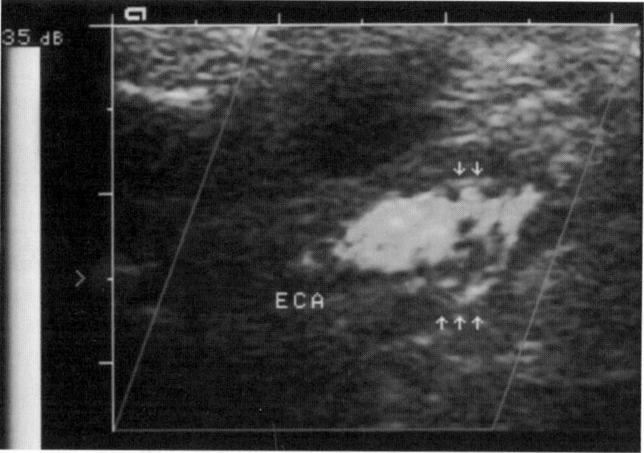

Fig. 16.4 Longitudinal section with 'power' Doppler, through the external carotid artery (ECA), which has branches (arrows) arising from this artery distinguishing it from the ICA. For colour, see Plate 16.4 (between pp. 308 and 309).

be used, usually a 7 MHz linear array probe is ideal, but some of the newer probes image dynamically between 5 and 10 MHz, providing very good resolution of near-field structures. The scan should be first performed in the transverse direction from the root of the neck to the angle of the mandible, to ascertain the level of the bifurcation, the tortuosity of the vessels and the ideal plane to examine the vessels in the longitudinal direction. At this stage a rapid assessment of the presence of flow in the vessels can be made with colour Doppler, angling the probe slightly cephalad to allow the vessel to fill with colour. An occluded vessel will be picked up at this stage allowing the focus of the examination to alter.

It is best to estimate the area reduction of a stenosis of the ICA in the transverse plane with the probe in a perpendicular direction to the vessel wall, without colour Doppler, as colour images will underestimate the degree of vessel narrowing due to the tendency to 'leak' out of the vessel. Not all ICA luminal narrowing will be amenable to assessment in this manner, and a measurement of the velocity of flow in the longitudinal direction is invariably required.

Grey-scale imaging in the longitudinal direction precedes colour Doppler imaging for the same reasons outlined above. The CCA is imaged as far proximally as possible and then followed distally up the neck to the level of the bifurcation. A note is made of the presence, location and type of plaque seen. In most patients it is not possible to examine the ECA, ICA and carotid bulb simultaneously, and therefore each of these vessels are examined in turn. The ECA is identified by the criteria as discussed above. It may be possible to identify the region of maximal narrowing of the ICA on grey-scale images allowing placement of the pulsed Doppler sample volume, but without colour

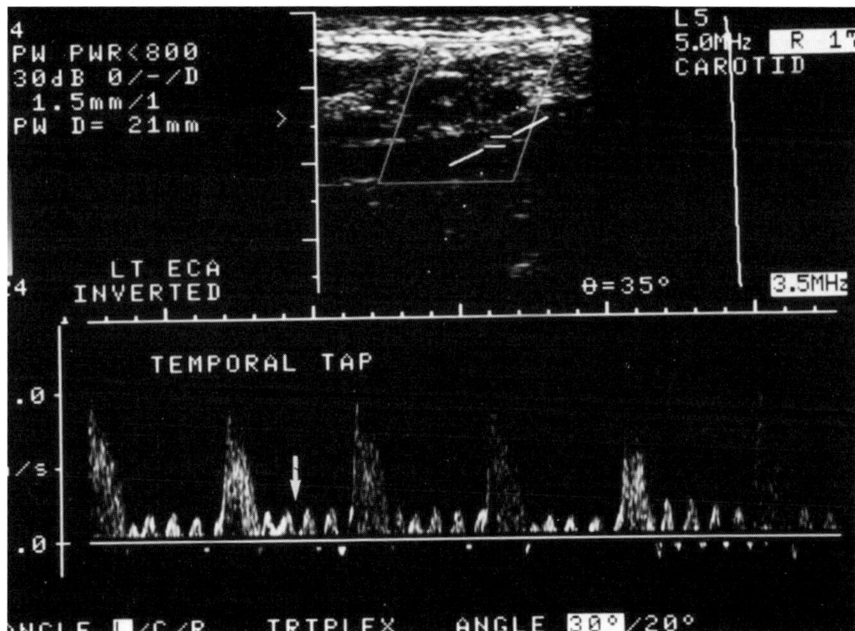

Fig. 16.5 When the area anterior to the ear is tapped by the examiner's finger, the so-called 'temporal tap', a pulsation, is transmitted to the spectral Doppler waveform of the ECA (arrow) and helps to distinguish this artery from the ICA.

Doppler the sample volume must be moved carefully through the entire lumen of the vessel. However, colour Doppler will allow rapid assessment of a stenosis, which manifests as an area of colour turbulence, allowing accurate placement of the pulsed Doppler sample volume and has greatly improved the sensitivity and speed of the examination [23,24].

By normal convention the arterial system is imaged in red and the venous system in blue. Duplex Doppler allows velocity measurements to be taken at the level of the proximal CCA and ICA. The site of greatest colour turbulence indicates the position of greatest narrowing and the pulsed wave Doppler sample volume is placed here to record a spectral waveform from which a velocity measurement can be taken. It is important that the angle of insonnation remains constant (usually between 45 and 60°) when measuring velocities in the ICA and CCA, as small changes in the angle may affect absolute velocity readings and as such give misleading results. Measurements are made of the peak systolic and the end-diastolic velocities in the CCA and ICA in order to calculate the degree of narrowing of the vessel. Spectral broadening represents a wide range of velocities and is an indirect indication of turbulent stenotic flow. It is important to identify and record the spectral waveform in the ECA, so that it is clear that the velocities have been measured in the correct vessels. It is normal to see flow reversal, manifest by colour change from red to blue separated by a thin black line, in the carotid bulb opposite to the origin of the ECA and should not be mistaken for turbulence.

Vertebral artery

By moving the probe laterally beyond the CCA, the vertebral arteries can be identified between the spinous processes of the cervical spine. The VA can normally be examined in three segments: the proximal (pretransverse) portion, the intertransverse portion and the atlas loop [25]. The VA joins with its fellow to form the basilar artery, and then supplies the circle of Willis, and therefore will return a low resistance spectral waveform pattern. The more anteriorly located vertebral vein should also be easily identified on spectral and colour Doppler. Failure to show the VA may be due to absence or occlusion which will not be clear from the ultrasound examination. The VA is absent in 7% of the general population more often on the left and segments of hypoplasia may persist. Very rarely a VA when absent, may be replaced by the primitive trigeminal artery, providing a connection between the ICA and basilar artery. VA calibre may be asymmetrical in up to 25% of normal individuals, the left usually the larger [26].

Normal haemodynamics

The normal spectral waveform patterns of the CCA, ICA, ECA and the VA are shown in Fig. 16.1. The principle that the morphology of the waveform corresponds to the vascular bed supplied, gives rise to the low resistance pattern of the ICA and the VA which directly supply the brain parenchyma and contrasts with the high resistance pattern of the ECA which supplies the facial muscles and scalp. Thus the ICA and VA have a wide systolic peak and high levels of forward diastolic flow, while the ECA has a narrow systolic peak and flow reversal in diastole. The CCA has a narrow systolic peak with more forward diastolic flow than the ECA and flow reversal in diastole may be absent.

Measurement of stenosis

Arteriographic measurements

Although the NASCET and ECST trials confirmed benefits of carotid endarterctomy, the methods employed to assess the degree of narrowing in the ICA have been criticized [21,27]. Arteriography was used to calculate the degree of stenosis and, although it is accepted as the standard against which other methods are usually compared, there are a number of variables which lead to significant intra- and interobserver variation in measurement. In other words arteriography, just like Doppler ultrasound, is operator and interpreter dependent. The NASCET study calculated the degree of stenosis on selective carotid arteriography by a linear measurement of the diameter in the region of greatest narrowing as the numerator and the normal distal ICA lumen as the denominator. ECST assessed the degree of narrowing from linear measurements, on a single angiographic view, with the narrowest point as the numerator and the estimated linear carotid bulb diameter as the denominator. This implies that the outline of the carotid bulb was guessed at. However, the carotid bulb size is variable and on occasion almost insignificantly larger than the distal CCA (Fig. 16.6).

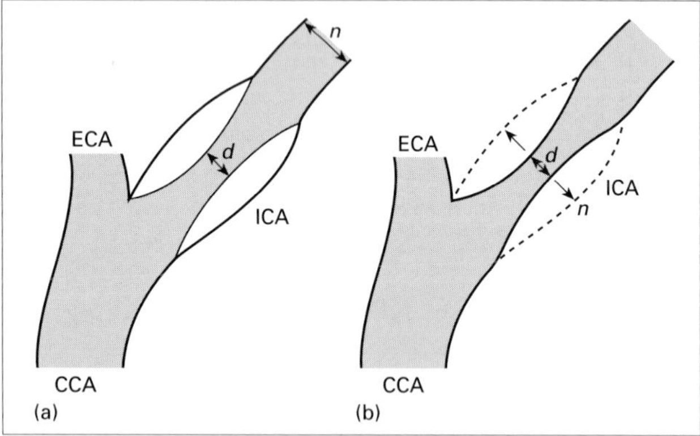

Fig. 16.6 Diagrams showing methods used by (a) the NASCET and (b) the ECST trial for estimating diameter reduction of the internal carotid artery (ICA) on angiography. *d* is the diameter of the residual lumen at angiography and *n* is an estimation of the normal vessel diameter. CCA, common carotid artery; ECA, external carotid artery. (Redrawn from Alexandrov *et al.*, 1993 [27] with permission, © 1993 American Heart Association.)

It is obvious that the results of the trials are not directly comparable. With these two methods, an 80% ECST diameter reduction is equivalent to 50% NASCET diameter reduction, implying a different management strategy, although the lesions are anatomically identical. Therefore the NASCET study conclusions are based on patients with a more stenosed carotid lesion. In a study assessing calculations of stenosis, the reliability of the linear method, the area reduction method, direct visual estimation ('eyeballing') of the angiogram and duplex ultrasound were compared with pathological specimens, and ultrasound was found to be highly accurate [27]. Therefore a calculated 70% diameter reduction on Doppler ultrasound will, with reasonable accuracy, reflect the true *in vivo* lumen narrowing.

Ultrasound measurements and criteria

Measuring the Doppler shift frequency is dependent on the frequency of the probe used and angle of insonation, whereas velocity measurements are calculated from the frequency shift by the Doppler equation and provide a standard criteria that allows comparison of results between different examination techniques and different equipment [28]. However, it should be borne in mind that the accuracy and reproducibility of velocity measurements between different ultrasound equipment may vary, with differences of up to 15% being found when the same stenosis was measured on different machines [29]. Velocity measurements and not Doppler shift frequencies should always be used.

Many velocity measurements have been suggested, including the internal carotid peak systolic velocity (ICPSV) and internal carotid end-diastolic velocity (ICEDV) [30–32]; the common carotid peak systolic velocity (CCPSV) and common carotid end-diastolic velocity (CCEDV) [33]; the ICPSV to CCPSV ratio [34], the ICEDV to CCEDV ratio [35] and the ICPSV to CCEDV ratio [36]. The multicentre study of Bluth *et al.* [35] was the first attempt at standardization of the Doppler criteria for a stenosis, they suggested that the peak systolic and end-diastolic velocity measurements in the ICA were only significant in the 60–90% stenosis range, and advocated that image measurement be used to quantify stenosis below 60% (Fig. 16.7).

In the light of the requirement for accuracy in the 60–70% diameter reduction range, these previous parameters have been reassessed. A retrospective study of 138 carotid bifurcations by Hunink *et al.* addressed this problem by comparing a variety of measurement parameters with the results of angiography [37]. The authors conclude that the single most useful measurement is the ICPSV, which, when greater than a measurement of

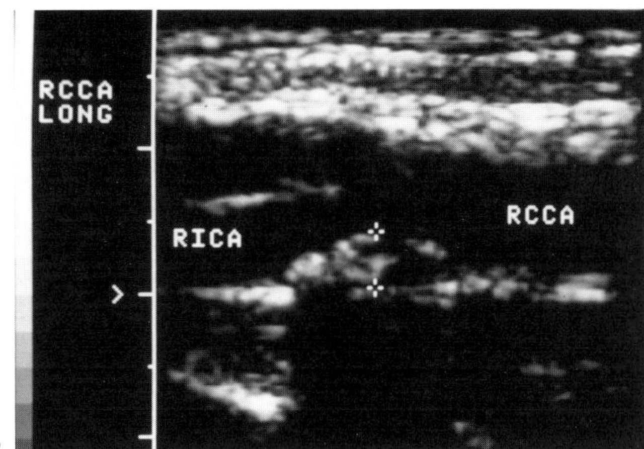

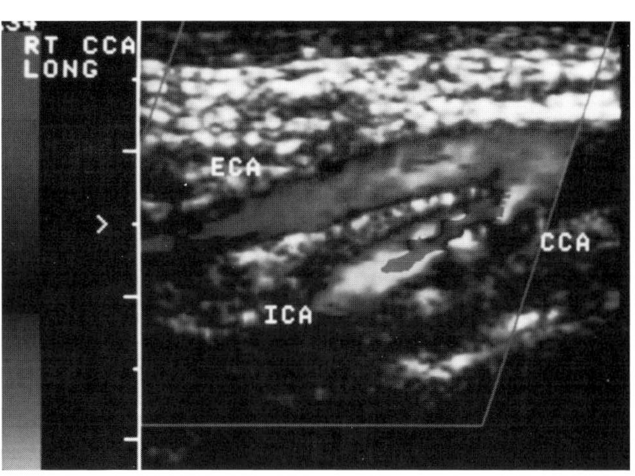

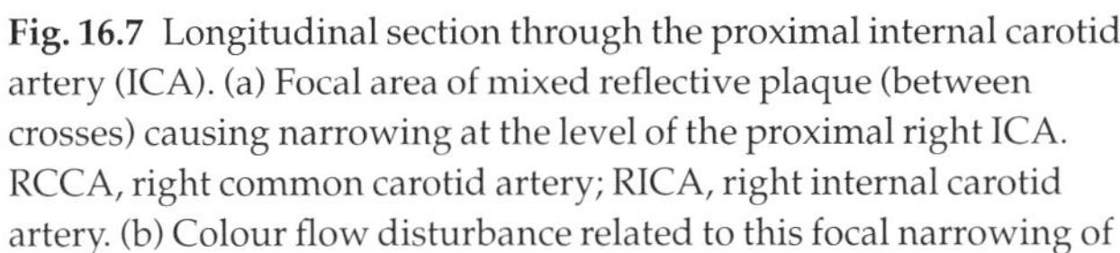

Fig. 16.7 Longitudinal section through the proximal internal carotid artery (ICA). (a) Focal area of mixed reflective plaque (between crosses) causing narrowing at the level of the proximal right ICA. RCCA, right common carotid artery; RICA, right internal carotid artery. (b) Colour flow disturbance related to this focal narrowing of plaque formation. The sample volume gate should be placed at the site of maximum colour disturbance in order to record the peak systolic velocity. CCA, common carotid artery; ECA, external carotid artery. For colour, see Plate 16.7 (between pp. 308 and 309).

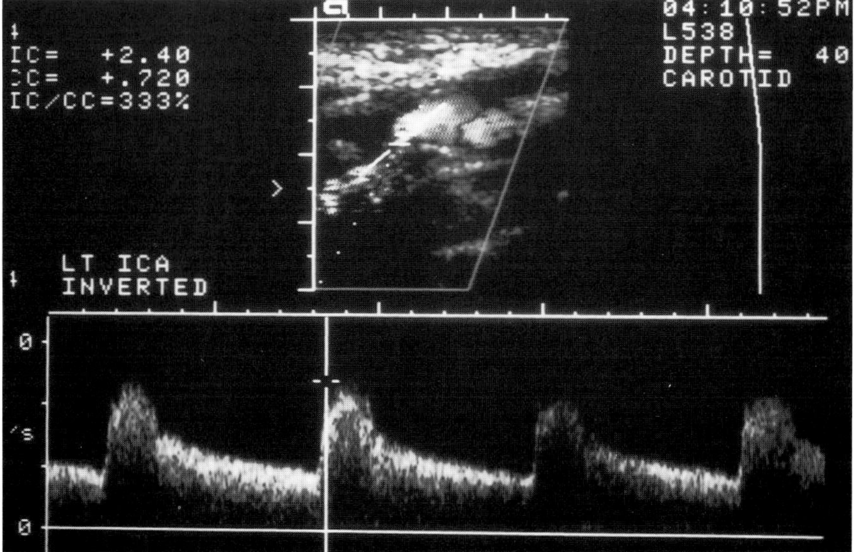

Fig. 16.8 Doppler spectral waveform analysis allows an angle corrected peak systolic velocity measurement of 240 cm s^{-1} to be recorded from the focal narrowing in the ICA, which according to the criteria in Table 16.3, suggests a diameter reduction of greater than 70%. Note the high end-diastolic velocity and a ICPSV to CCPSV ratio of 3.3. Some spectral broadening is present.

230 cm s^{-1}, indicates that a diameter reduction of over 70% is present (Fig. 16.8). Moneta *et al.* prospectively studied 100 angiograms, measuring the degree of diameter reduction by the NASCET method and correlating this with the duplex Doppler findings [38]. An ICPSV to CCPSV ratio of greater than 4.0 provided the best combination of sensitivity, specificity, positive predictive value, negative predictive value and overall accuracy for detection of a 70–99% diameter reduction (Fig. 16.9). An ICPSV of greater than 130 cm s^{-1} and an ICPSV to CCPSV ratio of greater than 3.2 would suggest a diameter reduction of greater than 60%. A guide to these measurement indices is shown in Table 16.3.

In practice, these figures should only be the basis from which to develop criteria specific for individual vascular ultrasound departments and the type of equipment used. Ideally each centre should be constantly auditing duplex Doppler findings, comparing these to angiographic appearances where available and the diameter reduction assessed at surgery, so that the basic criteria can be adapted to suit local conditions. The particular criteria chosen to assess a stenosis should be carefully considered.

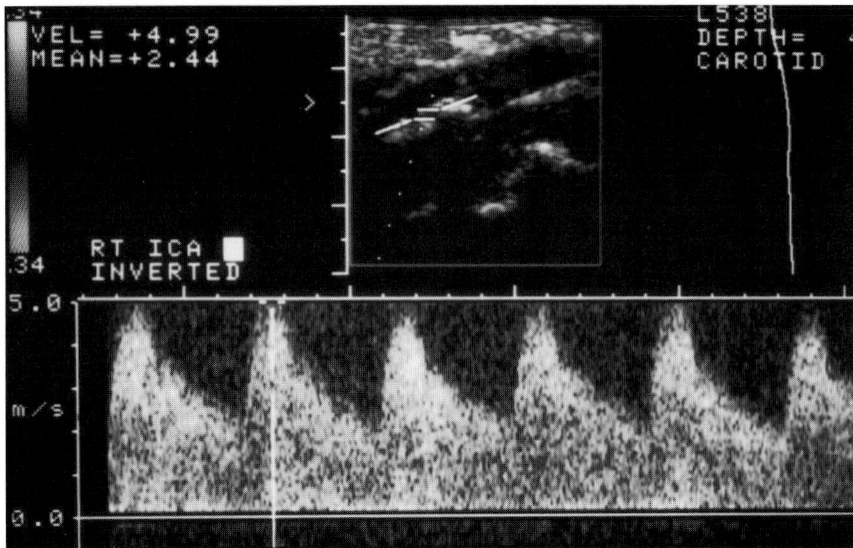

Fig. 16.9 Doppler spectral waveform analysis allows an angle corrected peak systolic velocity measurement of 499 cm s^{-1}, and end-diastolic velocity in excess of 200 cm s^{-1} to be recorded from the focal narrowing in the ICA, which according to the criteria in Table 16.3, suggests a diameter reduction of between 80 and 95%. Note the prominent spectral broadening.

Table 16.3 Suggested duplex Doppler ultrasound criteria for grading ICA diameter reduction, based on figures derived from references [37,38]. PSV, peak systolic velocity; EDV, end-diastolic velocity; PSV_{ICA} to PSV_{CCA}, ratio of the velocities. Velocity measurements are in cm s^{-1}

Diameter reduction (%)	PSV	EDV	PSV_{ICA} to PSV_{CCA} ratio
0–29	<100	<40	<3.2
30–49	110–130	<40	<3.2
50–59	>130	<40	<3.2
60–69	>130	40–110	3.2–4.0
70–79	>230	110–140	>4.0
80–95	>230	>140	>4.0
96–99	'String flow'	'String flow'	
100	'No flow'	'No flow'	

For example, employing a single ICPSV measurement instead of a ratio measurement does not eliminate problems of variable cardiac output, cardiac arrhythmia, the presence of a proximal CCA narrowing (the 'tandem' lesion) and interval changes of myocardial function. Often a combination of measurements will increase the accuracy of estimation of the stenosis. In addition all examination reports should include the Doppler examination angle as well as the velocity and whenever possible a standard examination angle, as near as possible to 60°, should be used.

Other imaging methods

Arteriography, magnetic resonance arteriography (MRA) and contrast-enhanced dynamic computed tomography (CT) provide an assessment of the luminal size but are unable to characterize the vessel wall or associated plaque. Early plaque formation is accompanied by compensatory arterial enlargement, a phenomenon seen both in the coronary arteries [39] and the carotid arteries [40], with considerable plaque formation occurring before luminal narrowing is seen on arteriography. Direct comparison between ultrasound and arteriography in 900 patients demonstrated that half the 345 arteries considered normal at arteriography were shown to have a lesion at ultrasound [41]. Ultrasound provides an effective means of evaluating atherosclerosis within the carotid arteries but is limited by several inherent problems particularly by the presence of calcification in complicated lesions.

The accuracy of colour Doppler ultrasound in comparison with conventional angiography is not disputed [24,42]. MRA, although an accurate method for detection of stenosis, is not widely available, does not give information about the arterial wall and is not cost-effective at present [43].

Pitfalls and problems of carotid Doppler ultrasound

Calcification

When there is extensive plaque disease present in a vessel, and if much of it is calcified, insonnation of the area distal to the calcification is difficult due to the acoustic shadowing produced (Fig. 16.10). A significant narrowing of the underlying vessel may be present, but the high velocity jet is not seen. Scanning from a different direction, e.g. posteriorly may help, but very often the examination is inconclusive and another form of imaging is necessary. Sometimes it may be possible to infer from the flow in the vessel distal to a significant stenosis, that a narrowing is present beneath an area of calcified plaque, but this may only be possible 1 to 2 cm postvessel narrowing and is unreliable [44].

High bifurcation

When the bifurcation does not lie at the level of C4, difficulty may be encountered in obtaining adequate images due to the presence of the mandible. This may in some patients be overcome by imaging from a posterior position, but in most cases it may be impossible to visualize the bifurcation.

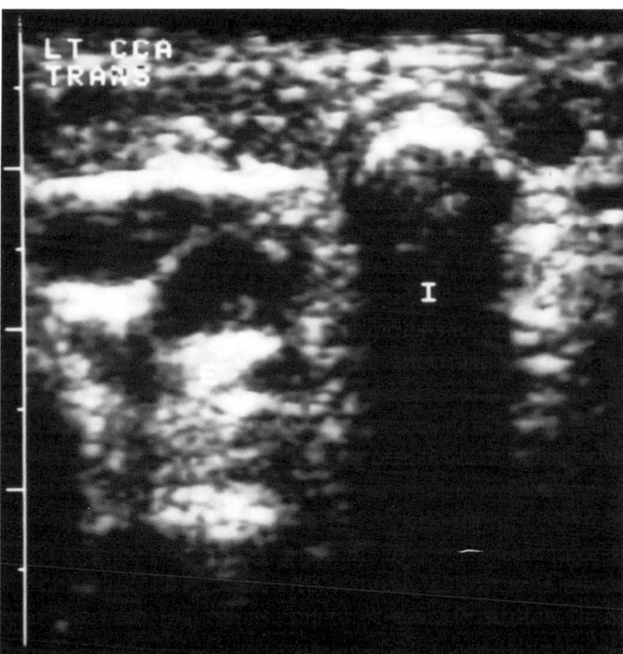

Fig. 16.10 Extensive calcification at the level of the carotid bulb in this transverse view precludes an accurate assessment of the degree of narrowing of the artery at this level, and the patient needs to undergo another form of imaging to evaluate this area. I, internal carotid artery.

Tortuous vessel

When the vessel under examination is tortuous and makes a sharp turn, a false impression of an increase in velocity may be inferred. This is less of a problem with colour Doppler imaging when the vessel is completely filled with colour and no narrowing is detected.

Aliasing

This may be reduced by a change in the position of the probe, increasing the Doppler angle or lowering the Doppler frequency. If aliasing persists, a measurement of the diastolic velocity may be used, as this is much less affected than the peak systolic velocity on spectral tracings.

Detection of carotid occlusion

To distinguish between a total occlusion and a 99% diameter reduction is crucial, as complete obstruction is a contraindication to surgery due to progressive thrombus forming above the occluded plaque, extending superiorly beyond the operating field to the next major branch such as the ophthalmic artery [45]. High grade ICA lesions cause a reduction in volume flow therefore causing the velocity measured at the stenosis to decrease, and velocity criteria will no longer apply.

ICA occlusion can be inferred on the basis of the lack of pulsation or expansion of vessel walls but this is an unreliable method [46]. Success in diagnosing occlusion on the basis of detecting a thrombus-filled lumen, the absence of wall motion characteristics and the lack of Doppler flow signal has been reported to a level of accuracy of 96% (Fig. 16.11) [47]. A characteristic flow reversal may be present in the patent vessel just proximal to the occlusion, with a generalized damping of flow in the CCA. Furthermore, with a long-standing occlusion, the ECA may become 'internalized' with the development of collaterals, particularly around the orbit, producing a hypertrophied ECA with a high forward diastolic component to the spectral waveform pattern. The ipsilateral VA may then become dominant.

Colour Doppler ultrasound has minimized the difficulty of duplex ultrasound in distinguishing between an occlusion and a severe stenosis by allowing a narrow channel to be identified, but technical difficulties remain (Fig. 16.12). The accuracy of detection of a very narrow patent channel of a severe stenosis and the distinction from a total occlusion is likely to improve in the future

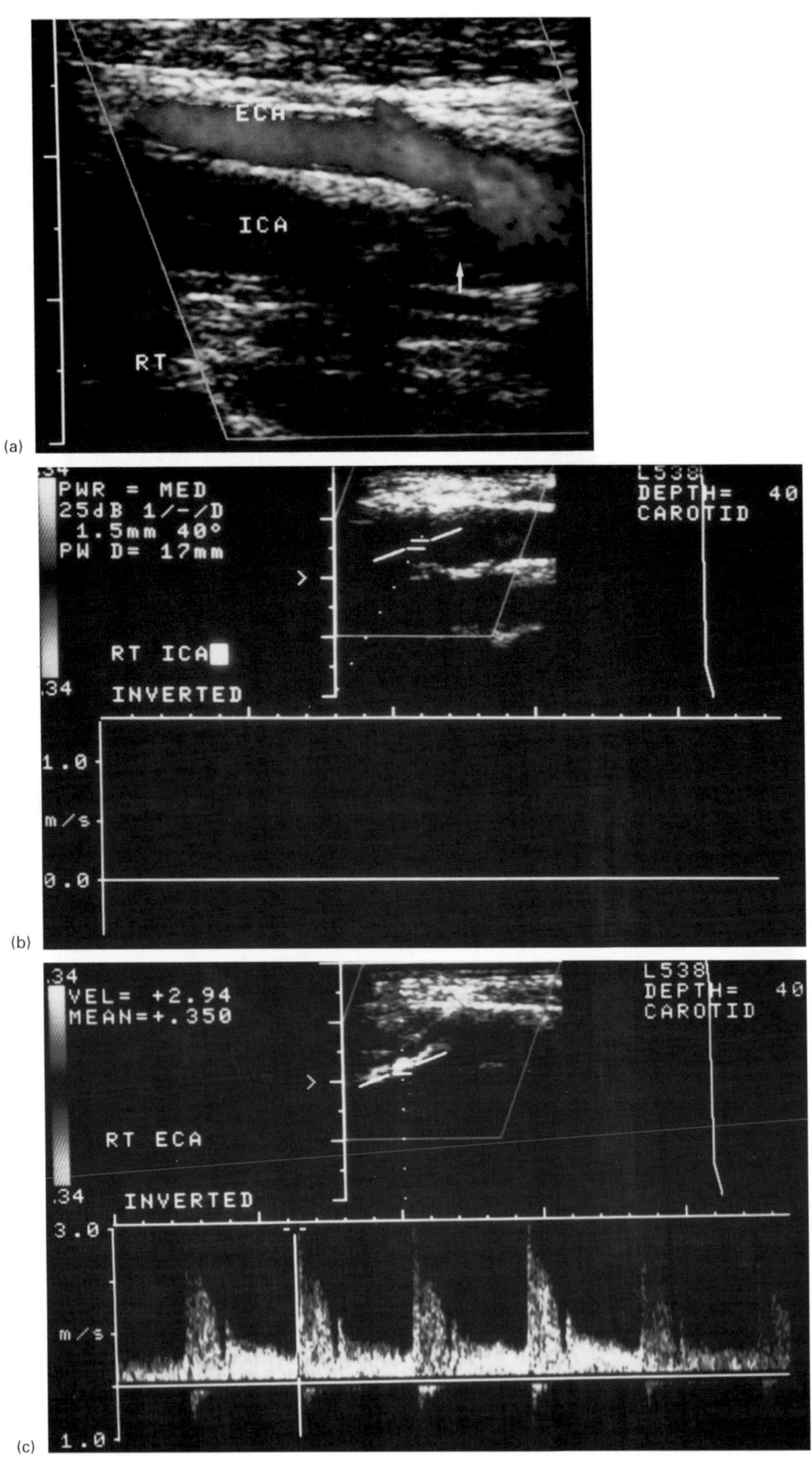

Fig. 16.11 (a) Longitudinal section through the bifurcation with colour Doppler showing no colour flow in the internal carotid artery (ICA) (arrow) which is filled with low reflective material and is occluded. ECA, external carotid artery; RT, right. (b) No spectral waveform is obtained on Doppler from the occluded ICA. (c) The ECA is 'internalized' with a peak systolic velocity of 294 cm s^{-1} and high diastolic forward flow. For colour, see Plate 16.11 (between pp. 308 and 309).

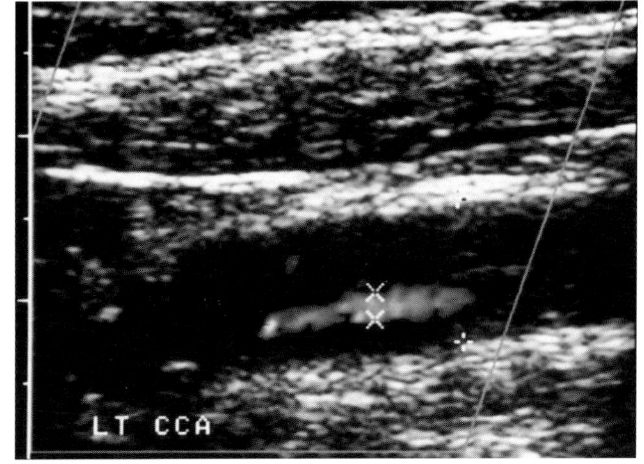

(a)

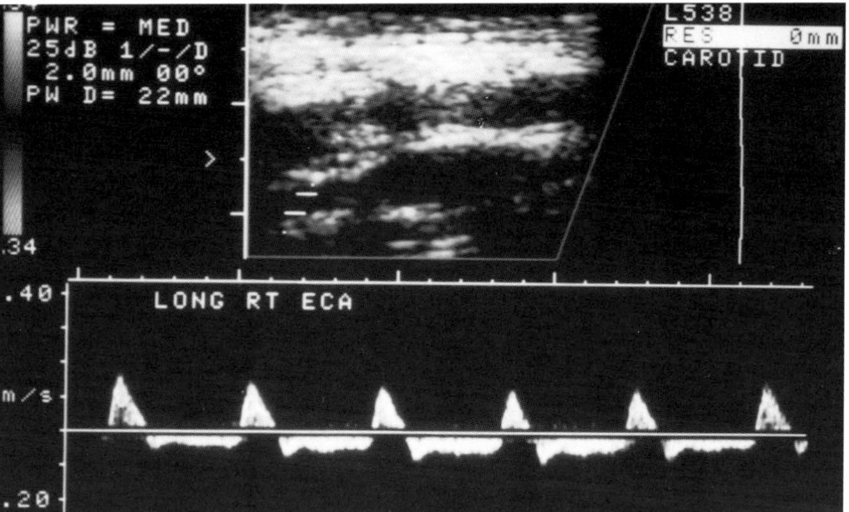

(b)

Fig. 16.12 (a) Longitudinal section through the left common carotid artery (CCA) (between crosses, +) using colour Doppler demonstrates a narrow channel of colour flow, the 'string sign' or 'pseudo-occlusion' (between crosses, ×). (b) In a different patient, the presence of a CCA occlusion has given rise to diastolic flow reversal in the external carotid artery (ECA), which supplies a patent ICA. For colour, see Plate 16.12 (between pp. 308 and 309).

with the use of 'power' Doppler and intravenous ultrasound contrast media [48].

Postendarterectomy follow-up

The incidence of restenosis after endarterectomy is low and is due to neointimal hyperplasia if it occurs within 2 years and to the recurrence of atherosclerotic disease if it occurs after 2 years [49]. The appearance of the ICA on grey-scale imaging reveals a vessel stripped of its intimal layer, and the spectral waveform assumes a rather prolonged systolic peak, suggesting an alteration of vessel wall elasticity (Fig. 16.13).

Vertebral artery abnormalities

Reversal of blood flow in the VA ipsilateral to a proximal subclavian artery stenosis was first demonstrated in 1960 by Contorni [50] and Reivich *et al.* [51], and termed the subclavian steal syndrome by Fisher [52] (Fig. 16.14). This situation occurs when there is a tight stenosis or occlusion of the subclavian artery proximal to the origin of the VA. The arm is then supplied by blood siphoning from the contralateral VA into the ipsilateral VA and down into the subclavian artery distal to the diseased segment, in effect stealing blood from the basilar artery. Most commonly this abnormality is a result of atheromatous disease, but may be caused by Takayasu arteritis, trauma, congenital causes as with interruption of the aortic arch proximal to the subclavian artery, or after a surgical procedure such as Blalock–Taussig anastomosis [53]. The lesions are predominantly left sided, reflecting the more acute angle at the origin of the left subclavian artery.

The incidence of subclavian or innominate artery stenosis, as found on angiography, is estimated at between 17 and 23%, with reversal of flow in the ipsilateral VA seen on arteriography in between 2.5 and 6% of these patients. The male to female ratio is 4 to 1 [54]. It has been suggested

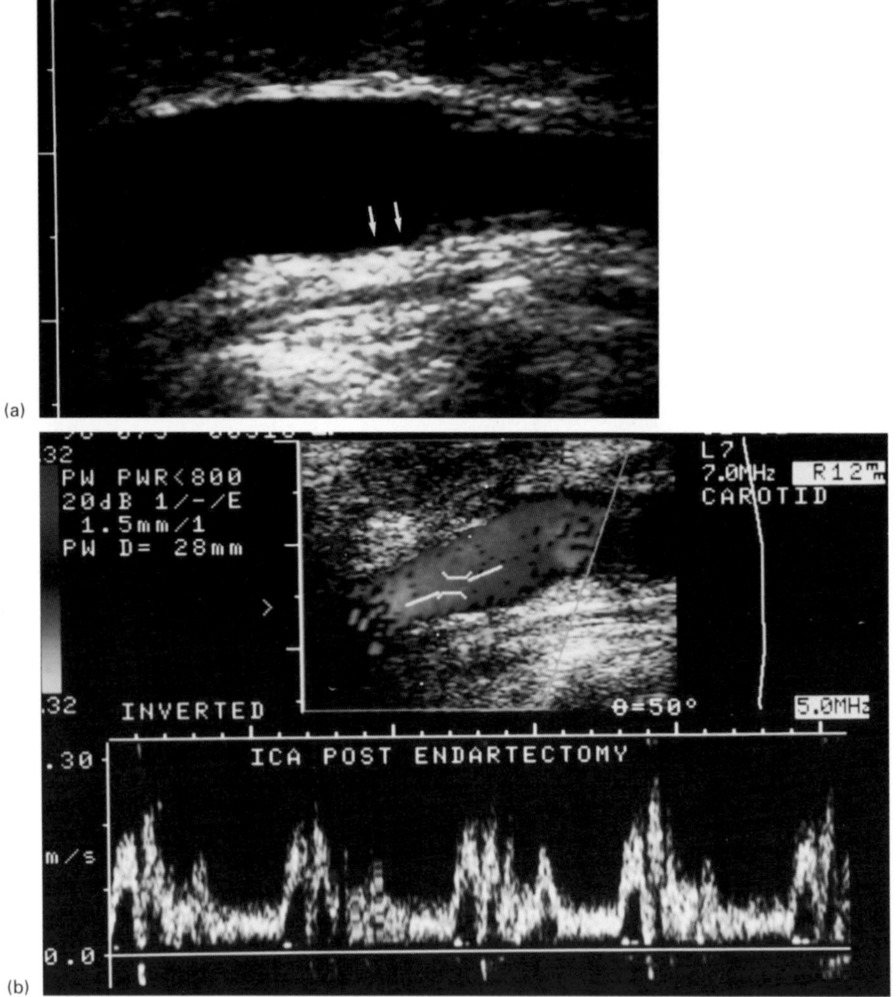

Fig. 16.13 (a) Longitudinal section through the carotid bifurcation following an endarterectomy demonstrates the changes in the appearance of the inner arterial wall when the intimal–medial layer has been stripped (arrows). (b) The corresponding spectral Doppler waveform shows a prolonged systolic peak suggesting changes in the elasticity of the artery postsurgery. ICA, internal carotid artery. For colour, see Plate 16.13 (between pp. 308 and 309).

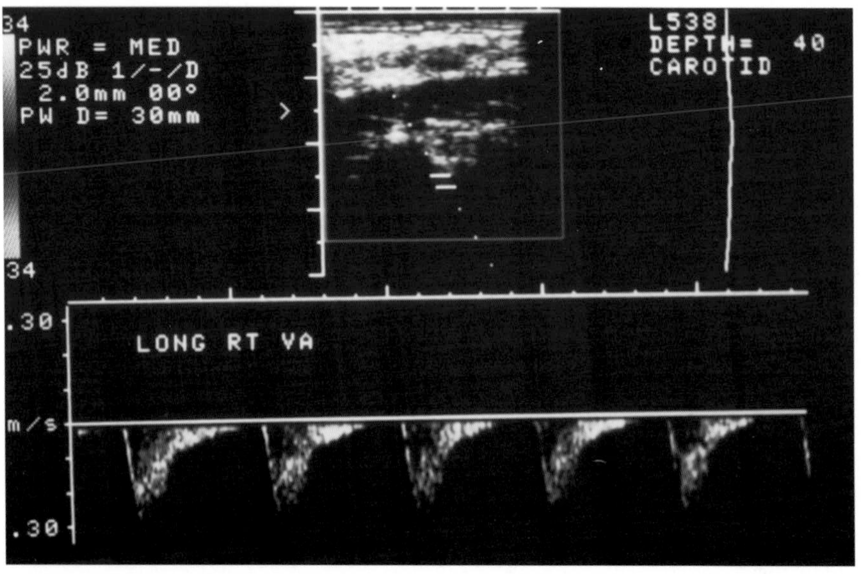

Fig. 16.14 Flow reversal in the VA in the subclavian steal syndrome. The spectral waveform tracing is below the baseline indicating flow away from the transducer and thus in a reverse direction to the normal direction of flow. RT VA, right vertebral artery.

that abnormalities are only apparent in the VA when the stenosis in the innominate artery exceeds 60%.

Initially a large spectrum of symptoms were thought to be a result of this disorder, arising from brainstem ischaemia and stroke; these were considered to occur spontaneously, or secondary to arm exercise [55]. More recent observations have raised doubts as to the significance of retrograde VA flow in producing cerebrovascular events and like ICA stenosis, the subclavian steal phenomenon represents generalized atherosclerosis and may be a harmless haemodynamic phenomenon [56,57].

Demonstration of reversal of VA flow by duplex Doppler ultrasound is now commonly accepted practice and replaces arteriography as the first-line investigation of suspected subclavian steal syndrome, although arteriography will sometimes still be necessary to delineate the proximal stenotic lesion [58]. Routine examination of the vertebral arteries during a carotid ultrasound examination is generally rapid and easily determines the presence of VA flow reversal.

The detection of reversal or biphasic flow at rest in the VA allows the diagnosis of subclavian steal to be made without any further investigation. In some cases steal from the basilar artery does not occur at rest and blood flow to the arm must be increased to demonstrate vertebral flow reversal. The most convenient way to do this is to inflate a blood pressure cuff on the upper arm to above systolic pressure for a few minutes, with reactive hyperaemia on release of the cuff providing maximal arterial flow to the arm. In normal individuals a slight decrease in the amplitude of the flow signal is seen, but in individuals with a steal phenomenon, vertebral flow reversal or a biphasic pattern may be seen [25].

Stenosis and occlusion of the innominate artery proximal to the right CCA occurs infrequently. Direct examination of the innominate artery in the right supraclavicular fossa is not always possible, especially in an obese patient and indirect assessment of the poststenotic flow disturbance in the CCA, subclavian artery and the VA may be helpful in determining the severity of the innominate narrowing.

Vertebral artery ultrasound may be used to detect the presence and direction of flow as well as sampling turbulent areas or waveform dampening for stenosis. The relationship between the severity of a VA stenosis and the peak systolic velocity has not been studied as fully as it has for ICA stenoses (Fig. 16.15). The average peak systolic velocity in the normal VA is estimated at 56 cm s^{-1} (range 19–98 cm s^{-1}) [26], and a focal velocity measurement of greater than 100 cm s^{-1}, accompanied by disturbed flow is suggestive of a stenosis. In a study of VA disease, when a moderately dampened waveform ('tardus-parvus appearance') was found on VA Doppler ultrasound, angiography showed a greater than 50% stenosis proximal to the region of insonnation [59]. It must be stressed, however, that ultrasound of the vertebral arteries has not been fully explored because of the lack of clinical interest in the vertebral arteries, and arteriography, which gives information of the basilar artery, continues to be accepted as the standard imaging modality, with MRA assuming an increasingly important role. Transcranial ultrasound is able to image the distal vertebral arteries to the level of the basilar artery and this may extend the value of ultrasound in the assessment of the posterior fossa circulation [60].

Dissections of the carotid and vertebral arteries

Carotid dissections may be divided into (a) traumatic, when a clear history of trauma is obtained; (b) spontaneous, when no trauma is evident; or (c) as an extension from a dissection of the aortic arch. Spontaneous dissections of the ICA, first described by Jentzer in 1954 [61], are not as rare as was initially thought with dissection causing between 0.4 and 2.5% of all strokes in the general population, and between 5 to 20% of strokes under the age of 45 years [62]. The presenting clinical features of ICA dissection vary widely. Acute neurological deficits (hemiparesis, dysphasia and visual loss) predominate but neck and head pain, Horner's syndrome and pulsatile tinnitus also occur. The pathophysiology of a dissection is attributed to a break in the intima, followed by passage of blood along a cleavage plane, usually sited deep within the media but sometimes extending into the zone between the media and adventitia [63]. Alternatively, haemorrhage may occur directly into the arterial wall from damaged vasa vasorum, giving rise to a haematoma, which can then dissect through the media, causing lumen narrowing, or in the subadventitial plane resulting in the formation of an aneurysm [64].

The most common angiographic feature is a tapered stenosis (Fig. 16.16). Complete occlusion, or an isolated aneurysm, are seen less often [65]. Initially management was directed towards surgical intervention at an early stage in the belief that dissections tended to progress and would lead eventually to total occlusion [66,67]. However, serial angiography of these patients shows that the lumen often returns to normal over a period of time, making the use of anticoagulant therapy more appropriate than surgical intervention [68,69].

Ultrasound is capable of imaging and analysing the flow dynamics of a dissection and the patency of a false lumen, it will also delineate the extent of thrombus in the

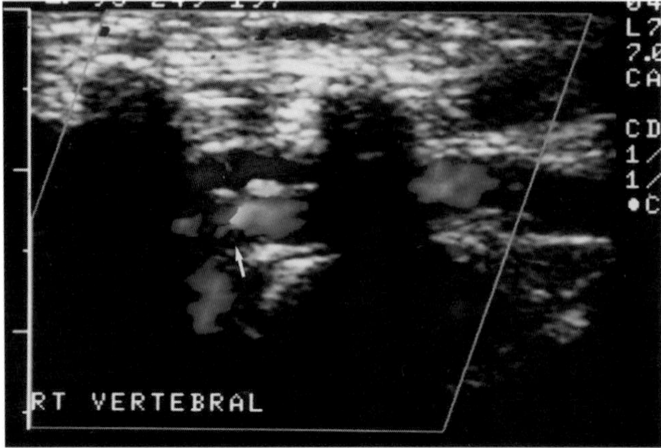

(a)

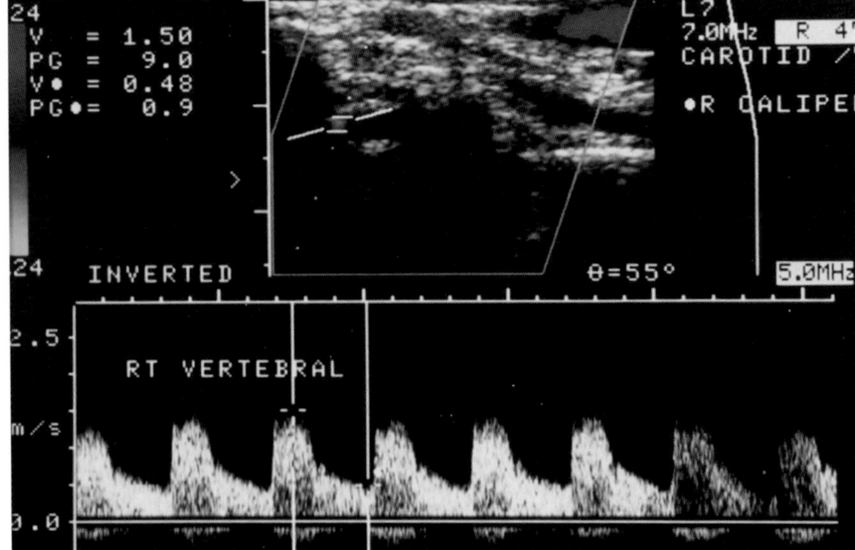

(b)

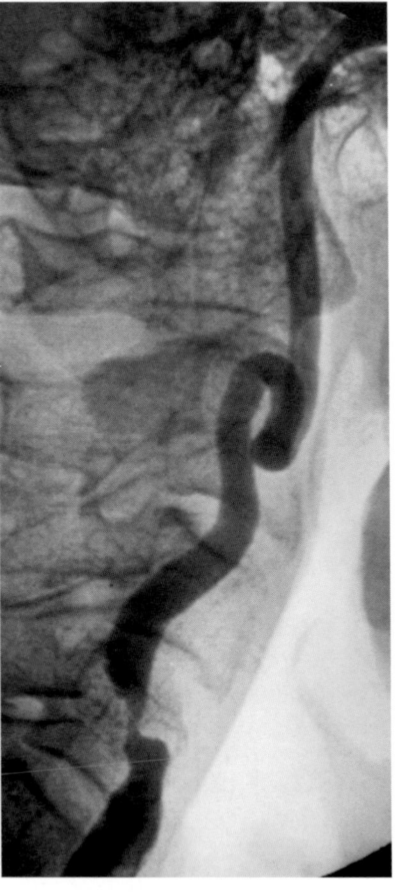
(c)

Fig. 16.15 (a) Longitudinal section through the VA demonstrates a focal area of colour flow disturbance representing a narrowed lumen caused by an area of plaque (arrow). (b) The corresponding spectral waveform allows the angle corrected peak systolic velocity to be measured at 150 cm s^{-1}, which is much higher than the normal mean value of 56 cm s^{-1}. (c) The selective vessel angiographic image of the VA confirms the presence of a focal narrowing. For colour, see Plate 16.15 (between pp. 308 and 309).

vessel wall. Imaging with dynamic contrast-enhanced spiral CT and magnetic resonance imaging (MRI) show promise as non-invasive methods but these modalities do not allow the interrogation of the flow dynamics of a dissection as does ultrasound. MRI and CT rely on demonstrating the presence of a periarterial rim of intramural haematoma, surrounding either a normal or narrowed flow void [70].

Two large series of ICA dissections have shown that the commonest spectral Doppler findings in the affected ICA are either a bidirectional high resistance pattern or absence of a signal in a total occlusion [71,72]. Both these

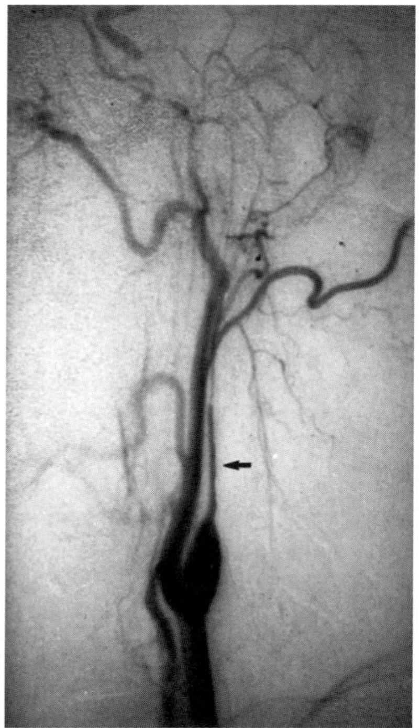

(a)

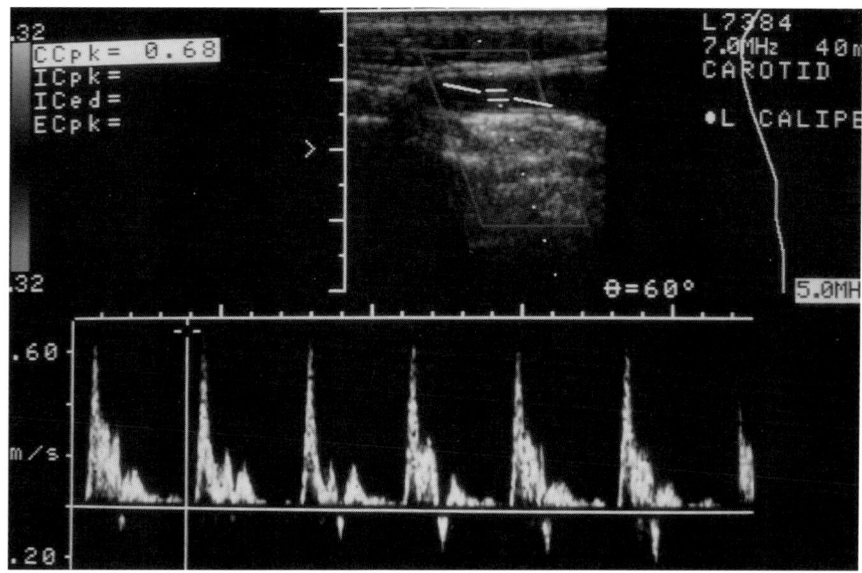

Fig. 16.16 (a) Selective vessel angiogram of the CCA demonstrates the presence of the classic 'rat's tail' appearance of a dissection of the ICA (arrow). These appearances are caused by the formation of thrombus in the false lumen expanding and compressing the true lumen. (Reproduced from Sidhu *et al.*, 1997 [25] with permission.) (b) The resultant spectral waveform reflects the narrowed channel and the high resistance pattern with flow reversal in diastole is a frequently encountered pattern.

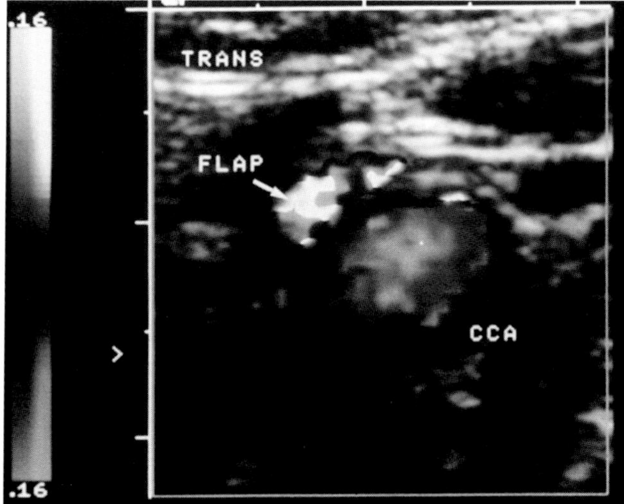

Fig. 16.17 Transverse section through the distal common carotid artery (CCA) demonstrates an area of colour turbulence in the patent flap (arrow) of a CCA dissection. For colour, see Plate 16.17 (between pp. 308 and 309).

studies demonstrated that recanalization of dissections occurs in a high proportion of patients—68% over a mean time of 51 days. Patency of the false lumen has been demonstrated (Fig. 16.17). A report using Doppler and colour ultrasound of two CCA dissections arising from an extension of an aortic arch dissection demonstrated the presence of a flap with flow reversal in the false lumens [73]. Bidirectional flow in the false lumen has been demonstrated, and attributed to the movement of the weak wall of the flap through the cardiac cycle, systole producing flow reversal when the wall expands into the false lumen, forward flow in the false lumen returning when the wall falls away during diastole [74]. Forward flow in the false lumen during the cardiac cycle has also been reported [75].

Vertebral artery dissections are less common, occurring secondary to neck trauma as well as spontaneously. Patients experience pain, and may develop subarachnoid haemorrhage, brainstem syndromes and ophthalmic manifestations, and these dissections tend to occur in a younger age group [76]. VA dissection is thought to be an important cause of Wallenberg's syndrome, where occlusion of the posterior inferior cerebellar artery manifests as ipsilateral loss of temperature and pain sensations of the face and contralateral loss of these sensations of the extremities and trunk, ipsilateral ataxia, dysphagia, dysarthria and nystagmus [77]. VA dissections have been analysed using both transcranial and extracranial ultrasound: patterns seen include absent flow signal, severely reduced systolic velocity, no diastolic flow, bidirectional flow and a stenosis signal but none was characteristic for VA dissection [78,79].

Other vascular abnormalities

A non-specific response to terminal ICA occlusion of any cause is the development of a fine system of collateral vessels around the base of the brain, the angiographic features described as a 'puff of smoke'. Classically these appearances are associated with moyamoya disease, a progressive disease of unknown aetiology characterized by spontaneous occlusion of the distal ICA and proximal anterior and middle cerebral arteries [80]. Similar appearances have been described in a number of acquired conditions detailed in Table 16.4 [81–83].

In an assessment of the ultrasound appearances associated with moyamoya disease, abnormal spectral waveforms were obtained from the ipsilateral ICA showing either no flow or a high resistance flow pattern. Low flow velocities were obtained from the ipsilateral intracranial ICA and middle cerebral artery on transcranial Doppler, while the contralateral intracranial vessels demonstrated high velocities [84].

Takayasu's disease is a chronic inflammatory arteriopathy of unknown cause mainly affecting the aorta and its major branches including the vessels of the neck [85]. With ultrasound a characteristic circumferential arterial wall thickening of the carotid arteries is seen, described as a 'macaroni-like' diffusely thickened intimal–medial complex [86]. Ultrasound was found to be superior to arteriography in delineating this abnormality, and therefore able to detect disease at an earlier stage. Furthermore, ultrasound was found to be more sensitive than MRI in resolving wall thickening and spectral Doppler usually shows a high resistance pattern [87]. Follow-up with ultrasound allows the monitoring of the regression of the wall abnormalities while on treatment, greatly reducing the need for repeated angiography.

Pulsatile lumps

Aneurysms of the extracranial carotid arteries are rare, arising commonly as a result of trauma [88], or as a consequence of atherosclerotic disease [89] but they may be mycotic in drug addicts and can also occur with infection following head and neck surgery [90]. Carotid aneurysms are also associated with congenital diseases of the arterial wall such as Marfan's disease [91] or Ehlers–Danlos syndrome [92]. Carotid aneurysms involve the common and internal segments with a similar frequency [93]. The symptoms and signs are a neck mass, cervical pain, dysphasia, hoarseness and cerebrovascular events. Clinical presentation in infected aneurysms may be through life-threatening bleeding into the pharynx, ear or nose [94]. Ultrasound examination is usually diagnostic in extracranial aneurysms, and it has been suggested that an aneurysm be defined as a carotid diameter at the level of the bulb of greater than twice the proximal ICA, or a dilated ICA 1.2 times the normal ICA diameter [95]. Vertebral artery aneurysms are exceedingly rare, presenting as a palpable mass with pain and cerebrovascular symptoms, mostly arising from trauma and located at the C1/C2 level [96].

An enlarged lymph node in the cervical region may present as a pulsatile lump (Fig. 16.18). Normal lymph nodes are rarely seen on ultrasound but reactive or metastatic lymph nodes are usually larger, hypoechoic and easier to detect [97]. Metastatic nodes show a more rounded configuration than non-metastatic nodes, and in the cervical region, nodes greater than 8 mm in the axial direction suggest metastatic disease (normal 2–5 mm).

A carotid chemodectoma (carotid body tumour) is a rare tumour than has an equal sex incidence occurring in the fourth and fifth decades. Slow growing and locally invasive it can metastasize to local lymph nodes. Treatment with radiotherapy alone or in combination with surgery is often successful [98]. Ultrasound diagnosis is possible in

Table 16.4 Causes of the development of the 'moyamoya' appearance on cerebral angiography

Tuberculous meningitis
Hypoplasia of the ICA
Leptospirosis
Neurofibromatosis
Postradiotherapy
Atherosclerosis
ICA fibromuscular hyperplasia

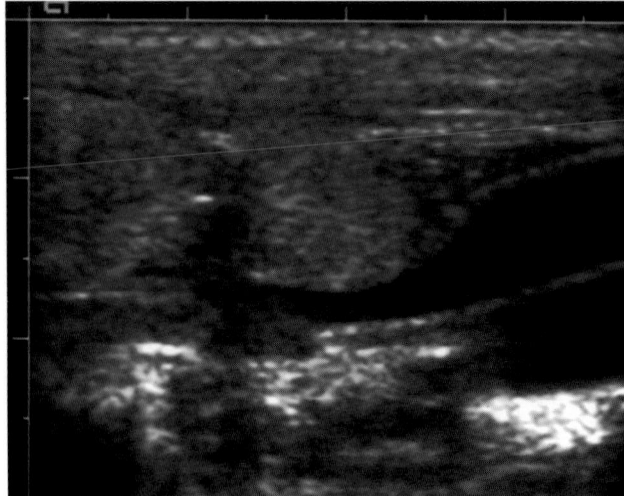

Fig. 16.18 Longitudinal section through a 'pulsatile neck mass' demonstrates enlarged lymph nodes transmitting pulsations from the underlying carotid artery.

a high proportion of cases. The tumours are usually solid, slightly heterogeneous, ranging in size from 1.2 to 5.0 cm and located within the carotid bifurcation. Colour Doppler shows a vascular tumour and spectral Doppler waveform analysis from blood flow within these lesions is usually of a low resistance pattern, helping to differentiate chemodectomas from other solid, non-vascular masses [99].

Arterial wall changes: intimal–medial thickness

The development of plaque disease and the consequent encroachment on the arterial lumen, giving rise to arterial luminal narrowing, are late manifestations of disease that has its beginnings in minor changes at the level of the inner arterial wall, the intima–media complex (Fig. 16.19). Early detection is important as early arterial wall changes are a marker for the future development of atherosclerosis. MRI techniques for imaging plaque morphology are unable to resolve arterial wall changes [100], leaving B-mode ultrasound as the only current imaging modality with sufficient resolution to image the arterial wall. The boundaries of the layers of the arterial wall can be imaged with clarity on ultrasound, as first described by James *et al.* in 1982 [101]. The inner echogenic line represents the luminal–intima interface and the outer echogenic line represents the media–adventitia interface, with the distance between the two lines being a measure of the thickness of the intima and media combined [102]. These interfaces can be seen on both the near and far walls of larger arteries when the ultrasound beam is at right angles to the wall, but more clearly on the far wall in vessels running parallel to the skin surface, such as the CCA. An increase in the distance between these two lines, the intima–media thickness (IMT), is associated with atherosclerosis in other vessels, especially the coronary arteries [103].

(a)

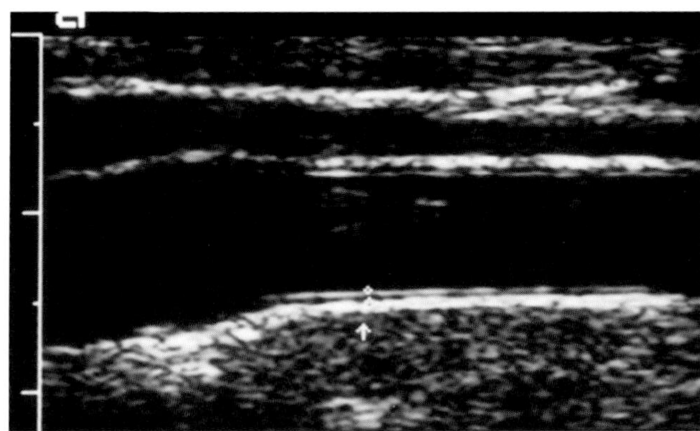

(b)

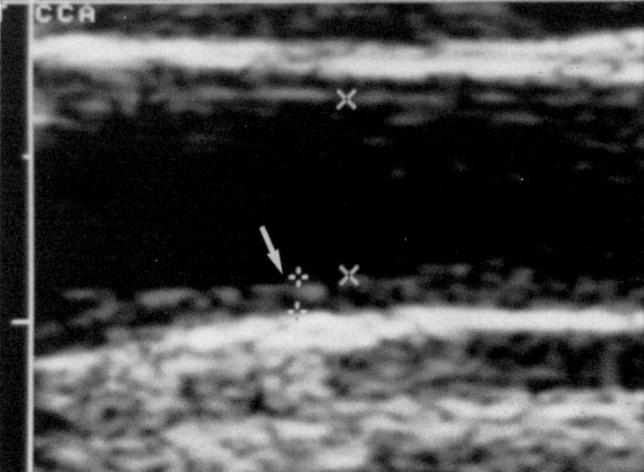

Fig. 16.19 (a) Normal IMT. The IMT is the distance between the inner and outer echogenic lines, seen more clearly on the far wall of the distal carotid artery (arrow; between crosses). The IMT measures 0.6 mm in this patient, which is normal. (b) The IMT in this patient measures 1.0 mm (arrow; between crosses, +), indicating abnormal thickening of the IMT. The arterial lumen is indicated with crosses (×).

A number of risk factors have been associated with an increased IMT in the carotid artery. Patients with hypercholesterolaemia are at higher risk of developing cardiovascular disease and elevated levels of cholesterol, independent of other risk factors, have been related to increased IMT measurements [104,105]. Various other factors have been linked to increased IMT measurements, and these are detailed in Table 16.5 [104–112]. In addition, it has also been demonstrated that high density lipoprotein (HDL) cholesterol levels have a negative correlation with IMT measurements suggesting a protective effect at the arterial wall level [113].

The relationship between IMT, as measured in the carotid arteries, and coronary heart disease has been documented. An increase in IMT has been found in middle-aged adults with prevalent cardiovascular disease [114], is associated with the presence of severe angiographically proven coronary heart disease [106] and has been related to the presence of coronary artery calcification, itself a marker of early coronary artery disease, detected by elec-

Table 16.5 Risk factors for an increase in IMT of the inner arterial wall as seen on ultrasound

Age
Familial hypercholesterolaemia
LDL cholesterol
Lipoprotein (a)
Active and passive smoking
Homocysteine
Chronic exposure to elevated levels of serum angiotensin-converting enzyme
Hypertension
Diabetes mellitus

tron beam CT [115]. The presence of any atherosclerotic finding in the carotid arteries was associated with a threefold risk of an acute myocardial infarction and for each 0.1 mm of common carotid IMT increase, the risk of an acute myocardial infarction increased by 11% [103]. Furthermore, a short follow-up study reported that non-focal IMT increase of the CCA was associated with a 2.17-fold risk of acute myocardial infarction compared with subjects with no structural changes of the carotid artery wall [116]. More recently the measurement of IMT has been used to document the regression of atherosclerotic disease in patients treated with a new class of lipid-lowering drugs, the 3-hydroxy-3-methylglutaryl coenzyme A (HMG CoA) reductase inhibitors, such as lovastatin [117]. This finding demonstrates that lowering the serum cholesterol has a direct effect on the arterial wall, paving the way for future studies to use IMT as a marker of regression and progression of atherosclerosis.

Measurement of IMT

There is, at present, no agreement on the precise location in the carotid arterial system where measurements of IMT should be recorded. In routine radiological practice it would seem appropriate to measure at a site that is readily visualized to allow accurate and repeatable measurements to be made in longitudinal studies, which can be performed by different observers. Ideally, multiple measurements should be taken at several sites and averaged, as the mean of the maximum IMT in the CCA and ICA at several sites is more reproducible than single measurements at any individual site [118]. Alternatively, three measurements of the IMT can be made on the far wall of the CCA on each side, within 1 cm proximal to the carotid bulb, averaging the six measurements for the final value [119].

The median wall thickness in adults ranges between 0.5 and 1.0 mm, with the measurement increasing with advancing age. IMT is also thicker in men than women. It has been claimed that fewer than 5% of the general population have a measurement of greater than 2.0 mm [120]. Values of 1.0 mm or greater are taken to be abnormal by most authors [121], although in some epidemiological studies a measurement of 1.2 mm is taken to be abnormal [122].

Ultrasound classification of atherosclerotic plaques

J.P. WOODCOCK, S. GORMAN & N. PUGH

Plaque morphology

The relationship between the ultrasound appearance of plaque and plaque histology has been an active area of investigation. Early studies described the ultrasound appearances of plaque as either homogeneous, where the range of echoes was uniform, or heterogeneous, where these were mixed high and low level echoes. It was suggested that homogeneous echoes may represent fibrosis or calcification indicating plaque stability or healing [123], and heterogeneous or predominantly echolucent ultrasound appearance, may indicate intraplaque haemorrhage [123–125]. Lipid loaded plaques have a similar appearance [126].

Merritt and Bluth [127] reviewed a large number of publications which looked for correlations between homogeneity and heterogeneity, haemorrhage and ulceration. Their conclusions are that the results are very variable and that, in general, it is not possible reliably to predict either haemorrhage or ulceration from a visual description of the ultrasound appearance.

White *et al.* [128] carried out a comparative study of 148 ultrasound images with the corresponding histology, made by two observers and a pathologist. The aim of the study was to look for correlations between seven visual ultrasound features and seven tissue types. The hypothesis to be tested was that a mixed granular, echogenic dots feature would correlate with normal tissue, a dense echogenic feature should correlate with calcification, coarse soft granular with cholesterol, mixed granular/ragged with internal proliferation, fine granular/loose with fibrous tissue, lucency with haemorrhage, condensing/granular with elastic tissue, and homogeneous with elastic tissue. Inter and intraobserver variability was investigated, as was bias, i.e. the tendency for one observer to note a particular feature more frequently than another. The results show that there was reasonable intraobserver agreement for calcification only, but very poor agreement between observers or with actual histology identified by a pathologist. Grouping of ultrasound features gave little significant improvement for features other than calcification, although there were weak positive correlations with normal tissue and negative correlations with intimal proliferation. There is clearly a major problem with reproducibility between observers and within observers. Subjectivity plays a major role in the visual description of plaque echogenicity and as a result, it is very difficult reliably to describe plaque histology. In order to achieve this the subjective element must be minimized.

Plaque movement

The movement of the atherosclerotic plaque over the cardiac cycle was first described in 1988 [129]. On real-time ultrasound images various types of movement were detected, namely, differential sliding between inner and outer layers of the artery wall, pulsation of the plaque with the arterial wall, movement of the proximal part of the plaque with the distal end being fixed, and finally, the plaque itself being fixed but the arterial wall both proximal and distal to it, showing movement. It was postulated that the relative movement, particularly within the plaque would produce differences in stress within the plaque which would contribute to its disruption. The first attempt to quantitate this was by Chan in 1990 [130]. The following sections show how the statistical texture feature analysis, and the quantitation of plaque movement have been achieved, and their success in describing plaque classification objectively.

Objective method of plaque classification

Two methods have been developed to classify plaque structure using ultrasound. The first is based on a statistical texture analysis of the grey-scale distribution in plaque images, and the second quantifies relative movement of the plaque over the cardiac cycle.

Texture analysis

Texture is thought of as describing properties such as smoothness, coarseness and regularity.

STATISTICAL TECHNIQUES

Statistical texture analysis aims to characterize texture by calculating statistics from the spatial distribution of echo intensities. These have been shown to be good for characterizing regions of interest as smooth, coarse, grainy, and so on, but they should also differentiate between textures of very similar appearance. Although statistical techniques were selected, it is important to realize that other methods of texture analysis are available. Most of them were developed for the interpretation of texture from satellite images of the earth's resources, and can be summarized as shown below.

STRUCTURAL TECHNIQUES

The structural approach regards texture as a repeating pattern and describes such patterns in terms of the rules for generating them. It is not expected to find a regular structure within most soft tissues at the resolutions available, but these techniques may help in the discrimination of very low level and homogeneous texture such as that from blood.

SPECTRAL TECHNIQUES

Spectral techniques are based on the properties of the Fourier spectrum and are used to detect global periodicity in an image by identifying high energy narrow peaks in the spectrum. It is not anticipated that at present levels of resolution, regular structures will be found within soft tissues.

Since statistical models are relatively easy to implement and manipulate, the statistical approach to texture analysis has been favoured.

Spatial grey-level co-occurrence matrices

The theory underlying ultrasound texture analysis has been reviewed by McCarty [131]. As a result of this work it was decided that the co-occurrence matrix is one of a small number of statistical descriptors of texture that might be relatively independent of equipment variables. Grey-level co-occurrence matrices contain information about the spatial distribution of grey-scale levels in an image. The basic assumption behind their use is that the texture–context information in an image is contained in the overall or average spatial relationship of the grey levels in the image relative to one another.

The pixels in a region of interest are examined in different directions as shown in Fig. 16.20. If there are strongly directionally dependent structures in the texture, there would be striking differences between the matrices derived from different directions. The spatial grey-level co-occurrence matrix is generated by examining all possible pairs of pixels separated by a certain specified spacing.

An example of the method is illustrated in Fig. 16.21. For simplicity, imagine a succession of pixels with grey levels from 0 to 3, and suppose that the array is scanned from left to right. The matrix is set up by beginning with zero grey-scale level on the far left and moving along the array from left to right looking for a data sample of intensity 0 to the immediate right of a data sample of intensity

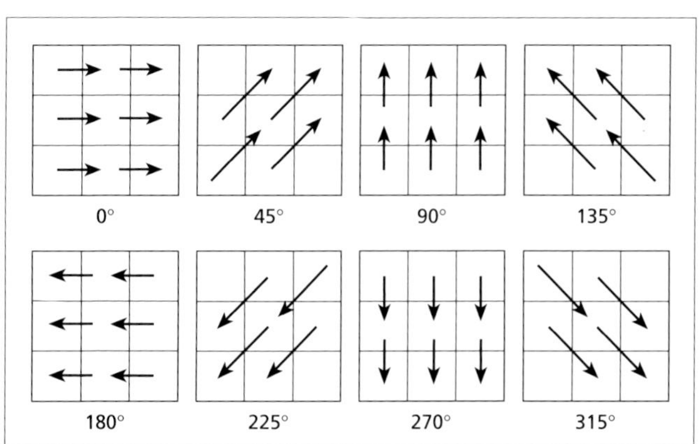

Fig. 16.20 Pixel matrix showing the possible directions of investigation if the intersample distance is limited to one pixel. Arrows indicate direction of pixel examination.

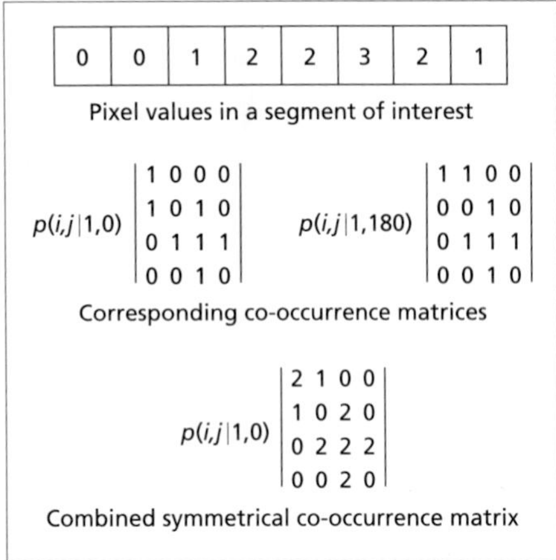

Fig. 16.21 Example of a one-dimensional pixel array where the grey-scale levels vary from 0 to 3. The array is read from left to right.

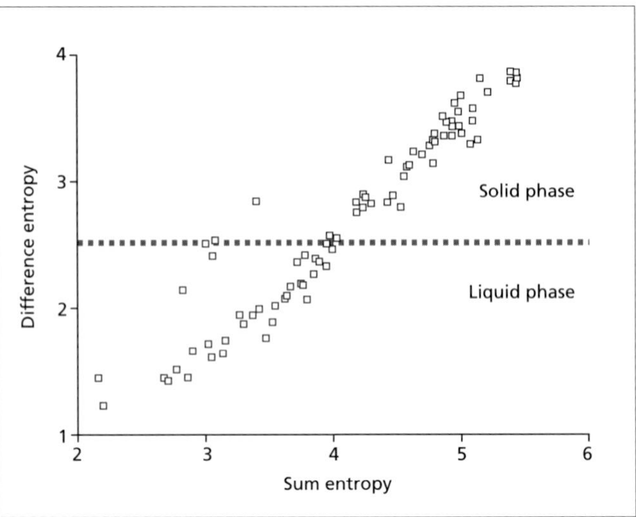

Fig. 16.22 Objective characterization of the co-occurence matrix derived from blood clotting *in vitro*. Note the liquid and solid phases. The ordinate and abscissa are two parameters derived from the statistics of the grey-scale distribution.

0. By inspection it can be seen that this occurs only once along the array of data points and so a 1 is put in the top left-hand corner of the matrix. The next step is to see how many times a 1 is to the immediate right of a zero as the array is scanned from left to right. This does not occur at all and so a zero is placed in the second position of the first row of the matrix. This procedure is repeated for intensity level 2 and 3 to produce the third and fourth values in the first row of the matrix. The second row is constricted by repeating this process but starting with the intensity level 1 and looking for how many zeros there are to the right of a 1, and so on. In this way a co-occurrence matrix is built up.

In reality the pixel arrays are two-dimensional and co-occurrence matrices are constructed from data obtained by scanning in all the directions shown in Fig. 16.20. Various descriptions can then be derived from the matrices which quantitate the statistics of grey-scale variation across an image, e.g. sum entropy, difference entropy, and so on.

Measurement of plaque movement

A method for investigating plaque movement has been developed based on speckle tracking. Speckle is the interference between wavelets from scatterers within the same resolution cell which can result in constructive or destructive interference. This results in a granular pattern in the image which is not related to the actual tissue microstructure. The method is based on the ability to detect a given speckle pattern in one ultrasound frame and to define where this particular pattern has moved to in the second frame. In order to do this the grey-scale statistics must be calculated for the reference region and then these statistics are looked for in the new frame of information. The reference region is stepped across the search region and in every position an error between the measured and reference statistics is calculated. A graph is then drawn of the x and y position of the reference region against the calculated error in statistics. This produces an error surface and the minimum value of this is taken as the x and y co-ordinates of the original speckle pattern in the new image. The movement that has occurred between the ultrasound frames is then known.

Results

Texture analysis of thrombus

The first area in which the texture analysis was applied was in the investigation of thrombus formation *in vitro* and *in vivo*. The *in vitro* results indicated in Fig. 16.22 show how the texture changes during the clotting process. During the 'liquid-phase', which lasted about 8 h, no change in structure was visible in the image. During the solid phase, which lasted over about 5 days, the thrombus grew in size and complexity of echo patterns.

The *in vivo* data consisted of a patient with a jugular vein thrombus (Fig. 16.23) who, during the course of the investigations, developed a second. Thrombus texture analysis of the old thrombus, new thrombus and surrounding tissue, showed a very similar pattern to the results obtained *in vitro*. It looks from these results that it may be possible to age thrombi. The next stage is to investigate thrombus formation associated with plaques.

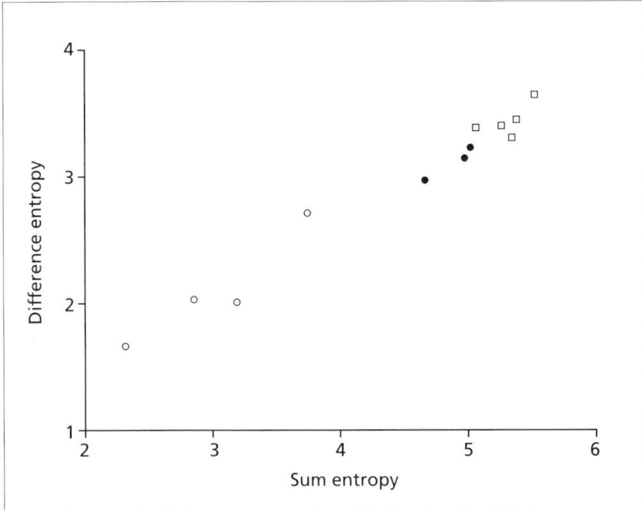

Fig. 16.23 Results derived from *in vivo* jugular vein thrombi. □, surrounding tissue; •, older thrombus; ○, new thrombus. (Courtesy of Dr D.E. Fitzgerald.)

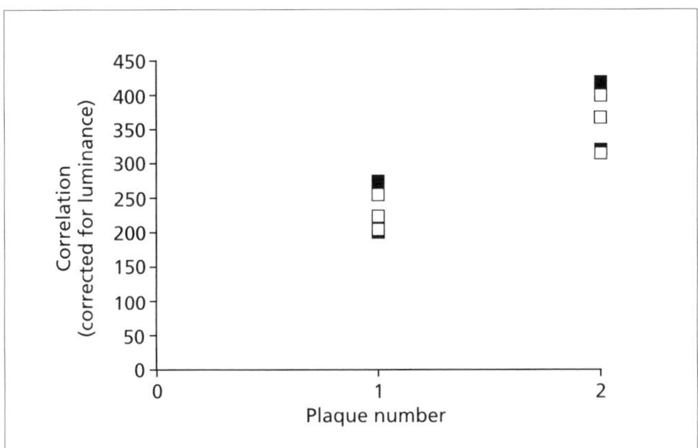

Fig. 16.24 Parameters derived from an objective statistical texture analysis of two visually similar plaques. The texture analysis shows that although they appear similar by eye, they have different textures.

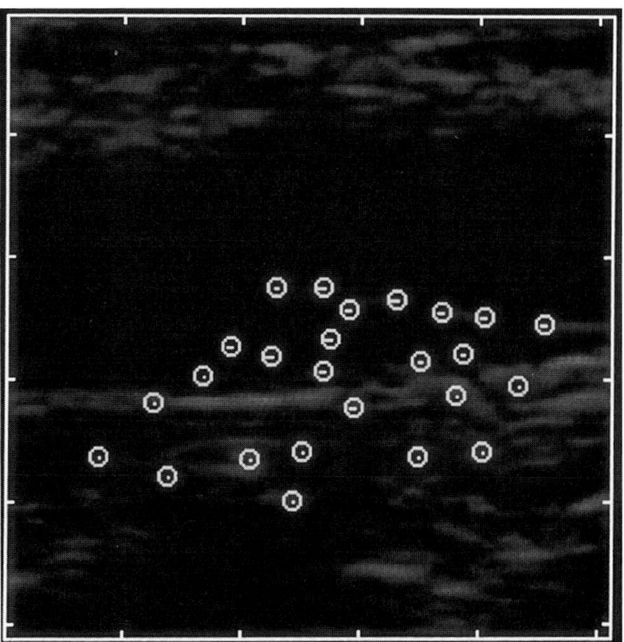

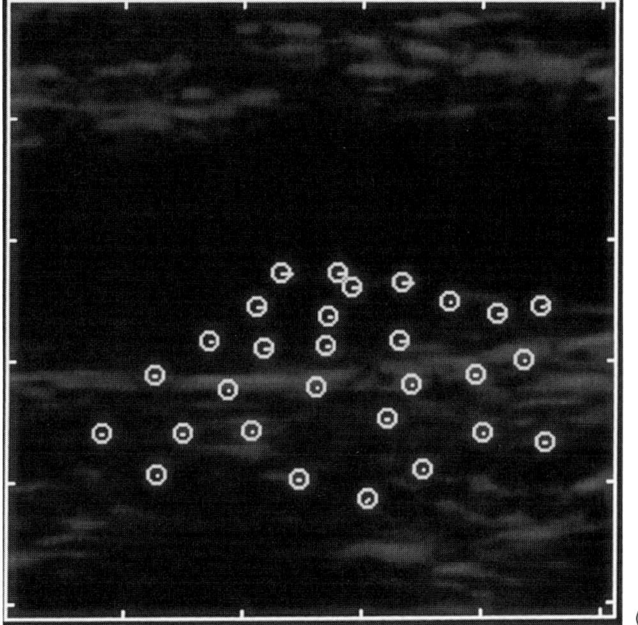

Fig. 16.25 (a) Movement of plaque from right to left during two frames in systole and (b) movement from left to right in diastole. See text for explanation.

Texture analysis of plaque structure

These methods were then applied to atherosclerotic plaques to investigate whether plaques which appear similar by eye have different textures when measured objectively. An example of the results from two similar plaques are shown in Fig. 16.24. It can be seen that statistical texture features do distinguish between plaques of similar appearance.

Plaque movement

An example of plaque movement is shown in Fig. 16.25. Speckle tracking was carried out as described previously, and the movement between two frames in systole (Fig. 16.25a) and two frames in diastole (Fig. 16.25b) are shown. The centres of the circles define the positions in frame 1, which have moved to the end of the line in frame 2. It can be seen that the movement is from right to left in systole, which is the direction of the blood flow, and from left to right in diastole. It can also be seen that there is no translational movement of the outer arterial wall indicated by the posterior, longitudinal, bright echo.

Discussion and conclusion

In order to characterize atherosclerotic plaque objectively, both the texture and movement should be quantified. It has been shown that methods based on the use of the co-occurrence matrix may objectively age thrombus, and distinguish between similar looking plaques by means of their texture. Speckle tracking methods can be used to investigate relative movement in plaques and may be used to discriminate between plaques on the basis of their dynamic properties.

Correlations between texture and histology may make it possible to detect lipid in plaques objectively. These methods could then be used to investigate the effect of lipid-lowering agents on plaque structure. Furthermore, if identification of the various components of plaque structure is possible then this information could be used to develop finite element analysis models of plaque, which will calculate the stresses involved in various positions within the plaque. Using these models, it should be possible to show the reduced risk of fracture as a result of removing lipid from the plaque. This may result in ways of measuring plaque stabilization as a result of pharmacological intervention. The information available in the future, by linking ultrasound texture and movement with finite element analysis models, could radically alter the management of atherosclerosis in the carotid arteries.

References

1 Pickering, G.W. (1948) Transient cerebral paralysis with hypertensive cerebral embolism. *Journal of the American Medical Association* **137**, 848–853.

2 Fisher, C.M. (1954) Occlusion of the carotid arteries: further experience. *Archives of Neurology* **72**, 187–204.

3 Eastcott, H.H.G., Pickering, G.W., Rob, C.G. (1954) Reconstruction of internal carotid artery in a patient with intermittent attacks of hemiplegia. *Lancet* **ii**, 994–996.

4 Whisnant, J.P., Sandok, B.A., Sundt, T.M. (1983) Carotid endarterectomy for unilateral carotid system transient cerebral ischemia. *Mayo Clinic Proceedings* **58**, 171–175.

5 Brott, T.G., Labutta, R.J., Kempczinski, R.F. (1986) Changing patterns in the practice of carotid endarterectomy in a large metropolitan area. *Journal of the American Medical Association* **225**, 2609–2612.

6 Theron, J.G., Payelle, G.G., Coskun, O., *et al.* (1996) Carotid artery stenosis: treatment with protected balloon angioplasty and stent placement. *Radiology* **201**, 627–636.

7 Warlow, C.P. (1984) Carotid endarterectomy: does it work? *Stroke* **15**, 1068–1076.

8 Dyken, M.L. (1986) Carotid endarterectomy studies: a glimmering of science. *Stroke* **17**, 355–358.

9 European Carotid Surgery Trialists Collaboration Group (1991) MRC European Carotid Surgery Trial: interim results for symptomatic patients with severe (70–99%) or with mild (0–29%) carotid stenosis. *Lancet* **337**, 1235–1243.

10 North American Symptomatic Carotid Endarterectomy Trial Collaborators (1991) Beneficial effect of carotid endarterectomy in symptomatic patients with high-grade carotid stenosis. *New England Journal of Medicine* **325**, 445–453.

11 Excutive Committee for the Asymptomatic Carotid Atherosclerosis Study (1995) Endarterectomy for asymptomatic carotid artery stenosis. *Journal of the American Medical Association* **273**, 1421.

12 O'Leary, D.H., Person, A.V., Clouse, M.E. (1981) Noninvasive testing for carotid artery stenosis: 1. Prospective analysis of three methods. *American Journal of Neuroradiology* **2**, 437–442.

13 Barber, F.E., Baker, D.W., Nation, A.W.C., *et al.* (1974) Ultrasonic duplex echo-Doppler scanner. *IEEE Transactions Biomedical Engineering* **21**, 109–113.

14 Polak, J.F., Dobkin, G.R., O'Leary, D.H., *et al.* (1989) Internal carotid artery stenosis: accuracy and reproducibility of color-Doppler assisted duplex imaging. *Radiology* **173**, 793–798.

15 Hankey, G.J., Warlow, C.P., Sellar, R.J. (1990) Cerebral angiographic risk in mild cerebrovascular disease. *Stroke* **21**, 209–222.

16 Hankey, G.J., Warlow, C.P. (1990) Symptomatic carotid ischaemic events: safest and most cost effective way of selecting patients for angiography, before carotid endarterectomy. *British Medical Journal* **300**, 1485–1491.

17 Stevens, J.M., Barters, S., Kerslake, R., *et al.* (1989) Relative safety of intravenous digital subtraction angiography over other methods of carotid angiography, and impact on clinical management of cerebrovascular disease. *British Journal of Radiology* **62**, 813–816.

18 Pujia, A., Gnasso, A., Cortese, C., *et al.* (1993) Early extracoronary atherosclerosis and coronary heart disease risk factors in a sample of civil servants in Southern Italy. *Atherosclerosis* **102**, 1–7.

19 Wiebers, D.O., Whisnant, J.P., Sandok, B.A., *et al.* (1990) Prospective comparison of a cohort with asymptomatic carotid bruit and a population-based cohort without carotid bruit. *Stroke* **21**, 984–988.

20 Zwiebel, W.J., Knighton, R. (1990) Duplex examination of the carotid arteries. *Seminars in Ultrasound, CT, and MRI* **11**, 97–135.

21 Toole, J.F., Castaldo, J.E. (1994) Accurate measurement of carotid stenosis. Chaos in methodology. *Journal of Neuroimaging* **4**, 222–230.

22 Kliewer, M.A., Freed, K.S., Hertzberg, B.S., *et al.* (1996) Temporal artery tap: usefulness and limitations in carotid sonography. *Radiology* **201**, 481–484.

23 Hallam, M.J., Reid, J.M., Cooperberg, P.L. (1989) Color-flow Doppler and conventional duplex scanning of the carotid bifurcation: prospective, double-blind, correlative study. *American Journal of Roentgenology* **152**, 1101–1105.

24 Steinke, W., Kloetzsch, C., Hennerici, M. (1990) Carotid artery disease assessed by color Doppler flow imaging: Correlation with standard Doppler sonography and angiography. *American Journal of Roentgenology* **154**, 1061–1068.

25 Zwiebel, W.J. (1992) Duplex vertebral examination. In: Zwiebel, W.J. (ed.) *Introduction to Vascular Ultrasound* (3rd edn). WB Saunders, New York, pp. 133–143.

26 Trattnig, S., Hubsch, P., Schuster, H., *et al.* (1990) Color-coded Doppler imaging of normal vertebral arteries. *Stroke* **21**, 1222–1225.

27 Alexandrov, A.V., Bladin, C.F., Maggisano, R., *et al.* (1993) Measuring carotid stenosis. Time for a reappraisal. *Stroke* **24**, 1292–1296.

28 Jacobs, N.M., Grant, E.G., Schellinger, D., *et al.* (1985) Duplex carotid sonography: criteria for stenosis, accuracy, and pitfalls. *Radiology* **154**, 385–391.

29 Hoskins, P.R. (1996) Accuracy of maximum velocity estimates made using Doppler ultrasound systems. *British Journal of Radiology* **69**, 172–177.

30 Spencer, M.P., Reid, J.M. (1979) Quantification of carotid stenosis with continous-wave (CW) Doppler ultrasound. *Stroke* **10**, 326–330.

31 Roederer, G.O., Langlois, Y.E., Jaeger, K.A. (1984) A simple parameter for accurate classification of severe carotid disease. *Bruit* **8**, 174–178.

32 Moneta, G.L., Taylor, D.C., Zierler, R.E., *et al.* (1989) Asymptomatic high-grade internal carotid stenosis: is stratification to risk factors or duplex spectral analysis possible? *Journal of Vascular Surgery* **10**, 475–483.

33 Vaisman, U., Wojciechowski, M. (1986) Carotid artery disease: new criteria for evaluation by sonographic duplex scanning. *Radiology* **158**, 253–255.

34 Keagy, B.A., Pharr, W.F., Thomas, D., *et al.* (1982) Evaluation of peak frequency ratio (PFR) measurement in the detection of internal carotid artery stenosis. *Journal of Clinical Ultrasound* **10**, 109–112.

35 Bluth, E.I., Wetzner, S.M., Stavros, A.T., *et al.* (1988) Carotid duplex sonography: a multicenter recommendation for standardized imaging and Doppler criteria. *Radiographics* **8**, 487–506.

36 Knox, R.A., Breslau, P.J., Strandness, D.E. (1982) A simple parameter for accurate detection of severe carotid disease. *British Journal of Surgery* **69**, 230–233.

37 Hunink, M.G.M., Polak, J.F., Barlan, M.M., *et al.* (1993) Detection and quantification of carotid artery stenosis: efficacy of various Doppler velocity parameters. *American Journal of Roentgenology* **160**, 619–625.

38 Moneta, G.L., Edwards, J.M., Chitwood, R.W., *et al.* (1993) Correlation of North American Symptomatic Carotid Endarterectomy Trial (NASCET) angiographic definition of 70–99% internal carotid artery stenosis with duplex scanning. *Journal of Vascular Surgery* **17**, 152–159.

39 Glagov, S., Weisenberg, E., Zarins, C.K., *et al.* (1987) Compensatory enlargement of human atherosclerotic coronary arteries. *New England Journal of Medicine* **316**, 1371–1375.

40 Crouse, J.R., Goldbourt, U., Evans, G., *et al.* (1994) Arterial enlargement in the atherosclerosis risk in communities (ARIC) cohort. *In vivo* quantification of carotid arterial enlargement. *Stroke* **25**, 1354–1359.

41 Ricotta, J.J., Bryan, F.A., Bond, M.G., *et al.* (1987) Multicenter validation study of real-time (B-mode) ultrasound, arteriography, and pathologic examination. *Journal of Vascular Surgery* **6**, 512–520.

42 Erickson, S.J., Mewissen, M.W., Foley, W.D., *et al.* (1989) Stenosis of the internal carotid artery: assessment using color Doppler imaging compared with angiography. *American Journal of Roentgenology* **152**, 1299–1305.

43 Young, G.R., Humphrey, P.R.D., Shaw, M.D.M., *et al.* (1994) Comparison of magnetic resonance angiography, duplex ultrasound, and digital subtraction angiography in assessment of extracranial internal carotid artery stenosis. *Journal of Neurology, Neurosurgery and Psychiatry* **57**, 1466–1478.

44 Baxter, G.M., Polak, J.F. (1994) Variance mapping in colour flow imaging: what does it mean? *Clinical Radiology* **49**, 262–265.

45 Berman, S., Devine, J., Erodes, L. (1997) Distinguishing carotid artery pseudo-occlusion with color flow Doppler. *Stroke* **26**, 434–438.

46 Thiele, B.L., Jones, A.M., Hobson, R.W., *et al.* (1992) Standards in noninvasive cerebrovascular testing. Report from the Committee on Standards for Noninvasive Testing of the Joint Council of the Society for Vascular Surgery and the North American Chapter of the International Society for Cardiovascular Surgery. *Journal of Vascular Surgery* **15**, 495–503.

47 Lee, T.H., Ryu, J.E., Chen, S.T., *et al.* (1992) Comparison between carotid duplex sonography and angiography in the diagnosis of extracranial internal carotid artery occlusion. *Journal of the Formosa Medical Association* **91**, 575–579.

48 Sitzer, M., Furst, G., Siebler, M., *et al.* (1994) Usefulness of an intravenous contrast medium in the characterization of high-grade internal carotid stenosis with color Doppler-assisted duplex imaging. *Stroke* **25**, 385–389.

49 Palmaz, J.C., Hunter, G., Carson, S.N., *et al.* (1983) Postoperative carotid restenosis due to neointimal fibromuscular hyperplasia. *Radiology* **148**, 699–702.

50 Controni, L. (1960) Il circolo collaterale vertebro-vertebro nell' obliterazione dell'arteria succlavia alla sua origine. *Minerva Chirurgia* **15**, 268–271.

51 Reivich, M., Holling, H.E., Roberts, B., *et al.* (1961) Reversal of blood flow through the vertebral artery and its effect on cerebral circulation. *New England Journal of Medicine* **265**, 878–885.

52 Fisher, C.M. (1961) A new vascular syndrome 'the subclavian steal'. *New England Journal of Medicine* **265**, 912–913.

53 Sidhu, P.S., Morarji, Y. (1995) Case report: a variant of the subclavian steal syndrome. Demonstration by duplex Doppler imaging. *Clinical Radiology* **50**, 420–422.

54 Fields, W.S., Lemak, N.A. (1972) Joint study of extracranial occlusion. VII. Subclavian steal—a review of 168 cases. *Journal of the American Medical Association* **222**, 1139–1143.

55 Herring, M. (1977) The subclavian steal syndrome: a review. *American Surgeon* **43**, 220–228.

56 Borstein, N.M., Norris, J.W. (1986) Subclavian steal: a harmless haemodynamic phenomenon? *Lancet* **ii**, 303–305.

57 Hennerici, M., Klemm, C., Rautenberg, W. (1988) The subclavian steal phenomenon: a common vascular disorder with rare neurologic deficits. *Neurology* **38**, 669–673.

58 Walker, D.W., Acker, J.D., Cole, C.A. (1982) Subclavian steal syndrome detected with duplex pulsed Doppler sonography. *American Journal of Neuroradiology* **3**, 615–618.

59 Bendick, P.J., Jackson, V.P. (1986) Evaluation of the vertebral arteries with duplex sonography. *Journal of Vascular Surgery* **3**, 523–530.

60 Schoning, M., Walter, J. (1992) Evaluation of the vertebrobasilar-posterior system by transcranial color duplex sonography in adults. *Stroke* **23**, 1280–1286.

61 Jentzer, A. (1954) Dissecting aneurysm of the left internal carotid artery. *Angiology* **5**, 232–234.

62 Biller, J., Hingtgen, W.L., Adams, H.P., *et al.* (1986) Cervicocephalic arterial dissections. A ten-year experience. *Archives of Neurology* **43**, 1234–1238.
63 Ehrenfeld, W.K., Wylie, E.J. (1976) Spontaneous dissection of the internal carotid artery. *Archives of Surgery* **111**, 1294–1301.
64 Anson, J., Crowell, R.M. (1991) Cervicocranial dissection. *Neurosurgery* **29**, 89–96.
65 Fisher, C.M., Ojemann, R.G., Roberson, G.H. (1978) Spontaneous dissection of cervico-cerebral arteries. *Canadian Journal of Neurological Sciences* **5**, 9–19.
66 O'Dwyer, J.A., Moscow, N., Trevor, R., *et al.* (1980) Spontaneous dissection of the carotid artery. *Radiology* **137**, 379–385.
67 Houser, O.W., Mokri, B., Sundt, T.M., *et al.* (1984) Spontaneous cervical cephalic arterial dissection and its residuum: angiographic spectrum. *American Journal of Neuroradiology* **5**, 27–34.
68 Hart, R.G., Easton, J.D. (1985) Dissections. *Stroke* **16**, 925–927.
69 McNeill, D.H., Dreisbach, J., Marsden, R.J. (1980) Spontaneous dissection of the internal carotid artery: its conservative management with heparin sodium. *Archives of Neurology* **37**, 54–55.
70 Zuber, M., Meary, E., Meder, J.F., *et al.* (1994) Magnetic resonance imaging and dynamic CT scan in cervical dissections. *Stroke* **25**, 576–581.
71 Sturzenegger, M., Mattle, H.P., Rivoir, A, *et al.* (1995) Ultrasound findings in carotid artery dissection: analysis of 43 patients. *Neurology* **45**, 691–698.
72 Steinke, W., Rautenberg, W., Schwartz, A., *et al.* (1994) Noninvasive monitoring of internal carotid artery dissection. *Stroke* **25**, 998–1005.
73 Bluth, E.I., Shyn, P.B., Sullivan, M., *et al.* (1989) Doppler color flow imaging of carotid artery dissection. *Journal of Ultrasound in Medicine* **8**, 149–153.
74 Kotval, P.S., Babu, S.C., Fakhry, J., *et al.* (1988) Role of the intimal flap in arterial dissection: sonographic demonstration. *American Journal of Roentgenology* **150**, 1181–1182.
75 Sidhu, P.S., Jonker, N.D., Khaw, K.T., *et al.* (1997) Spontaneous dissections of the internal carotid artery: appearances on color Doppler ultrasound. *British Journal of Radiology* **70**, 50–57.
76 Hinse, P., Thie, A., Lachenmayer, L. (1991) Dissection of the extracranial vertebral artery: a report of four cases and a review of the literature. *Journal of Neurology, Neurosurgery and Psychiatry* **54**, 863–869.
77 Hosoya, T., Watanabe, N., Yamaguchi, K., *et al.* (1994) Intracranial vertebral artery dissection in Wallenberg syndrome. *American Journal of Neuroradiology* **15**, 1161–1165.
78 Sturzenegger, M., Mattle, H.P., Rivoir, A., *et al.* (1993) Ultrasound findings in spontaneous extracranial vertebral artery dissection. *Stroke* **24**, 1910–1921.
79 Hoffmann, M., Sacco, R.L., Chan, S., *et al.* (1993) Noninvasive detection of vertebral artery dissection. *Stroke* **24**, 815–819.
80 Suzuki, J., Kodama, N. (1983) Moyamoya disease: a review. *Stroke* **14**, 104–109.
81 Matthew, N.T., Abraham, J., Chandy, J. (1970) Cerebral angiographic features in tuberculous meningitis. *Neurology* **20**, 1015–1023.
82 Poor, G., Gias, G. (1974) The so-called 'moyamoya disease'. *Journal of Neurology* **37**, 370–377.
83 Ashleigh, R.J., Weller, J.M., Leggate, J.R.S. (1992) Fibromuscular hyperplasia of the internal carotid artery. A further cause of the 'moyamoya' collateral circulation. *British Journal of Neurosurgery* **6**, 269–274.
84 Muppala, M., Castaldo, J.E. (1994) Unilateral supraclinoid internal carotid artery stenosis with moyamoya like vasculopathy. *Journal of Neuroimaging* **4**, 11–16.
85 Pariser, K.M. (1994) Takayasu's arteritis. *Current Opinion in Cardiology* **9**, 575–580.
86 Maeda, H., Handa, N., Matsumoto, M., *et al.* (1991) Carotid lesions detected by B-mode ultrasonography in Takayasu's arteritis: 'macaroni sign' as an indicator of the disease. *Ultrasound in Medicine and Biology* **17**, 695–701.
87 Buckley, A., Southwood, T., Culham, G., *et al.* (1991) The role of ultrasound in evaluation of Takayasu's arteritis. *Journal of Rheumatology* **18**, 1073–1080.
88 Sharma, S., Rajani, M., Mishra, N., *et al.* (1991) Extracranial carotid artery aneurysms following accidental injury: ten years experience. *Clinical Radiology* **43**, 162–165.
89 Zwolak, R.M., Whitehouse, W.M., Knake, J.E., *et al.* (1984) Atherosclerotic extracranial artery aneurysms. *Journal of Vascular Surgery* **1**, 415–422.
90 Ledgerwood, A.M., Lucas, C.E. (1974) Mycotic aneurysm of the carotid artery. *Archives of Vascular Surgery* **109**, 496–498.
91 Ohyama, T., Ohara, S., Momma, F. (1992) Aneurysm of the cervical internal carotid artery associated with Marfan's syndrome-case report. *Neurologica Medico-Chirurgica* **32**, 965–968.
92 Ruby, S.T., Kramer, J., Cassidy, S.B., *et al.* (1989) Internal carotid artery aneurysm: a vascular manifestation of type IV Ehlers–Danlos syndrome. *Connecticut Medicine* **53**, 142–144.
93 Schechter, D.C. (1979) Cervical carotid aneurysms. *New York State Journal of Medicine* **79**, 892–901.
94 Mokri, B., Piepgras, D.G., Sundt, T.H., *et al.* (1982) Extracranial internal carotid artery aneurysms. *Mayo Clinic Proceedings* **57**, 310–321.
95 DeJong, K.P., Zondervan, P.E., Van Urk, H. (1989) Extracranial carotid artery aneurysms. *European Journal of Vascular Surgery* **3**, 557–562.
96 Davidson, K.C., Weiford, E.D., Dixon, G.D. (1975) Traumatic vertebral artery pseudoaneurysm following chiropractic manipulation. *Radiology* **115**, 651–652.
97 Marchal, G., Oyen, R., Verschakelen, J., *et al.* (1985) Sonographic appearance of normal lymph nodes. *Journal of Ultrasound in Medicine* **4**, 417–419.
98 Powell, S., Peters, N., Harmer, C. (1992) Chemodectoma of the head and neck: results of treatment in 84 patients. *International Journal of Radiation Oncology, Biology, Physics* **22**, 919–924.
99 Derchi, L.E., Serafini, G., Rabbia, C., *et al.* (1992) Carotid body tumours: ultrasound evaluation. *Radiology* **182**, 457–459.
100 Skinner, M.P., Yuan, C., Mitsumori, L., *et al.* (1995) Serial magnetic resonance imaging of experimental atherosclerosis detects lesion fine structure, progression and complications *in vivo*. *Nature Medicine* **1**, 69–73.
101 James, E.M., Earnest, F., Forbes, G.S., *et al.* (1982) High resolution dynamic ultrasound of the carotid bifurcation: a prospective evaluation. *Radiology* **144**, 853–858.
102 Pignoli, P., Tremoli, E., Poli, A., *et al.* (1986) Intimal plus medial thickness of the arterial wall: a direct measurement with ultrasound imaging. *Circulation* **74**, 1399–1406.
103 Salonen, J.T., Salonen, R. (1993) Ultrasound B-mode imaging in

observational studies of atherosclerotic progression. *Circulation* **87**, II-56 to II-65.

104 Poli, A., Tremoli, E., Colombo, A., *et al.* (1988) Ultrasonographic measurement of the common carotid artery wall thickness in hypercholesterolemic patients. *Atherosclerosis* **70**, 253–261.

105 Wendelhag, I., Wiklund, O., Wikstrand, J. (1992) Arterial wall thickness in familial hypercholesterolaemia. Ultrasound measurement of the intima-media thickness in the common carotid artery. *Atherosclerosis and Thrombosis* **12**, 70–77.

106 Geroulakos, G., O'Gorman, D.J., Kalodiki, E., *et al.* (1994) The carotid intima–media thickness as a marker of the presence of severe symptomatic coronary artery disease. *European Heart Journal* **15**, 781–785.

107 Pauciullo, P., Iannuzzi, A., Sartorio, R., *et al.* (1994) Increased intima–media thickness of the common carotid artery in hypercholesterolaemic children. *Arteriosclerosis and Thrombosis* **14**, 1075–1079.

108 Sinclair, A.M., Hughes, A.D., Geroulakos, G., *et al.* (1995) Structural changes in the heart and carotid arteries associated with hypertension in humans. *Journal of Human Hypertension* **7**, 1–13.

109 Howard, G., Burke, G.L., Szklo, M., *et al.* (1994) Active and passive smoking are associated with increased carotid wall thickness. The Atherosclerosis Risk in Communities Study. *Archives of Internal Medicine* **154**, 1277–1282.

110 Malinow, M.R., Nieto, J., Szklo, M., *et al.* (1993) Carotid artery intimal–medial wall thickening and plasma homocyst(e)ine in asymptomatic adults. The Atherosclerosis Risk in Communities Study. *Circulation* **87**, 1107–1113.

111 Bonithon-Kopp, C., Ducimetiere, P., Touboul, P.J., *et al.* (1994) Plasma angiotensin-converting enzyme activity and carotid wall thickening. *Circulation* **89**, 952–954.

112 Veller, M., Fisher, C., Nicolaides, A. (1993) Measurement of the ultrasonic intima–media complex thickness in normal subjects. *Journal of Vascular Surgery* **17**, 719–725.

113 Sidhu, P.S., Naoumova, R.P., Maher, V.M.G., *et al.* (1996) The extracranial carotid artery in familial hypercholesterolaemia: relationship of intimal–medial thickness and plaque morphology with plasma lipids and coronary heart disease. *Journal of Cardiovascular Risk* **3**, 61–67.

114 Burke, G.L., Evans, G.W., Riley, W.A., *et al.* (1995) Arterial wall thickness is associated with prevalent cardiovascular disease in middle-aged adults. *Stroke* **26**, 386–391.

115 Sidhu, P.S., Naoumova, R.P., Forbat, S.M., *et al.* (1995) The association of intima–media thickening and plaque morphology of the extracranial carotid arteries with coronary artery calcificaton in hypercholesterolaemia. *British Journal of Radiology* **68**, 803(abstract).

116 Salonen, R., Salonen, J.T. (1991) Ultrasonographically assessed carotid morphology and the risk of coronary heart disease. *Atherosclerosis and Thrombosis* **121**, 1245–1249.

117 Furberg, C.D., Adams, H.P., Applegate, W.B., *et al.* (1994) Effect of lovastatin on early carotid atherosclerosis and cardiovascular events. Asmptomatic Carotid Artery Progression Study (ACAPS) Research Group. *Circulation* **90**, 1679–1687.

118 Crouse, J.R., Harpold, G.H., Kahl, F.R., *et al.* (1986) Evaluation of a scoring system for extracranial carotid atherosclerosis extent with B-mode ultrasound. *Stroke* **17**, 270–275.

119 Sidhu, P.S., Desai, S.R. (1997) A simple and reproducible method of assessing intimal–medial thickness of the common carotid artery. *British Journal of Radiology* **70**, 85–89.

120 Howard, G., Sharrett, A.R., Heiss, G., *et al.* (1993) Carotid artery intimal–medial thickness distribution in general populations as evaluated by B-mode ultrasound. *Stroke* **24**, 1297–1304.

121 Shah, E. (1994) Use of B-mode ultrasound of peripheral arteries as an end point in clinical trials. *British Heart Journal* **72**, 501–503.

122 Salonen, R., Seppanen, K., Rauramaa, R., *et al.* (1988) Prevalence of carotid atherosclerosis and serum cholesterol levels in Eastern Finland. *Arteriosclerosis* **8**, 788–792.

123 Lusby, R.J., Ferrell, L.D., Ehrenfeld, W.R., Stoney, R.J., Wylie, W.J. (1982) Carotid plaque haemorrhage. its role in the production of cerebral ischaemia. *Archives of Surgery* **117**, 1479–1488.

124 Weinburger, J., Marks, S.J., Gaul, J.J., *et al.* (1987) Atherosclerotic plaque at the carotid artery bifurcation. Correlation of ultrasonographic imaging with morphology. *Journal of Ultrasound Medicine* **6**, 363–366.

125 Rudofsky, G., Ranft, J., Hirche, H. (1991) Das Duplexverfahren in der Prävention der Arteriosklerose. *Vasa* **33**, (suppl.) 59–61.

126 Bock, R.W., Lusby, R.J. (1992) Carotid plaque morphology and interpretation of the echolucent lesion. In: Labs, K.H., Jäger, K.A., Fitzgerald, D.E., Woodcock, J.P., Neuerburg-Heusler, D. (eds) *Diagnostic Vascular Ultrasound*. Edward Arnold, London, pp. 225–236.

127 Merritt, C., Bluth, E.I. (1992) Ultrasound identification of plaque composition. In: Lab, K.H., Jäger, K.A., Fitzgerald, D.E., Woodcock, J.P., Neuerburg-Heusler, D. (eds) *Diagnostic Vascular Ultrasound*. Edward Arnold, London, pp. 213–224.

128 White, A.D., Carolan, G.S., Newcombe, R.G., Wilkus, P., Woodcock, J.P., Pathy, J. (1997) Problems in the comparison of ultrasound morphology and histology of carotid artery atheromatous plaques. *Journal of Vascular Investigation* (in press).

129 White, A.D., McCarty, K., Morgan, R., Wilkens, P., Woodcock, J.P. (1988) Investigation of carotid plaque motility. In: Price, R., Evans, J.A. (eds) *Blood Flow Measurement in Clinical Diagnosis*. Biological Engineering Society, pp. 109–115.

130 Chan, K.L. (1993) Two approaches to motion analysis of the ultrasound image sequence of carotid atheromatous plaque. *Ultrasonics* **31**, 117–123.

131 McCarty, K. (1992) Ultrasound texture analysis of thrombus using the co-occurrence matrix: preliminary results. In: Lab, K.H., Jäger, K.A., Fitzgerald, D.E., Woodcock, J.P., Neuerburg-Heusler, D. (eds) *Diagnostic Vascular Ultrasound*. Edward Arnold, London, pp. 264–272.

Chapter 17: Transcranial Doppler ultrasound

J.M. Wardlaw

Transcranial Doppler (TCD) ultrasound was developed by Rune Aaslid in 1982 using a low frequency, high power output, portable Doppler ultrasound machine. This was capable of obtaining spectral Doppler signals from the arteries around the base of the brain through the intact skull in adults. Since then, analysis of the spectral waveform has improved, position-sensitive probe holders have become available for three-dimensional (3D) mapping of the basal intracranial arteries, emboli counting has developed and, more recently, real-time colour flow Doppler images of the brain and arteries through the intact skull of adults has been developed. TCD is a useful tool allowing non-invasive assessment of cerebral arterial blood vessels both in research and, increasingly, in clinical practice.

Equipment

Equipment suitable for spectral TCD in adults operates at around 2 MHz. Depth discrimination enabling sampling at sites 25–100 mm from the probe surface is achieved using a pulsed Doppler signal and range-gated transducer which is also directionally sensitive to distinguish flow towards and away from the probe. The sample volume is generally between 3 and 6 mm.

The simplest spectral TCD instruments automatically calculate the pulsatility index and time-averaged mean velocity from the Doppler waveform. Many modern spectral TCD instruments are linked to a microcomputer for sophisticated analysis of the frequency/power spectrum of the Doppler waveform and to assist emboli counting.

Colour flow TCD imaging is now available on many of the general purpose ultrasound machines with the addition of a low frequency probe (about 2 MHz or less), increase in power output above the normal soft tissue imaging limit (for penetration of the adult skull) and appropriate software upgrades. Several modern instruments produce satisfactory real-time transcranial colour flow imaging of the basal intracranial arteries superimposed on a grey-scale image of the brain. 'Power' Doppler is also used for transcranial imaging, and probably improves vessel identification over conventional colour Doppler. Other technical factors include high persistence.

Technique of examination

Transcranial Doppler requires good understanding of the anatomy of the structures through which the beam is passing, particularly of the arteries in the base of the brain. Considerable practice is required to become proficient. Operator skill is essential for correct interpretation of the information obtained, whether it be spectral or colour TCD, as there are many pitfalls [1].

It is simplest to perform the examination with the patient supine and resting comfortably as this helps to ensure that the head stays still. Points of access to the basal intracranial arteries through the adult skull—'bone windows'—are the temporal bones (immediately above the zygomatic arch between the outer canthus of the eye and the tragus), the foramen magnum and the orbits (Fig. 17.1). The temporal bone window gives access to the middle, anterior and posterior cerebral arteries (MCA, ACA and PCA, respectively), the anterior communicating artery (ACoA), posterior communicating artery (PCoA), intracranial internal carotid artery (ICA) and basilar artery (BA). The BA and intracranial portions of the vertebral arteries (VA) may be insonated through the foramen magnum by positioning the probe in the midline on the back of the neck at the hairline and directing the beam anteriorly and superiorly. The ICA siphons, ophthalmic arteries and ACAs can be insonated through the orbits, but the power output must be reduced to less than 10% of maximum in order to prevent damage to the eye. In addition, the ICA can be examined in the upper neck by positioning the spectral probe inferior to the angle of the mandible and angling superiorly, medially and posteriorly. The VAs can be insonated in the upper neck by positioning the probe immediately posterior to the mastoid process and directing the beam medially [1].

On spectral TCD the arteries are identified by knowledge of their positions in relation to each other through each bone window. Careful attention to the audible

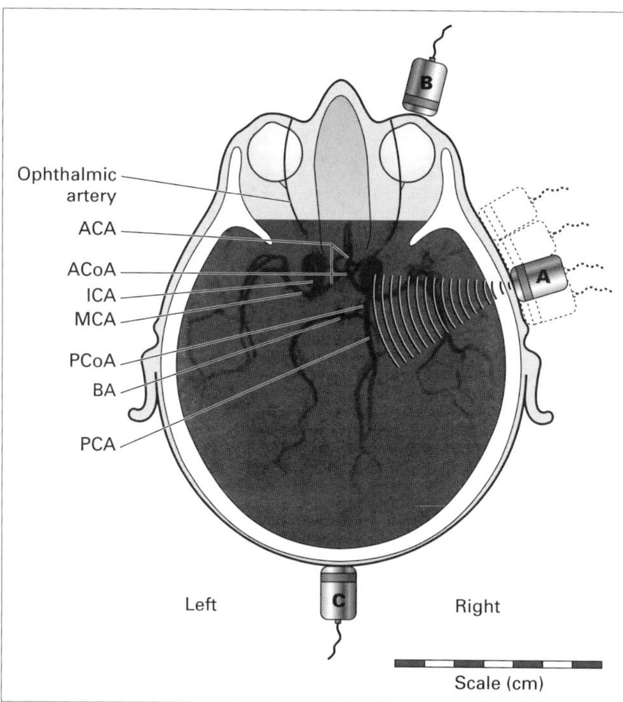

Fig. 17.1 Composite image from a magnetic resonance angiogram of the circle of Willis superimposed on the outline of the skull as viewed from the vertex with the ultrasound beam focused at a depth of 65 mm from the temporal skin surface on the terminal internal carotid artery (ICA) bifurcation. A, B and C indicate the access 'windows' through the skull (not shown are the submandibular approach to the ICA in the neck and the postmastoid approach to the VA as it arches over the first cervical vertebra). Note in (A) the theoretical anterior, middle and posterior temporal bone windows and how the angle of insonation will vary depending on the bone window used, the tortuosity of the arteries and the depth of insonation. Note the tortuosity of the arteries, and consequently the angle of insonation must be altered slightly to examine the anterior, middle and posterior carotid arteries (ACA, MCA and PCA) at each depth. Note that in this patient the right PCA arises direct from the ICA therefore a strong signal will be obtained from the right PCoA, whereas on the left the PCA arises from the basilar artery (BA) so no PCoA signal will be detected.

Doppler signal is helpful as well as to the spectral image on the instrument monitor. Wearing headphones helps to cut out background noise (a frequent problem in busy wards), making full use of the auditory signal to help identify the arteries.

On colour TCD imaging, the grey-scale image of the brain is of assistance in finding the basal intracranial arteries with the sphenoid wing, midbrain, third ventricle and suprasellar cisterns as visible landmarks [2]. The ability to obtain a good grey-scale image indicates that the bone window is adequate (Fig. 17.2), whereas failure to obtain even a grey-scale image indicates a poor bone window.

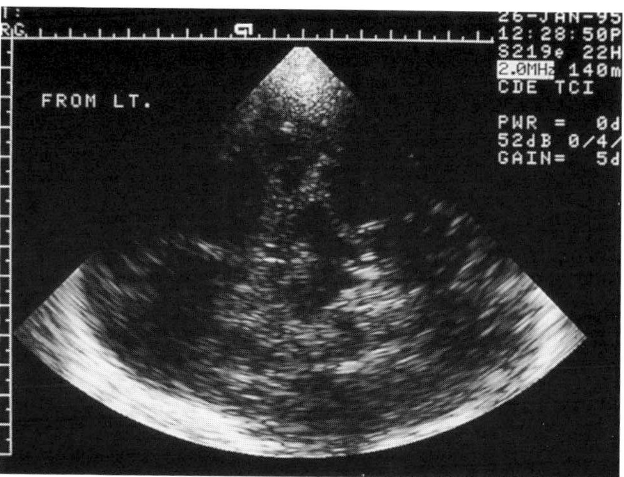

Fig. 17.2 Grey-scale image of the brain obtained axially through the temporal bone window with a 2 MHz probe on an Acuson 128XP10V. The front of the head is to the left of the image and the back to the right. All subsequent images are orientated similarly.

Colour flow TCD allows real-time visualization of the basal intracranial arteries, aids positioning of the cursor to obtain a spectral Doppler signal, correction of the angle of the artery to the beam to ensure accurate velocity readings and probably helps to reduce errors in correct identification of the arteries due to technical factors which occur with spectral TCD.

The spectral TCD examination is best started using the temporal bone window and sample depth set at 65 mm. Position the probe so that the beam is directed medially in the axial plane towards the centre of the head. It is useful to have an image of the skull base and circle of Willis in one's mind. By making small adjustments to the probe angle and position on the skin surface it is usually possible to pick up an arterial signal. The most useful signal to identify first is the ICA bifurcation, usually at 65 mm depth, which gives a strong bidirectional signal (Fig. 17.3). The signal towards the probe is from the MCA and that going away is the ACA. From there, the MCA may be followed superficially to a depth of approximately 35 mm with only minor changes in probe angulation. The ACA may be tracked medially from the ICA bifurcation by angling the probe anteriorly and either slightly inferiorly or superiorly in relation to the MCA position, to a depth of 75 mm where the ACoA may be identified as a high velocity signal. The PCA is identified immediately posterior to, and in a similar craniocaudad position to, the MCA origin at between 55 and 80 mm depth, with flow directed towards the probe. At 80 mm depth, a bidirectional signal is identified from the tip of the BA and contralateral PCA. The intracranial ICA is identified at approximately 65 mm

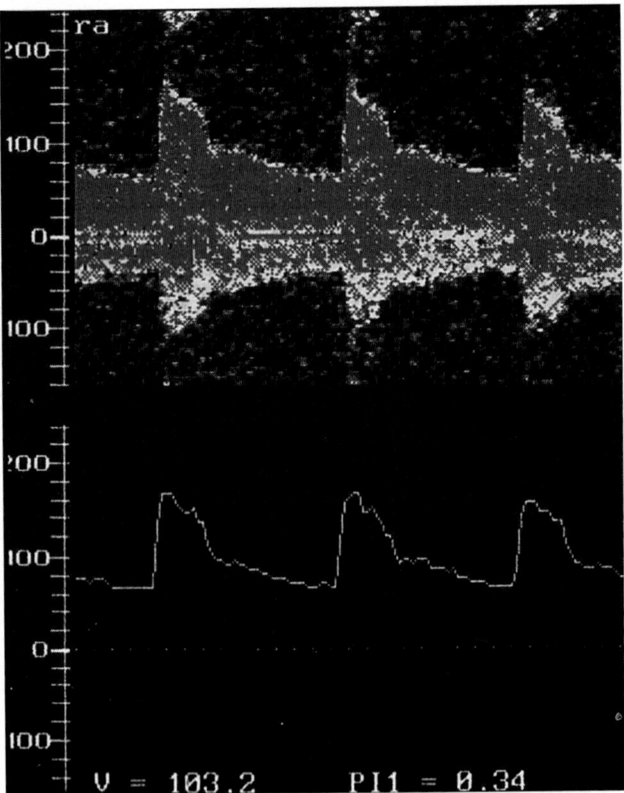

Fig. 17.3 Normal spectral TCD signal obtained from the terminal ICA through the temporal bone window—the top part of the image shows the 'raw' signal with the ipsilateral MCA signal above the baseline (directed towards the probe) and the ipsilateral ACA signal below the baseline (directed away from the probe); the lower part of the image shows the computer-derived tracing of the outline of the MCA waveform from which the peak and mean velocity and pulsatility index are derived. For colour, see Plate 17.3 (between pp. 308 and 309).

Table 17.1 Normal values for blood velocities in the basal intracranial arteries [1]

	Age	Mean	Range (±2SD)
MCA			
Peak velocity	<40	94.5	67.3–121.7
Peak velocity	40–60	91.0	57.2–124.8
Peak velocity	>60	78.1	58.1–108.1
Mean velocity	<40	58.4	41.6–75.2
Mean velocity	40–60	57.7	34.7–80.7
Mean velocity	>60	44.7	22.6–66.9
Pulsatility index	20–45	0.71	0.51–0.91
Pulsatility index	46–63	0.94	0.66–1.22
ACA			
Peak velocity	<40	76.4	42.6–110.2
Peak velocity	40–60	86.4	46.2–126.6
Peak velocity	>60	73.3	32.7–113.9
Mean velocity	<40	47.3	21.3–73.3
Mean velocity	40–60	53.1	32.1–74.1
Mean velocity	>60	45.3	18.3–72.3
PCA			
Peak velocity	<40	53.2	30.6–75.8
Peak velocity	40–60	60.1	19.1–101.0
Peak velocity	>60	51.0	27.2–74.8
Mean velocity	<40	34.2	18.6–50.0
Mean velocity	40–60	36.6	17.0–56.4
Mean velocity	>60	29.9	11.3–48.5

depth as a bidirectional low velocity signal caudad to its bifurcation.

The BA is identified through the foramen magnum at between 65 and 100 mm depth in the midline with flow directed away from the probe towards the vertex. The terminal VAs are identified more superficially and laterally to the BA at the craniocervical junction.

The ophthalmic arteries are identified through the orbits at between 35 and 60 mm depth with flow directed towards the probe. The ICA siphon may be identified at around 65 mm depth through the orbit posterior to the ophthalmic arteries. The contralateral ACA is identified by moving the probe to the lateral part of the orbit and angling medially—the ACA gives a signal directed towards the probe usually at a higher velocity than the ICA siphon. It is vital to remember to *reduce* the power output to less than 10% of maximum if examining through the orbit.

It is usual to examine both MCAs and both ACAs. The PCAs and BA are more difficult to examine reliably. The ophthalmic arteries and ICAs can supply additional useful information depending on clinical circumstances. The range of normal values for each basal intracranial artery is shown in Table 17.1. As the sample volume is generally larger than the diameter of the vessel insonated, a broad spectrum of velocities is normally detected rather than the crisp narrow signal band found on Doppler ultrasound of peripheral arteries.

Cerebral arterial blood velocities are influenced by age, posture, respiration ($Pa\text{CO}_2$) and therefore hyperventilation, haematocrit, blood viscosity and intracranial pressure (ICP), all of which should be taken into consideration in the interpretation of the TCD signal. In practice, the age of the patient and their respiration are the most important [1]. Normally the MCA blood velocity signals should be symmetrical in amplitude with no more than 20% difference in mean velocity between the two sides. The ACA and PCA are more variable because of the normal variability in anatomy of the circle of Willis, but generally there should be no more than 25% difference between the ACAs and 22% difference between the PCAs. Usually the velocity in the ACA is slightly lower than the ipsilateral MCA, but it may be higher (and still be normal) if one ACA (A1 segment) supplies both distal ACAs (A2 segments) when the contralateral ACA is hypoplastic or absent. Similarly, if the PCA arises from the ipsilateral ICA via a dominant PCoA, and the connection with the BA is absent (persistent 'fetal pattern'), then the PCA signal will only be detected going away from the probe at around 55–65 mm depth. These 'normal' and frequent anatomical variants must be kept in mind when interpreting the TCD examination.

With colour TCD, the grey-scale image and colour Doppler information help correct identification of the basal intracranial arteries (Fig. 17.4), but considerable operator skill is still required [2]. It is also possible to identify aneurysms (Fig. 17.5), arteriovenous malformations, venous signals and arterial displacement from masses. The grey-scale image can yield some information about haematomas, infarcts, areas of brain oedema, tumours and calcification. 'Power' Doppler yields more information by making the arteries more visible and showing them in greater detail; it is the author's preferred mode of examination. Intraoperative transcranial ultrasound is gaining in acceptance and usefulness in neurosurgery, but is beyond the scope of this chapter.

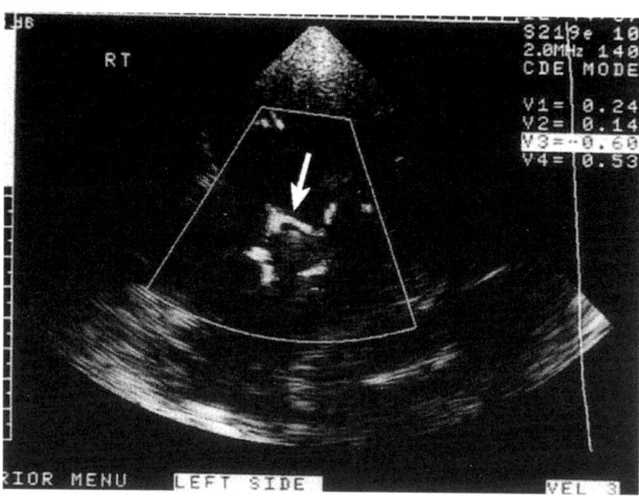

(a)

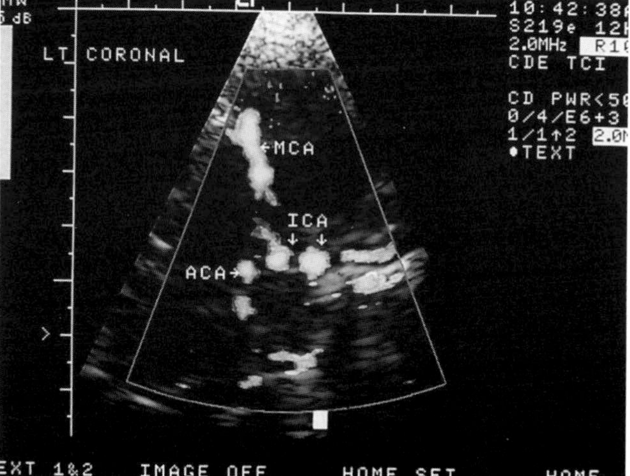

(b)

Fig. 17.4 Colour TCD image of the normal circle of Willis: (a) with PCoA (arrow); (b) another view in a different patient. ACA, MCA, anterior and middle cerebral arteries; ICA, internal carotid artery. For colour, see Plate 17.4 (between pp. 308 and 309).

Pitfalls

There are numerous traps for the unwary, inexperienced, TCD operator but careful attention to detail and to the few basic principles outlined above should help to ensure correct artery identification and avoid important errors. On spectral TCD it is essential to obtain the best arterial velocity signal at each sample point (best amplitude and highest velocity) because this is likely to represent the best angle of incidence and therefore the most accurate velocity reading. A good amplitude signal with crisp outline assists the computer analysis of the mean velocity and pulsatility index. Weak signals result in miscalculated mean velocities and pulsatility indices. In order to obtain the best signal through the temporal bone window it may be necessary to track all over the temporal area remembering that there are three imaginary windows (see Fig. 17.1), but that in any individual patient the true window may be extremely small. It may be necessary to go as far posteriorly as the tragus, as far anteriorly as the outer canthus of the eye, as well as inferiorly to the zygomatic arch and superiorly to the upper margin of the masseter insertion. Small slow movements of the probe are best as it takes a moment for the TCD apparatus to detect and compute the returning ultrasound beam into the Doppler signal. Too rapid movement of the probe over the skin surface can lead to confusion about the arterial position and may increase the time taken to identify the artery correctly.

The depths given above at which the MCA, ACA and PCA are identified are very rough guides and may vary in patients with very narrow or very broad heads. In general, the PCA should never be identified more superficially than 55 mm depth. Only the MCA is usually identified more superficially than 55 mm depth, therefore to ensure correct MCA identification it is necessary to trace the MCA superficially to 45 or even 35 mm depth. The ICA syphon should not be confused with the ACA. The ACA velocity is usually higher than that in the ICA but slightly less than that in the MCA (see Table 17.1).

In patients with occlusive cerebrovascular disease the direction of flow in the arteries may be reversed, for example proximal MCA occlusion may result in reversed,

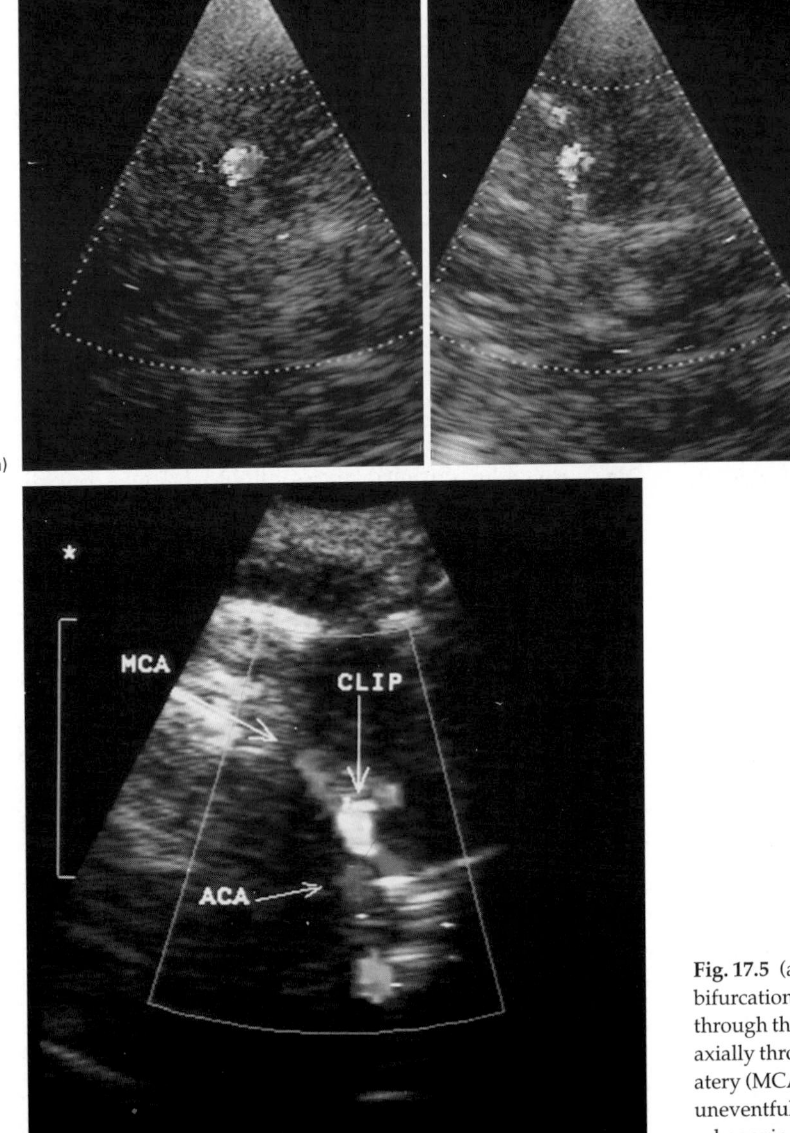

Fig. 17.5 (a) Colour flow TCD images of an asymptomatic MCA bifurcation aneurysm. The image was obtained in the axial plane through the temporal bone window. (b) Colour flow TCD image axially through the temporal bone window of the middle cerebral atery (MCA) mainstem and proximal branches following an uneventful clipping of an MCA bifurcation aneurysm. Note the echogenic aneurysm clip. ACA, anterior cerebral artery. For colour, see Plate 17.5 (between pp. 308 and 309).

damped flow in the more superficial MCA. To avoid confusion in such circumstances it is essential to examine all the basal intracranial arteries including the ophthalmc arteries. The arterial blood velocity and direction of flow in one artery cannot be interpreted in isolation from the other arteries.

Remember that the A1 (proximal) segment of the ACA is hypoplastic or absent in approximately 20% of normal people. The ACoA is absent in 9% of the population. The PCA arises predominantly from the ICA syphon in approximately 30% of the population and from the BA, with or without some communication from the ICA, in the remainder. Variation in the VA territory is even more common. Compression tests may be useful in assisting in identification of each artery but care should be taken when employing these techniques in patients with ischaemic cerebrovascular disease.

Clinical applications of TCD ultrasound

Detection of vasospasm following subarachnoid haemorrhage

'Vasospasm' leading to cerebral ischaemia is responsible for approximately one-third of the morbidity and mortality after subarachnoid haemorrhage (SAH). 'Spasm' of the basal intracranial arteries can be detected easily with TCD as a rise in peak and mean velocity above the upper limit of normal (see Table 17.1; Fig. 17.6). A mean velocity over approximately 120 cm s^{-1} in the MCA correlates with early angiographic vasospasm. The higher the velocity, the worse the vasospasm [3]. Clinical deficits occur when the MCA or ACA mean velocities reach 180–200 cm s^{-1} or greater. Usually the blood velocities rise in the first week after SAH reaching a peak at about 7 days and thereafter gradually declining. However, velocities can rarely rise very rapidly (i.e. within the first 24 h after SAH) or not rise significantly until much later in the course of the disease (i.e. after 10 days). The majority of patients will have some elevation of blood velocities in the first 2 weeks after SAH although only a proportion of those patients will develop symptoms of cerebral ischaemia. Ischaemia is not just due to vasospasm but may be compounded by raised ICP, dehydration or hypotension even if apparently mild. The cerebral arterial blood velocities should not therefore be read in isolation (see below for effect of ICP). Numerous studies have attempted to increase the specificity of TCD for detecting patients at high risk of ischaemic neurological deficit secondary to vasospasm presymptomatically. In general the patients with highest velocities (over 200 cm s^{-1} mean) and patients whose velocities rise very rapidly in the first few days after SAH (between 30 and 50 cm s^{-1} per day rise in mean velocity) are at greatest risk. When using TCD to detect 'vasospasm' it is essential to ensure that the very highest velocity is detected. As the vasospasm worsens, not only does the mean velocity rise but the intensity of the ultrasound signal may decrease making it more difficult to detect the very high velocities sometimes found in patients with severe spasm. Care is essential to ensure correct identification of the peak velocity.

Colour TCD imaging has been used to identify intracranial aneurysms (see Fig. 17.5), with reasonable sensitivities and specificity, but is still undergoing evaluation so it is too early to know its true reliability.

Atherosclerotic ischaemic cerebrovascular disease

In acute ischaemic stroke, where there is occlusion of the mainstem of one of the basal intracranial arteries or major branch occlusion, the blood velocity in the symptomatic artery is usually reduced in comparison with the opposite side [4]. In a typical MCA mainstem occlusion the velocity may be reduced to less than half of that on the normal side, or even to zero. The ipsilateral ACA and/or PCA velocities may be increased in comparison with the asymptomatic side due to supply of collateral flow to the symptomatic MCA territory. Frequently the velocity in the symptomatic artery will rise over the week following the

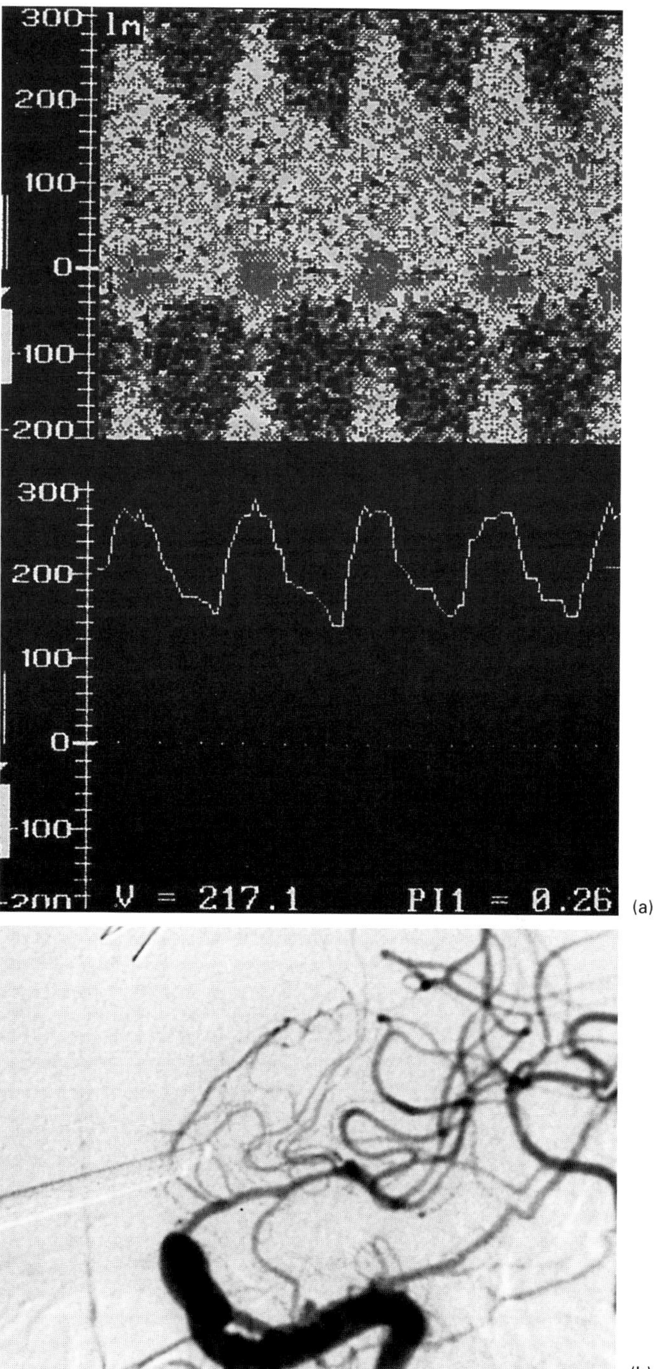

Fig. 17.6 (a) Middle cerebral artery blood velocity and (b) cerebral angiogram 1 week after SAH showing high mean blood velocity (217 cm s^{-1}). In the MCA and corresponding marked spasm. Note how pale the spectral signal is in (a)—compare with Fig. 17.3—due to fewer red cells passing along the narrowed artery and consequently diminished echo amplitude. Note also the turbulence (dark red signal near the baseline) in keeping with severe spasm. For colour, see Plate 17.6 (between pp. 308 and 309).

stroke as the arterial occlusion spontaneously recanalizes, and may even rise above that on the normal side if there is a period of hyperaemia following recanalization (Fig. 17.7). TCD is useful in the diagnosis of major cerebral artery occlusion following an acute ischaemic stroke but at present there is little clinical use for this information, so TCD is largely a research tool. Colour TCD imaging probably improves the accuracy of identification of occluded arteries by increasing the operator's confidence that the 'missing' artery has not simply been overlooked.

(a)

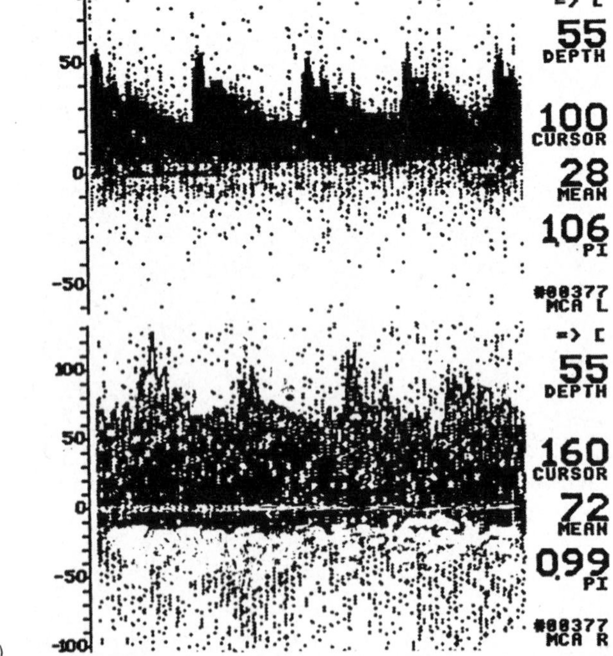

(b)

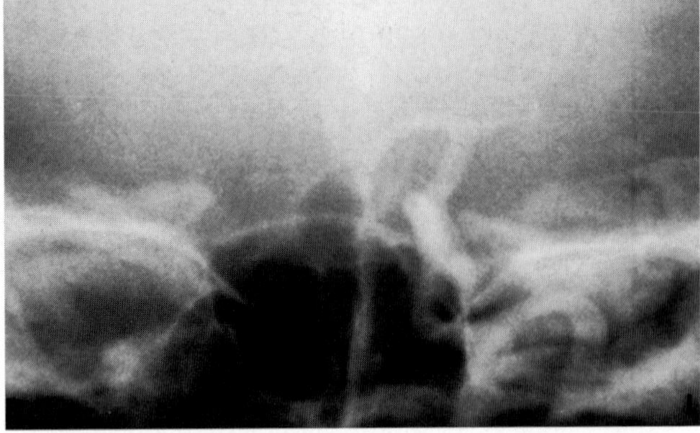

Fig. 17.7 (a) Spectral TCD waveform from the left (top) and right (bottom) MCA obtained within 6 h of onset of an acute ischaemic stroke due to occlusion of the left MCA mainstem. Note the left MCA velocity is reduced (28 cm s^{-1}) although still clearly detectable . The right MCA velocity is normal (72 cm s^{-1}). (b) Corresponding left ICA angiogram showing occlusion of the left MCA mainstem. The author has often found that the blood velocity is still detectable even in the presence of angiographically demonstrated complete occlusion.

In patients with transient ischaemic attacks, TCD may provide information to supplement Doppler ultrasound of the cervical carotid arteries. TCD is sensitive to stenoses in the MCAs (which may be a cause of stroke or TIA) by detecting a focal area of increased blood velocity (Fig. 17.8). The detection of stenosis or occlusion of the ACA and PCA is less reliable than of the MCA in view of the greater variability of the anatomy of these arteries. In patients with tight cervical ICA stenosis or occlusion, reversed flow in the ipsilateral ophthalmic artery and ACA, and increased velocity in the ipsilateral PCA may be detected indicating supply of collateral blood flow to the ipsilateral hemisphere.

TCD has also been used to assess patients with stenosis of the cervical ICA prior to carotid endarterectomy, by examining the response of the MCA blood velocity to changes in arterial CO_2 concentrations ($Paco_2$). Failure to respond to increased $Paco_2$ (e.g. by rebreathing exhaled air) suggests that the arteries are already maximally vasodilated, therefore the ICA lesion is haemodynamically significant. However, many carotid surgeons do not require this information when deciding on whether or not to operate on a carotid stenosis, or on the technique of surgery (e.g. whether to shunt or not).

Intraoperative monitoring

TCD has been variably used to monitor patients during carotid endarterectomy to look for significant reduction in the ipsilateral MCA blood velocity following clamping of the carotid artery in the neck as a guide to the use of intraoperative shunts and also for detection of embolic material passing into the cranial circulation. There is no general consensus on this use; however, some surgeons routinely using TCD, others never.

Diagnosis of brain death

Brain death following head injury or other intracranial event is associated with very high ICP and stasis of the arterial blood flow into the head. These changes are mirrored in the blood velocity waveform detected in the basal intracranial arteries [5]. Characteristic changes in MCA velocity waveform occur with increasing levels of ICP. Pulsatility increases and mean velocity decreases as ICP rises. When the ICP reaches extremely high levels, diastolic flow ceases or reverses and a brief burst of forward flow occurs only during systole. This pattern occurs consistently in brain death (Fig. 17.9). However, in the UK the diagnosis of brain death is based on clinical criteria not TCD findings. TCD may be useful for monitoring patients with head injury, SAH or other severe intracranial problem as pulsatility changes may provide useful warning of changes in ICP. This is non-specific and may

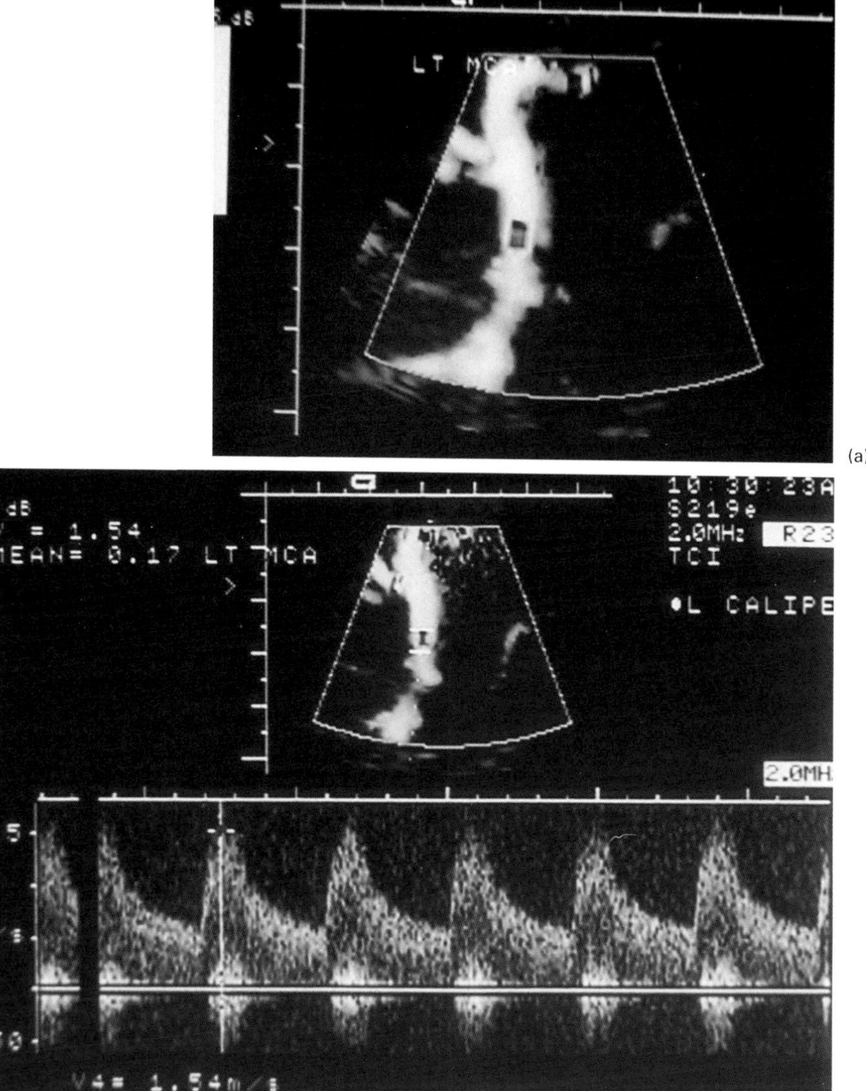

Fig. 17.8 Colour TCD of an MCA stenosis. (a) Colour 'power' Doppler image shows the MCA and its major branches with a calcified plaque causing stenosis in its mainstem. (b) Velocity waveform from the region of the stenosis shows high, turbulent velocity. For colour, see Plate 17.8 (between pp. 308 and 309).

be due, for example, to hydrocephalus, diffuse brain swelling, rebleed following subarachnoid haemorrhage, enlarging haematoma, and so on. The absolute value of the ICP cannot yet be predicted from TCD recordings at any one time (direct ICP monitoring is still required) but the trend in TCD velocity and pulsatility may be a useful warning of rising ICP.

Detection of emboli

Transcranial Doppler is very sensitive to embolic material in the cerebral circulation, whether air bubbles or particulate matter [6]. Air emboli tend to produce low amplitude, high frequency multiple showers or 'blips' in the Doppler trace, whereas particulate matter tends to produce discrete, solitary, higher amplitude 'blips' superimposed on the Doppler waveform and identified as an audible 'popping' noise. It is not possible to identify the nature of the embolus conclusively from the appearance or noise on the Doppler waveform as yet (Fig. 17.10).

Air emboli have been detected during cerebral angiography, cardiac surgery and catheterization, and during carotid endarterectomy. Presumed particulate emboli have been detected in patients with prosthetic cardiac valves (in both MCAs) and in unilateral tight carotid stenosis (in the ipsilateral MCA only). Embolic noises are frequent in patients with mechanical prosthetic valves such as the Starr–Edwards or Bjork Shiley valves, but the majority of these are now known to be due to gas bubbles (not particulate emboli) sucked out of the blood by the powerful negative pressure induced by the valve motion. These last long enough to reach the intracranial circula-

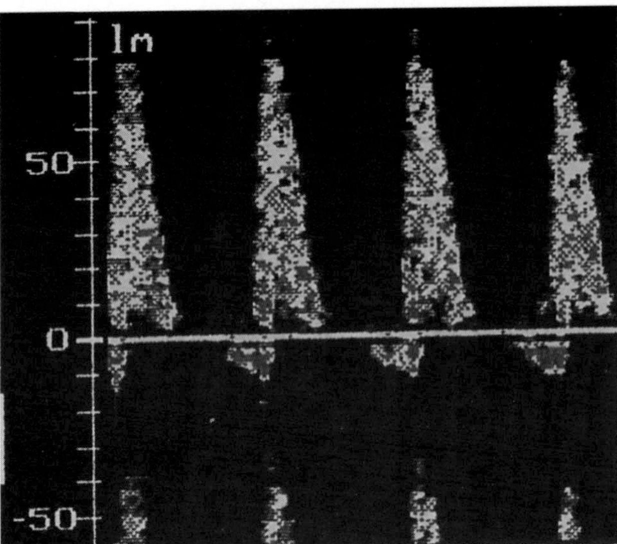

Fig. 17.9 Low velocity, high pulsatility waveform with reversal of flow during diastole obtained from the MCA of a patient with very high ICP diagnosed clinically as brain dead. For colour, see Plate 17.9 (between pp. 308 and 309).

tion before redissolving into the blood (Fig. 17.11). Early studies have suggested that there is a correlation between the frequency of detection of emboli and the risk of future stroke but further study is required.

The ability of TCD to detect emboli can usefully be used to identify patients with right-to-left intracardiac defects such as patent foramen ovale and atrial septal aneurysms (increasingly recognized as sources of embolic material in young patients with stroke) by injecting well-aerated normal saline in the anticubital vein and monitoring one of the MCAs for air bubbles [7]. Air bubbles should be extracted in the lungs so detection of bubbles in the MCA indicates a right-to-left cardiac shunt. This was previously possible also with early ultrasonic contrast agents which did not pass through the lungs. Unfortunately, modern ultrasonic contrast agents do, so cannot be used for this purpose.

Emboli counting is very time-consuming and requires considerable expertise. It is not suited to routine use at present. Periods of monitoring of up to 1 h from each artery on at least two occasions are required. Although many manufacturers say that their equipment is capable of automatic embolus detection, in fact few are accurate enough to be reliable. At present a human observer is required to detect the emboli either in real-time or from an audiotape recording. Finally, as yet, there is no clear clinical use for emboli counting so for the moment it remains a research tool. It will need to be much quicker and more reliable before it could be used in busy clinics.

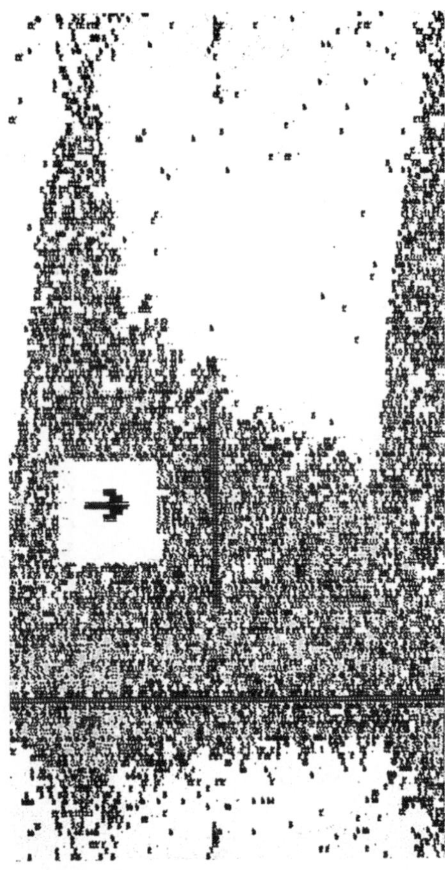

Fig. 17.10 Spectral Doppler. Example of a probable particulate embolus detected in the MCA in a patient with a prosthetic heart valve but no symptoms of cerebrovascular disease. Note the high intensity, discrete signal from the embolus (arrow) superimposed on the normal MCA velocity waveform. (Courtesy of Dr D. Grossart, Institute of Neurological Sciences, Glasgow.) For colour, see Plate 17.10 (between pp. 308 and 309).

Arteriovenous malformations

Transcranial Doppler has been used to monitor response of arteriovenous malformations to treatment [8]. Usually, significant arteriovenous malformations are associated with increased velocity in the major supplying arteries. Successful treatment is associated with decrease towards normal in the velocity in the supplying artery. This, however, is extremely non-specific and does not replace angiography or even contrast-enhanced computed tomography (CT).

Colour TCD: other aspects

Colour TCD can be used in all the applications discussed above [2]. In addition it may be possible to identify intracranial aneurysms (see Fig. 17.5), arteriovenous mal-

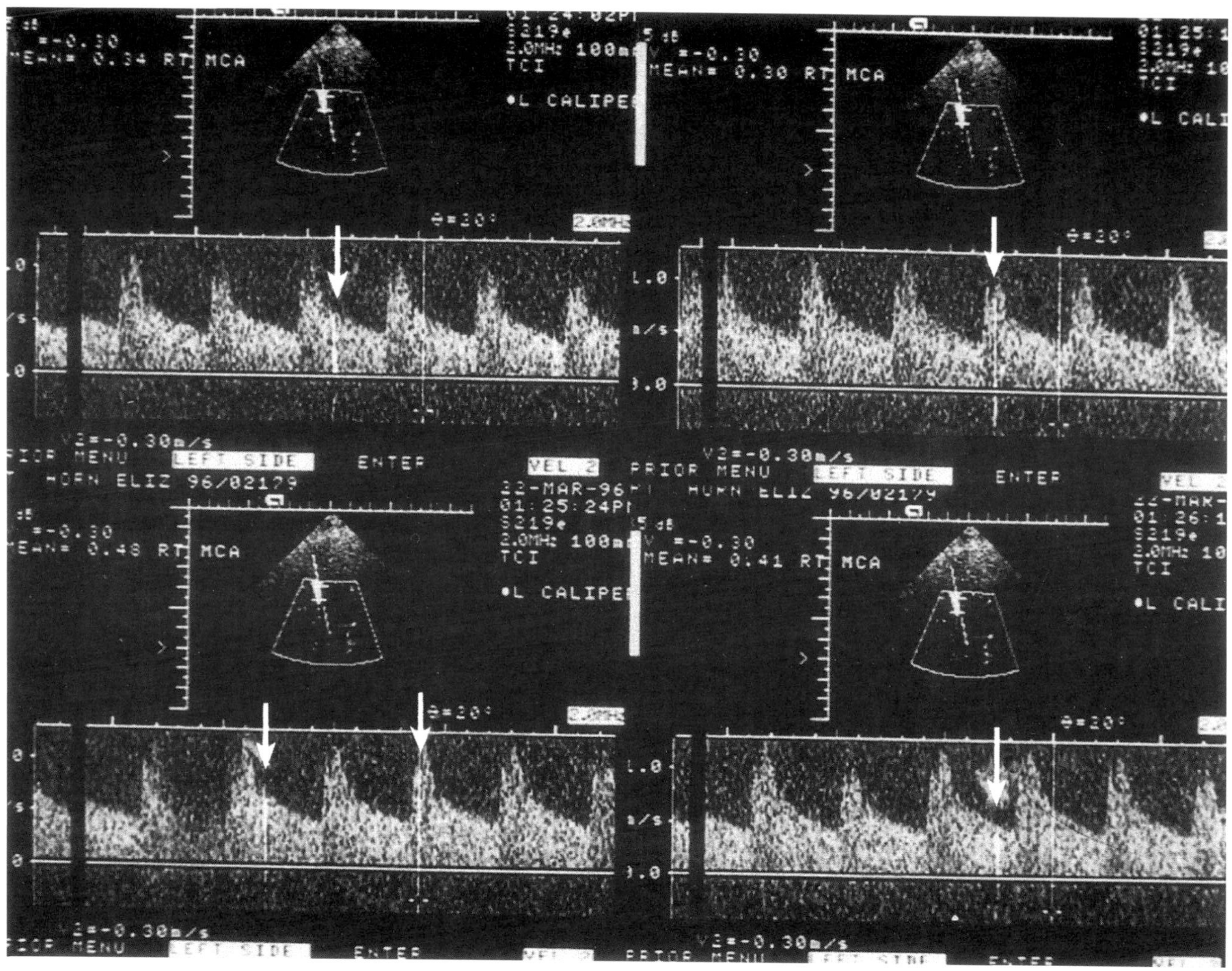

Fig. 17.11 Colour TCD image and spectral waveform from the MCA in a patient with a mechanical prosthetic heart valve. Note the frequent high amplitude signals occurring in the Doppler waveform (arrows) which are very probably due to gas bubbles sucked from the dissolved gas in the blood by the strong negative pressure of the valve motion. For colour, see Plate 17.11 (between pp. 308 and 309).

formations and possibly tumour vascularity. The brain parenchymal changes occurring in cerebral infarction, haematomas and tumours may be detected as alterations in the grey-scale image of the brain. Acute infarction is associated with swelling in the affected tissue, loss of brain pulsation in the territory in the affected vessel and, in the later stages, increased echo density corresponding with the hypodensity visible on a CT scan. Intraparenchymal haemorrhage appears as an area of increased echo density with sharp margins. Tumours appear as areas of hyper- and hypoechoic tissue associated with some swelling replacing normal brain. However, in adults, the view of the brain is rather restricted so ultrasound is of limited use for brain parenchyma imaging.

Research and future applications

At present TCD is a useful research tool in many aspects of the neurosciences and of clinical use in a few areas. It has only been possible to touch very briefly on most of these topics and the interested reader is referred to the publications listed for further details. TCD is widely used in research on SAH, ischaemic cerebrovascular disease, head injury, monitoring patients during cardiac surgery, assessing cerebral perfusion reserve and trying to improve the identification of patients at risk of stroke from embolic sources. Colour flow TCD offers further possibilities of developing all of these uses with the advantage of also providing mobile, non-invasive, grey-scale imaging of part of the brain.

References

1 Adams, R.J., Nichols, F.T., Hess, D.C. (1992) Normal values and physiological variables. In: Newell, D.W., Aaslid, R., (eds) *Transcranial Doppler*. Raven Press, New York, pp. 41–48.

2 Becker, G., Bogdahn, U. (1993) Transcranial colour-coded real-time ultrasonography in adults. In: Babikian, V.L., Wechsler, L.R. (eds) *Transcranial Doppler Ultrasonography*. Mosby-Year Book, St Louis, pp. 51–66.

3 Aaslid, R., Huber, P., Nornes, H. (1984) Evaluation of cerebrovascular spasm with transcranial Doppler ultrasound. *Journal of Neurosurgery* **60**, 37–41.

4 Ringelstein, E.B. (1988) Transcranial Doppler ultrasonography. In: Poeck, K., Ringelstein, E.B., Hacke, W. (eds) *New Trends in Diagnosis and Management of Stroke*. Springer-Verlag, Berlin, pp. 3–28.

5 Petty, G.W., Mohr, J.P., Pedley, T.A., *et al.* (1990) Role of transcranial Doppler in confirming brain death. *Neurology* **40**, 300–303.

6 Markus, H.S., Brown, M.M. (1993) Differentiation between different pathological cerebral embolic materials using transcranial Doppler in an *in vitro* model. *Stroke* **24**, 1–5.

7 Teague, S.M., Sharma, M.K. (1991) Detection of paradoxial cerebral echo contrast embolisation by transcranial Doppler ultrasound. *Stroke* **22**, 740–745.

8 Hassler, W., Burger, R. (1992) Arteriovenous malformations. In: Newell, D.W., Aaslid, R. (eds) *Transcranial Doppler*. Raven Press, New York, pp. 123–136.

Chapter 18: The peripheral arterial system

P.L.P. Allan & G.M. Baxter

The peripheral arteries

P.L.P. ALLAN

The arteries of the arms and legs supply blood to the muscles and tissues of the limbs; a variety of changes can interfere with this function and ultrasound can be used in the diagnosis and assessment of many of these problems. The majority of work is related to the lower limbs and the first section of this chapter therefore concentrates on these aspects but relevant applications in the upper limb are also covered.

Atheroma affects arteries throughout the body but the degree of severity varies to some extent for different vascular territories; in addition, disease in some territories such as the brain, heart and legs, will produce more noticeable signs and symptoms than disease in other territories, such as the arms or gut. The prevalence of symptoms of intermittent claudication varies with age, geography and sex; reported rates varying between 0.3 and 7.7% [1]. It is important to distinguish between clinically significant disease and haemodynamically significant disease in the lower limbs, where the potential to form collateral routes of supply around diseased segments is greater than can occur in relation to a diseased carotid artery. Two patients may each have a stenosis producing 80% diameter reduction but one can play a round of golf whereas the other can only walk 50 yards; the difference being that the former stenosis developed slowly, allowing collaterals to form but the latter stenosis developed acutely, so that no significant collateral channels exist.

Indications

Doppler ultrasound can be used for the assessment of several aspects of peripheral artery disease, the main uses are shown in Table 18.1.

Patients with signs and symptoms of severe, or limb-threatening ischaemia will normally be referred directly for arteriography; patients with mild symptoms will usually be treated conservatively and observed. Between these two groups lies a number of patients with moderate to marked symptoms; ultrasound can be used to identify those who might benefit from percutaneous angioplasty and distinguish them from those who will need a bypass graft. Once these treatments have been carried out ultrasound is of value in identifying potential problems, so that remedial treatment can be undertaken before the function of the artery, or the graft is significantly compromised. The value of ultrasound in the diagnosis and treatment of pseudoaneurysms and the assessment of dialysis shunts is discussed elsewhere.

Lower limb

Anatomy

The common iliac arteries arise at the bifurcation of the aorta and pass down and around the pelvic wall; the internal iliac artery branches off to supply the pelvic and perineal structures. The external iliac artery carries on to the inguinal ligament where it becomes the common femoral artery; this divides into the profunda femoris artery, which supplies the muscles of the thigh, and the superficial femoral artery, which passes down through the medial thigh to the adductor canal and the popliteal region, where it becomes the popliteal artery as it emerges from the adductor canal to lie behind the lower femur. The popliteal artery gives rise to five genicular branches which supply tissues around the knee and the sural arteries, which supply the calf muscles. The popliteal artery divides behind the upper tibia into the anterior tibial artery and the tibioperoneal trunk; the tibioperoneal trunk divides after a short distance into the posterior tibial artery and the peroneal artery. The posterior tibial artery runs down the deep, medial aspect of the calf; the anterior tibial artery penetrates the interosseous membrane and then runs distally on the anterior aspect of this membrane; the peroneal artery runs down the centre of the calf immediately behind the fibula and the interosseous membrane.

At the ankle the posterior tibial artery passes behind the

Table 18.1 Uses of ultrasound in relation to the peripheral arteries

Diagnosis and assessment of disease in patients with ischaemic symptoms
Follow-up of surgical bypass graft procedures and angioplasty
Diagnosis and treatment of false aneurysms and other pulsatile masses
Assessment of dialysis fistulae

medial malleolus and divides into the medial and lateral plantar arteries. The anterior tibial artery passes in front of the lower tibia and crosses the ankle joint to become the dorsalis pedis artery.

Technique

The examination usually begins at the groin, unless iliac disease is suspected from the clinical picture. The patient lies in a supine position and a 5–10 MHz transducer is used. The external iliac artery is identified as it passes anteriorly from the pelvis to pass behind the inguinal ligament, the origins of the profunda and superficial femoral arteries are located. Colour Doppler will identify any areas of abnormal flow which will need further assessment with spectral Doppler; if no abnormal areas of flow are seen, then a representative spectral display is recorded from the common femoral artery; this should be assessed for any changes which may indicate the presence of significant iliac disease, if this is suspected the iliac vessels will require examination (see below). The origin and proximal 5 cm of the profunda artery are examined as this may be a major collateral pathway in patients with severe superficial femoral artery disease, or it may be required as a point of origin for a bypass graft.

The proximal and mid-superficial femoral artery is examined with colour Doppler and spectral Doppler with the patient lying supine. The transducer is then moved down the course of the vessel in short steps in order to obtain a continuous assessment of the vessel. In addition to investigating any areas of abnormal colour flow with spectral Doppler, spectral displays should be obtained every 5–10 cm for assessment of any changes which may indicate significant disease in the vicinity and which have appeared as the transducer is moved along the limb.

The superficial femoral artery passes posteriorly behind the medial aspect of the femur in the lower thigh as it passes through the adductor canal. This region is better examined with the patient in a decubitus position so that the medial aspect of the knee being examined is facing upwards; in this position the adductor canal, popliteal fossa, together with the upper and medial aspects of the calf can be examined. Again, colour Doppler is performed with spectral Doppler sampling at areas of abnormal flow; routine upper and lower popliteal artery spectral traces can be obtained if no particular areas of abnormal flow are seen on colour Doppler.

The popliteal artery is followed down into the upper calf, the bifurcation into the tibioperoneal trunk and anterior tibial artery is identified and examined. The calf arteries may require a full examination if disease in them is considered to be relevant to the patient's symptoms and subsequent management. Alternatively, a brief examination to confirm, or exclude patency and obtain an assessment of the run-off may be all that is required if an angioplasty, or proximal bypass graft is being considered.

Examination of the iliac vessels is required if the patient's signs and symptoms suggest disease in these vessels, or if the appearances of the waveform at the groin suggest an abnormal segment of vessel proximally. The external iliac artery is scanned in a cranial direction as far as it remains visible; firm pressure with the transducer and moving the patient into different degrees of obliquity may help in allowing visualization of the iliac arteries. In those cases when they become obscured by overlying bowel gas the transducer should be moved to the umbilical region and the lower aorta located, the bifurcation and common iliac artery can then be located and the artery followed distally as far as possible. In most patients all or most of the iliac arteries can be examined in this way. In patients with an obscured segment of the iliac arteries it is important to assess the waveform above and below the segment concerned in order to identify any changes which suggest disease in the obscured segment; conversely, similar velocities and waveform characteristics above and below the obscured segment makes the presence of significant disease unlikely.

Upper limb

Anatomy and technique

The subclavian arteries arise from the innominate artery on the right and the arch of the aorta on the left. Each artery crosses the first rib and is then called the axillary artery; this runs down through the axilla becoming the brachial artery on leaving the axilla to pass down the medial aspect of the upper arm. Just below the elbow joint it divides into the radial and ulnar arteries, which run down the forearm to the wrist joint and into the hand where they form the deep and superficial palmar arches which supply the tissues of the hand and digits.

A 5–10 MHz transducer can be used for the examination as the artery lies superficially for most of its length, although the lower innominate artery and the origin of the left subclavian artery cannot be seen on ultrasound as they lie within the mediastinum. The upper limb arteries can be located as they leave the thoracic inlet by scanning down from above and behind the medial clavicle, the artery will be seen emerging from the mediastinum posterior to the vein. The artery is followed laterally to the clavicle and the transducer is then moved to a subclavicular position and the artery followed out through the axilla. This is facilitated if the patient is asked to abduct their arm to 90°, it is helpful if the arm can be supported in this position. The artery can then be followed through the axilla and along the medial aspect of the upper arm to the antecubital fossa, from where the radial and ulnar arteries are tracked down to the wrist. If these smaller branches are difficult to locate, scanning transversely at the wrist using colour or power Doppler can usually identify the arteries at this level; from here they can be traced back up the forearm.

In cases where thoracic outlet compression syndromes are suspected, the artery can be examined in the region of the clavicle and first rib with the arm in different positions of abduction and rotation. The point of compression may be seen directly, or changes in the waveform beyond the point of compression may provide indirect evidence of compression [2].

Assessment of peripheral vascular disease

In the assessment of carotid disease there is a strong correlation between the severity of the stenosis and the clinical significance of the disease. This is less true for disease in the peripheral arteries, where the opportunity is much greater for collateral circulation to develop and thus reduce the clinical significance of a stenosis which is haemodynamically significant. This means that the findings of the ultrasound examination must be taken in conjunction with the whole clinical picture and not be considered in isolation.

Direct measurement

Direct measurement, either diameter or area reduction, is used less frequently in the peripheral arteries than in the carotids as the vessels are smaller and lie more deeply, so that visualization and accurate placement of the callipers is more difficult. Nevertheless, disease in the lower external iliac and common femoral arteries can be measured directly if it can be clearly defined. Area measurements are better as they account more accurately for asymmetrical distribution of plaque around the circumference of the vessel, although they are marginally more time-consuming to perform. If diameter measurements are used, then the plaque must be examined in both longitudinal and transverse planes so that the most appropriate diameter is measured; this is usually the shortest diameter.

Doppler changes

POWER DOPPLER

Power Doppler is useful for locating arteries which may be difficult to identify due to a deep location, as in the adductor canal; because of disease reducing the lumen significantly; or a combination of both these factors.

COLOUR DOPPLER

Colour Doppler is of value in identifying abnormal segments of the artery which have disturbed flow as a result of disease (Fig. 18.1) [3]. Whilst experience and familiarity with the colour maps used will allow some assessment of the severity of a stenosis, these areas of abnormal flow must be interrogated subsequently with spectral Doppler in order to measure the velocity changes and use these to predict the degree of lumen narrowing.

SPECTRAL DOPPLER AND WAVEFORM CHANGES

The main changes in the waveform associated with disease are given in Table 18.2. The normal waveform in the resting lower limb has three, sometimes four components (Fig. 18.2): the initial forward flow in systole is followed by a short period of reversed flow; this is then succeeded by a further short period of forward flow, which may then be followed by a very short period of further reversed flow in younger fit patients. These variations in the resting lower limb waveform are produced by the pressure wave from one systolic episode being reflected back up the artery to interact with the subsequent pressure wave travelling down the artery. Exercise dilates the distal arterioles and capillary bed so that this reflection of the pressure wave does not occur and there is forward flow throughout the cardiac cycle (Fig. 18.2). Distal disease also affects the reflection of the pressure wave back up the artery so that loss of the normal third and/or second components is a non-specific sign of pathological changes downstream.

Proximal stenoses of haemodynamic significance will result in loss of the normal laminar flow in the artery and

Table 18.2 Changes in the spectral waveform associated with disease

Loss of the third and then the second components of the waveform
Spectral broadening
Widening of the systolic complex
Increase in the acceleration time
Damping of the waveform
Absent flow in occlusion

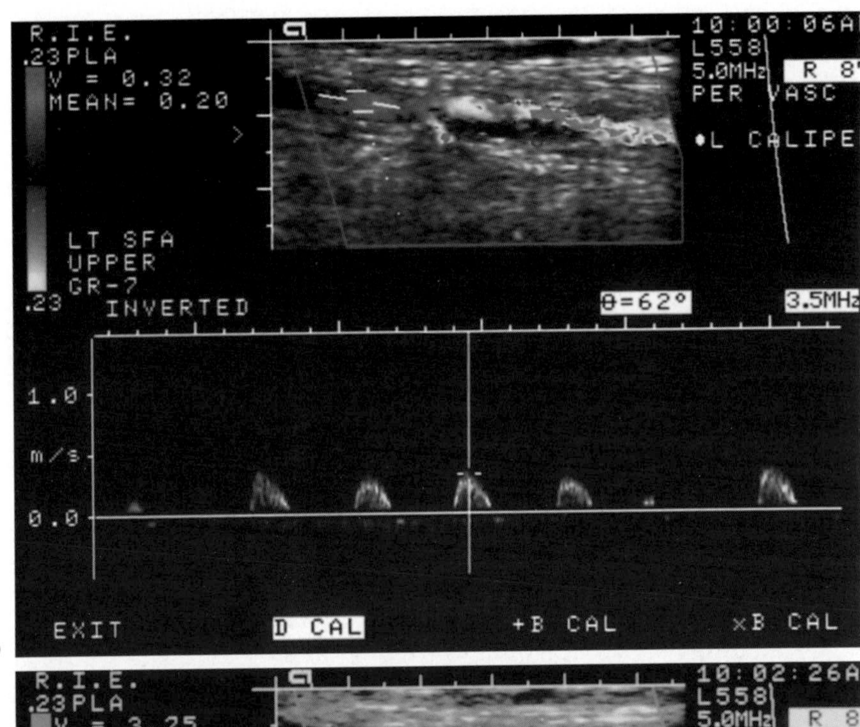

(a)

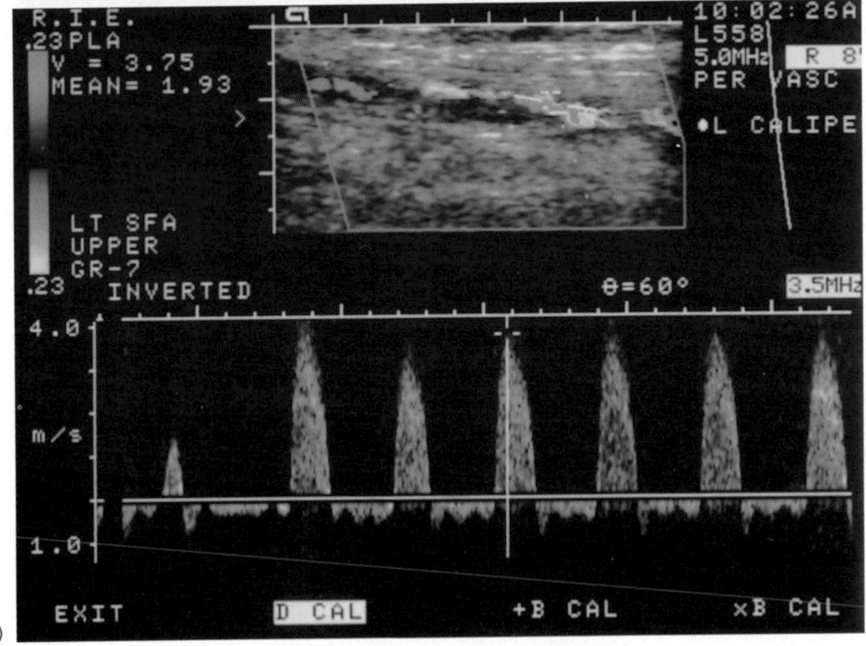

(b)

Fig. 18.1 A severe stenosis in the superficial femoral artery. (a) Measurement of a peak systolic velocity of 0.32 m s^{-1} above the stenosis; a collateral vessel is also visible. (b) A peak systolic velocity of 3.75 m s^{-1} at the level of the stenosis, which is also shown by the aliasing in the colour display. For colour, see Plate 18.1 (between pp. 308 and 309).

the generation of turbulence; these changes will affect the shape and character of the waveform beyond the stenosis. Normal laminar flow is regained over a length of several centimetres and along this segment of the artery there is decreasing turbulence which manifests as spectral broadening of the waveform. Instead of most of the blood travelling at a similar speed, which is the case in laminar flow, the turbulence results in a variety of velocities and directions of flow within the vessel which are reflected in the spectrum as a widening of the range of Doppler shifts detected (Fig. 18.3).

The presence of disease also affects the speed at which the pressure wave travels along the artery. This results in a widening of the systolic complex and an increase in the acceleration time as measured by the slope of the systolic upswing of the complex. Proximal disease can also result in the non-specific sign of loss of the second and third components of the waveform.

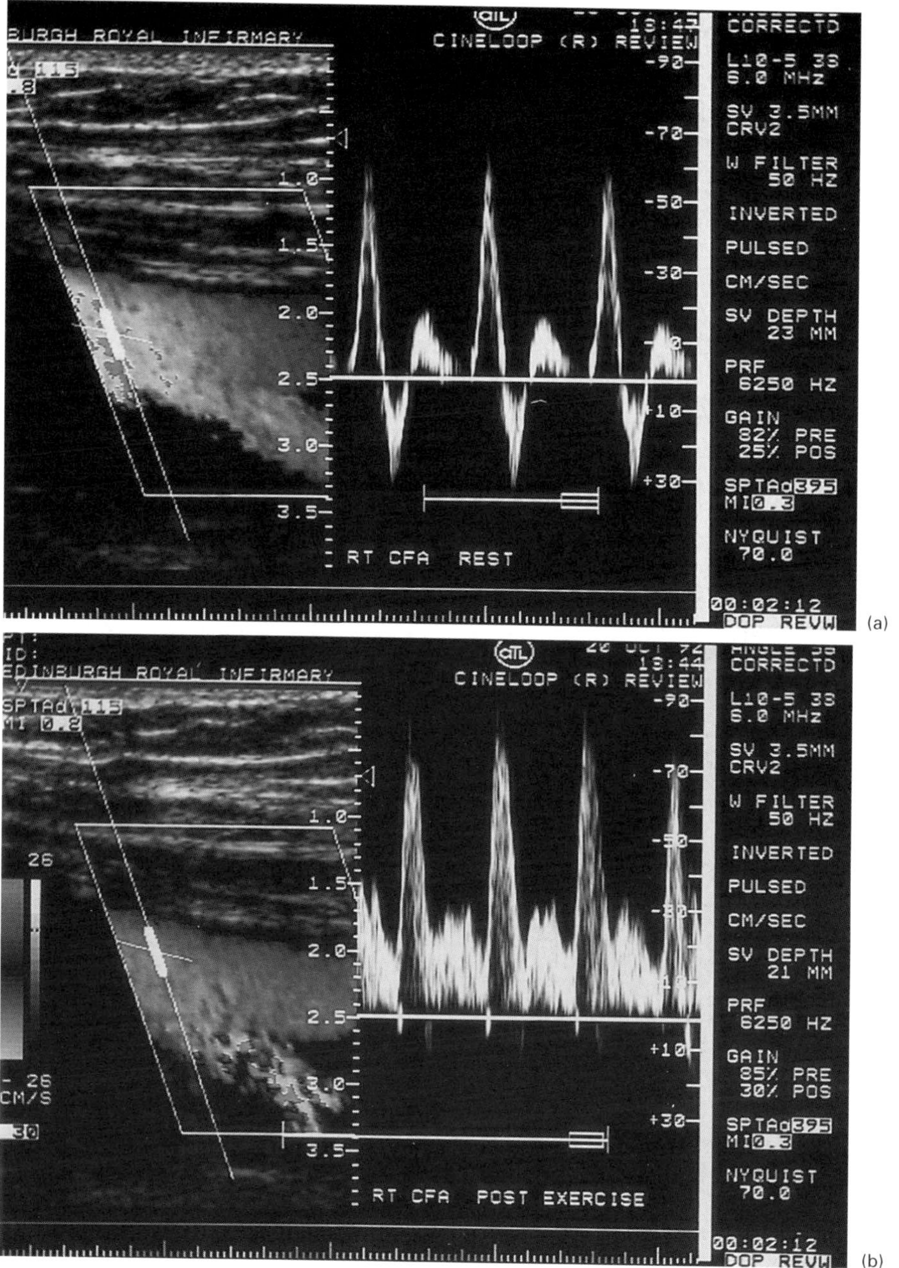

Fig. 18.2 (a) The waveform in the common femoral artery at rest. A forward, reverse and second forward phase are seen. (b) The effects of exercise with loss of reverse flow and increased diastolic flow. For colour, see Plate 18.2 (between pp. 308 and 309).

In the presence of severe disease in proximal segments with a very tight stenosis, or an occluded segment, the blood and the pressure wave pass through collateral channels. This results in marked dissipation of the velocity and pressure so that the waveform becomes very broad and flattened; this is also known as a damped waveform (see Fig. 18.3).

Identification of these waveform changes indicates that there is likely to be significant disease proximal to the point of measurement and careful examination of the proximal arteries must then be undertaken to identify the cause of these changes. This is most often the case when examination of the common femoral artery at the groin shows changes which will have arisen from disease in the iliac arteries.

SPECTRAL DOPPLER AND VELOCITY CHANGES

In addition to the qualitative changes in the waveform described above, quantitative changes in the velocity of the blood can be measured using spectral Doppler. The exact criteria used may vary depending on the equipment

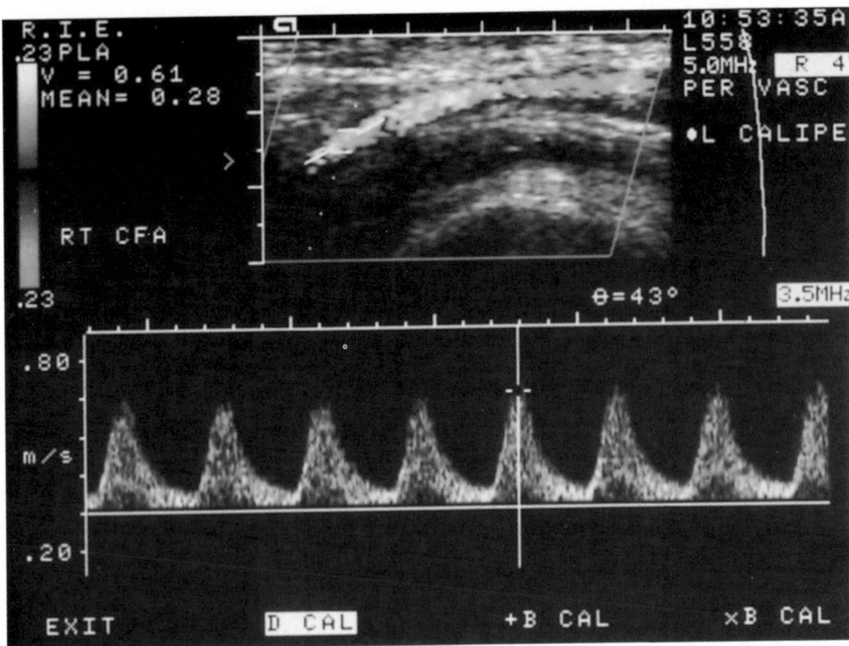

Fig. 18.3 The common femoral artery below an iliac stenosis. There is turbulence with spectral widening and some damping of the waveform. For colour, see Plate 18.3 (between pp. 308 and 309).

Table 18.3 Velocity criteria for arterial stenosis in the lower limb [4]

Stenosis (%)	Peak systolic velocity ($m\,s^{-1}$)	Velocity ratio
Normal	<1.5	<1.5:1
0–49	1.5–2.0	1.5–2:1
50–75	2.0–4.0	2–4:1
>75	>4.0	>4:1
Occlusion	—	—

and the technique employed and it is important that each department assesses carefully its results and uses those criteria which are most accurate in their hands. The criteria which this author has found to be most relevant to his practice are those published by Cossman *et al.* in 1989 [4], these are shown in Table 18.3. The velocity is measured in the usual way with the peak Doppler shift at the stenosis being located and measured; this is then converted to a velocity by obtaining the angle correction factor which allows the system to calculate the estimated velocity. As in other areas it is sound technique if the Doppler angle is kept as low as possible, and it must be less than 70° for the calculated velocity to be considered of value.

The velocity ratio is obtained by calculating the peak velocity at the stenosis and dividing it by the peak systolic velocity obtained 1–2 cm above the stenosis in a normal segment of the artery.

Accuracy of Doppler in the detection of stenosis or occluded segments

The value of ultrasound and Doppler techniques in predicting the state of the lower limb arteries has been assessed by several authors. Polak reviewed five studies performed between 1989 and 1992 [5], including the study by Cossman *et al.* [4] quoted in Table 18.3. The overall sensitivity of colour Doppler compared to arteriography for the detection of a stenosis greater than 50% diameter reduction was 87.5% (316 of 361 segments), for an occluded segment the sensitivity was 92.6% (403 of 435) and the overall specificity for the identification of normal segments was 97% (1247 of 1282). These are encouraging figures and suggest that Doppler has a useful role in the diagnosis and assessment of peripheral artery disease.

Follow-up of surgical bypass grafts and angioplasty procedures

Bypass grafts

There is a variety of surgical techniques which may be used to bypass diseased or abnormal segments of artery. The preferred option is to use autologous vein, usually the long saphenous vein, either *in situ* or reversed; alternatively, various types of synthetic material can be used, such as Goretex or polytetrafluoroethylene (PTFE). Both types of graft are at risk of failure but if the abnormality leading to failure can be identified and treated prior to graft failure then the long-term outcome for the graft is significantly better than if the graft is allowed to fail before efforts at salvage are commenced.

Early graft failure, occurring in the first 6–8 weeks after surgery, is often related to surgical technical problems or inadequate run-off; 3–5% of grafts will fail during this period, which is approximately 25% of all graft failures [6]. Failures developing in the period beginning 3 months and extending to 2 years after surgery are usually due to myointimal hyperplasia; 12–37% of grafts may fail during this period, which is approximately 70–80% of all graft failures, most of these failures will occur in the first 12 months [6]. More than 2 years after surgery a small number of failures may occur, usually due to the progression of atheroma affecting either the graft itself or the native artery. Problems other than stenosis may affect the graft and compromise its function, including dehiscence or false aneurysm at the origin or insertion, arteriovenous fistulae, infected collections and compression or kinking. Haemodynamic graft failure is said to occur if the graft remains patent but the distal circulation fails to improve and tissue ischaemia persists. An adequate programme of postoperative graft surveillance should identify problems with the graft before failure occurs and allow appropriate intervention; this reduces significantly the number of graft failures and increases the number of long-term functioning grafts [7].

The timing of scans in a surveillance programme will therefore be based on these patterns of failure. Usually the first scan is performed 4–6 weeks after surgery, subsequently a scan is done at 3 months and then at 3-monthly intervals until the end of the first year. It is not usually necessary to continue beyond this if no cause for concern exists, as the majority of failures will occur in the first year. If there are any problems which cause concern then 3-monthly scans are continued for a further 6–12 months. Grafts should also be examined whenever relevant symptoms occur as these may herald the imminent development of graft failure.

TECHNIQUE

It is useful if the request form gives details of the surgery performed, the type of graft used and the route of the graft. The origin of the graft is located using a transducer of 5–10 MHz and the native artery above the graft, the area of the anastomosis and the upper graft are examined using colour Doppler (Fig. 18.4). Any abnormal areas of flow shown on colour Doppler are assessed using spectral Doppler; if no specific areas of abnormal flow are detected velocities are recorded from the native artery above the graft, the anastomotic area and the upper graft.

The body of the graft is then examined with colour Doppler. Synthetic grafts tend to develop problems at the origin and insertion, focal problems along the graft are less common. Vein grafts may also develop stenoses at sites of incomplete valve avulsion, sites where communicating and perforating veins have been tied, or clamps applied to the vessel. In addition, *in situ* vein grafts may develop arteriovenous fistulae if a small communicating

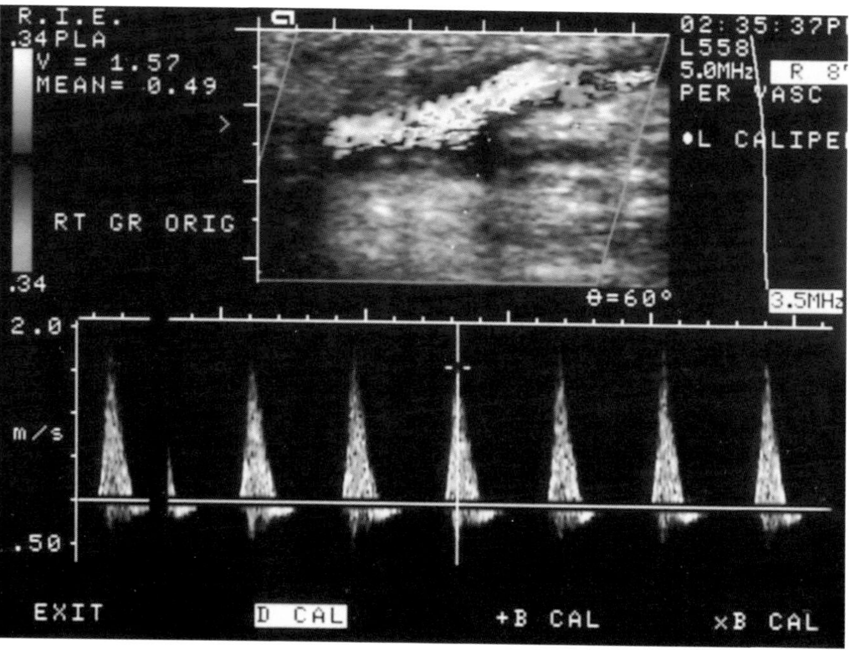

Fig. 18.4 Origin of a femorodistal graft from the common femoral artery. For colour, see Plate 18.4 (between pp. 308 and 309).

vein is overlooked at the time of surgery. It is therefore important to examine vein grafts carefully along their length and assess any abnormal areas seen on colour Doppler with spectral Doppler. If no abnormal areas are identified, routine velocity measurements are made in the upper, mid and lower segments of the graft.

The lower anastomosis, where the graft is inserted into the native artery, is then examined in a manner similar to that employed at the origin of the graft; the native artery for 3–5 cm distal to the insertion should be included in this assessment.

Sometimes collections of fluid are seen along the course of the graft; these are usually sterile collections of lymphatic fluid and will resolve spontaneously over a period of several weeks. If there is any suggestion of possible infection, aspiration using a 20–22 gauge needle can be performed for diagnostic purposes, although care must be taken not to infect a sterile collection.

CRITERIA FOR A GRAFT AT RISK

The main criteria for a graft at risk are shown in Table 18.4. The presence of a stenosis of >50% (Fig. 18.5) is a cause for concern and intervention might be considered, depending on the clinical situation. A stenosis of >70%, especially if it is associated with symptoms, or a fall in the ankle brachial pressure index (ABPI) of >0.15, is strongly associated with a graft at risk [6]. A velocity of <40–45 cm s^{-1} along the graft is also associated with subsequent graft failure. Sometimes velocities of this level are found in the last few centimetres of a long graft and appear to be of less significance but any graft with such low velocities over a significant segment must be considered at risk and any possible cause sought on ultrasound; however, it may be that an inadequate run-off is responsible.

Angioplasty procedures

In addition to identifying patients with disease who may benefit from angioplasty [8], ultrasound is also of value during the procedure and in the assessment of patients who develop problems following angioplasty, atherectomy and stent placement. Routine follow-up of angioplasty patients is not usually indicated unless there are particular concerns, or the patient develops symptoms

Table 18.4 Criteria for a graft at risk [7]

Direct measurement of stenosis	Moderate >50%, severe >70%
Peak systolic velocity changes	>1.5 m s^{-1} = 50–70% >2.5 m s^{-1} = >70% diameter stenosis
End-diastolic velocity	>0.2 m s^{-1} = >70% diameter stenosis
Velocity ratio	>2.5 = >50% >3.5 = >70% diameter stenosis
Peak systolic velocity	<45 cm s^{-1} in narrowest segment

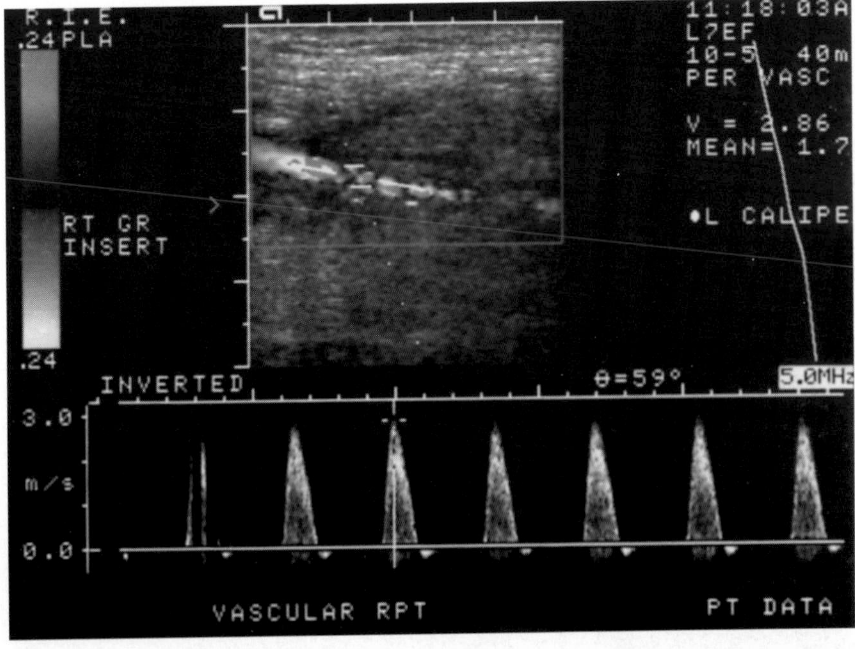

Fig. 18.5 Stenosis at a graft insertion, there is aliasing and a significantly increased velocity of 2.86 m s^{-1}, compared with 0.6 m s^{-1} in the graft above the insertion. For colour, see Plate 18.5 (between pp. 308 and 309).

which suggest restenosis. In these circumstances ultrasound allows a rapid examination of the segment which has been treated and any recurrence of stenosis can be identified and quantified, allowing appropriate management decisions to be reached. Ultrasound has been shown to be comparable to arteriography in the detection of restenosis or occlusion following recanalization of segmental occlusions in the femoropopliteal segments [9].

Other applications

Whilst atheroma is the main pathology affecting the arteries and the majority of ultrasound examinations are related to this, other abnormalities can be investigated with the technique.

Pulsatile lumps

Pulsatile lumps can be assessed rapidly using ultrasound. False aneurysms are considered elsewhere but other causes of pulsatile masses include true aneurysms, adjacent masses with transmitted pulsation and cystic adventitial disease. True aneurysms develop more commonly in the popliteal artery but may occur anywhere along the major arteries. As with other aneurysms the rate of enlargement can be followed using ultrasound. They may act as a source of emboli to the distal arteries, or result in thrombosis and occlusion, leading to distal ischaemia.

Cystic adventitial disease is a condition in which a cystic area develops in the wall of the vessel. It is a rare condition, usually occurring in the popliteal artery, or superficial femoral artery in the adductor canal; it is found in younger patients, more commonly males (Fig. 18.6). The aetiology of these cysts is unclear and various theories, including repeated trauma, ectopic synovial tissue or a congenital abnormality linking the cyst to the adjacent knee joint space or to adjacent tendons have been proposed.

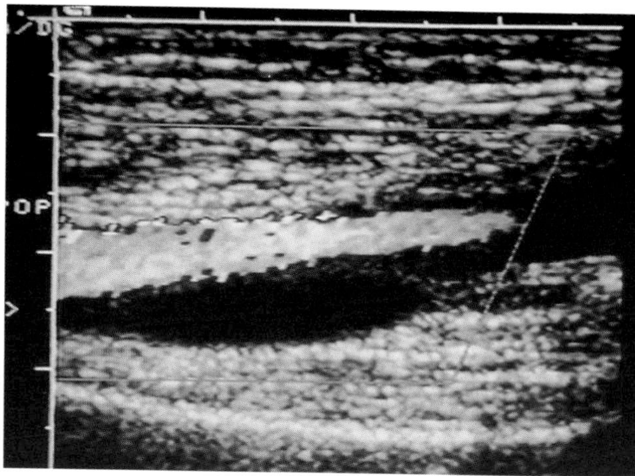

Fig. 18.6 Cystic adventitial disease of the upper popliteal artery showing the cystic degeneration posteriorly. For colour, see Plate 18.6 (between pp. 308 and 309).

Entrapment syndromes

The limb arteries may become entrapped by adjacent structures, particularly the subclavian and popliteal arteries. In patients with suspected thoracic outlet entrapment the artery can be examined as it passes over the first rib, or a cervical rib (Fig. 18.7); the arm is moved into different positions of abduction and elevation and any narrowing of the vessel, or disturbance of the spectral waveform is noted [2]. In many patients the compression of the artery will be demonstrated on abducting the arm in the supine position, although the fibrous band responsible may not be identified, colour Doppler will show the change in the velocity of the blood as the arm is elevated; in some patients, however, compression may be shown only with the patient in the vertical position. Even if the point of compression is not seen, a change in the waveform shape may suggest significant proximal obstruction on moving the arm to different positions.

In cases of suspected entrapment of an artery or graft in the adductor canal or popliteal fossa, direct examination of the vessel is often restricted by the limited access to the popliteal fossa with the knee flexed. However, careful examination of the lower popliteal artery or posterior tibial artery with the knee in different positions of flexion will demonstrate changes in the arterial waveform resulting from compression.

Conclusion

Ultrasound and the associated Doppler techniques allows many aspects of the peripheral arteries and their disorders to be assessed. In addition to primary diagnosis of arterial disease, the technique is complementary to arteriography and may be used to assess the significance of changes seen on an arteriogram. Providing care is taken with the examination and the findings are assessed in the light of the clinical picture, the technique provides an accurate, relatively rapid and cheap method for assessing the peripheral arteries. The development of newer techniques using echo-enhancing agents, harmonic imaging and power Doppler applications enhances further the potential of ultrasound in the assessment of peripheral artery disease.

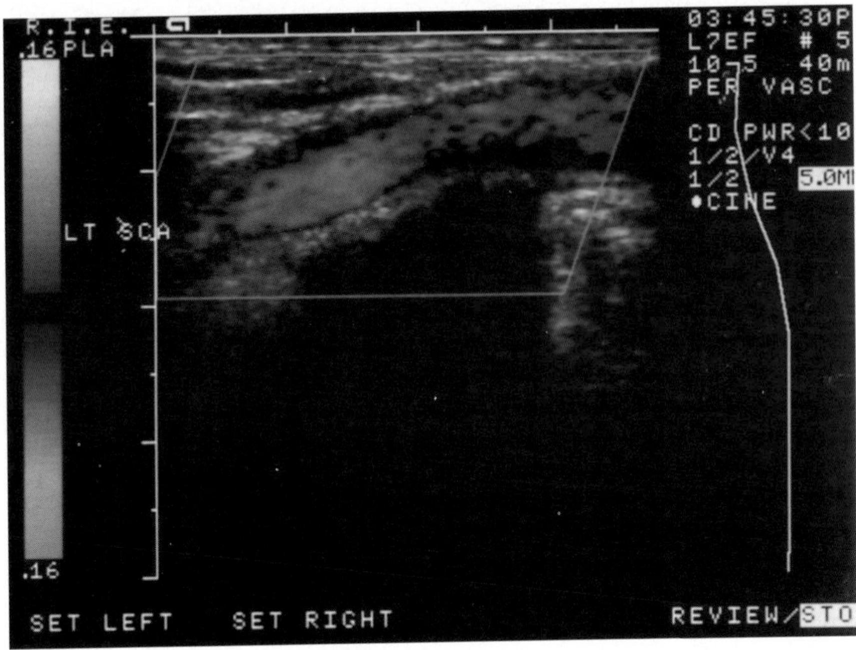

Fig. 18.7 The left subclavian artery passing over a shadowing structure corresponding to a cervical rib. For colour, see Plate 18.7 (between pp. 308 and 309).

Iatrogenic vascular injury

G.M. BAXTER

Postcatheterization pseudoaneurysms

The incidence of postcatheterization pseudoaneurysms is largely unknown although it is a relatively infrequent complication following angiography. The reported frequency varies between 0.02 and 1% [10–12] and is increasing [13,14]. Many predisposing factors exist [15] and include the use of peri- and postangiographic anticoagulation, the use of large catheters and sheaths up to 10 F in size, low femoral artery puncture and recent advances in coronary arteriography and angioplasty.

A pseudoaneurysm is a haematoma that contains flow via a persistent communication with the punctured artery. The diagnosis can be made on clinical grounds, by the presence of a pulsatile mass with an associated excessive or expanding haematoma; however, it may be difficult to diagnose especially when the groin is tender or swollen.

The diagnostic criteria are now well established with colour flow Doppler. Using this technique haematoma can be easily differentiated from pseudoaneurysm [16,17] and indeed from other angiographic complications including arteriovenous fistula [18,19]. Diagnostic features include flow outwith the confines of the artery, swirling flow in the pseudoaneurysm sac, the presence of a jet and the 'to and fro' or 'yin yang' sign in the pseudoaneurysm jet on spectral examination (Fig. 18.8). The source vessel may or may not be identified.

Historically treatment was early surgical repair. Serial ultrasound studies, however, have documented spontaneous thrombosis in up to 58% [20–22]. The main drawback of this 'wait and see' policy is that the time to complete resolution is variable, and may take up to 6 weeks. Furthermore, it is not possible to predict which pseudoaneurysms will heal although those with long jets and a tendency to form centripetal thrombus have a high incidence of spontaneous thrombosis [22]. Any decision to observe such a lesion must be balanced against the potential complications which include enlargement, compression neuropathy and rupture—a potentially life-threatening event.

Ultrasound-guided compression repair (UGCR) has resolved this dilemma in the majority. The success of this new procedure is dependent upon the elimination of blood flow within the pseudoaneurysm jet, and consequently the pseudoaneurysm sac with the induction of haemostasis and the conversion of the injury into a simple haematoma (Fig. 18.9).

Initial success rates were 71%. However, with experience and more aggressive sedation policies, this has increased to approximately 93% [23]. As with any sedation technique monitoring of the patient's vital signs is essential. Intravenous access is mandatory to allow intravenous sedation and fluid administration. Reported compression times vary significantly from less than 1 h to 2–3 h. Long compression times can be related to the continued administration of anticoagulant therapy although a recent study suggested no such relationship [24]. Solu-

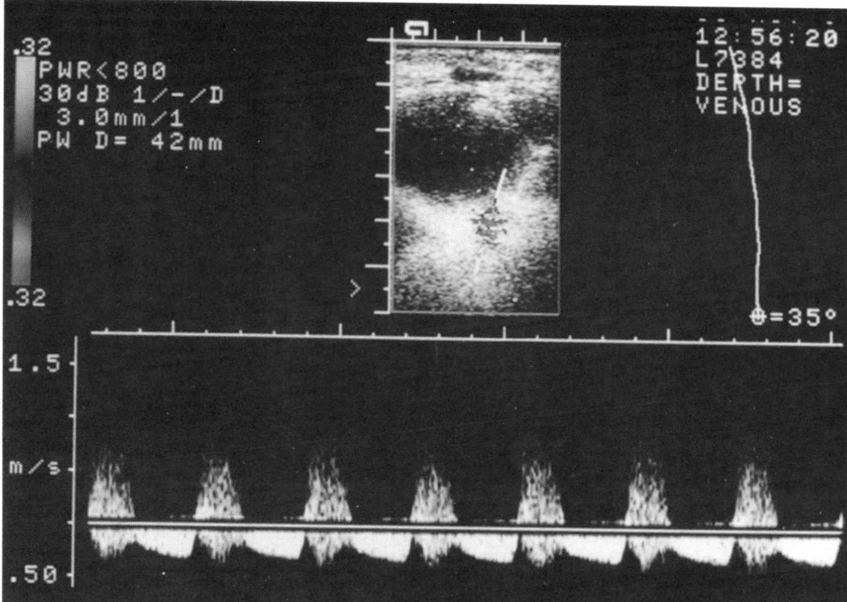

Fig. 18.8 Doppler spectrum sampled through the neck of a pseudoaneurysm demonstrating the 'to and fro' or 'yin yang' sign. Bidirectional flow is present. Blood flows into the pseudoaneurysm during systole and out during diastole. The jet velocity has no predictive value in relation to either spontaneous thrombosis or successful compression-guided ultrasonic repair.

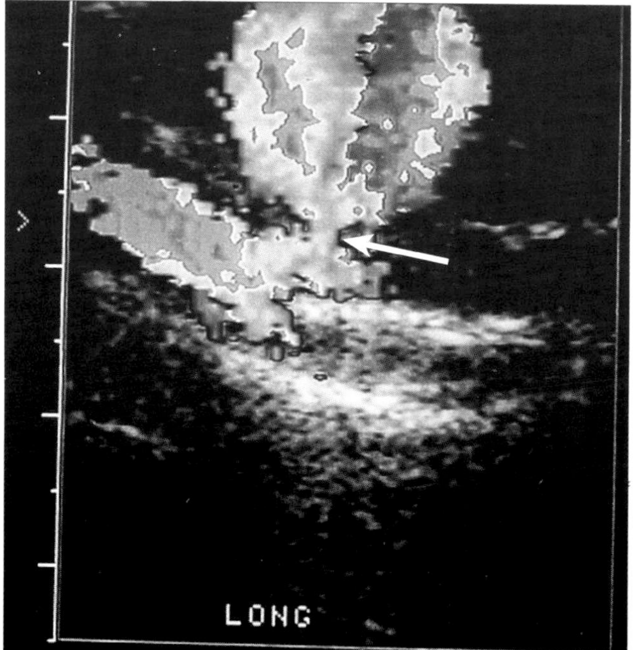

(a)

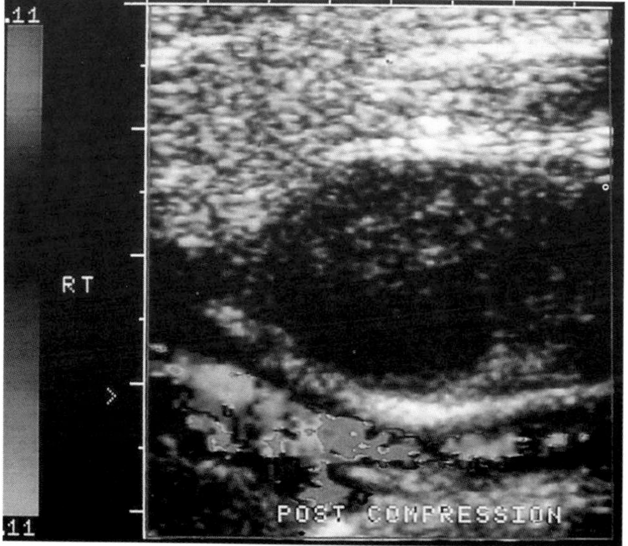

(b)

Fig. 18.9 (a) Initial colour flow ultrasound of the femoral artery bifurcation in the longitudinal axis. There is a postcatheterization pseudoaneurysm arising from the superficial femoral artery. The communicating jet is well demonstrated (arrow) whilst mixing and swirling of colour is seen within the sac itself. Following the administration of intravenous analgesia and sedation, UGCR was performed. (b) Complete obliteration of the pseudoaneurysm was achieved in 30 min with conversion into a haematoma. For colour, see Plate 18.9 (between pp. 308 and 309).

tions to this problem have included a 'tag team' approach and the development of a mechanical C-clamp device to position the ultrasound probe in the groin [25]. Complications of the technique are very rare; however, one case of femoral artery occlusion has been described [26].

In conclusion, this technique is a non-invasive, successful, cost-effective and acceptable procedure. All patients should undergo a trial of UGCR, and surgery should now only be reserved for unsuccessful repairs.

Postcatheterization arteriovenous fistula

The incidence of traumatic arteriovenous fistulae is small at less than 0.5%. Although most likely to occur following arterial catheterization, they are much less common than pseudoaneurysms [13].

The major predisposing factors include low femoral artery puncture and simultaneous catheterization of the femoral artery and vein. Their presence is normally suspected by the clinical palpation of a 'thrill'. This physical sign is thought to arise from high velocity signals hitting the venous wall, with the resultant vibration being transmitted to the surrounding soft tissues.

The diagnosis is usually made with colour Doppler imaging. The vein, most commonly the femoral, is distended and Doppler spectral analysis will show an arterialized or pulsatile venous waveform [13]. Extrinsic compression may also cause high velocity venous flow and care should be taken in distinguishing this from an arteriovenous fistula. Turbulent flow is generally more marked in the fistula (Fig. 18.10). The distinguishing acid test is the Valsalva manoeuvre. The Doppler venous signal will cease if there is extrinsic compression, whilst it will persist if there is a large arteriovenous communication.

Changes may also be present in the feeding artery. The femoral artery waveform may be monophasic due to the direct communication with the low vascular resistance vein. In isolation, such a waveform may also reflect severe proximal atheromatous disease, i.e. aortoiliac occlusion.

A communicating jet between the artery and vein can often be identified. This is best achieved with the probe in a transverse plane. Searching for such a communication without the aid of colour is time-consuming and unrewarding.

Perivascular colour artefact may be prominent in an arteriovenous fistula (Fig. 18.11), the colour signals extending beyond the vessel lumen and into the surrounding soft tissues [18,27]. This is thought to reflect soft tissue vibration secondary to the impact of the fistulous jet against the vein wall.

Small arteriovenous fistulae can be studied at regular intervals, e.g. 10–14 days. Loss of the arterialized venous signal during the Valsalva manoeuvre signifies a strong probability of spontaneous closure often within 4 weeks; however, if this persists at 1 month then surgical repair is normally required.

The technique of ultrasound-guided pseudoaneurysm repair has also been modified in an attempt to accelerate healing in arteriovenous fistulae. Only small numbers have been attempted; however, presently it is a much less successful technique than pseudoaneurysm repair [28].

The upper limb

G.M. BAXTER

Normal anatomy and technique

The subclavian artery arises from the innominate artery on the right and directly from the aorta on the left. Both subclavian arteries can be visualized via a sonographic

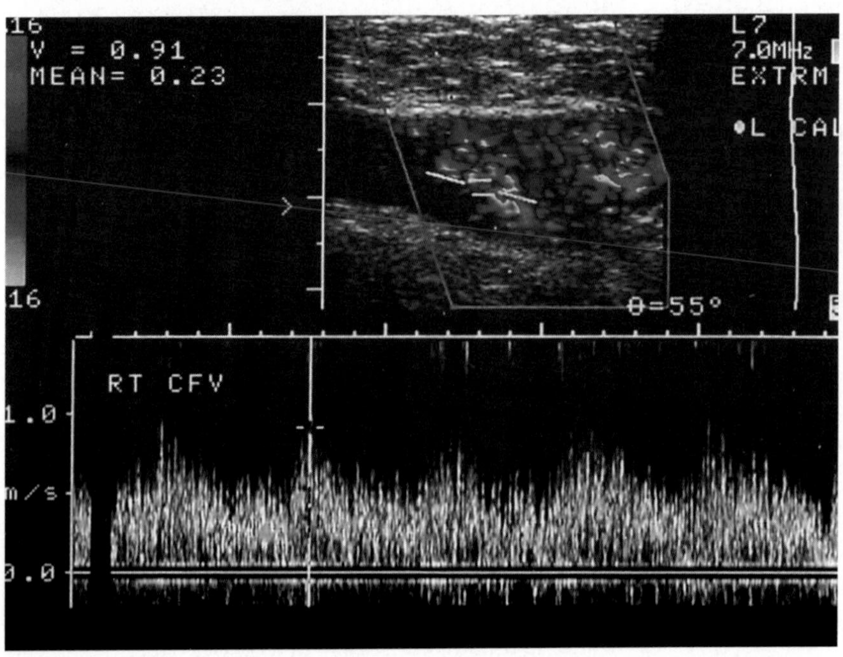

Fig. 18.10 Femoral vein Doppler waveform in a known case of postcatheterization arteriovenous fistula. The waveform within the femoral vein is arterialized and shows marked turbulent flow indicative of a fistula. For colour, see Plate 18.10 (between pp. 308 and 309).

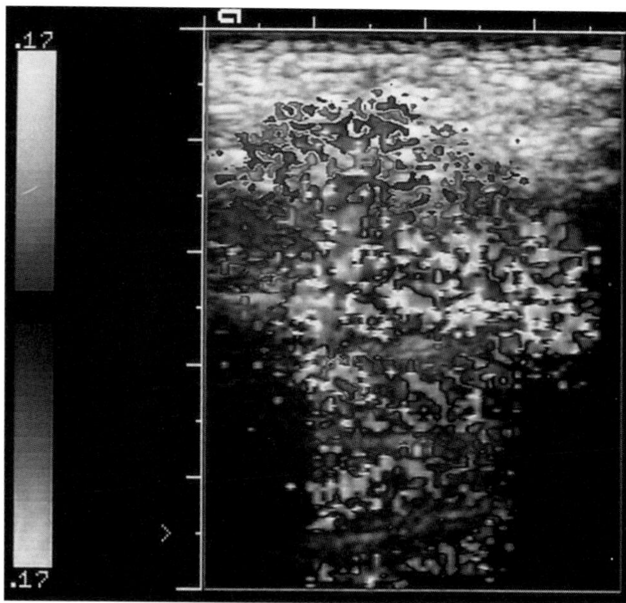

Fig. 18.11 Colour flow image of a large subcutaneous arteriovenous fistula showing marked perivascular tissue vibration. This is thought to be secondary to transmitted vibration from the vein wall. This vibration is detected as movement by the colour Doppler software and consequently coded as such. When this appearance is present it should alert the ultrasonologist to the possibility of an arteriovenous fistula. For colour, see Plate 18.11 (between pp. 308 and 309).

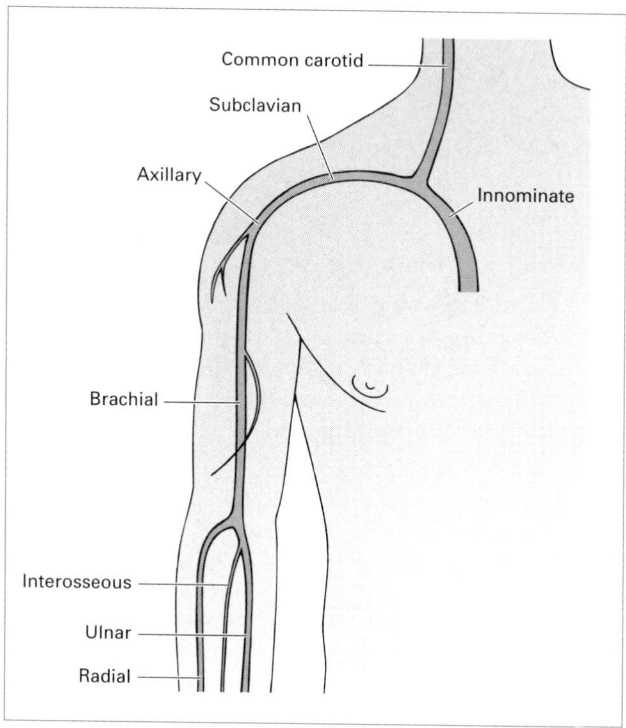

Fig. 18.12 Arterial anatomy of the upper limb.

window just superior to the sternoclavicular joints. In this position the transducer is held transversely and angled towards the feet, the subclavian artery lying superficial to the vein. On moving laterally, the subclavian artery can be visualized beneath the clavicle, the artery now lying deep to the subclavian vein and followed as the axillary artery over the humeral head into the axilla and down the arm to become the brachial artery. At the anticubital fossa the brachial artery trifurcates into the radial, ulnar and interosseous branches, respectively (Fig. 18.12). Although these small vessels can be followed to the wrist there are very few indications for performing this procedure. In the normal healthy state the Doppler spectral waveform is characteristically triphasic throughout the upper limb as these vessels supply a high impedence system distally (Fig. 18.13).

Clinically significant stenoses of the upper limb are relatively rare. The main application of colour Doppler imaging in the upper limb is in the detection of post-catheterization complications, evaluating haemodialysis shunts and detecting focal stenosis and/or aneurysms in the thoracic outlet syndrome.

Vascular disease

For the detection of arterial stenosis the same criteria used in the lower limb apply to the upper limb, i.e. a doubling of the peak systolic velocity is taken to represent a 50% stenosis. The use of the peak systolic velocity ratio proximal to and within the stenosis can be used to give an indication of the severity of the stenotic lesion (Fig. 18.14). Both the absence of colour-coded flow within the arterial lumen and the absence of a Doppler waveform on spectral analysis are indicative of arterial occlusion.

Thoracic outlet syndrome

The most common physical finding in this syndrome is the presence of paraesthesia which occurs in up to 80% of affected individuals. The ulnar nerve is most commonly affected. This may arise secondary to a cervical rib or be secondary to extrinsic tissue compression. In the diagnosis of the thoracic outlet syndrome the patient is examined supine with the arm in the neutral position, in abduction, with the patient's head first in a neutral position and then turned to each side in turn. The effect of these different positions is to induce a significant velocity change in the subclavian artery indicative of a stenosis secondary to surrounding tissue compression or a cervical rib.

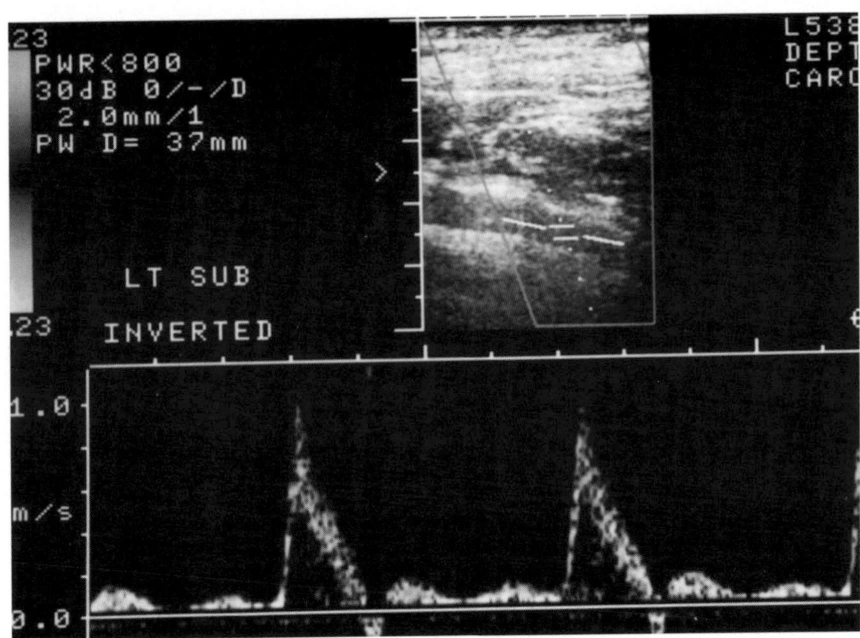

Fig. 18.13 Doppler waveform sampled from the distal subclavian artery showing a triphasic waveform. This waveform is typical of both the upper and lower limb arterial tree and is secondary to the high peripheral resistance of these limbs.

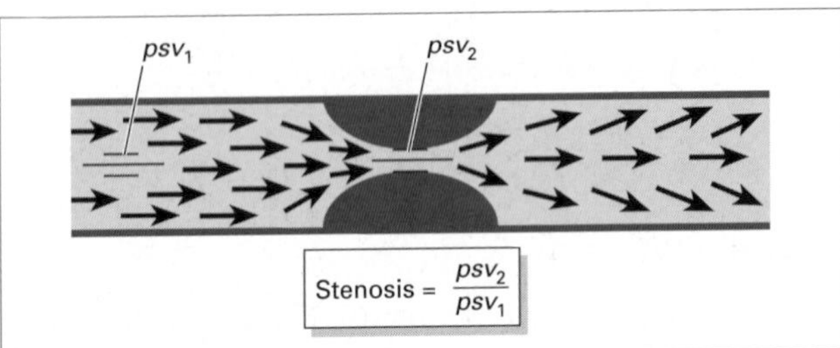

Fig. 18.14 Diagram demonstrating the relationship between the peak systolic velocity (*psv*) just prior to and within an arterial stenosis. By constructing a ratio of these two values as shown, the *psv* ratio can be used to give an indication of the severity of the lesion. A ratio of 2 to 4 is indicative of a 50–75% stenosis whilst a ratio >4.0 represents a stenosis of >75%.

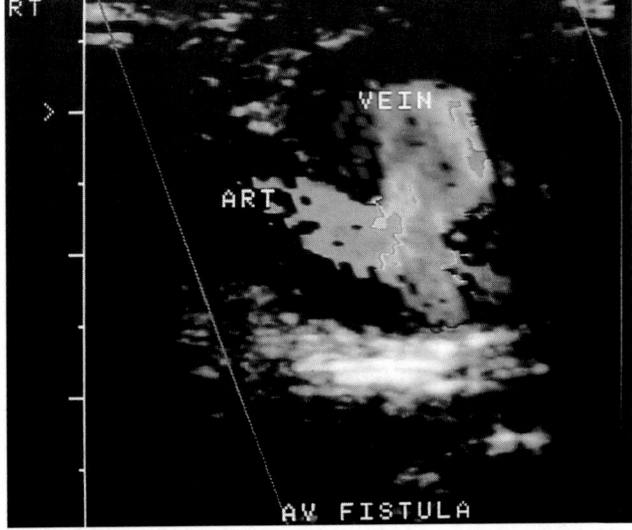

Fig. 18.15 Colour flow image of a haemodialysis fistula in the antecubital fossa demonstrating the surgical anastomosis of the brachial artery (ART) and basilic vein. This anastomosis is well demonstrated on this occasion. For colour, see Plate 18.15 (between pp. 308 and 309).

Iatrogenic complications

Complications of brachial or axillary arteriography can be easily monitored and documented using Doppler ultrasound. Suspected arterial occlusions can be confirmed or refuted and appropriate action taken depending on the ultrasonic findings. The presence of a pulsatile mass can be readily evaluated using this technique and large haematomas distinguished from aneurysms. Diagnostic arteriography in this situation is not required. If a pseudoaneurysm is confirmed then the first-line treatment option is UGCR, in a manner analogous to the lower limb. Although this technique has only been used on occasion in the upper limb, successful cases have been recorded [29].

Haemodialysis fistulae

G.M. BAXTER

Evaluation of dialysis arteriovenous fistulae can be performed using colour Doppler ultrasound as these communications are superficially situated and thus well imaged

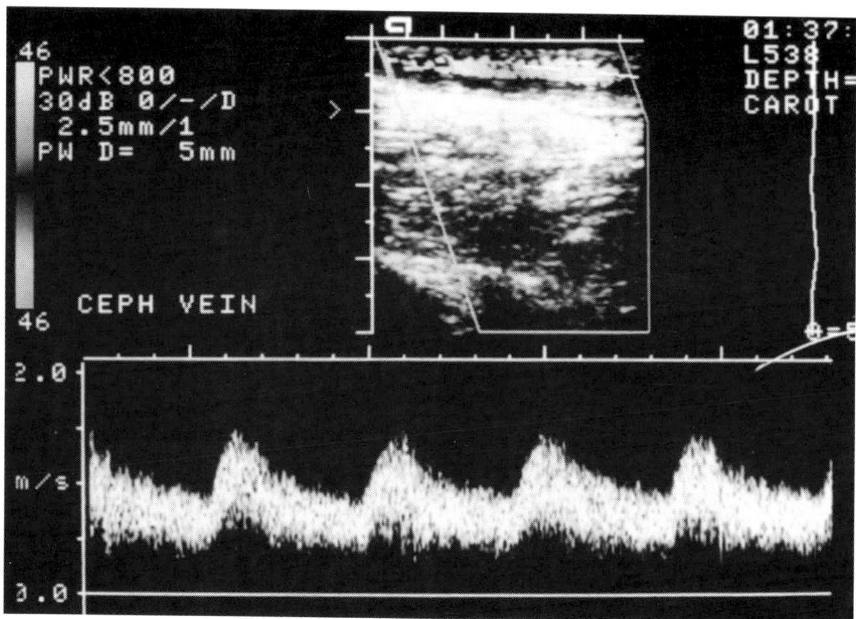

Fig. 18.16 Doppler waveform sampled from the venous side of a normally functioning haemodialysis fistula. This demonstrates marked arterialization and turbulence within the draining vein.

(Fig. 18.15). The most common site of fistula is the antecubital fossa the surgical anastomosis often being performed either between the brachial artery and the cephalic vein, or the brachial artery and basilic vein (Fig. 18.16). In addition fistulae can also be formed at the wrist using either the radial or ulnar arteries, or at the groin between the femoral artery and vein.

There are two types of surgically constructed fistulae, synthetic or autologous vein grafts. The latter is preferred. The potential complications are common to all surgically created arteriovenous fistulae and include small pseudoaneurysms, large aneurysms (Fig. 18.17), and arterial or vein stenoses. Some centres can detect stenoses with an accuracy close to 90% [30]; however, difficulty can arise when turbulent flow patterns are present which often arise secondary to tortuous and sharp bends this being a particular problem in the loop graft. However, in the straight segment of the efferent vein, the sensitivity for detecting stenoses is close to 95%. Colour Doppler ultrasound facilitates an easier examination especially for the detection of small pseudoaneurysms which although unlikely to require surgical revision in the absence of uncompromised dialysis, can be easily documented using this technique.

Haemodialysis grafts are of three main types, the Brescia–Cimino graft, straight interposition graft or loop interposition graft (Fig. 18.18). The first is a direct side-to-side connection, and the second a straight segment interposition between the artery and vein. The loop interposition graft is of a longer loop interposed between the two main vessels. The diagnostic accuracy for the detection of pseudoaneurysms is the same between the different shunt types; however, stenoses are detected with a higher degree of accuracy in the straight interposition graft due to the more complex haemodynamics within the loop graft.

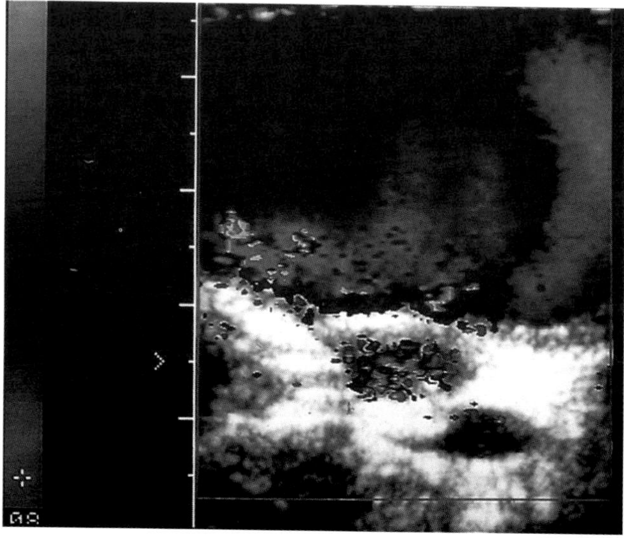

Fig. 18.17 One complication of an arteriovenous fistula is large aneurysm formation. This is easily demonstrated with colour Doppler ultrasound. A giant aneurysm sac with swirling flow is demonstrated on colour flow imaging in such a case. For colour, see Plate 18.17 (between pp. 308 and 309).

In addition to its diagnostic capability, ultrasound is the ideal non-invasive modality for the follow-up and

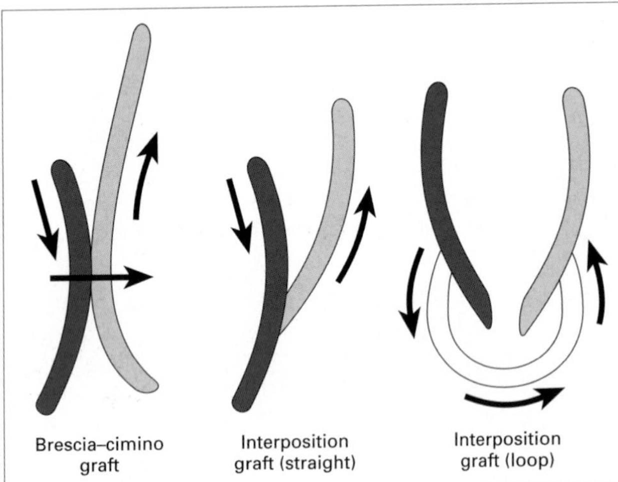

Fig. 18.18 The three main types of surgically created haemodialysis fistulae in common use. The loop interposition graft is the most difficult to image with colour Doppler ultrasound as not only is the velocity within a bend difficult to measure accurately but also flow within these surgical loops is extremely turbulent. Both of these factors make the detection of stenotic lesions difficult. ■, artery; □, vein.

monitoring of percutaneous procedures performed for the treatment of focal stenoses.

References

1 Leng, G.C., Evans, C.J., Fowkes, F.G.R. (1995) Epidemiology of peripheral vascular diseases. *Imaging* **7**, 85–96.

2 Longley, D.G., Schwabacher, S., Yedlicka, J.W., Hunter, D.W., Molina, E.J., Letourneau, J.G. (1992) Thoracic outlet syndrome: evaluation of the subclavian vessels by color duplex sonography. *American Journal of Radiology* **158**, 623–630.

3 Pellerito, J.S., Taylor, K.J.W. (1992) Peripheral arteries. In: Merritt, C.R.B. (ed.) *Clinics in Diagnostic Ultrasound*, vol. 27, Churchill Livingstone, London, pp. 97–112.

4 Cossman, D.V., Ellison, J.E., Wagner, W.H., *et al.* (1989) Comparison of contrast arteriography to arterial mapping with color-flow duplex imaging in the lower extremities. *Journal of Vascular Surgery* **10**, 522–529.

5 Polak, J.F. (1995) Peripheral arterial disease. Evaluation with color flow and duplex sonography. *Radiology Clinics of North America* **33**, 71–90.

6 Mills, J.L. (1993) Mechanisms of graft failure: the location, distribution and characteristics of lesions that predispose to graft failure. *Seminars in Vascular Surgery* **6**, 78–91.

7 Bandyk, D.F. (1993) Essentials of graft surveillance. *Seminars in Vascular Surgery* **6**, 92–102.

8 Elsman, B.H., Legemate, D.A., van der Heyden, F.W., de Vos, H., Mali, W.P., Eikelbloom, B.C. (1996) The use of color-coded duplex scanning in the selection of patients with lower extremity arterial disease for percutaneous transluminal angioplasty: a prospective study. *Cardiovascular and Interventional Radiology* **19**, 313–316.

9 Vroegindeweij, D., Tielbeek, A.V., Buth, J., van Kints, M.J., Landman, G.H., Mali, W.P. (1995) Recanalization of femoropopliteal occlusive lesions: a comparison of long-term clinical, color duplex US and arteriographic follow-up. *Journal of Vascular and Interventional Radiology* **6**, 331–337.

10 Halpern, P. (1964) Percutaneous transfemoral arteriography: an analysis of the complications in 1000 consecutive cases. *American Journal of Roentgenology* **92**, 918–934.

11 Hessel, S.J., Adams, D.F., Abrams, H.L. (1981) Complications of angiography. *Radiology* **138**, 273–281.

12 Rapoport, S., Sniderman, K.W., Morse, S.S., Proto, M.H., Ross, G.R. (1985) Pseudoaneurysm: a complication of faulty technique in femoral arterial puncture. *Radiology* **154**, 529–530.

13 Oweida, S.W., Roubin, G.S., Smith, R.B. IIIrd, Salam, A.A. (1990) Postcatheterisation vascular complications associated with percutaneous transluminal coronary angioplasty. *Journal of Vascular Surgery* **12**, 310–315.

14 Helvie, M.A., Rubin, J.M., Silver, T.M., Kresowik, T.F. (1988) The distinction between femoral artery pseudoaneurysms and other causes of groin masses; value of duplex Doppler sonography. *American Journal of Roentgenology* **150**, 1171–1180.

15 Altkin, R.S., Flicker, S., Naidech, H.J. (1989) Pseudoaneurysm and arteriovenous fistula after femoral artery catheterisation: association with low femoral punctures. *American Journal of Radiology* **152**, 629–631.

16 Mitchell, D.G., Needleman, L., Bezzi, M., *et al.* (1987) Femoral artery pseudoaneurysm: diagnosis with conventional duplex and color Doppler ultrasound. *Radiology* **165**, 687–690.

17 Sheikh, K.H., Adams, D.B., McCann, R., Lyerly, H.K., Sabiston, D.C., Kisslo, J. (1989). Utility of Doppler color flow imaging for identification of femoral arterial complications of cardiac catheterisation. *American Heart Journal* **117**, 623–628.

18 Igidbashian, V.N., Mitchell, D.G., Middleton, W.D., Schwartz, R.A., Goldberg, B.B. (1989) Iatrogenic femoral arteriovenous fistula: diagnosis with color Doppler imaging. *Radiology* **170**, 749–752.

19 Roubidoux, M.A., Hertzberg, B.S., Carroll, B.A., Hedgepeth, C.A. (1990) Color flow and image directed Doppler ultrasound evaluation of iatrogenic arteriovenous fistulas in the groin. *Journal of Clinical Ultrasound* **18**, 463–469.

20 Johns, J.P., Pupa, L.E. Jr, Bailey, S.R. (1991) Spontaneous thrombosis of iatrogenic femoral artery pseudoaneurysms: documentation with color Doppler and two dimensional ultrasonography. *Journal of Vascular Surgery*, **14**, 24–29.

21 Kotval, P.S., Khoury, A., Shah, P.M., Babu, S.C. (1990) Doppler sonographic demonstration of the progressive spontaneous thrombosis of pseudoaneurysms. *Journal of Ultrasound in Medicine* **9**, 185–190.

22 Paulson, E.K., Hertzberg, B.S., Paine, S.S., Carroll, B.A. (1992) Femoral artery pseudoaneurysms: value of color Doppler sonography in predicting which ones will thrombose without treatment. *American Journal of Roentgenology* **159**, 1077–1081.

23 Fellmeth, B.D., Baron, S.B., Brown, P.R., *et al.* (1992) Repair of postcatheterisation femoral pseudoaneurysms by color flow ultrasound guided compression. *American Heart Journal* **123**, 547–551.

24 Schwend, R.B., Hambsch, K.P., Kwan, K.W., Boyajian, R.A., Otis, S.M. (1993) Color duplex sonographically guided obliteration of pseudoaneurysm. *Journal of Ultrasound in Medicine* **12**, 609–613.

25 Fellmeth, B.D., Buckner, N.K., Ferreira, J.A., Rooker, K.T., Parsons, P.M., Brown, P.R. (1992) Postcatheterisation femoral

artery injuries: repair with color flow US guidance and C-clamp assistance. *Radiology* **182**, 570–572.

26 Fellmeth, B.D., Roberts, A.C., Bookstein, J.J., *et al.* (1991) Postangiographic femoral artery injuries: nonsurgical repair with US-guided compression. *Radiology* **178**, 671–675.

27 Middleton, W.D., Erickson, S., Melson, G.L. (1989) Perivascular color artifact: pathologic significance and appearance on color Doppler images. *Radiology* **171**, 647–652.

28 Wey, D., Delcour, C., Golzarian, J., Azancot, M., Grand, C., Struyven, J. (1991) Iatrogenic femoral pseudoaneurysm and arteriovenous fistula. Non-surgical treatment. *Journal of Radiology* **72**, 91–94.

29 Skibo, L., Polak, J.F. (1993) Compression repair of a postcatheterisation pseudoaneurysm of the brachial artery under sonographic guidance. *American Journal of Roentgenology* **160**, 383–384.

30 Middleton, W.D., Picus, D.D., Marx, M.V., Melson, G.L. (1989) Color Doppler sonography of hemodialysis vascular access: comparison with angiography. *American Journal of Roentgenology* **152**, 633–639.

Chapter 19: The peripheral venous system

G.M. Baxter

Lower limb venous imaging

There are 20 million cases per year of deep venous thrombosis (DVT) in the USA of which approximately 600000 will develop pulmonary thromboembolism, a potentially life-threatening condition. In the UK this condition is estimated to account for 25000 deaths per year from pulmonary thromboembolism [1]. This relatively common clinical condition is notoriously difficult to diagnose on clinical grounds alone, the diagnostic accuracy rarely exceeding 50%. Obviously with such a common and potentially life-threatening disease an accurate, reliable and reproducible test is required. Venography has fulfilled this role and until recently had been regarded as the 'gold standard' imaging modality. The disadvantages of the technique, which include its relative expense, discomfort, potential risk of contrast reaction and the risk of inducing phlebitis or thrombosis itself [2,3], are well known and this has led to an active search for a suitable non-invasive alternative.

Radioisotope scanning [4–6], impedance plethysmography [7] and thermography [8–10] have all been evaluated and results are extremely variable, questioning their reliability and reproducibility. Radioisotope scanning is particularly sensitive below the knee but not above [11], which negates its use as a clinical test.

Results of impedance plethysmography are variable. Localization of disease within the limb is not possible and false negative results may occur when thrombus is confined to the smaller veins. Difficulty in differentiating true DVT from superficial phlebitis, both of which may give rise to a temperature rise, led to a rapid decline in the use of thermography, this technique now being regarded as obsolete.

Real-time ultrasonic techniques have been evaluated in the diagnosis of venous disease and have been shown to be safe, reliable and reproducible [12–14]. There are three main ultrasonic techniques currently in use. The first, real-time imaging, is very effective, cheap and still widely used today. The second is Doppler ultrasound [15] and the most recent and popular is colour flow imaging [16,17]. All three techniques are reliable and accurate in the diagnosis of femoral and popliteal disease; however, the addition of colour technology allows calf vein visualization [18–20].

Colour flow imaging is rapidly becoming the first-line imaging modality in suspected venous occlusion, venography being reserved for inconclusive or unsuccessful colour flow examinations.

Anatomy

The venous system of the lower limb is divided into the deep, communicating and superficial systems (Fig. 19.1). There are three main sets of calf veins below the knee which join to form the popliteal vein which in turn drains into the main femoral vein. Duplications within the venous system are common and occur in up to 20% of the superficial femoral vein and 35% of popliteal veins.

The communicating veins which are prominent in the medial aspect of the lower leg, connect the posterior arch branch of the greater saphenous vein with the deep veins of the calf.

The superficial veins include the greater saphenous vein, which runs from the medial malleolus along the medial aspect of the lower limb and thigh to the saphenofemoral junction where it is commonly visualized at its site of entry into the femoral vein. The short saphenous vein runs along the lateral aspect of the calf and drains into the popliteal vein.

Technique

Lower limb venous ultrasound is performed using a 7.5 or 5MHz linear array probe, depending upon patient build. Real-time, pulsed Doppler or colour flow imaging may be used.

COLOUR FLOW ULTRASOUND

The examination is best carried out by an experienced ultrasonologist. All patients are examined in the supine position. The examination begins at groin level, the

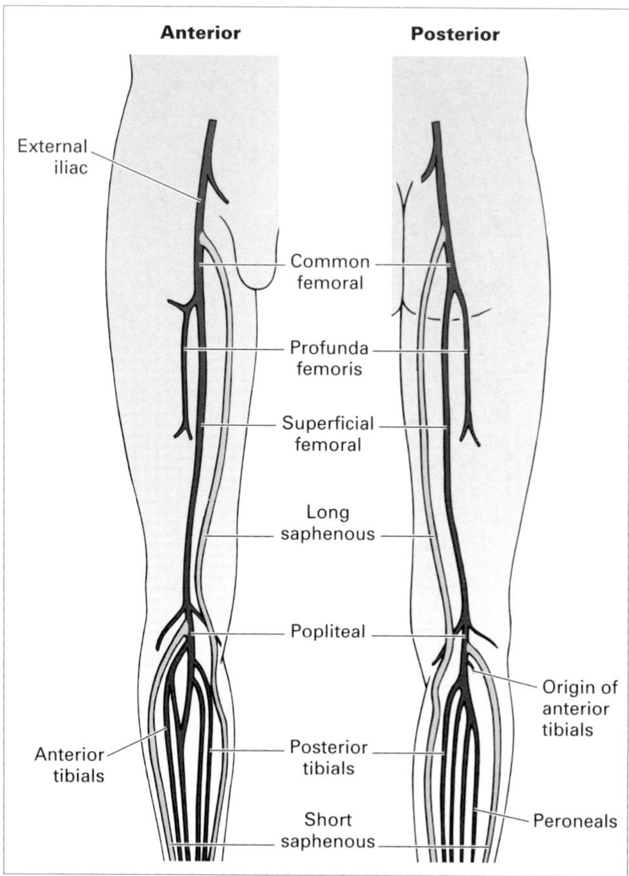

Fig. 19.1 Anatomy of both the superficial (□) and deep (■) venous system of the lower limb. The superficial system drains into the deep system and although anatomical variants exist, the major deep and superficial venous anatomy is fairly constant. Most anatomical variants within the deep venous system involve duplication of either the femoral or popliteal veins.

patient's leg being slightly abducted 10–15°. Acoustic jelly is applied to the skin at groin level and down the thigh along the course of the femoral vein to permit uninterrupted scanning. The probe is first positioned at groin level and the common femoral vein and accompanying artery identified in the transverse axis, the vein lying medial to the artery. The identification of each vessel is confirmed by placing the Doppler spectral gate over each of the vessels in turn. Phasic venous flow is easily differentiated from the triphasic waveform of the common femoral artery. It is important to remember that these vessels also have different audible properties, the venous waveform being analogous to a soft blowing wind whilst the artery is much sharper with systolic and diastolic components. At this point probe compression is applied to the common femoral vein to assess its compliance. In addition, a Valsalva manoeuvre is performed. Retardation of flow in the common femoral vein with a significant increase in the cross-sectional area (Fig. 19.2) is indicative of a patent iliac vein and inferior vena cava (IVC) [21].

The ultrasonic probe is now positioned at the groin in the longitudinal axis and the common femoral vein is followed proximal in order to visualize as much of the external iliac vein as possible, until it disappears deep into the pelvis. A Doppler spectral waveform is always obtained from the most proximal part of the external iliac or common femoral vein. At approximately the level of the inguinal ligament the common femoral vein divides into the superficial femoral vein which lies posterior to the superficial femoral artery, and the profunda femoris vein which is accompanied by the profunda femoris artery (Fig. 19.3). The remaining venous examination is performed in the longitudinal axis although some centres, especially in the USA, prefer the transverse axis. At groin level the profunda femoris vein is scanned for only 4–5 cm routinely. The superficial femoral vein is carefully followed from its origin to the adductor canal, it maintaining a constant position posterior to the superficial femoral artery. Flow within this vessel is spontaneous and should completely fill the lumen of the vein. Light touch should always be applied as excessive probe pressure may result in collapse of the vein, and the false impression of venous occlusion. Anatomical variants, e.g. duplicated veins, are common (Fig. 19.4) and care must be taken to exclude thrombosis in both. At the level of the adductor canal the femoral vein lies at its deepest and thus most difficult point to image and a good colour signal can be difficult to elicit. This signal can be augmented by the use of calf compression, or if this technique is unhelpful, then by pulling on the tendon of the hamstring muscles at the back of the thigh. This manoeuvre has the affect of bringing the vein closer to the surface and thus aiding visualization. In addition, with the probe in a transverse axis, a modified compression test can also be performed. Having completed the examination of the femoral vein the patient turns into a partial decubitus position with the knee flexed approximately 25° and the popliteal vein is examined.

The popliteal vein is examined in this manner as tension and stretch on the vein that may occur when the knee is locked is removed. Anatomically when examining from the popliteal fossa, the popliteal vein lies anterior to the artery. These vessels are identified initially using colour flow imaging in the transverse axis and confirmed by their specific Doppler spectral waveforms. Scanning then proceeds in a longitudinal axis, the popliteal vein being followed superiorly to the adductor canal and inferiorly to the proximal posterior tibial and common peroneal trunk. Once again flow in the popliteal vein is spontaneous. Augmentation of the venous Doppler waveform using distal

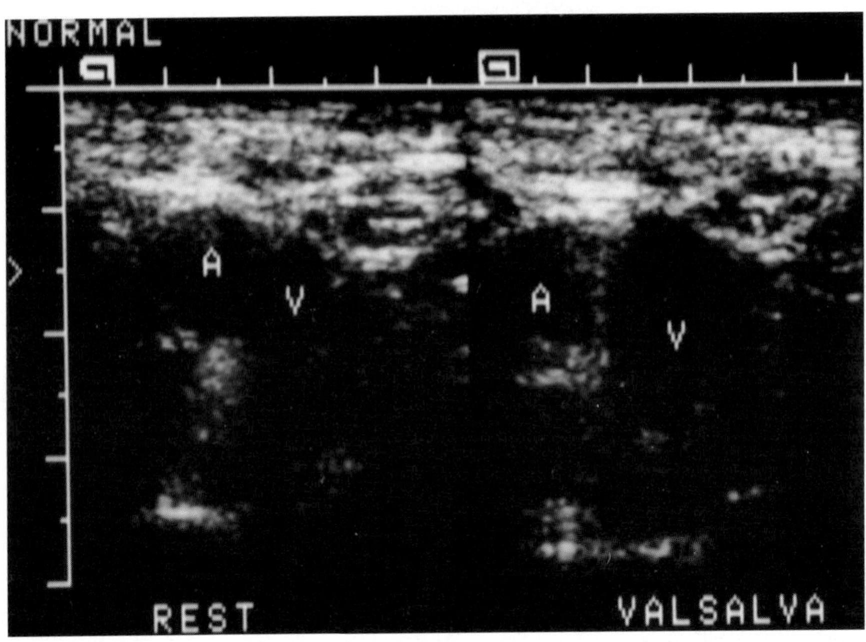

Fig. 19.2 Transverse ultrasonic image through the common femoral vein (V) and artery (A). The vein lies medial to the artery and is seen in a resting state (on the left) and following the Valsalva manoeuvre (on the right). A marked increase in venous diameter and cross-sectional area is noted within the common femoral vein. This is normally of at least 15 and 50%, respectively. This is a normal physiological response and is indicative of proximal venous patency. Imaging is always performed in the transverse axis when assessing the effects of this manoeuvre.

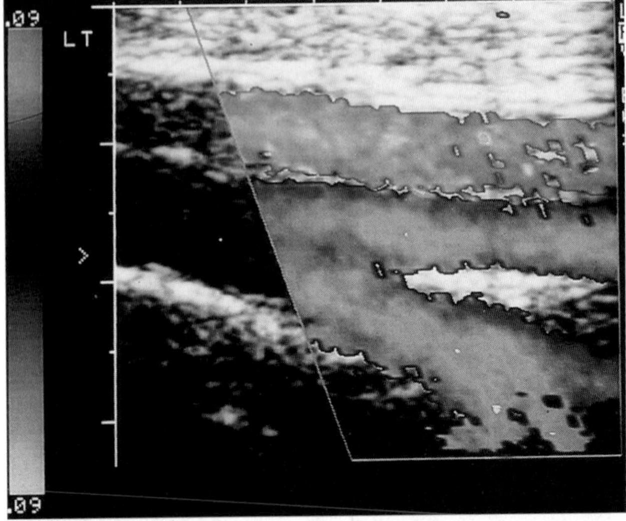

Fig. 19.3 Longitudinal colour Doppler image at groin level demonstrating the junction of the superficial femoral vein and the more deeply situated profunda femoris vein. The superficial femoral vein lies posterior to the superficial femoral artery. The common femoral vein is formed by the junction of the superficial femoral vein and the deeper profunda femoris vein. Flow at this level is entirely spontaneous. For colour, see Plate 19.3 (between pp. 308 and 309).

limb compression can be performed with the ultrasound probe at the popliteal vein—this, including pitfalls, is discussed in more detail below. The examination for above-knee thrombosis is thus complete, and only if required is examination of the calf veins undertaken.

CALF VEIN IMAGING

Calf vein analysis can only be performed using colour flow ultrasound. These veins have been studied in previous normal cohort studies and the evidence suggests that colour flow imaging may have a role in their assessment [22,23]. The paired posterior tibial and common peroneal veins are visualized in the medial aspect of the calf by imaging along the medial border of the tibia (Fig. 19.5). The vessels are identified by the recognition of the posterior tibial and common peroneal arteries and following distal limb compression, venous flow can be visualized in the accompanying calf veins (Fig. 19.6). Unlike the femoral and popliteal veins there is little or absent spontaneous venous flow, and distal manual compression or graded cuff compression is required for visualization.

The anterior tibial veins are thin and thought to be relatively unimportant in the diagnosis of major calf vein thrombosis [24] with the result that many centres do not now include these veins in their routine protocol.

Occasionally the common peroneal veins may be too deep to visualize from the medial approach, and in this situation, posterior imaging, or imaging from the anterolateral aspect of the calf, is usually successful.

REAL-TIME (COMPRESSION) ULTRASOUND

With regard to B-mode imaging, the femoral and popliteal veins are scanned with the patient supine in a similar manner. The main difference between this scanning technique and that of colour Doppler imaging is that with

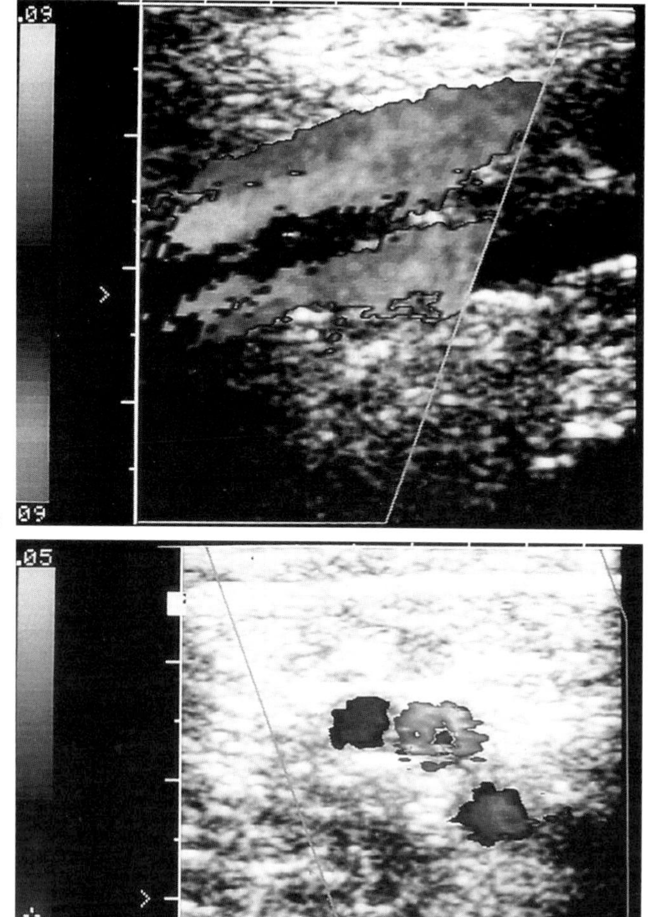

Fig. 19.4 (a) Colour Doppler image (longitudinal axis) through the popliteal fossa demonstrating a duplicated popliteal venous system. The popliteal artery is sandwiched between the veins; however, this is difficult to demonstrate completely on a still picture. (b) Transverse colour Doppler image in a different patient of a duplicated femoral venous system. Both femoral veins are seen on either side of the superficial femoral artery. Occasionally only one of these veins may be affected by thrombosis and this is a recognized pitfall both of this technique and venography but fortunately this is a relatively rare occurrence. For colour, see Plate 19.4 (between pp. 308 and 309).

real-time ultrasound all scanning is performed in the transverse plane. As a diagnosis of venous patency or occlusion is dependent on the response of the vein to probe compression it is much more reliable to perform this manoeuvre with the probe straddling the vein transversely. Although venous compressibility can be assessed

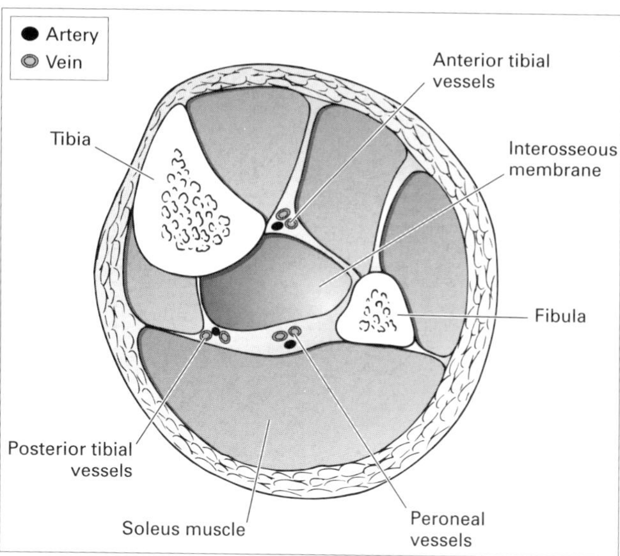

Fig. 19.5 Cross-sectional anatomy of the calf. There are three paired veins as shown (open), each pair being accompanied by an artery (black). The posterior tibial and common peroneal set of veins are normally visualized in the same scan plane medial to the tibia whilst the anterior tibial veins are visualized lateral to the tibia.

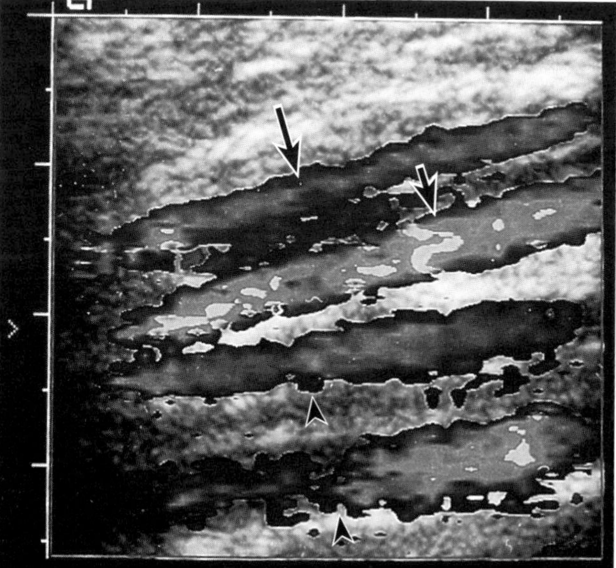

Fig. 19.6 Colour flow image of the posterior tibial and common peroneal set of calf veins in a longitudinal axis at mid calf level. The posterior tibial set are more superficial (arrows) than the common peroneal veins (arrowheads). Flow within these veins can only be appreciated with the aid of distal limb compression which can be achieved manually or by graded cuff compression. (Reproduced with permission from *Clinical Radiology* (1992), **46**, 198–201.) For colour, see Plate 19.6 (between pp. 308 and 309).

in the longitudinal plane, the probe may inadvertently slip off the vein giving a false impression of compressibility. With the real-time technique only the femoral and popliteal veins can be assessed.

DIAGNOSTIC CRITERIA OF COLOUR FLOW IMAGING

The following are a list of diagnostic criteria that should be addressed when performing colour flow imaging of the lower limb.

Spontaneous flow

Venous flow within the iliac, femoral and popliteal segments is spontaneous. This is normally obvious with complete filling of the vein lumen from the anterior to posterior wall (see Fig. 19.3). Occasionally although spontaneous flow may be present, venous filling may be incomplete. This is common in pregnancy where the increased abdominal pressure, secondary to the pregnant uterus, causes retardation of flow in the lower limb. In such cases distal compression will result in complete venous filling. Persistent absence of spontaneous flow above knee in the major deep veins suggests thrombus.

Presence of echogenic material within the vein lumen

The vein lumen is normally anechoic and is filled with colour-coded flow. The presence of echogenic material within the vein lumen is diagnostic of DVT.

Distal augmentation

The third characteristic of normal flow is an increase in the amplitude of the Doppler spectral waveform following distal limb compression (Fig. 19.7). Such manoeuvres imply that the venous system between the area of distal compression and the probe is patent; however, if a good collateral system is present, or thrombus is non-occlusive, normal venous augmentation may occur even in the presence of major vein thrombosis (Fig. 19.8). This manoeuvre is often performed to help obtain better visualization of the distal femoral vein or to assess the calf veins indirectly.

One of the potential dangers when squeezing the limb is that of dislodging thrombus and resultant pulmonary thromboembolism [25]. This complication is, however, extremely rare and is as likely to happen during venography as ultrasound. Nevertheless, if the diagnosis of DVT is obvious, then distal limb compression need not be performed.

Response to probe compression

This manoeuvre is applicable to both real-time and colour flow techniques as a patent vein will consistently respond to probe compression by complete apposition of the anterior and posterior vein walls (Fig. 19.9). The accompanying artery should not normally compress and if so only does so minimally, springing back extremely quickly following withdrawal of the probe. The artery should never be more than only minimally compressed or too much probe pressure has been applied.

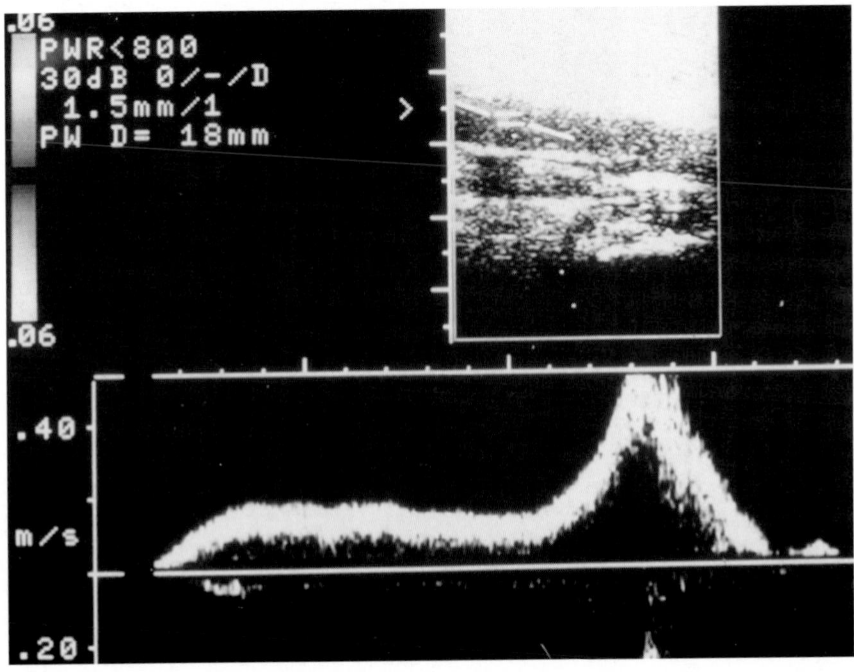

Fig. 19.7 Doppler waveform of the popliteal vein following distal manual compression of the calf. Marked augmentation of the venous waveform is noted following this manoeuvre. This is a normal response said to be indicative of venous patency between the level of distal compression and the ultrasonic probe. Whilst this is true in the majority of cases this test is not completely reliable and should not be used in isolation as a marker of venous patency. There are well-recognized pitfalls (see Fig. 19.9) and where possible direct visualization of the vein should be achieved.

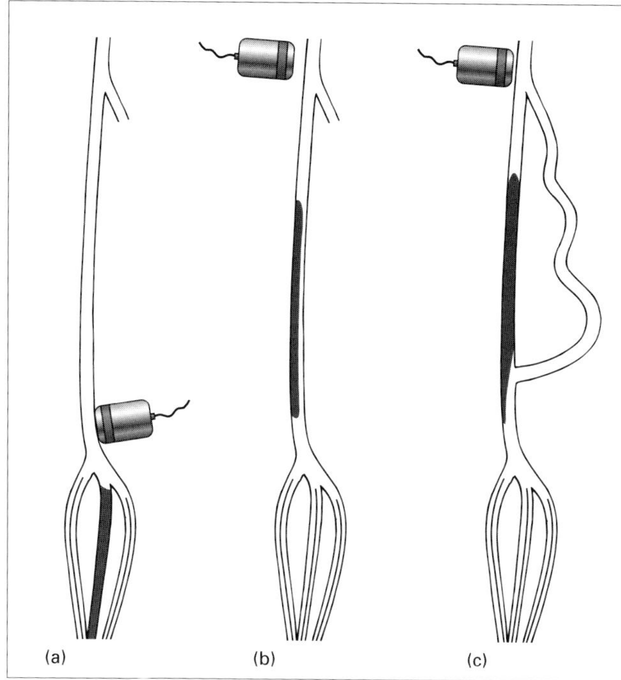

Fig. 19.8 Diagram demonstrating why thrombus may be missed if too great a reliance is placed only on the augmentation manoeuvre. Normally these augmentation manoeuvres are only performed with the probe positioned at either the popliteal or femoral vein. It is clear to see that with (a) thrombus confined to only one pair of calf veins, (b) with non-occlusive thrombus, or (c) thrombus with well-formed collateral vessels how a falsely reassuring response can be achieved.

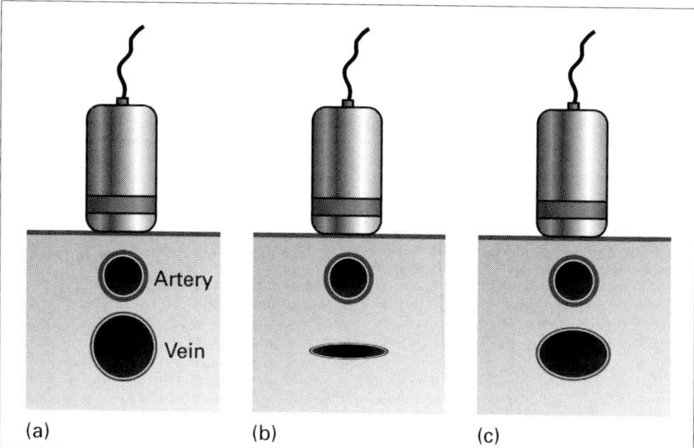

Fig. 19.9 Diagram demonstrating the effects of venous compression ultrasound on both a patent and occluded vein. The vein is visualized in the transverse plane posterior to the accompanying artery and is seen in the resting phase with little or no probe pressure (a). (b) If the vein is patent when probe pressure is applied the anterior and posterior vein walls are seen to completely oppose with obliteration of the vein lumen. (c) If the vein is occluded by thrombus then when probe pressure is applied there is failure of wall apposition. A further clue to the presence of thrombus is that often the affected vein will be distended. Normally the force applied to the probe should not be greater than that required to slightly deform the accompanying arterial wall.

Table 19.1 Ultrasonic criteria of venous patency of the femoral and popliteal veins using colour Doppler imaging

	Patent	Thrombosis
Spontaneous flow	Present	Absent
Augmentation of flow	Present	Absent*
Response to probe compression	Present	Absent or diminished
Doppler waveform	Present + phasic	Absent
Intraluminal echoes	Absent	Present
Colour flow imaging	Fills lumen completely	Absent or incomplete filling of lumen

* Beware of false negative results (see Fig. 19.10).

Phasic variation of the spectral waveform with respiration

The venous spectral Doppler waveform normally varies with respiration, flow normally decreasing upon inspiration secondary to increased intra-abdominal pressure during diaphragmatic descent with a rebound increase during expiration. The degree of phasic swing varies greatly from individual to individual (Fig. 19.10); however, a continuous venous flow signal with complete absence of respiratory variation in a major proximal vein should suggest the possibility of a more proximal obstructing lesion. Continuous non-phasic flow may also be seen in collateral veins, and in patients with low circulating blood volume.

Dilatation of the vein

Normally when a vein contains thrombus it dilates. This can be a useful sign of DVT and thus a helpful confirmatory sign especially when the thrombus is new and anechoic. It should be noted, however, that significant venous dilatation does not occur in all cases.

THROMBOSIS

It can be seen that a positive diagnosis of venous thrombosis using colour flow imaging depends upon a number of factors. These include lack of spontaneous flow,

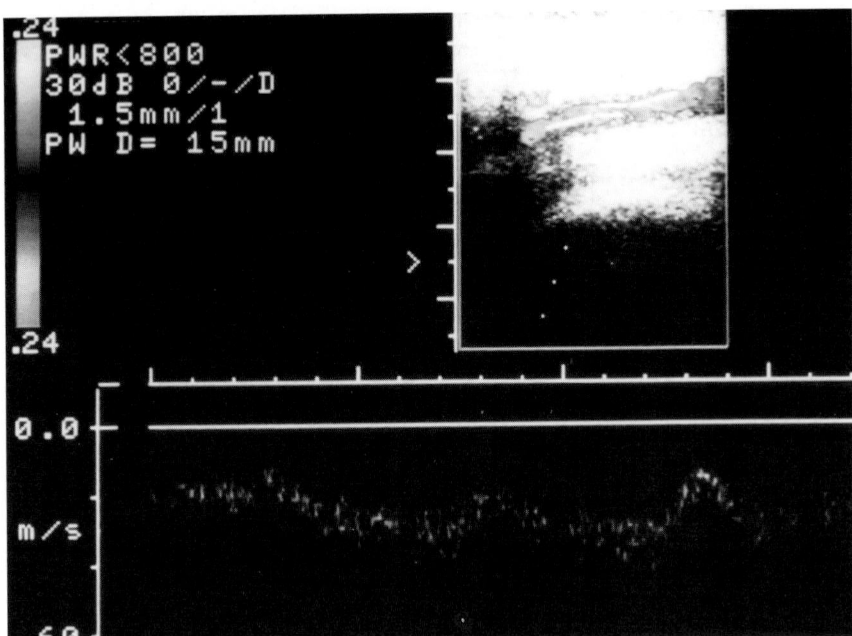

Fig. 19.10 Doppler waveform of the femoral vein demonstrating normal phasic flow with respiration indicative of a patent venous system. A small reduction in venous flow is noted on inspiration with an increase in flow on expiration.

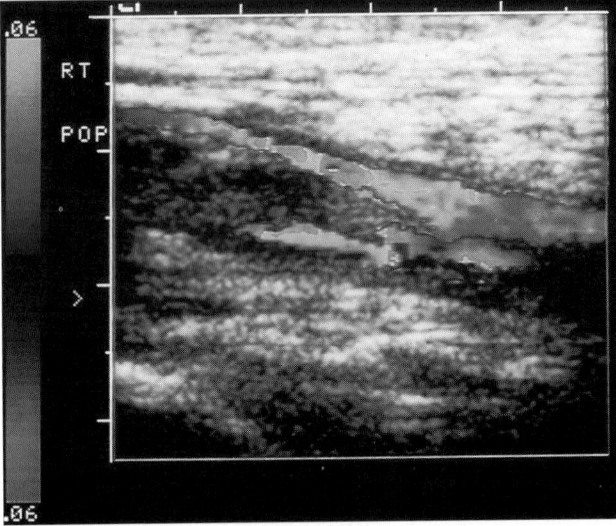

Fig. 19.11 Longitudinal colour Doppler image through the popliteal fossa demonstrating non-occlusive thrombus within the popliteal vein. The popliteal vein is slightly distended and contains a large amount of mixed echogenic thrombus. Some residual venous flow persists and this is seen both along the vein wall (analogous to the 'tram line' appearance on venography) and within the thrombus itself. For colour, see Plate 19.11 (between pp. 308 and 309).

presence of echogenic material within the vein lumen, absent or poor response to distal augmentation, non-compressibility of the vein, and an absent Doppler spectral waveform. With experience, using colour flow imaging, the diagnosis is so visual that spectral analysis is often unnecessary (Table 19.1) (Fig. 19.11).

Assessment of the iliac system and IVC

With regard to the iliac venous system, despite adequate patient preparation and many different techniques to aid visualization of these vessels, the iliac veins remain poorly visualized in at least 50% of individuals [26]. This is often due to a combination of patient build and the relatively deep position of these veins within the pelvis. In general, only the distal aspect of the external iliac vein can be visualized.

Indirect assessment of iliac patency thus depends on two factors, the presence of a normal phasic common femoral or external iliac Doppler waveform and the response of the common femoral vein to the Valsalva manoeuvre. In the latter a diameter increase of at least 15% or a 50% cross-sectional area increase of the common femoral vein in response to the Valsalva manoeuvre is normal. This can be difficult to judge and in conditions such as congestive cardiac failure, the response to this manoeuvre may be damped resulting in misinterpretation. In view of this, more reliance is often placed on the cessation of Doppler flow with return in expiration as being indicative of proximal patency.

Calf vein assessment

Calf vein flow is relatively slow and can only be identified using distal compression. Although multiple veins may

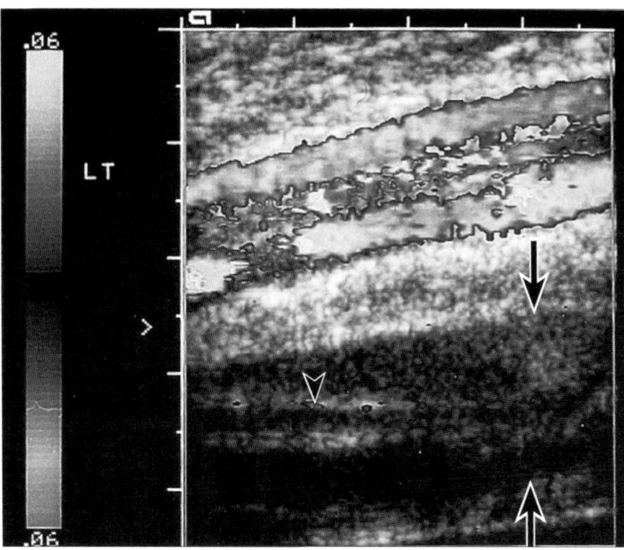

Fig. 19.12 Longitudinal colour Doppler scan through the medial aspect of the calf demonstrating patency of both posterior tibial veins with the posterior tibial artery sandwiched in between. The deeper situated common peroneal veins are distended and thrombosed (arrows) with complete absence of colour-coded flow. These ultrasonic findings were confirmed by venography. Small flashes of flow were seen within the common peroneal artery (arrowhead). For colour, see Plate 19.12 (between pp. 308 and 309).

Table 19.2 Potential sources of error of venous ultrasound

Infrapopliteal thombosis
Non-compressibility of vein, i.e. most commonly at adductor canal
Chronic DVT
Focal non-obstructing DVT
Venous duplication
Iliac vein thrombosis*
Profunda femoris DVT*

* Very uncommon.

be imaged in one plane, small changes in probe angulation may be necessary in order to visualize flow in each set of veins individually. As in the case of above-knee lesions, the absence of flow is indicative of thrombosis (Fig. 19.12). When multiple calf veins are involved, the diagnosis is usually straightforward using this technique. When one vein or one part of a vein are affected by this disease, the diagnosis may be missed using this technique; therefore equivocal scans or the presence of persistent symptoms may require venography.

Problems and pitfalls

There are many potential sources of error in imaging the lower limb venous system, some of which also apply when using real-time compression ultrasound as well as the colour flow technique, (Table 19.2). These potential sources of error include the following.

TECHNICAL

Technical settings of the colour Doppler machine must be optimized. The focal point should be at a depth at or just posterior to the vessels being imaged. The Doppler filter should be at a low setting so as not to remove essential venous information and the pulse repetition frequency (PRF) or colour velocity imaging scale should be set at a suitably low level in order to detect venous flow. A level of 6 cm s^{-1} is generally adequate for both above- and below-knee imaging although for assessment of the calf veins it is occasionally reduced to 3 cm s^{-1}.

ASSOCIATED MEDICAL CONDITIONS

The diagnosis of DVT is based on the criteria previously discussed (see Table 19.1); however, a few traps for the unwary remain. A diminished response of the common femoral vein to the Valsalva manoeuvre may occur normally in patients with congestive cardiac failure and this should not be misinterpreted as necessarily representing proximal thrombosis.

ANATOMICAL VARIANTS

Anatomical variants in the femoral and popliteal segments may lead to misinterpretation in the unwary and inexperienced [27]. Duplication of the femoral and popliteal veins may occur in up to 30% of individuals. This should be recognized as one limb of the duplication may be patent whilst the other is thrombosed. The difference in size of the two duplicated segments may also occasionally cause confusion as may their anatomical relationships to the accompanying arteries.

DISTAL AUGMENTATION

Reliability on the response of distal compression to reflect venous patency should never be taken in isolation. There can be complete thrombosis of the major deep veins with large surrounding collaterals with can result in a normal venous response and thus a false negative report (see Fig. 19.8). With colour flow imaging each venous segment must be examined carefully and colour-coded flow should normally fill the vein lumen. This can occasionally be difficult to achieve due to low velocity flow, depth of vessel or patient build. Distal augmentation may be useful in this situation to help increase flow within the venous segment under examination. Persistent partial non-filling may be representative of non-occlusive thrombus. In these difficult situations where there is poor filling of the vein with colour, even following augmentation, in a technically challenging patient, venous compressibility may be helpful.

COLLATERAL VESSELS

It is important not to confuse large collateral vessels with the major deep venous system although this is a relatively infrequent finding. These collaterals can normally be easily separated from the main venous tributaries as they bear little relationship to the major lower limb arteries.

Clinical applications

DIAGNOSIS OF ACUTE DVT

Colour flow imaging is generally regarded as the first-line imaging modality in patients with suspected acute lower limb DVT. It is rapid, portable, safe and accurate. This technique not only allows a diagnosis of venous thrombosis to be confirmed or excluded, but detects other conditions that may present with similar signs such as a ruptured Baker's cyst, subfascial haematoma or a pelvic malignancy. Inflammation of the greater or lesser saphenous veins, diagnostic of superficial thrombophlebitis, can also be easily differentiated from deep venous involvement and a decision to treat with anti-inflammatory or anticoagulant therapy can thus be made on a rational basis.

A clinical decision can be made and the majority of patients treated, if required, on the basis of a colour flow examination alone. The sensitivity and specificity of this technique has consistently been shown to be of the order of 95 and 100%, respectively (Table 19.3), for symptomatic DVT. In addition, the diagnosis of deep venous patency on ultrasound examination has been shown in long-term follow-up studies to be a reliable indicator of normality. Results, however, are less impressive for asymptomatic venous thrombosis with a reduction in sensitivity ranging from 35 to 86%, which is presumably due to a combination of increased technical difficulty, increased incidence of small non-occlusive thrombi and calf vein involvement. Whilst these results are slightly disappointing a reassessment of this patient group is required as there have been significant imaging improvements since many of these studies were performed.

Recent studies have demonstrated that the calf veins can be identified in normal individuals. Early clinical results indicate that the sensitivity and specificity of calf vein imaging is similar to that of above-knee imaging; however, the long-term debate on the relative importance of confined calf vein thrombosis and its propensity for proximal propagation continues [28,29].

Before calf veins can be confidently examined, there is undoubtedly a learning curve. One strategy that negates the need for calf vein imaging is to confine the examination to the femoral and popliteal veins and repeat the ultrasound scan in 2 days time, assuming the original scan is normal. This 48-h check excludes or confirms proximal venous propagation of clot from the calf veins. Although this practice is instituted in many American centres this delay is often unacceptable in the UK and if ultrasound is equivocal then venography is preferred. In addition, a role for venography remains, as not all patients are suitable for ultrasonic examination due to obesity and/or tissue oedema.

Once introduced into hospital practice, due to its free availability, non-invasive nature, high degree of accuracy and patient acceptability, the number of referrals significantly increase. Interestingly the positive diagnosis rate remains constant [30]. In conclusion, this test is both extremely accurate and cost-effective.

Table 19.3 Sensitivity and specificity of ultrasound in the diagnosis of deep venous thrombosis

Author	Sensitivity (%)	Specificity (%)	Distribution of thrombus	Ultrasonic technique
Aitken & Godden (1987) [12]	94	100	AK	RT
Cronan *et al.* (1987) [13]	89	100	AK	RT
Lensing *et al.* (1989) [14]	100	99	AK	RT
	36		BK	RT
Rose *et al.* (1990) [23]	96	100	AK	CDI
	73	86	BK	CDI
Baxter *et al.* (1991) [32]	95	100	AK + BK	CDI
Cronan *et al.* (1991) [48]	100	100	AK	DD + RT
Baxter *et al.* (1992) [22]	95	100	BK	CDI

AK, above-knee (iliac, femoral, popliteal) thrombosis; BK, below-knee (calf vein) thrombosis; CDI, colour Doppler imaging; DD, duplex Doppler ultrasound; RT, real-time compression ultrasound.

SUSPECTED PULMONARY THROMBOEMBOLISM

This technique can also be employed in patients with suspected pulmonary embolism to try and locate a possible venous source. Colour flow imaging may also be helpful to the clinician in those cases of suspected pulmonary thromboembolism where the ventilation perfusion lung scan is equivocal. Clearly if the diagnosis is positive for DVT then treatment can be confidently instituted as it is essentially the same for lower limb DVT as it is for pulmonary thromboembolism. Unfortunately life is always more complicated than this as even in those patients with high probability V:Q scans the lower limb venous scan is only positive in approximately 50%. It is important to remember that those patients with negative lower limb studies in the clinical setting of suspected pulmonary thromboembolism may well have had clinically significant pulmonary thromboembolisms despite the negative lower limb study. This is currently a very active area of research with many differing viewpoints. A search for a clinically useable algorithm is awaited.

MONITORING OF CLOT LYSIS

This technique could clearly be of use in the monitoring of the therapeutic response in venous occlusive disease, there already being provisional reports of faster, more complete clot lysis in those patients with non-occlusive thrombus when compared with those with occlusive thrombus [31]. Although standard therapy involves the use of heparin and oral anticoagulants such as warfarin, alternative therapeutic regimes exist, e.g. streptokinase, urokinase or tissue plasminogen activator (TPA). It would seem sensible that any therapeutic trial should now be performed using colour flow imaging to allow frequent temporal imaging.

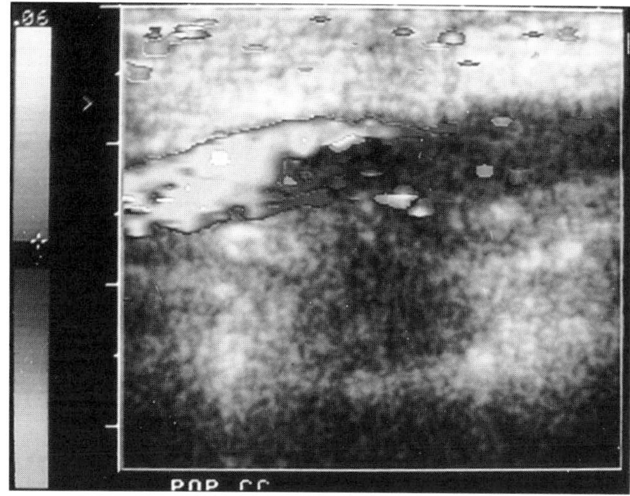

(a)

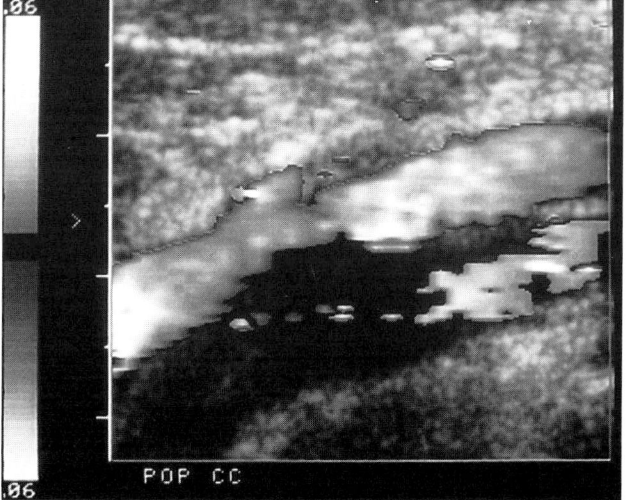

(b)

Fig. 19.13 Longitudinal colour Doppler scan of the popliteal vein (a) at the time of diagnosis of DVT and (b) 3 months later, subsequently showing complete recanalization of the vein. This only occurs in 50% of patients with acute DVT. For colour, see Plate 19.13 (between pp. 308 and 309).

CHRONIC VENOUS THROMBOSIS

It is well recognized that in the long-term follow-up of patients following DVT, approximately 50% will completely recanalize the deep venous system by 1 year (Fig. 19.13). In the remaining 50% venous abnormalities persist [32,33]. The exact incidence of chronic DVT is unknown; however, it is likely that following an acute episode the vast majority have residual wall or valve damage. Thus, should these patients represent with signs and symptoms similar to the primary episode or with additional symptoms, they will clearly represent a diagnostic dilemma.

There are certain ultrasonic patterns that help differentiate acute from chronic DVT (Table 19.4). These features, if classical, can be diagnostic, e.g. a small narrow major vein with thickened walls and of increased echogenicity with multiple surrounding collateral vessels is almost certainly chronic. Unfortunately, overlap of both acute and chronic DVT features are seen in the majority of patients in the healing phase following acute DVT, for up to 1–2 years following the primary insult. Therefore, the presence of intraluminal echogenic material, lack of spontaneous flow and incomplete vein compressibility are as likely to be chronic as they are acute, in the postphlebitic limb reflecting the normal recanalization process (Fig. 19.14). All this adds to the difficulty and challenge of imaging the postphlebitic limb.

Our experience and that of others suggest that attempts at ageing thrombi based on echogenicity are largely futile due to the wide variability [34]. It has been suggested that

Table 19.4 Ultrasonic features of acute and chronic venous thrombosis

		Chronic DVT	
	Acute DVT	Complete recanalization	Partial recanalization
Spontaneous flow	Absent	Reduced	Reduced
Augmented flow	Absent	Normal	Reduced
Vein wall thickening	Absent	Present	Absent
Response to probe compression	Absent	Normal or slightly reduced	Markedly reduced
Intraluminal echoes	Present	Absent	Present
Thrombus characteristics	Low echoes	—	Variable
Venous distension	Present	Absent	Variable
Collateral vessels	None, few	Variable	Variable

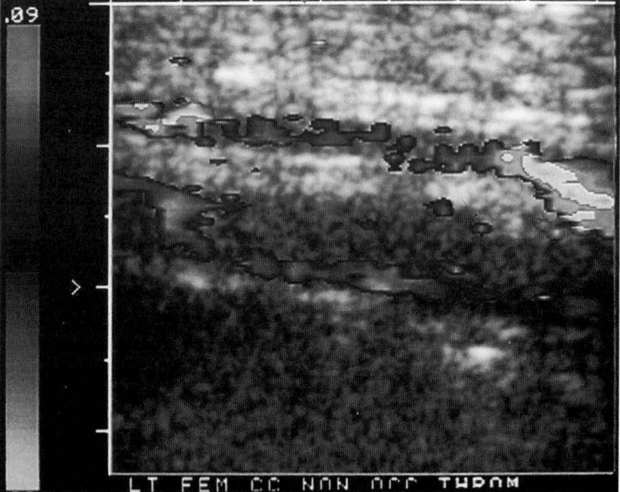

Fig. 19.14 Colour Doppler image of the femoral vein in a longitudinal axis 6 months following acute DVT. There has only been partial recanalization of the femoral vein with some peripheral flow within the lumen. Although this represents part of the spectrum of recanalization following the acute insult it leads to difficulty in imaging should there be a recurrence of symptoms as these ultrasonic appearances cannot be distinguished from acute non-occlusive thrombus. (Reproduced with permission from *Clinical Radiology* (1991), **43**, 301–304.) For colour, see Plate 19.14 (between pp. 308 and 309).

6-month scans be performed on all with previous DVT to allow a baseline comparison should these patients present again with similar signs and symptoms.

Patients with previous venous thrombosis present diagnostic difficulties. A normal scan is helpful but one with venous abnormalities should be interpreted with care and ultimately, may not in isolation aid clinical management.

Other techniques including venography, impedance plethysmography, thermography and radioisotope scanning are similarly of limited use. The clinical impression is very important with regard to the most appropriate mode of treatment.

VENOUS INSUFFICIENCY

The prevalence in the general population of venous insufficiency is approximately 3%. The symptoms are often chronic and manifest as pain, leg swelling, skin changes, obvious varicose veins and ulceration. Venous insufficiency may either be due to a defect in valve function or damage from previous DVT. In the latter, the incidence of the postphlebitic syndrome is related to the extent of previous thrombosis (Table 19.5).

Venous insufficiency can be confined to the superficial or deep system but very often it is a combination of both. The incidence of secondary venous insufficiency is related to the extent of previous deep venous involvement. Of patients with femoropopliteal DVT 75% will develop symptoms 5–6 years following an acute episode whilst only 20% of patients with calf thrombosis are affected [35–38].

Patients with varicose veins should be evaluated for the presence or absence of concomitant deep venous disease. Colour flow imaging is an extremely quick, easy and accurate method. If the deep venous system is normal then varicose veins are considered to be primary and therefore have a more favourable outcome. Conversely, patients

Table 19.5 The distribution of DVT and the incidence of postphlebitic symptoms

Distribution of DVT	Incidence of postphlebitic symptoms (%)
Popliteal and calf veins	17
Femoral, popliteal and calf veins	23
Iliac, femoral, popliteal and calf veins	34

with secondary varicose veins due to underlying deep venous disease, tend to run a more unsatisfactory course with significant oedema, dermatitis, ulceration and possible recurrent pulmonary embolism. Venous incompetence can be assessed using colour flow imaging in both the deep and superficial venous system as well as in the assessment of incompetent perforating veins [39]. This is done by applying compression and assessing the direction of venous flow. If venous flow reverses then there must be an incompetent valve at that level. Venous compression can be applied using either graded cuff compression or the free hand compression technique.

This is the basis of ultrasonic assessment of venous insufficiency. For assessment of both the superficial and deep system the patient can be examined on a tilt table with the couch 30–60° head up or the patient can be examined standing with most of their weight on the non-examined leg. The use of distal compression and assessment of flow retardation (normal) or reversal (incompetence) is the main method of examination and diagnosis. The patient can also be asked to perform a Valsalva manoeuvre. Any flow detected down the leg is abnormal (Fig. 19.15). This method is normally only suitable for assessing proximal long saphenous insufficiency. If reflux of blood is detected for greater than 0.5 s then the test is regarded as positive. If only brief reflux is seen (<0.5 s) then this is regarded as normal and is probably due to small amounts of flow associated with valve closure. These tests can be used for assessment of both the superficial and deep systems.

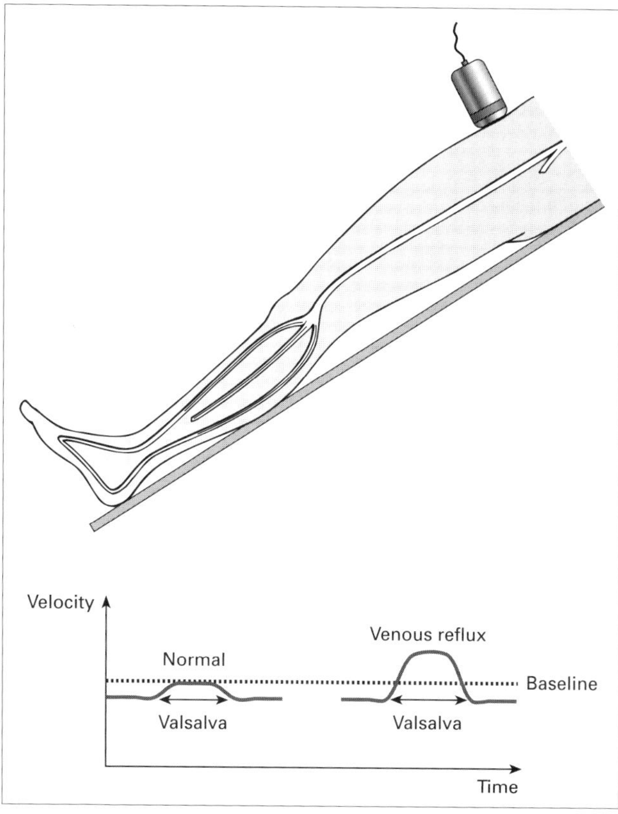

Fig. 19.15 Diagram demonstrating venous reflux during the Valsalva manoeuvre with the patient on a tilt table at an angle of approximately 20–25°. The normal response to the Valsalva manoeuvre is a cessation of venous flow; however, if the venous segment is incompetent then reverse flow will be seen.

VEIN MAPPING

This can be done to assess the long saphenous vein for suitability prior to bypass surgery, either coronary or lower limb. This examination is normally performed with the patient standing and the path of the long saphenous vein, its major tributaries and perforating veins can be mapped out on the skin surface with the use of a black felt pen. This is helpful to the surgeon when harvesting the vein for bypass.

ADVANCES

Power Doppler (Doppler energy) is a more sensitive technique for the detection of low velocity flow and therefore theoretically at least may be advantageous in DVT imaging. The major drawback of the technique is excessive flash artefact and lack of directional information although this is less relevant for venous imaging. It was originally thought that it may be of help in calf vein imaging; however, there is no study to date to support any of these early claims and currently this technique offers no significant advantage over conventional colour flow imaging in DVT. Its lack of directional information negates its use in the assessment of venous incompetence.

Contrast agents are also under development. As yet, there is no indication that these agents have a specific application in DVT imaging; however, progress in this field is so rapid that applications may soon arrive.

Upper limb venous imaging

Upper limb thrombosis is a relatively uncommon clinical condition and accounts for 1–2% of cases of DVT [40]. The reason for this relatively infrequent occurrence is ill understood although many reasons have been postulated including increased movement of the upper limb, reduced thrombogenic activity, and reduced number of values [41] when compared with the lower limb.

Central vein thrombosis may be of two types, primary or secondary. There are many predisposing conditions;

Table 19.6 Causes of central vein thrombosis

Traumatic
Venous catheterization
Fracture dislocation of clavicle or first rib
Irritants, e.g. contrast agents, chemotherapy
Stress (effort) thrombosis
Spontaneous
Idiopathic
Secondary to: congestive cardiac failure
malignancy
coagulopathies

however, by far the commonest is central vein catheterization (Table 19.6).

Anatomy and examination technique

The forearm veins are small, normally paired, and accompany the radial and ulnar arteries. Although these veins can be visualized there is little clinical indication for doing so. These veins join at the elbow to form the brachial vein which accompanies the brachial artery and runs along the medial aspect of the upper arm. In some, the brachial vein may be split into two separate trunks. As the brachial vein runs proximally it forms the axillary vein, which lies anterior to the artery, and can be followed up into the axilla (Fig. 19.16). At the junction of the brachial and axillary vein, the basilic vein, which is nearer to the skin surface, may be visualized along the posteromedial aspect of the upper arm. Examination of the upper arm is normally performed with the patient supine, and the arm raised to permit access to the axilla. The cephalic vein is superficially located and can be imaged as it runs along the anterior border of the biceps muscle. This vein is normally examined with the arm extended and abducted 90°.

With the examination of the upper arm complete, the arm is returned to the patient's side to lie in the anatomical position. Imaging of the subclavian and proximal axillary vein is then possible. These vessels have a fairly constant anatomical position, the subclavian and proximal axillary vein lying above the accompanying artery below the clavicle, whilst the subclavian vein lies deep to the artery above the clavicle. Very often only the proximal subclavian vein can be visualized beneath the clavicle. However, the more distal part can usually be visualized by examining superior to the clavicle and angling medially and inferiorly towards the sternoclavicular joint. There does, however, remain a small segment of non-visualized subclavian vein directly beneath the clavicle. This is known to be a common site of subclavian vein stenosis. The internal jugular vein can also be routinely visualized. In good subjects and with appropriate probe angulation, the proximal innominate vein can be visualized. The superior vena cara (SVC) and distal innominate veins cannot be visualized using this technique.

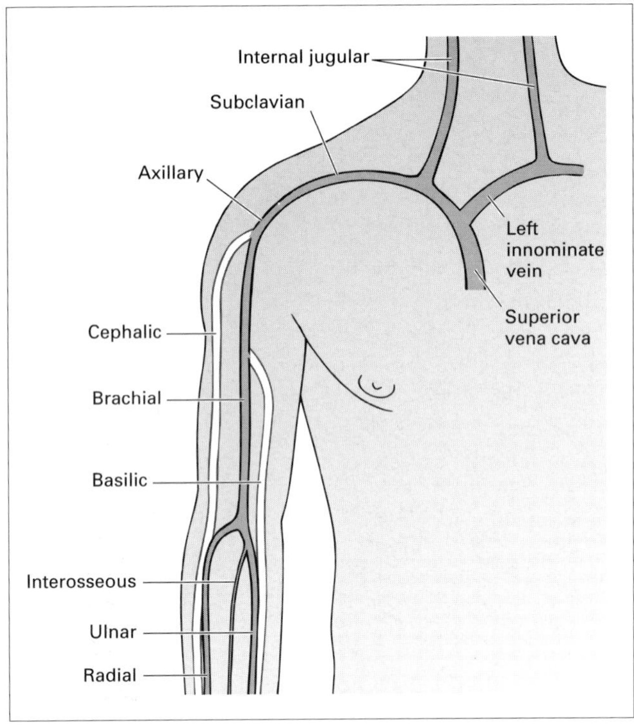

Fig. 19.16 Diagram of both the superficial (□) and deep (■) venous system of the upper limb. Variation in the anatomy of the superficial system in the antecubital fossa is common. The anatomy of the deep system is fairly constant in all, although duplications of the brachial vein is not uncommon.

Scanning of the upper limb is normally performed using a 7.5 MHz linear array probe with occasional recourse to a 5 MHz probe. As for the lower limb, the machine should be optimized and this means both a low filter and colour velocity scale. Scanning can be performed in both a transverse and longitudinal axis, although again the latter is preferred. The transverse axis, however, is very good in aiding vessel identification when beginning an examination.

Normal and thrombosed veins

Colour flow imaging is a useful method for the visualization of the upper limb veins and also reduces examination time when compared with real-time ultrasound or Doppler alone [42]. In addition it can identify collateral vessels some of which may be below the resolution of real-time ultrasound [43] adding confidence to the diagnosis.

Normal

The examination entails a complete assessment of the axillary vein, subclavian vein, internal jugular vein and proximal innominate vein. Scanning normally begins below the clavicle, the vessels being identified initially in the transverse plane. From this point onwards, imaging is normally performed in the longitudinal axis. The major upper limb veins exhibit spontaneous flow, colour filling the lumen completely from anterior to posterior wall (Fig. 19.17). Venous compressibility using the ultrasonic probe can only be applied with confidence to the axillary, brachial and internal jugular veins, the subclavian and innominate veins being largely inaccessible for this manoeuvre.

Doppler spectral analysis of these veins reveal two main types of waveforms, one is similar to that in the lower limb, whilst the other is more pulsatile reflecting cardiac pulsation and the opening and closure of the tricuspid valve (Fig. 19.18). A flat spectral Doppler waveform whilst indicative of patency may reflect previous thrombosis. This may also be seen in collateral vessels.

A patent subclavian vein responds to the Valsalva manoeuvre by dilating with a consequent reduction in flow, whilst sniffing collapses the vein and increases venous velocity [44]. With colour flow imaging these manoeuvres are rarely required to make the primary diagnosis.

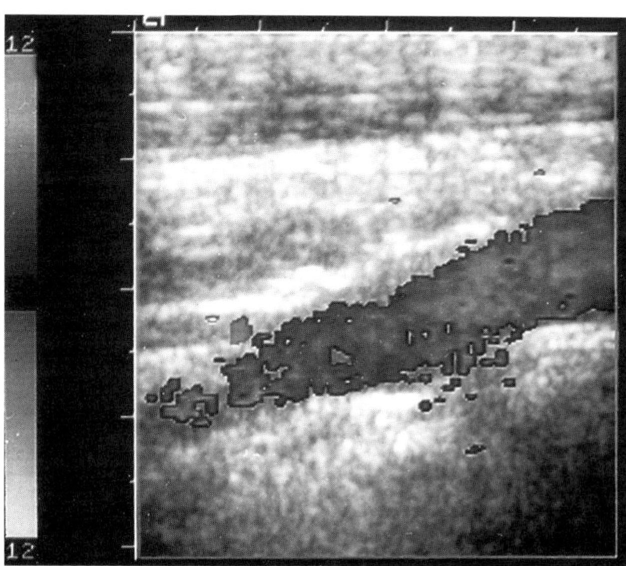

Fig. 19.17 Colour flow image in a longitudinal plane demonstrating a normal patent subclavian vein just below the clavicle. Flow is spontaneous and completely fills the vein lumen. (Reproduced with permission from the *British Journal of Radiology* (1991), **64**, 777–781.) For colour, see Plate 19.17 (between pp. 308 and 309).

Thrombosis

A diagnosis of thrombosis is made on a combination of poor or absent spontaneous flow, and the presence of intraluminal echogenic material (Fig. 19.19). Non-compressibility of the vein is an additional helpful diag-

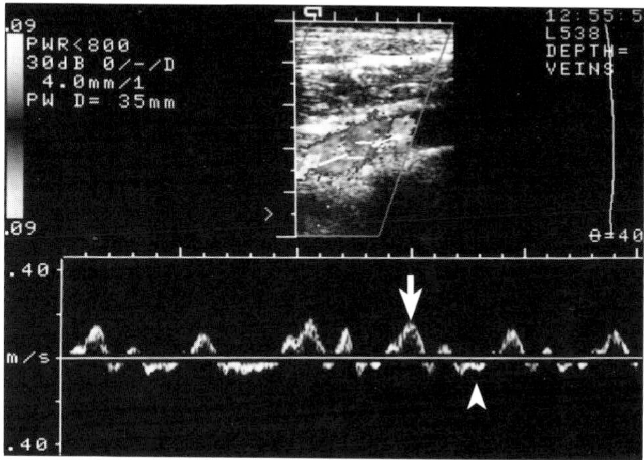

Fig. 19.18 Doppler spectrum from a normal subclavian vein demonstrating a more pulsatile, cyclical waveform reflective of cardiac pulsation. Peak flow occurs in mid diastole (arrow) whilst reversal of flow is maximum at tricuspid valve closure (arrowhead). The peak velocity also varies with the respiratory cycle being maximum on inspiration and minimum on expiration.

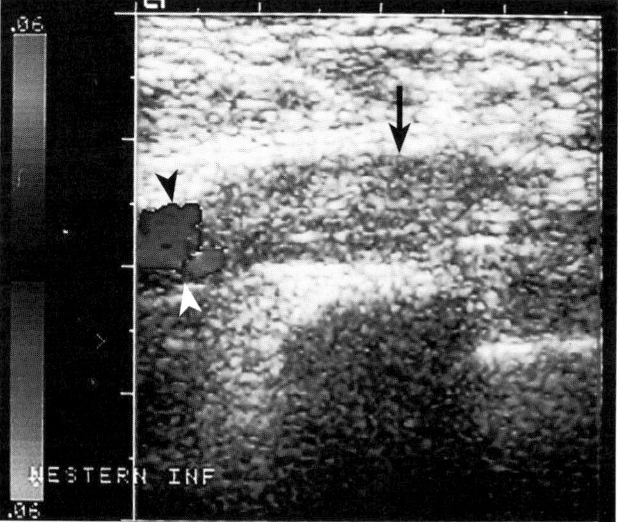

Fig. 19.19 Colour flow image in a longitudinal axis demonstrating acute thrombus within the distal axillary and lateral aspect of the subclavian vein (arrow). Some residual flow is noted laterally (arrowheads) but more medially there is complete absence of colour-coded flow indicative of thrombosis. (Reproduced with permission from the *British Journal of Radiology* (1991), **64**, 777–781.) For colour, see Plate 19.19 (between pp. 308 and 309).

nostic criterion. New thrombus may be difficult or even impossible to visualize; however, the absence of colour-coded flow in the lumen is diagnostic.

If no abnormality is identified in the subclavian or proximal axillary vein in the presence of a clinically swollen upper limb, the arm is raised to permit access to the axilla where the axillary and brachial veins are examined. Light probe pressure must be used at all times as excessive probe pressure will collapse the patent vein and result in misinterpretation.

A secondary sign of major vein thrombosis is collateral circulation and when present is further evidence of a primary thrombotic episode (Fig. 19.20).

In situations where a thrombosed venous segment may be older and the clot echogenic, the vein may blend in with background tissue and is often difficult or impossible to identify. The absence of a colour-coded vessel accompa-

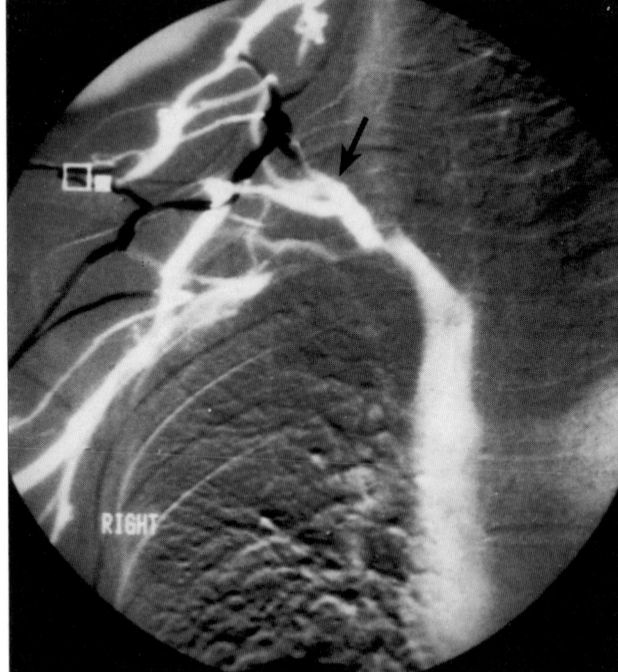

Fig. 19.20 (a) Demonstrates a secondary finding in upper limb thrombosis, namely the presence of a large collateral vein (arrow). This may add confidence to the initial diagnosis especially if the examination and/or anatomy is difficult to interpret. (b) This collateral (arrow) is clearly shown on an intravenous digital subtraction angiogram, the main subclavian vein being occluded. For colour, see Plate 19.20 (between pp. 308 and 309).

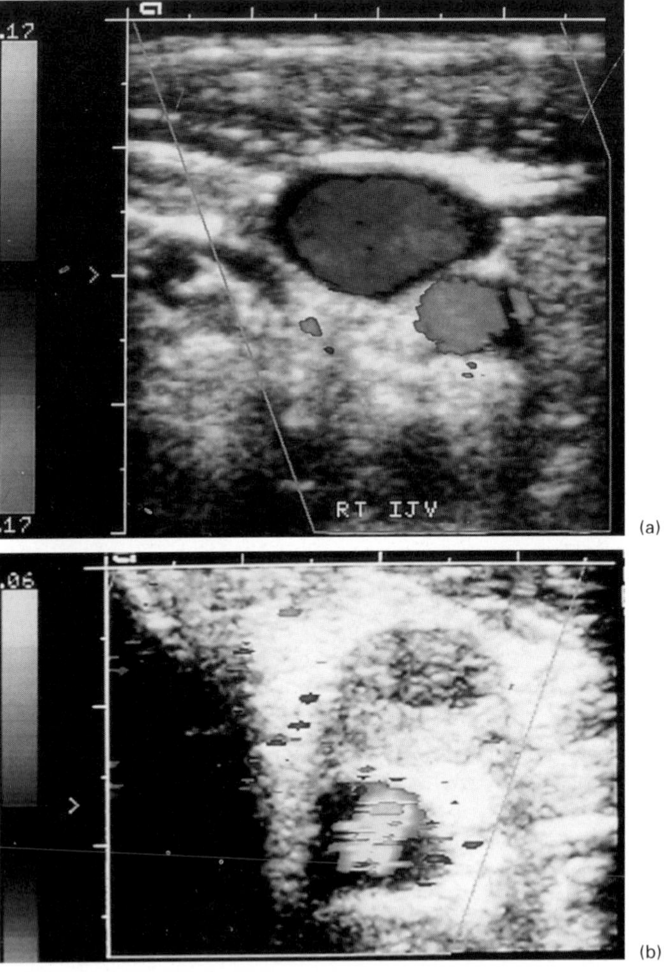

Fig. 19.21 (a) Transverse colour flow image of a patent internal jugular vein (IJV) lying anteriorly to the common carotid artery. (b) A thrombosed internal jugular vein in a different patient is shown for comparison. This scan has been performed in a similar image plane and once again the common carotid artery lies posteriorly. This vein is routinely imaged with colour Doppler imaging whereas it is not with intravenous contrast studies. This is one advantage of the non-invasive study. (Reproduced with permission from the *British Journal of Radiology* (1991), **64**, 777–781.) For colour, see Plate 19.21 (between pp. 308 and 309).

nying the adjacent artery is reassuring evidence of thrombosis and often adds confidence to the ultrasonic diagnosis.

Advantages and limitations of ultrasound

The advantages of ultrasound include safety, patient comfort, cost, and it is painless and radiation free. In the upper limb the internal jugular vein is routinely visualized and this may be of clinical importance if further sites for central venous catheterization are required [45] (Fig. 19.21). Venography of course does not routinely image this vein. Furthermore, follow-up and response to anticoagulant or lytic therapy can be easily monitored using this technique [46].

As a non-invasive technique, it has been used to help delineate problem areas in the upper limb, revealing some interesting results. Such an area is in the assessment of the postmastectomy swollen limb. Although this has always been attributed to lymphoedema, colour Doppler studies have shown that in this patient group the incidence of a significant venous abnormality may be in the order of 25% [47].

Limitations of the technique are those of any ultrasonic technique, i.e. access may be limited in the muscular, obese or severely oedematous patient. As mentioned previously, great care must be taken to ensure minimum pressure is applied to the probe as collapsing the vein may lead to misinterpretation. The distal innominate veins and SVC cannot be visualized using this technique and if a SVC syndrome is present clinically or there is a clinical indication that the lesion may be more centrally situated than the subclavian vein, then ultrasound is of no value and alternative imaging with computed tomography, magnetic resonance imaging or venography is more appropriate. As alluded to above, there is a blind spot of the mid-subclavian vein directly beneath the clavicle. Unfortunately, as many as 40% of postcatheterization vein stenoses occur here and ultrasound may miss these lesions [43]. Thus in patients with previous catheterization who present with a swollen limb, an ultrasound may exclude thrombosis but a venogram may still be required to exclude a stenotic lesion.

References

1 Kakkar, W. (1975) Deep vein thrombosis: detection and prevention. *Circulation* **51**, 8–19.

2 Lea Thomas, M., Keeling, F.P., Piaggio, R.B., Treweeks, P.S. (1984) Contrast agent induced thrombophlebitis following leg phlebography: iopamidol versus meglumine iothalamate. *British Journal of Radiology* **57**, 205–207.

3 Albrechtson, U., Olsson, C.G. (1976) Thrombotic side effects of lower limb venography. *Lancet* **i**, 723–724.

4 Christensen, S.W., Wille-Jorgensen, P., Kjaer, L., *et al.* (1987) Contact thermography, ^{99m}Tc-plasmin scintimetry and ^{99m}Tc-plasmin scintigraphy as screening methods for deep venous thrombosis following major hip surgery. *Thrombosis and Haemostasis* **58**, 831–833.

5 Gomes, A.S., Webber, M.M., Buffkin D. (1982) Contrast venography vs radionuclide venography: a study of their discrepancies and their possible significance. *Radiology* **142**, 719–728.

6 Zorba, J., Schier, D., Posmituck, G. (1986) Clinical value of blood pool radionuclide venography. *American Journal of Radiology* **146**, 1051–1055.

7 Ramchandani, P., Soulen, R.L., Fedullo L.M., Gaines, V.D. (1985) Deep vein thrombosis: significant limitations of non invasive tests. *Radiology* **156**, 47–49.

8 Pochaczevsky, R., Pillari, G., Feldman, F. (1982) Liquid crystal contact thermography of deep venous thrombosis. *American Journal of Radiology* **138**, 717–723.

9 Ritchie, W.G.M., Soulen, R.L., Lapayowker, M.S. (1979) Thermographic diagnosis of deep venous thrombosis. *Radiology* **131**, 341–344.

10 Sandler, D.A., Martin, J.F. (1985) Liquid crystal thermography as a screening test for deep vein thrombosis. *Lancet* **i**, 665–668.

11 Prescott, S.M., Tikoff, G., Coleman, R.E., *et al.* (1978) ^{131}I labelled fibrinogen in the diagnosis of deep venous thrombosis of the lower extremities. *American Journal of Roentgenology* **131**, 451–453.

12 Aitken, A.G.F., Godden, D.J. (1987) Real time ultrasound diagnosis of deep vein thrombosis: a comparison with venography. *Clinical Radiology* **38**, 309–313.

13 Cronan, J.J., Dorfman, G.S., Scola, F.H., Schepps, B., Alexander, J. (1987) Deep venous thrombosis: US assessment using vein compression. *Radiology* **162**, 191–194.

14 Lensing, A.W.A., Prandoni, P., Brandges, D., *et al.* (1989) Detection of deep venous thrombosis by real time B-mode ultrasonography. *New England Journal of Medicine* **320**, 342–345.

15 Lee Nix, M., Nelson, C.L., Harmon, B.H., Ferris, E.F., Barnes, R.W. (1989) Duplex venous scaning: image vs Doppler accuracy. *Journal of Vascular Technology* **13**, 123–126.

16 Baxter, G.M., MacKechnie, S., Duffy, P. (1990) Colour Doppler ultrasound in deep venous thrombosis: a comparison with venography. *Clinical Radiology* **42**, 32–36.

17 Foley, W.D., Middleton, W.D., Lawson, T.L., Erickson, S., Uiroz, F.A., Macrander, S. (1989) Colour Doppler ultrasound imaging of lower extremity venous disease. *American Journal of Radiology* **152**, 371–376.

18 van Bemmelin, P.S., Bedford, G., Strandness, D.E. (1990) Visualisation of calf veins by colour flow imaging. *Ultrasound in Medicine and Biology* **16**, 15–17.

19 Baxter, G.M., Duffy P. (1992) Calf vein anatomy and flow: implications for colour Doppler imaging. *Clinical Radiology* **46**, 84–87.

20 Polak, J.F., Culter, S.S., O'Leary D.H. (1989) Deep veins of the calf: assessment with colour Doppler flow imaging. *Radiology* **171**; 481–485.

21 Raghavendra, N., Rosen, R.J., Lam, S., Riles, T., Horii, S.C. (1984) Deep venous thrombosis: detection by high-resolution real time ultrasound. *Radiology* **152**, 789–793.

22 Baxter, G.M., Duffy, P., Partridge, E. (1992) Colour flow imaging of calf vein thrombosis. *Clinical Radiology* **46**, 198–201.

23 Rose, S.C., Zwiebel, W.J., Nelson, B.D., *et al.* (1990) Symptomatic lower extremity deep venous thrombosis: accuracy, limitations,

and role of colour duplex flow imaging in diagnosis. *Radiology* **175**, 639–644.

24 Nicolaides, A.N., Kakkar, W., Field, E.S., Renney, J.T.G. (1971) The origin of deep vein thrombosis: a venographic study. *British Journal of Radiology* **44**, 653–663.

25 Perlin, S.J. (1992) Pulmonary embolism during compression ultrasound of the lower extremity. *Radiology* **184**, 165–166.

26 Richardson, G.D., Beckwith, T.C., Sheldon, M. (1991) Ultrasound windows to abdominal and pelvic veins. *Phlebology* **6**, 125.

27 Quinn, K.L., Vandeman, F.N. (1990) Thrombosis of a duplicated superficial femoral vein. Potential error in compression ultrasound diagnosis of lower extremity deep venous thrombosis. *Journal of Ultrasound in Medicine* **9**, 235–238.

28 Lagerstedt, C.I., Olsson, C.G., Fagher, B.O., Oqvist, B.W., Albrechtsson, U. (1985) Need for long term anticoagulant treatment in symptomatic calf vein thrombosis. *Lancet* **ii**, 515–518.

29 Moser, K.M., LeMoine, J.R. (1981) Is embolic risk conditioned by location of deep venous thrombosis? *Annals of Internal Medicine* **94**, 439–444.

30 Vaccaro, J.P., Cronan, J.J., Dorfman, G.S. (1990) Outcome analysis of patients with normal compression US examinations. *Radiology* **175**, 645–649.

31 Meyerovitz, M.F., Polak, J.F., Goldhaber, S.Z. (1992) Short-term response to thrombolytic therapy in deep venous thrombosis: predictive value of venographic appearance. *Radiology* **184**, 345–348.

32 Baxter, G.M., Duffy, P., MacKechnie S. (1991) Colour Doppler ultrasound of the post-phlebitic limb: sounding a cautionary note. *Clinical Radiology* **43**, 301–304.

33 Cronan, J.J., Leen, V. (1989) Recurrent deep venous thrombosis: limitations of US. *Radiology* **170**, 739–742.

34 Murphy, T.P., Cronan, J.J. (1990) Evolution of deep venous thrombosis: a prospective evaluation with US. *Radiology* **177**, 543–548.

35 Sy, W.M., Seo, I.S. (1986) Radionuclide venography: imaging monitor in deep venous thrombosis of the pelvis and lower extremities. *British Journal of Radiology* **59**, 325–328.

36 Lea Thomas, M., McAllister, V. (1971) The radiological progression of deep venous thrombosis. *Radiology* **99**, 37–40.

37 Mudge, M., Hughes, L.E. (1978) The long term sequelae of deep vein thrombosis. *British Journal of Surgery* **65**, 692–694.

38 Lindner, D.J., Edwards, J.M., Phinney, E.S., Taylor, L.M., Porter, J.M. (1986) Long term haemodynamic and clinical sequelae of lower extremity deep vein thrombosis. *Journal of Vascular Surgery* **4**, 436–442.

39 Polak, J.F. (1992) Chronic venous thrombosis and venous insufficiency. In: Polak, J.F. *Peripheral Vascular Sonography: A Practical Guide*. Williams & Wilkins, Baltimore, pp. 232–245.

40 Coon, W.W., Willis P.W. (1966) Thrombosis of axillary and subclavian veins. *Archives of Surgery* **94**, 657.

41 Prescott, S.M., Tikoff, G. (1979) Deep venous thrombosis of the upper extremity: a reappraisal. *Circulation* **59**, 350–355.

42 Falk, R.L., Smith, D.L. (1987) Thrombosis of upper extremity thoracic inlet veins: diagnosis with duplex Doppler sonography. *American Journal of Roentgenology* **149**, 677–682.

43 Baxter, G.M., Kincaid, W., Jeffrey, R.F., Millar, G.M., Porteous, C., Morley, P. (1991) Comparison of colour Doppler ultrasound with venography in the diagnosis of axillary and subclavian vein thrombosis. *British Journal of Radiology* **64**, 777–781.

44 Hightower, D.R., Gooding, G.A.W. (1985) Sonographic evaluation of the normal response of subclavian veins to respiratory manoeuvres. *Radiology* **20**, 517–520.

45 Wing, V., Schieble, W. (1983) Sonography of jugular vein thrombosis. *American Journal of Roentgenology* **140**, 333–336.

46 Grassi, C.J., Polak, J.F. (1990) Axillary and subclavian venous thrombosis: follow up evaluation with colour Doppler flow ultrasound and venography. *Radiology* **175**, 651–654.

47 Svensson, W.E., Al-Murrani, B., Badger, C., *et al*. (1990) Is post mastectomy lymphoedema all lymphatic? Pulsed and color Doppler suggest a venous component. *British Journal of Radiology* **63**, 395–396.

48 Cronan, J.J., Froehlich, J.A., Dorfman, G.S. (1991) Image directed Doppler ultrasound: a screening technique for patients at high risk to develop deep vein thrombosis. *Journal of Clinical Ultrasound* **19**, 133–138.

Chapter 20: The abdominal vasculature

G.M. Baxter

Abdominal aorta

The abdominal aorta enters the abdomen through the diaphragm at approximately the 12th thoracic vertebrae and via its major branches, the coeliac axis, superior mesenteric artery (SMA), inferior mesenteric artery and renal arteries, supplies the abdominal viscera and bowel. It terminates at approximately the level of the fourth lumbar vertebral body and divides into the right and left common iliac systems. Although the iliac vessels are notoriously difficult to image both with real-time and colour flow Doppler, the abdominal aorta can be imaged in almost all individuals at some point within the abdomen and is only outwith the scope of ultrasound in the extremely obese or where there is an undue amount of bowel gas. Standard ultrasonic preparation is a 4–6-h fast although on many occasions this may be unnecessary.

Aortic aneurysm

The commonest disease of the abdominal aorta is the aortic aneurysm, with rupture accounting for approximately 1.7% of all deaths in males aged 65–74 years [1]. Although this diagnosis is often made on clinical examination, the most accurate, cheap and easy method is real-time ultrasound (Fig. 20.1), with a sensitivity of approximately 97–100% [2]. Doppler or colour Doppler ultrasound contributes little to the diagnosis.

The aneurysm is best sized in the transverse axis, the anteroposterior diameter being the most important for prognosis. The normal anteroposterior diameter is less than 2.5 cm. A localized bulge of the abdominal aorta is not classified as an aneurysm until this diameter is 3 cm or greater. The advantage of the longitudinal axis is in demonstrating its origin and distal extent. Most begin below the level of the renal arteries and terminate prior to the aortic bifurcation.

The relationship of the proximal aneurysm neck to the renal arteries is difficult to demonstrate in the majority. Involvement of these vessels by the aneurysm is important should surgery be contemplated. Although the renal arteries cannot be directly visualized they are known to lie approximately 1 cm below the level of the superior mesenteric artery, which can nearly always be visualized, and by utilizing this relationship the proximal extent of the aneurysm can often be inferred. Spiral computed tomography (CT) with coronal reconstruction and multiplanar magnetic resonance imaging (MRI) can convincingly demonstrate this relationship; however, as yet these modalities are not universally available. Angiography, of course, can show this relationship well but is invasive.

Growth rates of aneurysms vary between individuals and indeed from study to study. For an aneurysm less than 5 cm diameter anteroposteriorly, growth rates vary from 3 mm per year [3] to as much as 7 mm in 6 months [4]. In general terms, the larger the aneurysm the greater the rate of expansion [5]. It is clear that for aneurysms less than 5 cm diameter anteroposteriorly regular screening on a 6-monthly or yearly basis, depending on stability, is required. Once an aneurysm is greater than 5 cm the patient it is at increased risk of spontaneous rupture which, by definition, carries a high mortality rate [6–8]. Elective surgery, however, in the non-emergency situation reduces both morbidity and mortality considerably [9].

As a result of this, screening programmes have been advocated [10]. The cost-effectiveness of such a programme has still to be calculated and currently a nationwide screening programme is difficult to justify. Focusing a screening programme upon high risk patients to include the elderly, males, hypertensives, those patients with cardiovascular or peripheral vascular disease [11] or a family history of aortic aneurysm rupture [12] may be more rewarding initially. Screening programmes are currently under assessment; however, life-saving benefit has already been demonstrated [13].

RUPTURED AORTIC ANEURYSM

Any patient who presents with a pulsatile abdominal mass and hypotension does not normally require any form of imaging as the over-riding priority is to resuscitate and transport the patient to theatre where definitive

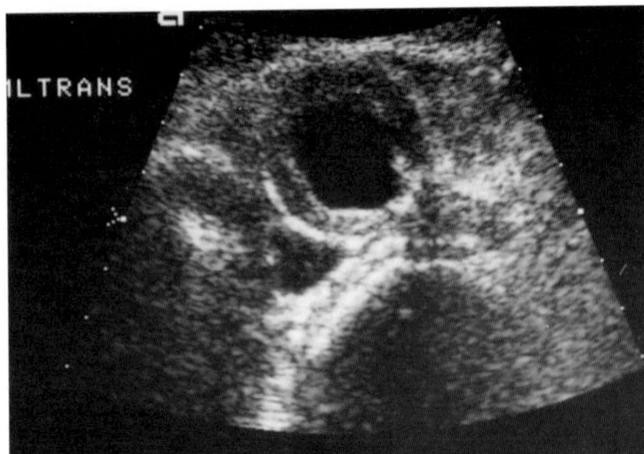

(a)

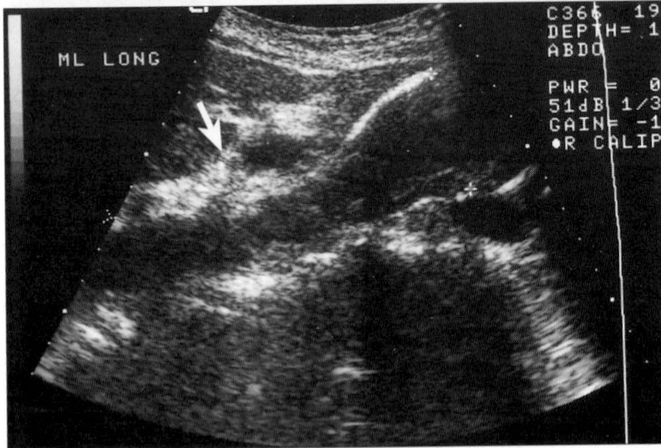

(b)

Fig. 20.1 (a) An aortic aneurysm in transverse section with an anteroposterior diameter of 3.6 cm. (b) In longitudinal section the same aneurysm can be seen to arise well below the level of the SMA (arrow) and presumably the renal vessels although these cannot be directly visualized.

surgery can be performed. When the rupture is less dramatic, abdominal ultrasound examination can be performed. This, however, will simply confirm the presence and size of the aneurysm. As ultrasound has an extremely poor sensitivity (4%) for the detection of periaortic fluid [14]. A clinical decision is required for overall patient management.

Aortic dissection

Aortic dissection is a catastrophic condition found in approximately 1 in 380 autopsies. It is most common in men over 50 years of age and predisposing conditions include hypertension, Marfan's syndrome, pregnancy, trauma, coarctation of aorta, bicuspid aortic valves and aortic valve repair.

The DeBakey classification is based upon the premise that 95% of dissections arise either in the ascending aorta within 2 cm of the aortic valve or in the descending aorta at the ligamentum arteriosum. There are three types of dissection (Fig. 20.2). Type I and II are treated surgically whilst type III is normally treated conservatively.

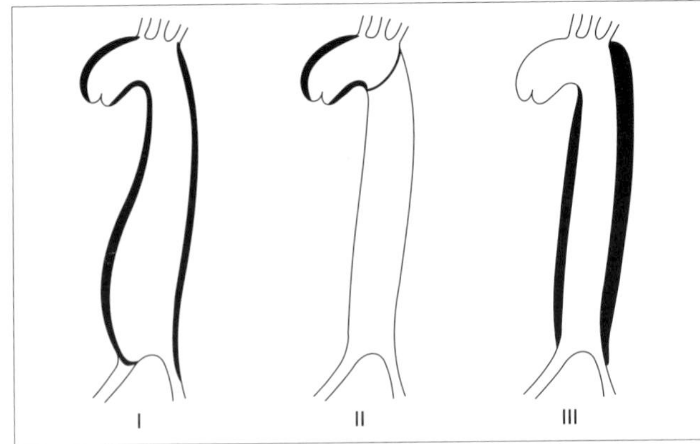

Fig. 20.2 Diagram of the DeBakey classification of acute aortic dissection. A type I dissection begins in the ascending aorta and propagates distally beyond the ligamentum arteriosum, whilst type II dissections are confined to the ascending aorta. Both type I and II dissections may involve the aortic root vessels. Type III dissections begin at or distal to the ligamentum arteriosum and spread distally. With this form of classification types I and II dissections are clinically managed surgically whilst type III dissections are managed conservatively with antihypertensive therapy.

Patients present with sudden tearing chest pain with radiation to the neck, back or arms. Hypertension is present in 50%. Conventional imaging strategies vary; however, MRI or transoesophageal echocardiography (TOE) are universally accepted as the most accurate imaging modalities. In addition, praecordial echocardiography is often used to visualize the proximal point of dissection as this may be difficult on TOE alone.

Although no one would recommend abdominal ultrasound in this condition as a primary diagnostic tool, an intimal flap can be visualized within the aortic lumen and involvement of the major visceral vessels can be detected using Doppler ultrasound [15].

Aortocaval fistula

This is a very rare condition where there is rupture, normally of an aneurysmal aorta, with direct communication between it and the inferior vena cava (IVC). Clinical presentation is rare and this condition is normally fatal. Rare case reports exist and identification of a fistulous communication with Doppler ultrasound [16] have been documented, mixed turbulent arterial and venous flow within the IVC being suggestive of this condition [17].

Renal artery stenosis

Background

The blood supply of the kidney is normally from a single renal artery but accessory vessels may occur in up to 20–30% of normal individuals. These vessels, although well demonstrated by angiography, are poorly visualized by ultrasound even with colour Doppler.

Renal artery stenosis (RAS) is a condition which results in narrowing of the proximal portion of the renal artery. Clinical presentation varies from hypertension resistant to standard therapy, to renal impairment, to a discrepancy in renal size on ultrasound. In some it may be an unexpected finding. Fibromuscular hyperplasia, which may involve the intrarenal branch vessels as well as the main renal artery, can present in a similar manner but classically affects young to middle-aged females.

Renal artery stenosis may respond to angioplasty; however, vascular stenting is often required especially in those with ostial lesions. Clinical outcome is variable and depends to a large extent upon patient selection. Cure is possible in up to only one-third of patients, a further one-third will improve or remain stable whilst the remaining third will deteriorate. Fibromuscular hyperplasia invariably responds well to angioplasty, and has a much better prognosis.

Technique

Although real-time ultrasound imaging of the kidneys is straightforward, Doppler and colour Doppler imaging is more difficult. Whilst the intrarenal branches and the renal artery at hilar level can be visualized and interrogated by spectral Doppler on most occasions (Fig. 20.3), the proximal main renal artery is extremely difficult to visualize. As most stenotic lesions occur in this area this creates a problem. Furthermore, the origin of the renal arteries subtend a very poor Doppler angle making absolute velocity measurements difficult.

Examination of the main renal artery

As alluded to earlier, direct examination of the main renal artery is an extremely difficult technique to master and numerous Doppler indices have been evaluated to help aid diagnosis. These include the peak systolic velocity within the main renal artery. This is normally below 1 m s^{-1} [18] and values do not become significant until this reaches ≥1.8 m s^{-1} this representing a 60% stenosis. Whilst peak systolic velocities greater than this value are indicative of more severe lesions no linear relationship exists. These values are clearly only of use if the entire length of the renal artery can be visualized. Technically inadequate examinations vary greatly between 9–16% of patients [19–21] to 31–42%, despite the use of colour Doppler [22,23]. The majority of these difficulties are due to obesity, bowel gas or poor Doppler angulation.

In order to try and overcome the anglulation problem, Doppler ratios including resistive and pulsatility index have been evaluated. Although these superficially appear to offer certain advantages, they have not been shown to be of any benefit in the diagnosis of this disease, as they require the contralateral kidney to be normal allowing comparison.

Further parameters have involved the use of the renal

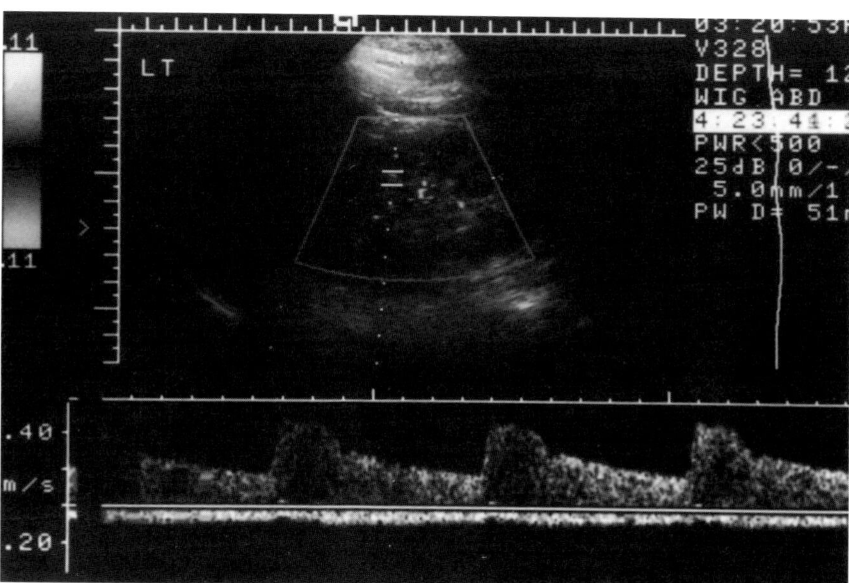

Fig. 20.3 Normal Doppler spectral waveform from an intrarenal branch of the renal artery. This waveform exhibits the characteristics of an artery that supplies a low impedance vascular bed with maintenance of high flow throughout diastole.

aortic ratio (RAR) in which the peak systolic velocity within the main renal artery is compared with that of the abdominal aorta. An RAR of greater than 3.5 is said to be indicative of a renal artery stenosis >60% [21]. This, however, assumes the entire length of the renal artery can be visualized and that a good spectral waveform can be obtained from both the abdominal aorta and renal artery, again a challenging feat. Results using this ratio vary from sensitivities of 79–91% and specificities of 73–93% [19–21] to much poorer results with sensitivities of 0%, the latter being with the aid of colour Doppler [22,23].

Many centres feel this technique, independent of which ratio or measurement is used, is too technically demanding to be used in routine practice. In addition, it is extremely time-consuming and very dependent upon patient cooperation.

Examination of the intrarenal vessels

An interesting concept and an alternative examination technique in RAS has now evolved. This involves Doppler spectral interrogation of the intrarenal vessels, normally the interlobar. The normal intrarenal waveform has a sharp systolic upstroke and a well-defined systolic peak. The presence of a dampened and rounded waveform, i.e. the 'parvus–tardus' effect, is indicative of a proximal stenosing lesion. This dampening of the spectral waveform is known to occur downstream from a significant arterial stenosis. 'Tardus' refers to a delayed or prolonged early systolic acceleration and 'parvus' to the diminished amplitude and rounding of the systolic peak. These changes can be quantified as an increased acceleration time (>0.07 s) and reduced acceleration index (<3 m s^{-2}) (Fig. 20.4). Initial studies showed these indices to be present in those arteries with a 60% or greater stenosis [24]. The initial sensitivity and specificity results were encouraging at 95 and 97%, respectively; however, more recently performed studies using similar techniques could only reproduce these findings for severely stenosed renal vessels (>80%) [25]. Indeed a more recent publication has suggested that the probability of a significant RAS does not approach 90% until the acceleration time is above 0.12 s [26].

In order for the 'parvus–tardus' effect to be present there are two criteria that are required. Firstly, there must be a significant stenosis; and secondly, the vessels downstream from the stenosis must be compliant. The latter of those considerations is thought to be the most important [27]. Indeed this loss of vessel compliance is thought to be responsible for the false negative scans that do occasionally plague this technique whilst the false positive scans generally reflect poor technique.

Despite some claims to the contrary this technique, although more user friendly than the direct method, is not a stand alone screening technique. Suboptimal scans still occur in up to 10% of patients and the issue of false positive and negative scans still has to be addressed [26].

Ultrasound's main role may well not be as a diagnostic screening test but in the follow-up and monitoring of renal artery angioplasty or stenting (Fig. 20.5). Early results would indicate that this is a useful application of the technique as long-term studies using these stents are few. Indeed another useful clinical role may also be in studying

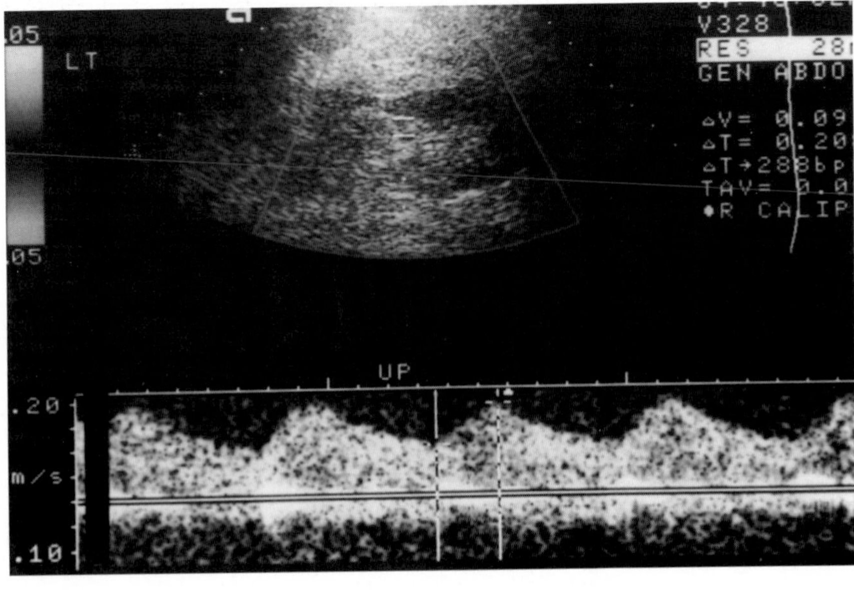

Fig. 20.4 Doppler waveform of an intrarenal vessel from a kidney with an angiographically proven 80% stenosis demonstrating a very damped waveform with a reduced acceleration index of 0.45 and prolongation of the acceleration time to 0.20 s. These features occur downstream from a more proximal stenosing lesion.

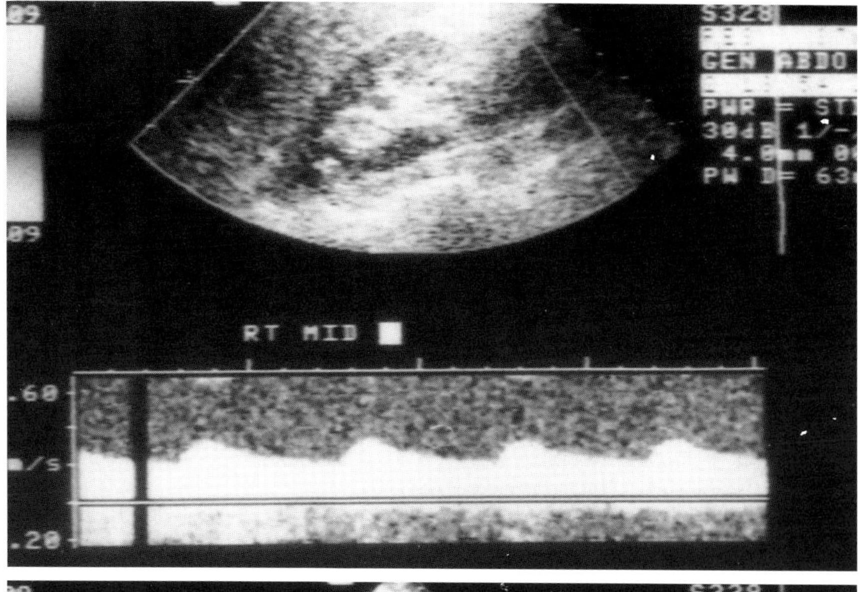

(a)

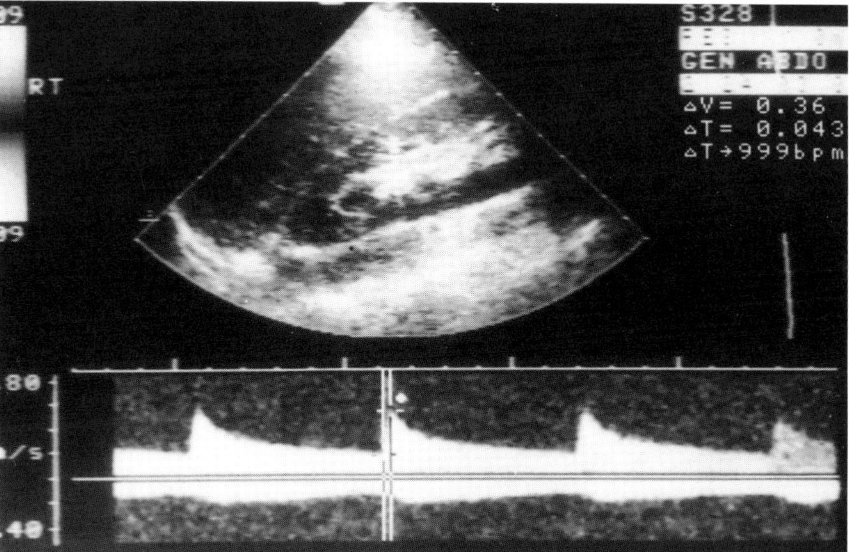

(b)

Fig. 20.5 (a) Doppler waveform from an intrarenal vessel in a kidney with an 85% proximal RAS. The waveform is markedly damped. The acceleration index is 0.83 and the acceleration time is 0.162 s. (b) Doppler examination was performed 24 h following successful angioplasty. Restoration of a normal intrarenal waveform, with a marked increase in acceleration index to 8.37 and a consequent reduction in acceleration time to 0.043 s, was noted.

those patients with 'borderline significant stenoses' on angiography to try and give more useful haemodynamic information.

With regard to the future of the technique, this may revolve around a combination of the colour and power flow techniques, harmonics and contrast agents.

Visceral vessels

The visceral vessels consist of the coeliac axis, the superior mesenteric artery (SMA) and inferior mesenteric artery. The inferior mesenteric artery is notoriously difficult to visualize and is not routinely interrogated by colour Doppler imaging. Many elderly patients, in fact, have long-standing occlusion of this vessel with no obvious detriment to health. The coeliac artery and SMA are best examined after at least a 6-h fast. This allows comparison between serial measurements as waveforms differ in the fasting and postprandial state [28].

Coeliac artery

EXAMINATION TECHNIQUE

Both the coeliac trunk and SMA arise from the aorta anteriorly (Fig. 20.6). The origin of the coeliac axis is best visu-

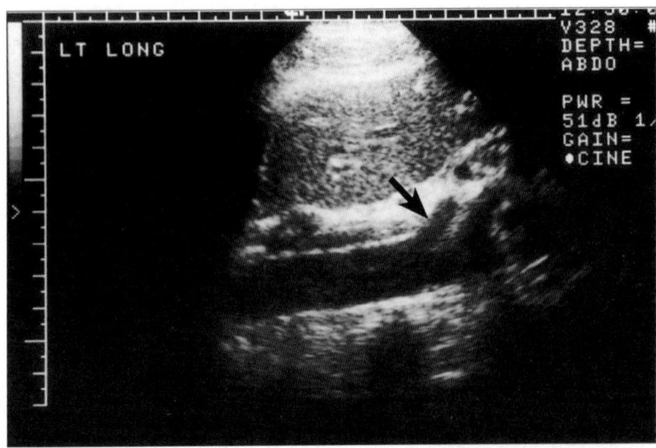

Fig. 20.6 Longitudinal section through the upper abdominal aorta demonstrating the origin of the coeliac axis (arrow) with the origin of the SMA immediately below. Both vessels can be visualized with real-time imaging and with the aid of colour and duplex Doppler can be assessed for evidence of significant stenoses.

alized in the transverse axis; alternatively, the coeliac axis can be imaged in the longitudinal plane either with the patient in the supine or right anterior oblique position. In this latter position a good angle is often obtained for absolute velocity measurements.

COELIAC ARTERY STENOSIS

This may occur secondary to atheromatous change and can present clinically, in the presence of multiple visceral vessel involvement as 'abdominal angina'. The coeliac axis can also narrow secondary to extrinsic compression, most often malignant. The peak systolic velocity in this vessel is normally <1 m s^{-1}. A peak systolic velocity greater than 2 m s^{-1} in the fasting condition is said to be diagnostic of a >70% coeliac artery stenosis [29].

Coeliac artery aneurysms

Both coeliac and superior mesenteric artery aneurysms, can occur in rare conditions like Ehlers–Danlos syndrome, and can be identified non-invasively using colour flow imaging [30,31].

Coeliac artery aneurysms only account for 4% of splanchnic artery aneurysms, are usually detected in the sixth decade of life and have no sexual predilection. They are often clinically silent or present with vague abdominal pain. As early diagnosis is now possible, fewer than 20% rupture due to elective surgical repair. Although atherosclerosis is the commonest cause, trauma, infection, inflammation, connective tissue disease and developmental causes have been implicated [32].

Splenic artery

The splenic artery is very rarely examined with colour Doppler imaging as very few pathologies affect flow significantly within this vessel. The splenic and hepatic arteries are, however, the most common site of pseudoaneurysm formation within the abdomen, normally as a result of abdominal trauma or pancreatitis.

Hepatic artery

The hepatic artery normally arises from the coeliac axis but anatomical variations are common. The right hepatic artery may arise from the superior mesenteric artery in 11% of cases and can be visualized posterior, rather than anterior, to the portal vein. The left hepatic artery may arise separately from the left gastric artery in 18% of cases and can be visualized within the ligamentum venosum. It should not be mistaken for a portocaval collateral pathway.

The hepatic artery is best interrogated with colour Doppler distal to the origin of the gastroduodenal branch. The main right hepatic branch can be visualized by a lateral intercostal approach as it accompanies the main right portal vein branch or the distal few centimetres of the main portal vein (Fig. 20.7). The left hepatic artery is visualized subcostally accompanying the left portal vein branch. Selective use of the colour velocity scale and post-processing colours and hues can help differentiate these vessels as they lie in close apposition.

There are very few situations in which Doppler examination of the hepatic artery has any direct clinical benefit. Although it has recently been demonstrated that the use of the hepatic perfusion index (HPI) may show change in both metastatic and overt metastatic liver disease [33,34], this work is in its infancy and collaborative studies have yet to confirm these findings.

Increased flow can be detected within the hepatic artery secondary to portal vein occlusion leading to the hypertrophied, more easily identified and aptly named corkscrew hepatic artery.

Flow within the hepatic artery itself is of little diagnostic benefit but it is of use in the monitoring of paediatric secondary biliary cirrhosis. Serial measurements in this condition do correspond with a response or non-response to steroid and steroid-sparing therapy, whilst flow reversal is a serious finding normally resulting in a more aggressive approach which includes transplantation.

The role of the hepatic artery following liver transplantation has been discussed but Doppler analysis is of little use in the monitoring of hepatic rejection [35]. Patency of the hepatic artery is essential following transplantation as if it occludes the transplant fails and therefore the main

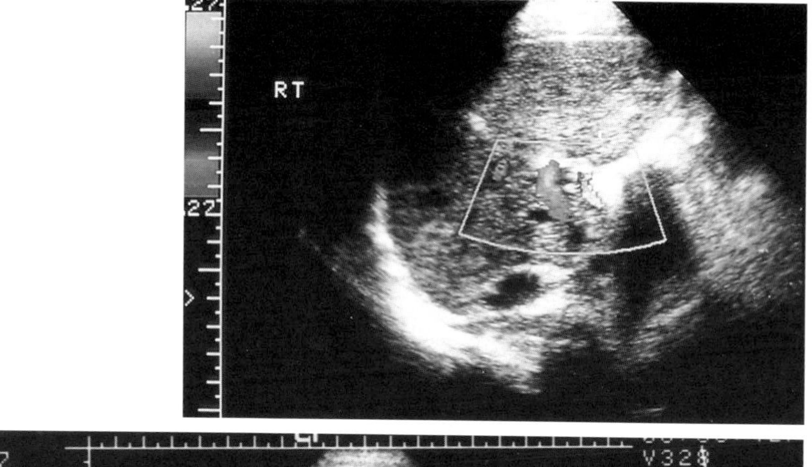

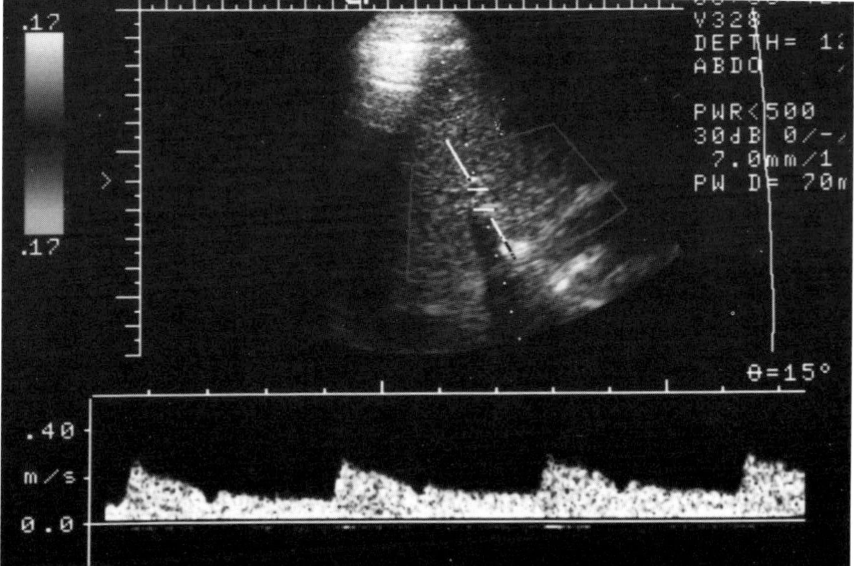

Fig. 20.7 (a) Colour flow image through a right intercostal approach demonstrating hepatopetal flow within the distal portal vein, the hepatic artery lying anteriorly. (b) A normal hepatic artery waveform is demonstrated on spectral analysis with maintenance of flow throughout diastole. For colour, see Plate 20.7 (between pp. 308 and 309).

role of ultrasound is to confirm vessel patency in the post-transplant period. The average rate of post-transplant hepatic artery thrombosis is in the order of 3–12%.

SMA

TECHNIQUE

The SMA arises just below the coeliac axis and can be visualized between the aorta posteriorly and portal vein anteriorly in the transverse axis. This scan plane, however, cannot be utilized to obtain an accurate Doppler velocity profile. This is normally done by scanning in a longitudinal plane with the patient supine or in a right anterior oblique position. Once again this vessel must be examined with the patient fasting as significant change occurs following the administration of food [36] (Fig. 20.8).

SUPERIOR MESENTERIC ARTERY STENOSIS

The peak systolic velocity is normally $<1.5\,m\,s^{-1}$ and the end-diastolic velocity $24 \pm 4\,cm\,s^{-1}$ [36]. A peak systolic velocity $>2.75\,m\,s^{-1}$ is said to be diagnostic of a $\geq 70\%$ stenosis [29]. An end-diastolic velocity $>45\,cm\,s^{-1}$ has been suggested as the best indicator of superior mesenteric artery stenosis of >50% [37]. Turbulence may also be noted downstream from the stenotic site and is another good indicator of a more proximal narrowed lesion.

The use of postprandial changes may also aid the diagnosis of intestinal ischaemia. Although patients with SMA stenosis may be identifiable on the fasting examination, others may have minor or non-diagnostic change. In the latter group, a food challenge may result in abnormal responses within the SMA [38].

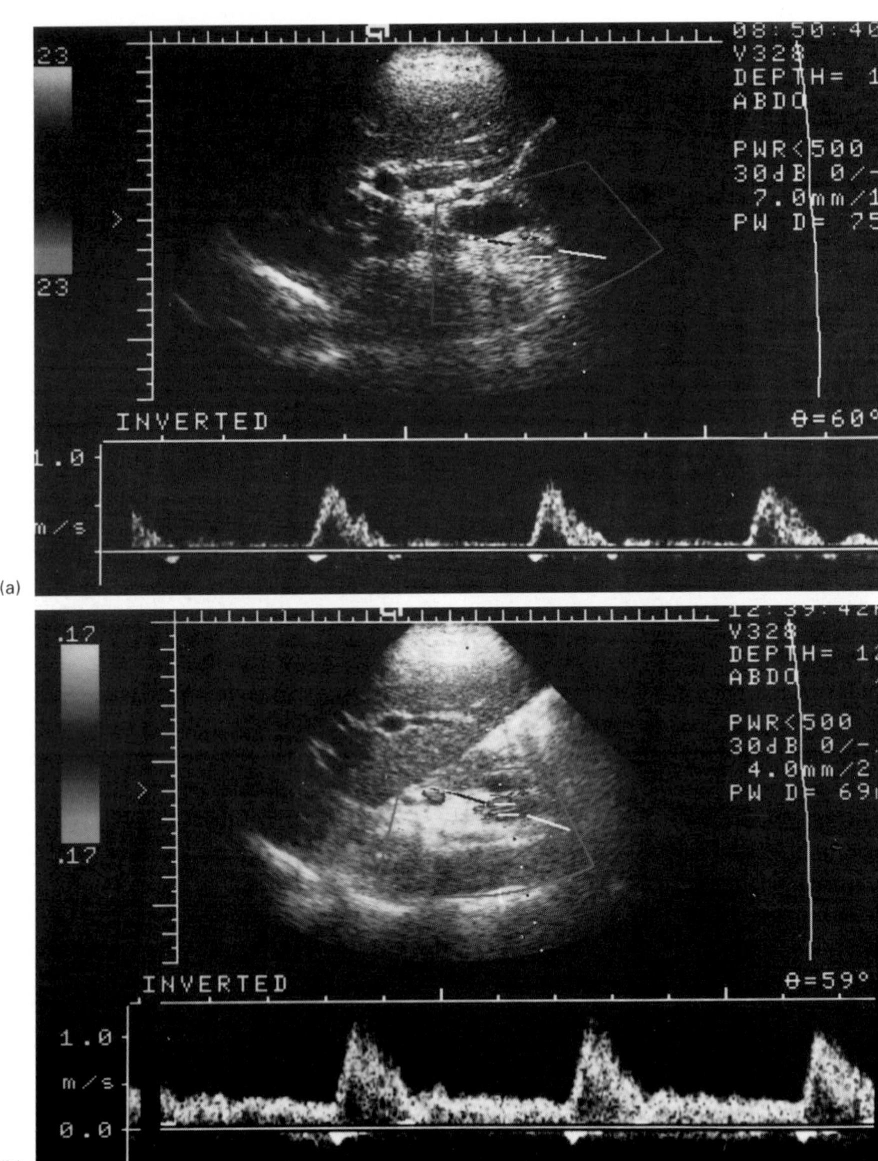

Fig. 20.8 (a) Doppler waveform of the SMA in the fasting state demonstrating little diastolic flow and a small reverse flow component. (b) Following a meal, there is a visible change in the waveform of the SMA with loss of reverse flow and a significant increase in diastolic flow.

SUPERIOR MESENTERIC ARTERY ANEURYSMS

See coeliac artery aneurysms (p. 298).

OTHER CONDITIONS AFFECTING THE VISCERAL VESSELS

Another potential use of Doppler ultrasound is in determining acute episodes of inflammatory bowel disease. Changes in velocity readings have been noted within the visceral vessels during periods of disease activity when compared with inactive disease and normal control groups [39]. As monitoring therapy response can be difficult on clinical grounds alone, and the barium findings have no correlation with disease activity, ultrasound may be useful in this role.

Colour Doppler imaging can monitor the affects of drugs not only directly on the portal venous system but through their secondary effects on the visceral and renal vessels. Velocity changes in the visceral vessels have been demonstrated following the administration of β-blockers such as propranolol, vasodilators such as isosorbide mononitrate and other drugs including somatostatin and its analogues [40]. Many of these drugs are used in the treatment of portal hypertension and bleeding varices, and a more clear understanding of their affects on local haemodynamics is possible using this technique.

IVC, renal and hepatic veins

The IVC begins at approximately the level of L4, lies to the right of the abdominal aorta and terminates at its entrance into the right atrial cavity. In addition to receiving the venous drainage of both lower limbs it receives the venous return from both kidneys and liver. Anatomical variants exist and a left-sided IVC (0.2%) is a well-recognized phenomenom. The IVC varies significantly in size depending on the phase of respiration and may even have a slit-like appearance [41] this being most marked at end expiration and following the Valsalva manoeuvre. These dramatic changes in diameter are normal.

All of these veins can be affected by various pathological processes; however, by far the commonest ones are those of venous thrombosis and tumour invasion.

Examination technique

The IVC is best examined with the patient in a fasting state to reduce the amount of bowel gas. With the patient lying supine or in a right anterior oblique position, the IVC can be scanned in both a transverse and longitudinal axis. In thin individuals this can usually be performed with little difficulty but this vessel does lie deep within the abdominal cavity and may be difficult and occasionally impossible to image successfully in well-built or obese individuals.

Examination of the renal veins is performed in a similar manner. Visualization is often best in the transverse axis, the left renal vein being sandwiched between the aorta posteriorly and the SMA anteriorly whilst the right renal vein runs a straighter course from the kidney. With some degree of patient obliquity a reasonable Doppler angle can often be obtained to allow a decision on venous patency.

All three hepatic veins, i.e. the left, middle and right, can be identified both on grey-scale and colour Doppler imaging. All drain into the IVC whilst the caudate lobe drains directly into the IVC. Once again these vessels are best examined with the patient fasting and for Doppler examination, in quiet respiration. If suspended respiration is used then this may alter the venous tracing and lead to misinterpretation of the spectral waveform.

IVC

Thrombus within the IVC may arise *de novo* or from secondary spread from the iliac veins. On real-time imaging this may be seen as an echogenic solid mass projecting into the normally anechoic lumen of the IVC. Colour Doppler ultrasound in such cases adds little to the examination apart from confirming the grey-scale findings (Fig. 20.9). Colour Doppler ultrasound may, however, be of help when thrombus is acute, i.e. anechoic as this may not be recognized on real-time imaging alone. Simple thrombus cannot be differentiated from tumour thrombus although tumour flow within the 'thrombus mass' itself has been demonstrated with colour [42]. Further trials are necessary to confirm this.

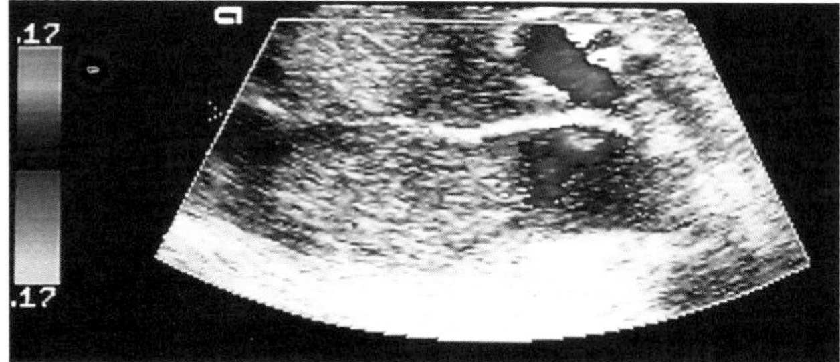

Fig. 20.9 Colour flow image of the IVC in longitudinal axis, demonstrating echogenic tumour thrombus within the lumen and some surrounding peripheral flow. The tumour had extended along the main renal vein secondary to a primary renal cell carcinoma. For colour, see Plate 20.9 (between pp. 308 and 309).

Colour flow imaging is also effective in confirming IVC and renal vein patency following IVC filter insertion. Good technique is important as poor examinations may be misleading and result in falsely reassuring scans [43]. Complications of caval filter insertion [43,44] include IVC thrombosis, filter malposition, filter angulation, pericaval haematoma and prong perforation. Although both CT and MRI have been shown to be more accurate in the definition of these complications this is in part due to their better technical success rate. When visualization with ultrasound is good, it is as accurate as CT and MRI in the diagnosis of caval thrombosis. Filter position and orientation is often best demonstrated by a simple plain abdominal film [45].

Intravascular ultrasound is in a very early stage of development but has been assessed in animal studies. The presence of intrafilter thrombi and filter position would seem to be well demonstrated with this technique giving additional information not available with conventional imaging [45]. Early clinical applications are also encouraging with better delineation of thrombus both within the IVC and filter in some cases [46].

Renal veins

Renal vein thrombosis

Renal vein thrombosis is most common in childhood, and relatively infrequent in the adult. The left renal vein is more frequently involved than the right. Many predispos-

Table 20.1 Conditions associated with renal vein thrombosis

Dehydration in neonates
diarrhoea
vomiting
sepsis
Nephrotic syndrome
Glomerulonephritis
Tumour
Trauma
Pregnancy
Systemic diseases
amyloidosis
systemic lupus erythematosus
diabetes

ing conditions exist (Table 20.1). Clinical presentation includes loin pain, haematuria, nephromegaly and evidence of thromboembolic phenomena elsewhere in the body.

Grey-scale changes depend upon the time since the initial insult. Initially, the kidney is enlarged, swollen and of decreased cortical echogenicity secondary to oedema; however, as time progresses, by 1–3 weeks there is an increase in cortical echogenicity with preservation of corticomedullary differentiation. These latter features are thought to correspond to a combination of cellular infiltrate and fibrosis. Finally, the late change of fibrosis, i.e. decreased renal size, increased cortical echogenicity and loss of corticomedullary differentiation, are noted [47]. As the grey-scale changes lag behind the initial insult, colour Doppler imaging at least potentially provides an earlier method of diagnosis. To date, this unfortunately has not been realized and as yet this has not influenced the outcome of this disease.

Tumours

Tumour infiltration of the renal vein is a well-recognized feature of renal cell carcinoma (Fig. 20.10) and is important to recognize, occurring in up to 23% of cases in one series [48]. This is of surgical importance as it can influence management. A transabdominal or retroperitoneal surgical approach is used if tumour thrombosis is confined to the renal vein or infradiagphragmatic IVC; however, if there is extension into the right atrium then atrial thrombectomy with possible cardiopulmonary bypass will be required [49] should this surgery be undertaken.

Various techniques including CT, MRI and ultrasound have all been used to assess renal vein extension. Results vary and it is not entirely clear which is the best method of assessment. On occasion CT has been shown to be more effective, the accuracy of CT being 74% in comparison to 65% for angiography and 63% for MRI [50]. Others have found MRI superior to CT [51,52] and ultrasound, with positive predictive values for real vein and IVC involvement for MRI of 95% and 100%, respectively. Overall CT and MRI are the favoured options.

Real-time ultrasound is hindered by suboptimal examinations and isoechoic tumour thrombus. Both of these reasons undoubtedly contribute to the relatively poor performance of this technique. Pulsed Doppler, although helpful, is time-consuming. Recently, colour Doppler imaging compared well with CT and MRI with an overall sensitivity of 95% in detecting venous involvement [53]. Limitations of this technique included bulky tumours which by causing local compression makes vascular assessment difficult.

Leiomyosarcoma

Leiomyosarcoma of the renal veins or IVC is an extremely rare tumour, there only being 106 cases reported to date. It is more common in females and arises from the smooth muscle wall lining the vein. Although a mass lesion can be seen with ultrasound it is impossible to differentiate from other causes of retroperitoneal masses. It has a very poor prognosis [54,55].

Hepatic veins

The hepatic veins can be visualized with grey-scale ultrasound adequately but the addition of colour Doppler ultrasound adds a new dimension to the amount information that is available.

The hepatic venous waveform has a more pulsatile feature than the normal continuous flow associated with other venous structures, e.g. the portal vein. Although the vast majority of flow occurs away from the probe, some does occur in the opposite direction, these fluctuations being secondary to right heart contraction (Fig. 20.11).

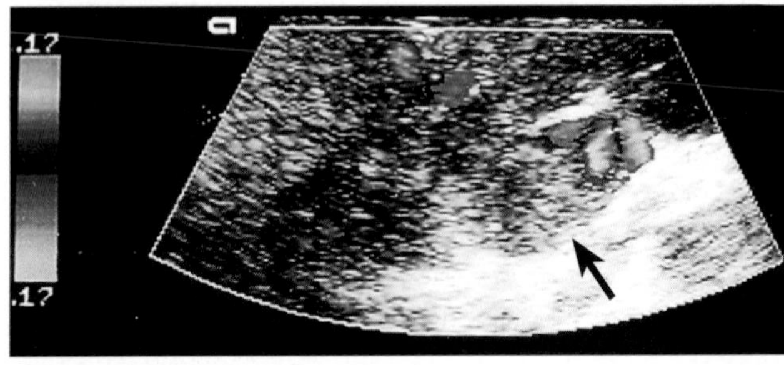

Fig. 20.10 Colour flow image demonstrating tumour thrombus (arrow) within a distended renal vein from a primary renal cell carcinoma. For colour, see Plate 20.10 (between pp. 308 and 309).

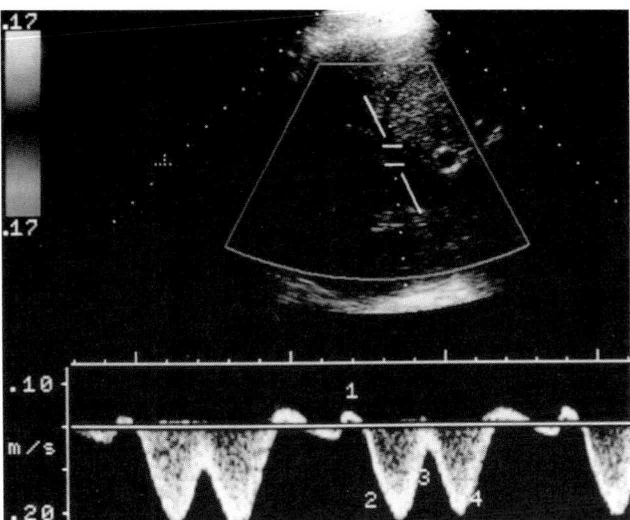

Fig. 20.11 Doppler spectral waveform of the hepatic vein showing marked fluctuation secondary to right heart contraction. The variations within the waveform reflect: (1) right atrial filling; (2) right atrial systole; (3) completion of right atrial systole; and (4) right ventricular contraction. It is important that when the hepatic veins are being sampled with Doppler that respiration is not suspended as this can dampen the waveform secondary to diaphragmatic splinting of the liver and lead to false interpretation.

This bidirectional flow may be affected by suspended respiration and it is therefore important that the examination is performed during quiet respiration, and with a wide Doppler gate to accommodate the movement of the hepatic vein with inspiration and expiration.

Right-sided heart disease may influence the hepatic venous waveform via an increase in right-sided heart pressure and conduction back to the IVC and hepatic veins [56,57]. In this situation, the value of the hepatic venous waveform is lost. Indeed, obtaining good information from the left hepatic vein is often difficult due to transmitted cardiac pulsation.

Changes in the spectral characteristics of the hepatic venous waveform may be secondary to a wide variety of hepatic insults. The most common of these is cirrhosis but any insult that results in decreased liver compliance, e.g. infiltrative diseases (glycogen storage diseases, Wilson's disease), widespread metastatic disease and hepatitis, will result in dampening, i.e. flattening of the waveform. Mild disease may simply cause a loss of bidirectional flow but as disease severity progresses the pulsatility of the hepatic waveform decreases until eventually a flat continuous waveform similar to the portal vein is obtained (Fig. 20.12). These changes in waveform correlate reasonably well with the severity of hepatic disease [58]. It is important to remember, however, that flattening of the hepatic venous waveform may also occur in suspended respiration in obese individuals and in patients with ascites, and in those groups of patients results should be interpreted with caution.

Budd–Chiari syndrome

Hepatic vein thrombosis (Budd–Chiari syndrome) can occur both spontaneously and secondary to many predisposing conditions (Table 20.2). It is a very uncommon condition with a prevalence of 0.061% in one autopsy series. Clinical features includes ascites (93%), hepatomegaly

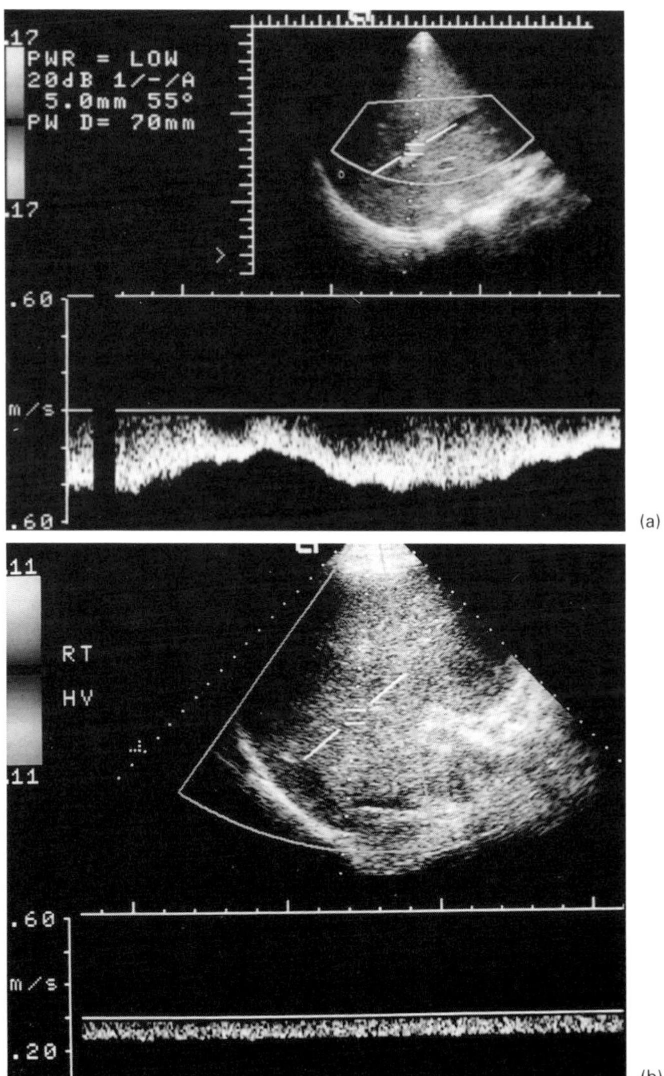

Fig. 20.12 Doppler waveform of the hepatic vein in a patient with (a) mild and (b) severe liver disease showing loss of the normal waveform pulsatility. The hepatic waveform in the latter case (b) is flat and continuous and is similar in appearance to the portal vein.

Table 20.2 Causes of hepatic vein thrombosis

Idiopathic
Hypercoagulable states, e.g. polycythaemia
Oral contraceptive
Tumours
hepatic
renal
Thrombophlebitis migrans
Congenital diaphragm of IVC

(70%), abdominal pain, oedema and dilated superficial veins. Occasionally, chronic Budd–Chiari syndrome can be accompanied by the complications of cirrhosis and portal hypertension and in some cases may even be asymptomatic.

This condition can affect the hepatic veins globally, pick out any combination of veins selectively and occasionally may involve the IVC. The pattern of ultrasonic findings therefore is extremely varied [59,60]. If all three hepatic veins are acutely involved then reverse flow may be visualized within the portal vein. A reduction in portal vein velocity is also a secondary finding in up to 70% of those affected, whilst portal vein thrombosis may occur in 10%.

As all patients share a common vascular abnormality, i.e. reduction or occlusion of hepatic venous outflow, then collateral pathways must be found. These include hepatic vein to portal vein collaterals (e.g. paraumbilical veins, oesophageal varices, recanalized umbilical vein), hepatic to systemic venous channels (e.g. via capsular veins to the azygous, intercostals, etc.) and hepatic to hepatic venous collaterals (spiderweb collaterals). On venography the so-called 'spiderweb' appearance is characteristic.

This condition is notoriously difficult to diagnose on ultrasound even with the aid of colour Doppler as the liver may already be chronically damaged and have an abnormal hyperechoic texture. Secondary effects from compression and distortion of abnormal liver architecture may result in thin hepatic veins that are difficult to visualize. It may be difficult to decide whether the appearances reflect technical factors, background liver changes or indeed true Budd–Chiari lesion. Colour flow ultrasound is said to aid this differentiation [61] by better delineation of the hepatic venous vasculature. Despite the aid of this tool diagnostic dilemmas remain.

Diagnostic criteria are generally non-specific. Absent flow, reverse flow or flattening of the hepatic venous waveform may all be seen in this disease. The situation may be complicated as flattening of the hepatic waveform can also occur secondary to obesity and ascites, both of which are common in the Budd–Chiari patient. Colour flow imaging can visualize the various collateral pathways, including small capsular vessels, many of which are either below the resolution of real-time imaging—in this way it may help confirm the diagnosis. Other complementary imaging modalities can also be utilized to help make the diagnosis. Isotope scanning may show sparing of the caudate lobe—again an indirect diagnostic sign. CT, MRI or hepatic venography may be required to make the definitive diagnosis.

Portosystemic shunts

Portosystemic shunts may be used to treat patients with portal hypertension at high risk of bleeding usually from oesophageal varices. The normal sites of vascular anastomoses are end-to-side and side-to-side portacaval shunts, mesocaval and proximal and distal splenorenal shunts. The distal splenorenal shunt was designed to decompress a high pressure splanchnic bed and decrease hepatic encephalopathy. Although the porta and mesocaval shunts are effective in reducing portal hypertension they have the undesirable secondary effect of being likely to increase the risk of encephalopathy.

Doppler ultrasound [62], and more recently colour Doppler ultrasound, can be used to visualize these shunts directly and determine the direction of flow within the shunt and within the cava itself. In addition, if the shunt itself cannot be directly visualized then the presence of reverse flow (hepatofugal) within the portal vein is a reliable indirect sign of shunt patency. These surgically created shunts are now very rarely performed and their use has been usurped by the less invasive transjugular intrahepatic portosystemic shunt (TIPS) procedure.

TIPS

With the advent of the TIPS procedure in which a metallic stent is placed between the portal and hepatic vein after artificially creating a communication between them, there has been a consequent reduction in the number of surgical shunts performed. The two commonest indications for performing a TIPS procedure are portal hypertension at high risk of actively bleeding and resistant ascites. This is a relatively new but seemingly successful technique with good short-term results.

Colour flow ultrasound has a role both prior to stent insertion to confirm patency of the portal vein and in the assessment of shunt patency following the procedure. Shunt patency can be accurately assessed [63] but specific velocity values within the shunt vary considerably leading to some confusion of their interpretation. Velocity values within the TIPS is generally high and normally functioning shunts will have peak values over $1.0\,m\,s^{-1}$.

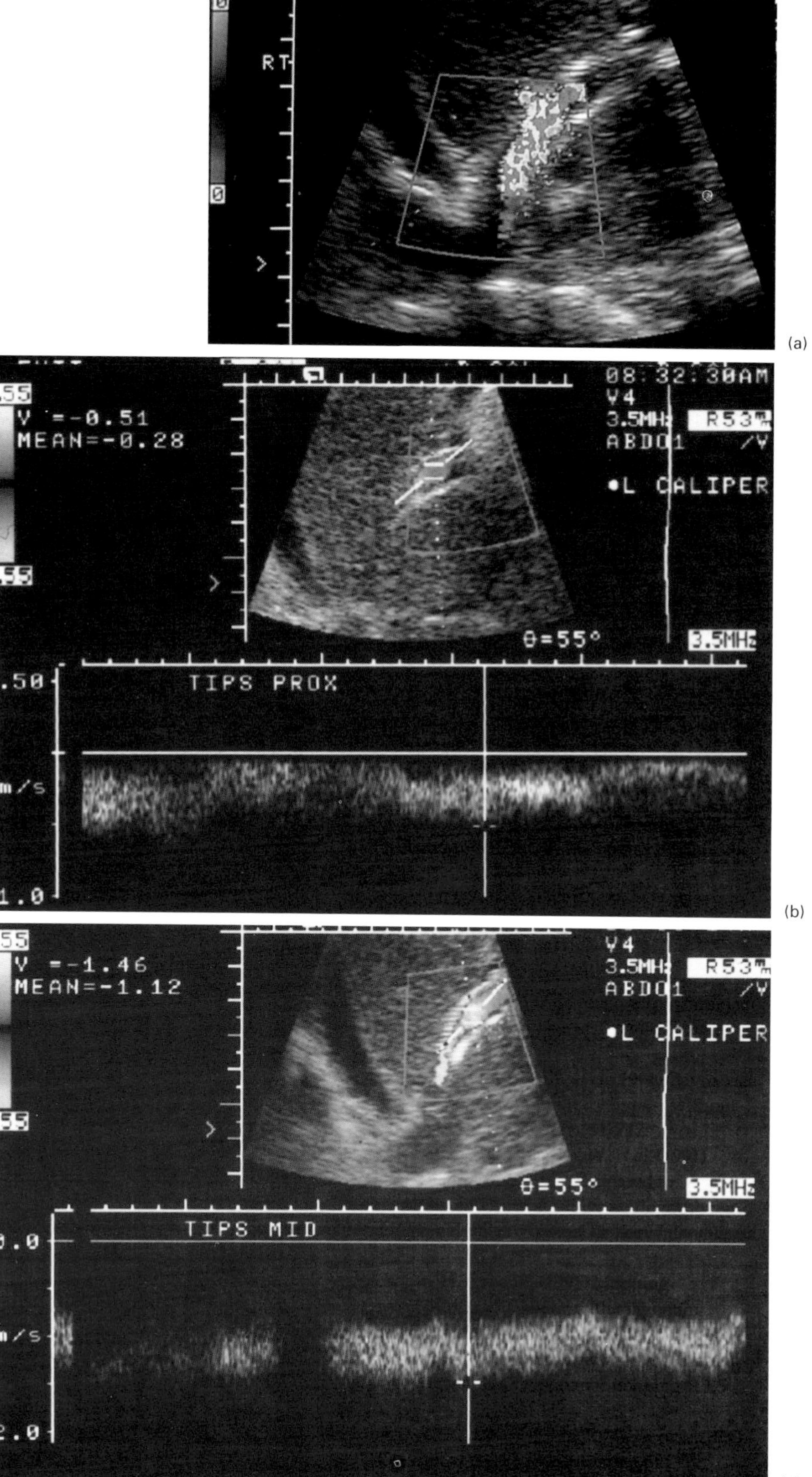

Fig. 20.13 (a) Colour Doppler image at the mid to hepatic end of a TIPS stent demonstrating marked aliasing despite an appropriate high pulse repetition frequency. The flow from the proximal to mid stent segments did not show any aliasing and the overall colour flow appearances are highly suggestive of a mid to distal TIPS stent stenosis. (b) Doppler spectral waveform from the proximal to mid part of the TIPS stent. This demonstrated a peak velocity of 51 cm s^{-1}. (c) Doppler spectral waveform from the distal TIPS stent at the site of previously demonstrated aliasing. The peak velocity has increased significantly by almost three times to 1.46 m s^{-1} consistent with a TIPS stenosis. This was confirmed angiographically. For colour, see Plate 20.13 (between pp. 308 and 309).

Furthermore, if the direction of portal vein flow prior to the TIPS is known to be hepatopetal and the flow direction of the intrahepatic portal vein and possibly its right and left branches reverse following the procedure, this can also be used to assess shunt function indirectly. Should the direction of portal venous flow revert to hepatopetal this implies shunt malfunction and should alert the sonographer to the possibility of a stent stenosis.

As with any metallic stent there is a tendency to intimal hyperplasia which predisposes to shunt stenoses which may occur in up to 17–50% at 6 months [64]. Shunt stenoses invariably occur at the mid to hepatic vein side of the shunt. Detection of these stenoses is difficult with ultrasound and the wide variation of velocity values even within normally functioning stents adds to the difficulty of interpretation. It is now generally accepted that a shunt stenosis should be suspected if the peak systolic velocity is $<60–90\,\text{cm}\,\text{s}^{-1}$ or there is a doubling of velocity values within the stent [64] (Fig. 20.13). Treatment of such lesions is normally with angioplasty in the first instance.

Veno-occlusive disease

Veno-occlusive liver disease results from intensive chemotherapy and radiotherapy in patients undergoing allogenic or autologous bone marrow transplantation. It normally presents in the first few weeks following transplantation with weight gain, tender hepatomegaly and deranged liver function tests. Differentiation of veno-occlusive disease from other forms of liver dysfunction including graft-versus-host disease is necessary.

Various abnormalities have been noted on real-time ultrasound with this disease process and these include ascites, thickening of the gallbladder wall, hepatomagaly, altered liver texture and hepatofugal portal vein flow.

In veno-occlusive disease, the hepatic veins, IVC and their venous flow patterns on Doppler examination are normal. Recently elevation of the resistive index of the hepatic artery has been noted [65] although no definitive explanation exists.

Paediatric transplant rejection

The hepatic venous waveform may also be a useful indicator of liver transplant rejection in children [66]. The criteria of loss of hepatic vein pulsatility, reflecting poor liver compliance secondary to the inflammatory infiltrate that is associated with rejection, has a sensitivity of 92% and specificity of 100%. Although Doppler may contribute to the diagnosis of acute rejection it is important to realize that accurate assessment cannot be made in those patients with flat waveforms throughout the postoperative period and in those with right heart problems. These spectral waveform changes may occur prior to any clinical or biochemical evidence of rejection.

References

1 Collin, J. (1988) The epidemiology of abdominal aortic aneurysm. *British Journal of Hospital Medicine* **40**, 64–67.

2 Nevitt, M.P., Ballard, D.J., Hallett, J.W. (1989) Prognosis of abdominal aortic aneurysms: a population based study. *New England Journal of Medicine* **321**, 1009–1014.

3 Walsh, A.K., Briffa, N., Nash, J.R., Callum, K.G. (1990) The natural history of small abdominal aortic aneurysms: an ultrasound study. *European Journal of Vascular Surgery* **4**, 459–461.

4 Collin, J., Araujo, L., Walton, J. (1989) How fast do very small abdominal aortic aneurysms grow? *European Journal of Vascular Surgery* **3**, 15–17.

5 Zollner, N., Zoller, W.G., Spengel, F., Weigold, B., Schewe, C.K. (1991) The spontaneous course of small abdominal aortic aneurysms. Aneurysmal growth rates and life expectancy. *Klinische Wochenschrift* **69**, 633–639.

6 Guirguis, E.M., Barber, G.G. (1991) The natural history of abdominal aortic aneurysms. *American Journal of Surgery* **162**, 481–483.

7 Kaufman, J.A., Bettmann, M.A. (1991) Prognosis of abdominal aortic aneurysms: a population based study. *Investigative Radiology* **26**, 612–614.

8 Glimaker, H., Holmberg, L., Elvin, A., *et al.* (1991) Natural history of patients with abdominal aortic aneurysm. *European Journal of Vascular Surgery* **5**, 125–130.

9 Dalla Costa, F., Sogaro, F., Previato Schiesari, A., Picchi, G., Morelli, I. (1988) Ruptured aneurysms of the abdominal aorta. *Italian Journal of Surgery and Science* **18**, 75–78.

10 Kullmann, G., Wolland, T., Krohn, C.D., Staxrud, L.E., Kroese, A., Kvernebo, K. (1992) Ultrasonography for early diagnosis of abdominal aortic aneurysm. *Tiddsskr Nor Laegeforen* **112**, 1825–1826.

11 Quill, D.S., Colgan, M.P., Sumner, D.S. (1989) Ultrasonic screening for the detection of abdominal aortic aneurysms. *Surgical Clinics of North America* **69**, 713–720.

12 Webster, W., Ferrell, R.E., St Jean, P.L., Majumder, P.P., Fogel, S.R., Steed, D.L. (1991) Ultrasound screening of first degree relatives of patients with an abdominal aortic aneurysm. *Journal of Vascular Surgery* **13**, 9–13.

13 Collin, J., Araujo, L., Walton, J., Lindsell, D. (1988) Oxford screening programme for abdominal aortic aneurysm in men aged 65 to 74 years. *Lancet* **ii**, 613–615.

14 Shuman, W.P., Hastrup, W., Kohler, T.R., *et al.* (1988) Suspected leaking abdominal aortic aneurysms: use of sonography in the emergency room. *Radiology* **168**, 117–119.

15 Thomas, E.A., Dubbins, P.A. (1990) Duplex ultrasound of the abdominal aorta—a neglected tool in aortic dissection. *Clinical Radiology* **42**, 330–334.

16 Cook, A.M., Dyet, J.F., Mann, S.L. (1990) Ultrasonic and comparative angiographic appearances of a spontaneous aorto-caval fistula. *Clinical Radiology* **41**, 286–288.

17 Bolognesi, R., Tsialtas, D., Manca, C. (1991) Diagnosis of an aorto-caval fistula by echo 2D color Doppler flow imaging and echocardiographic probe. *Cardiology* **79**, 151–155.

18 Desberg, A.L., Paushter, D.M., Lammert, G.K., *et al.* (1990) Renal artery stenosis: evaluation with color Doppler flow imaging. *Radiology* **177**, 749–753.
19 Avasthi, P.S., Voyles, W.F., Greene, E.R. (1984) Noninvasive diagnosis of renal artery stenosis by echo-Doppler velocimetry. *Kidney International* **25**, 824–829.
20 Kohler, T.R., Zierler, R.E., Martin, R.L., *et al.* (1986) Noninvasive diagnosis of renal artery stenosis by ultrasonic duplex scanning. *Journal of Vascular Surgery* **4**, 450–456.
21 Taylor, D.C., Kettler, D., Moneta, G.L., *et al.* (1988) Duplex ultrasound scanning in the diagnosis of renal artery stenosis: a prospective evaluation. *Journal of Vascular Surgery* **7**, 363–369.
22 Berland, L.L., Koslin, D.B., Routh, W.D., Keller, F.S. (1990) Renal artery stenosis: prospective evaluation of diagnosis with color Duplex US compared with angiography. *Radiology* **174**, 421–423.
23 Desberg, A.L., Pauschter, D.M., Lammert, G.K., *et al.* (1990) Renal artery stenosis; evaluation with color Doppler flow imaging. *Radiology* **177**, 749–753.
24 Stavros, A.T., Parker, S.H., Yakes, W.F., *et al.* (1992) Segmental stenosis of the renal artery: pattern recognition of tardus and parvus abnormalities with duplex sonography. *Radiology* **184**, 487–492.
25 Kliewer, M.A., Tupler, R.H., Carroll, B.A., *et al.* (1993) Renal artery stenosis: analysis of Doppler waveform parameters and tardus–parvus pattern. *Radiology* **189**, 779–787.
26 Baxter, G.M., Aitchison, F., Sheppard, D., *et al.* (1996) Colour Doppler ultrasound in renal artery stenosis: intrarenal waveform analysis. *British Journal of Radiology* **69**, 810–815.
27 Bude, R.O., Rubin, J.M., Platt, J.F., Fechner, K.P., Adler, R.S. (1994) Pulsus–tardus: its cause and potential limitations in detection of arterial stenosis. *Radiology* **190**, 779–784.
28 Sieber, C., Beglinger, C., Jager, K., Stalder, G.A. (1992) Intestinal phase of superior mesenteric artery blood flow in man. *Gut* **33**, 497–501.
29 Moneta, G.L., Yeager, R.A., Dalman, R., Antonovic, R., Hall, L.D., Portland, O.R. (1991) Duplex ultrasound criteria for diagnosis of splachnic artery stenosis or occlusion. *Journal of Vascular Surgery* **14**, 511–520.
30 Verma, B.S., Bose, A.K., Bhatia, H.C., Katoch, R. (1991) Superior mesenteric artery branch aneurysm diagnosed by ultrasound. *British Journal of Radiology* **64**, 169–171.
31 Cremers, P.T., Busschner, D.L., MacFarlane, J.D. (1990) Ultrasound demonstration of a superior mesenteric artery aneurysm in a patient with Ehlers–Danlos syndrome. *British Journal of Rheumatology* **29**, 482–444.
32 Junewick, J.J., Grant, T.H., Weiss, C.A., Piano, G. (1993) Celiac artery aneurysm: color Doppler evaluation. *Journal of Ultrasound in Medicine* **12**, 355–357.
33 Leen, E., Goldberg, J.A., Robertson, J., *et al.* (1991) Detection of hepatic metastasis using duplex/colour Doppler sonography. *Annals of Surgery* **214**, 599–604.
34 Leen, E., Goldberg, J.A., Robertson, J., Sutherland, G.R., McArdle, C.S. (1991) The use of duplex sonography in the detection of colorectal hepatic metastasis. *British Journal of Cancer* **63**, 323–325.
35 Longley, D.G., Skolnick, M.L., Sheahan, D.G. (1988) Acute allograft rejection in liver transplant recipients: lack of correlation with loss of hepatic artery flow. *Radiology* **169**, 417–420.
36 Schaberle, W., Seitz, K. (1991) Duplex ultrasound measurement of blood flow in the superior mesenteric artery. *Ultraschall-Med* **12**, 277–282.
37 Bowersox, J.C., Zwolak, R.M., Walsh, D.B., *et al.* (1991) Duplex ultrasonography in the diagnosis of celiac and mesenteric artery occlusive disease. *Journal of Vascular Surgery* **14**, 780–786.
38 Muller, A.F. (1992) Role of duplex Doppler ultrasound in the assessment of patients with post prandial abdominal pain. *Gut* **33**, 460–465.
39 Bolondi, L., Gaiani, S., Brignola, C., *et al.* (1992) Changes in splanchnic haemodynamics in inflammatory bowel disease. Non-invasive assessment by Doppler ultrasound flowmetry. *Scandinavian Journal of Gastroenterology* **27**, 501–507.
40 Cooper, A.M., Braatvedt, G.D., Qamar, M.I., *et al.* (1991) Fasting and post prandial splanchnic blood flow is reduced by somatostatin analogue (octreotide) in man. *Clinical Science* **81**, 169–175.
41 Rak, K.M., Hopper, K.D., Tyler, H.N. (1991) The slit infrahepatic IVC: pathologic entity or normal variant? *Journal of Clinical Ultrasound in Medicine* **19**, 399–403.
42 Hubsch, P., Schurawitzki, H., Susani, M., *et al.* (1992) Color Doppler imaging of inferior vena cava: identification of tumor thrombus. *Journal of Ultrasound in Medicine* **11**, 639–645.
43 Kim, D., Edelman, R.R., Margolin, C.J., *et al.* (1992) The Simon nitinol filter: evaluation by MR and ultrasound. *Angiology* **43**, 541–548.
44 Guglielmo, F.F., Kurtz, A.B., Wechsler, R.J. (1990) Prospective evaluation of computed tomography and duplex sonography in the evaluation of recently inserted Kimray–Greenfield filters into the inferior vena cava. *Clinical Imaging* **14**, 216–220.
45 Marx, M.V., Tauscher, J.R., Williams, D.M., Greenfield, L.J. (1991) Evaluation of the inferior vena cava with intravascular ultrasound after Greenfield filter placement. *Journal of Vascular and Interventional Radiology* **2**, 261–268.
46 McCowan, T.C., Ferris, E.J., Carver, D.K. (1990) Inferior vena caval filter thrombi: evaluation with intravascular ultrasound. *Radiology* **177**, 783–788.
47 Rosenfield, A.T., Zeman, R.K., Cronan, J.J., Taylor, K.J.W. (1980) Ultrasound in experimental and clinical renal vein thrombosis. *Radiology* **137**, 735–741.
48 Kallman, D.A., King, B.F., Hattery, R.R., *et al.* (1992) Renal vein and inferior vena cava tumor thrombus in renal cell carcinoma: CT, US, MRI and venocavography. *Journal of Computed Assisted Tomography* **16**, 240–247.
49 Stewart, J.R., Carey, J.A., McDougal, W.S., *et al.* (1991) Cavoatrial tumor thrombectomy using cardiopulmonary bypass without circulatory arrest. *Annals of Thoracic Surgery* **51**, 717.
50 Constantinides, C., Recker, F., Bruehlmann, W., *et al.* (1991) Accuracy of magnetic resonance imaging compared to computerised tomography and renal selective angiography in preoperatively staging renal cell carcinoma. *Urology International* **47**, 181.
51 Weese, D.L., Applebaum, H., Taber, P. (1991) Mapping intravascular extension of Wilms' tumour with magnetic resonance imaging. *Journal of Paediatric Surgery* **26**, 64.
52 Amendola, M.A., King, L.R., Pollack, H.M., *et al.* (1990) Staging of renal cell carcinoma using magnetic resonance imaging at 1.5 Tesla. *Cancer* **66**, 40.
53 McGahan, J.P., Lindsey, C.B., deVere White, R., Gerscovich, E.O., Brant, W.E. (1993) Color flow songraphic mapping of intravascular extension of malignant renal tumors. *Journal of*

Ultrasound in Medicine **12**, 403–409.
54 Farah, M.C., Shirkhoda, A., Ellwood, R.A., Bernacki, E., Farah, H. (1989) Leiomyosarcoma of the renal vein: radiologic pathologic correlation. *Clinical Imaging* **13**, 323–326.
55 Cacoub, P., Piette, J.C., Weschler, B., *et al.* (1991) Leiomyosarcoma of the inferior vena cava. Experience with seven patients and literature review. *Medicine (Baltimore)* **70**, 293–306.
56 von Bibra, H., Schober, K., Jenni, R., Busch, R., Sebening, H., Blomer, H. (1989) Diagnosis of constrictive pericarditis by pulsed Doppler echocardiography of the hepatic vein. *American Journal of Cardiology* **63**, 483–488.
57 Abu-Yousef, M.M. (1991) Duplex Doppler sonography of the hepatic vein in tricuspid incompetence. *American Journal of Roentgenology* **156**, 79–83.
58 Bolondi, L., Li Bassi, S., Gaiani, S., *et al.* (1991) Liver cirrhosis: changes of Doppler waveform of hepatic veins. *Radiology* **178**, 513–516.
59 Grant, E.G., Perrella, R., Tessler, F.N., Lois, J., Busutill, R. (1989) Budd–Chiari syndrome: the results of duplex and color Doppler imaging. *American Journal of Roentgenology* **152**, 377–381.
60 Hosoki, T., Kuroda, C., Tokunaga, K., Marukawa, T., Masuike, M., Kozuka, T. (1989) Hepatic venous outflow obstruction; evaluation with pulsed duplex sonography. *Radiology* **170**, 733–737.
61 Ralls, P.W., Johnson, M.B., Radin, D.R., Boswell, Jr W.D., Lee, K.P., Halls, J.M. (1992) Budd–Chiari syndrome: detection with color Doppler sonography. *American Journal of Roentgenology* **159**, 113–116.
62 Lafortune, M., Patriquin, H., Pimier, G., *et al.* (1987) Hemodynamic changes in portal circulation after portosystemic shunts: use of duplex sonography in 43 patients. *American Journal of Roentgenology* **149**, 701–706.
63 Ferral, H., Foshager, M.C., Bjarnason, H., *et al.* (1993) Early sonographic evaluation of the transjugular intrahepatic portosystemic shunt (TIPS). *Cardiovascular and Interventional Radiology* **16**, 275–279.
64 Saxon, R.R., Barton, R.E., Keller, F.S., Rosch, J. (1995) Prevention, detection and treatment of TIPS stenosis and occlusion. *Seminars in Interventional Radiology* **12**, 4.
65 Herbetko, J., Grigg, A.P., Buckley, A.R., Phillips, G.L. (1992) Venoocclusive liver disease after bone marrow transplantation: findings at duplex sonography. *American Journal of Roentgenology* **158**, 1001–1005.
66 Britton, P.D., Lomas, D.J., Coulden, R.A., Farman, P., Revell, S. (1992) The role of hepatic vein Doppler in diagnosing acute rejection following paediatric liver transplantation. *Clinical Radiology* **45**, 228–232.

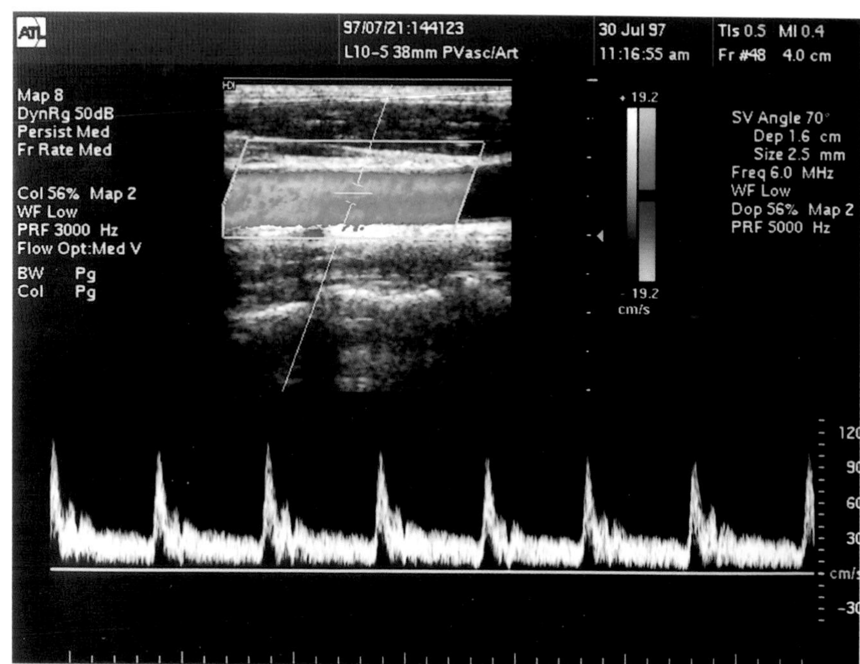

Plate 4.6 Triplex display of carotid artery with spectral display.

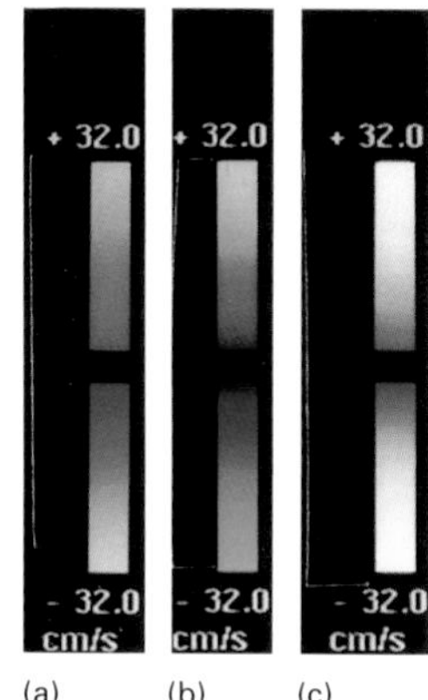

Plate 4.7 Velocity colour maps. (a, b) Broad range maps. (c) Rapidly saturating map.

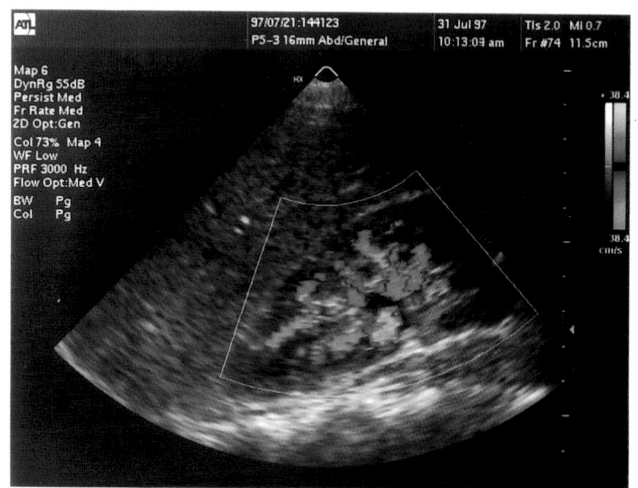

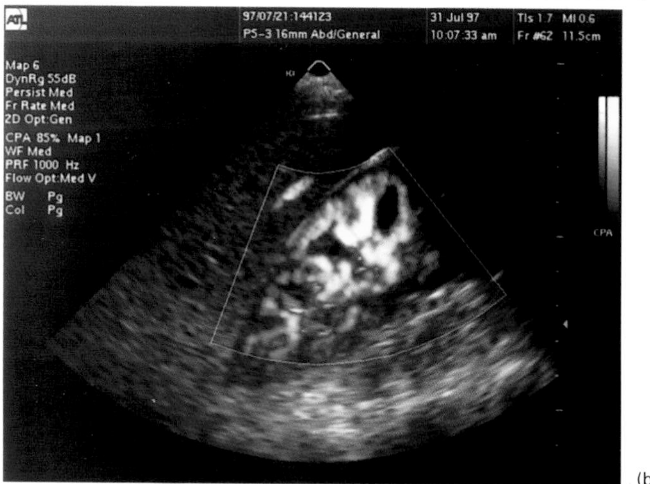

Plate 4.8 (a) Velocity and (b) power colour flow images of a normal kidney.

(a)

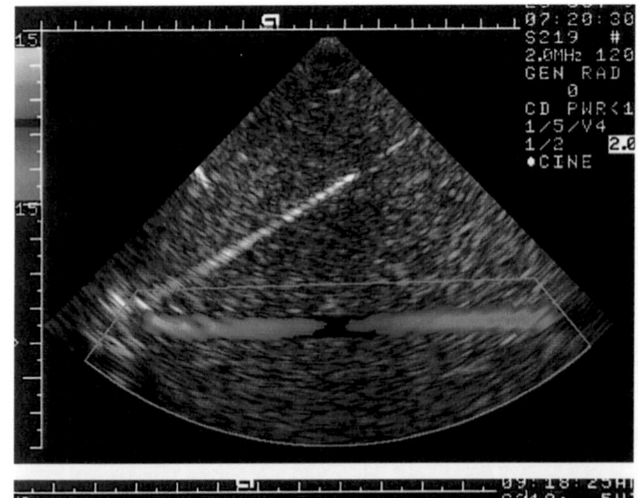

(b)

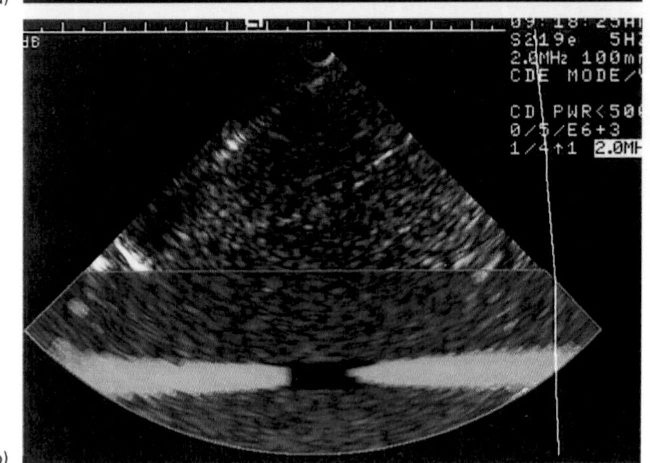

Plate 4.9 Images from a flow phantom using a convex probe showing (a) colour Doppler images showing variation in colour with beam–vessel angle across scan; and (b) a power Doppler image showing no variation except near to 90°.

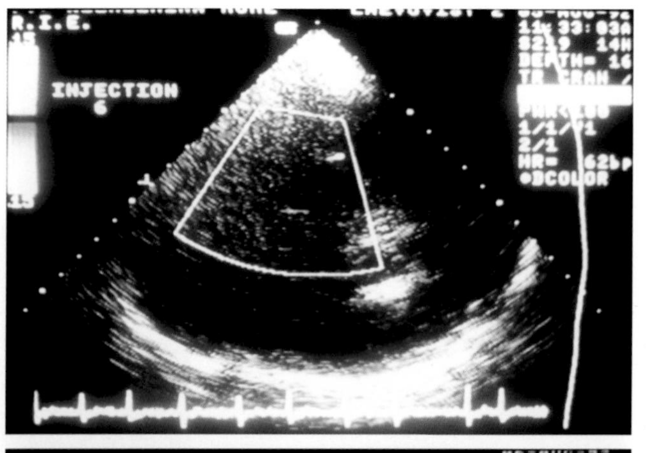

(a)

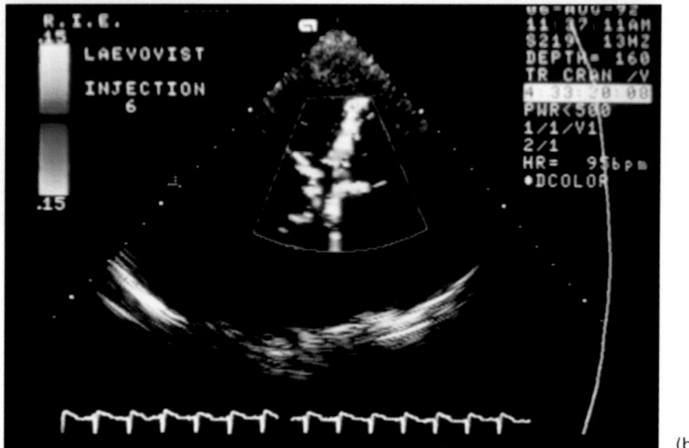

(b)

Plate 7.6 (a) Transcranial colour Doppler scan prior to injection of Levovist. (b) Same scan after injection of Levovist. Notice the circle of Willis clearly enhanced. (Courtesy of P. Allan, Edinburgh.)

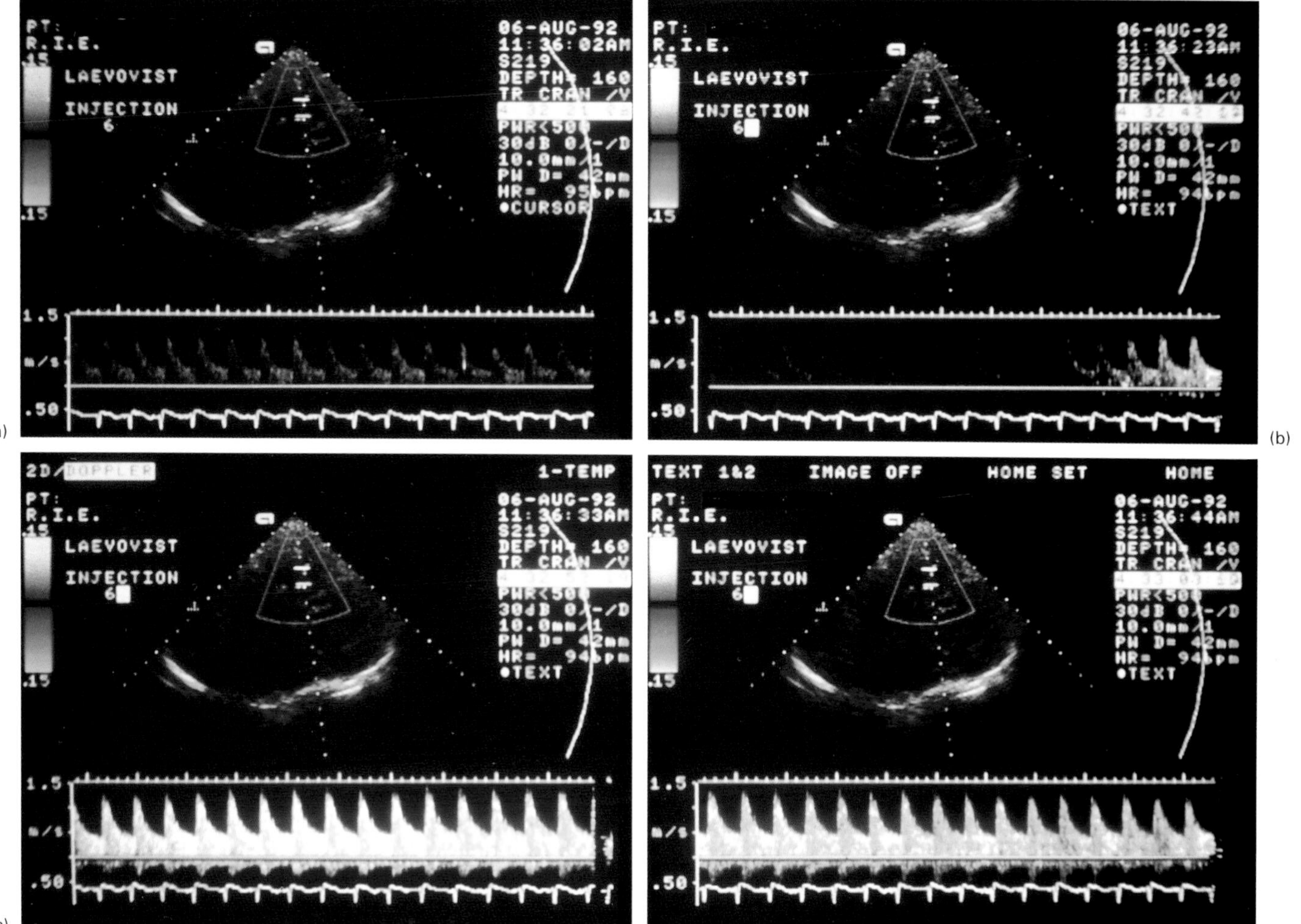

Plate 7.7 Transcranial colour Doppler M-mode (a) prior to, (b, c) during, and (d) after an injection of Levovist. (Courtesy of P. Allan, Edinburgh.)

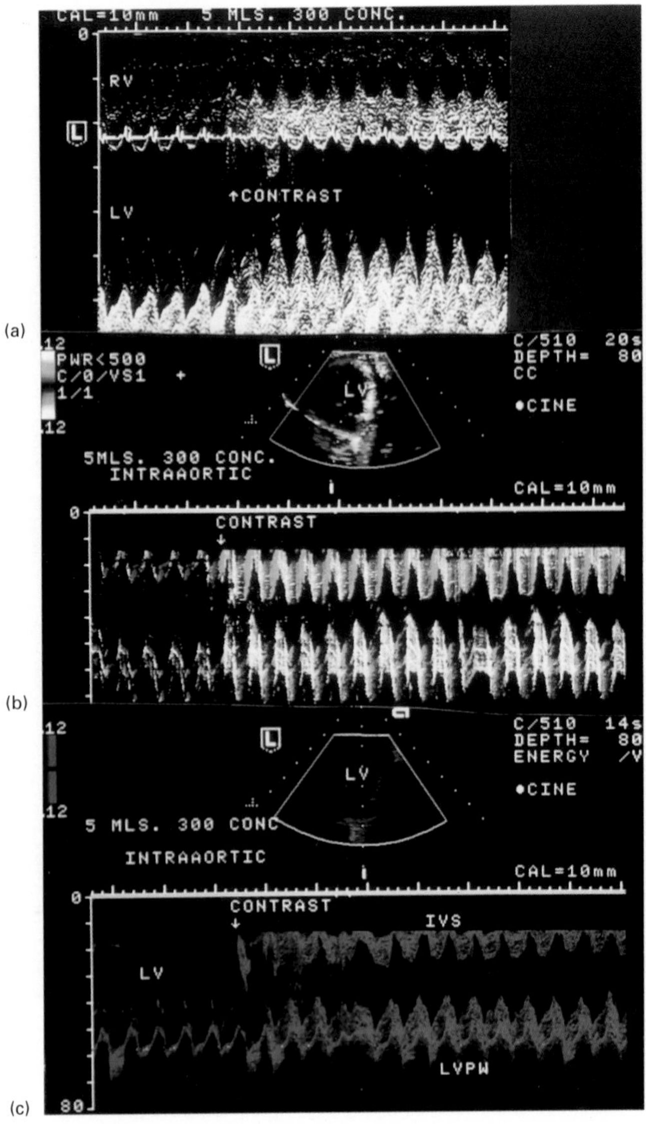

Plate 7.8 Open-chest pig study after intra-aortic injection of Levovist. (a) Standard grey-scale M-mode through the left ventricle; (b) the same M-mode using Doppler tissue velocity imaging, and (c) an M-mode using the Doppler energy map.

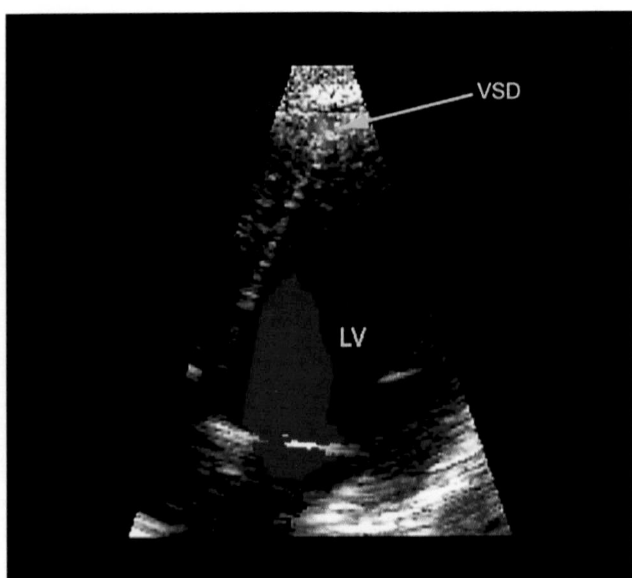

Plate 8.5 Apical view in systole of a child with a very small apical ventricular septal defect (VSD) which is so small and anterior it is difficult to image, but colour Doppler highlights its position. LV, left ventricle.

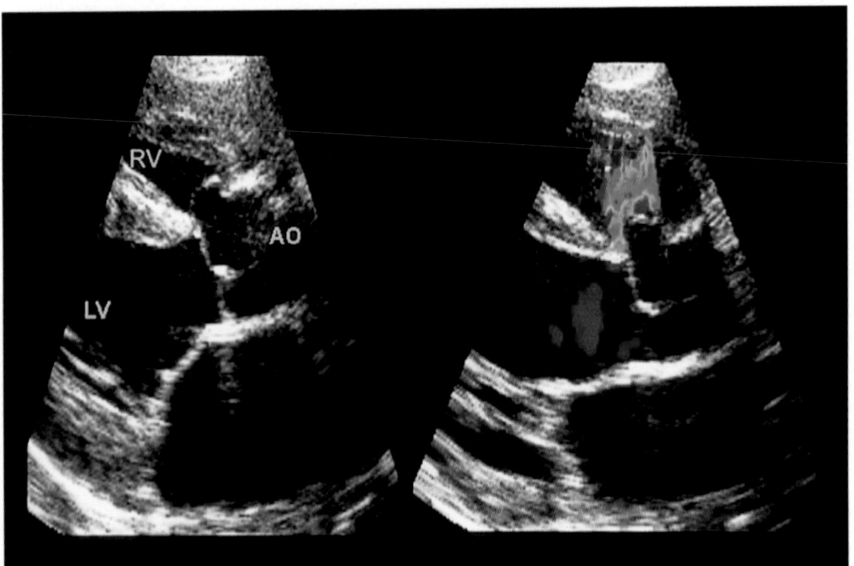

Plate 8.3 Long axis views with and without colour of a patient with a subaortic ventricular septal defect and aortic valve prolapse. The defect is between the upper edge of the septum and the aortic margin. In this diastolic frame it is partially closed by the prolapsed right coronary cusp. AO, aorta; LV, left ventricle; RV, right ventricle.

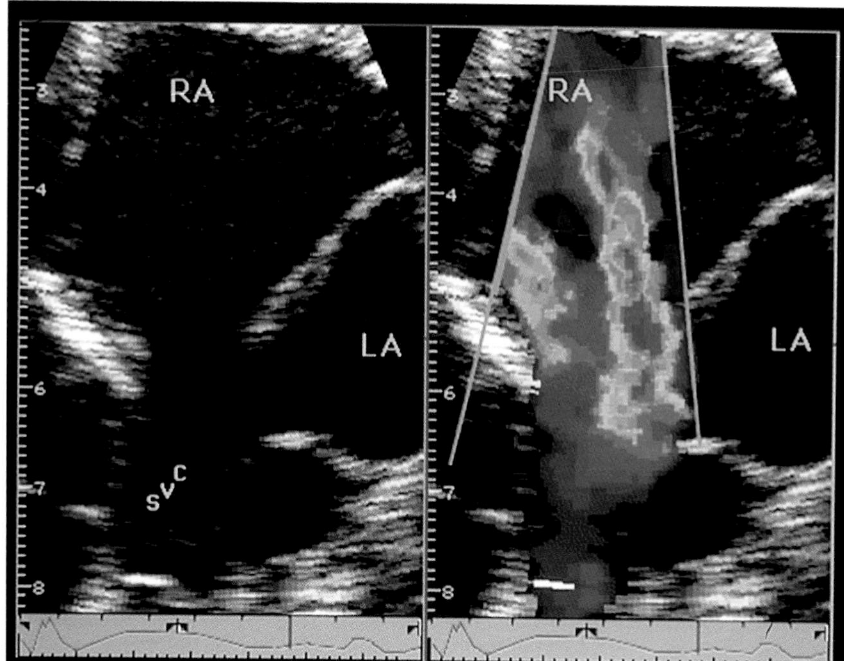

Plate 8.10 Subcostal images of a patient with sinus venosus atrial septal defect. The scanning plane is tilted up from a subcostal position to show the upper margin of the right atrium and the sinus venosus defect with apparent overriding of the superior vena cava (SVC). The right image shows flow from both the SVC and left atrium (LA) into the right atrium (RA).

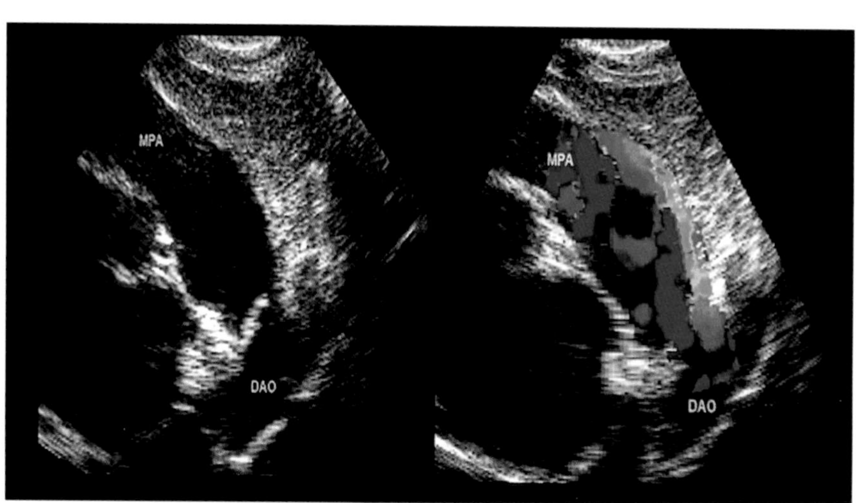

Plate 8.13 Left parasagittal images of a patient with an arterial duct. The colour image shows acceleration into the mouth of the duct with the jet passing along the superior wall of the main pulmonary artery (MPA). DAO, descending aorta.

(a)

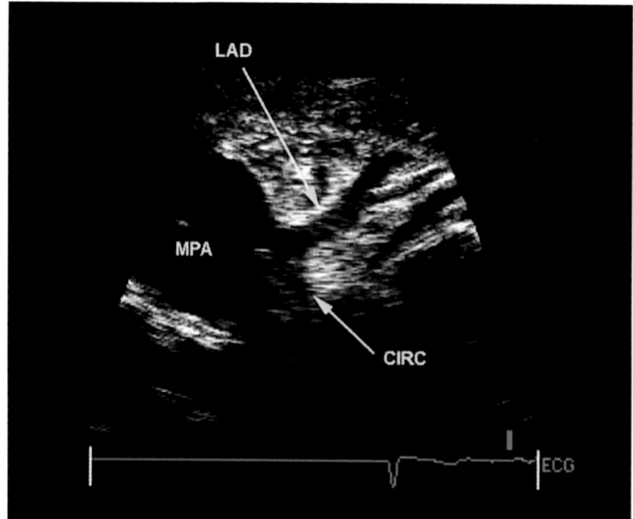

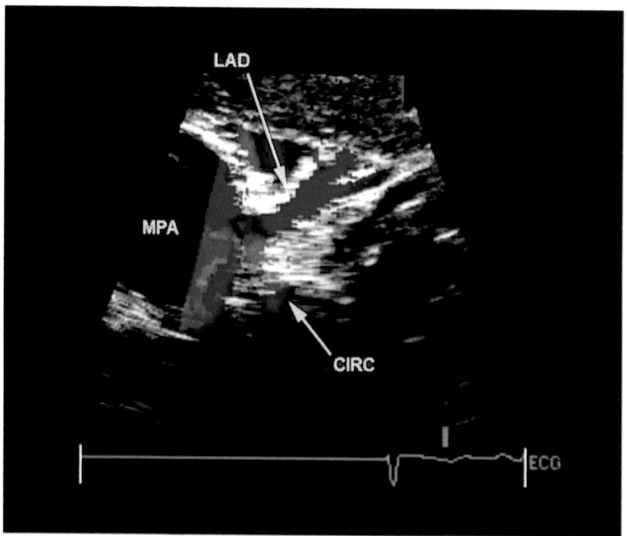

(b)

Plate 8.26 Views from an infant with anomalous origin of the left coronary artery from the pulmonary artery. (a) The left anterior descending (LAD) and circumflex (CIRC) branches are seen, and (b) in the colour image retrograde flow is shown in the coronaries towards the main pulmonary artery (MPA).

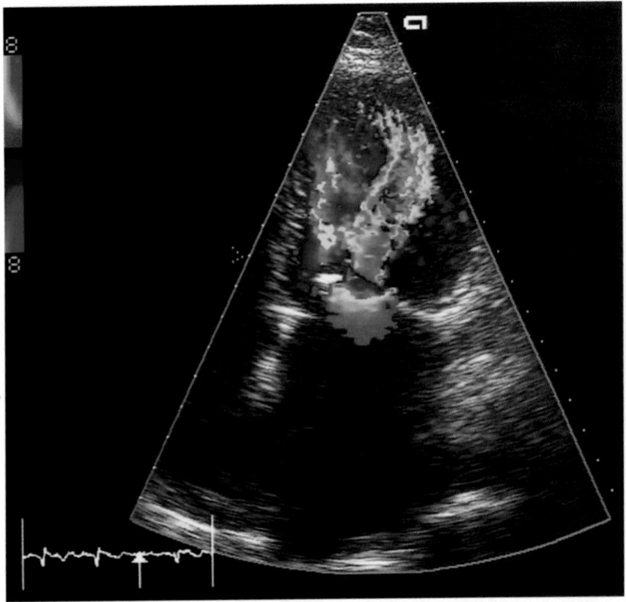

Plate 9.7 Colour flow Doppler record from stenotic rheumatic mitral valve in diastole (see text).

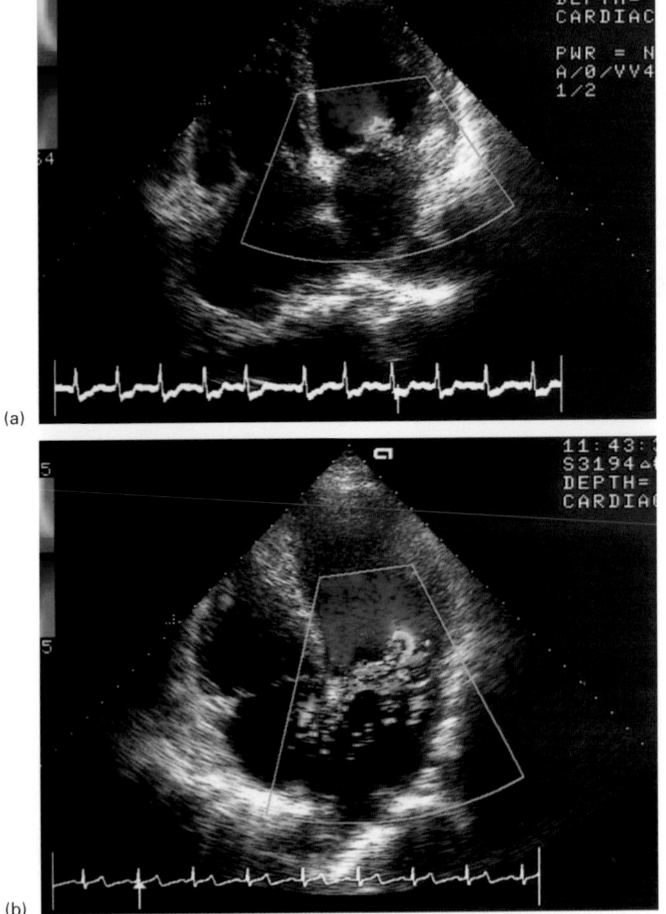

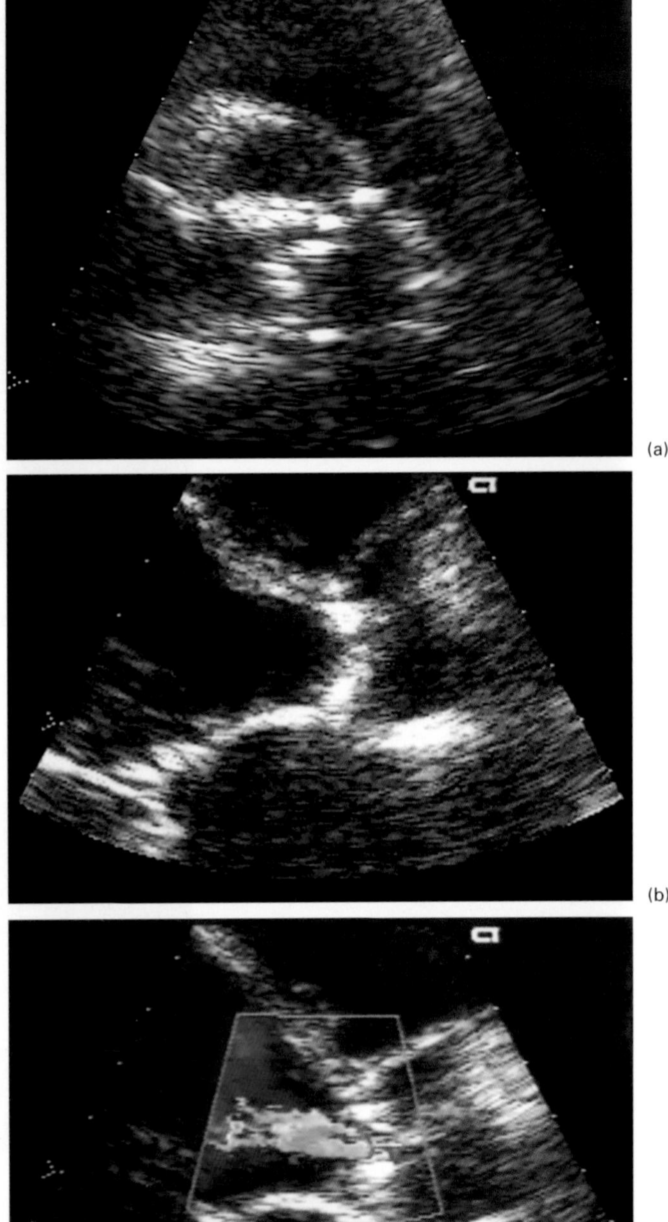

Plate 9.18 Rheumatic aortic valve. (a) Parasternal short axis showing thickening and calcification of the edge of the leaflets. The long axis images in (b) systole and (c) diastole demonstrate the rigidity of the leaflets, the stenotic orifice and, with colour flow, a central regurgitant jet.

Plate 9.14 (*left*) Colour flow Doppler records (apical four chamber, systole) from floppy mitral valves with (a) mitral anterior leaflet prolapse, and (b) mitral posterior leaflet prolapse. In (a) the regurgitant jet is directed laterally and in (b) medially towards the interarterial septum. Acceleration of flow as it approaches the mitral valve on its ventricular side, more obvious in (b), is in keeping with severe regurgitation.

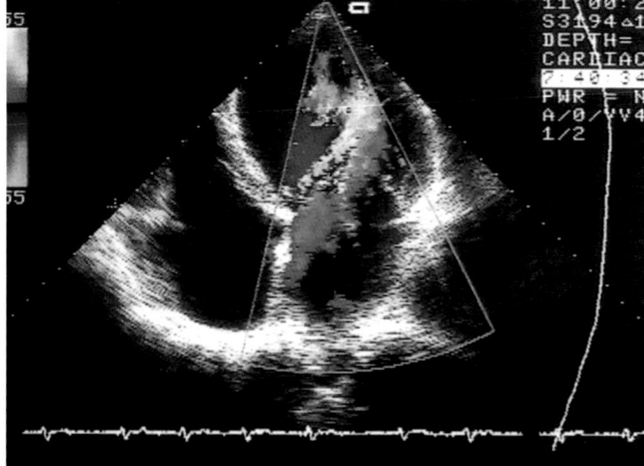

(a)

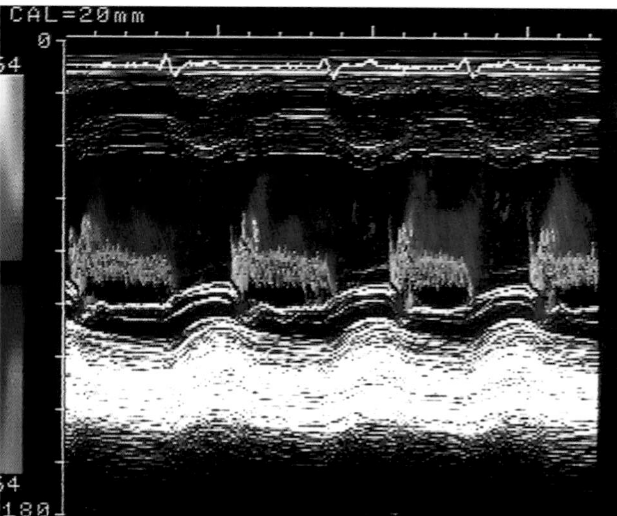

(b)

Plate 9.20 (a) Apical four-chamber diastolic image. Turbulent aortic regurgitant flow extends across the front of normal mitral anterior leaflet to mix with mitral forward flow. (b) Colour M-mode shows the aortic regurgitant flow producing diastolic oscillation of the mitral anterior leaflet.

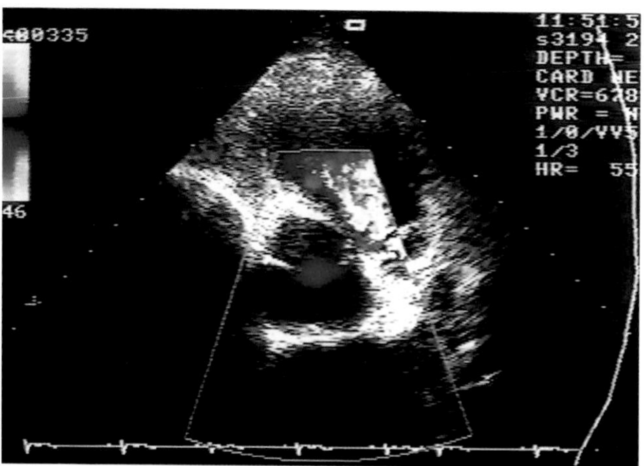

Plate 9.30 Colour flow Doppler showing wide regurgitant jet in patient with carcinoid disease and significant pulmonary regurgitation. The valve is thick.

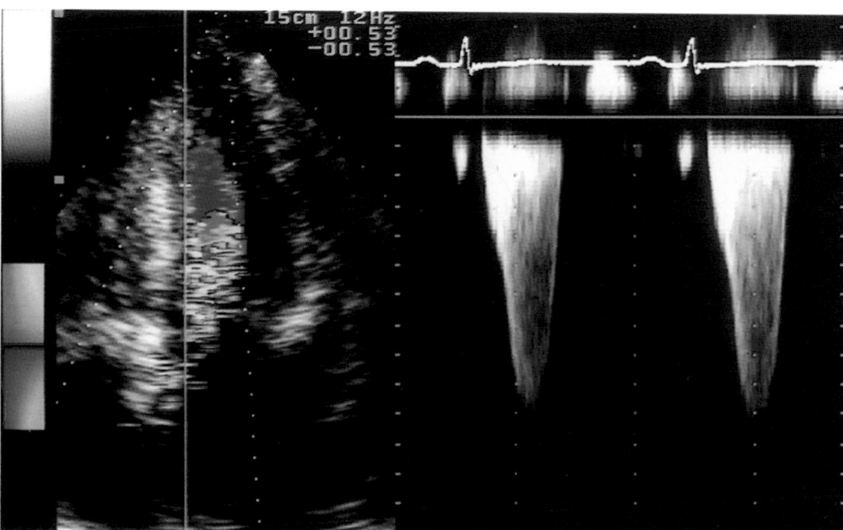

Plate 11.10 Apical four-chamber view with colour flow imaging of the left ventricle showing aliasing in mid left ventricle indicating a ventricular gradient. Doppler analysis at the same level shows a slow and later peak of flow compared to what is seen in aortic stenosis.

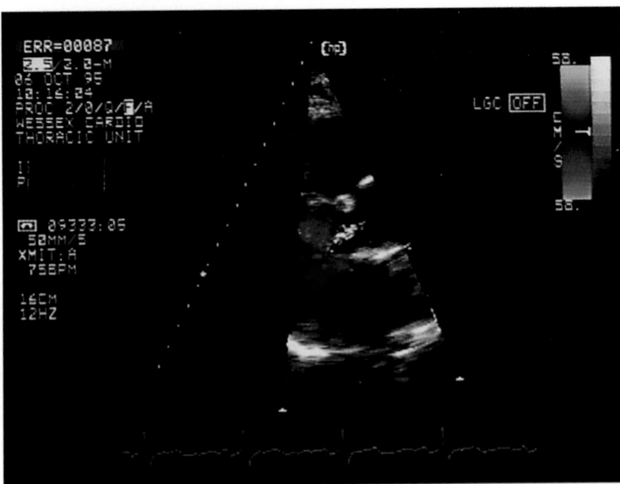

Plate 12.6 Regurgitation through an otherwise normal aortic homograft. This was present postoperatively and did not represent structural valve degeneration.

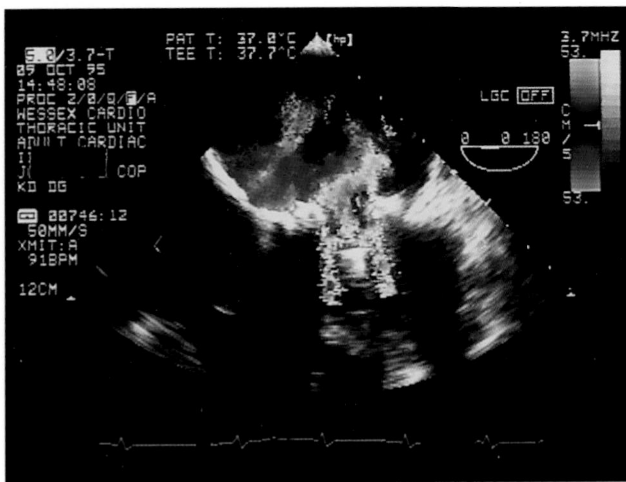

Plate 12.12 Doppler colour flow mapping of normal forward flow through a caged ball prosthesis.

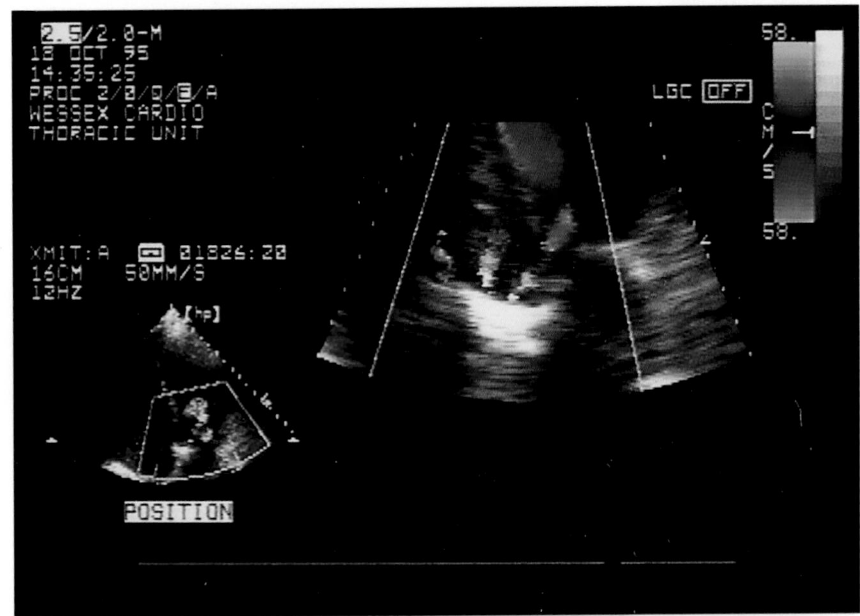

Plate 12.13 Transthoracic imaging of normal regurgitant flow through an aortic bileaflet prosthesis.

(a)

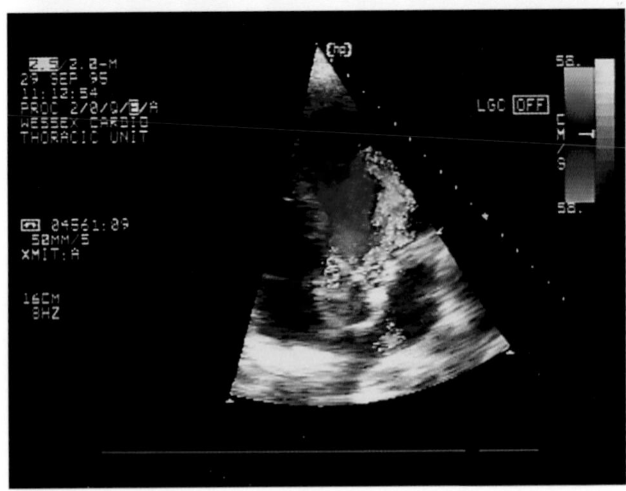

(b)

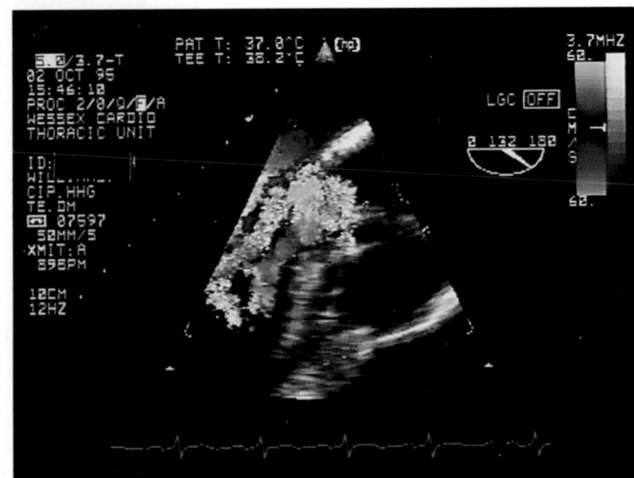

Plate 12.14 Significant regurgitation due to structural valve degeneration of an aortic homograft from (a) transthoracic and (b) transoesophageal windows.

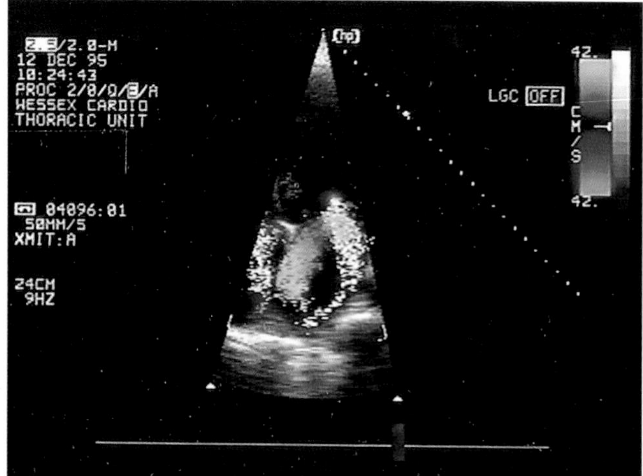

Plate 12.15 Eccentric wall jet of severe paraprosthetic mitral regurgitation.

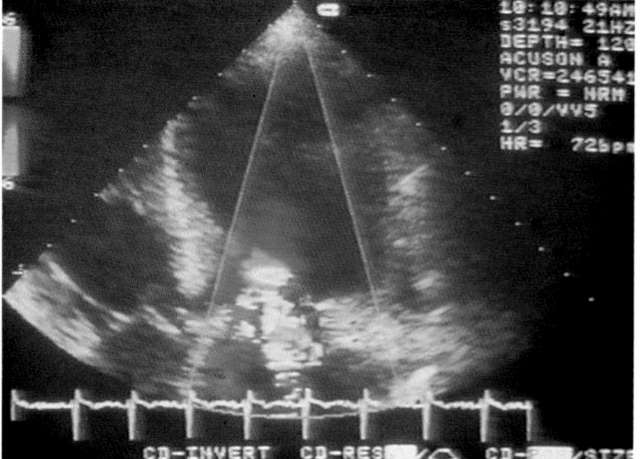

Plate 12.16 Region of colour flow convergence on the ventricular aspect of a severely regurgitant mitral valve.

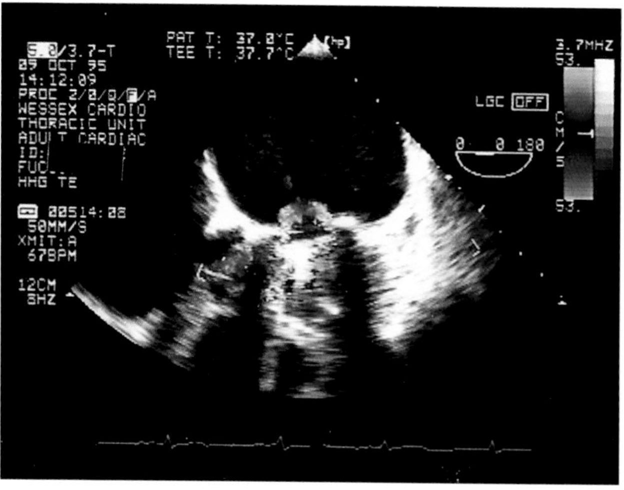

Plate 12.17 Normal regurgitant flow through a mitral bileaflet prosthesis.

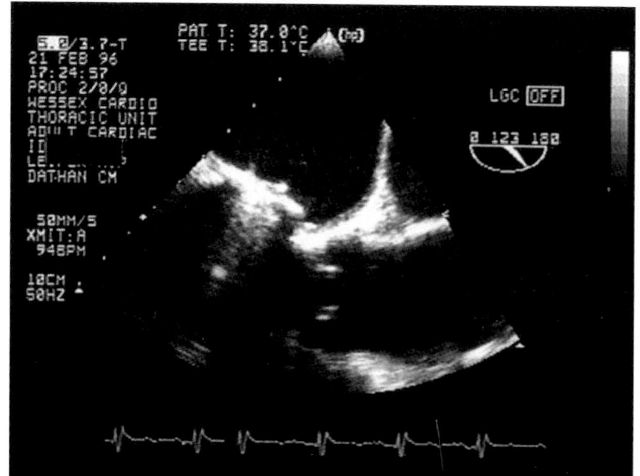

(a)

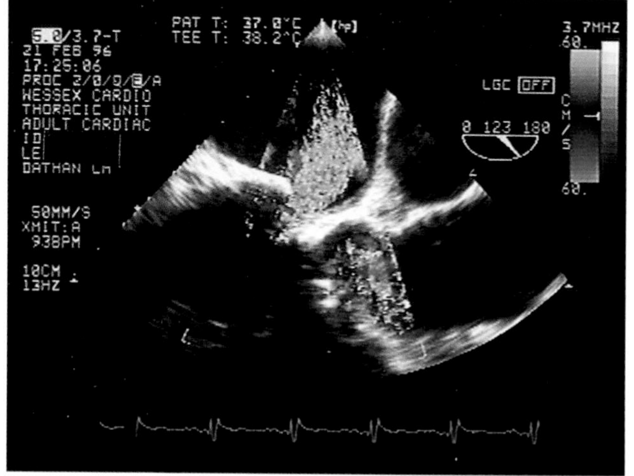

(b)

Plate 12.18 Paraprosthetic mitral regurgitation: (a) a region of partial valve dehiscence, and (b) a broad regurgitant jet.

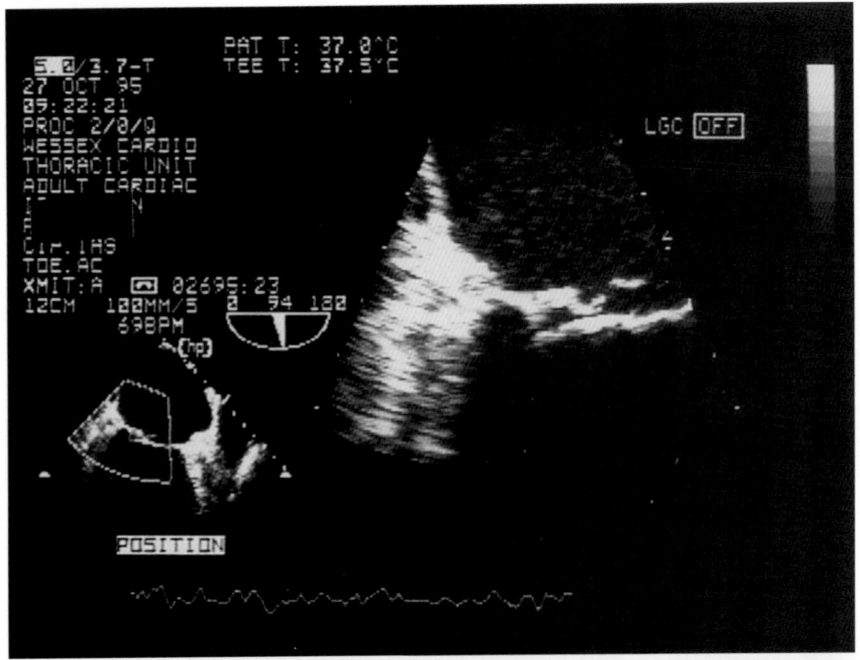

(a)

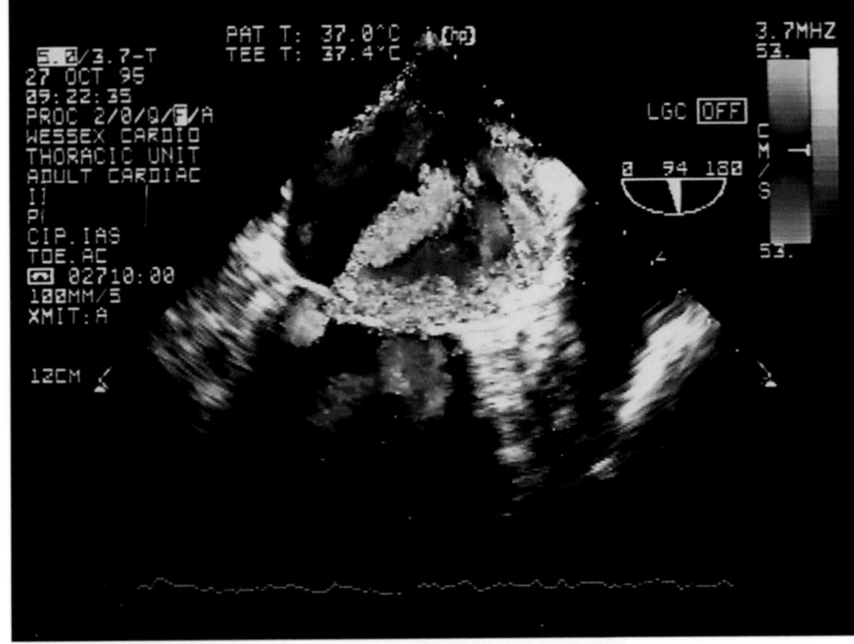

(b)

Plate 12.24 A flail posterior mitral valve leaflet due to ruptured chordae (a), with a broad jet of regurgitation (b).

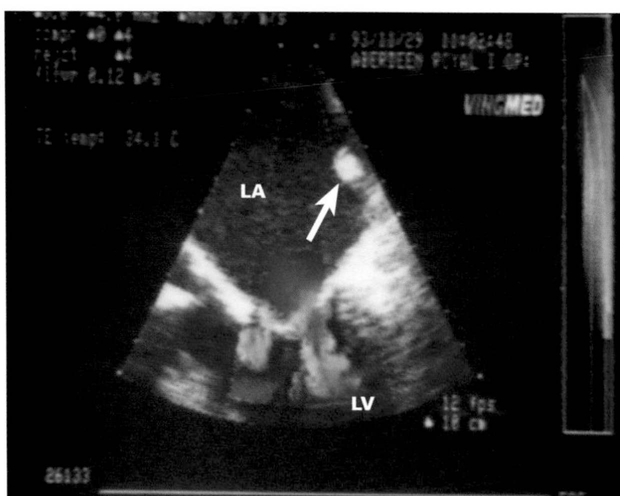

Plate 13.4 Transoesophageal echocardiographic view of a thrombus in the left atrial appendage (arrow) in a patient with mitral stenosis as shown by the colour jet into the left ventricle (LV). LA, dilated left atrium.

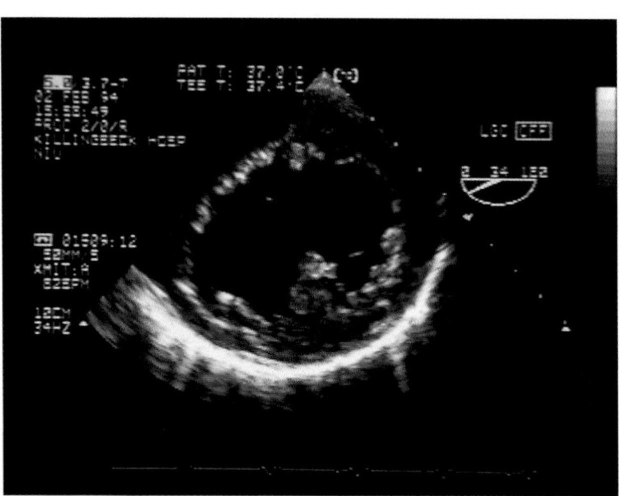

(a)

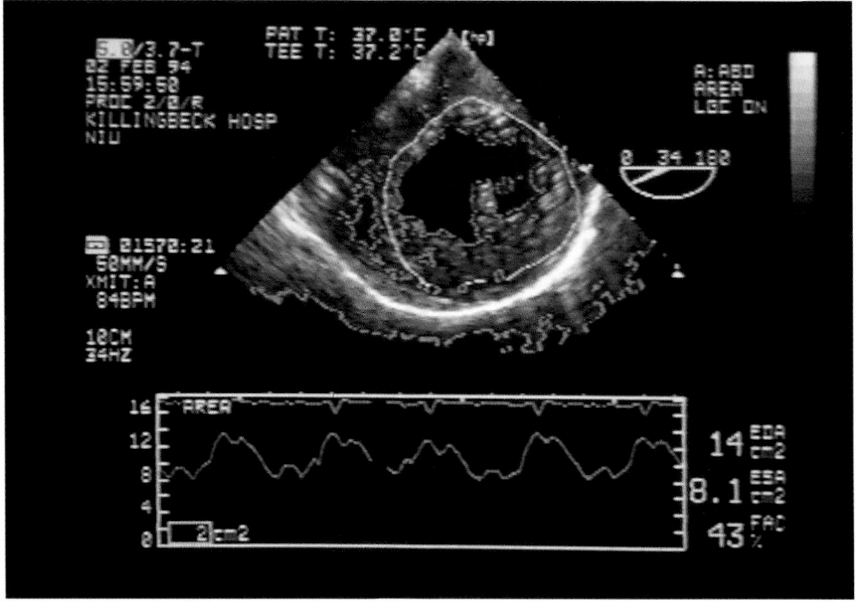

(b)

Plate 14.3 (a) Cross-sectional view of the left ventricle taken from the gastric fundus and (b) illustrating the use of automated boundary location in the measurement of area changes between diastole and systole.

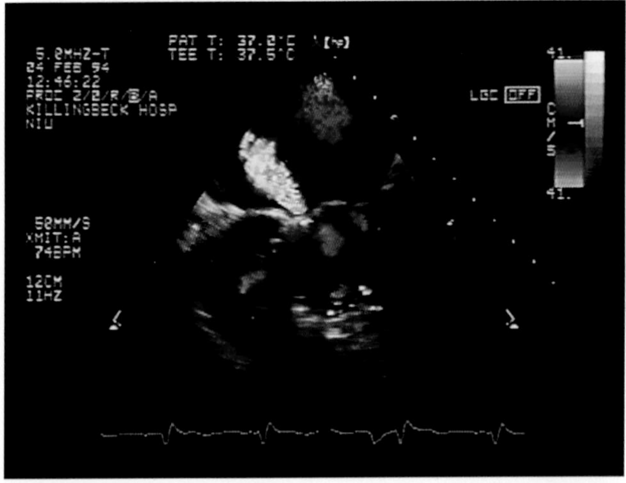

Plate 14.8 View of a mechanical aortic prosthesis and a jet of mitral regurgitation through a hole at the base of the anterior mitral leaflet, a result of the aortic valve surgery.

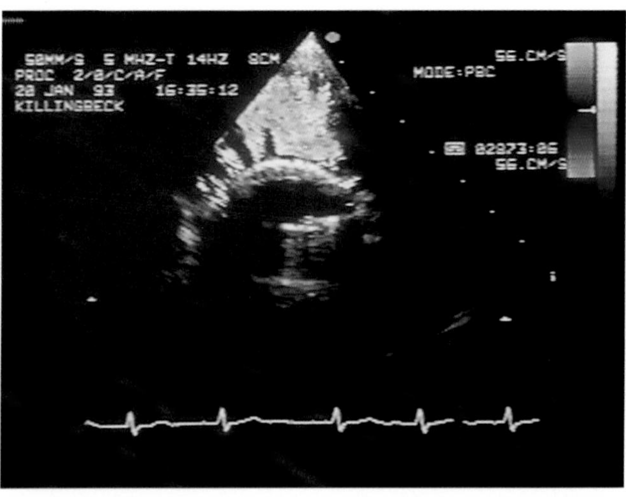

Plate 14.12 Short axis view of a prosthetic mitral valve with an extensive paraprosthetic leak illustrated by colour flow Doppler.

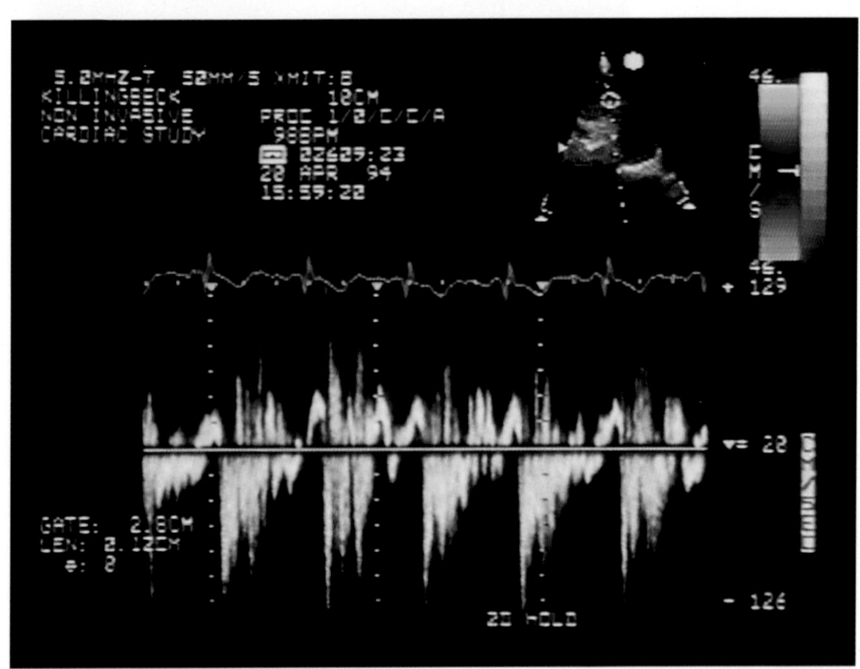

Plate 14.9 Pulsed wave Doppler trace from the left lower pulmonary vein in a patient with severe mitral regurgitation. Note the reversed systolic flow.

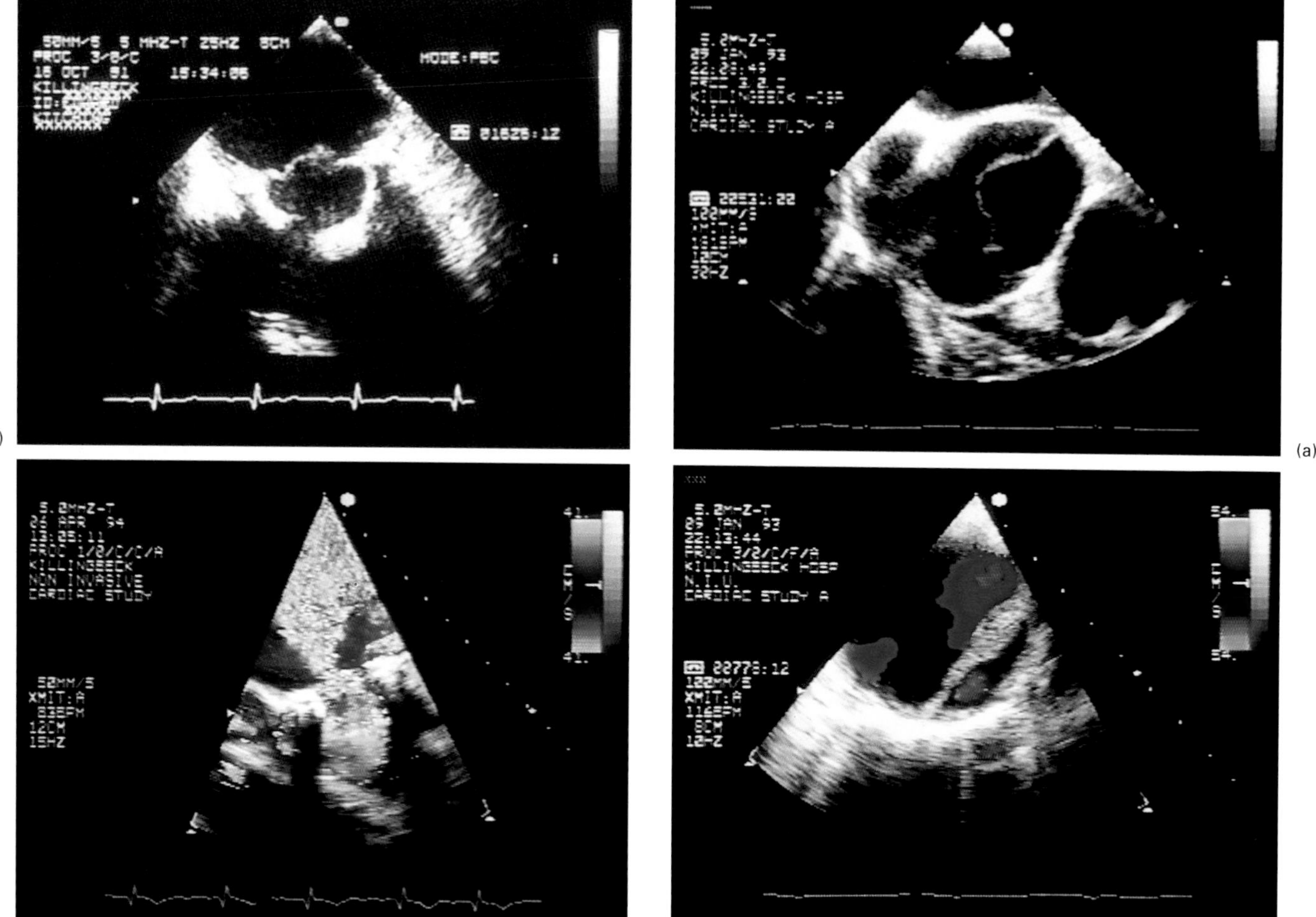

Plate 14.14 (a) View of mitral bioprosthesis with prolapse of a torn leaflet back into the left atrium during systole and (b) the same valve with severe mitral regurgitation illustrated by a broad-based colour jet extending to the posterior atrial wall.

Plate 14.15 (a) Type 1 aortic dissection with intimal flap easily identified in the aortic root and (b) seen extending into the descending aorta where colour flow Doppler helps differentiate the true from the false lumen.

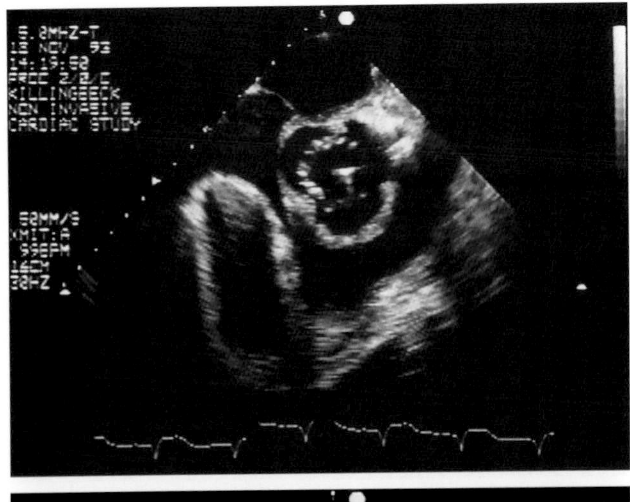

(a)

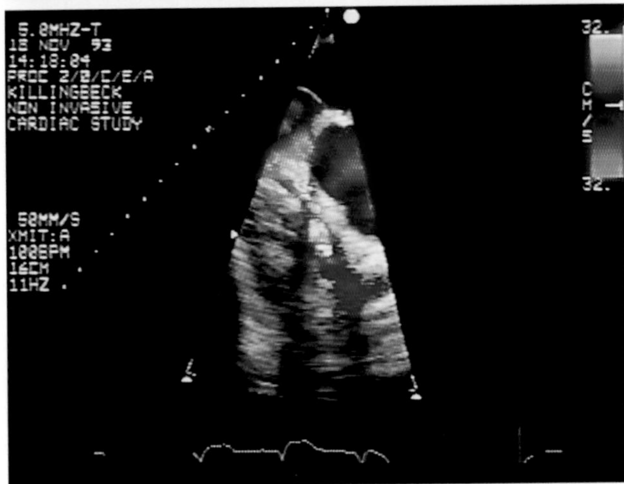

(b)

Plate 14.24 (a) Aortic prosthetic valve in short axis with compression of the right heart by a localized postoperative pericardial collection in a patient with clinical signs of pericardial tamponade; (b) colour flow Doppler shows turbulent high velocity flow here confirming limitation of flow through the right heart.

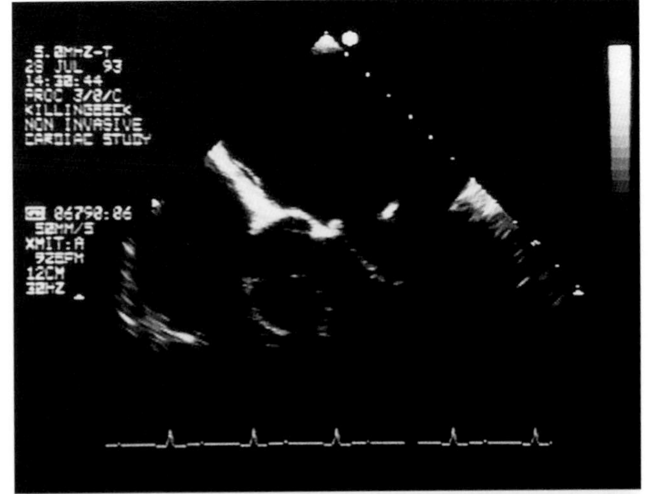

(a)

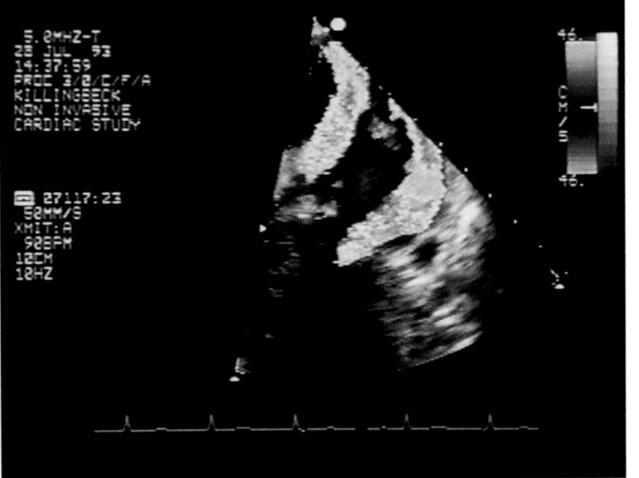

(b)

Plate 14.26 (a) Following a mitral valve repair the flexible Duran ring has become separated from the mitral annulus at the base of the posterior mitral leaflet resulting in two significant regurgitant jets as seen with colour flow Doppler (b).

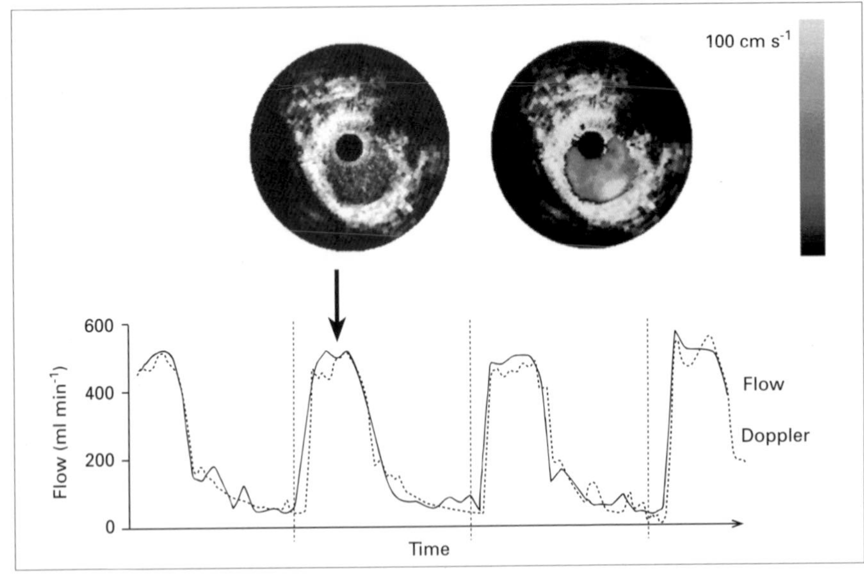

Plate 15.11 Volume flow (—) in a renal artery obtained with the described RF method and compared to a Doppler measurement (---). The instantaneous velocity is colour-coded. For comparison the regular image is shown.

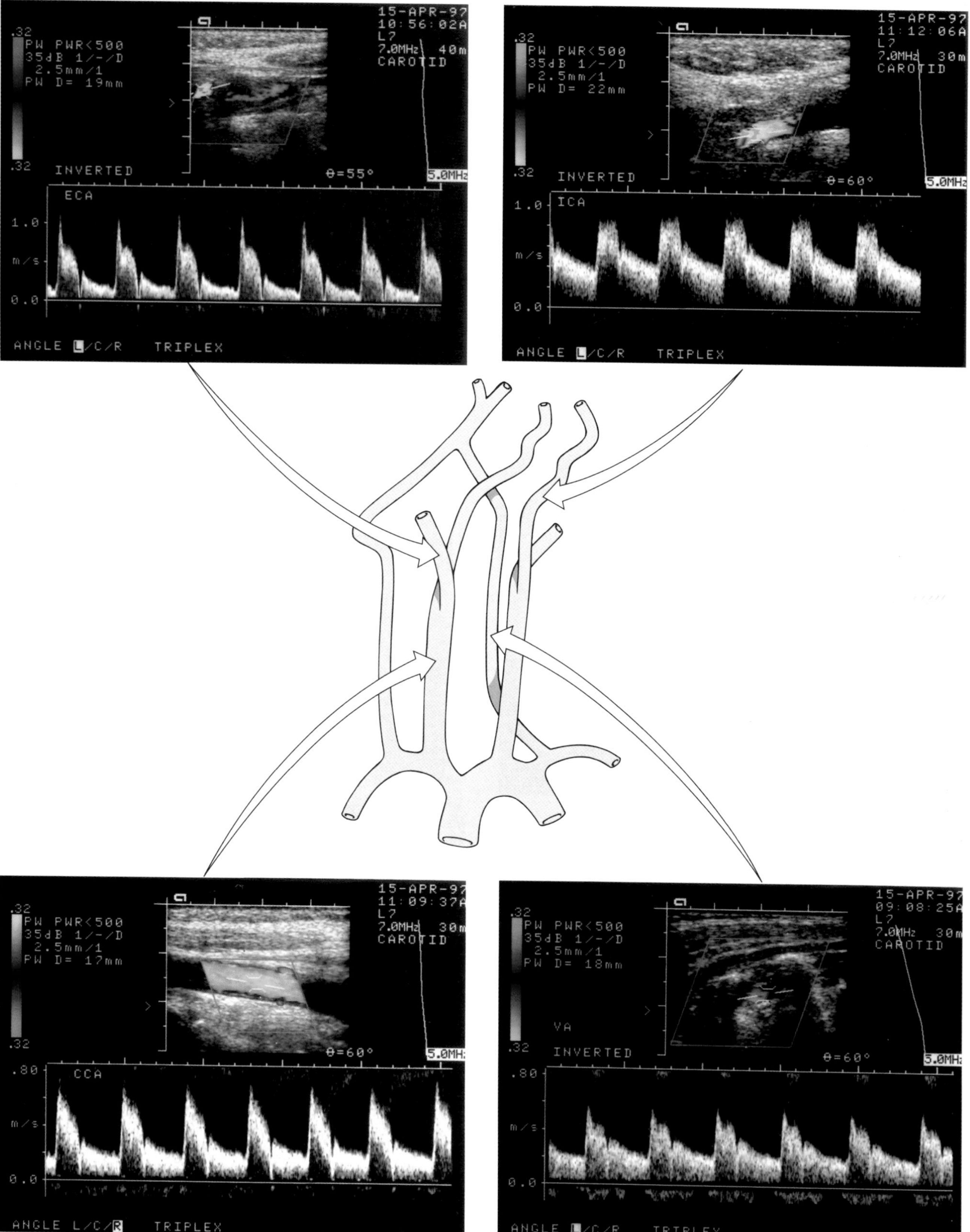

Plate 16.1 Diagram of the normal anatomy of the extracranial carotid arterial system arising off the aortic arch. The normal spectral Doppler waveform pattern for each artery is indicated. CCA, common carotid artery; ECA, external carotid artery; ICA, internal carotid artery; VA, vertebral artery.

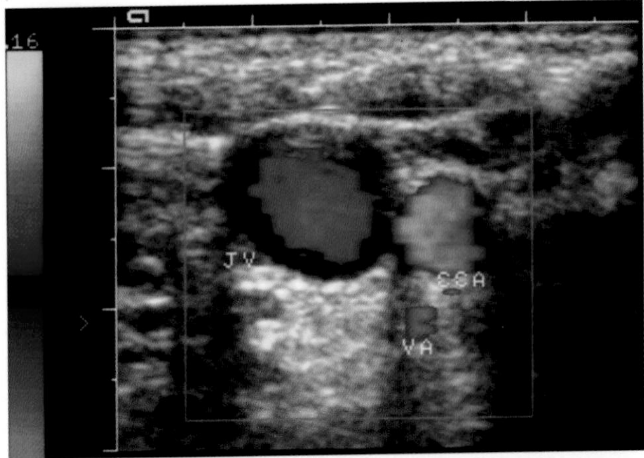

Plate 16.2 Transverse section through the root of the neck, showing the common carotid artery (CCA), jugular vein (JV) and vertebral artery (VA).

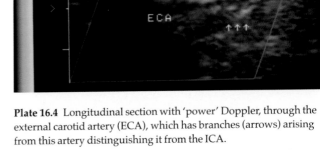

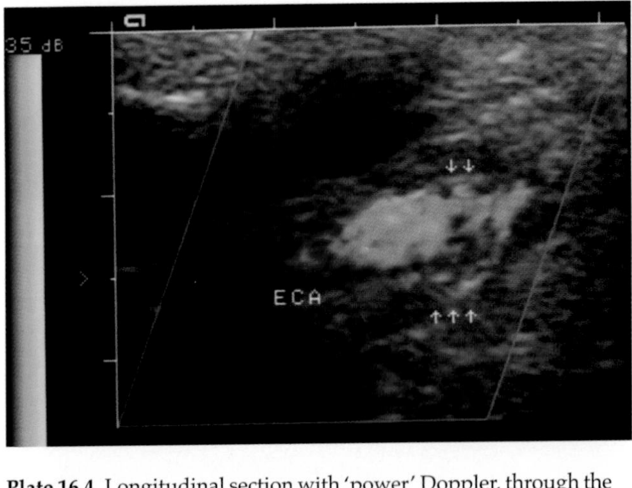

Plate 16.4 Longitudinal section with 'power' Doppler, through the external carotid artery (ECA), which has branches (arrows) arising from this artery distinguishing it from the ICA.

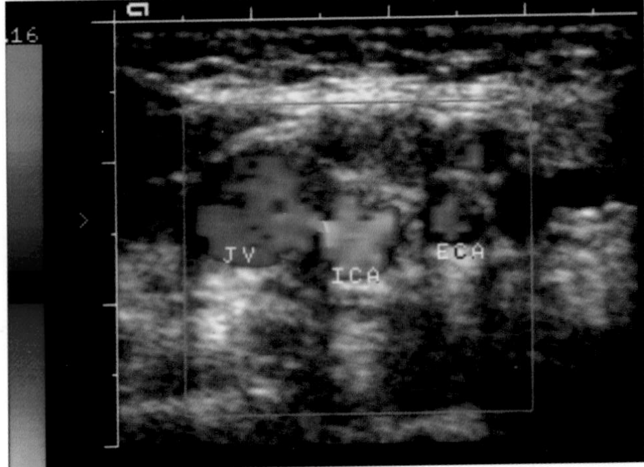

Plate 16.3 Transverse section at the level of the bifurcation of the common carotid artery into the internal carotid artery (ICA) laterally and the external carotid artery (ECA) medially. JV, jugular vein.

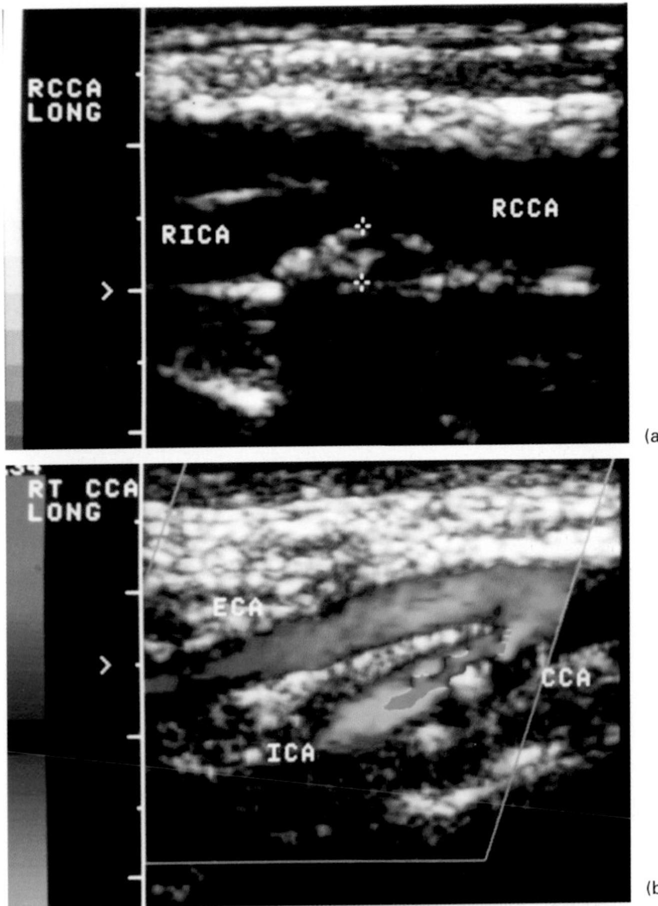

Plate 16.7 Longitudinal section through the proximal internal carotid artery (ICA). (a) Focal area of mixed reflective plaque (between crosses) causing narrowing at the level of the proximal right ICA. RCCA, right common carotid artery; RICA, right internal carotid artery. (b) Colour flow disturbance related to this focal narrowing of plaque formation. The sample volume gate should be placed at the site of maximum colour disturbance in order to record the peak systolic velocity. CCA, common carotid artery; ECA, external carotid artery.

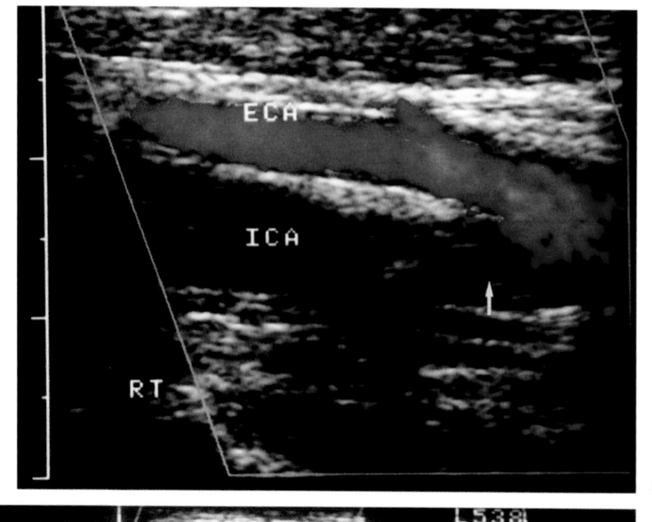

(a)

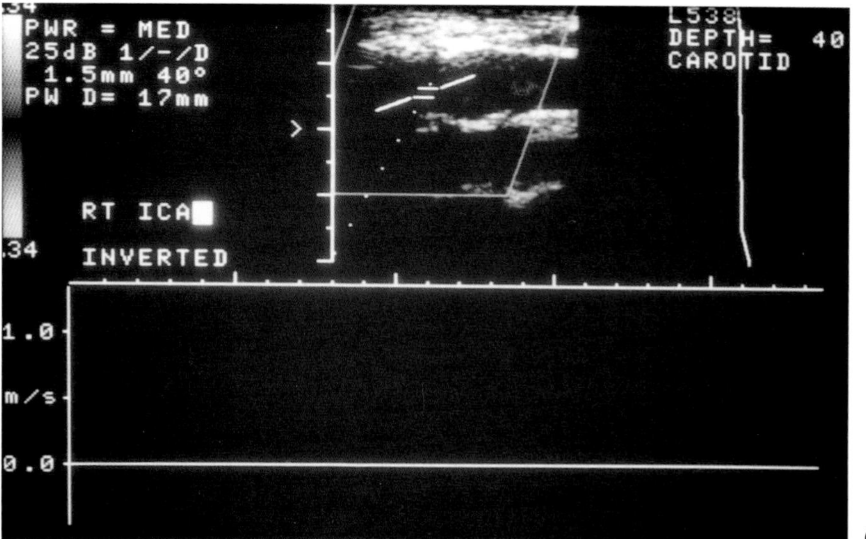

(b)

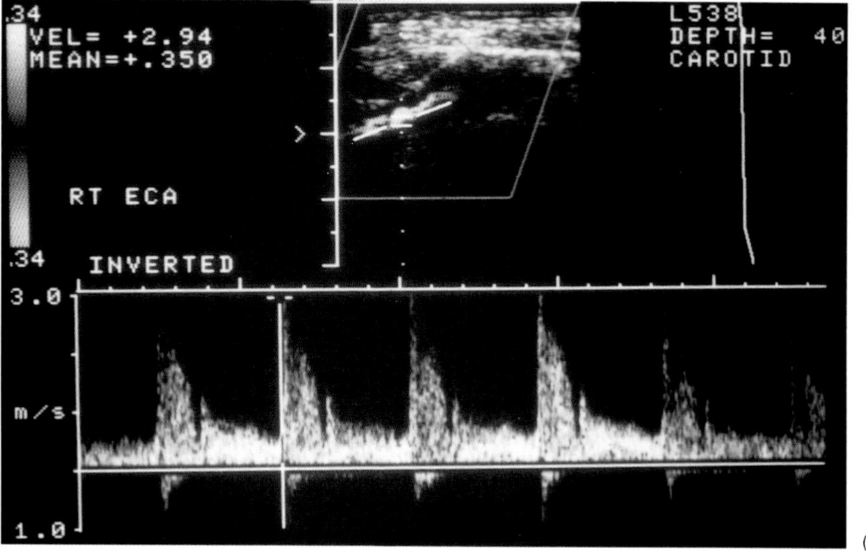

(c)

Plate 16.11 (a) Longitudinal section through the bifurcation with colour Doppler showing no colour flow in the internal carotid artery (ICA) (arrow) which is filled with low reflective material and is occluded. ECA, external carotid artery; RT, right. (b) No spectral waveform is obtained on Doppler from the occluded ICA. (c) The ECA is 'internalized' with a peak systolic velocity of 294 cm s^{-1} and high diastolic forward flow.

(a)

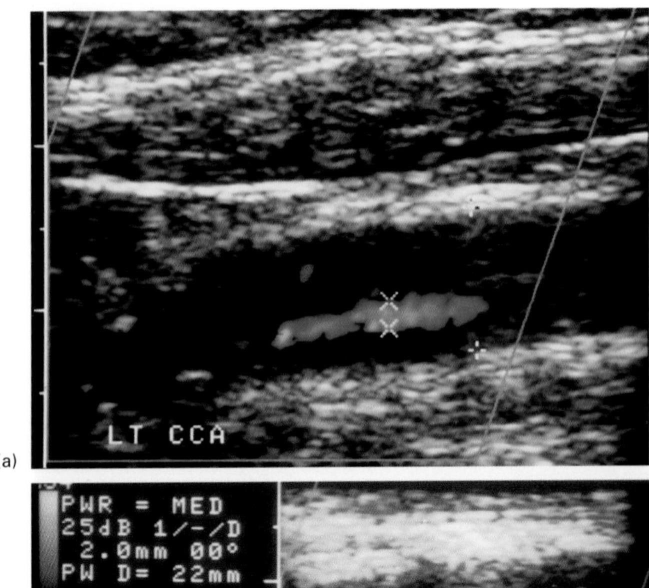

(b)

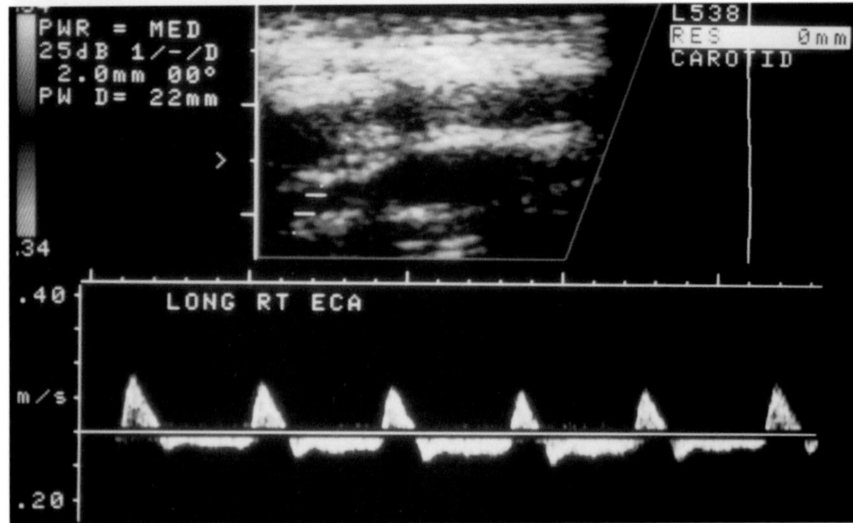

Plate 16.12 (a) Longitudinal section through the left common carotid artery (CCA) (between crosses, +) using colour Doppler demonstrates a narrow channel of colour flow, the 'string sign' or 'pseudo-occlusion' (between crosses, ×). (b) In a different patient, the presence of a CCA occlusion has given rise to diastolic flow reversal in the external carotid artery (ECA), which supplies a patent ICA.

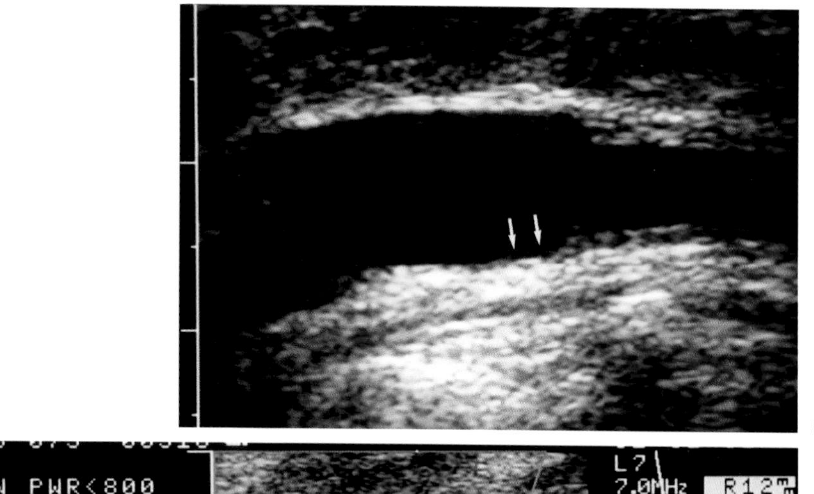

(a)

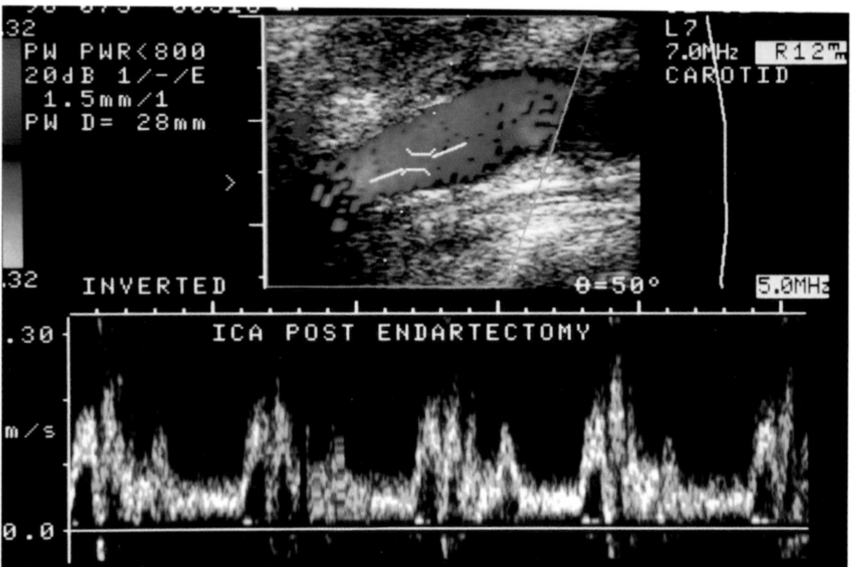

(b)

Plate 16.13 (a) Longitudinal section through the carotid bifurcation following an endarterectomy demonstrates the changes in the appearance of the inner arterial wall when the intimal–medial layer has been stripped (arrows). (b) The corresponding spectral Doppler waveform shows a prolonged systolic peak suggesting changes in the elasticity of the artery postsurgery. ICA, internal carotid artery.

(a)

(b)

(c)

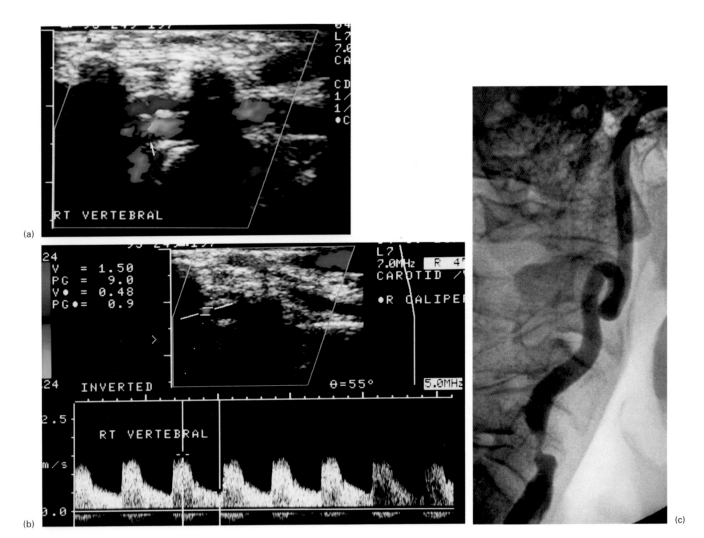

Plate 16.15 (a) Longitudinal section through the VA demonstrates a focal area of colour flow disturbance representing a narrowed lumen caused by an area of plaque (arrow). (b) The corresponding spectral waveform allows the angle corrected peak systolic velocity to be measured at 150 cm s^{-1}, which is much higher than the normal mean value of 56 cm s^{-1}. (c) The selective vessel angiographic image of the VA confirms the presence of a focal narrowing.

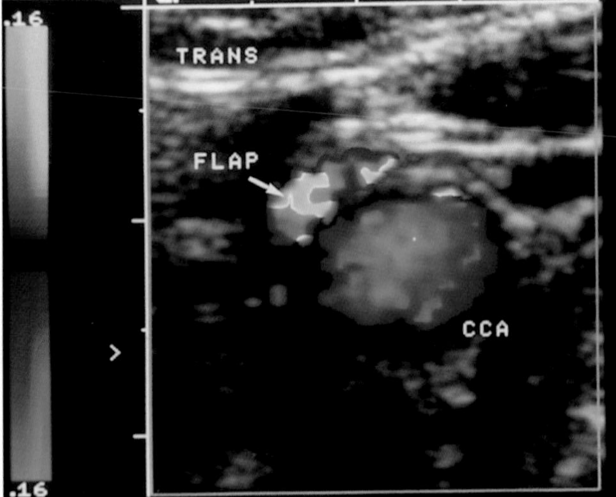

Plate 16.17 Transverse section through the distal common carotid artery (CCA) demonstrates an area of colour turbulence in the patent flap (arrow) of a CCA dissection.

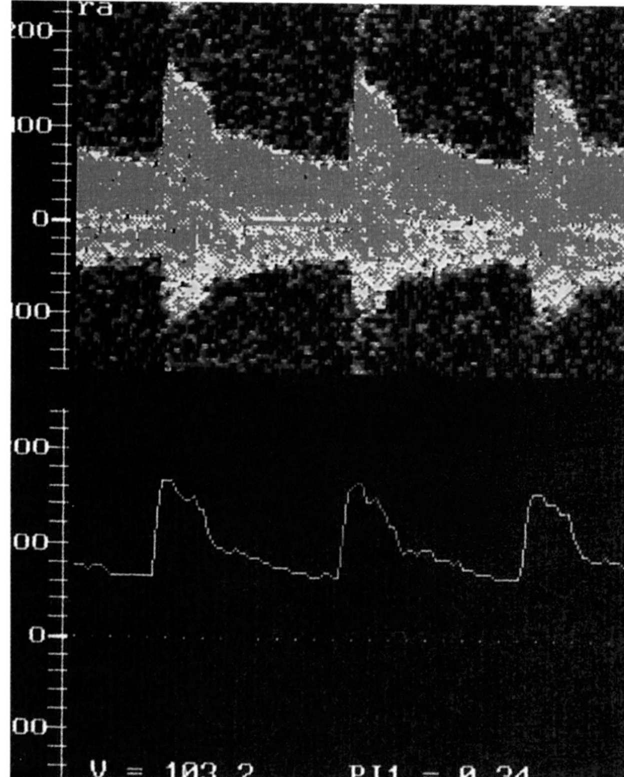

Plate 17.3 Normal spectral transcranial Doppler signal obtained from the terminal ICA through the temporal bone window—the top part of the image shows the 'raw' signal with the ipsilateral MCA signal above the baseline (directed towards the probe) and the ipsilateral ACA signal below the baseline (directed away from the probe); the lower part of the image shows the computer-derived tracing of the outline of the MCA waveform from which the peak and mean velocity and pulsatility index are derived.

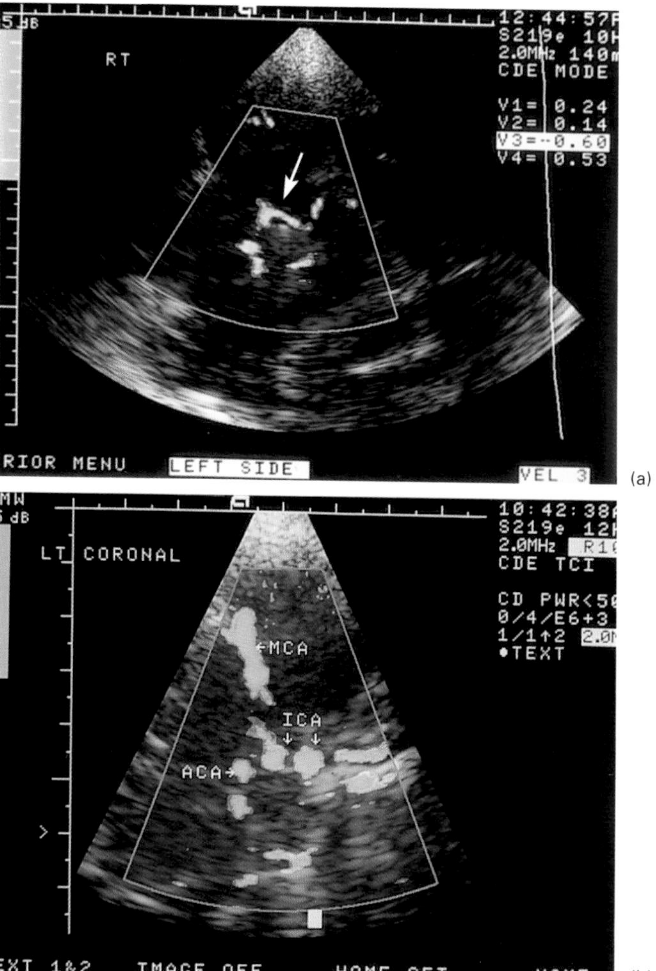

Plate 17.4 Colour transcranial Doppler image of the normal circle of Willis: (a) with PCoA (arrow); (b) another view in a different patient. ACA, MCA, anterior and middle cerebral arteries; ICA, internal carotid artery.

(a)

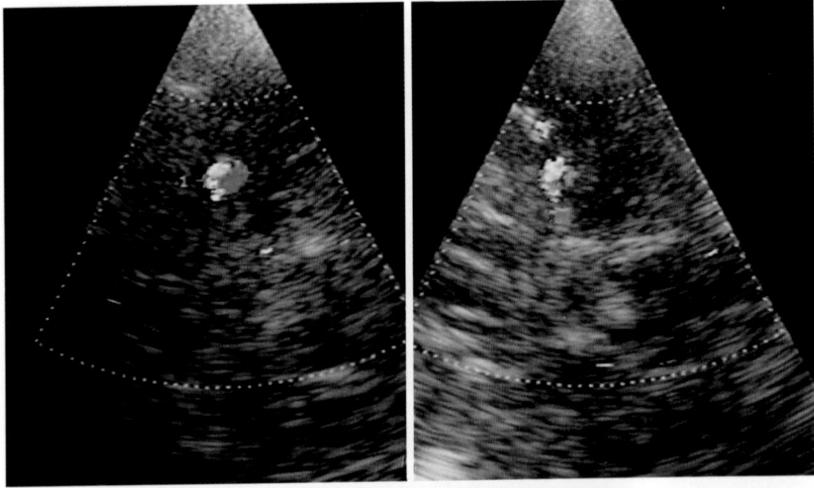

(b)

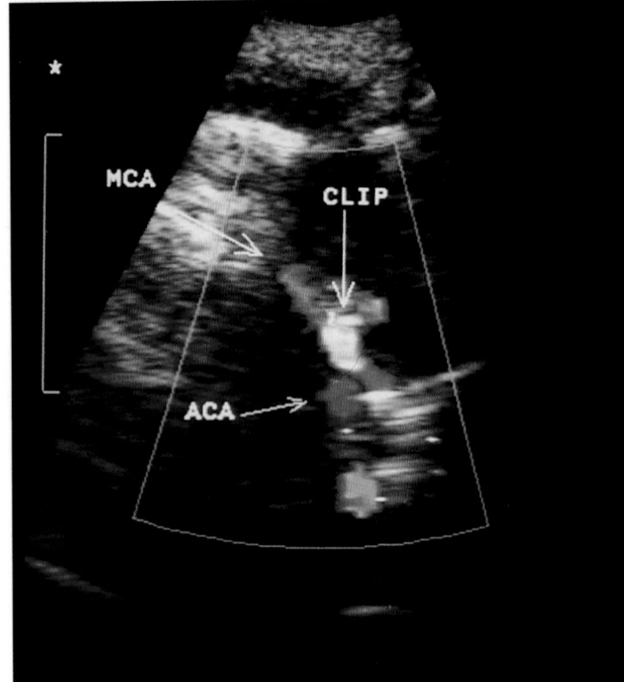

Plate 17.5 (a) Colour flow transcranial Doppler images of an asymptomatic MCA bifurcation aneurysm. The image was obtained in the axial plane through the temporal bone window. (b) Colour flow transcranial Doppler image axially through the temporal bone window of the middle cerebral artery (MCA) mainstem and proximal branches following an uneventful clipping of an MCA bifurcation aneurysm. Note the echogenic aneurysm clip. ACA, anterior cerebral artery.

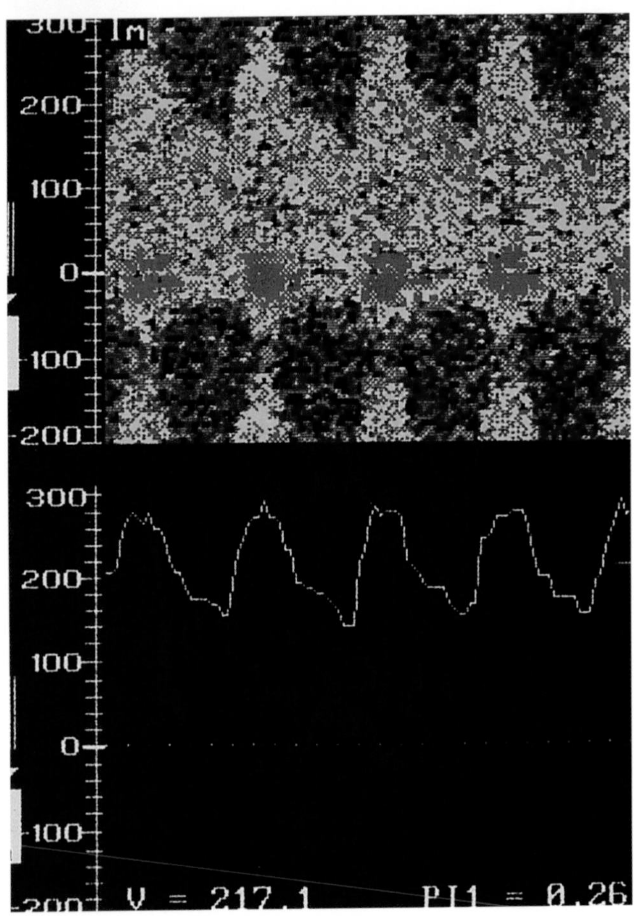

(a)

Plate 17.6 (a) Middle cerebral artery blood velocity and (b) cerebral angiogram 1 week after subarachnoid haemorrhage showing high mean blood velocity (217 cm s^{-1}) in the MCA and corresponding marked spasm. Note how pale the spectral signal is in (a)—compare with Plate 17.3— due to fewer red cells passing along the narrowed artery and consequently diminished echo amplitude. Note also the turbulence (dark red signal near the baseline) in keeping with severe spasm.

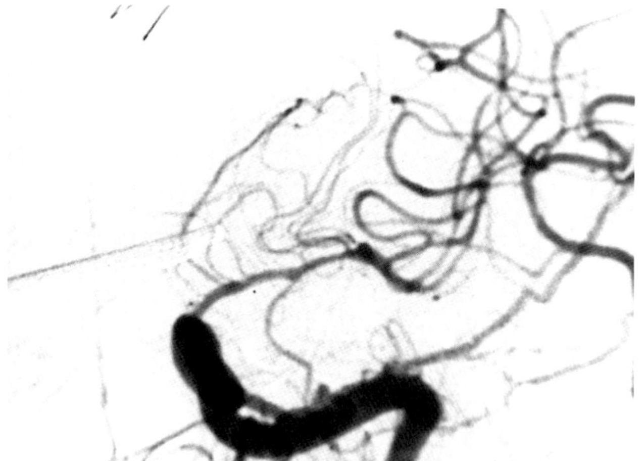

(b)

Plate 17.6 *Continued.*

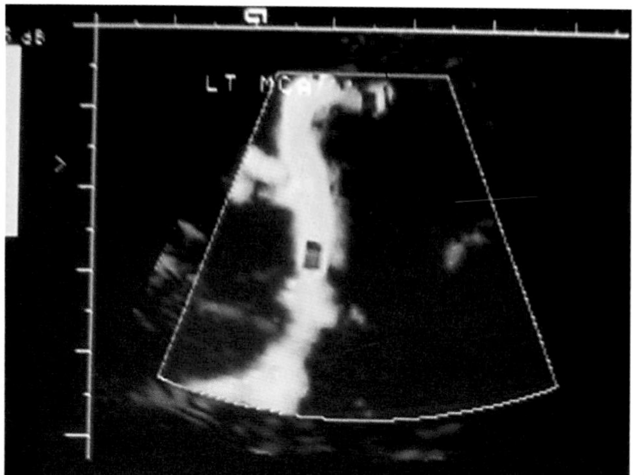

(a)

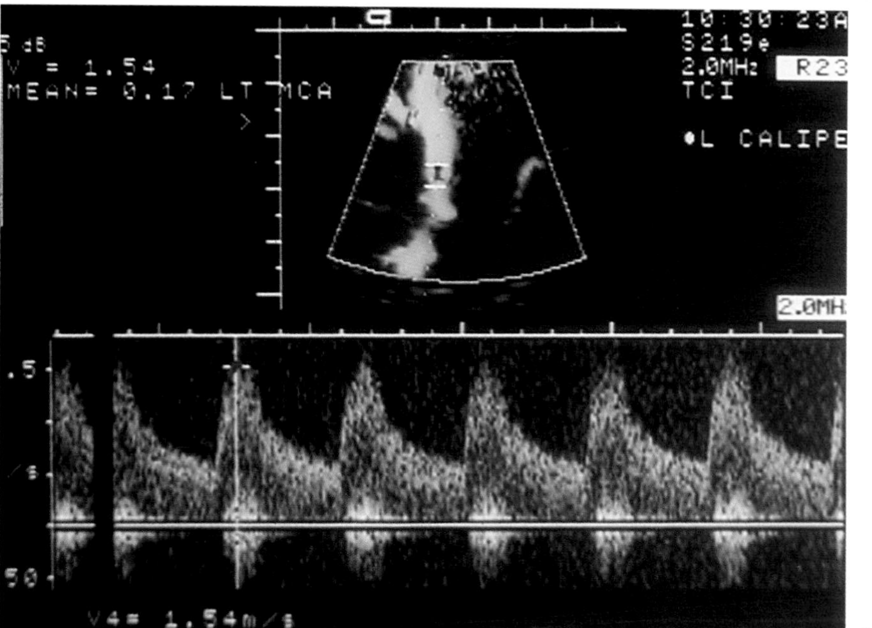

(b)

Plate 17.8 Colour transcranial Doppler of an MCA stenosis. (a) Colour 'power' Doppler image shows the MCA and its major branches with a calcified plaque causing stenosis in its mainstem. (b) Velocity waveform from the region of the stenosis shows high, turbulent velocity.

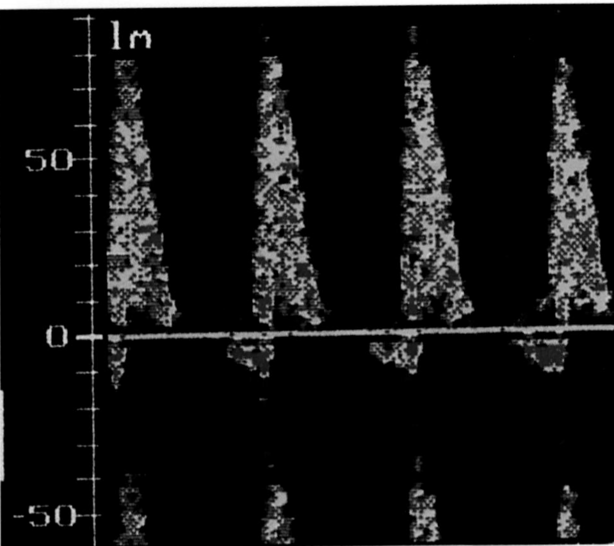

Plate 17.9 Low velocity, high pulsatility waveform with reversal of flow during diastole obtained from the MCA of a patient with very high intracranial pressure diagnosed clinically as brain dead.

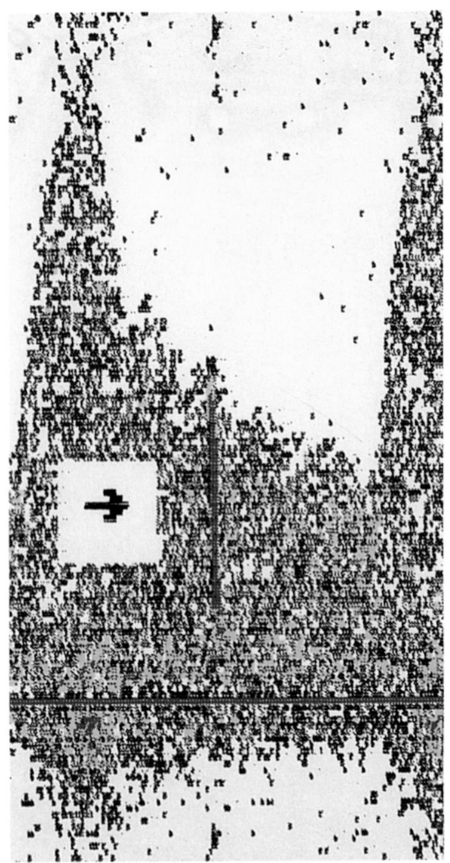

Plate 17.10 Spectral Doppler. Example of a probable particulate embolus detected in the MCA in a patient with a prosthetic heart valve but no symptoms of cerebrovascular disease. Note the high intensity, discrete signal from the embolus (arrow) superimposed on the normal MCA velocity waveform. (Courtesy of Dr D. Grossart, Institute of Neurological Sciences, Glasgow.)

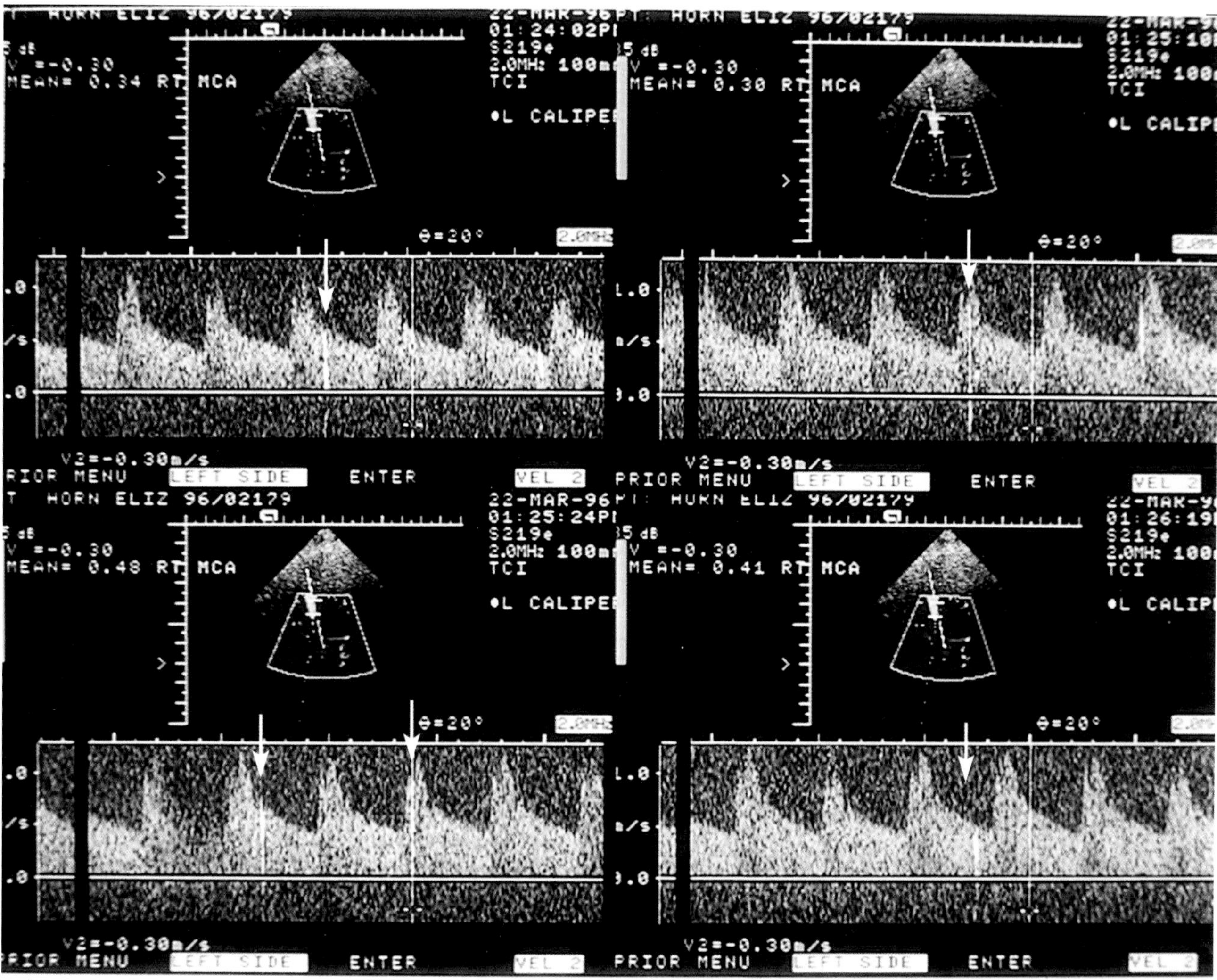

Plate 17.11 Colour transcranial Doppler image and spectral waveform from the MCA in a patient with a mechanical prosthetic heart valve. Note the frequent high amplitude signals occurring in the Doppler waveform (arrows) which are very probably due to gas bubbles sucked from the dissolved gas in the blood by the strong negative pressure of the value motion.

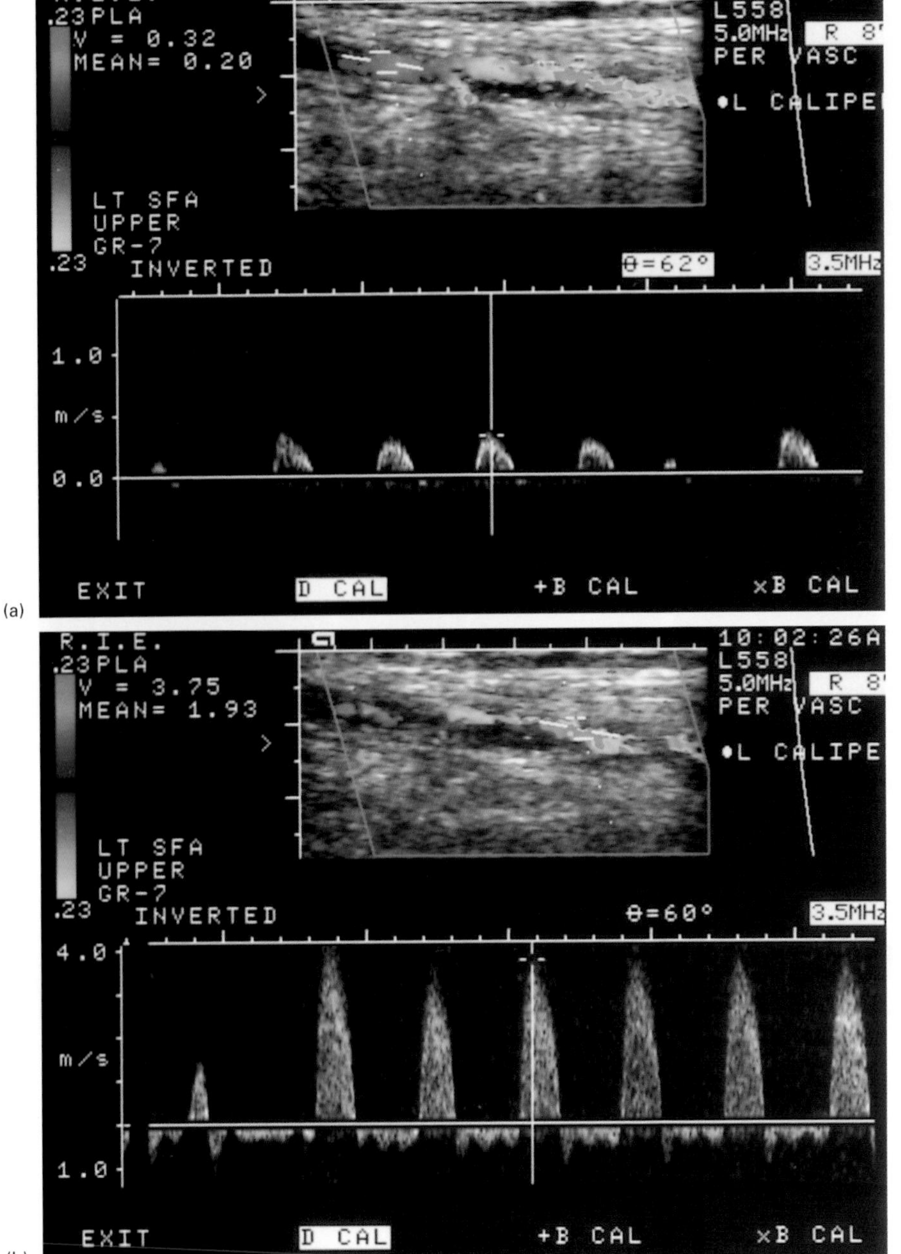

Plate 18.1 A severe stenosis in the superficial femoral artery. (a) Measurement of a peak systolic velocity of 0.32 m s^{-1} above the stenosis; a collateral vessel is also visible. (b) A peak systolic velocity of 3.75 m s^{-1} at the level of the stenosis, which is also shown by the aliasing in the colour display.

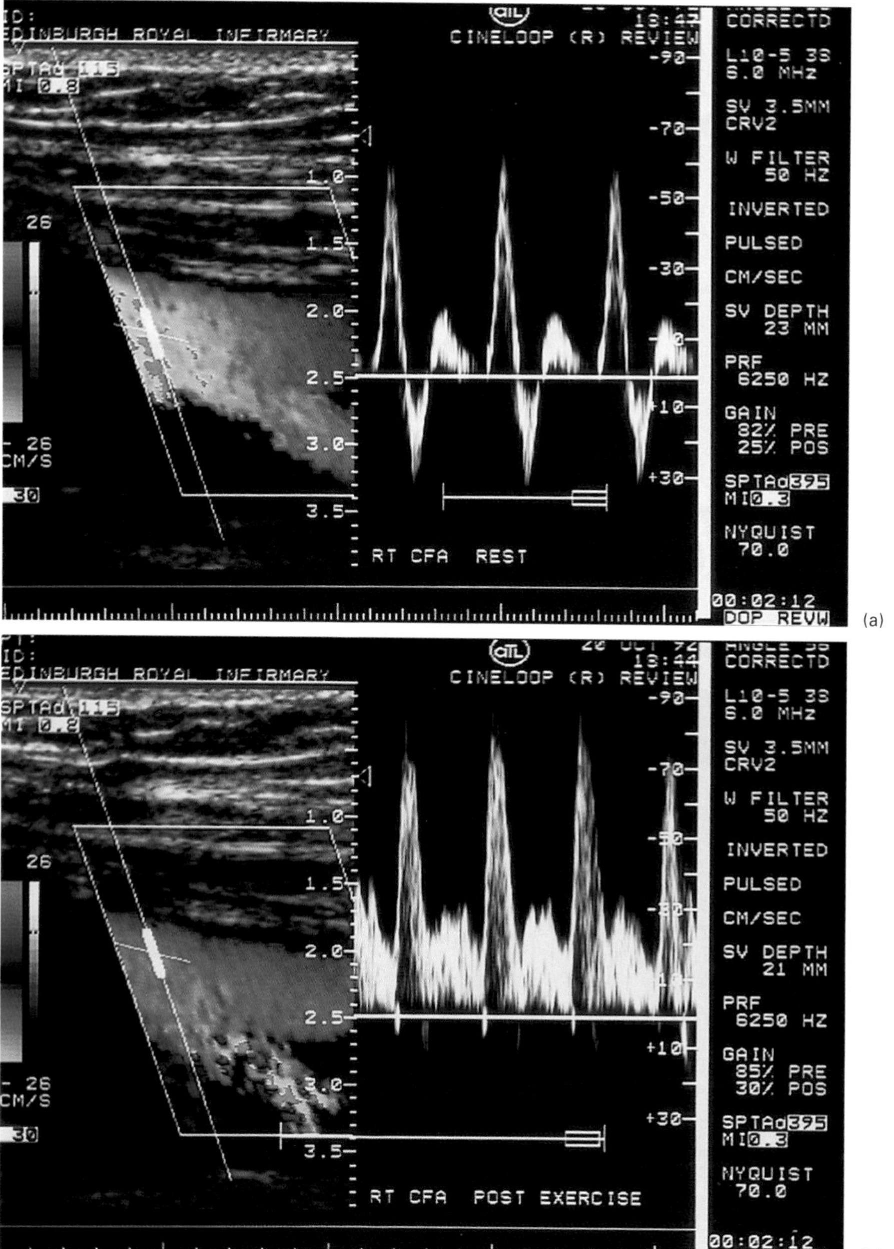

Plate 18.2 (a) The waveform in the common femoral artery at rest. A forward, reverse and second forward phase are seen. (b) The effects of exercise with loss of reverse flow and increased diastolic flow.

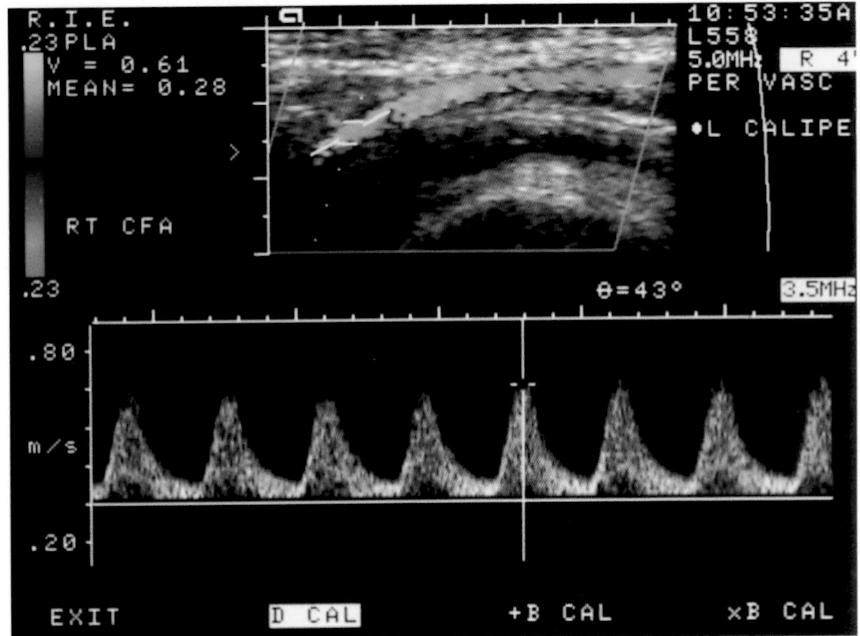

Plate 18.3 The common femoral artery below an iliac stenosis. There is turbulence with spectral widening and some damping of the waveform.

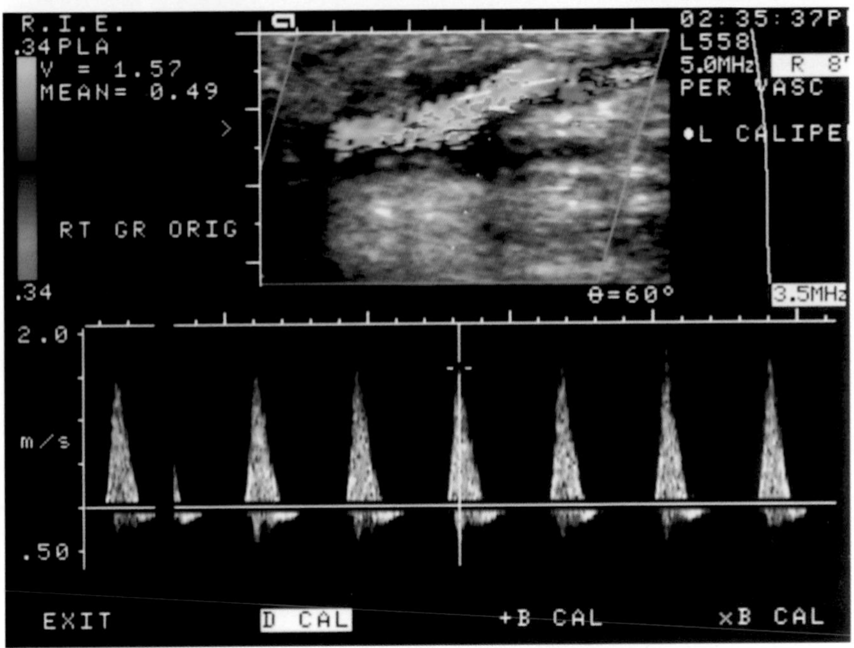

Plate 18.4 Origin of a femorodistal graft from the common femoral artery.

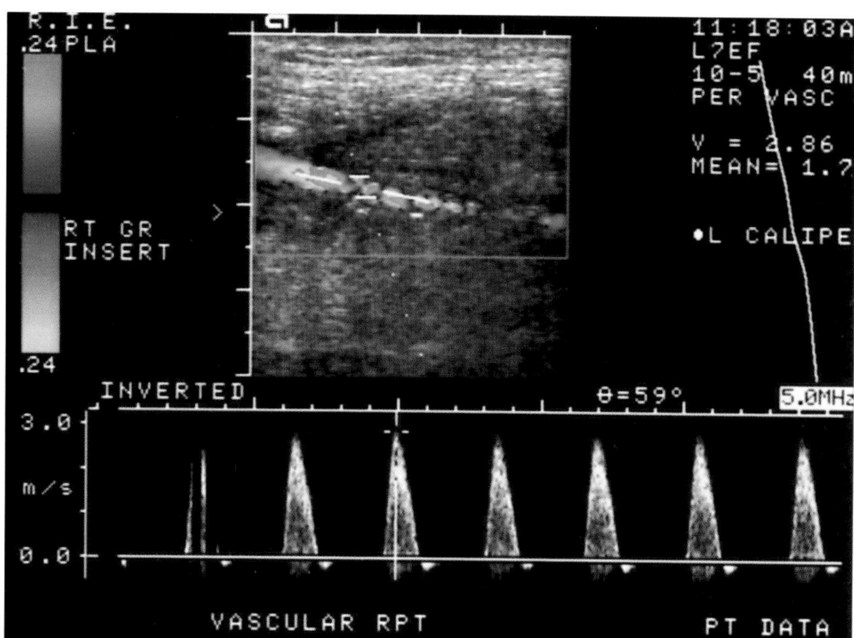

Plate 18.5 Stenosis at a graft insertion, there is aliasing and a significantly increased velocity of 2.86 m s^{-1}, compared with 0.6 m s^{-1} in the graft above the insertion.

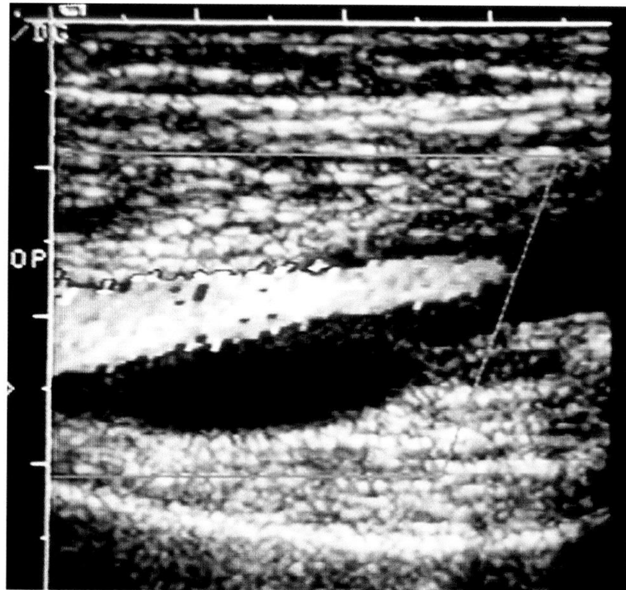

Plate 18.6 Cystic adventitial disease of the upper popliteal artery showing the cystic degeneration posteriorly.

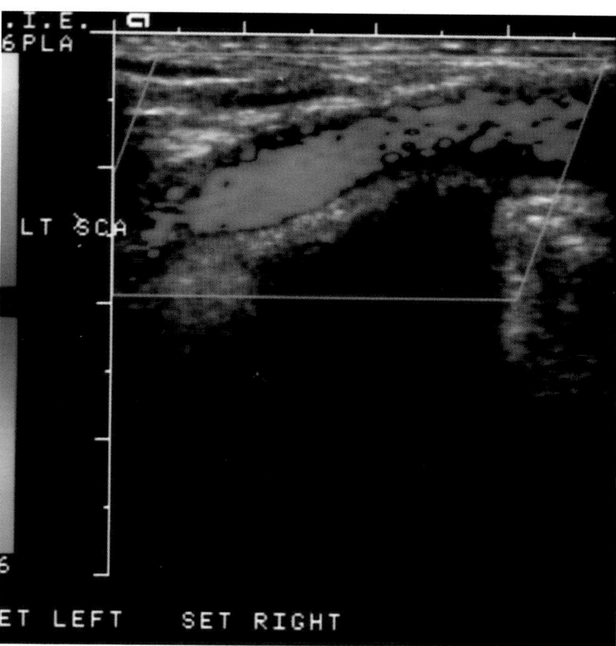

Plate 18.7 The left subclavian artery passing over a shadowing structure corresponding to a cervical rib.

(a)

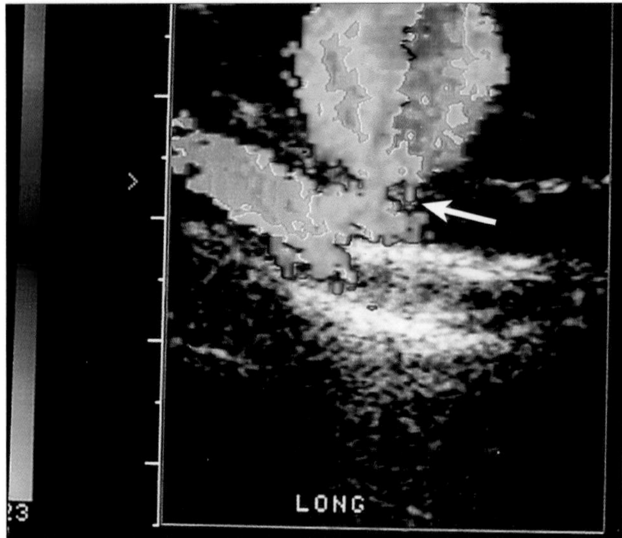

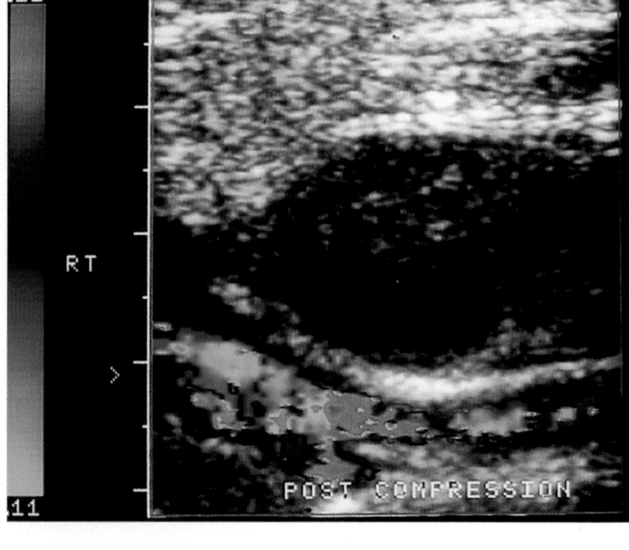

(b)

Plate 18.9 (a) Initial colour flow ultrasound of the femoral artery bifurcation in the longitudinal axis. There is a postcatheterization pseudoaneurysm arising from the superficial femoral artery. The communicating jet is well demonstrated (arrow) whilst mixing and swirling of colour is seen within the sac itself. Following the administration of intravenous analgesia and sedation, ultrasound-guided compression repair was performed. (b) Complete obliteration of the pseudoaneurysm was achieved in 30 min with conversion into a haematoma.

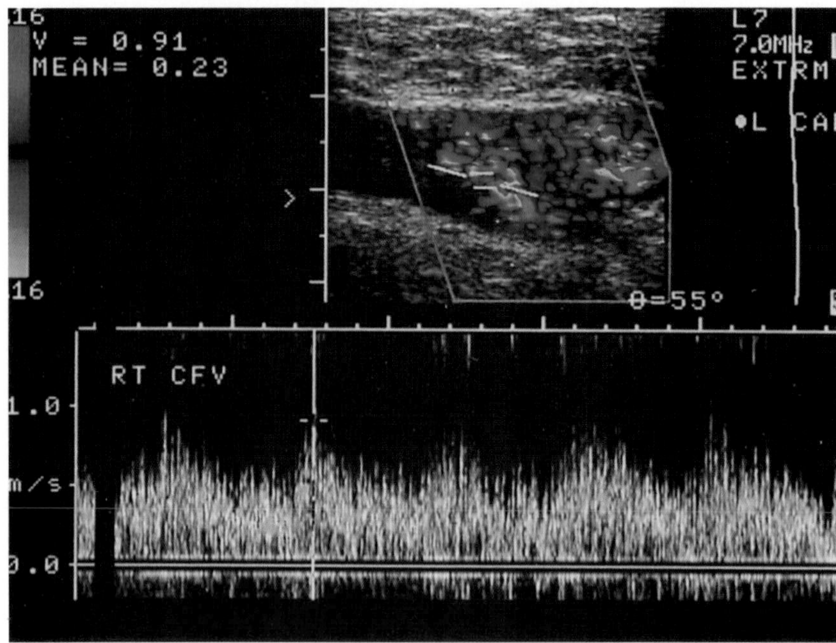

Plate 18.10 Femoral vein Doppler waveform in a known case of postcatheterization arteriovenous fistula. The waveform within the femoral vein is arterialized and shows marked turbulent flow indicative of a fistula.

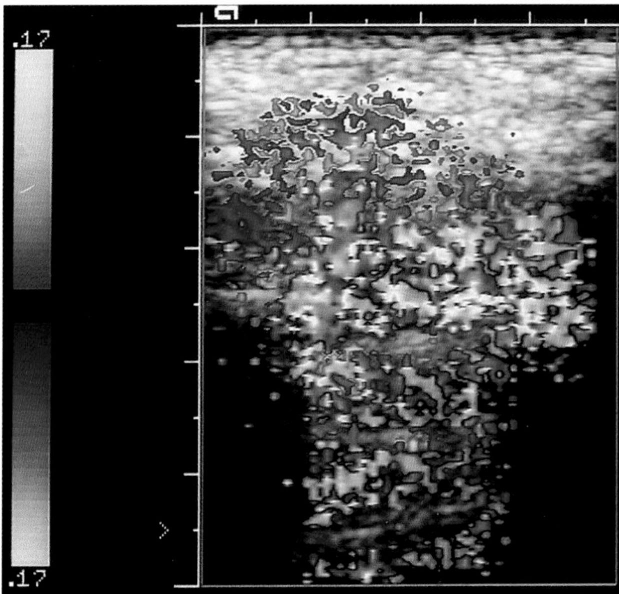

Plate 18.11 Colour flow image of a large subcutaneous arterioveneous fistula showing marked perivascular tissue vibration. This is thought to be secondary to transmitted vibration from the vein wall. This vibration is detected as movement by the colour Doppler software and consequently coded as such. When this appearance is present it should alert the ultrasonologist to the possibility of an arteriovenous fistula.

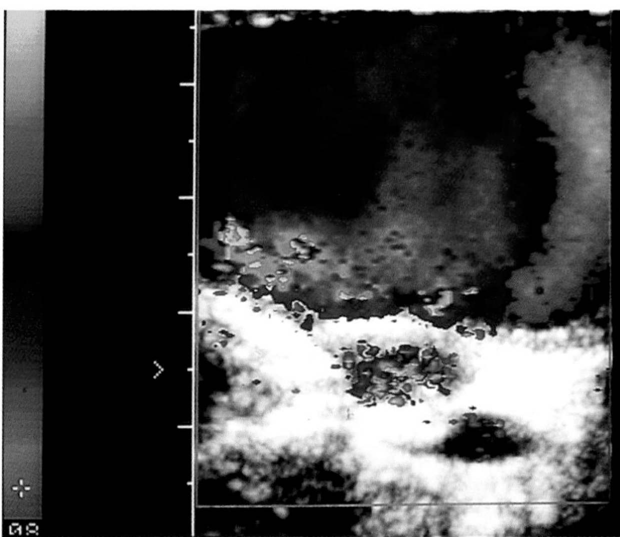

Plate 18.17 One complication of an arteriovenous fistula is large aneurysm formation. This is easily demonstrated with colour Doppler ultrasound. A giant aneurysm sac with swirling flow is demonstrated on colour flow imaging in such a case.

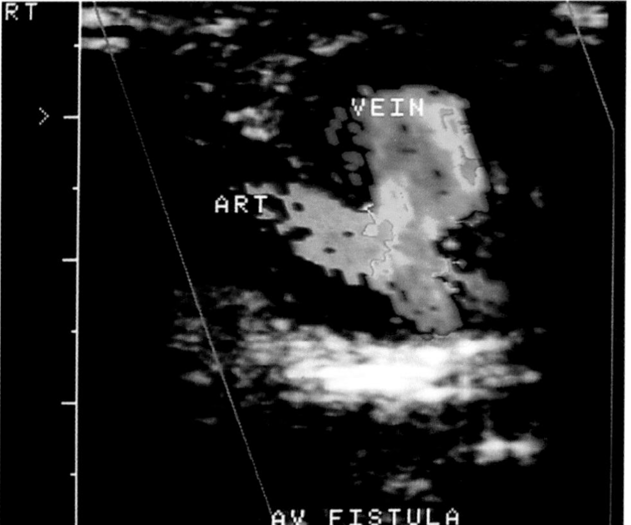

Plate 18.15 Colour flow image of a haemodialysis fistula in the antecubital fossa demonstrating the surgical anastomosis of the brachial artery (blue) and basilic vein (red). This anastomosis is well demonstrated on this occasion.

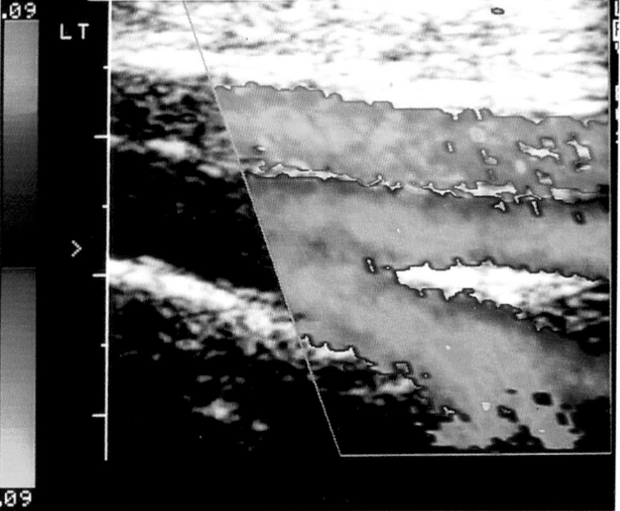

Plate 19.3 Longitudinal colour Doppler image at groin level demonstrating the junction of the superficial femoral vein and the more deeply situated profunda femoris vein (colour-coded in blue). This superficial femoral vein lies posterior to the superficial femoral artery (colour-coded in red). The common femoral vein is formed by the junction of the superficial femoral vein and the deeper profunda femoris vein. Flow at this level is entirely spontaneous.

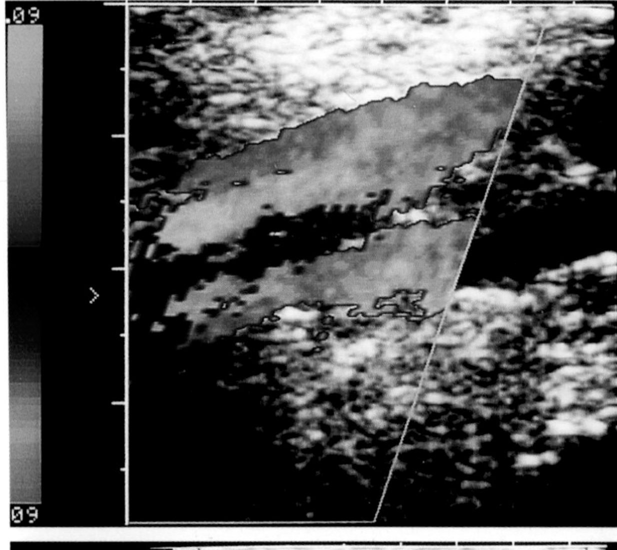

(a)

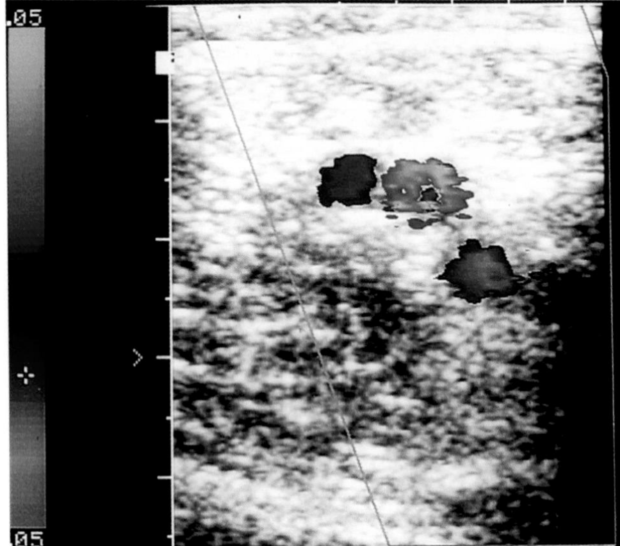

(b)

Plate 19.4 (a) Colour Doppler image (longitudinal axis) through the popliteal fossa demonstrating a duplicated popliteal venous system (colour-coded in blue). The popliteal artery is sandwiched between the veins; however, this is difficult to demonstrate completely on a still picture. (b) Transverse colour Doppler image in a different patient of a duplicated femoral venous system. Both femoral veins (blue) are seen on either side of the superficial femoral artery (red). Occasionally only one of these veins may be affected by thrombosis and this is a recognized pitfall both of this technique and venography but fortunately this is a relatively rare occurrence.

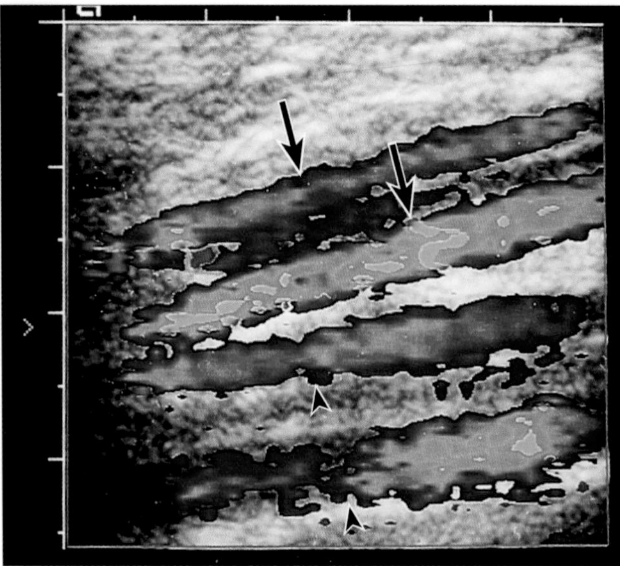

Plate 19.6 Colour flow image of the posterior tibial and common peroneal set of calf veins in a longitudinal axis at mid calf level. The posterior tibial set are more superficial (arrows) than the common peroneal veins (arrowheads). Flow within these veins can only be appreciated with the aid of distal limb compression which can be achieved manually or by graded cuff compression. (Reproduced with permission from *Clinical Radiology* (1992), **46**, 198–201.)

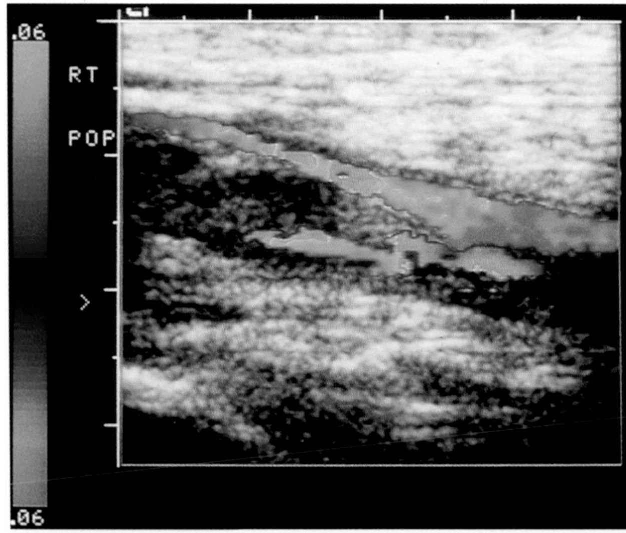

Plate 19.11 Longitudinal colour Doppler image through the popliteal fossa demonstrating non-occlusive thrombus within the popliteal vein. The popliteal vein is slightly distended and contains a large amount of mixed echogenic thrombus. Some residual venous flow persists and this is seen both along the vein wall (analogous to the 'tram line' appearance on venography) and within the thrombus itself.

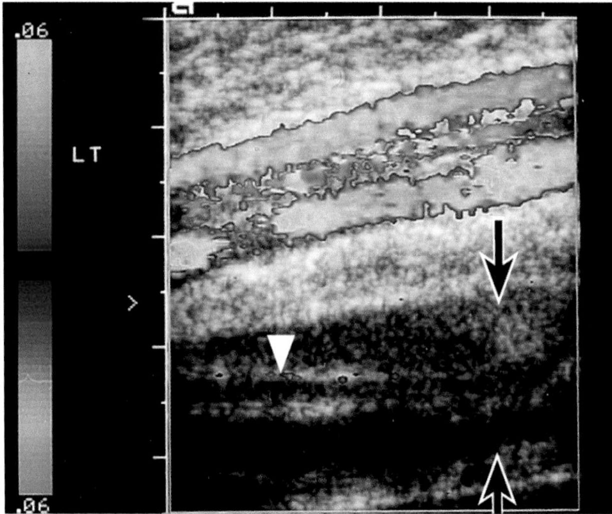

Plate 19.12 Longitudinal colour Doppler scan through the medial aspect of the calf demonstrating patency of both posterior tibial veins (blue) with the posterior tibial artery (red) sandwiched in between. The deeper situated common peroneal veins are distended and thrombosed (arrows) with complete absence of colour-coded flow. These ultrasonic findings were confirmed by venography. Small flashes of flow were seen within the common peroneal artery (arrowhead).

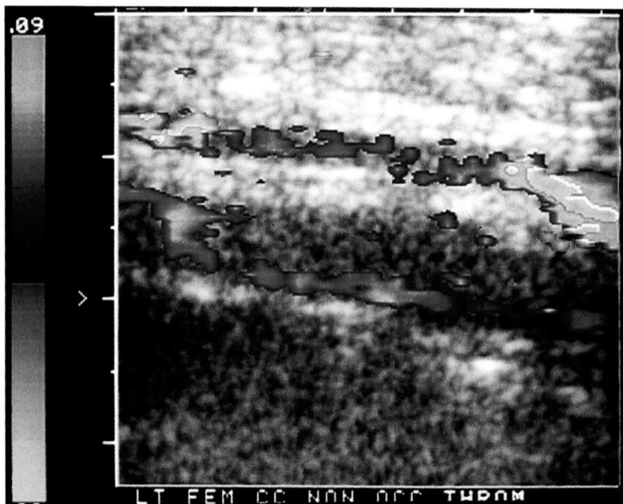

Plate 19.14 Colour Doppler image of the femoral vein in a longitudinal axis 6 months following acute DVT. There has only been partial recanalization of the femoral vein with some peripheral flow within the lumen. Although this represents part of the spectrum of recanalization following the acute insult it leads to difficulty in imaging should there be a recurrence of symptoms as these ultrasonic appearances cannot be distinguished from acute non-occlusive thrombus. (Reproduced with permission from *Clinical Radiology* (1991), **43**, 301–304.)

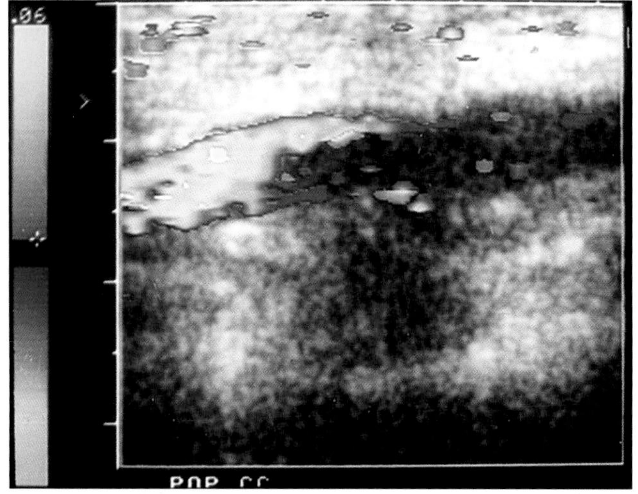

(a)

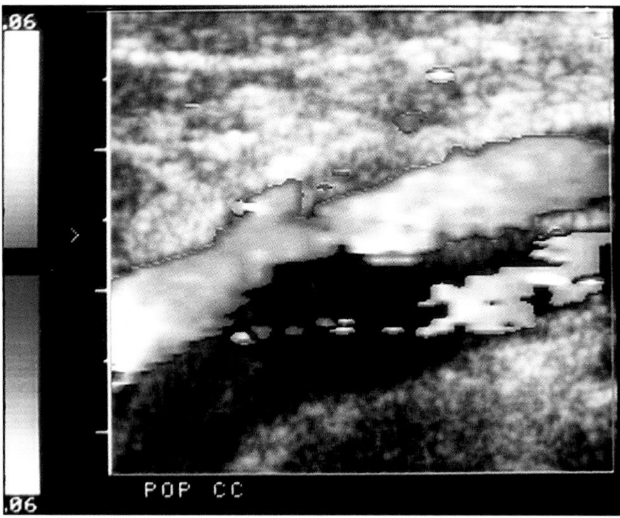

(b)

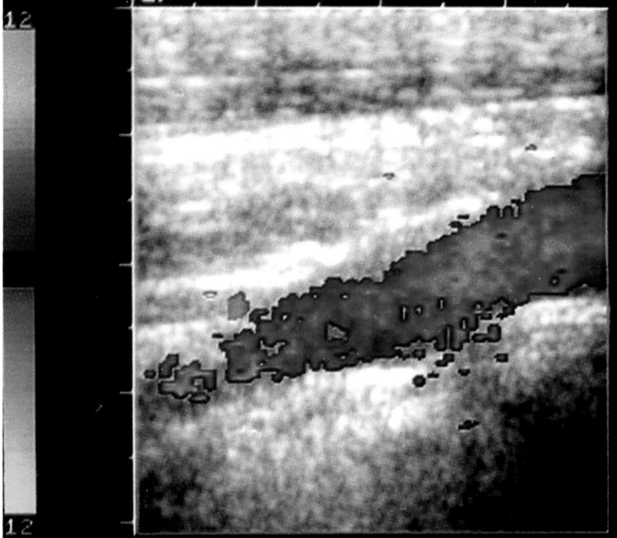

Plate 19.17 Colour flow image in a longitudinal plane demonstrating a normal patent subclavian vein just below the clavicle. Flow is spontaneous and completely fills the vein lumen. (Reproduced with permission from the *British Journal of Radiology* (1991), **64**, 777–781.)

Plate 19.13 (*left*) Longitudinal colour Doppler scan of the popliteal vein (a) at the time of diagnosis of DVT and (b) 3 months later, subsequently showing complete recanalization of the vein. This only occurs in 50% of patients with acute DVT.

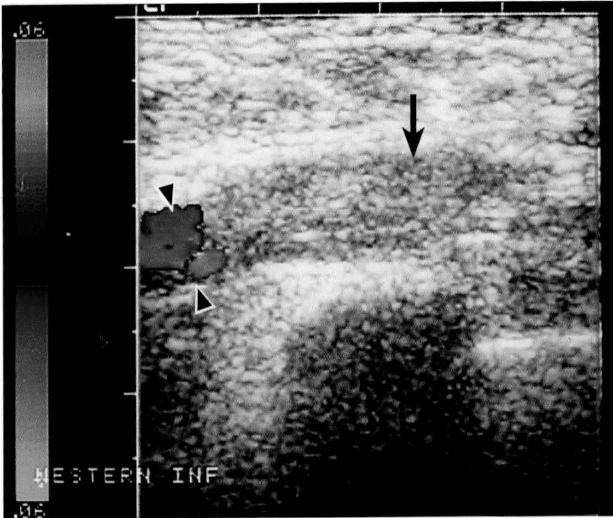

Plate 19.19 Colour flow image in a longitudinal axis demonstrating acute thrombus within the distal axillary and lateral aspect of the subclavian vein (arrow). Some residual flow is noted laterally (arrowheads) but more medially there is complete absence of colour-coded flow indicative of thrombosis. (Reproduced with permission from the *British Journal of Radiology* (1991), **64**, 777–781.)

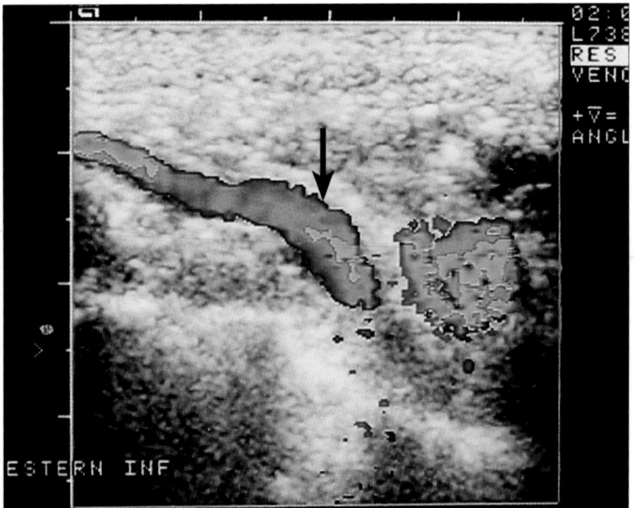

(a)

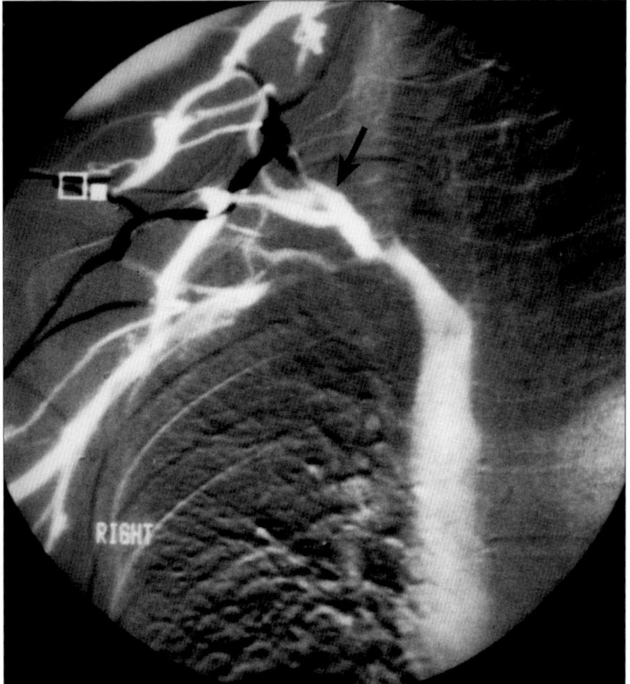

(b)

Plate 19.20 (a) Demonstrates a secondary finding in upper limb thrombosis, namely the presence of a large collateral vein (arrow). This may add confidence to the initial diagnosis especially if the examination and/or anatomy is difficult to interpret. (b) This collateral (arrow) is clearly shown on an intravenous digital subtraction angiogram, the main subclavian vein being occluded.

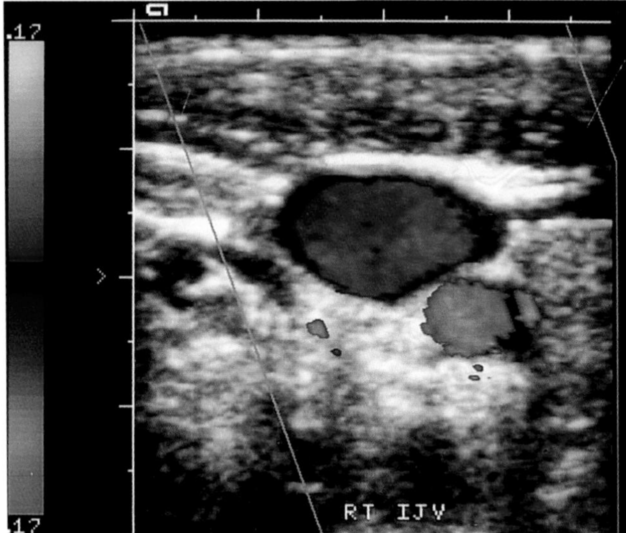

(a)

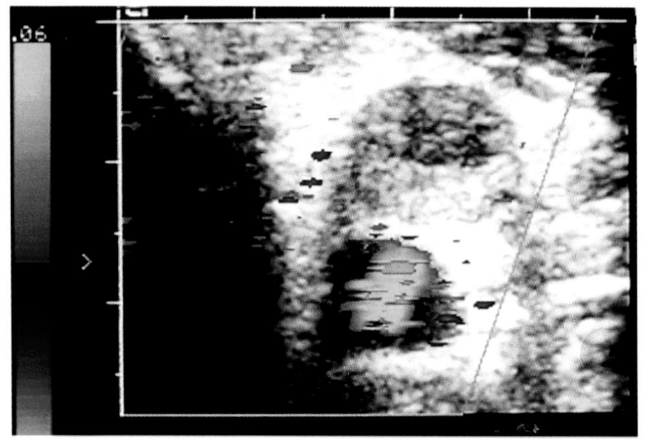

(b)

Plate 19.21 (a) Transverse colour flow image of a patent internal jugular vein (IJV) (blue) lying anteriorly to the common carotid artery (red). (b) A thrombosed internal jugular vein in a different patient is shown for comparison. This scan has been performed in a similar image plane and once again the common carotid artery (red) lies posteriorly. This vein is routinely imaged with colour Doppler imaging whereas it is not with intravenous contrast studies. This is one advantage of the non-invasive study. (Reproduced with permission from the *British Journal of Radiology* (1991), **64**, 777–781.)

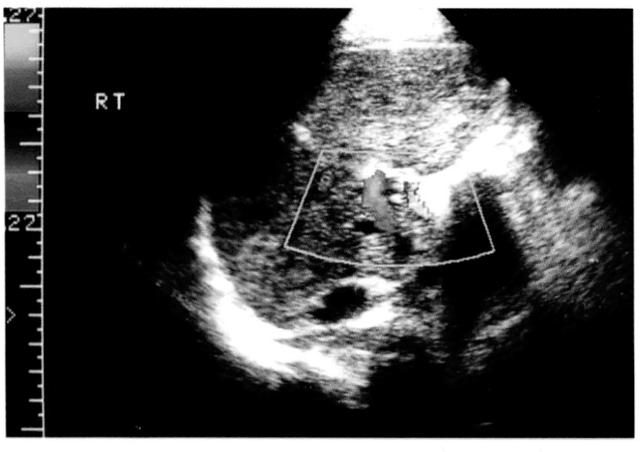

(a)

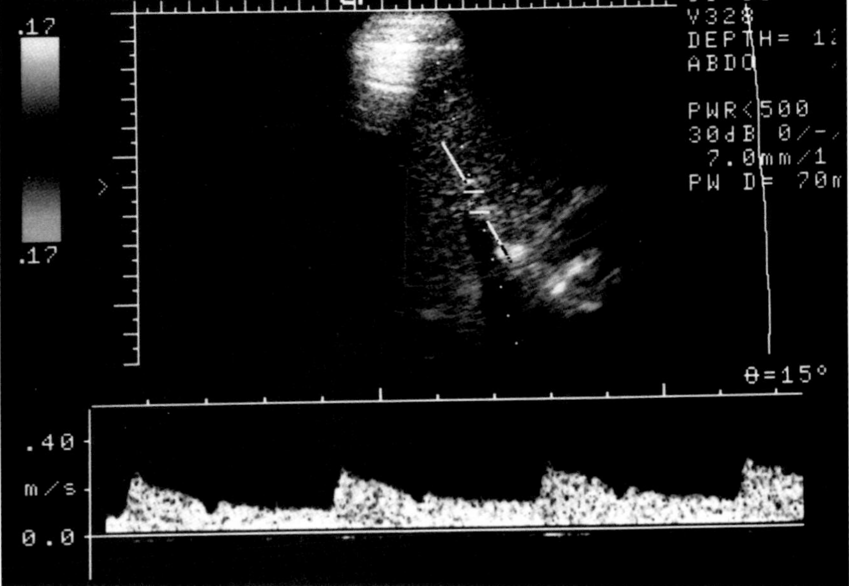

(b)

Plate 20.7 (a) Colour flow image through a right intercostal approach demonstrating hepatopetal flow within the distal portal vein, the hepatic artery lying anteriorly. (b) A normal hepatic artery waveform is demonstrated on spectral analysis with maintenance of flow throughout diastole.

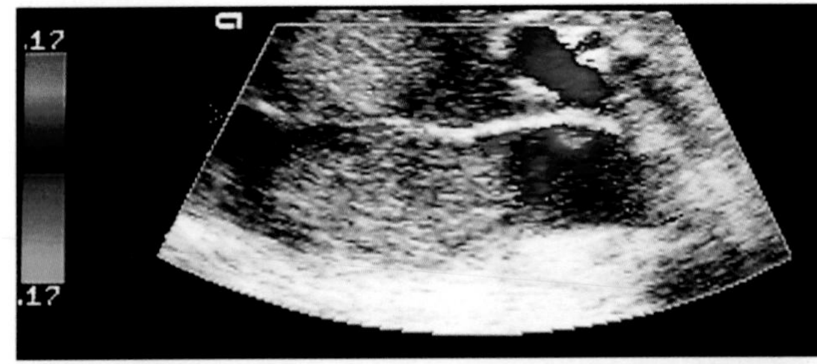

Plate 20.9 Colour flow image of the IVC in longitudinal axis, demonstrating echogenic tumour thrombus within the lumen and some surrounding peripheral flow. The tumour had extended along the main renal vein secondary to a primary renal cell carcinoma.

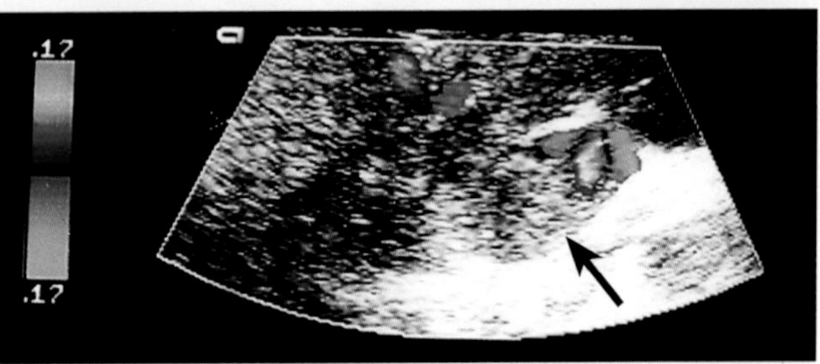

Plate 20.10 Colour flow image demonstrating tumour thrombus (arrow) within a distended renal vein from a primary renal cell carcinoma.

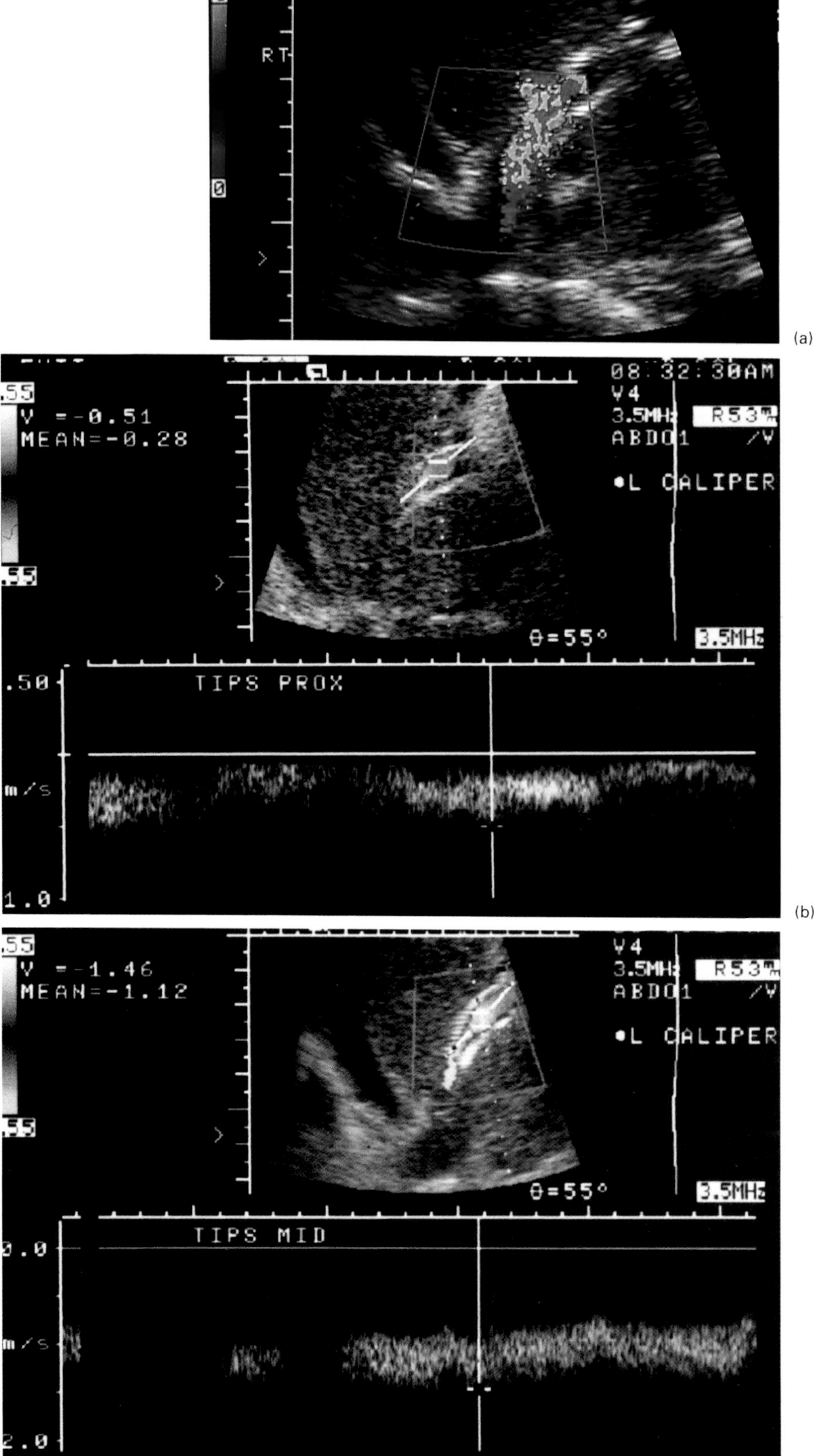

Plate 20.13 (a) Colour Doppler image at the mid to hepatic end of a TIPS stent demonstrating marked aliasing despite an appropriate high pulse repetition frequency. The flow from the proximal to mid stent segments did not show any aliasing and the overall colour flow appearances are highly suggestive of a mid to distal TIPS stent stenosis. (b) Doppler spectral waveform from the proximal to mid part of the TIPS stent. This demonstrated a peak velocity of 51 cm s^{-1}. (c) Doppler spectral waveform from the distal TIPS stent at the site of previously demonstrated aliasing. The peak velocity has increased significantly by almost three times to 1.46 m s^{-1} consistent with a TIPS stenosis. This was confirmed angiographically.

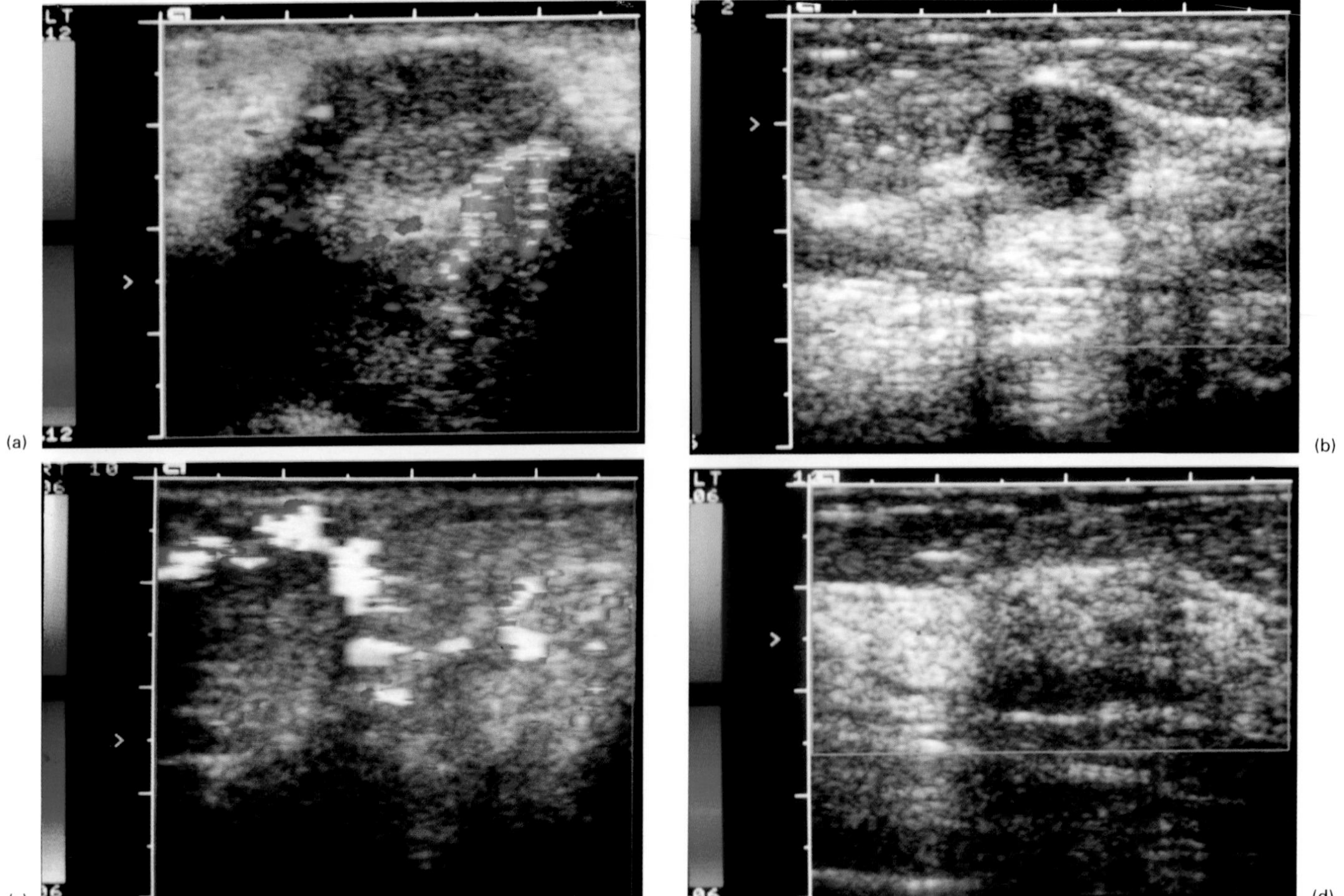

Plate 21.1 Colour Doppler of breast lesions. The power of colour Doppler is that it combines the anatomical information of an ultrasound scan with the haemodynamic information of an angiogram. (a) Numerous vessels are seen within this large carcinoma. The alternating colours indicate fast or disturbed flow, both characteristic of neovascularization. The 12 mm lesion in (b) has all the features of a fibroadenoma on the grey-scale image but the vascularization is suspicious; an infiltrating carcinoma was found on excision biopsy. (c) Inflammatory carcinomas have prolific vascularization, a feature that is diagnostic when it calls attention to a diffuse lesion that may be undetectable on the grey-scale scan. (d) Generally benign processes are avascular, as with this focal region of benign breast change (the scanty blue colours are from normal breast vessels). Rapidly growing fibroadenomas and inflammatory processes are exceptions.

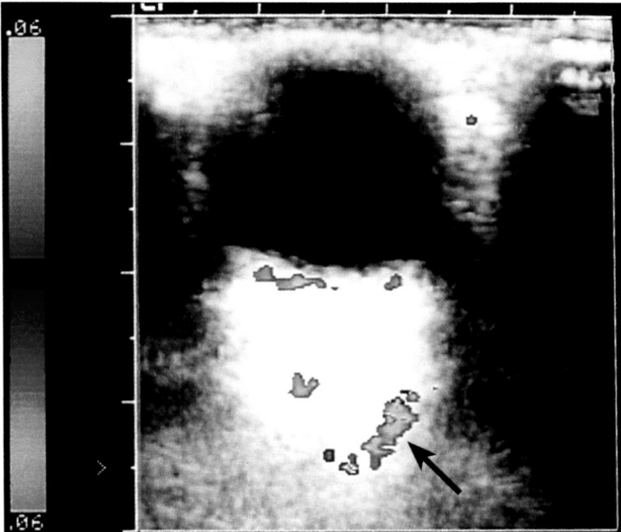

Plate 24.27 Colour Doppler image of the ophthalmic artery. The ophthalmic artery crosses the optic nerve in the posterior aspect of the orbit and gives a large nasal branch (arrow) which occupies a constant anatomical position and as such is suitable for Doppler analysis.

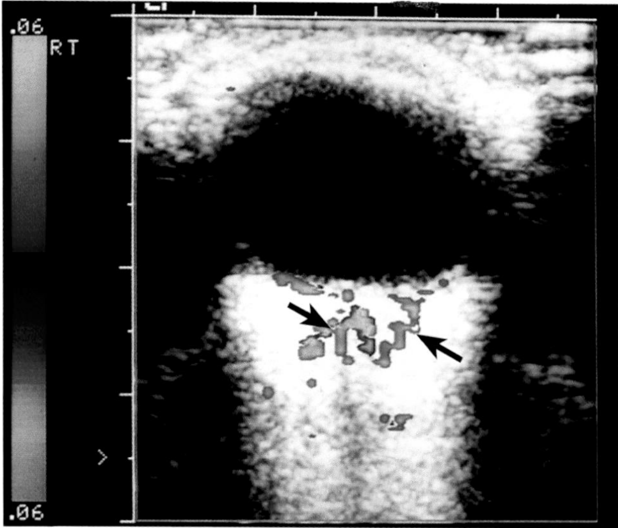

Plate 24.30 Colour flow image of the vessels at and around the optic nerve head. The central retinal artery (red) and central retinal vein (blue) are seen centrally within the optic nerve head whilst the peripapillary vessels on either side are the posterior ciliary arteries (arrows). These latter vessels appear as short flashes of colour flow and although seen during a dynamic examination are difficult to capture on still film.

(a)

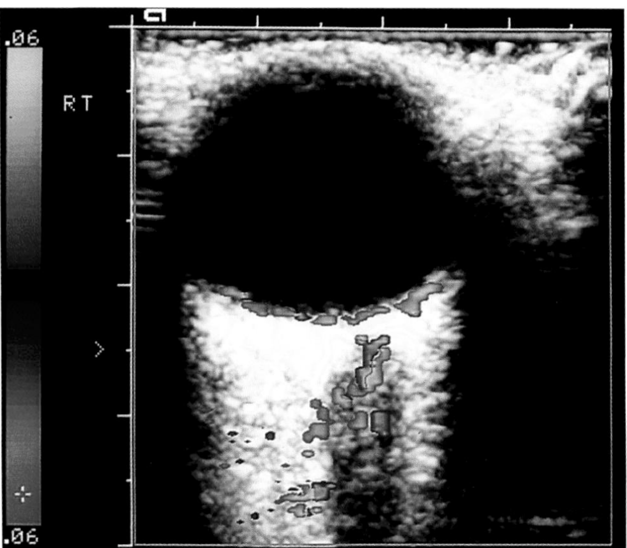

(b)

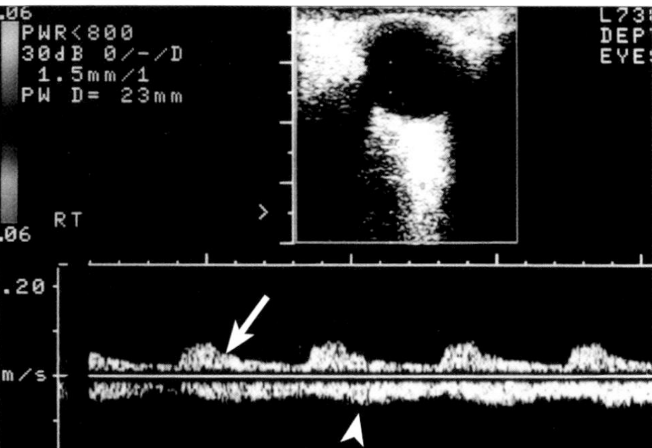

Plate 24.28 (a) Colour flow image just posterior to the choroid demonstrating flow within both the central retinal vein and central retinal artery. Flow within the artery is towards the probe and is colour-coded in red, whilst flow in the vein is in the opposite direction and is colour-coded in blue. Both these vessels lie within the intraneural portion of the optic nerve head. (b) Typical Doppler waveforms of both these vessels are shown. The arterial waveform has both systolic and diastolic components (arrow) whilst the venous waveform is more phasic (arrowhead).

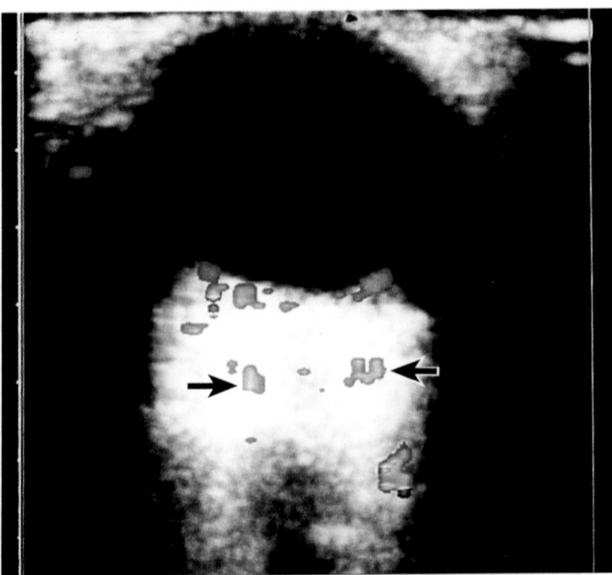

Plate 24.31 Colour Doppler image just behind the choroid demonstrating complete absence of the central retinal artery (CRA) with maintenance of the posterior ciliary vessels on either side of the optic nerve (arrows). This patient presented clinically with an acute CRA occlusion which was confirmed on fluorescein angiography, the ultrasound scan being performed within 24 h of presentation. (Reproduced with permission from *Eye* (1993), **7**, 74–79.)

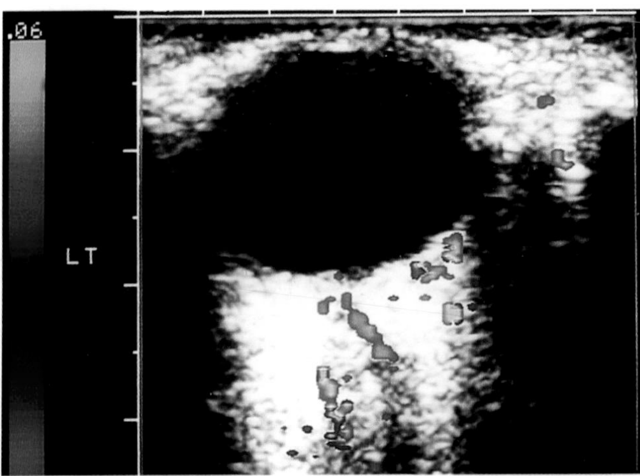

Plate 24.33 Colour flow image of a patient with ischaemic central retinal vein (CRV) occlusion. The CRA is still visualized (in red); however, the CRV is absent as it is occluded. The venous signal was absent on both colour flow and Doppler analysis.

(a)

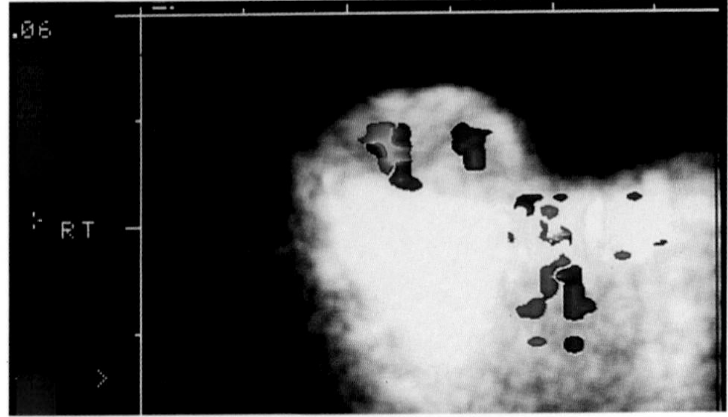

(b)

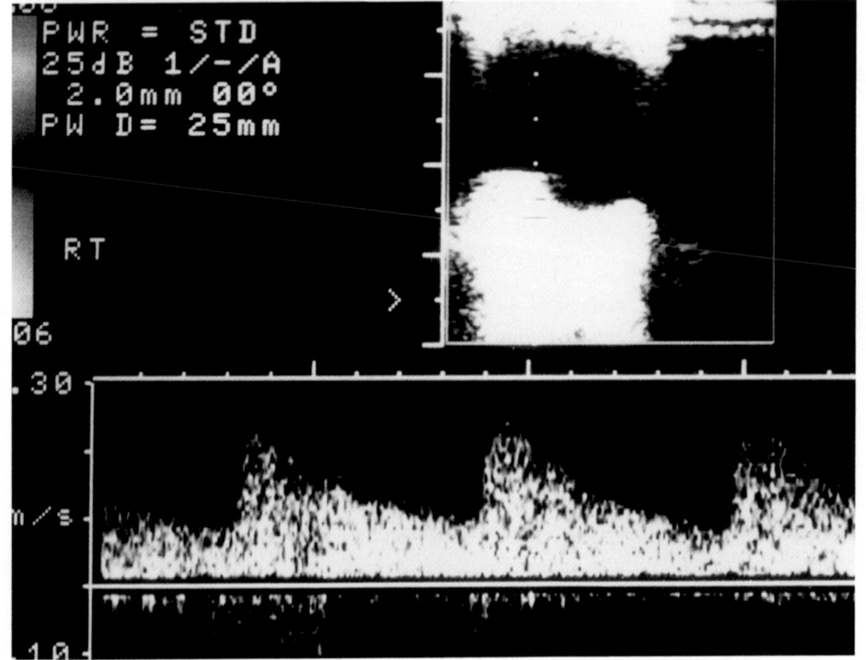

Plate 24.34 (a) Colour flow image of a malignant melanoma demonstrating intratumoral flow. (b) This can be quantified using spectral analysis and velocity and Doppler indices measured in the usual manner.

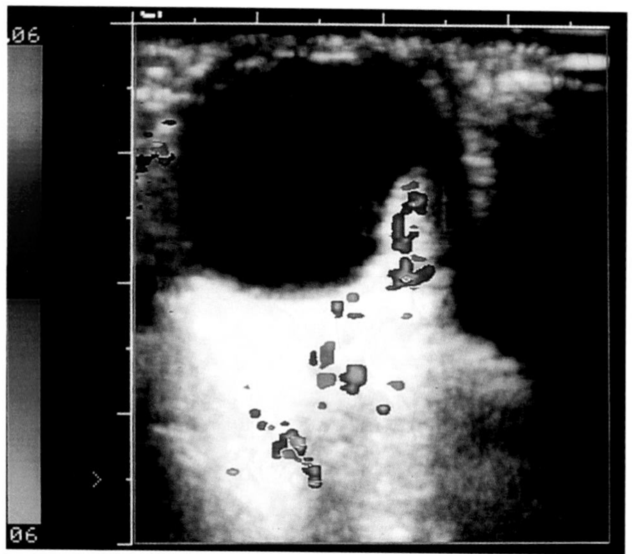

(a)

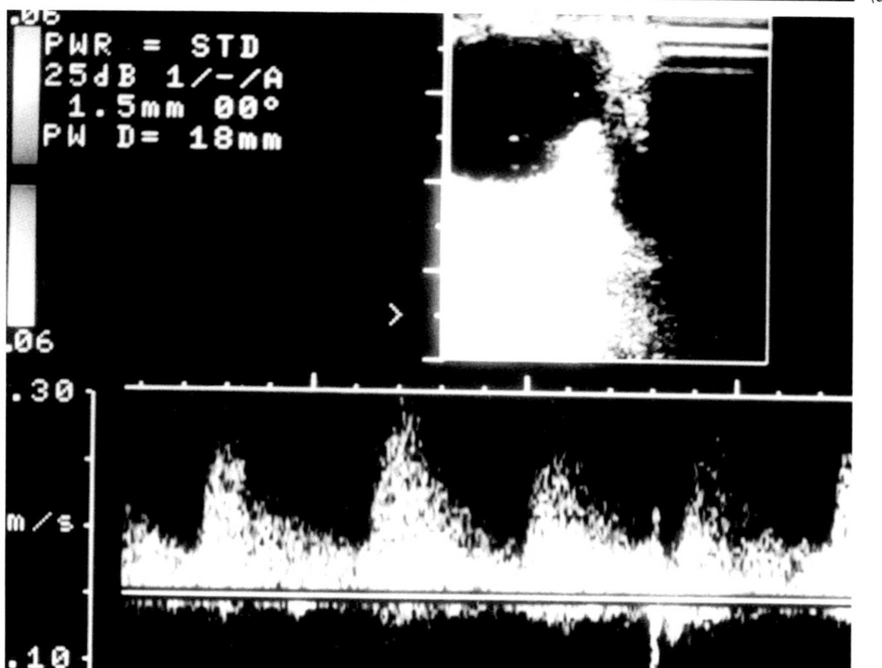

(b)

Plate 24.35 (a) Colour flow image of a capillary haemangioma. Again flow within the mass is demonstrated using colour flow imaging whilst further analysis is possible using spectral Doppler (b). Although some differences have been demonstrated between caplliary haemangiomas and malignant melanomas there is an overlap in Doppler measurements between the two groups and therefore they cannot be differentiated on Doppler analysis.

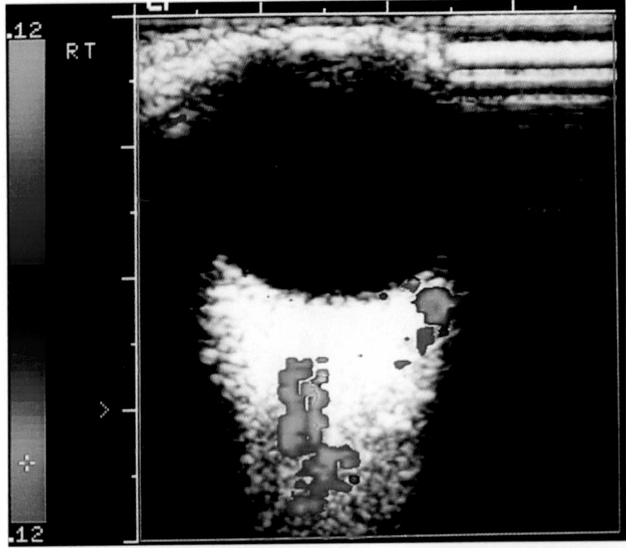

(a)

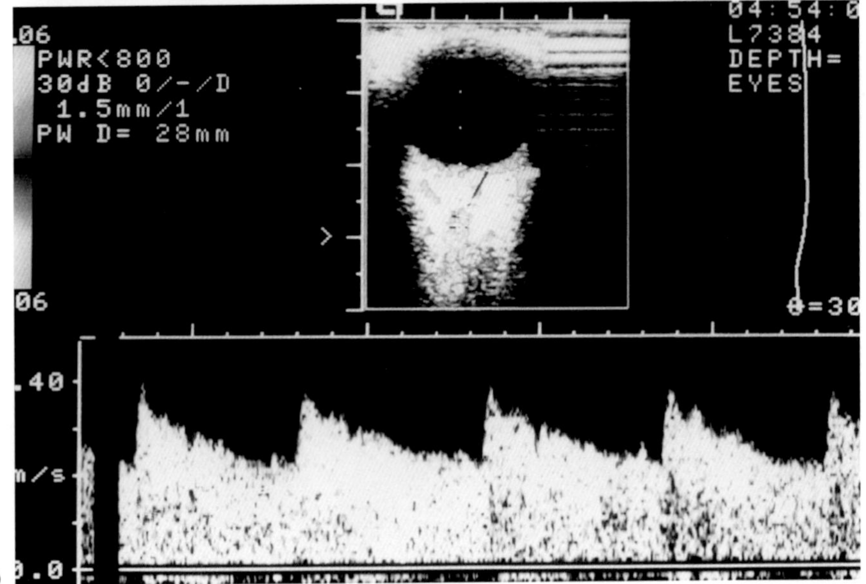

(b)

Plate 24.37 (a) Colour flow image of a patient with a caroticocavernous fistula showing marked enlargement of the ophthalmic artery. (b) Doppler analysis of the ophthalmic artery shows marked increase in diastolic flow with a consequent reduction in resistive index.

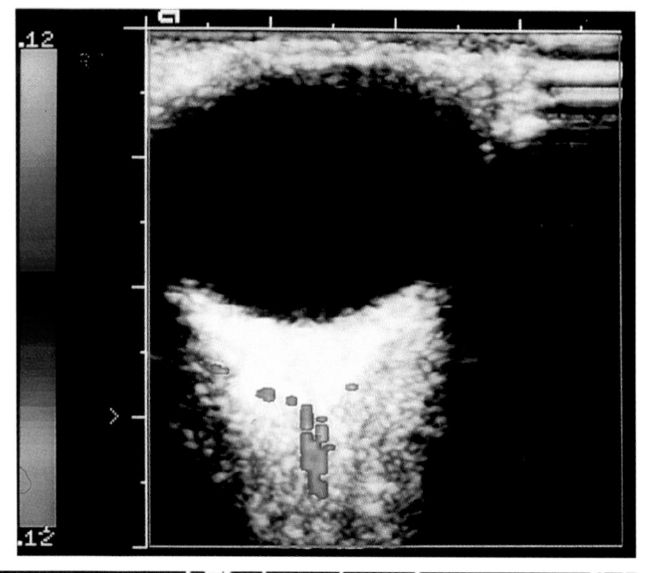

(a)

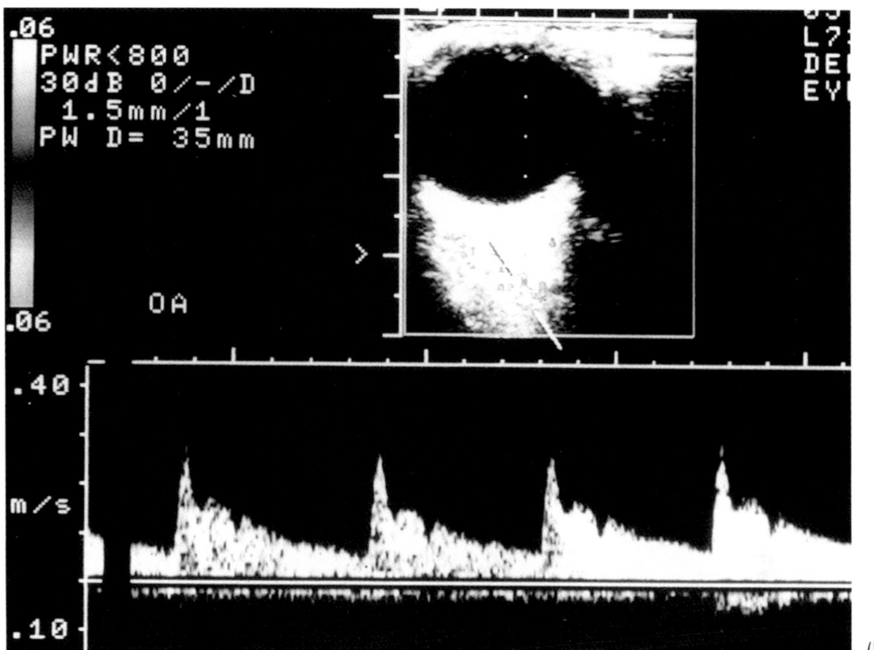

(b)

Plate 24.38 (a) The opposite eye of the same patient as in Plate 24.37 showing a normal appearance on colour flow imaging of the ophthalmic artery. (b) Similarly the Doppler spectrum of the ophthalmic artery is normal with significantly less diastolic flow when compared with Plate 24.37b.

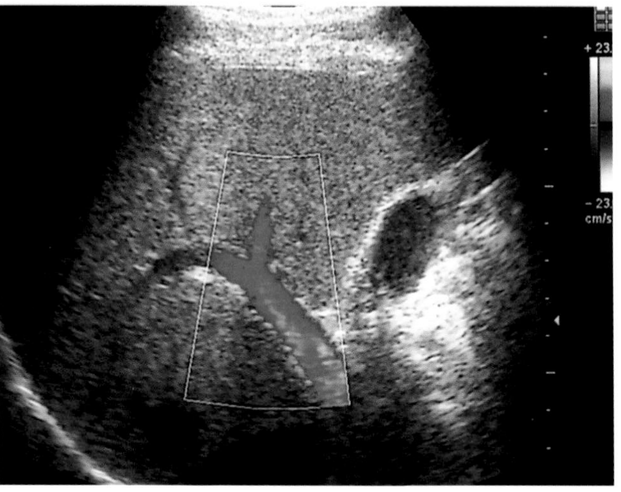

Plate 25.27 Colour Doppler of the portal vein. Portal vein patency and flow direction is readily confirmed by a right lateral intercostal colour Doppler study.

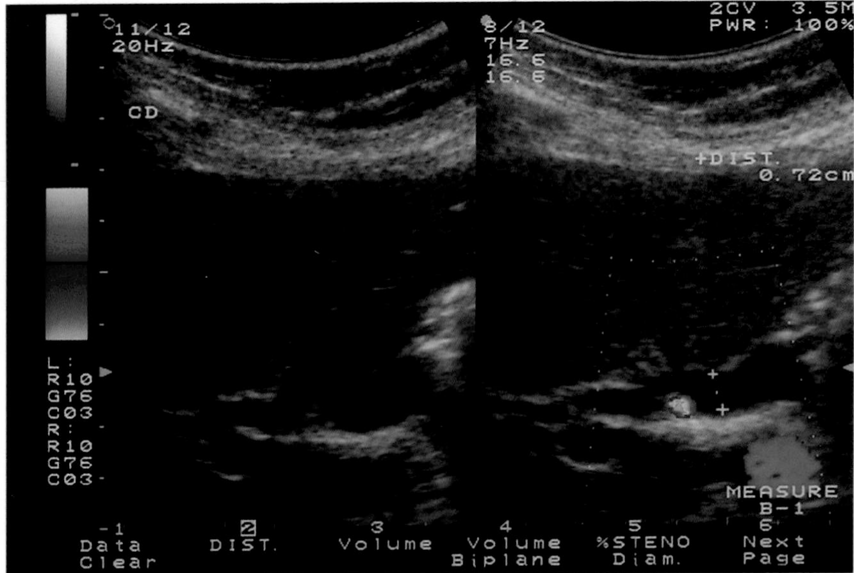

Plate 26.1 Normal anatomy at the porta hepatis. Right hepatic artery crossing between the portal vein (posteriorly) and a slightly dilated common duct (7 mm) might be mistaken for a filling defect in the duct but this is a tubular structure on scanning along its length. Colour Doppler imaging (on the right) demonstrates arterial pulsation in the right hepatic artery.

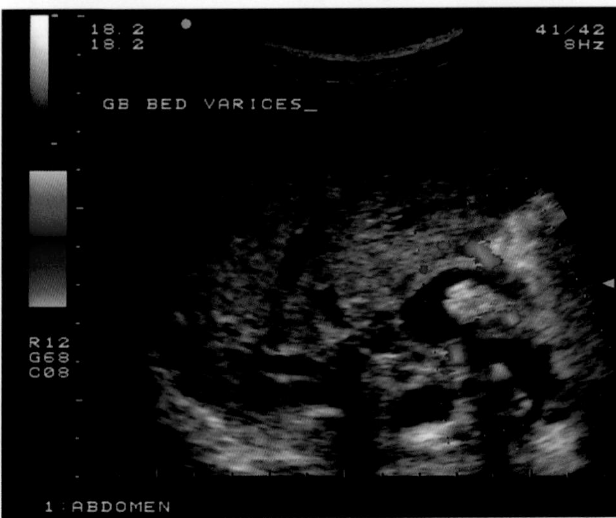

Plate 26.11 Gallbladder varices. Multiple serpiginous anechoic channels were seen around the gallbladder in this patient with portal vein thrombosis. Colour Doppler imaging shows flow within these venous collaterals.

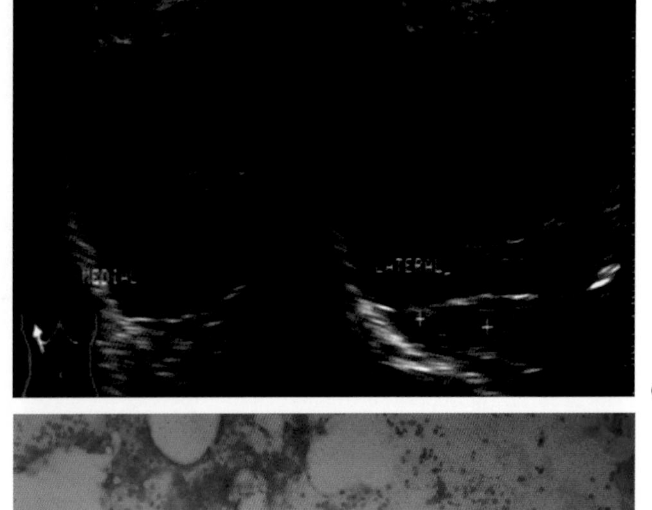

(a)

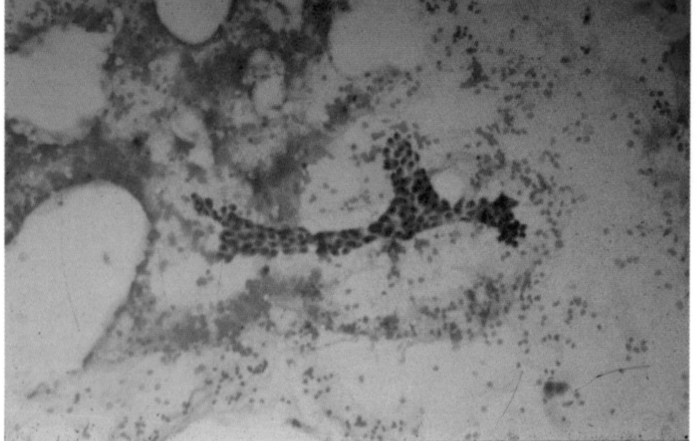

(b)

Plate 29.3 (a) Sagittal and transverse scans through an enlarged right adrenal gland in a patient with a primary bronchial carcinoma. (b) The fine-needle aspiration cytology sample from the adrenal gland shows a cluster of malignant cells confirming a metastatic deposit.

Plate 31.3 Power Doppler image of a normal transplant kidney. The intrarenal vasculature is well visualized with flow demonstrated as far as the cortical margin. Good colour flow visualization allows accurate placement of the spectral gate to obtain spectral Doppler waveforms and reduces examination time to a minimum.

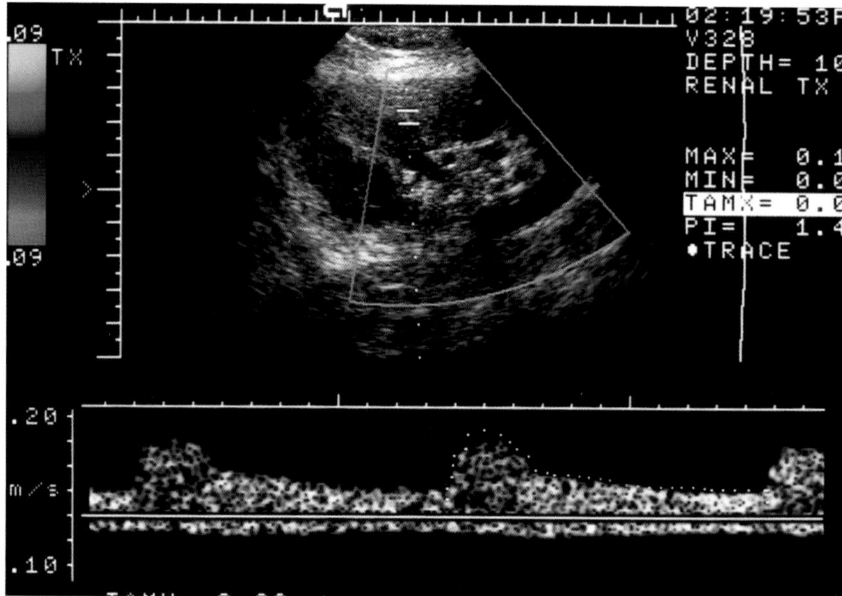

Plate 31.4 Normal Doppler waveform from an interlobar artery. The systolic peak rises sharply with a generalized reduction in velocity throughout diastole. This has been termed the 'ski slope' appearance. The end-diastolic velocity is approximately one-third or more of the peak systolic velocity.

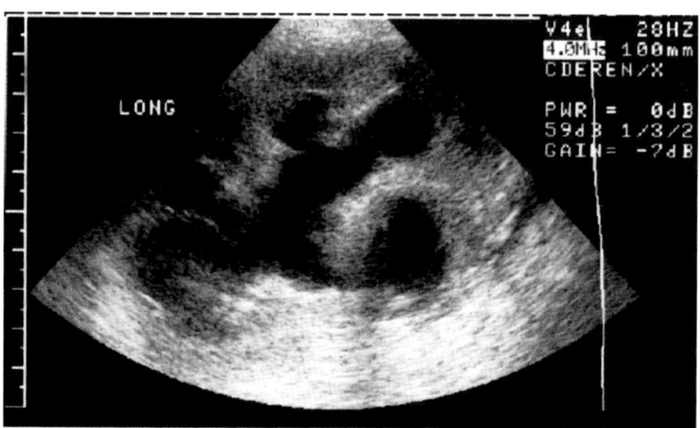

(a)

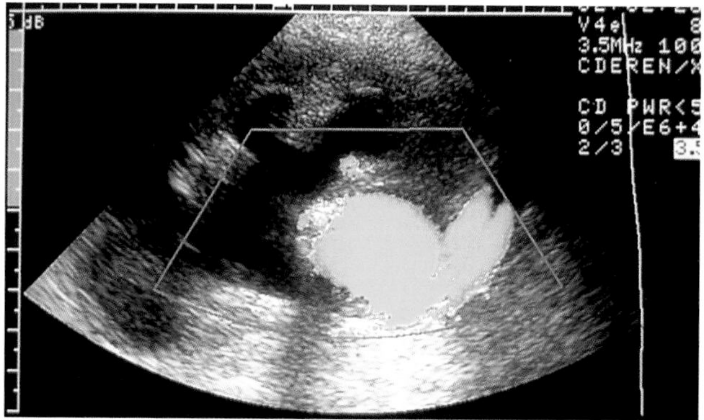

(b)

Plate 31.7 (a) Real-time image of a transplant kidney with fairly typical features of hydronephrosis, i.e. the renal sinus is opened up by the dilated minor and major calyces and renal pelvis. There is, however, a separate less well-circumscribed cystic area with a thick margin to it. (b) Power Doppler image of the iliac vessel showing flow within the focal cystic area at the iliac artery consistent with a pseudoaneurysm. Hydronephrosis noted as in (a).

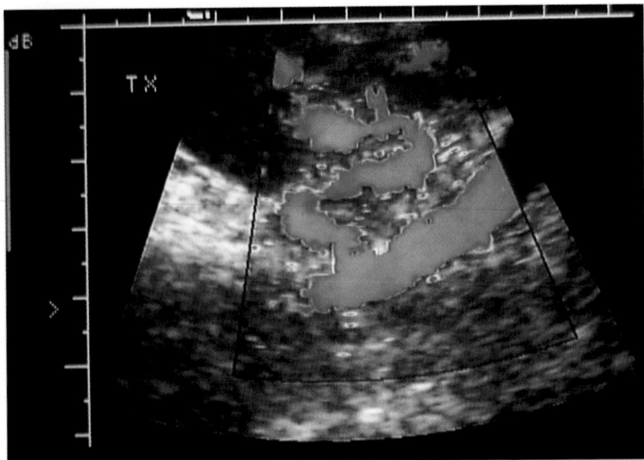

Plate 31.9 Power Doppler scan of a transplant renal artery. The marked vessel tortuosity can be easily appreciated, this being a very common finding. Clearly, good visualization of this vessel is required to allow accurate Doppler vessel angle correction when interrogating it for suspected renal artery stenosis.

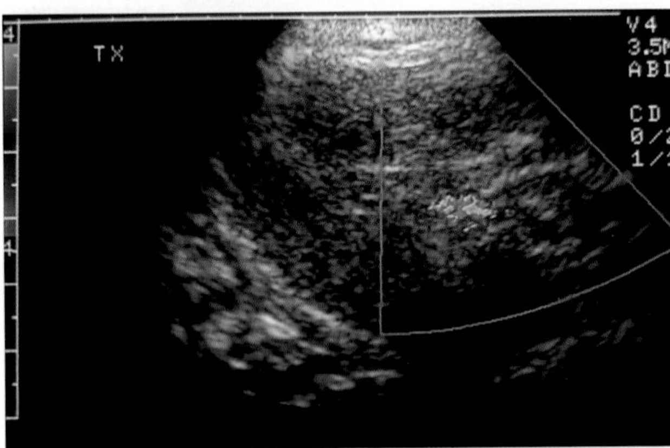

Plate 31.11 Colour flow image of a transplant kidney with a small focal flow abnormality towards one pole. The colour velocity scale was increased to a level where normal intrarenal flow could not be visualized. This area is clearly an abnormal area of high flow representative of an arteriovenous fistula.

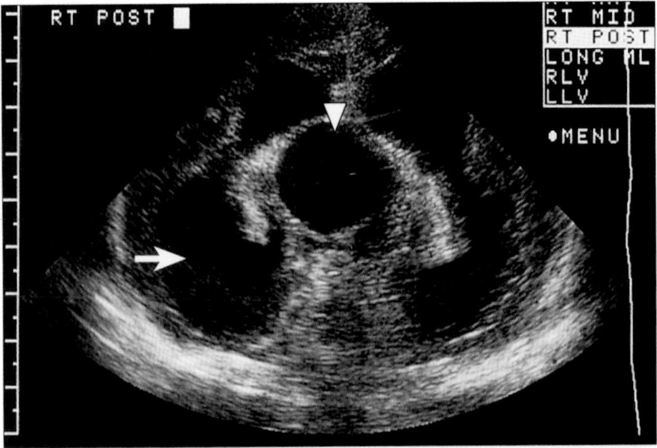

(a)

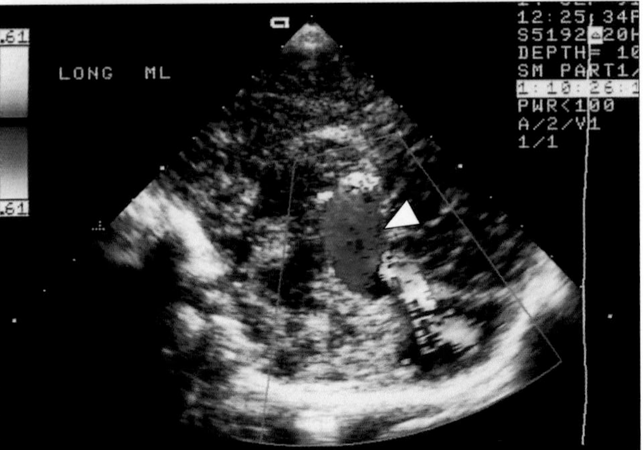

(b)

Plate 44.13 (a) Vein of Galen malformation. A posterior coronal scan performed on the first day of life shows the mid line dilated vein of Galen (arrowhead) associated with hydrocephalus (arrow). This malformation had been diagnosed antenatally. (b) Colour Doppler ultrasound of a 2-day-old male infant presenting with intractable cardiac failure. The sagittal scan demonstrates a dilated vein of Galen (arrowhead) with an enlarged straight sinus and transverse sinus.

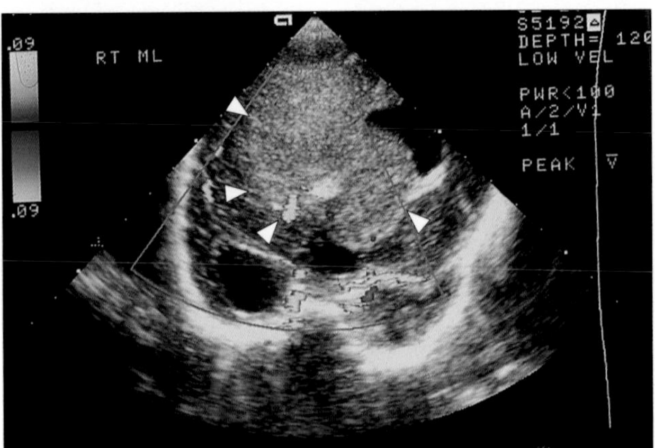

(a)

Plate 44.18 (a) Mid line coronal scan of a 1-day-old infant with a congenital pineal tumour (arrowheads). Antenatal ultrasound in the third trimester had shown this large mid line solid cerebral tumour.

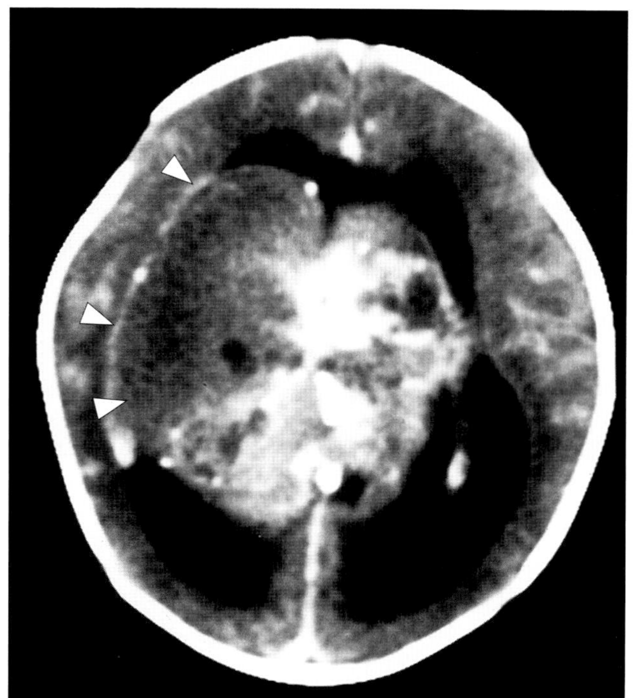
(b)

Plate 44.18 *Continued*. (b) CT scan of the brain confirms centrally placed cerebral tumour (arrowheads). Biopsy was performed but the pineal tumour was considered inoperable.

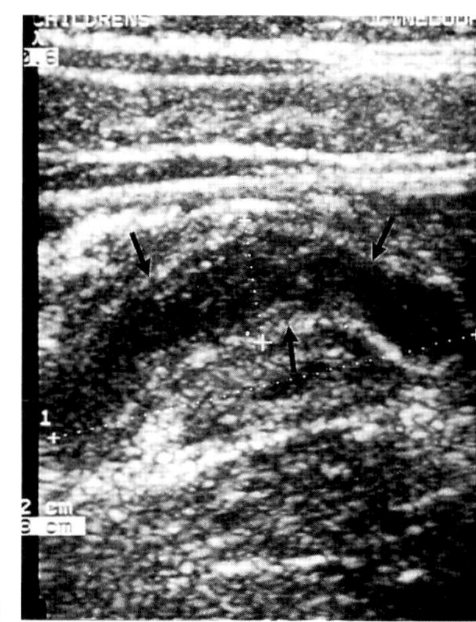
(a)

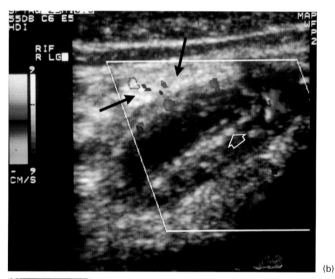

(b)

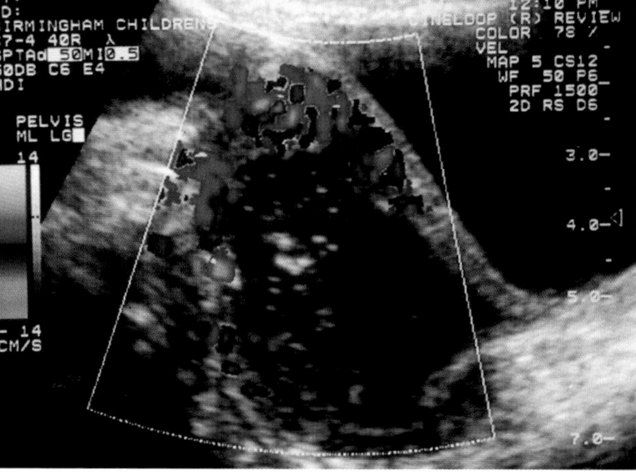

(c)

Plate 45.3 Acute appendicitis. (a) Longitudinal scan with compression using a linear 5–10 MHz probe in the right lower quadrant. A non-compressible, blind-ending, distended and fluid-filled appendix is shown with its echogenic mucosa (arrows). (b) Longitudinal scan. There is some increased vascularity in the inflammed appendix (the normal appendix has no demonstrable colour flow on Doppler imaging). Note the prominent echogenic pericaecal fat due to inflammation (black arrows) and echogenic appendiceal mucosa (open arrow). (c) Appendiceal abscess. Longitudinal scan showing a pelvic abscess from a perforated appendix with peripheral hypervascularity around the collection. Appendiceal abscesses can be limited to the right lower quadrant or extend into the pelvis or upper abdomen.

(a)

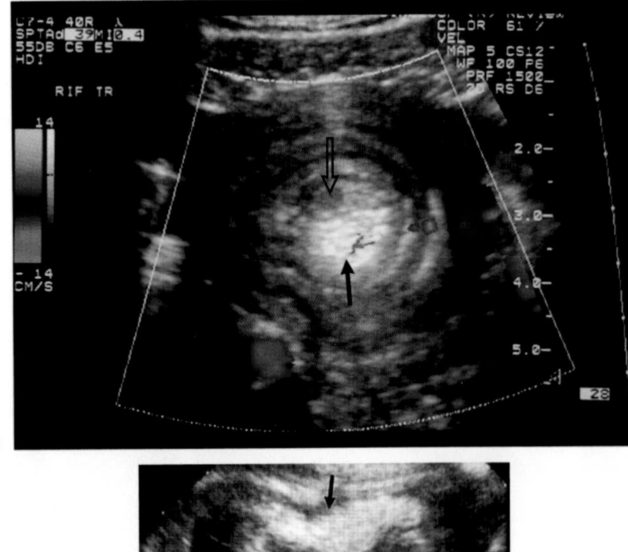

(b)

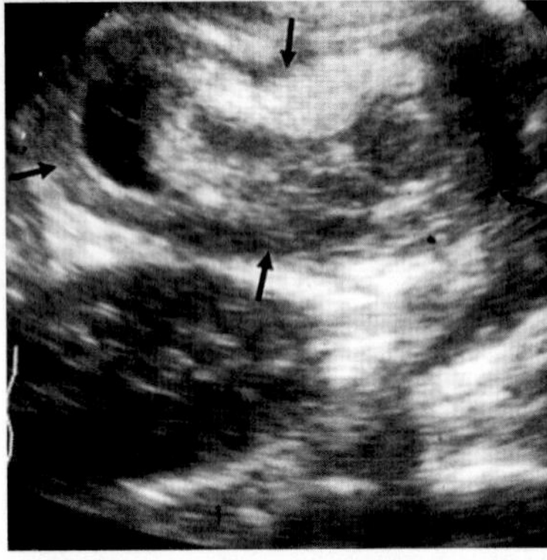

Plate 45.4 Intussusception. (a) Transverse colour Doppler scan with typical target sign of multiple layers and concentric rings due to the invagination of the bowel wall. The reflectivity and number of concentric rings depends on the degree of oedema and impaction of mucosal and serosal layers. An invaginated echogenic mesentery is shown (black arrow). Fluid trapped in the mesentery (open arrow) can look like a cyst. Blood flow in the intussusception is in keeping with a viable bowel. (b) Longitudinal scan showing a reniform or 'pseudo-kidney' shape to the intussusception (arrows).

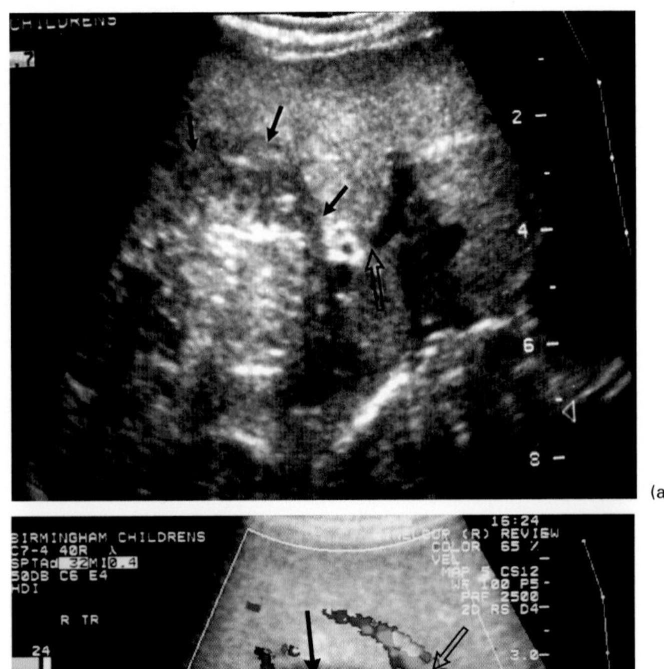

(a)

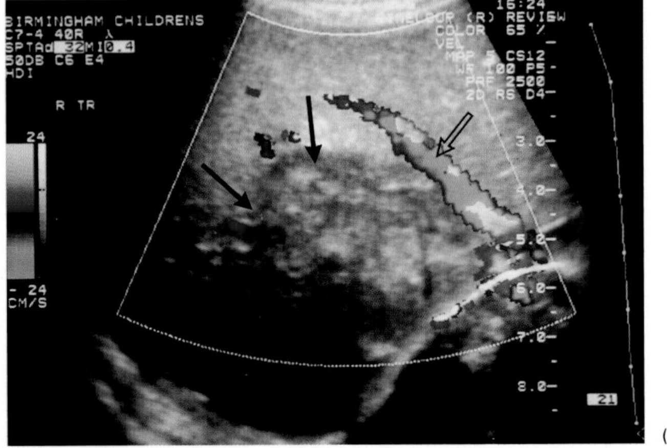

(b)

Plate 45.12 Hepatoblastoma. (a) Transverse scan showing an echogenic tumour in the right liver with partially ill-defined margins (black arrows). The left portal vein is truncated and involved by tumour (open arrow). (b) Large right hepatic tumour (black arrows). There is no tumour on the left side of the middle hepatic vein (open arrow). No right hepatic vein is seen—it is likely that tumour is compressing rather than invading it.

Part 4
Small Parts

Chapter 21: The breast

D.O. Cosgrove

Ultrasound has become increasingly applied to breast diagnosis, mainly because of the development of practical and convenient ultrasound scanners. It has in fact been used for the breast for more than three decades [1] and was one of the first clinical applications of ultrasound.

The earliest scanners were experimental devices employing a water bath between the transducer and the skin of the breast [2]. They were cumbersome, expensive machines; most could only be used for the breast and so, though good results were reported, they did not gain wide acceptance.

Real-time hand-held systems overcome most of these limitations and, in addition, provide a whole new family of dynamic diagnostic features based on observing the movement or deformation of the tissues in real-time as they are compressed by the probe [3]. They also allow application of Doppler techniques. Their only drawback is the small field of view (some 3–6 cm long) which makes for difficulties when comparing one region with another.

Technique

Since the anatomy to be studied often lies within a few centimetres of the skin, good superficial resolution and a wide field of view at the skin are acquired. A high frequency linear away with good near field in imaging is probably the ideal transducer. Frequencies of 7 MHz or higher give the required resolution without sacrificing penetration. An alternative is a mechanical sector system incorporating a small water bath to lift the transducer off the skin, thus producing a trapezoidal field of view and placing the skin at the focal zone. Such systems can be cheap and small enough to consider their location in the breast clinic to address immediate problems.

The patient is lain supine, slightly rotated to the left with the right arm elevated for the right breast and vice versa for the left. This position has the effect of flattening the breast on the chest wall, so that the depth of tissue is reduced. It is also reasonably reproducible, a consideration for serial studies. Using liberal amounts of contact jelly, the probe is scanned slowly and systematically across the entire breast, including the axillary tail, using light pressure. Any suspicious region and any palpable mass or thickening are studied from multiple angles. Since the nipple often casts a shadow, the retroareolar region must be examined from the side, angling the probe to direct the beam into the otherwise shadowed region. As appropriate, the node-bearing regions in the axilla and upper parasternal spaces are also examined.

Any suspicious region is also studied dynamically, using probe pressure to observe the compressibility of the lesion [4]. In addition, the mobility of the lesion is observed as it is shifted with the fingers of the other hand. Dynamic tests add significantly to the morphological features of the ultrasound image by confirming the presence of a doubtful lesion and indicating its consistency and fixity.

Doppler has become a practical technique with the recent introduction of colour Doppler (Fig. 21.1) [5]. Though still cumbersome for screening, colour Doppler is well suited to interrogate suspicious areas and is sensitive enough to detect small tumour vessels no more than 1 mm in diameter. It forms a useful (if expensive) extension of ultrasound imaging that improves specificity.

Localization techniques

Ultrasound can be used to guide a needle or localize wire into a lesion, an application for which the interactive nature of real-time is particularly helpful [6]. Needle guides are not needed for the breast, the procedure being simpler using the free-hand approach in which the probe is held in one hand and the needle and syringe in the other, puncturing the breast skin a little to one side of the lesion. Masses as small as a few millimetres in diameter can be targeted in this way and, where a suspicious region from only part of the lesion (e.g. an irregularity on the wall of a cyst), this can be sampled precisely. The only difficulties encountered are with hard and mobile masses such as some cysts and fibroadenomas that move away from the needle tip.

In the same way, localization wires can be placed with

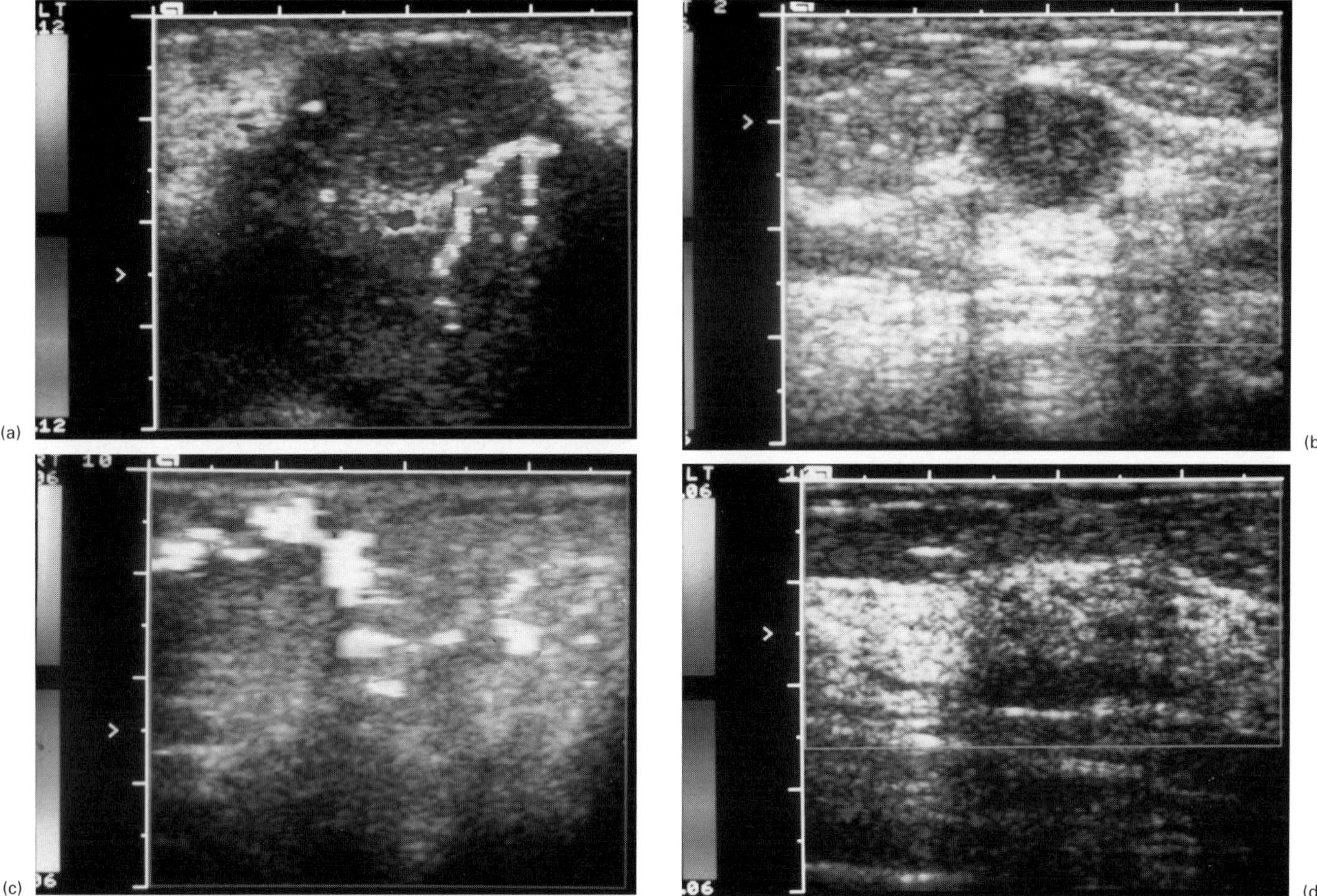

Fig. 21.1 Colour Doppler of breast lesions. The power of colour Doppler is that it combines the anatomical information of an ultrasound scan with the haemodynamic information of an angiogram. (a) Numerous vessels are seen within this large carcinoma. The alternating colours indicate fast or disturbed flow, both characteristic of neovascularization. The 12 mm lesion in (b) has all the features of a fibroadenoma on the grey-scale image but the vascularization is suspicious; an infiltrating carcinoma was found on excision biopsy. (c) Inflammatory carcinomas have prolific vascularization, a feature that is diagnostic when it calls attention to a diffuse lesion that may be undetectable on the grey-scale scan. (d) Generally benign processes are avascular, as with this focal region of benign breast change (the scanty blue colours are from normal breast vessels). Rapidly growing fibroadenomas and inflammatory processes are exceptions. For colour, see Plate 21.1 (between pp. 308 and 309).

the hook precisely within the lesion to be excised. Where relevant, the path of the wire can be sited to correspond with the proposed incision, e.g. entry at the margin of the areola with an oblique path into the lesion where a good cosmetic result is important. Since the patient is supine for the procedure, it is much better tolerated than the sitting position with compression for mammographic localization and it is also usually quicker. Obviously, this form of localization can only be used for abnormalities that are detectable by ultrasound.

Normal appearances

The glandular tissue is typically seen as a cone-shaped region of uniform and relatively intense echoes lying between the subcutaneous and retromammary fat layers which are echo-poor (Fig. 21.2) [7]. Within the glandular tissue, ducts may be detected as echo-poor tubular structures 1 mm or so in diameter, converging to the nipple; under the areola they expand into the lactiferous sinuses and are more easily detected. The skin, muscle and blood vessels can also be identified. The precise appearance of the gland varies physiologically and with age atrophy (Fig. 21.3). In the adolescent and young adult there is very little fat and the gland itself is less echogenic. In pregnancy, hyperplasia of the gland occurs at the expense of the fat and the ducts become prominent, forming a sponge-like mottled pattern (Fig. 21.4). During lactation the engorged ducts may be identified as tubular structures widest near the nipple. After menopause the glandular

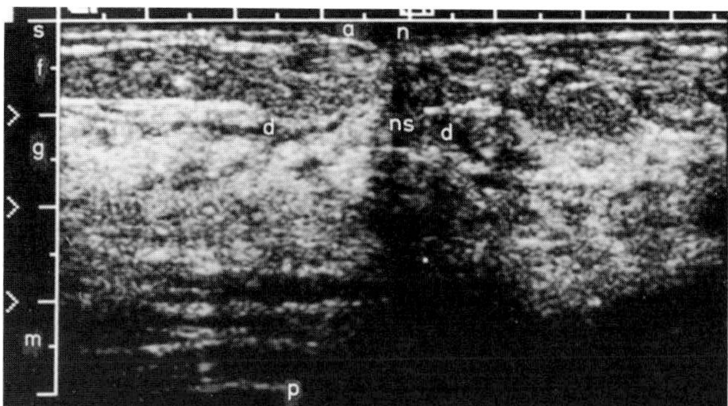

Fig. 21.2 Ultrasound of normal breast. In a section taken through the nipple, the glandular cone of the breast is seen as a reflective region 'floating' between the echo-poor fat in the subcutaneous and retromammary spaces. The areola is thicker than the surrounding skin and the nipple commonly absorbs sufficient ultrasound to produces an acoustic shadow, seen as a dark band. The larger portions of the ducts are demonstrable in the subareolar region. (Note: the image is a side-by-side montage of two adjacent scans; the longer slice that this presentation allows facilitates appreciation of the anatomy or pathology to be demonstrated.) a, areola; d, duct; f, subcutaneous fat; g, gland; m, pectoralis muscle; n, nipple; ns, nipple shadow; p, pleura; s, skin.

portion atrophies progressively, to be replaced by fat, so that eventually the entire breast is echo-poor except for fine linear echogenic steaks that represent the residual gland and Cooper's ligaments. The rate of this atrophy is very variable such that there may be surprising amounts of persisting glandular tissue in a 60-year-old subject, and even later in women on hormone replacement therapy.

The pattern of atrophy in fat replacement is usually fairly uniform but sometimes one lobe persists longer: though this may be worrying when palpated against the softer background of fat, the surviving gland retains its normal appearance on ultrasound and this can be very reassuring. Sometimes the fat replacement is more marked in one site to produce a localized fatty region enclosed by gland (Fig. 21.5). This appearance, the so-called 'fat island', is confusing initially as it simulates an echo-poor mass but its fluid consistency on probe palpation demonstrates its true nature. Usually also, these islands do actually communicate with the subcutaneous fat layer at least at one point—demonstration of this 'peninsula' is also reassuring.

The region immediately deep to the nipple is difficult to image because the connective tissue it contains causes marked shadowing (see Fig. 21.2). This region must be scanned from close to the areola with angling of the probe.

Normal nodes in the breast are seen as small, rounded echo-poor structures (Fig. 21.6) but when buried in the fat of the axilla or internal mammary space, they cannot be detected [8].

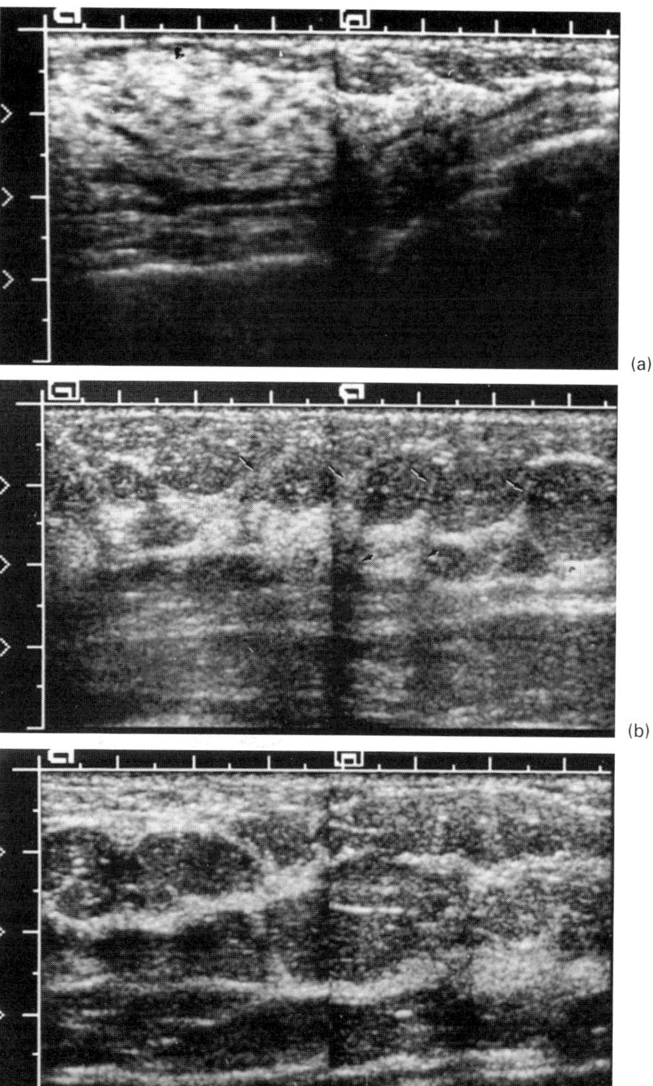

Fig. 21.3 Varying patterns with age atrophy. (a) In the young breast glandular tissue predominates and the scan has a generally high level of echoes sandwiched between layers of echo-poor subcutaneous and retromammary fat. The fine mottled pattern within the gland is probably caused by the relatively immature lobular structure. (b) As the gland atrophies with age the echogenic portions occupy less of the scan and the Cooper's ligaments that tether it to the skin can be seen as curved reflective lines (arrows). Many give rise to fine bands of shadowing (arrowheads). (c) In the predominantly fatty breast at and after menopause only strands of reflective tissue remain; they represent the residual glandular tissue together with Cooper's ligaments.

Normal variants

The commonest variant is an accessory lobe usually lying superolateral to the axillary tail. It is seen as a region with the same echotexture as the normal breast. In lactation, milk may accumulate to produce an echo-poor mass, though the affected tissue often looks entirely normal on

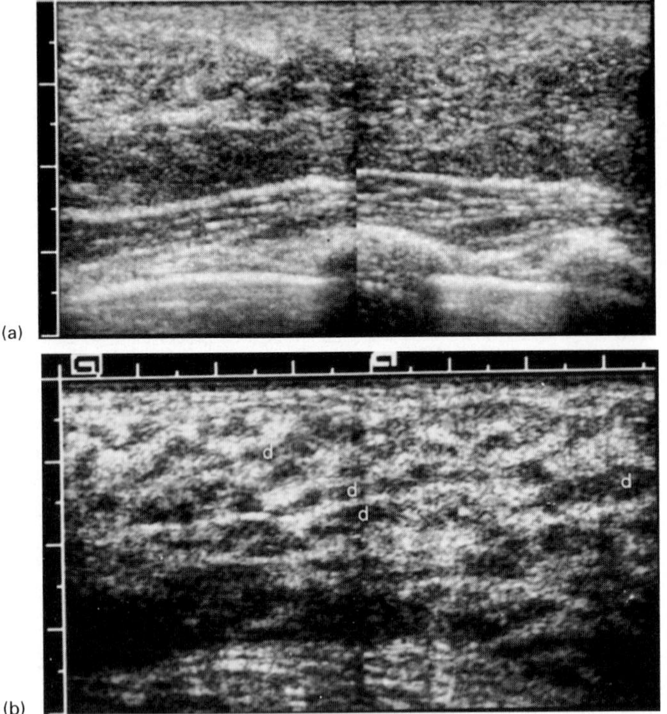

Fig. 21.4 The breast in pregnancy and lactation. During pregnancy (a) the marked increase in the amount of glandular tissue gives a relatively homogeneous and reflective appearance ('ground glass pattern'). The dilated ducts in lactation (b) are seen as tubular or mottled appearances, more obvious closer to the nipple. d, ducts.

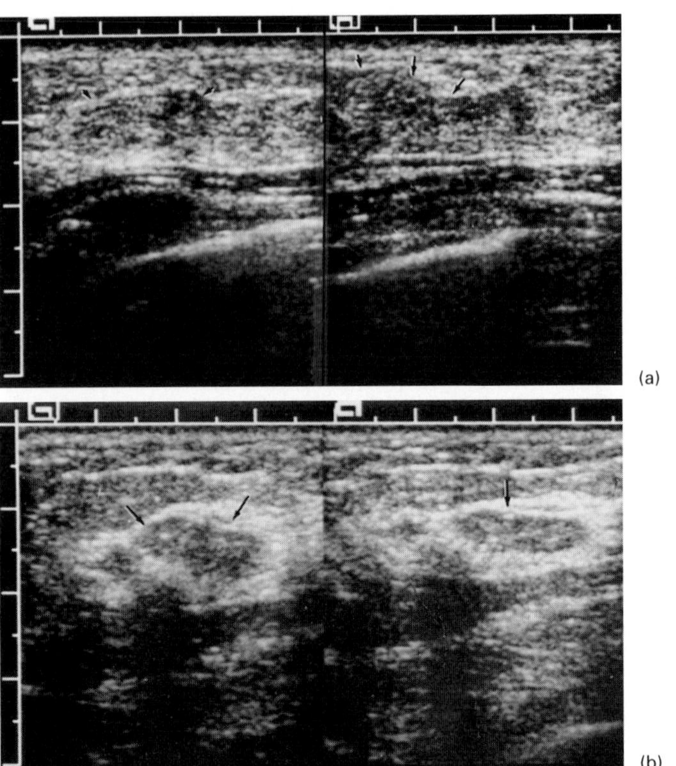

Fig. 21.5 Fat island. (a) Localized fatty regions sometimes produce confusing appearances (arrowheads on left). Usually they are not truly isolated as islands but are peninsular extensions of the fat into the glandular tissue. This continuity can be demonstrated by scanning from a variety of angles (arrows on right). (b) In addition, the liquid consistency of fat at body temperature can be demonstrated on real-time scanning with compressing the tissues by the probe. The fat (arrows) is readily compressed (with a light touch on the left and under probe compression on the right).

ultrasound because milk is as reflective as the glandular tissue.

The common situation where one lobe is thickened is easily diagnosed on ultrasound since it is seen as an entirely normal portion of the gland, though often somewhat elongated and with a radial orientation.

Prostheses

Prostheses are well visualized in ultrasound [9]; typically they are entirely echo-free with strong echoes from the retaining bag (Fig. 21.7). Sometimes, degeneration of the content or foldings of the pouch gives linear internal echoes. An interesting artefact, due to the fact that ultrasound is conducted very slowly through silicone, leads to their depth appearing as approximately twice the true value.

With ultrasound, imaging of the surrounding and overlying breast tissue is unaffected by a prosthesis, so that coexisting lesions can be detected whereas with mammography the density of the prosthesis causes difficulty. If biopsy of an adjacent abnormality is required, ultrasound can be used to check that the prosthesis is not punctured.

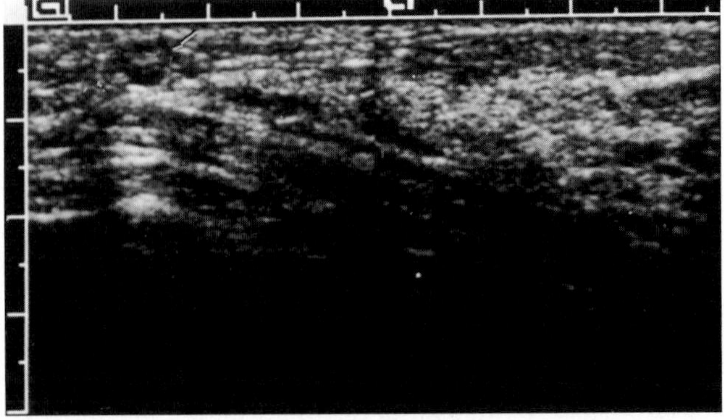

Fig. 21.6 Intramammary lymph node. Normal nodes (arrow) can only be detected when they lie in the glandular portion of the breast; in the axilla they blend with the surrounding fat. Malignant nodes, however, are often obvious, even when small.

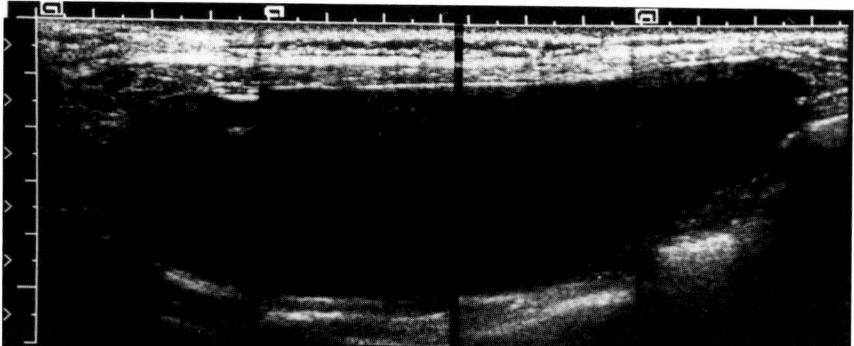

Fig. 21.7 Breast prosthesis. While the plastic envelope of a prosthesis gives strong echoes. the silicone expander is generally echo-free. Note that the surrounding tissues are well seen: the quality of an ultrasound examination is not impaired by the presence of a prosthesis. (Montage of four contiguous scans.)

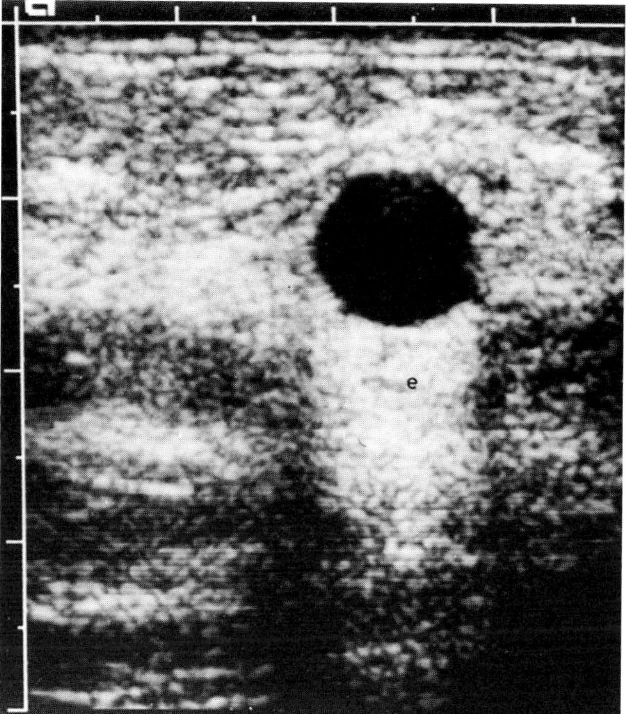

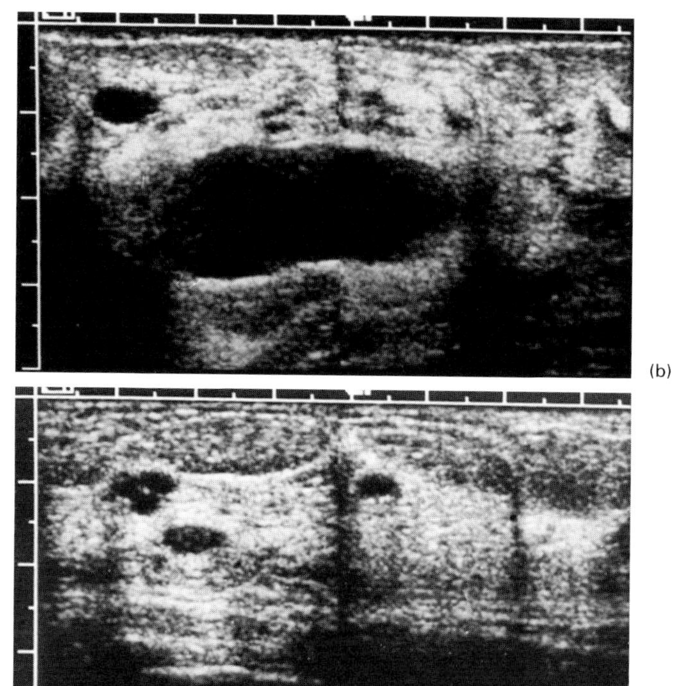

Fig. 21.8 Cysts. (a) Typical cysts are characterized by being echo-free with well-defined walls. They show distal enhancement (e) because the clear cyst fluid absorbs less ultrasound than the surrounding tissues. (b) They are rounded when tense but may be flattened when lax; this type tend to be compressible. (c) They are often found to be multiple even when only one or a few are palpable or demonstrated on mammography.

Benign breast changes and cysts

These are respectively the most difficult and the most straightforward ultrasound diagnoses [10].

Cysts are seen as very well-defined echo-free spaces with distal accentuation of the echoes (acoustic enhancement) and smooth wall (Fig. 21.8) [11]. They are spherical when tense but flattened when lax and often form in bunches. Since they arise from the ductal and glandular structures, they are attached to the surrounding breast tissue and therefore are only partially mobile.

Ultrasound can detect cysts as small as 1–2 mm in diameter with confidence. Provided all the diagnostic criteria are fulfilled, the diagnosis is completely reliable and no further investigation is required, needling only being used to relieve pain or sometimes for reassurance, either of the patient or of the attending doctors. Any cyst that departs from these strict criteria must be needled for cytology because it may represent an intracystic tumour or, more rarely, a necrotic carcinoma or one that has arisen adjacent to a cyst. Thickening or irregularity of the wall are particularly worrying (Fig. 21.9). These appearances can be mimicked exactly by bleeding into a cyst after fine-needle aspiration: wherever possible, ultrasound (and mammo-

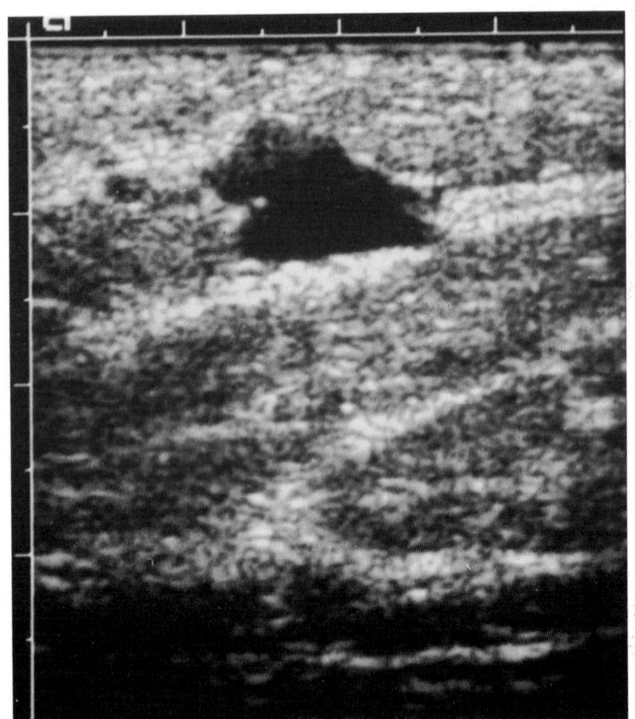
(a)

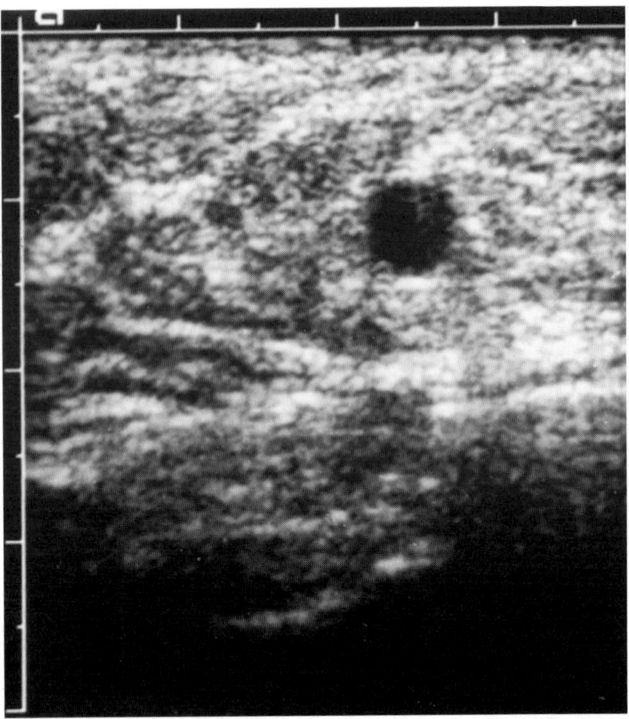
(b)

Fig. 21.9 Atypical cysts. (a) Irregularity of the wall of a cyst could be due to a cancer and such lesions require aspiration for cytology. (b) The rounded lesion seems to be a cyst but it does not show the typical bright band of distal acoustic enhancement; on needling, inspissated sebaceous material was aspirated. These 'cheesy' cysts can pose a diagnostic problem but their rounded shape suggests their true nature.

graphy) should precede needling. Some simple cysts contain low level echoes due to sebaceous contents; typically these echoes are very uniform and the cyst is small, tense and spherical—cheesy or oily material is aspirated and this need not be sent for cytology unless there is blood-staining.

Benign breast changes produce a spectrum of appearances, in keeping with their varied pathological features. Often the ultrasound scan is entirely normal or merely shows regional thickening of the gland, typically affecting the upper outer quadrant. There may be generalized or segmental ductal changes in which the ducts become prominent with a fine echo-poor cuff surrounding them. This produces a sponge-like or mottled appearance which is not necessarily pathological, being encountered also in asymptomatic women. None of these appearances is worrying but, when the benign mammary change is localized, and particularly when there is fibrosis, an incompressible echo-poor ill-defined region with suspicious distal shadowing that suggests a carcinoma (Fig. 21.10) is seen. Differentiation may be impossible but, because the lesion is not a true mass, it may be traversed by ductal elements, whereas they are deviated by a true mass. Demonstration of these is reassuring. A feature that may also be helpful is the fact that such 'benign shadowing' reduces or disappears when the lesion is compressed by the probe. Absence of vascularity on colour Doppler is another typical feature—carcinomas are almost always vascular (see Fig. 21.1). Despite these helpful features, this type of benign mammary change can be very worrying and biopsies are often required.

Fibroadenomas

Most fibroadenomas have a very typical appearance on ultrasound, producing well-defined lesions with an oval or polygonal contour (occasionally lobulated) and uniform internal echoes of about the same intensity as the subcutaneous fat (Fig. 21.11) [12,13]. There is often acoustic enhancement—fibroadenomas only attenuate if they are calcified, which produces obvious intensely reflective regions. There is no reaction from the surrounding tissues, the lesions seeming to float within the breast tissue. In keeping with their clinical epithet as 'breast mice', the mobility of fibroadenomas is a very obvious ultrasound feature that may even lead to their being missed if they skip rapidly across the field of view as the probe is swept across the tissues. They are only slightly compressible. Fibroadenomas tend to lie with their long axis parallel to the skin as they accommodate themselves

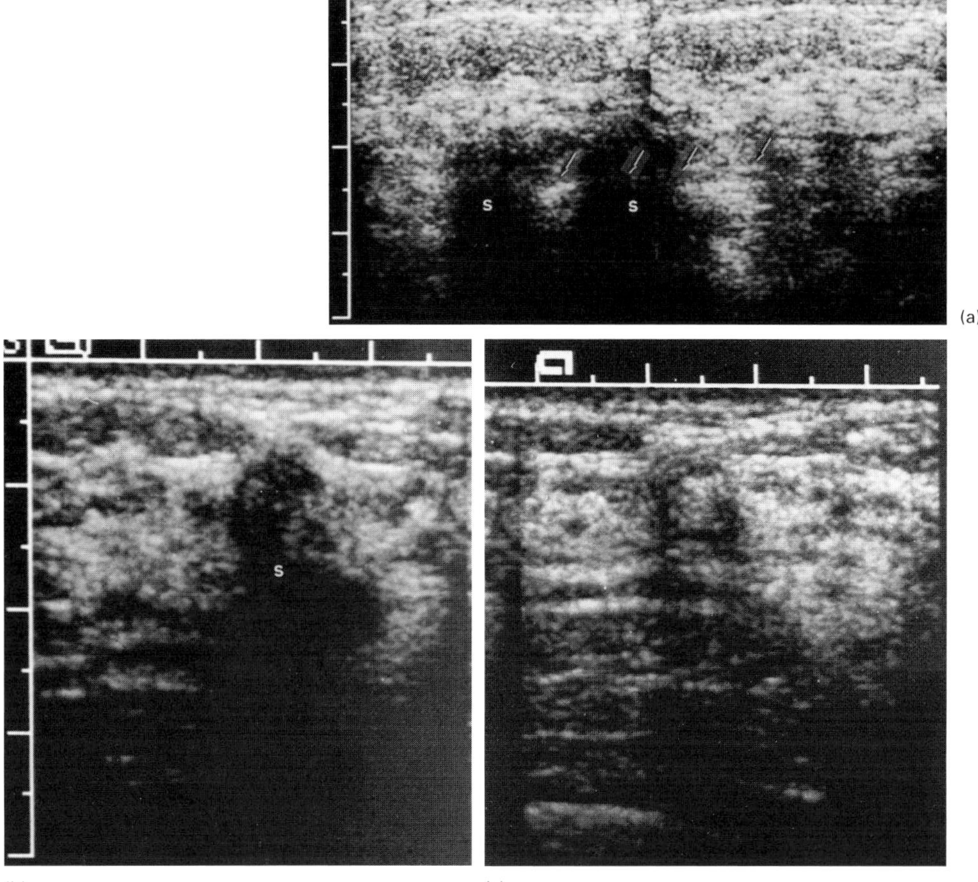

Fig. 21.10 Localized benign breast changes. (a) This ill-defined disturbance of the local architecture with distal shadowing (s) is a suspicious finding. However, close study reveals ductal elements (arrows) that traverse the 'lesion', making it unlikely to be a true space-occupying mass. (b) In another even more localized example, the disappearance of the shadowing when probe pressure is applied (c) is a reassuring feature. Both were regions of benign breast changes with fibrosis.

to the local anatomy defined by the breast lobules and Cooper's ligaments. Larger fibroadenomas may be moderately vascular, one or two vessels being demonstrated on a colour Doppler study.

The distinctive features of fibroadenomas usually allow a confident diagnosis, but with very small solid lesions, where the appearances of carcinomas may converge, there is often some doubt. A large fibroadenoma may also suggest a phyloides tumour (the younger age group of patients with large fibroadenomas is helpful here). Occasionally, the uniform echoes of an inspissated cyst may falsely suggest a fibroadenoma but the spherical shape and relative immobility are distinguishing features.

Invasive carcinoma

Invasive carcinomas have a range of ultrasound appearances, but the most typical is as an echo-poor central nidus (less reflective than fat), often somewhat heterogeneous, with distal shadowing that is often intense and characteristically variable across the lesion (Fig. 21.12) [14–16]. The nidus tends to 'sit proud' with its long axis in the antero-posterior direction, reflecting its invasive behaviour as it grows across the internal boundaries of the gland, though this is by no means an invariable finding [17]. Around the nidus is an echogenic 'halo' representing the infiltrating edge of the carcinoma. It has ill-defined outer margins and typically is more obvious at the sides of the lesion than anteriorly (probably because here the invading columns of cells run along the ultrasound beam rather than across it, and so do not present such strong interfaces). Calcification is commonly seen within the nidus; the foci range in size from clumps several millimetres in diameter that cast acoustic shadowing to non-shadowing punctate echogenicities (microcalcifications). The lesion is incompressible and relatively fixed to the adjacent breast tissues which can be seen to be dragged along with it when the tumour is moved by the finger. In the same way, invasion into the pectoralis muscle may be demonstrated.

There may also be characteristic changes in the surrounding breast: thickening of Cooper's ligaments, for example, due to invasion, provides a tell-tale stellate pattern when they shorten. Skin thickening, not necessarily confined to the area immediately overlying the

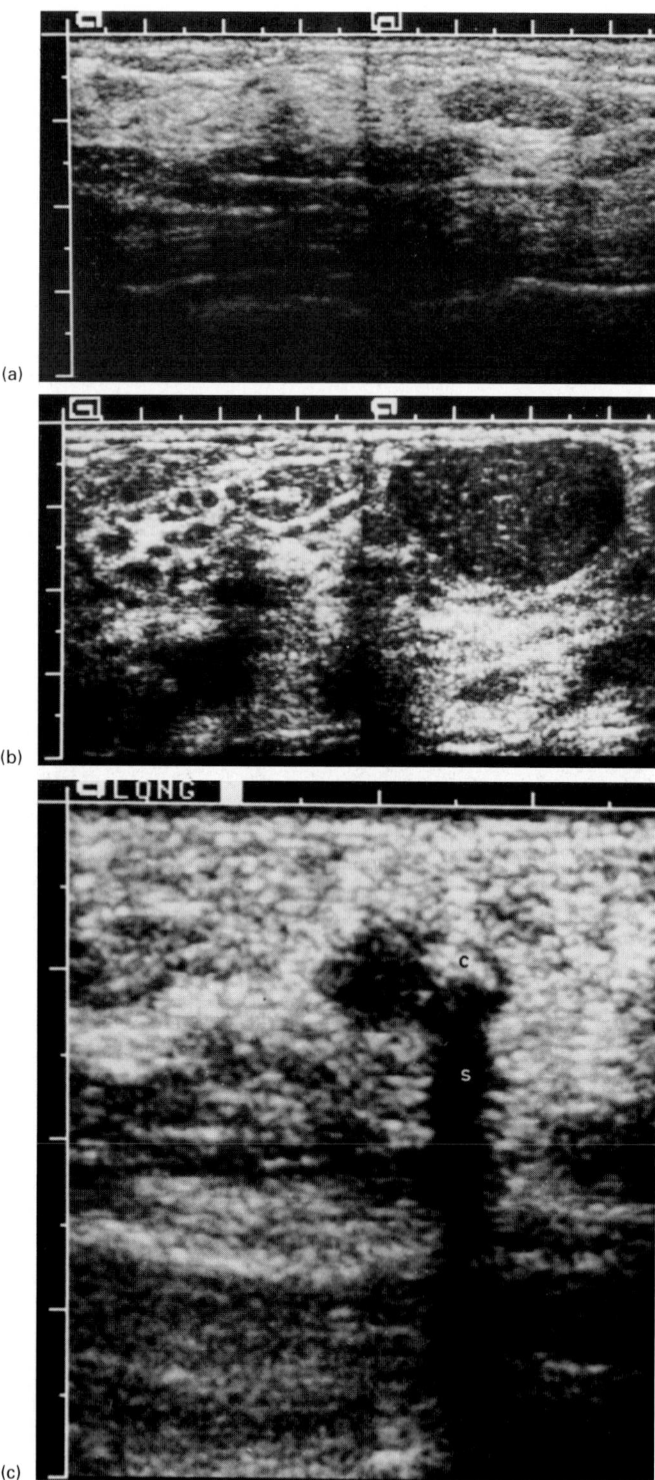

Fig. 21.11 Fibroadenomas. (a, b) A well-defined mass of about the same reflectivity as the subcutaneous fat and a uniform echo texture is typical of a fibroadenoma. They are often oval in shape with their long axis parallel to the skin and, on real-time, are highly mobile. They may show distal enhancement but shadowing occurs if they are hyalinized or calcify. (c) A characteristic feature is the absence of disturbance to the surrounding breast architecture which is simply displaced to one side. c, calcification; s, shadow.

tumour, results from invasion or oedema. Dilated ducts are sometimes seen; when caused by tumour invasion the downstream portion may be dilated. Enlarged regional nodes are often obvious (Fig. 21.13).

As well as such typical lesions, a variety of other patterns is less commonly encountered, some of which correspond to histological variants. Where there is little fibrous tissue, shadowing is less apparent so that very cellular carcinomas may even show distal enhancement (e.g. medullary carcinoma) (Fig. 21.14) [18]. The halo is absent if the tumour does not invade locally. The echogenicity of the nidus is occasionally higher and may even match that of the subcutaneous fat—in this case the tumour may be invisible on the scan if it lies within the fatty layer though it can be picked out by its harder consistency as demonstrated by probe compression (Fig. 21.15). This pattern is seen typically with colloid carcinomas [19]. While patchy necrosis is not uncommon with larger lesions, extensive necrosis is rare (except after chemotherapy); when seen, it produces a mainly cystic lesion, but the 'cyst' walls are irregular so that these lesions are more likely to be mistaken for a haematoma or abscess than a simple cyst. Coexistence of a cyst and a carcinoma is well recognized, as is the presence of a fibroadenoma in the carcinoma: in both cases the ultrasound features of the malignant component is usually typical.

Two important types of carcinoma are particular diagnostic problems for ultrasound. Small lesions (less than 5 mm), while usually having the characteristic malignant appearances, sometimes mimic fibroadenomas exactly and, at present, there is no way these can be differentiated with confidence on ultrasound [20]. The limitation, presumably, is one of resolution: better detail might reveal the infiltrating margin of smaller lesions and allow an earlier differential diagnosis. Even more problematical are widely infiltrating carcinomas that do not form a discrete mass. Even when extensive (e.g. inflammatory carcinomas), they may not be obvious on the ultrasound scan, though in this case the hardness of the affected portion of the breast and the associated skin thickening (peau d'orange) are obvious (Fig. 21.16). Smaller infiltrating carcinomas without a mass may be completely undetectable on ultrasound or may cause only subtle architectural disturbance or acoustic shadowing which should raise suspicion if it persists on probe compression.

The neovascularization that is always present in carcinomas larger than a few millimetres in diameter can be demonstrated on colour Doppler (see Fig. 21.1). Often the increased vascularity with numerous tortuous vessel is very obvious and provides an important additional sign of malignancy, especially where the typical features are not seen, e.g. in inflammatory or non-mass-forming carcinomas. However, the limited sensitivity of colour

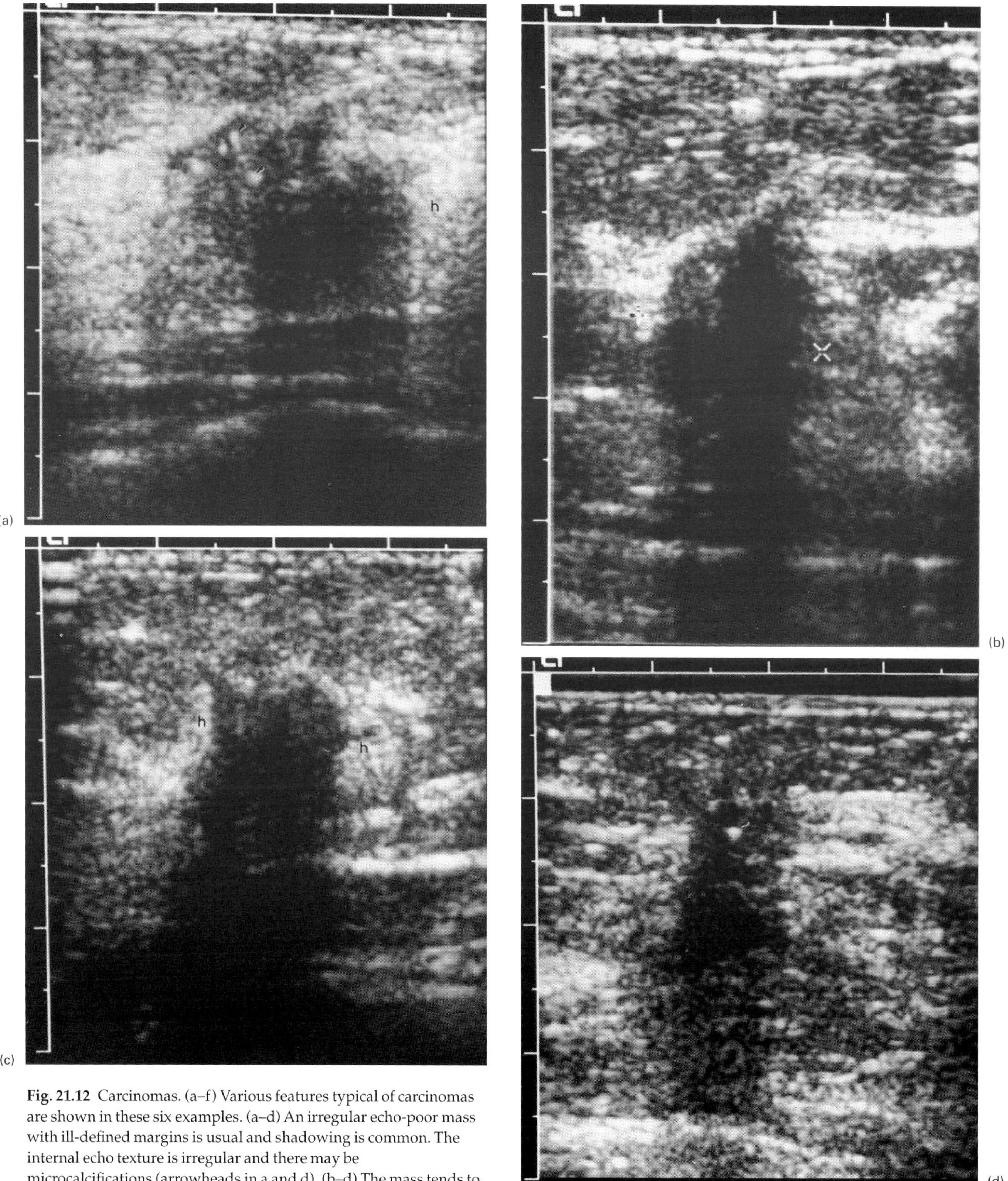

Fig. 21.12 Carcinomas. (a–f) Various features typical of carcinomas are shown in these six examples. (a–d) An irregular echo-poor mass with ill-defined margins is usual and shadowing is common. The internal echo texture is irregular and there may be microcalcifications (arrowheads in a and d). (b–d) The mass tends to lie with its long axis in the anteroposterior direction. The surrounding breast architecture is disturbed, often forming a reflective halo (h) that is thicker to the sides of the mass (a and c).

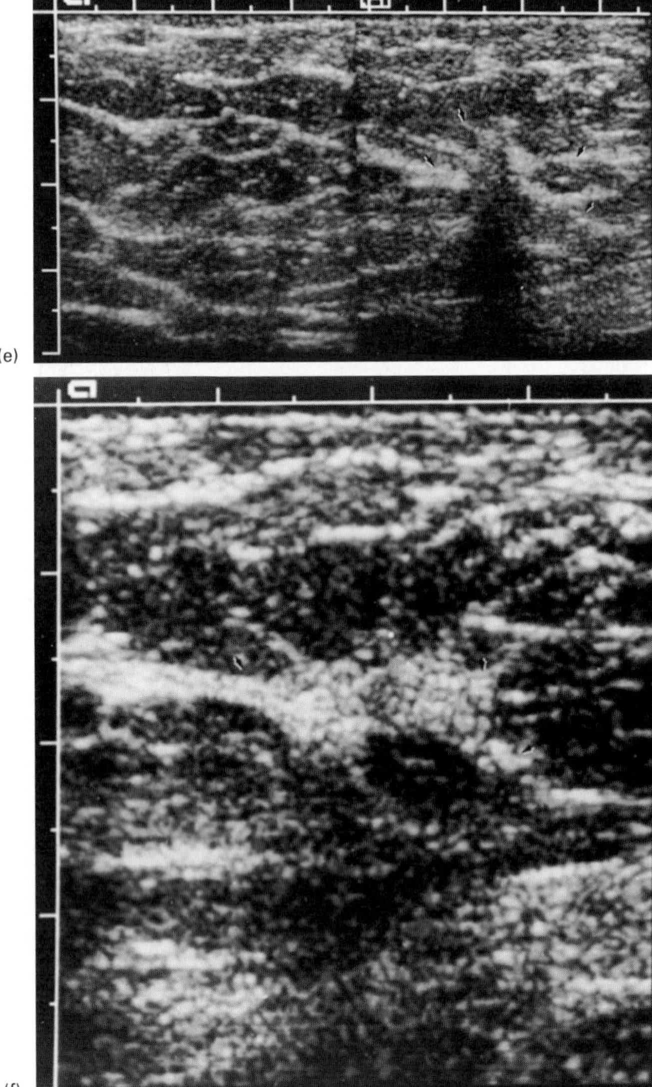

Fig. 21.12 *Continued* Indrawing of the Cooper's ligaments so that they converge on the lesion may draw attention to the tumour (arrowheads in e and f). (e) For very small lesions the mass itself may be less obvious than the architectural disturbances it causes (indrawing of the ligaments, shadowing).

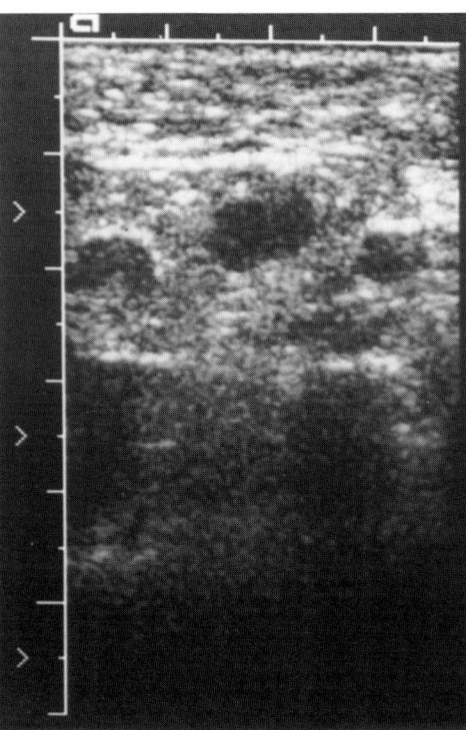

Fig. 21.13 Axillary lymphadenopathy. Involved nodes stand out as echo-poor nodules in contrast with the axillary (or internal mammary) fat.

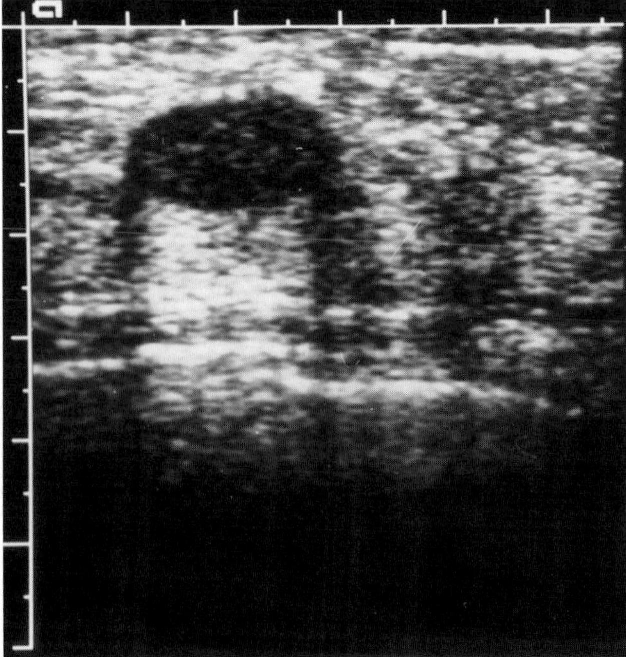

Fig. 21.14 Medullary carcinoma. When a carcinoma is of low invasiveness and lacks fibrous tissue, many of the features that are typical of malignancy may be missing, giving the lesion a benign appearance. This mass is well defined and shows acoustic enhancement, suggesting the diagnosis of a fibroadenoma. However, its reflectivity is lower than that of the subcutaneous fat and suspicion was increased when vascularity was demonstrated on colour Doppler.

Doppler systems means that the vessels in smaller carcinomas may be less obvious so that apparent lack of vascularization in small lesions is not useful in differential diagnosis, though the demonstration of numerous vessels is highly suspicious. Benign masses may also be vascularized (up to two-thirds of adenomas and, rarely also, benign mammary change), but in these the vessels are sparse and lack the tangled pattern of malignant vessels.

Carcinoma *in situ*

Non-invasive carcinoma cannot be detected reliably by ultrasound, usually no abnormality being apparent though occasionally a subtle architectural disturbance is noted [21].

Calcification

Benign-type clumps of calcification are readily demonstrated on ultrasound as intensely echogenic foci with distal shadowing (see Fig. 21.11) [22]. Microcalcification is also seen as echogenic puncta but without shadowing (they are smaller than the beam width so some sound passes alongside them) (see Fig. 21.12). However, these echogenic puncta are difficult to detect in tissue which is itself echogenic, such as the glandular part of the breast, because they merge with the background structure, though they are obvious against a dark background such as within the nidus of a tumour. This means that calcification is not a practically useful feature for ultrasound, either for detection of abnormalities or for differential diagnosis. It is one of the main limitations of ultrasound in screening.

Intraduct tumours

A solid nodule within a 'cyst' or dilated duct is the typical appearance of an intraduct tumour (Fig. 21.17) [23,24]; distinction from a debris-containing cyst is not always possible but a definite texture within the 'lesion' and its rounded or irregular margins are distinct from the uniform echoes and layering of debris. If flow is demonstrated within the lesion on colour Doppler, the distinction is certain because debris is avascular; otherwise biopsy is needed and here ultrasound guidance is useful

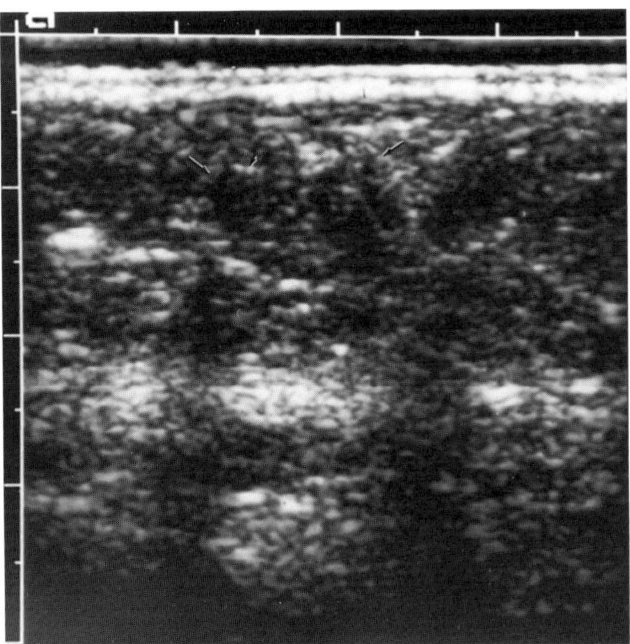

Fig. 21.15 A 'non mass-forming' carcinoma. Although the probe has been positioned directly over a palpable 1 cm lesion, it was almost impossible to delineate on the frozen image, because its reflectivity matches the subcutaneous fat almost exactly. On real-time its incompressibility made it a little more obvious (arrows) and there is a fleck of calcification (arrowhead), though this is not sufficiently distinctive to allow a diagnosis of malignancy.

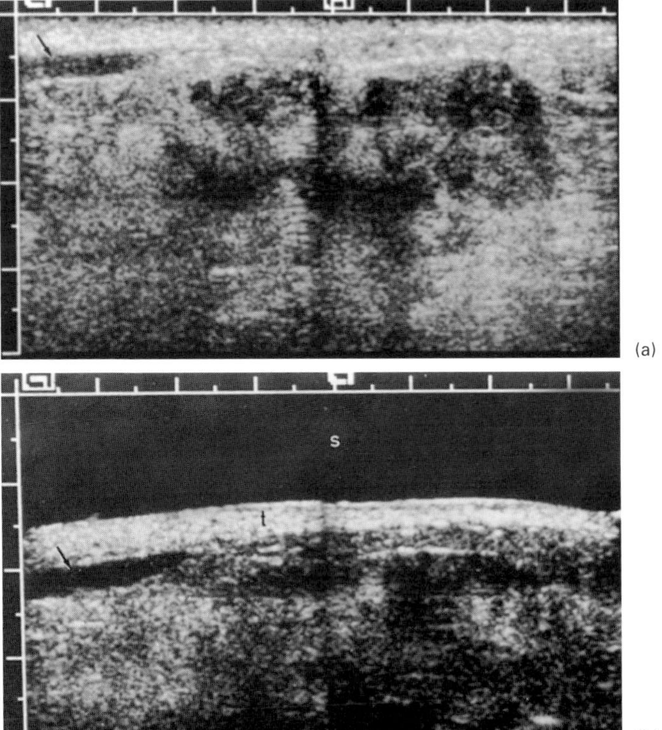

Fig. 21.16 Inflammatory carcinoma. (a) The marked vacularity of inflammatory carcinomas may lead to prominent vessels (arrows) while the typical skin thickening is best demonstrated when a stand-off block is used (b). s, stand-off block; t, thickened skin.

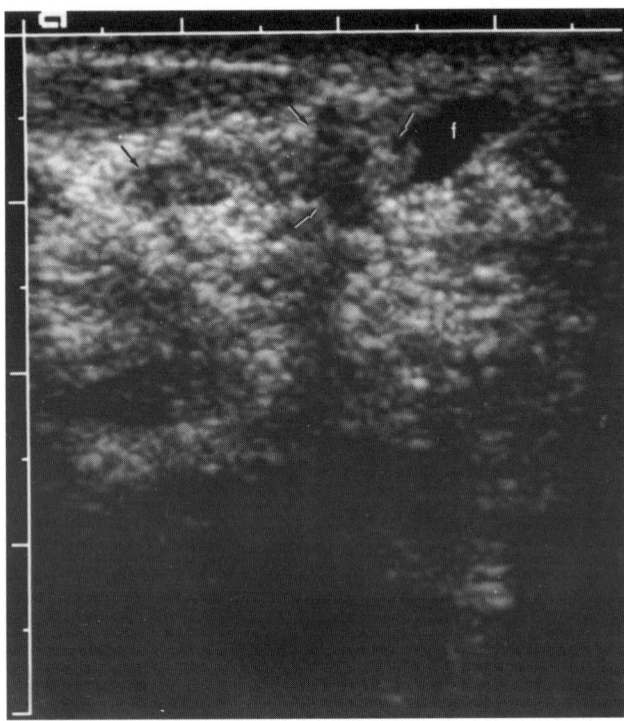

Fig. 21.17 Intraduct tumour. A solid mass (arrows) is seen within this dilated duct. It is much more easily discerned where it lies adjacent to the duct fluid (f)—if this had been expressed immediately prior to the scan, the mass would probably have been missed.

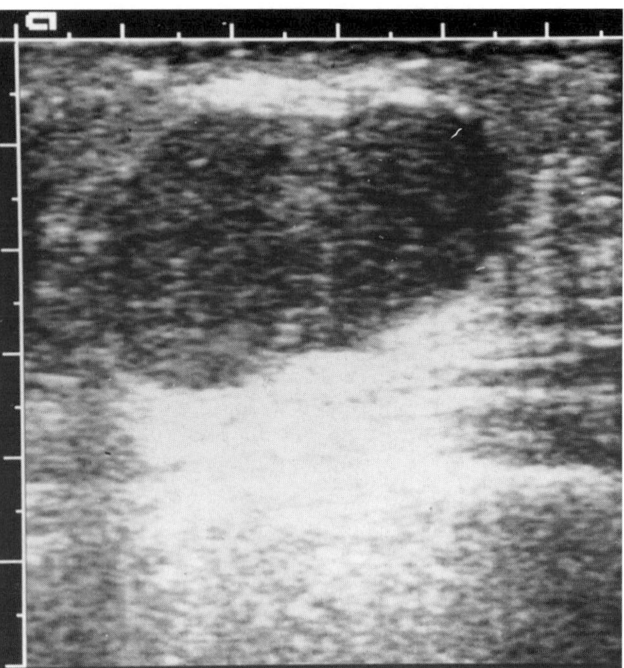

Fig. 21.18 Phylloides tumour. With a pattern very similar to a large fibroadenoma, the diagnosis of a phylloides tumour may be suggested if there are fluid clefts and by their marked vascularity on colour Doppler.

to ensure that the appropriate portion of the lesion is sampled. Ultrasound cannot distinguish between intraduct papilloma and carcinoma.

Phylloides tumours

These lesions have a similar appearance to large fibroadenomas with well-defined margins and distal enhancement (Fig. 21.18) [25]. However, their size may be suggestive, especially when considered in relation to the patient's age (giant fibroadenomas mainly occur in younger women), and the otherwise uniform internal echoes are usually broken up by fluid spaces. Phylloides tumours are typically vascular on colour Doppler.

Metastases

Metastases to the breast tend to be better defined than infiltrating carcinomas so that they lack the echogenic halo (Fig. 21.19) [26]. Otherwise they have similar appearances, with low level heterogeneous echoes. They are also incompressible and often are very vascular.

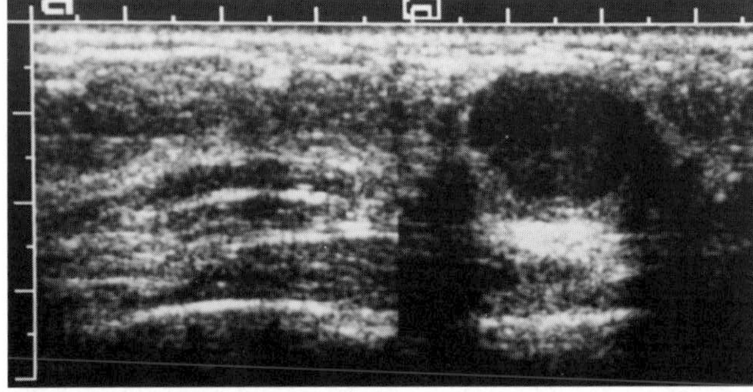

Fig. 21.19 Metastasis. Metastases tend to have more clearly defined margins than primary carcinomas but their internal echoes are more heterogeneous than is typical of a fibroadenoma.

Trauma, scars and granulomas

Trauma to the breast produces two patterns of change. Haematomas are seen as shaggy-walled cavities containing echogenic fluid in which the debris and blood products may be seen to move with posture (Fig. 21.20) [27]. An interesting variant occurs when there is associated fat spill producing an oil cyst because the oil, which is echogenic, floats over the watery component to produce a fluid level which is upside down by comparison with the usual layering due to dependent debris [28].

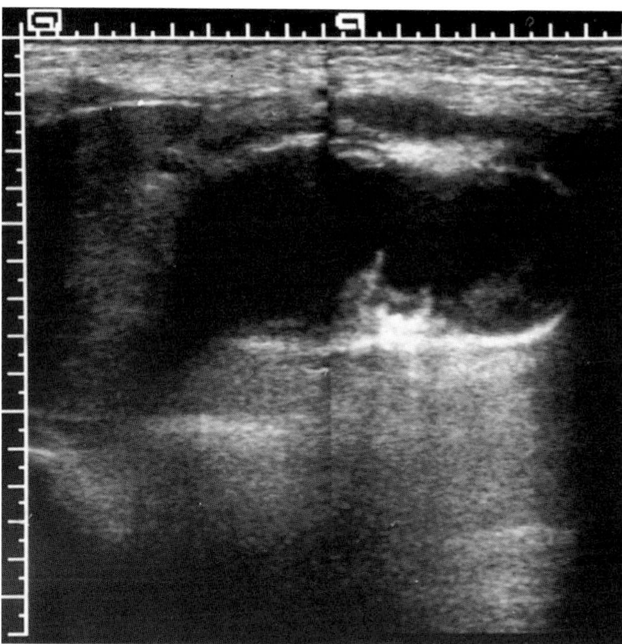

Fig. 21.20 Haematoma. The shaggy wall and internal debris, which may be mobile on repositioning, are typical of a haematoma. Abscesses have the same appearances but are markedly vascular on colour Doppler. In both cases, ultrasound is useful for guiding aspiration.

A fibrous scar is seen as a fine, linear echo-poor structure more obvious for its shadowing than of itself (Fig. 21.21) [29]. Any widening is suspicious of tumour recurrence, though innocent widening occurs where there is excessive fibrosis as in a keloid or around sutures. Colour Doppler is negative in mature scarring, a point which may be very helpful distinguishing them from local recurrence of a carcinoma. A confusing feature is that the scar in the glandular layer need not lie under the skin scar since the incision may have been made at a cosmetic site, remote from the mass to be excised.

Radial scars produce ill-defined echo-poor regions with shadowing and distortion of the surrounding breast consisting of indrawing of the Cooper's ligaments to which they are fixed. Apart from being avascular, these are all the features of a carcinoma and the distinction is impossible on ultrasound imaging.

Granulomas have a characteristic appearance as small masses with high intensity echoes [30]. Apart from calcium and gas, no other lesion in the breast has echoes more intense than the gland itself. The commonest site to encounter them is at the periphery of a prosthesis where they produce a striking 'snow-storm' pattern that contrasts with the echo-free 'lake' of the silicone. Since they may produce suspicious nodules, this clear distinction on ultrasound is clinically useful. While the demonstration of

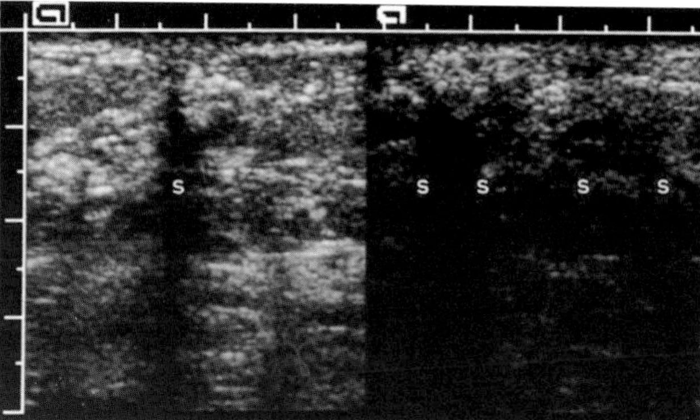

Fig. 21.21 Scar. Often the scar itself is relatively inapparent but the shadowing it produces is obvious. A characteristic is that it forms a fine band when scanned across its length (left) but, when the scan is aligned with the scar (right), the shadowing (s) is more extensive.

granulomas is reliable evidence of silicone leakage, intracapsular rupture may not produce ultrasonic abnormalities and cannot be excluded.

Infection

Abscesses have the same general appearances as haematomas: a cavity with shaggy walls (see Fig. 21.20) [31]. Usually the distinction is obvious clinically but if in doubt specific features such as the presence of echogenic gas bubbles and intense colour signals at the hyperaemic periphery are useful.

Accuracy of ultrasound

Ultrasound is extremely reliable in the diagnosis of cysts: the only errors with simple cysts are operator mistakes. Complex cysts, i.e. those with internal echoes, can usually also be distinguished, though with somewhat lower confidence.

For solid lesions, the reliability of ultrasound is less good, mainly because the features of fibroadenomas may overlap those of carcinomas, especially for subcentimetre lesions [32]. Benign breast change is occasionally also a problem, sometimes simulating malignancy where there is focal fibrosis. Nevertheless, accuracies of 90–95% have been reported and confirmed in several series with false positives and false negatives in about equal proportions [16,33–36]. This is about the same as the quoted figures for X-ray mammography but there is an important difference: X-ray mammography retains this accuracy in a screening content where ultrasound has not been tested but almost certainly would do less well because of its lack of sensitivity to microcalcification.

Role of ultrasound

If it is accepted that ultrasound has no role in screening for malignancy (because it seems evident that it is insensitive to microcalcification) then the discussion as to its diagnostic role focuses on further evaluation of a presenting mass or problem, where all tests are ancillary to the clinical examination [37,38]. Essentially the potential use of ultrasound here depends on the philosophy of the physician or surgeon. At one hypothetical extreme, the surgeon who removes every lump has no need for any further investigation (including cytology). A more realistic stance is to try to avoid removing simple cysts; here the reliability of ultrasound (no false diagnoses, some complex cysts mistaken for solid lesions) makes it the obvious test of choice. If the surgeon prefers not to remove all solid lesions (i.e. to try to keep the benign to malignant biopsy rate down to 1.5 or less), then ancillary tests such as X-ray mammography, ultrasound and cytology are needed. The choice between X-ray and ultrasound mammography remains open, both having high overall accuracy in this context but both with weaknesses. One sensible approach is to choose ultrasound first in the younger women (less than 40 years of age), in whom the dense mammographic appearance is difficult to interpret and one would prefer to limit radiation exposure, and to choose X-ray mammography for the older women. In either case there should be no hesitation in using both tests, together with cytology, where there is conflict or doubt. In practice, since the contralateral breast needs a screening mammogram when surgery is contemplated for a presumed cancer, all such patients need X-ray mammography.

Special situations where ultrasound is undoubtedly the most reliable imaging test are when there is a prosthesis present and in the dense breast (both these have no effect on the ultrasound image quality but degrade X-ray mammography). For safety reasons, ultrasound is preferred during pregnancy and the same argument may be proposed where repeated examinations are planned for young women, e.g. with benign breast disease and a follow-up.

Ultrasound is often useful in interventional and localization procedures: they are often simple and quicker and the precision is better under ultrasound than under X-ray control. Where a lesion can be visualized on ultrasound (i.e. not microcalcification) this should be the first choice guidance method.

Deployment and skills

As ultrasound scanners have become smaller and cheaper while retaining adequate image quality, the possibility of having dedicated machines placed in each breast clinic has become practical. The great advantage is that problems that might otherwise require repeated clinic visits can be solved at once, with a major saving in patient anxiety and in financial terms.

Two crucial quality questions remain: they concern the machine and the operator. Several high resolution scanners are now available [39] which, though not equaling the superb images and additional features such as colour Doppler provided by high end machines, are adequate for differentiating cystic from solid lesions and for providing the reassurance that a region of thickening consists of ultrasonically normal breast tissue. Care and advice in choice of scanner from those familiar with the available equipment is important.

Operator skill is a more difficult problem, exacerbated by the apparent simplicity of the technique whereby an image appears as soon as the probe is contacted onto the skin. However, in reality mastering the scanner controls to avoid disastrous errors due to mis-set gain controls, understanding the myriad artefacts to which ultrasound is prone and achieving a grasp of the wide range of variants and pathologies that must be considered, is anything but simple. The learning process can, however, be taken in stages: fundamental is a practical grasp of the principles of ultrasound and of the controls, following which some pathologies are easily recognized, at least in their typical forms, notably cysts. Achieving this kind of skill at a safe level might take an ultrasound naive operator with the right abilities and motivation some 3 months of steady application in a daily clinic. To proceed to the next level, i.e. achieving 95% accuracy in the differential diagnosis of solid lesions, is much more taxing in all aspects; a not unreasonable proposal is that one needs to see at least 100 cancers before being safe at this level, so that a few years' experience is likely to be needed.

Based on these considerations, there are serious misgivings about the potential for disasters in the rush to place a scanner in every clinic; these can be avoided by insisting on adequate training and by a cautious, graded approach to the types of problems that can safely be tackled in the clinic initially with expert back-up from the ultrasound department [40,41]. Given this, the full potential of ultrasound in the diagnosis and management of breast diseases could be realized.

References

1 Wild, J.J., Reid, J.M. (1952) Further pilot echographic studies on the histological structure of tumours of the living intact human breast. *American Journal of Pathology* **28**, 839–861.

2 Vilaro, M.M., Kurtz, A.B., Needleman, L., *et al.* (1989) Hand-held and automated sonomammography: clinical role relative to X-ray mammography. *Journal of Ultrasound Medicine* **8**, 95–100.

3 Hilton, S.V.W., Leopold, G.R., Olson, L.K., Willson, S.A. (1986)

Real-time breast sonography: application in 300 consecutive patients. *American Journal of Roentgenology* **147**, 479–486.
4 Ueno, E., Tohno, E., Soeda, S., *et al*. (1988) Dynamic tests in real-time breast echography. *Ultrasound in Medicine and Biology* **14** (suppl. 1), 53–57.
5 Cosgrove, D.O., Bamber, J.C., Davey, J.B., *et al*. (1990) Colour Doppler signals from breast tumours. *Radiology* **176**, 175–180.
6 Kopans, D.B., Meyer, J.E., Lindfors, K.K., Bucchianeri, S.S. (1984) Breast sonography to guide cyst aspiration and wire localisation of occult solid lesions. *American Journal of Roentgenology* **143**, 489–492.
7 Schneck, C.D., Lehman, D.A. (1982) Sonographic anatomy of the breast. *Seminars in Ultrasound* **3**, 13–33.
8 Scatarige, J.C., Hamper, U.M., Sheth, S., Allen, H.A. (1989) Parasternal sonography of the internal mammary vessels: technique, normal anatomy, and lymphadenopathy. *Radiology* **172**, 453–457.
9 Cole-Beuglet, C., Schwartz G., Kurtz, A.B., *et al*. (1983) Ultrasound mammography for the augmented breast. *Radiology* **146**, 737–742.
10 Sickles, E.A., Filly, R.A., Callen, P.W. (1984) Benign breast lesions: ultrasound detection and diagnosis. *Radiology* **151**, 467–470.
11 Jellins, J., Kossoff, G., Reeve, T.S. (1977) Detection and classification of liquid-filled masses in the breast by gray scale echography. *Radiology* **125**, 205–212.
12 Jackson, V.P., Rothschild, P.A., Kreipke, D.L., *et al*. (1986) The spectrum of sonographic findings of fibroadenoma of the breast. *Investigative Radiology* **21**, 34–40.
13 Fornage, B.D., Longan, J.G., Andry, E. (1989) Fibroadenoma of the breast: sonographic appearance. *Radiology* **172**, 671–675.
14 Vlaisavljevic, V. (1988) Differentiation of solid breast tumors on the basis of their primary echographic characteristics as revealed by real-time scanning of the uncompressed breast. *Ultrasound in Medicine and Biology* **14** (suppl. 1), 59–73.
15 Ueno, E., Tohno, E., Hirano, Y., *et al*. (1986) Ultrasound diagnosis of breast cancer. *Journal of Medical Imaging* **6**, 178–188.
16 Cole-Beuglet, C., Soriano, R.Z., Kurtz, A.B., Goldberg, B.B. (1983) Ultrasound analysis of 104 primary breast carcinomas classified according to histologic type. *Radiology* **147**, 191–196.
17 Adler, D.D., Hyde, D.L., Ikeda, D.M. (1991) Quantitative sonographic parameters as a means of distinguishing breast cancers from benign solid breast masses. *Journal of Ultrasound Medicine* **10**, 505–508.
18 Meyer, J.E., Amin, E., Lindfors, K.K., *et al*. (1989) Medullary carcinoma of the breast: mammographic and US appearance. *Radiology* **170**, 79–82.
19 Sakuma, H., Nagasaki, H., Fujii, Y., Kasumi, F. (1985) Ultrasonographic findings of mucinous carcinoma of the breast. *Japan Society for Ultrasound in Medicine, Proceedings* **47**, 169–170.
20 Fornage, B.D., Sneige, N., Faroux, M.J., Andry, E. (1990) Sonographic appearance and ultrasound-guided fine-needle aspiration biopsy of breast carcinomas smaller than 1 cm^3. *Journal of Ultrasound Medicine* **9**, 559–568.
21 Tochio, H., Konishi, Y., Hashimoto T., *et al*. (1989) Ultrasonographic features of noninvasive breast cancer. *Japan Society for Ultrasound in Medicine, Proceedings* **16** (suppl. II), 534–543.
22 Kasumi, F., Tanaka, H. (1983) Detection of microcalcifications in breast carcinoma by ultrasound. In: Jellins, J., Kobayashi, T. (eds) *Ultrasonic Examination of the Breast*. John Wiley, pp. 89–97.
23 Reuter, K., D'Orsi, C.J., Reale, F. (1984) Intracystic carcinoma of the breast: the role of ultrasonography. *Radiology* **153**, 233–234.
24 Cilotti, A., Bagnolesi, P., Napoli, V., Lencioni, R., Bartolozzi, C. (1991) Solitary intraductal papilloma of the breast. An echographic study of 12 cases. *Radiology Medicine* **82**, 617–620.
25 Cole-Beuglet, C., Soriano, R., Kurtz, A.B., *et al*. (1983) Ultrasound, X-ray mammography, and histopathology of cystosarcoma phylloides. *Radiology* **146**, 481–486.
26 Toombs, B.D., Kalisher, L. (1977) Metastatic disease to the breast: clinical, pathologic, radiologic features. *American Journal of Roentgenology* **129**, 673–676.
27 Wolf, G., Hohenberg, G. (1984) Mammographic and sonographic appearances of traumatic changes in the female breast. *Roentgen Forschung* **141**, 204–208.
28 Morgan, C.L., Trought, W.S., Peete, W. (1978) Xeromammographic and ultrasonic diagnosis of a traumatic oil cyst. *American Journal Roentgenology* **130**, 1189–1190.
29 Leucht, W.J., Rabe, D.R. (1988) Sonographic findings following conservative surgery and irradiation for breast carcinoma. *Ultrasound in Medicine and Biology* **14** (suppl. 1), 27–41.
30 Herzog, P. (1989) Silicone granulomas: detection by ultrasonography. *Plastic Reconstruction Surgery* **84**, 856–857.
31 Hayes, R., Michell, M., Nunnerley, H.B. (1991) Acute inflammation of the breast—the role of breast ultrasound in diagnosis and management. *Clinical Radiology* **44**, 253–256.
32 Harper, A.P., Kelly-Fry, E., Noe, J.S., *et al*. (1983) Ultrasound in the evaluation of solid breast masses. *Radiology* **146**, 731–736.
33 Leucht, W.J., Rabe, D.R., Humbert, K.D. (1988) Diagnostic value of interpretative criteria in real-time sonography of the breast. *Ultrasound in Medicine and Biology* **14** (suppl. 1), 59–73.
34 Heywang, S.H., Lipsit, E.R., Glassman, L.M., Thomas, M.T. (1984) Specificity of ultrasonography in the diagnosis of benign breast masses. *Journal of Ultrasound Medicine* **3**, 453–461.
35 Sickles, E.A., Filly, R.A., Callen, P.W. (1982) Breast cancer detection with sonography and mammography: comparison using state-of-the-art equipment. *American Journal of Roentgenology* **140**, 843–845.
36 Smallwood, J.A., Guyer, P., Dewbury, K., *et al*. (1986) The accuracy of ultrasound in the diagnosis of breast disease. *Annals of the Royal College Surgeons (Eng)* **68**, 19–22.
37 Schmidt, W., Van Kaick, G., Müller, A., *et al*. (1983) Ultrasonic diagnosis of malignant and benign human breast lesions. *Ultrasound Medicine and Biology* (suppl. 2), 407–414.
38 Tohno, E., Ueno, E., Hirano, Y., *et al*. (1986) Sonographic diagnosis of breast diseases: comparison with other diagnostic methods. *Japan Society for Ultrasound in Medicine, Proceedings* **48**, 493–494.
39 Dempsey, P.J. (1988) The importance of resolution in clinical application of breast sonography. *Ultrasound in Medicine and Biology* **14** (suppl.), 43–48.
40 Jackson, V.P. (1990) The role of ultrasound in breast imaging. *Radiology* **177**, 305–311.
41 Feig, S.A. (1989) The role of ultrasound in a breast imaging center. *Seminars in Ultrasound, CT and MRI* **10**, 90–105.

Further reading

Tohno, E., Cosgrove, D.O., Sloane, J. (1993) *Ultrasound Atlas of Breast Diseases*. Churchill Livingstone, Edinburgh.

Chapter 22: Thyroid, parathyroid and salivary glands

K.C. Dewbury

Technique

The neck is ideally suited to evaluation by high frequency ultrasound. Access is unhampered in the majority of patients although a heavy beard may limit the utility of the examination. A 7–10 MHz transducer allows clear demonstration of the normal anatomical structures and subtle changes in the normal pattern. Typically a linear array transducer is used to optimize the near-field visualization. A small stand-off gel pad may occasionally be of value to eliminate near-field artefacts and improve skin contact. A combination of transverse, longitudinal and oblique planes as necessary to optimize complete visualization of the various structures are undertaken as routine.

Anatomy

Thyroid

The thyroid gland is located in the anterior part of the neck inferior to the thyroid cartilage. The lateral lobes lie on either side of the trachea connected across the midline by an isthmus. The pyramidal lobe which extends upward from the isthmus is described in some 25% of subjects but whilst this may be imaged in children and adolescents it undergoes progressive atrophy and it is unusual to image in adults. In an obese patient the thyroid may lie more caudal in position and so be more difficult to image. In the longitudinal plane the lateral thyroid lobes have an oval shape with an elongated upper pole and a more bulbous inferior pole. The length and thickness of the lateral lobes vary considerably with body habitus, but the more reliable index of thyroid size is usually considered to be its thickness. A thickness up to 2 cm is considered normal and over 2.5 cm definitely enlarged. The normal thyroid texture is even and high in reflectivity relative to surrounding tissues. The main superior and inferior thyroid vessels are routinely imaged piercing the gland. Colour Doppler shows the thyroid gland to be a highly vascular organ. Small focal alterations in the parenchymal pattern are seen as part of the normal range of appearances and these include tiny 2–3 mm anechoic areas representing colloid collections, isolated calcifications and reflective bands of fibrous tissue.

Parathyroids

In most people the parathyroid glands lie adjacent to the posterior surface of the thyroid gland, in the tracheo-oesophageal groove, in relationship to the recurrent laryngeal nerve which itself is posterior to the glands. However, many other possible locations for the glands are described which may make their location extremely difficult. Normal parathyroid glands are very thin and small, less than 5 mm. They have the same reflectivity as the thyroid gland and are not detectable with current ultrasound equipment.

Salivary glands

The parotids are the largest salivary glands. These lie inferior to the external auditory meatus overlying the ascending ramus of the mandible with an anterior extension over the masseter muscles and a posterior process between the mastoid and the sternomastoid muscle. The margins of the gland are not well defined and the deeper portions of the gland are not adequately evaluated with ultrasound. Small portions of the parotid duct may occasionally by visualized. The gland is artificially divided into a superior and deeper portion by the facial nerve of particular importance when surgical procedures are to be undertaken. The intraglandular portion of the facial nerve can be recognized in a proportion of patients. The overall reflectivity of the gland is greater than the surrounding muscles. Small intraglandular lymph nodes are not infrequently seen and are demonstrated as echo-poor oval areas within the parotid. If a reflective hilum can be identified this confirms the diagnosis. With inflammatory change lymph nodes may become slightly enlarged.

The submandibular glands lie beneath the mandible in close relationship to the mylohyoid and hyoglossus muscles which can be seen medial to them. The glands have an oval or triangular shape with a similar reflectivity to the parotid glands. The facial artery loops anteriorly within the gland and this is easily identified using colour Doppler images. The anechoic tubular structures should not be mistaken on grey-scale imaging for the duct. The normal duct is not routinely visualized. A small intraparenchymal branch of the facial vein may also be mistaken for the duct.

The sublingual glands are the smallest of the salivary glands and most deeply situated. Each gland lies on the floor of the mouth between mandible and close to the submandibular duct; they are not routinely identified.

Pathology

Thyroid

The term goitre is commonly used to describe thyroid enlargement which may have numerous causes; the term, however, should be reserved for thyroid enlargement which is neither neoplastic nor inflammatory. Hyperplasia either nodular or diffuse is the commonest cause of a goitre. The main role of ultrasound assessment of the thyroid gland is to determine whether the patient has a generalized parenchymal abnormality, multinodularity of the gland or a solitary nodule. A combination of any of these three basic types of process may occur. When thyroid nodules are identified they should be carefully evaluated noting their reflectivity in relationship to the normal parenchyma, the presence of calcification or cystic change, the definition of the lesion margins and the vascularity on colour Doppler.

Hyperplasia

Hyperplasia is the most commonly observed pathology of the thyroid gland. It may be familial, due to iodine difficiency or to compensatory hypertrophy. It may involve one or both lobes and cause a goitre when most of the gland becomes enlarged. Hyperplasia may have a diffuse or nodular pattern. When nodules are present these differ widely in size (Fig. 22.1). Hyperplasia without nodules gives rise to a diffuse inhomogeneity of the parenchymal texture although the level of reflectivity is similar to normal. The more common nodular hyperplasia is usually identified as multiple discrete nodules varying in size and number separated by normal parenchyma and varying in reflectivity. The main role of ultrasound here is to confirm that multiple nodules are present when only one may be palpable, making it more likely that this is a benign process. The incidence of neoplastic lesions in a clinically multinodular gland is low. The nodules in hyperplasia may be of similar reflectivity to the normal gland but it is quite common for them to be of greater reflectivity and it is also common for areas of cystic or colloid degeneration to be present within the centre of the lesion. Calcification is often present, these may be peripheral and curvilinear but they may also be rather coarser and more punctate. Colour Doppler does not show nodules to be highly vascular.

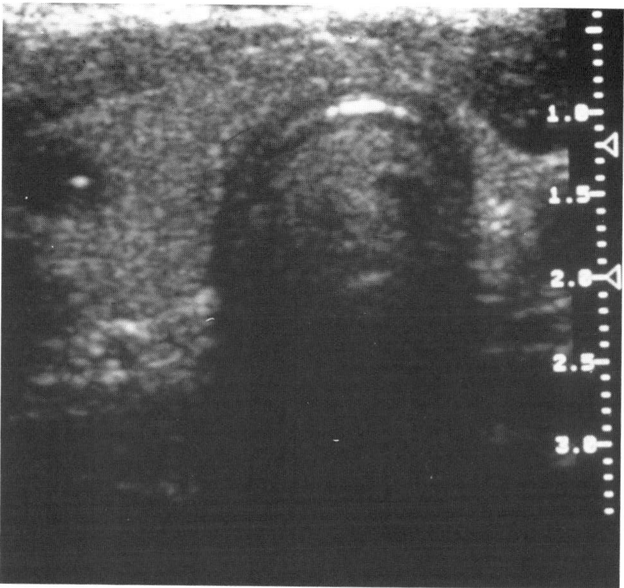

Fig. 22.1 Transverse thyroid ultrasound showing a small colloid nodule in the right lobe of the gland.

Solitary nodules

Thyroid adenomas and carcinomas are the thyroid pathologies which usually manifest themselves as a solitary nodule. Follicular adenomas have the same ultrasound appearances as hyperplastic nodules and both may undergo cystic degeneration and haemorrhage producing a poorly reflective centre (Fig. 22.2). Adenomas may become autonomous and toxic, producing thyrotoxicosis. Traditionally adenomas are described as having a well-defined peripheral halo. In reality the appearances of adenomas overlap the appearances of carcinomas and for histological diagnosis a fine-needle cytology or surgical removal of solitary nodules is required.

Malignant neoplasms of the thyroid are uncommon, the most common malignant thyroid tumour is the papillary carcinoma accounting for 65% of all cases. The incidence of papillary carcinoma shows two peaks, one in young adults and the other in elderly patients. The incidence is greater in females. Papillary cancer characteristically spreads via the lymphatics to regional lymph nodes and

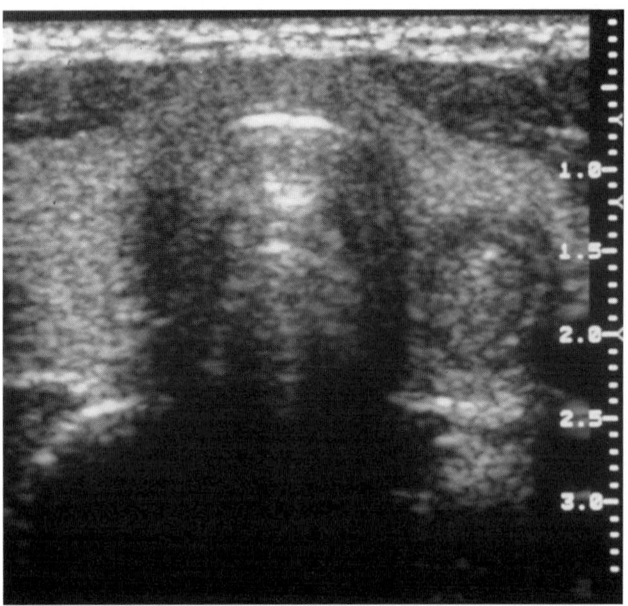

Fig. 22.2 A well-defined thyroid adenoma in the left lobe of the gland.

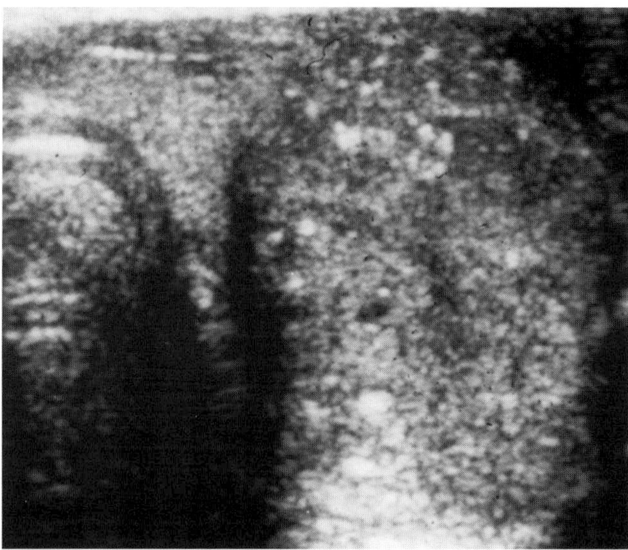

Fig. 22.3 Large slightly irregular papillary carcinoma containing small flecks of microcalcification.

so a careful search for nodal enlargement particularly containing fine calcifications should be made (Fig. 22.3).

Follicular carcinoma accounts for 15% of thyroid cancers and is more frequent in older patients. The spread is via the blood stream so that distant metastases to lung and bone are more common.

Anaplastic thyroid carcinoma accounts for 10% of all thyroid cancers and is primarily a disease of the elderly, this is a more aggressive tumour. Medullary carcinoma comprises of only 10% of all thyroid malignancies, but it may be familial and occur in association with multiple endocrine neoplasia. It has slow growth and spreads via the lymphatics to nearby lymph nodes. It may be diagnosed by the presence of the hormone marker calcitonin in the serum (Fig. 22.4).

On ultrasound imaging the great majority of malignant thyroid neoplasms are predominantly poorly reflective in relationship to the normal thyroid parenchyma. Careful evaluation of the margins of focal lesions are particularly important, the majority of cancers show a poorly marginated lesion with an irregular heterogeneous echo pattern. Microcalcification is a particularly useful diagnostic feature in papillary carcinoma of the thyroid and this microcalcification may also be seen within the nodal metastases. Colour Doppler shows a rich vascularity within the centre of the solid lesion in a typical carcinoma. Evidence of infiltration of structures around the thyroid and metastases are diagnostic features of malignancy.

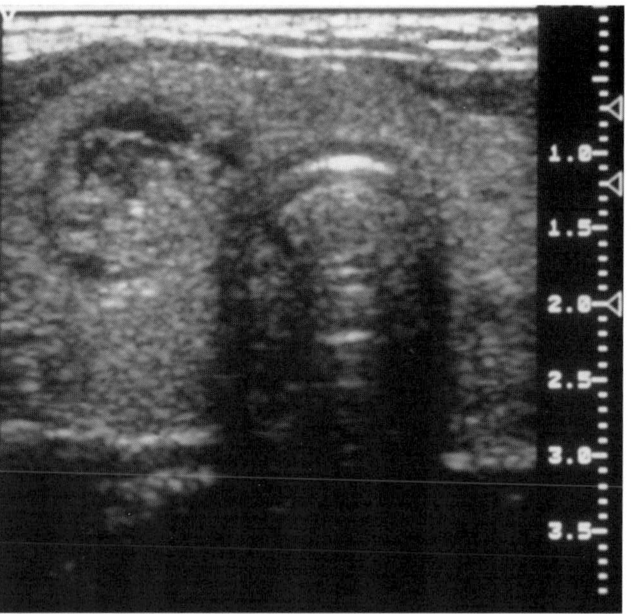

Fig. 22.4 Well-defined medullary carcinoma of the right lobe of the thyroid, diagnosed following discovery of raised serum calcitonin.

Thyroiditis

Thyroiditis may occur as an acute condition or in a chronic form. Acute thyroiditis may have a viral or bacterial aetiology. The clinical features are usually diagnostic and ultrasound is only required to evaluate the extent or presence of parenchymal involvement and to monitor abscess formation, which is extremely unusual. The typical

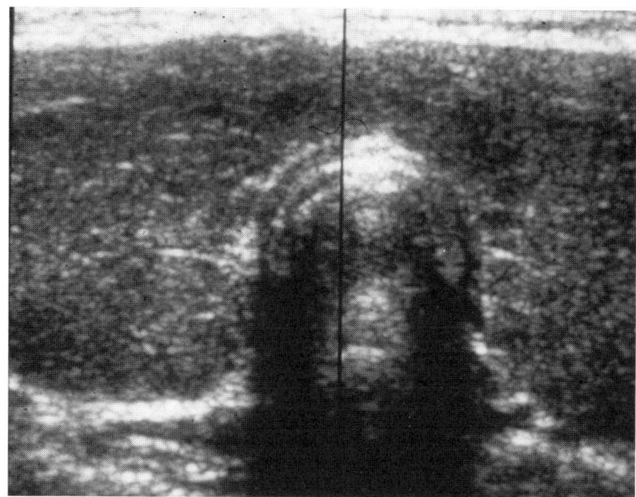

Fig. 22.5 Acute thyroiditis, the thyroid gland is enlarged and rather low in reflectivity with accentuation of the fibrous bands. Colour Doppler showed a marked increase in vascularity.

appearances on ultrasound are of a diffuse glandular enlargement with an overall reduction in reflectivity but accentuation of the fibrous stroma of the gland. Colour Doppler characteristically shows a marked uniform increase in vascularity which is very characteristic (Fig. 22.5).

Chronic thyroiditis may be caused by Hashimoto's disease. In the hypertrophic stage there is diffuse glandular enlargement with irregular rather lobular margins. There is a generalized decrease in parenchymal reflectivity with particularly prominent accentuation of the reflective fibrous bands. As with acute thyroiditis in the early stages it is common to show an overall increase in vascularity on colour Doppler imaging. With successful treatment of the condition the vascularity may be shown to diminish.

Parathyroid glands

In biochemically proven hyperparathyroidism ultrasound may be of value in attempting to localize parathyroid tumours. Abnormal glands become enlarged and poorly reflective. If the glands are in a normal position behind the thyroid they may be identified, hence directing surgical exploration. If the glands cannot, however, be identified in the neck, ultrasound is unlikely to be of any great further value (Fig. 22.6).

All imaging tests of the parathyroids are compromised by their great variations in number and locations. Instead of the normal four a few individuals may have two, three, five or even six glands while ectopic glands may occur anywhere in the neck or mediastinum.

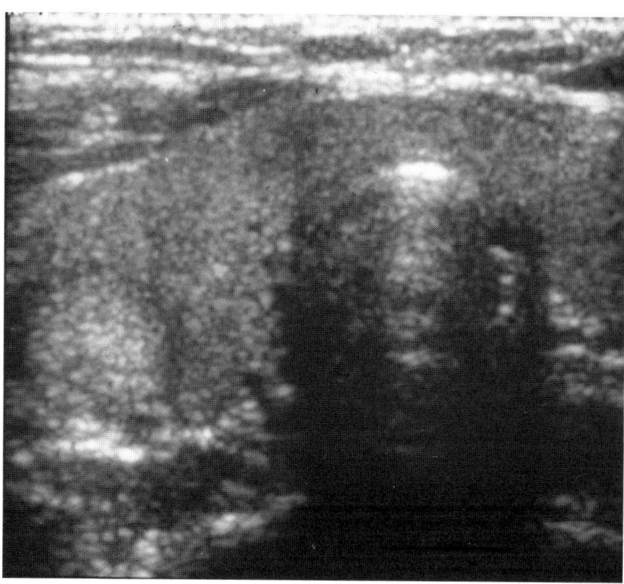

Fig. 22.6 Transverse view of the neck showing a normal thyroid and a slightly unusual reflective parathyroid adenoma lying posterior to the right lobe of the thyroid gland.

Salivary glands

Hypertrophy

Hypertrophy produces an enlarged gland with a normal shape and structure. This may be due to obesity or racial factors and may be observed associated with diabetes, liver cirrhosis or uraemia.

Inflammation and calculi

The role of ultrasound in demonstration of adenitis is limited. In acute inflammation the salivary gland is enlarged, rather poorly reflective and slightly heterogeneous. Tiny echo-poor foci may be observed within the gland and attributed to microabscesses. Acute changes usually return to normal. In chronic inflammation such as in Sjögren's syndrome there is little to see of diagnostic value on ultrasound. Sialography remains the best method for evaluating the fine detail of the intraglandular ducts in this condition.

Possibly the most useful role of ultrasound in patients with symptoms of acute inflammation of the salivary glands is to rule out duct stones. Ultrasound has been shown to be extremely sensitive in this regard in the demonstration of the duct stones (Fig. 22.7). Sialography should be reserved for patients with equivocal ultrasound findings or when ultrasound is negative but the clinical suspicion remains extremely strong. Salivary calculi are

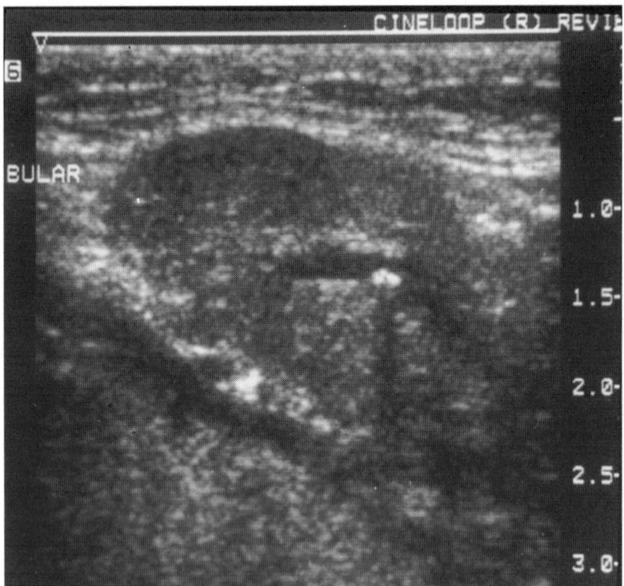

Fig. 22.7 Longitudinal view of the submandibular gland showing a typical calculus within a slightly dilated duct.

seen as highly reflective foci with distal acoustic shadowing. Demonstration of the calculi should be within dilated ducts.

Tumours

In patients with a palpable mass in the region of the salivary glands ultrasound is used to confirm the presence of a mass and to differentiate between intra- and extraglandular masses ultrasound may suggest the nature of the mass by analysis of texture and the margins of the lesion. Masses outside the salivary gland are most commonly enlarged lymph nodes.

Tumours of the salivary glands are relatively rare but are much more common in the parotid (85%) than in the submandibular glands 15%. Benign lesions account for 85–90% of all parotid tumours. Submandibular gland tumours, however, should be considered suspicious as malignancy is more frequent comprising 35% of all submandibular solid masses. The most common tumour of salivary glands is the pleomorphic adenoma also termed the mixed parotid tumour. It is a benign, sometimes multicentric, slow growing tumour composed of epithelial cells and varying proportions of mucoid, chondroid and myxoid tissue. Approximately 90% of these tumours occur in the superficial lobe of the parotid gland and thus ultrasound is an ideal method by which to image it. The imaging features are of a relatively homogeneous, solid, poorly reflective mass. The margins are well defined but often slightly lobular. There may be a small amount of distal acoustic enhancement (Fig. 22.8). Enlarged cervical lymph nodes are not found in association with these masses. Colour Doppler shows a predominantly peripheral type of flow although some vascularity will be seen within the lesion attesting to its solid nature.

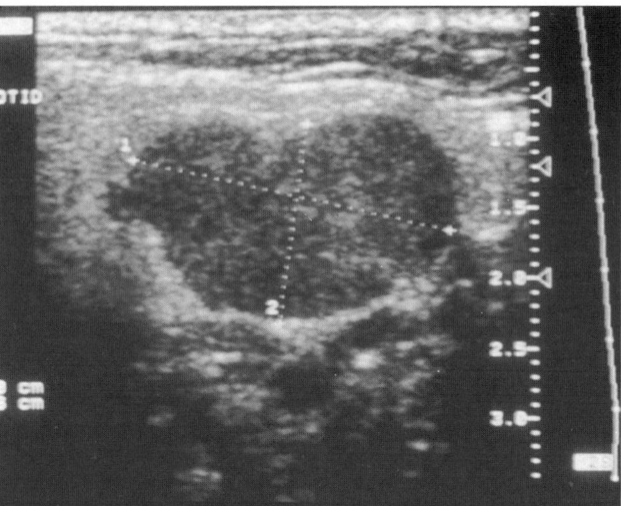

Fig. 22.8 A well-defined slightly lobular pleomorphic adenoma of the parotid gland.

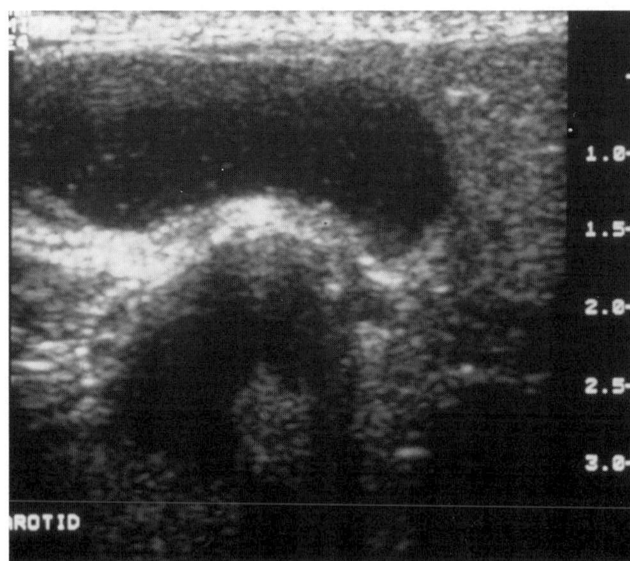

Fig. 22.9 Adenolymphoma of the left parotid.

Adenolymphoma (Warthin's) tumour accounts for 5–10% of all salivary gland tumours. The imaging appearances are of a poorly reflective almost cystic mass (Fig. 22.9). The margins are well defined, the echo pattern is mixed and distal acoustic enhancement is more prominent. Other rare benign tumours of salivary glands include lipomas and haemangiomas. A variety of malig-

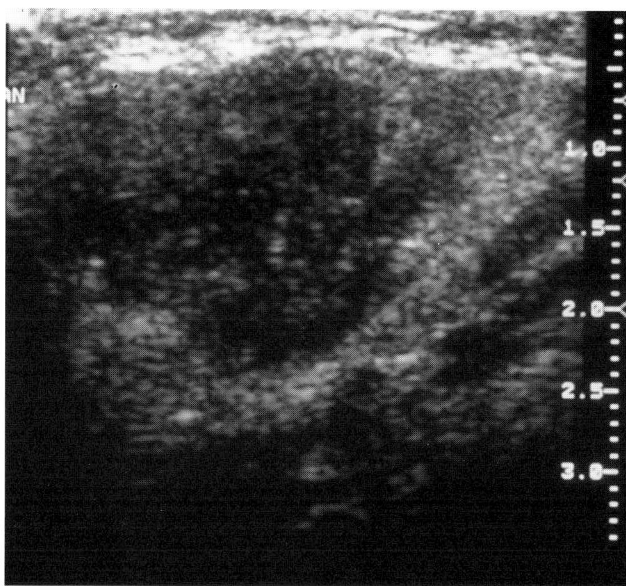

Fig. 22.10 Carcinoma of the right submandibular gland. Note a rather irregular heterogeneous poorly marginated tumour mass which showed a marked increase in vascularity on colour Doppler imaging.

nant tumours can develop in the salivary glands including mucoepidermoid carcinomas, cylindromas epidermoid carcinoma and undifferentiated carcinoma. Metastases and lymphomas occur rarely. Clinically all malignant tumours present as fixed hard masses possibly associated with ipsilateral cervical lymph node enlargement, typical of malignant lesions the margination is usually poorly defined and vascularity is typically increased and is bizarre in pattern (Fig. 22.10).

Further reading

Ajayi, B.A., Pugh, N.D., Carolan, G. (1992) Salivary gland tumours: is colour Doppler imaging of added value in their preoperative assessment? *European Journal of Surgery and Oncology* **18**, 463–469.

Bradley, M.J., Ahuja, A., Metreweli, C. (1991) Sonographic evaluation of the parotid ducts; its use in tumour localization. *British Journal of Radiology* **64**, 1092.

Bruneton, J.N., Normand, F., Santini, N., Balu-Maestro, C. (1987) Salivary glands. In: Bruneton, J.N. (ed.) *Ultrasonography of the Neck*. Springer-Verlag, Berlin, pp. 64–80.

Carrol, B.A. (1982) Asymptomatic thyroid nodules: incidental sonographic detection. *American Journal of Roentgenology* **133**, 499–501.

Derchi, L.E., Solbiati, L. (1993) Salivary glands. In: Cosgrove, D., Meire, H., Dewbury, K. (eds) *Abdominal and General Ultrasound*. Churchill Livingstone, Edinburgh, pp. 677–681.

Gorman, B., Charboneau, J.W., James, E.M., *et al.* (1987) Medullary thyroid carcinoma: roles of high resolution US. *Radiology* **162**, 147–150.

Graif, M., Itzchak, Y., Strauss, S., Dolev, E., Mohr, R., Wolfstein, I. (1987) Parathyroid sonography: diagnostic accuracy related to shape, location and texture of the gland. *British Journal of Radiology* **60**, 439–443.

Gritzmann, N. (1989) Sonography of the salivary glands. *American Journal of Roentgenology* **153**, 161–166.

Hatabu, H., Kasagi, K., Yamamoto, K. *et al.* (1992) Undifferentiated carcinoma of the thyroid gland: sonographic findings. *Clinics in Radiology* **45**, 307–310.

Hay, I.D. (1990) Papillary thyroid carcinoma. *Endocrinology Metabolism Clinics of North America* **19**, 545–576.

James, E.M., Charnoneau, J.W., Hay, I.D. (1991) The thyroid. In: Rumack, C.M., Wilson, S.R., Charboneau, J.W. (eds) *Diagnostic Ultrasound*. Mosby, St Louis, pp. 507–523.

Kerr, L. (1994) High resolution thyroid ultrasound: the value of colour Doppler. *Ultrasound Quarterly* **12**, 21–43.

Martinoli, C., Derchi, L.E., Solbiati, L., Giannoni, M. (1994) Colour Doppler imaging of salivary glands. *American Journal of Roentgenology* **163**, 933–941.

Ralls, P.W., Mayekawa, D.S., Lee, K.P., *et al.* (1988) Colour flow Doppler sonography in Graves' disease 'thyroid inferno'. *American Journal of Roentgenology* **150**, 781–784.

Randel, S.B., Gooding, G.A.W., Clark, O.H., Stein, R.M., Winkler, B. (1987) Parathyroid variants: US evaluation. *Radiology* **165**, 191–194.

Solbiati, L., Ballarati, E., Cioffi, V., *et al.* (1990) Microcalcifications: a clue in the diagnosis of thyroid malignancies. *Radiology* **177**, 140.

Solbiati, L., Ballarati, E., Cioffi, V. (1991) Contribution of colour flow mapping to the differential diagnosis of thyroid nodules. *Radiology* **181**, 177.

Solbiati, L., Cioffi, V., Ballarati, E. (1992) Ultrasonography of the neck. *Radiology Clinics of North America* **30**, 941–954.

Solbiati, L., Croce, F., Derchi, L.E. (1993) The neck. In: Cosgrove, D., Meire, H., Dewbury, K. (eds) *Abdominal and General Ultrasound*, vol. II. Churchill Livingstone, Edinburgh, pp. 659–694.

Sostre, S., Reyes, M.M. (1991) Sonographic diagnosis and grading of Hashimoto's thyroiditis. *Journal of Endocrinology Investigations* **14**, 115–121.

Chapter 23: The testes and scrotum

K.C. Dewbury

Ultrasound is the mainstay for imaging of the scrotum. The diagnosis of intrascrotal abnormalities should always be based on a combination of ultrasound and clinical findings. Most ultrasound departments have noticed a huge increase in demand for scrotal ultrasound over recent years, probably arising from the well-documented increase in the incidence of primary testicular tumours in young men in Europe and the UK and the associated publicity afforded to this. Coincidentally improvements in ultrasound technology have resulted in a new generation of high frequency transducers producing exquisite greyscale detail of the scrotal structures and physiological information regarding the vascularity.

Examination technique

Scrotal ultrasound is generally performed with the patient supine. A towel is placed over the penis and the patient requested to tension the towel to draw the penis away from the scrotum and to present the scrotum in a suitable position for contact scanning. Direct contact scanning is most commonly performed but a flexible gel stand-off may be useful to prevent distortion of very superficial structures and in patients with a very tender scrotum. Optimum results are achieved with high frequency linear array transducers operating at around 10 MHz. Doppler parameters are usually adjusted to the most sensitive settings. The scrotal contents are mobile and it is important to ensure that the testis and epididymis on each are identified as completely as possible. They should be compared for symmetry and size, texture and vascularity.

Normal anatomy and variance

The scrotum is divided by a midline septum into two halves, each containing a testis and associated structures. The tunica vaginalis has two layers, the outer parietal and inner visceral layer which covers the testis; these are separated by a small volume of fluid. In most men this fluid is normally detected around the upper pole of the testis and the head of the epididymis. The visceral layer of the tunica vaginalis is adherent to the tunica albuginea, a fibrous capsule that surrounds the testis. The fold of the tunica albuginea forms the mediastinum of the testis. A mature testis consists of approximately 250 cone-shaped lobules which are separated by thin fibrous septae. There are between one and four tortuous seminiferous tubules within each lobule. These join the tubuli recti that connect them to the rete testis. The rete testis is a network of epithelium-lined spaces that are inbedded in the fibrous stroma of the mediastinum testis and drain into the epididymis via 10–15 efferent ductules. The mediastinum is almost always visualized on ultrasound as a reflective linear band in the long axis of the testis on the same side as the epididymis. There is considerable variation in the prominence of the mediastinal reflectivity which has no particular diagnostic implications. The less reflective rete lies adjacent to this and extending from this region the fine fibrous septations of the testicular lobules may just be appreciated with the best equipment (Fig. 23.1). Apart from this fine detail the testes are almost homogeneous ovoid structures measuring approximately 4.5 × 3.5 × 3 cm. In infants and children the testis is less reflective than in adults, the increase in reflectivity occurring during puberty.

The epididymis lies adjacent to the mediastinum and closely envelops the testis. The head is usually the most easily visualized portion but the body and tail will usually also be demonstrable with modern equipment and careful scanning. The normal appendix testis will be regularly visualized in many patients (Fig. 23.2). The vas deferens is a tubular structure and runs close to the epididymis before joining the spermatic cord above the epididymal head. The pampiniform plexus of draining veins is formed around the upper half of the epididymis in a variable fashion. The main blood supply of the testis is via the testicular artery with deferential and cremesteric arteries mainly supplying the epididymis and peritesticular tissues. The testicular artery penetrates the tunica albuginea and gives off capsular arteries which in turn give off centripetal arteries running along the fibrous septal divisions. In up to 50% of men a large transtesticular or trans-

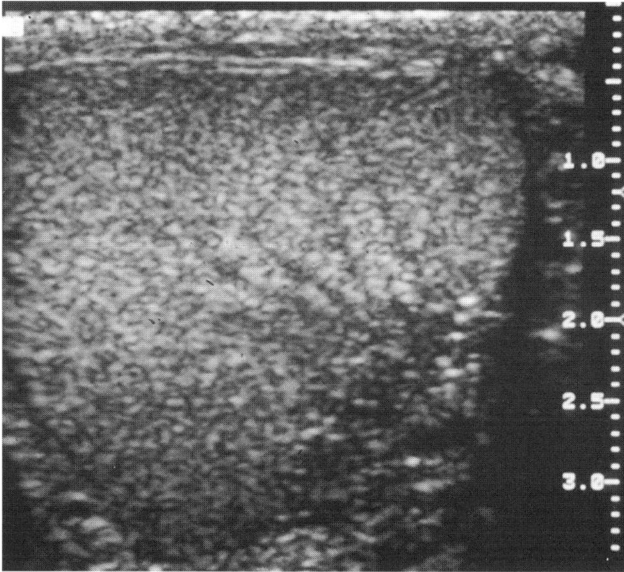

Fig. 23.1 A transverse scan of a normal testis showing the region of the mediastinum and rete testis and fine septal divisions of the testicular lobules.

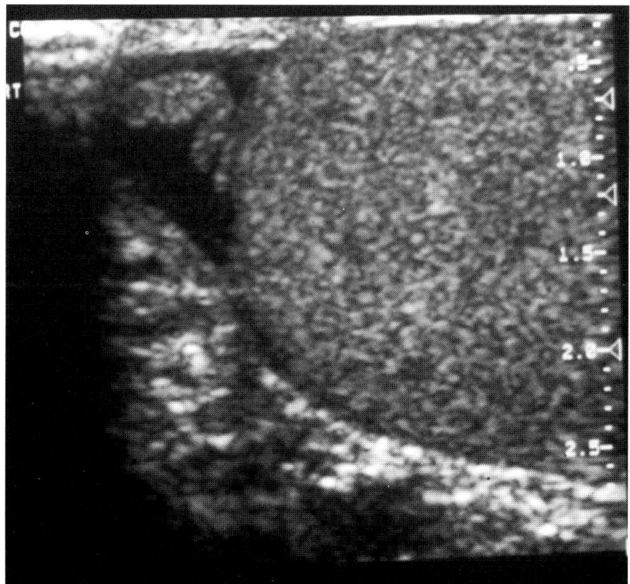

Fig. 23.2 A longitudinal view showing the normal appendix testis.

mediastinal artery is present (Fig. 23.3). It is routinely possible to identify the vascular supply as described in adults but the smaller vessels in children are not so reliably identified. Venous outflow is through the pampiniform plexus that flows into the cremesteric and internal spermatic veins and subsequently the ipsilateral testicular vein.

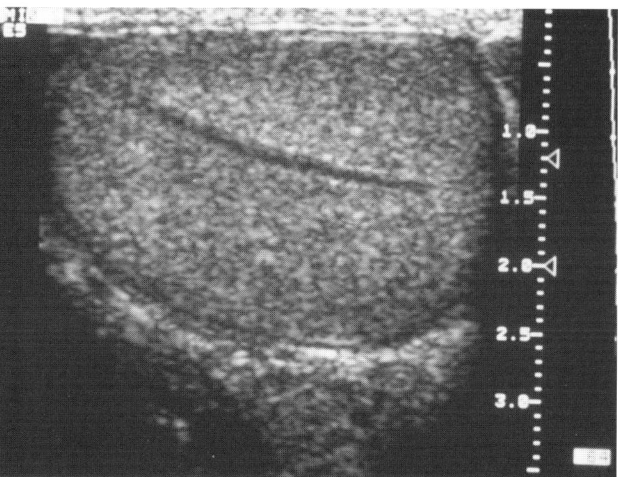

Fig. 23.3 A longitudinal scan of the testis showing a transtesticular artery.

Undescended testis

A testis that lies in the normal path of testicular descent is an undescended testis whereas a testis descended to a wrong location is called an ectopic testis. The latter is rare, the most common ectopic sites being femoral or perineal. Undescended testis is found in 40% of full-term infants: the testis is usually within the scrotum within 4–6 weeks only 0.8% of males at the age of 1 year have true cryptorchidism. Infertility and cancer of the testis are the major risk for these patients. The risk of cancer has been estimated to be five to 10 times as high as for healthy men. The risk of infertility is reduced if surgical orchiopexy is carried out before 3 years of age but this does not eliminate the risk of malignant change. In about 80% of patients the undescended testis is in the inguinal canal and is easily demonstrable with ultrasound and may be palpable. In the remainder of patients the testis is in the abdomen but may not always be demonstrable. An undescended testis in adults differs in ultrasonic appearance from a normal intrascrotal testis. It is small and frequently poorly reflective but remains homogeneous unless tumour has developed.

Indications for ultrasound

The main clinical indication for ultrasound scanning of the scrotum are scrotal masses and pain. Palpable scrotal masses are always demonstrable with ultrasound which allows their separation into intratesticular or extratesticular masses. This may not always be clinically obvious. Solid intratesticular masses are usually malignant with few exceptions. Extratesticular masses are most often benign. Masses that are clearly extratesticular on clinical examination are almost all benign and it could be argued that they do not need scanning; however, the current trend is to scan all palpable scrotal masses. Pain may be caused by epididymitis or torsion and ultrasound has a useful role in this differential diagnosis. Other indications for ultrasound include as a follow-up to trauma, in the investigation of infertility and in tumour screening in groups of high risk patients.

Fluid collections

A hydrocele is an abnormal fluid collection between the parietal and visceral layers of the tunica vaginalis (Fig. 23.4). They may be idiopathic or secondary to inflammation, torsion or trauma. Hydroceles in association with tumours are uncommon but when present are more usually associated with tumours in the paediatric age group.

The ultrasound appearance is of an anechoic fluid collection partly surrounding the testis and usually displacing it posteriorly and medially. Chronic hydroceles may develop low level mobile echoes probably due to cholesterol crystals. Haematoceles and pyoceles are 'complex' hydroceles usually complicating trauma and inflammation. Low level echoes, debris and septations are demonstrated within (Fig. 23.5). A hydrocele is usually clinically obvious. With a very tense hydrocele there may be diagnostic confusion and it may be reassuring to demonstrate the underlying testis as normal, particularly in younger patients where the incidence of malignancy is higher.

Inflammatory conditions

The diagnosis of scrotal inflammatory disease is often clinically clear cut and does not require ultrasound. In atypical or severe cases, however, ultrasound is appropriate to assess potential complications such as abscess formation and to differentiate painful inflammatory conditions from torsion of the testis. Epididymitis and epididymo-orchitis are the most common infections involving the scrotum and are the most common cause of acute scrotal pain. Epididymitis occurs in two distinct groups of patients. Men below the age of 40 years have a high incidence of sexually transmitted pathogens particularly *Chlamydia trachomatis* and *Neisseria gonorrhoea*. Older men have a high association with urinary tract pathology. With the causative organism often being *Escherichia coli*. Epididymitis may also be caused by testicular trauma, ischaemia and may arise secondary to tumour as previously noted. The clinical symptoms range from a severe febrile illness to mild discomfort. Pyuria is frequently present. The lower pole is usually affected first and typical appearances are of a swollen, poorly reflective epididymis which may be focal or global. In severe cases, haemorrhagic change may also occur producing an increase in overall reflectivity on ultrasound. The reactive hydrocele is a common association. Severe epididymitis may progress to abscess formation. This is more commonly seen with a more unusual gonococcal or tuberculous infection. Spread of infection to the adjacent testis may occur. This may initially be seen as patchy areas of low reflectivity within the testis. More severe infections may lead to the development of infarction or abscess formation within the testis producing quite a dramatic appearance. Swelling of the scrotal skin in also a feature of inflammatory change and is not often seen with malignancy. With inflammatory conditions there is a marked increase in vascularity which is a valuable diagnostic feature and is well

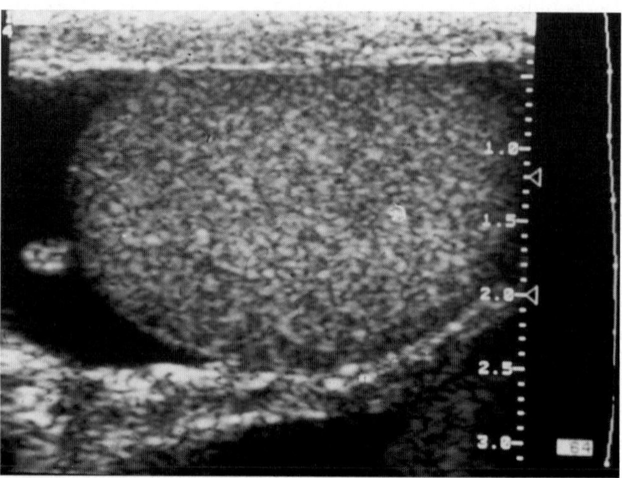

Fig. 23.4 A small hydrocele. Note outlining of the rather globular appendix testis in this patient.

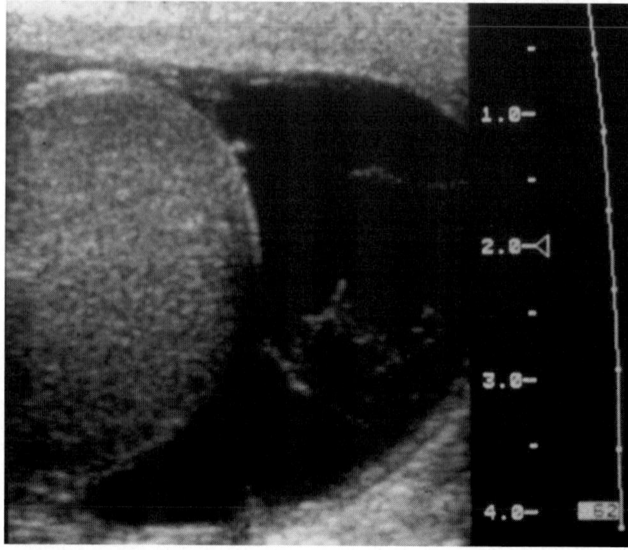

Fig. 23.5 A large pyocele. Note the septations within the fluid.

demonstrated with highly sensitive modern ultrasound equipment. Increase in vascularity may occur extremely early in the clinical course of the disease and may persist thereafter.

Orchitis alone is often the result of a specific pathogen such as the mumps causing paramyxovirus. Severe infection may lead to atrophy or even infarction of the infected testis.

Among the specific forms of epididymitis tuberculous epididymitis is of particular importance, its diagnosis, however, is primarily based on the clinical presentation, laboratory findings and bacteriological tests. The imaging appearances are non-specific but an important clinical clue may be a lack of response to standard treatment. Calcification in the epididymis and tunica may be a later sequela. Secondary involvement of the testis—epididymo-orchitis—is more common than was once appreciated. This is particularly well demonstrated by a marked increase in vascularity of both testes and epididymis on colour Doppler imaging. The change in reflectivity of the testis may range from a generalized reduction in reflectivity, patchiness often conforming to the septal architecture of the testis (Fig. 23.6) to areas of infarction or frank abscess formation as previously mentioned.

Following vasectomy, morphological changes of the epididymis occur in up to 45% of all men (Fig. 23.7). These include generalized enlargement, inhomogeneous echo texture and cystic change. This may be cystic tubular dilatation or epididymal cysts. Sperm granuloma are also a well-recognized complication, due to extravasation of sperm into epididymal tissues, causing inflammatory change and later granuloma formation and fibrosis.

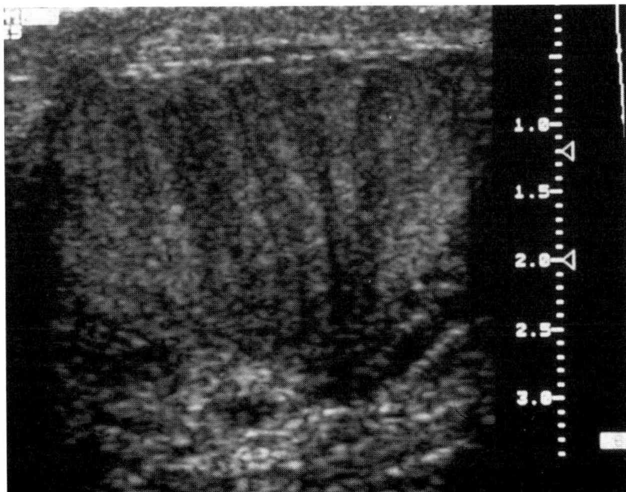

Fig. 23.6 Florid postorchitic change 6 months following a clinically severe epididymo-orchitis. Note the patchiness of the testicular texture conforms to the septal architecture of the testis.

Epididymal masses

The most common epididymal mass is a simple cyst, these vary in size and are most commonly found in the head of the epididymis (Fig. 23.8). Spermatoceles are large cystic dilatations of the ductal system also most commonly arising in the epididymal head. Spermatoceles are more common after vasectomy and are only distinguishable

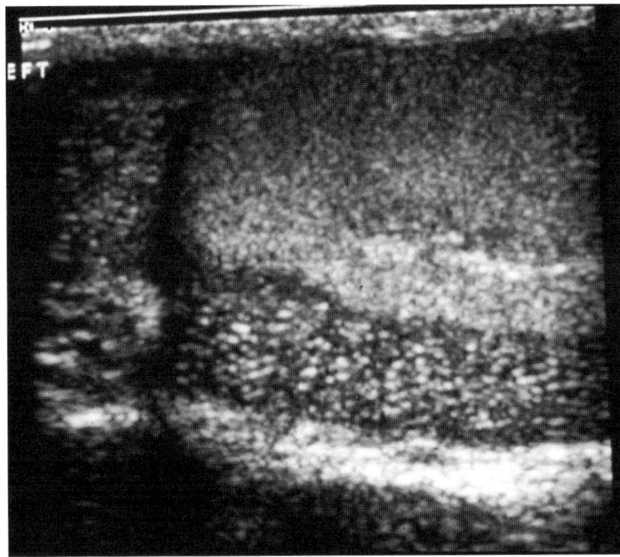

Fig. 23.7 Enlargement of the epididymis with a little minor cystic tubular dilatation in a patient who has had a vasectomy.

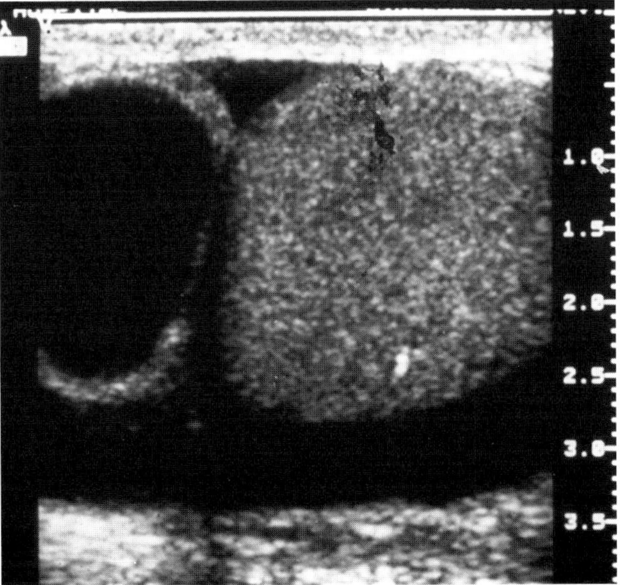

Fig. 23.8 A large simple epididymal cyst and an associated hydrocele.

from simple epididymal cysts by the low level echoes generated by the spermatic debris within the spermatocele.

The majority of solid epididymal lesions are benign and include adenomatoid tumours and lipomas. Inflammatory sperm granulomas have been previously described and may be clinically difficult to distinguish from benign tumours. Sarcomas are the most common malignant epididymal tumours but these are rare (Fig. 23.9).

Testicular masses

Tumours

Overall, testicular cancer accounts for approximately 1% of all cancers in men and is the most common malignancy amongst 15–30 year olds. The vast majority of testicular tumours are of germ cell origin but lymphoid tumours and secondary tumours are described.

The most common symptom of testicular cancer is a lump or painless swelling of the testis. Scrotal pain if present is usually dull and heavy in nature. Approximately 25% of patients complain of scrotal pain confirming that the presence of pain does not exclude the diagnosis of testicular cancer. In a smaller proportion of patients testicular cancer is associated with acute pain usually caused by haemorrhage or infarction mimicking torsion or epididymitis. A significant number of patients are aware of a testicular mass for a significant period of time before seeking medical advice.

The normal even texture of the testis represents an excellent background for the detection of intratesticular lesions. Small tumours are displayed as focal lesions and larger tumours may destroy the testicular architecture (Figs 23.10, 23.11). Tumour margins may be smooth or irregular. Most testicular tumours are poorly reflective but they also may display mixed reflectivity including calcification. Anechoic areas within tumours may correspond to haemorrhage or necrosis. The majority of semi-

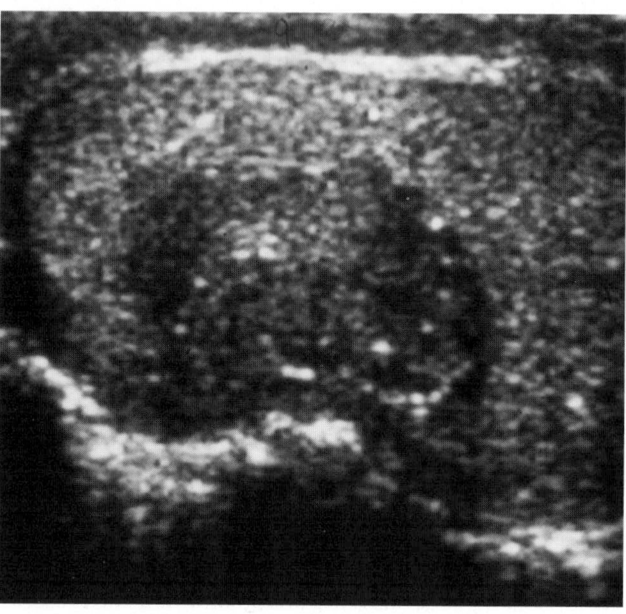

Fig. 23.10 A small teratoma of the testis. There is a slightly heterogeneous texture, one or two small flecks of calcification are noted within the mass which is not distorting the outline of the testis.

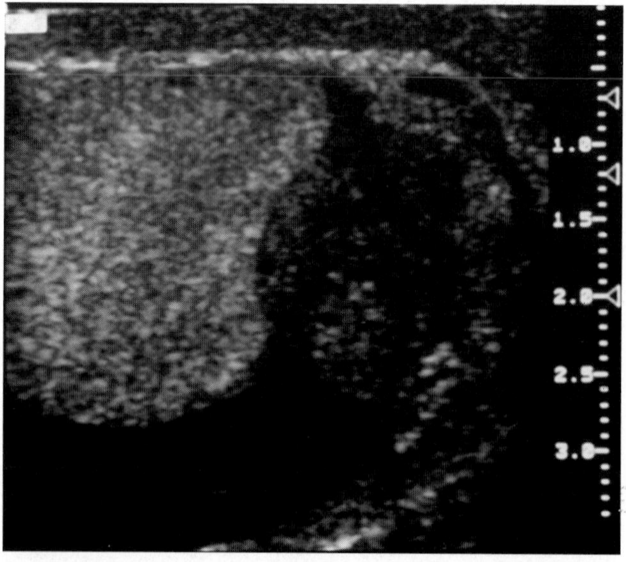

Fig. 23.9 An irregular solid mass in the tail of the epididymis; this is a sarcoma of the epididymis.

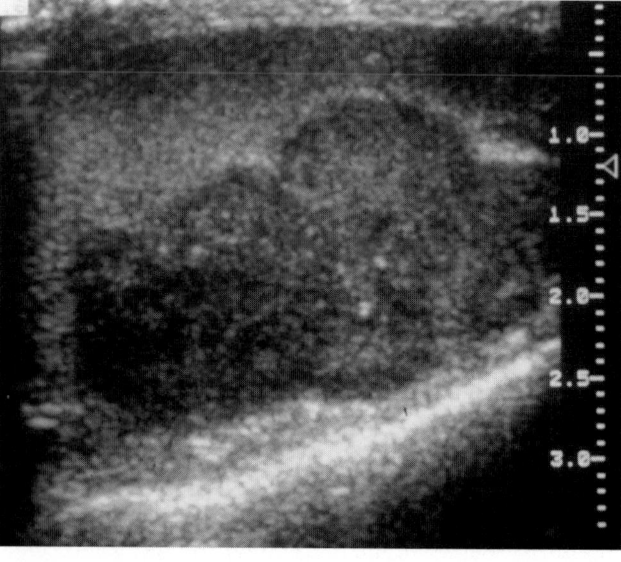

Fig. 23.11 A large seminoma of the testis causing enlargement and distortion of the testicular outline.

nomas show an even low reflectivity, teratomas characteristically are more heterogeneous and may contain areas of calcification. Lesions of under 5 mm which are nonpalpable can be reliably demonstrated with ultrasound. Patients presenting with retroperitoneal metastases, from an unknown primary tumour, should undergo systematic scrotal ultrasound to search for a primary. In cases of burnt-out testicular tumours palpation may be normal but ultrasound will demonstrate tumour scars frequently in the form of small highly reflective foci. Leukaemic infiltration or lymphoma of the testis produces a rather nonspecific appearance, sometimes with bilateral changes. The use of colour Doppler adds relatively little to the diagnosis of testicular tumours. Larger tumours frequently do show an increased vascularity with a bizarre pattern but the diagnosis has already usually been clearly established from the grey-scale imaging appearances.

Benign masses

Standard teaching is that solid focal lesions within the testis are considered malignant until proven otherwise, exceptions include rare benign tumours, focal orchitis and haematomas. Benign testicular tumours are reported and these include Sertoli and Leydig cell tumours which may produce secondary hormonal affects. They are indistinguishable from malignant tumours on the basis of their ultrasound appearances. Epidermoid tumours are rare benign testicular tumours which typically have a very characteristic appearance on ultrasound which may lead to a fairly confident preoperative diagnosis and hence appropriate conservative management. The tumours are easily 'shelled out' of the testis. This characteristic appearance comprises of a reflective ring, and concentric ring like appearance similar to an onion on the ultrasound scan (Fig. 23.12).

Simple testicular cysts which used to be regarded as rare have been more frequently detected as more scrotal ultrasound is undertaken. Cysts of the testis may present a diagnostic dilemma since testicular neoplasm may contain anechoic spaces; however, strict criteria for the diagnosis of these cysts should be employed as elsewhere in the body. Several types of simple cysts may be identified, the first is the very small cysts of the tunica albuginea (Fig. 23.13). These are palpable as firm masses of small pin head or small pea size. Ultrasound demonstrates these as small marginally located and sharply demarcated cysts without structural disturbance of the adjacent testicular parenchyma. Simple intratesticular cysts are most commonly located near the mediastinum and are shown to originate from the rete testis; however, simple intratesticular cysts do occur elsewhere in the testis (Fig. 23.14).

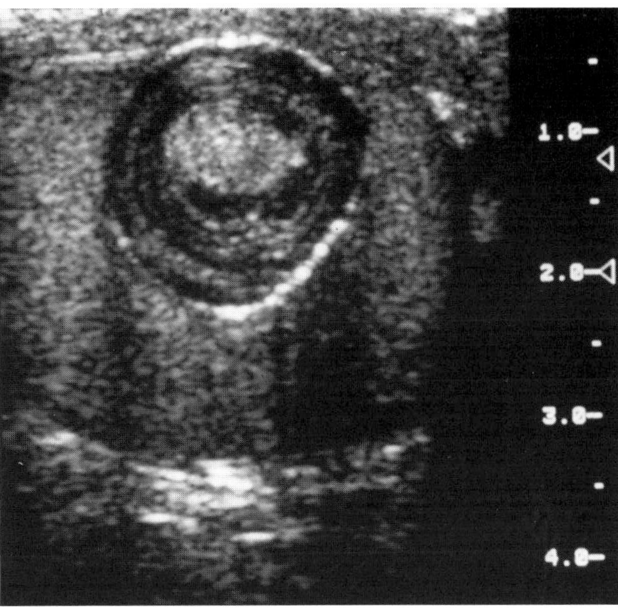

Fig. 23.12 A typical epidermoid tumour showing the concentric rings classic of this benign tumour.

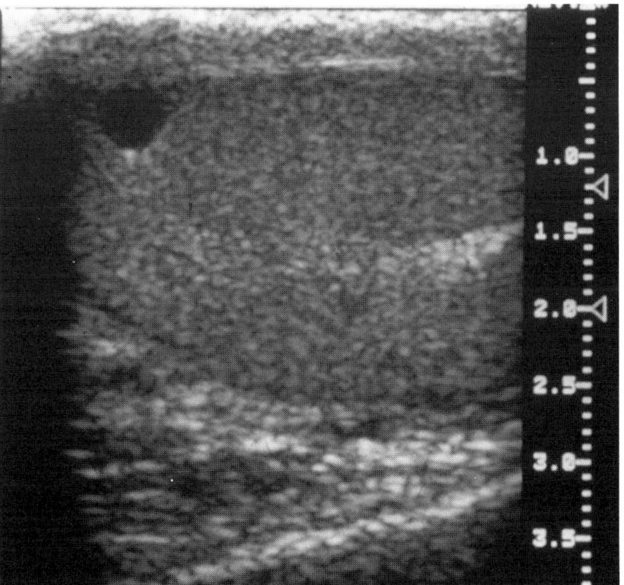

Fig. 23.13 Small cyst of the tunica albuginea.

Vascular conditions

Varicoceles are abnormal dilatation of the veins draining the testis and pampiniform plexus (Fig. 23.15). They are most commonly seen in the lower pole of the left testis and more than 90% occur here. They commonly occur being reported in more than 10% of men. They are important indicators of three main conditions:

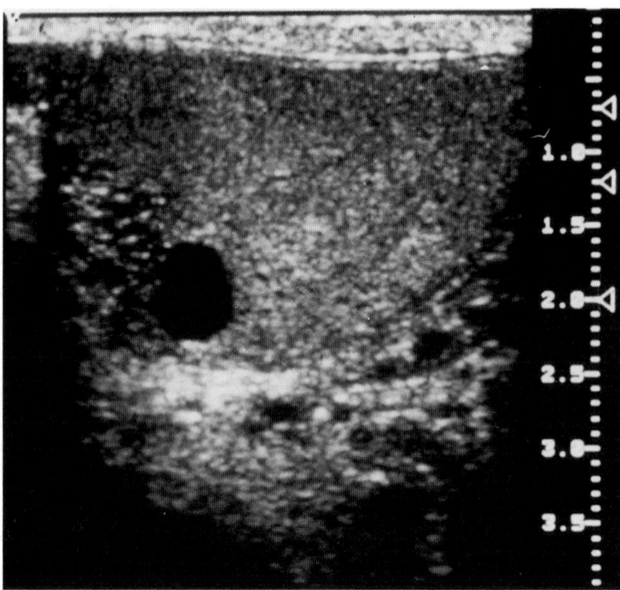

Fig. 23.14 A small intratesticular cyst adjacent to the rete testis and with some associated tubular dilatation in this region.

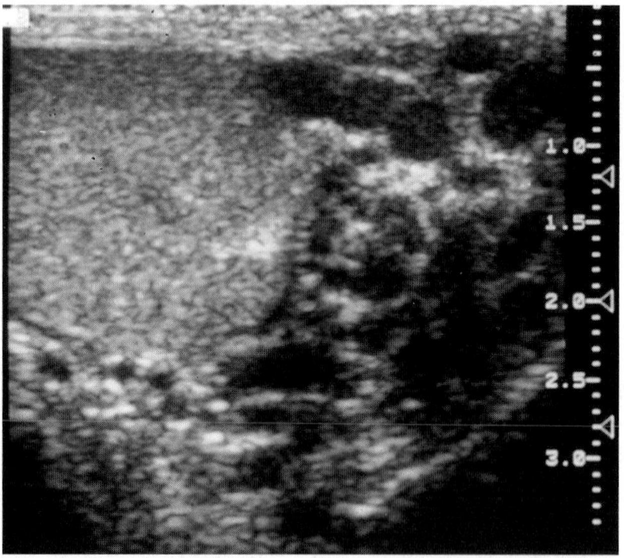

Fig. 23.15 A large left varicocele.

1 as a cause of ache or pain;
2 as a cause of infertility; and
3 associated with renal carcinoma.

If a varicocele suddenly appears, rapidly enlarges or is on the right side, renal ultrasound should be performed to exclude renal carcinoma. The ultrasound appearances are of multiple interconnecting tubular structures with slow venous flow demonstrated on colour Doppler. Torsion in the scrotum may involve the appendix testis or the spermatic cord both presenting with severe acute pain. Appendiceal torsion is not reliably diagnosed by ultrasound imaging. Torsion of the cord results from abnormal movement of the testis relative to the epididymis and cord compromising the blood supply. The ischaemia produced is critical and prompt diagnosis and treatment is essential. The grey-scale ultrasound appearances may be identical to those found in epididymo-orchitis but Doppler ultrasound is a very useful diagnostic aid in adults. Unfortunately in prepubertal boys intratesticular vessels may be too small to detect confidently with colour Doppler equipment. In this group diagnosis may be excluded by Doppler studies but not confirmed. The diagnosis depends on the exclusion of normal flow in intratesticular vessels. In adults specificity and sensitivity are in the order of 95–99%. False negatives may be found in incomplete torsion and in spontaneous detorsion. In cases of incomplete torsion spectral analysis of the Doppler signal will reveal absent or reversed diastolic flow.

Trauma

Owing to the mobility of the testis and the protective covering of the scrotal wall true ruptures of the testes are rare. Most injuries are treated conservatively. If surgical repair is required it must be performed within 3 days; early surgery reduces the rate of orchidectomy from 50 to 5%. Its diagnosis is therefore of great importance. Irregularity of testicular contour and either areas of high or low reflectivity are characteristic of testicular injury. However, direct visualization of the fracture line is rare. The most important role of ultrasound is to demonstrate the integrity of the tunica albuginea, in which case conservative management is appropriate.

Haemtomas are readily demonstrated with ultrasound (Fig. 23.16). The diagnosis of haematocele is established on the basis of a hydrocele-like fluid collection containing numerous low level reflectors.

Miscellaneous conditions

Hernia

A scrotal hernia is secondary to an inguinal hernia; this is mostly indirect via the inguinal canal. The majority of scrotal hernias are easily and correctly diagnosed by clinical examination. Chronic hernias may be irreducible and mimic a scrotal mass and the diagnosis may not always be obvious. The hernia usually shows as a heterogeneous mass that can be traced to the inguinal canal. Omental hernias are usually highly reflective. Chronic hernias can cause compression of the normal scrotal contents and produce consequent testicular atrophy.

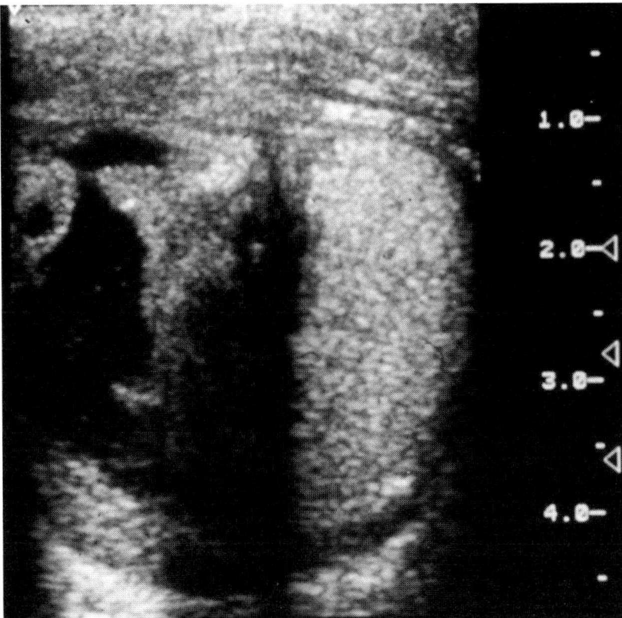

Fig. 23.16 A large haematoma occupying much of the scrotum and deforming the normal testis.

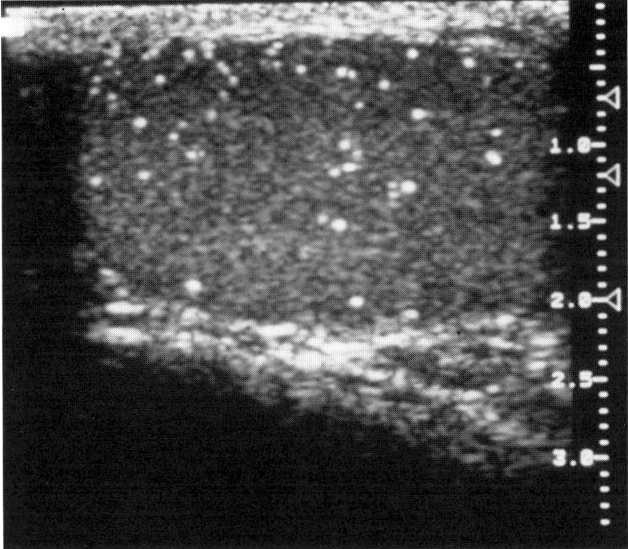

Fig. 23.17 Microlithiasis testis.

Microlithiasis

Testicular microlithiasis is a benign but possibly premalignant condition. On ultrasound it appears as bilateral symmetrical highly reflective foci of a millimetre or two in diameter producing a 'shimmering' appearance as the testis is scanned by the ultrasound beam (Fig. 23.17). The condition is rare, asymptomatic and non-progressive. It is usually idiopathic but an association has been identified between microlithiasis and certain conditions such as Klinefelter's syndrome, undescended testis and male pseudohermaphroditism. Histologically microcalcifications are seen within the seminiferous tubules. In patients shown to have testicular microlithiasis on ultrasound there is a high incidence of malignancy which is well reported in the literature. It is not clear whether this correlation is related to a high incidence of tumours in patients referred for ultrasound or whether this is a true association. There is no doubt that it remains an interesting incidental observation in many cases. To date there have been no reports of a case of microlithiasis testis subsequently developing a tumour. Nonetheless common policy in many centres is to be cautious and to perform serum estimations of tumour markers and rescan after an interval of 12 months paying particular attention to the texture of the testis.

Further reading

Albert, N.E. (1980) Testicular ultrasound for trauma. *Journal of Urology* **124**, 558.

Atkinson, G.O., Patrick, L.E., Ball, T.I., Stephenson, C.A., Broeckner, B.H., Woodard, J.R. (1992) The normal and abnormal scrotum in children: evaluation with colour Doppler sonography. *American Journal of Roentgenology* **158**, 613–617.

Backus, M.L., Mack, L.A., Middleton, W.D., King, B.F., Winter, T.C., True, L.D. (1994) Testicular microlithiasis: imaging appearances and pathologic correlation. *Radiology* **192**, 781–785.

Bird, K., Rosenfield, A.T., Taylor, K.J.W. (1983) Ultrasonography in testicular torsion. *Radiology* **147**, 527.

Burks, D.D., Markey, B.J., Burkhand, T.K., *et al.* (1990) Suspected testicular torsion and ischaemia: evaluation with colour Doppler sonography. *Radiology* **175**, 815.

Comiter, C.V., Benson, C.J., Capelouto, C.C., *et al.* (1995) Non palpable intratesticular masses detected sonographically. *Journal of Urology* **154**, 1367–1369.

Erden, M.I., Ozbek, S.S., Aytac, S.K., Adsan, O., Suzer, O., Safak, S.M. (1993) Colour Doppler imaging in acute scrotal disorders. *Urology International* **50**, 39–42.

Fitzgerald, S.W., Erickson, S., de Wire, D.M., *et al.* (1992) Colour Doppler sonography in the evaluation of the adult acute scrotum. *Journal of Ultrasound in Medicine* **11**, 543–548.

Friedland, G.W., Chang, P. (1988) The role of imaging in the management of the impalpable undescended testis. *American Journal of Roentgenology* **151**, 1107.

Gooding, G.A., Leonhardt, W., Stein, R. (1987) Testicular cysts: US findings. *Radiology* **163**, 537–538.

Hamm, B., Fobbe, F. (1995) Maturation of the testis: ultrasound evaluation. *Ultrasound in Medicine and Biology* **21**, 143–147.

Hamm, B., Fobbe, F., Loy, V. (1988) Testicular cysts: differentiation with US and clinical findings. *Radiology* **168**, 19–23.

Hobarth, K., Susani, M., Szabo, N., Kratzik, C. (1992) Incidence of testicular microlithiasis. *Urology* **40**, 464–467.

Holden, A., List, A. (1994) Extratesticular lesions: a radiological and pathological correlation. *Australasia Radiology* **38**, 99–105.

Horstman, W.G., Melson, G.L., Middleton, W.D., Andriole, G.L. (1992) Testicular tumours: findings with colour Doppler US. *Radiology* **185**, 733–737.

Hricak, H., Hamm, B., Kim, B. (1995) *Imaging of the Scrotum*. Raven Press, New York.

Jarvis, L.J. Dubbins, P.A. (1989) Changes in the epididymis after vasectomy: sonographic findings. *American Journal of Roentgenology* **152**, 531–534.

Johnson, K.A., Dewbury, K.C. (1996) Ultrasound imaging of the appendix testis and appendix epididymis. *Clinical Radiology* **51**, 335–337.

Kim, S.H., Pollack, H.M., Cho, K.S., Pollack, M.S., Han, M.C. (1993) Tuberculous epididymitis and epididymo-orchitis: sonographic findings. *Journal of Urology* **150**, 80–84.

Langer, J.E. (1993) Ultrasound of the scrotum. *Seminars in Roentgenology* **28**, 5–18.

Learch, T.J., Hansch, L.P., Ralls, P.W. (1993) US of ballistic scrotal trauma. *Radiology* **189**, 156.

Lentini, J.F., Benson, C.B., Richie, J.P. (1989) Sonography of the male genital tract. *American Journal of Roentgenology* **153**, 705–713.

Lerner, R.M., Mevorach, R.A., Hulbert, W.C., Rabinowitz, R. (1990) Colour Doppler US in the evaluation of acute scrotal disease. *Radiology* **176**, 355–358.

Makarainen, H., Tammela, T., Karttunen, T., Mattila, S., Hellstrom, P., Kontturi, M. (1993) Intrascrotal adenomatoid tumours and their ultrasound findings. *Journal of Clinical Urology* **21**, 33–37.

Marth, D., Scheideggar, J., Studer, U.E. (1990) Ultrasonography of testicular tumours. *Urology International* **45**, 237.

Maxwell, A.J., Mantora, H. (1990) Sonographic appearance of epidermoid cysts of the testis. *Journal of Clinical Ultrasound* **18**, 188.

Pryor, J.A., Walson, L.R., Day, D.L., *et al*. (1994) Scrotal US for evaluation of subacute testicular torsion: sonographic findings and adverse clinical applications. *Journal of Urology* **151**, 693–697.

Ralls, P.W., Larsen, D., Johnson, M.B., Lee, K.P. (1991) Colour Doppler sonography of the scrotum. *Seminars in Ultrasound, CT, MRI* **12**, 109–114.

Sanderson, A.J., Birch, B.R., Dewbury, K.C. (1995) Multiple epidermoid cysts of the testes—the ultrasound appearances. *Clinical Radiology* **50**, 414–415.

Tartar, V.M., Trambert, M.A., Balsara, Z.N., Mattrey, R.F. (1993) Tubular ectasia of the testicle: sonographic and MR imaging appearances. *American Journal of Roentgenology* **160**, 539–542.

Thomas, R.D., Dewbury, K.C. (1993) Appearances of rete testis. *Clinical Radiology* **47**, 121–124.

Weiss, A.J., Kellman, G.M., Middleton, W.D., Kirkemo, A. (1992) Intratesticular varicocele: sonographic findings in two patients. *American Journal of Roentenology* **158**, 1061–1063.

Whitaker, R.H. (1992) Undescended testis: the need for a standard classification. *British Journal of Urology* **70**, 1–6.

Wilbert, D.M., Schaerfe, C.W., Stern, W.D., Strohmaier, W.L., Bichler, K.H. (1993) Evaluation of the acute scrotum by colour-coded Doppler ultrasonography. *Journal of Urology* **149**, 1474–1477.

Wood, A., Dewbury, K.C. (1995) Paratesticular rhabdomyosarcoma—colour Doppler appearances. *Clinical Radiology* **50**, 130–131.

Chapter 24: The eye and orbit

N.C. McMillan & G.M. Baxter

The eye and orbit

N.C. MCMILLAN

General principles

Early methods of examining the eye by ultrasound relied on the A-scan display and required the use of a water bath or other transonic material to enable the anterior structures to be seen. Technological progress has produced high frequency transducers with small heads which can be placed directly onto the surface of the closed lid with a coupling gel. Some of these probes incorporate a stand-off effect to allow the anterior chamber to be within the focus of the ultrasound beam. Some manufacturers supply dedicated eye ultrasound machines which are appropriate for exclusive use in ophthalmic departments, but for the occasional examination in a district general hospital it is more efficient to have a general purpose machine with a small parts probe which is capable of imaging the eye and other superficial organs. With appropriate training and experience direct contact ultrasound of the eye through the closed lid can be performed by a radiologist in such a department [1].

Most ultrasound imaging of the eye and orbit can be satisfactorily achieved with a transducer operating at a frequency of 7.5–10 MHz. This is sufficient to provide the necessary resolution for the detection of intraocular pathology while allowing adequate penetration to show abnormalities in the orbit. While there are numerous references in the literature to the A-scan method, the author utilizes the B-scan method for all ultrasound examinations of the eye.

Ultrasound remains poor at imaging the structures at the apex of the orbit and suspected disease in this area is best examined by magnetic resonance imaging (MRI) or computed tomography (CT).

Technique

With direct contact scanning the patient may be examined seated or lying supine. In most cases it is a matter of preference of the operator; however, there are some instances in which the position of the patient will influence the quality of the images obtained, e.g. the presence of intraocular silicone or air, both of which prevent the normal transmission of sound. They are both less dense than vitreous and therefore float on the vitreous surface.

After the application of a non-irritant coupling gel the transducer is gently applied to the front of the closed eyelid. It is simpler to scan initially in the transverse plane, with the maximum area of the posterior segment visualized by scanning while the patient is asked to look slowly from side to side. A lesion which lies peripheral to the posterior pole of the eye will be better seen if the gaze is directed towards the side of the pathology. The examination can then be repeated in the sagittal or relevant oblique planes.

It is often difficult to image the superior quadrant as some patients find upward gaze awkward while being scanned. It may also be difficult to assess the inferior part of the eye or orbit if the patient has a prominent orbital rim. For the measurements of an intraocular mass it is important to scan in the most appropriate plane or obliquity for accurate assessment of the size of the lesion. If possible the sound wave should be perpendicular to the surface of the tumour.

Dynamic scanning (real-time visualization of intraocular structures during repeated regular eye movements) allows the operator to study the motion characteristics of any underlying pathology. In complex cases this can facilitate the differentiation between vitreous and retinal detachments, or between haemorrhage and a solid tumour.

Direct contact scanning allows an examination to be performed safely soon after acute trauma, accidental or surgical; however, a very gentle approach is required to prevent any further damage.

Normal anatomy

Figure 24.1 shows the appearances of a normal eye and orbit. The anterior and posterior chambers are normally

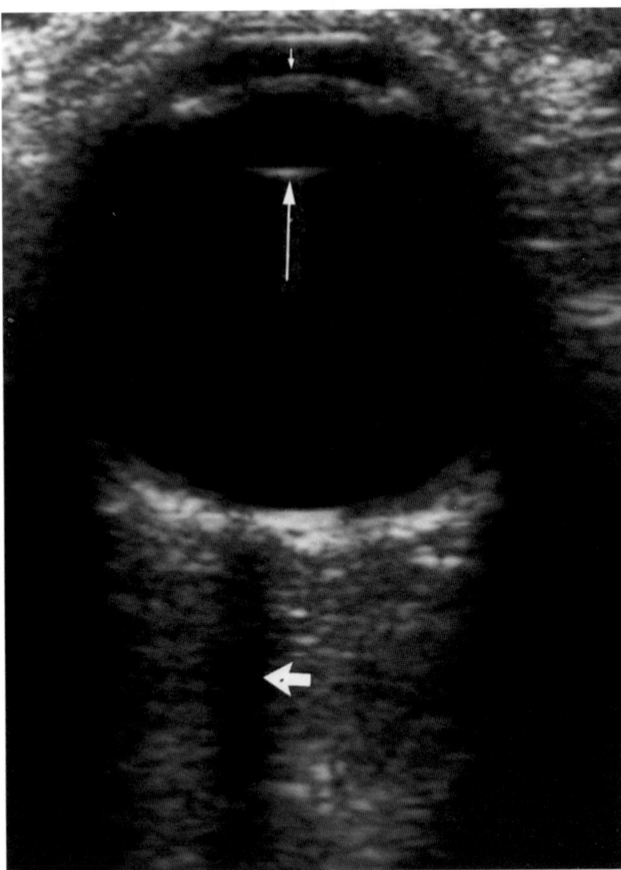

Fig. 24.1 Normal eye and orbit. Note anterior lens echo (small thin arrow), posterior lens echo (long thin arrow) and optic nerve (short thick arrow).

transonic; however, from middle-age the vitreous often contains diffuse low reflectivity echoes due to shrinkage caused by diminished water content and loss of elasticity. This appearance is such a common finding that it may simply be due to the normal ageing process in the eye.

The anterior and posterior surfaces of the lens are highly reflective but the central part of the lens is normally sonolucent.

It is not possible to separate individually the retina, choroid and sclera on a B-scan in the normal eye with transducer frequencies of 7–10 MHz. Dedicated machines incorporating standardized echography and much higher probe frequencies provide a detailed A-scan in addition to a B-scan image for diagnosis. A-scan methods of imaging are almost never used by the general radiologist, and although their value in the differential diagnosis of choroidal tumours is well established [2], the availability of colour flow Doppler (CFD) imaging is likely to be a more readily applicable technique to those involved in non-specialist units [3].

The retrobulbar region consists mainly of the extraocular muscles, optic nerve and orbital blood vessels. These are all hypoechoic structures and are readily identified within the highly reflective retrobulbar fat. CFD techniques enable blood flow within arteries and veins to be visualized and quantified. Potential uses include the assessment of flow in tumours before and after treatment (see below).

It is appropriate to discuss the role of ultrasound in ophthalmic disease by looking at the eye and orbit as two separate anatomical regions. The general indications for orbital ultrasound are outlined in Table 24.1.

Table 24.1 Indications for orbital ultrasound

Reduced visual acuity, due to opaque media
cataract
intraocular blood
Vitreous haemorrhage
extent
density
position
Retinal detachment
nature (serous, solid, fixed, mobile)
Intraocular tumour
position
size
echo pattern
Trauma
extent of damage
foreign body localization
Acute pain in a chronically blind eye
may indicate underlying tumour
Proptosis
unilateral
bilateral
CFD assessment
Biometry

The eye

Anatomically the eye is divided into anterior and posterior chambers which are separated by the iris and lens. The anterior chamber is readily examined clinically whereas the posterior segment may be obscured by opaque media such as cataract or vitreous haemorrhage. Ultrasound is particularly useful for the assessment of pathology in the posterior segment of the eye. It is appropriate to consider the separate structures of the eye and how they may be affected by disease.

Lens

In normal healthy individuals this is a biconvex transonic structure which is readily identified by its anterior position and high reflectivity echoes from its anterior and posterior surfaces. There are few conditions which affect the lens and require ultrasound examination.

In cataract the lens becomes progressively opaque with the clear central echolucency replaced by varying degrees of abnormal internal echoes. Ultrasound has no specific role in the assessment of cataract although it is increasingly requested preoperatively to exclude occult posterior segment pathology which cannot be directly visualized, e.g. retinal detachment or tumour. Ultrasound is sometimes helpful in assessing the position of a dislocated lens after trauma, although the damage is often so extensive that the lens cannot be identified within the multiple vitreous echoes resulting from haemorrhage.

Intraocular lens implants for cataract do not prevent ultrasound examination but some materials produce a typical acoustic reverberation artefact (Fig. 24.2)

Iris

The iris is the most anterior structure of the uveal tract. Inflammatory changes are clinically apparent and do not require imaging. Tumours of the iris are uncommon but are usually pigmented lesions such as naevi or melanoma. These lesions are usually small and can be visualized by standard ophthalmic examination. Ultrasound is helpful in determining the posterior extent of any mass prior to surgical excision and in distinguishing between a solid and cystic pathology [4].

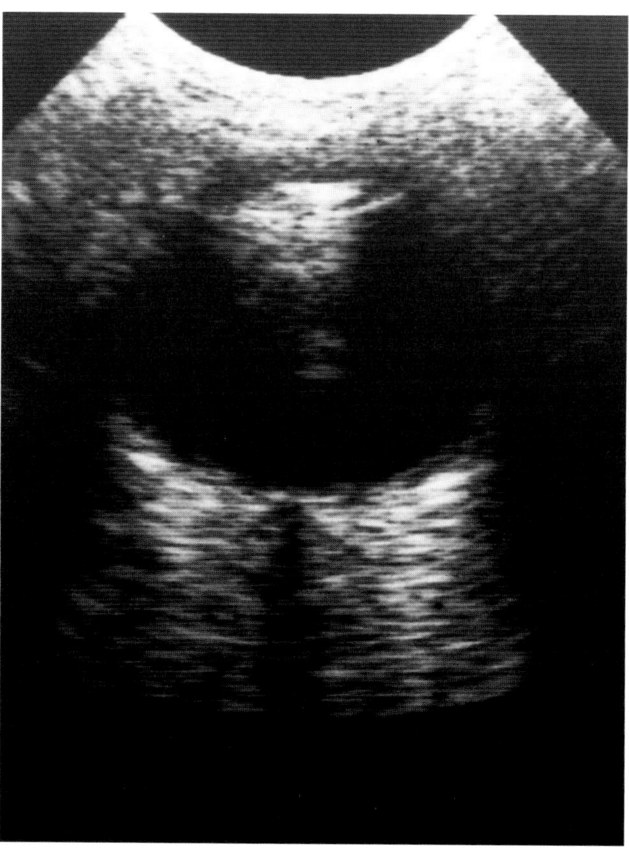

Fig. 24.2 Intraocular lens implant. Typical reverberation echoes.

Melanomas of the iris have a better prognosis than those arising elsewhere in the uveal tract [5]. This is partly due to their earlier detection, even when they are small, and the need for less invasive surgery. Ultrasound is rarely able to provide a diagnosis due to the small size of these tumours, and the similar echo characteristics of metastatic tumour and melanoma in this location. It is important to look for posterior extension of an iris melanoma into the ciliary body as this may influence the surgical approach.

Vitreous

DETACHMENT

The vitreous is a firm jelly-like material made up of fluid in a fine collagen matrix. It is normally echolucent but with age the vitreous loses elasticity and shrinks causing it to detach posteriorly (Fig. 24.3). Scanning during side to side eye movements will elicit a slow 'delayed action' swirling appearance of any contained echoes. These non-haemorrhagic multiple low reflectivity echoes cause no significant visual impairment.

HAEMORRHAGE

Vitreous haemorrhage is a common problem and even if slight can result in a marked loss of visual acuity. Bleeding may occur diffusely into the vitreous substance (intragel; see Fig. 24.3), or into the potential space behind the vitreous (retrogel or subhyaloid; Fig. 24.4). The latter appearance is more usually seen in diabetic patients in which the haemorrhage is secondary to a retinopathy and neovascularization posteriorly.

Fibrous bands may form as a consequence of previous haemorrhage, and can be detected by ultrasound. It is important to note the presence or absence of mobility as a fixed, taut band may cause a traction detachment of the retina.

ASTEROID HYALOSIS

This is an uncommon, usually unilateral, condition of the vitreous, in which there are multiple small calcific opacities present within the gel. It is an incidental clinical finding in an otherwise healthy eye, and does not cause any loss of visual acuity. It has a characteristic ultrasonic

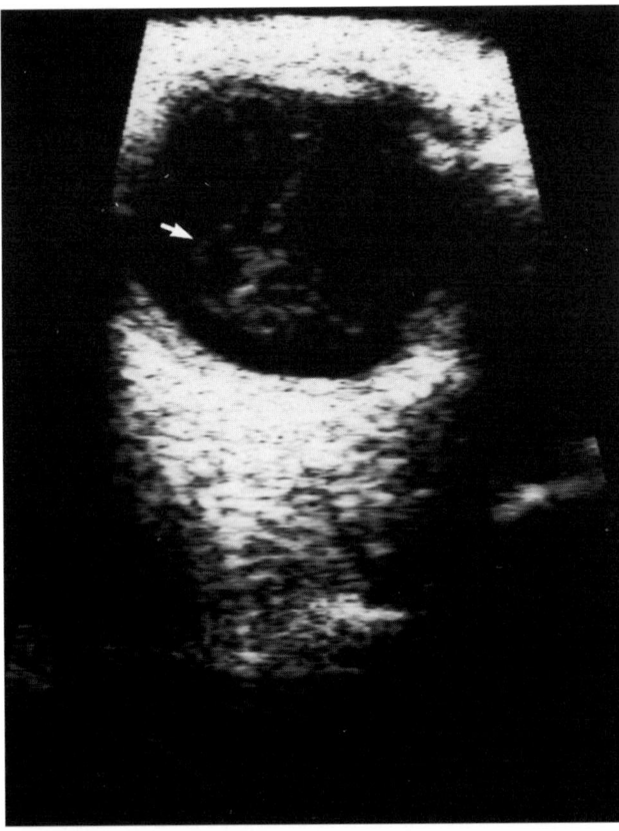

Fig. 24.3 Vitreous haemorrhage—intragel. Associated posterior vitreous detachment shown by arrow.

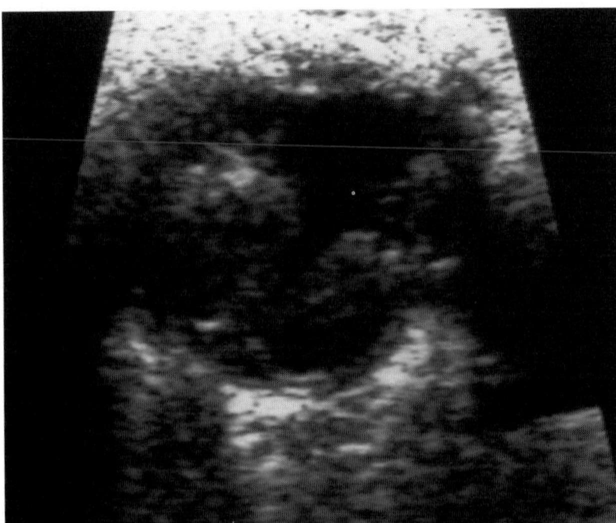

Fig. 24.4 Vitreous haemorrhage—retrogel or subhyaloid collection. Normal vitreous is the echo-free zone anteriorly.

appearance of numerous small highly reflective echoes in the posterior chamber which move within the vitreous (Fig. 24.5).

Additional causes of abnormal echoes in the vitreous include debris as a result of previous inflammation or intraocular spread of tumour from a melanoma. The ultrasound findings in such pathologies may be indistinguishable from haemorrhage.

PERSISTENT HYPERPLASTIC PRIMARY VITREOUS

This is a developmental abnormality resulting from incomplete regression of the embryonic hyaloid vascular system with failure of the vitreous to form completely as a single entity. It is a unilateral condition and typically presents in young children with leukocoria, microphthalmia and lens opacity. On ultrasound it appears as a single echogenic strand running behind the lens to the optic disc (Fig. 24.6).

Retina

This is the neural layer between the vitreous and choroid, extending from the ora serrata to the optic nerve head. In

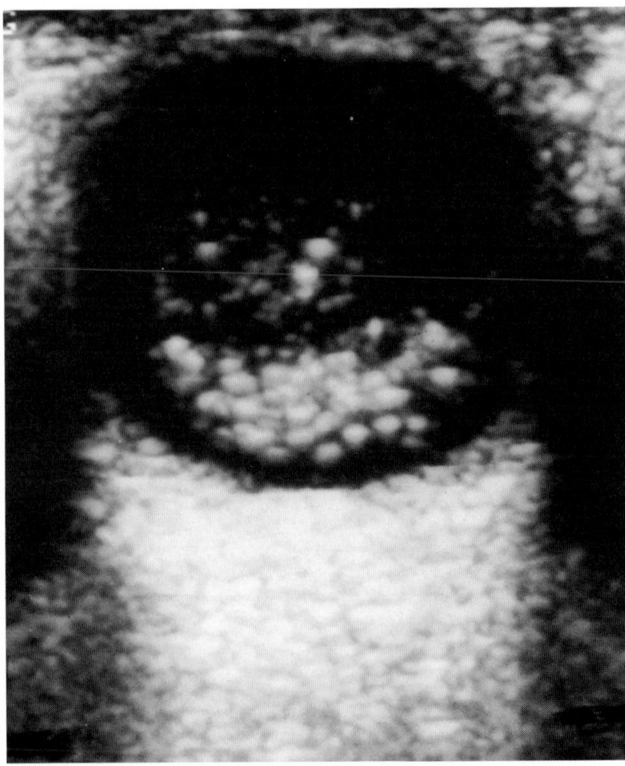

Fig. 24.5 Asteroid hyalosis of the vitreous.

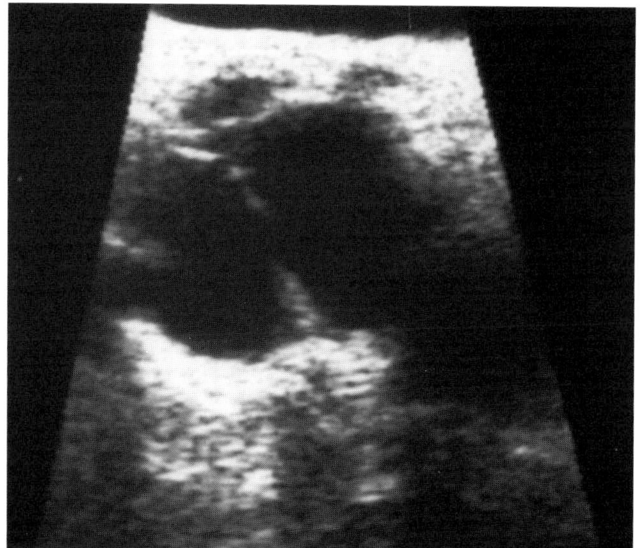

Fig. 24.6 Persistent hyperplastic primary vitreous.

its normal position the retina cannot be identified separately from choroid on conventional B-scans.

DETACHMENT

Clinical suspicion of retinal detachment is a common reason for performing eye ultrasound. It may occur as a primary complication as a result of a tear in the retina (rhegmatogenous) or be secondary to an underlying mass. The degree of detachment may be localized to one area of the posterior quadrant, or involve the entire retina (Fig. 24.7).

The retina is fixed posteriorly at the optic disc where the neural fibres form the optic nerve. In early detachment and in the absence of severe trauma the retina is usually mobile and this can be shown on dynamic scanning. Long-standing detachments may cause the retina to fibrose and thicken and ultimately become funnel-shaped (Fig. 24.8). Such end-stage disease does not permit any real prospect of restoration of vision. In some cases of long-standing detachment focal cystic degeneration may occur. Haemorrhage into such cysts, although rare, can mimic a solid tumour.

Surgical treatment may involve the placing of a strap ('plomb') around the globe to approximate the retina to the eye wall. This has a typical appearance of a highly reflective indentation of the globe on ultrasound (Fig. 24.9).

RETINOPATHY OF PREMATURITY

This is a bilateral retinal disease which occurs in premature infants. It causes total blindness and is due to pro-

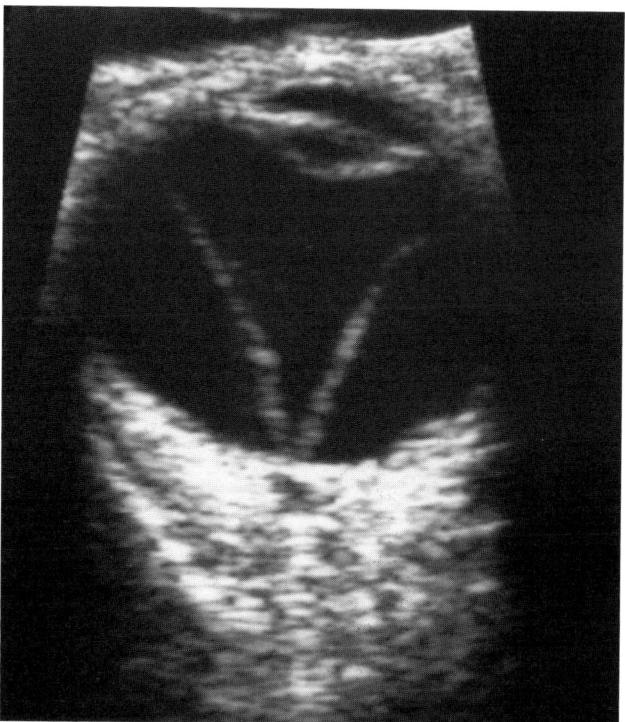

Fig. 24.7 Total detachment of the retina, rhegmatogenous.

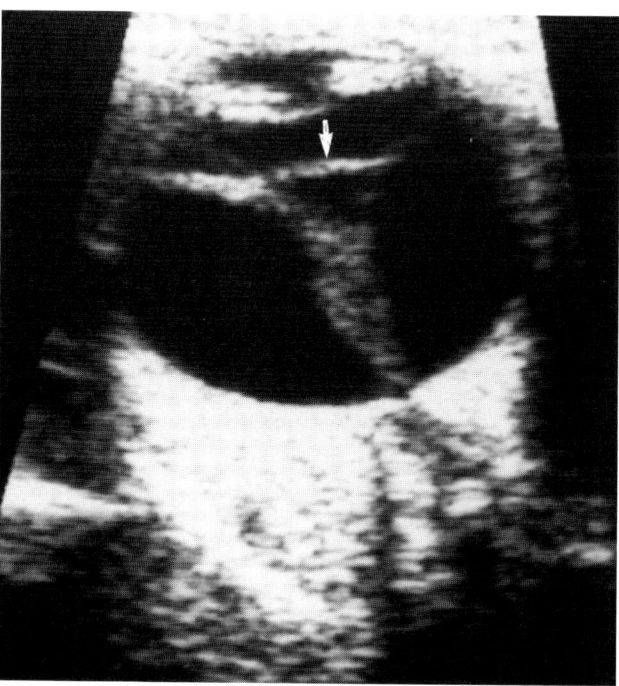

Fig. 24.8 Funnel detachment of the retina. This is typically associated with an anterior cyclitic membrane (arrow).

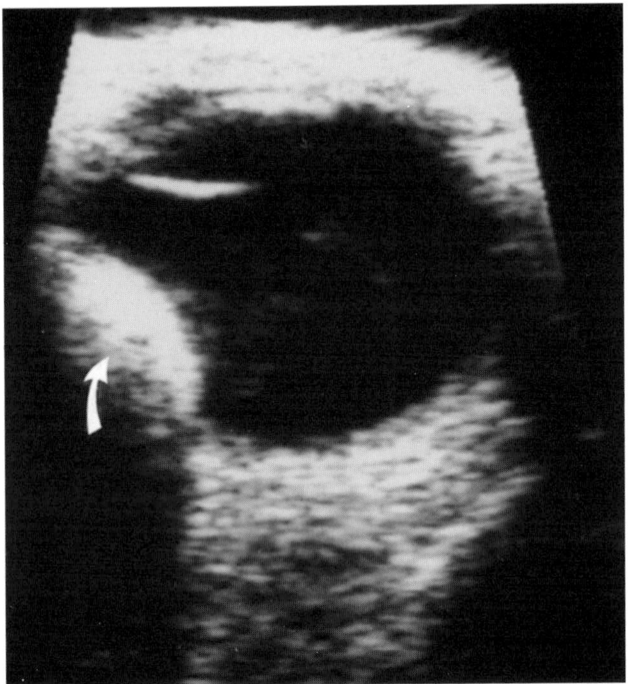

Fig. 24.9 Retinal plomb. The highly reflective buckle is shown (arrow).

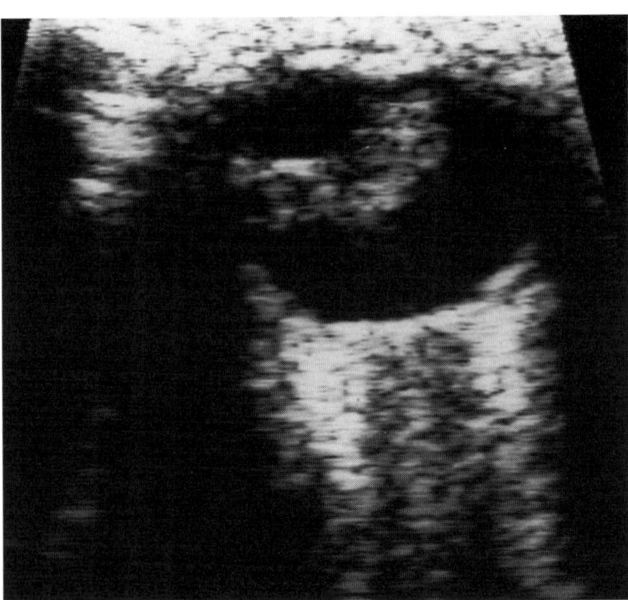

Fig. 24.10 Retinopathy of prematurity.

longed exposure to high concentrations of oxygen in early life. Improvements in neonatal care have markedly reduced the incidence of the condition. Vascular spasm and oedema of the immature retina are followed by fibrovascular proliferation into the vitreous and subsequent retinal detachment. The ultrasound findings usually reflect the end-stage of the process with a diffusely thick layer of echoes immediately behind the normal lens (Fig. 24.10).

RETINAL TUMOURS

Retinoblastoma

This is the most common malignant eye tumour in children [6]. The patient usually presents in the first few years of life with leukocoria ('white pupil'), and often has an eye which has gone blind but remained undetected by the child or parent.

Clinical examination of the eye usually reveals a large intraocular mass which can be readily confirmed by ultrasound. The tumours are moderately reflective, and the invariable presence of areas of highly reflective echoes due to internal calcification is highly suggestive of retinoblastoma (Fig. 24.11). In some cases there is only dense surface calcification. Retinoblastomas arise in eyes which are normal or slightly enlarged. This can be helpful in the differential diagnosis as both persistent hyperplastic primary vitreous (PHPV) and retinopathy of prematurity occur in small eyes.

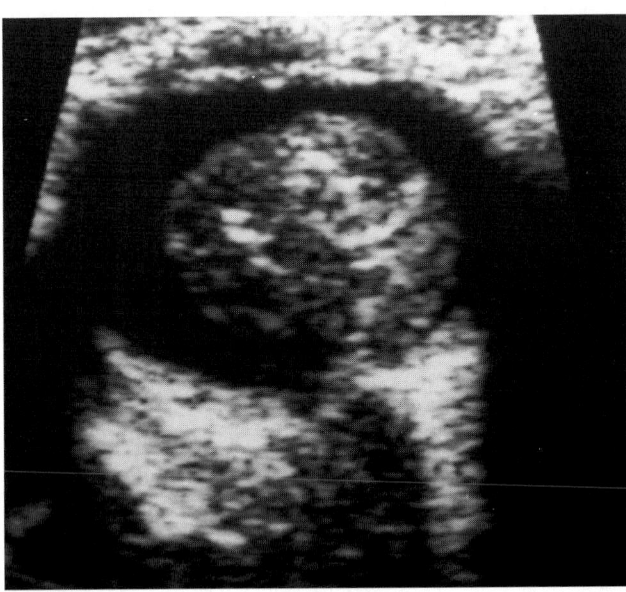

Fig. 24.11 Retinoblastoma. Note the multiple small central areas of high reflectivity due to calcification within the tumour.

Retinoblastoma has a genetic influence being more common in children with a family history. In 30% of patients the tumour is bilateral and examination of the 'normal' eye is advisable if there is any clinical concern. Other causes of leukocoria include Coats' disease and *Toxocara* infection.

Retinal angioma

This benign tumour occurs in adults and rarely grows to a size greater than a few millimetres in diameter. It may calcify and be visible only as a small echogenic mass. In some patients it is associated with similar renal angiomas of von Hippel–Lindau syndrome.

Choroid

This is the pigment layer of the eye and is only detectable on conventional B-scans when abnormally thickened or detached. The main pathological processes involving the choroid for which ultrasound examination may be useful include detachment due to effusion or haemorrhage, inflammatory conditions and neoplasms.

DETACHMENT

Detachment of the choroid has a characteristic sonographic appearance. There is separation of the peripheral choroid but with fixation posteriorly where the four vortex veins (one per quadrant) are attached. This results in the biconcave picture seen in Fig. 24.12. In a choroidal effusion the fluid underneath the detachment is transonic, whereas in haemorrhage it contains multiple echoes. This situation may be caused by a sudden reduction in intraocular pressure following trauma or as a complication of surgery.

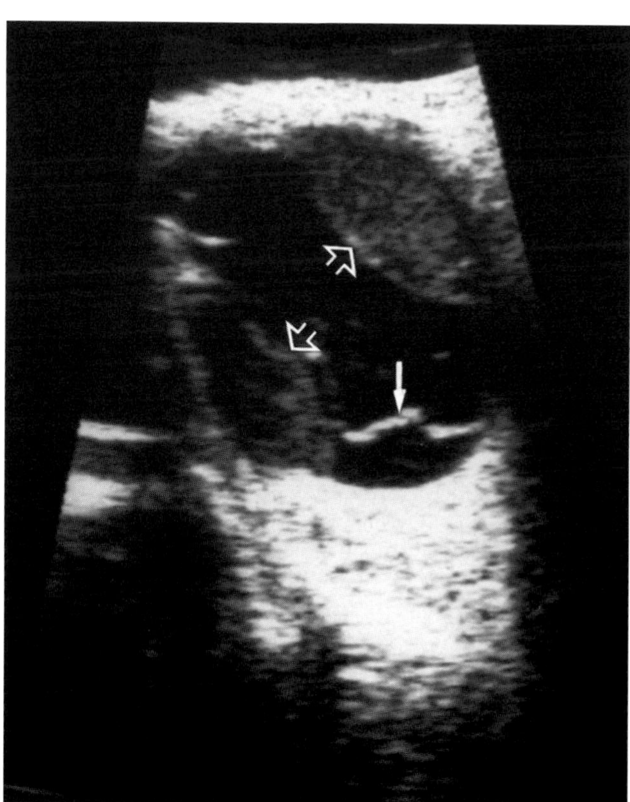

Fig. 24.12 Choroidal haemorrhage (open arrows). Note co-existent retinal detachment (white arrow).

CHOROIDITIS

This is usually part of a more generalized uveitis, and may be associated with systemic diseases such as sarcoidosis or seronegative arthropathies. The ultrasound features are often normal but some patients have evidence of thickening of the choroidoretinal layer (Fig. 24.13). The examination is most useful in determining a baseline measurement on which to assess the effects of therapy. There is often little sonographic change over a period of many months despite clinical improvement.

CHOROIDAL TUMOURS

Melanoma

This is the commonest primary malignant intraocular tumour in adults and typically arises in the pigment epithelium of the choroid although it can develop anywhere within the uveal tract. the location and size of the tumour are the prime determinants of the possible treatment options. Although these tumours are normally pig-

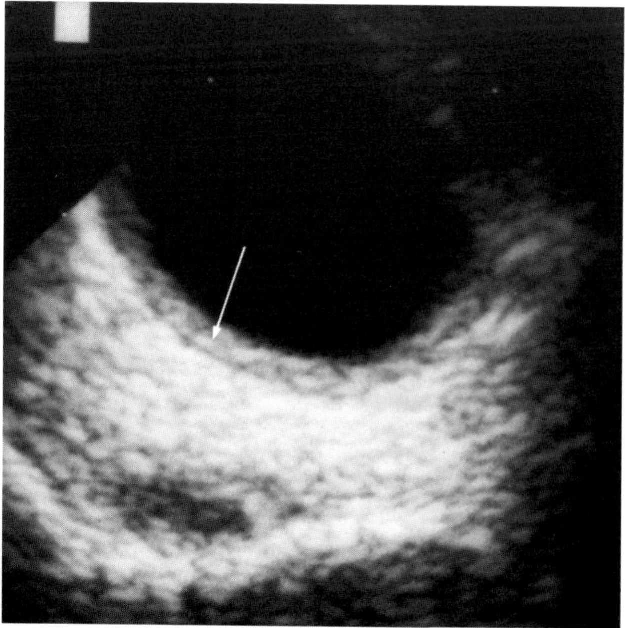

Fig. 24.13 Uveitis—thickened choroidal layer within the eye (arrow).

mented a minority of them are amelanotic. This may cause some diagnostic difficulty on clinical examination.

Melanomas of the ciliary body have a similar prognosis to those of the choroid. The cell type of the tumour is thought to be the most significant factor in the estimation of prognosis [7]. This cannot yet be determined reliably by any standard imaging method. The largest tumour diameter is another critical prognostic factor, this being relatively good if it is less than 10 mm [8]. Ultrasound can provide a fairly accurate indication of the size and position of these tumours and is essential in determining their suitability for surgery.

Melanomas have a relatively low reflectivity as a consequence of the densely packed nature of the cells within the tumour. This reduces the number of tissue interfaces and causes greater sound attenuation through the mass. The majority of melanomas are found in the pigment epithelium of the choroid. Most cause an elliptical elevation of the overlying retina (Fig. 24.14). Some tumours become narrowed towards the base and adopt a 'mushroom' or 'collar-stud' shape (Fig. 24.15). This appearance is due to tumour breaking through Bruch's membrane and is pathognomonic of melanoma. Melanomas that involve the optic disc are important to detect as therapy options become very limited. Some lesions that arise from a small base in the peripheral choroid are suitable for excision; however, this may not be apparent at ophthalmoscopy where the tumour may appear to overlap the optic disc.

Treatment options include local excision, radiotherapy by ruthenium plaque or proton beam, or photocoagulation by laser. Combinations of these methods are also used. Enucleation of the eye or orbital exenteration may occasionally be necessary in advanced locally invasive orbital disease or in tumours directly involving the optic disc and nerve.

Small lesions, e.g. <3 mm thick, are often observed over a period of months and years for any evidence of growth before definitive treatment is planned.

Amelanotic melanomas can cause diagnostic difficulty and may be confused with choroidal metastases. The ultrasound features are similar to the more typical pigmented lesions and aid the diagnosis. Metastases in the choroid rarely grow to a thickness greater than 3 mm and if irradiated they typically show a very rapid reduction in size, unlike melanoma.

Melanoma may spread within the orbit, usually by direct extension through the sclera. Their low reflectivity is clearly visible in the bright retrobulbar fat (Fig. 24.16).

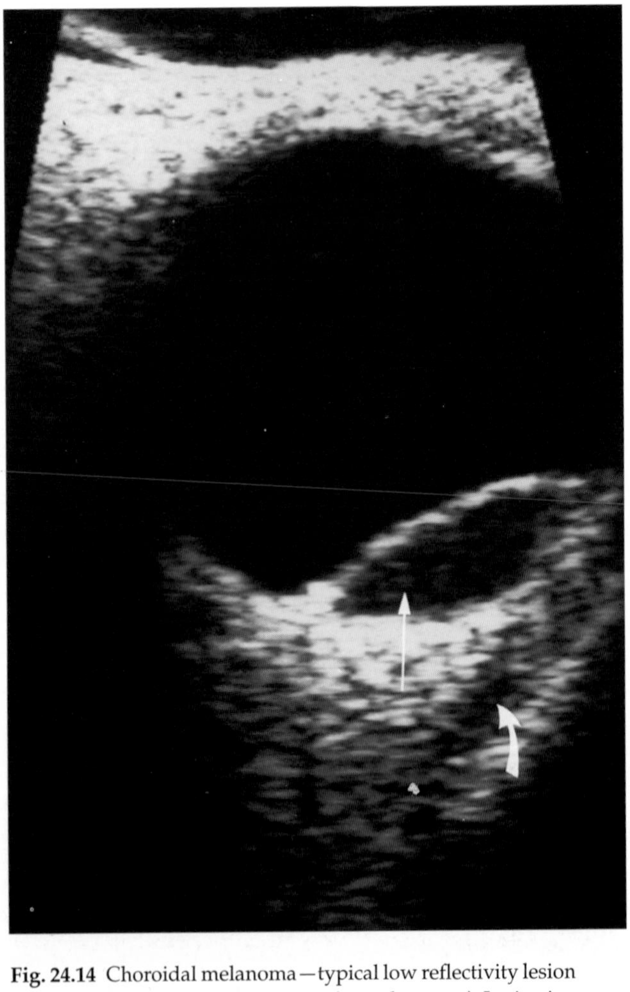

Fig. 24.14 Choroidal melanoma—typical low reflectivity lesion causing elliptical elevation of retina (straight arrow). Lesion is separate from adjacent rectus muscle (curved arrow).

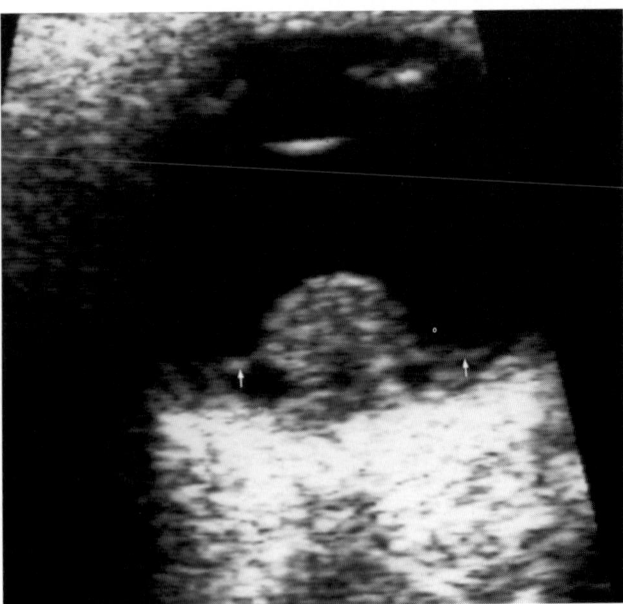

Fig. 24.15 Choroidal melanoma—classic 'collar-stud' configuration. The arrows illustrate the elevated retina.

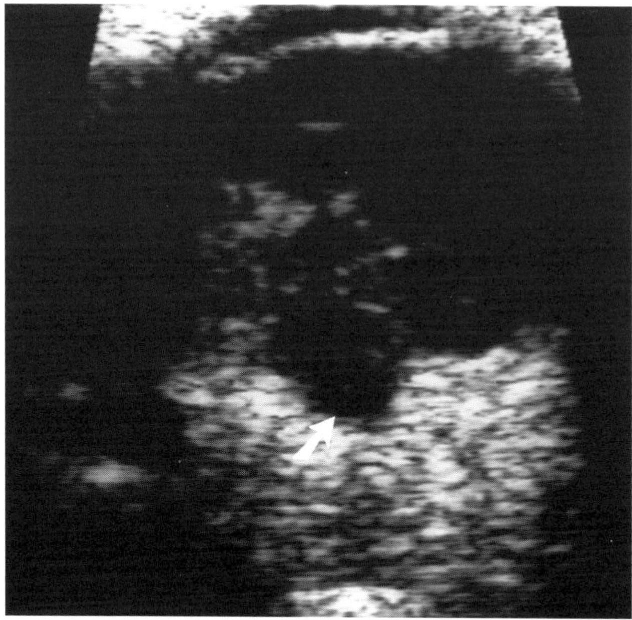

Fig. 24.16 Choroidal melanoma—extrascleral extension (arrow).

This is usually a late development but is more common in association with diffuse choroidal involvement which may be difficult to determine by ultrasound.

The accuracy of placement of a radioactive plaque can be assessed by ultrasound. The plaque is surgically attached to the sclera over the tumour for a sufficient time to give the required radiation dose, but it is sometimes necessary to confirm by ultrasound that the plaque adequately overlaps the tumour margins.

Haemangioma

This benign primary choroidal tumour may appear similar to a melanoma on clinical examination. There are significant ultrasonic differences in internal reflectivity between the two pathologies. Haemangiomas have multiple high intensity echoes within the mass reflecting the tissue interfaces between blood and the vessel walls (Fig. 24.17). They are typically elliptical in shape and are rarely thicker than 5 mm.

Choroidal naevus

These are usually flat or only minimally elevated and frequently not detectable by ultrasound. Those that are visible may not be distinguishable from a melanoma and a more confident diagnosis may only be made after long-term follow-up measurements indicating a lack of growth.

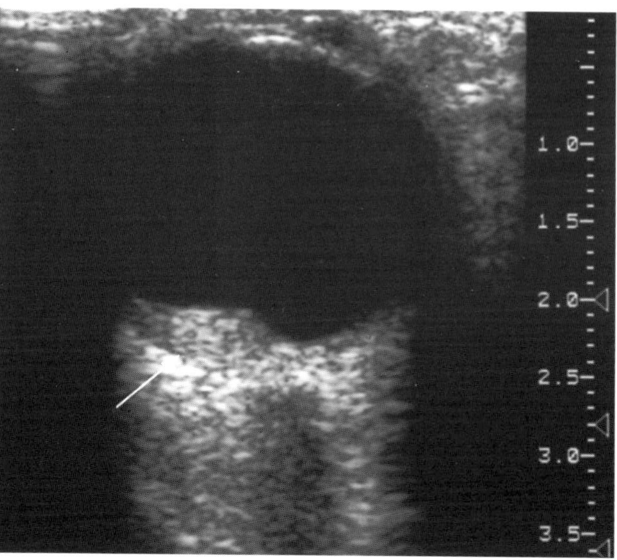

Fig. 24.17 Choroidal haemangioma (arrow). Note the much higher internal echoes compared with Fig. 24.14.

Senile macular degeneration (disciform lesion)

This occurs in the elderly and is a major cause of visual loss in this age group. It is usually diagnosed clinically but in acute cases may present with macular oedema which may mimic a choroidal mass on ultrasound. The diagnosis is supported by the presence of variable echoes within the lesion representing haemorrhage, and its typical macular position (Fig. 24.18). A disciform may be several millimetres in diameter but it is rarely more than a few millimetres thick. They usually decrease in size over a period of months.

Drusen

These are small calcified nodules which develop at the optic nerve head. They cause slight elevation of the optic disc but are distinguished ultrasonically by their highly echogenic appearance.

Staphyloma

These are localized bulges of the eyeball lined with scleral tissue. They may be congenital or occur following trauma or inflammation. They can arise in several sites; an example of a posterior staphyloma is shown in Fig. 24.19.

Ocular trauma

This often results in minor superficial injury to the eye and imaging is not required. In severe ocular trauma ultra-

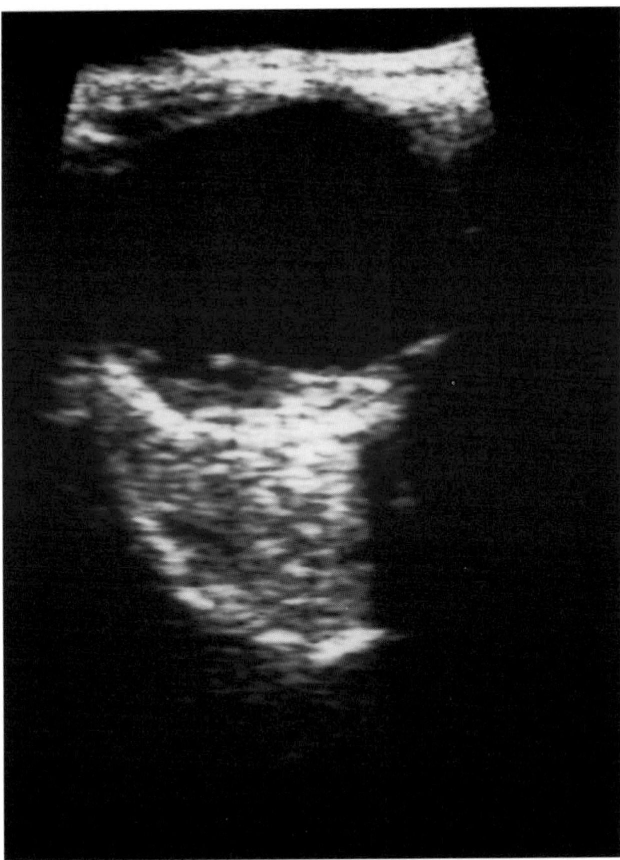

Fig. 24.18 Disciform lesion.

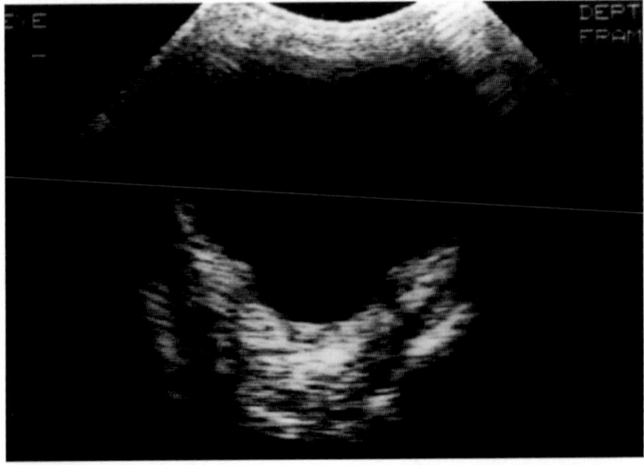

Fig. 24.19 Staphyloma. Note the bulge in the posterior wall of the globe.

sound or CT may be helpful. In possible globe rupture the pressure required to apply the probe to the eye for a satisfactory ultrasound examination may be hazardous and CT is preferable.

Non-metallic foreign bodies can occasionally be identified by ultrasound, but its main indication is to assess the state of the vitreous and retina after penetrating trauma. Severe vitreous haemorrhage may render early retinal assessment impossible and a repeat study after a few days is recommended.

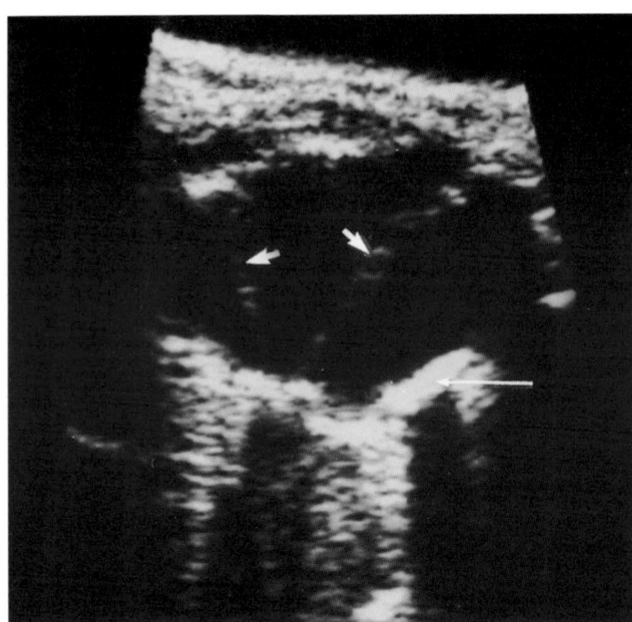

Fig. 24.20 Ocular phthisis. Dense posterior calcification (long arrow). Chronic retinal detachment (small arrows).

PHTHISIS

Chronic changes after trauma may result in globe shrinkage (phthisis); this often results in calcification of the posterior layers of the globe which is detectable by ultrasound (Fig. 24.20). A retinal detachment is often present as a consequence of the initial injury.

SUBRETINAL HAEMORRHAGE

This is an uncommon occurrence but is a recognized postoperative complication. It is often mild but when marked can have ultrasonic appearances similar to a tumour. The recent history and nature of the surgery are important clues to the diagnosis.

OTHER ARTEFACTS

After eye surgery the vitreous may be replaced with a silicone gel or air, in order to keep the eye distended and prevent retinal detatchment. It is important to note that any air must be fully resorbed before the patient undertakes any air travel.

Silicone oil may be injected into the eye at the end of an operation to maintain intraocular pressure. This has a lower sound velocity than the normal eye tissues and the eye consequently appears much larger than expected. The attenuation of sound is markedly affected and the resultant image is often non-diagnostic.

The orbit

Imaging of the orbit is now optimally performed by CT or MRI. Ultrasound is limited because of its inability to penetrate to the orbital apex with satisfactory resolution, although it is a useful screening test for gross retrobulbar pathology in patients with proptosis.

Proptosis

This is the term for abnormal forward displacement of the eyeball. The most frequent causes are shown in Table 24.2.

Dysthyroid eye disease is the most common cause of exophthalmos, unilateral or bilateral. This typically results in thickening of the rectus muscles, with the inferior and medial recti more commonly affected. Ultrasound examination of the medial rectus has been shown to be an accurate method of evaluating the orbits in patients with Graves' disease [9]. However, extraocular muscle thicknesses show a wide variability between individuals and results of ultrasonic measurements should be interpreted cautiously. Studies of normal volunteers comparing ultrasound with MRI have confirmed this and a wide range of maximum thicknesses for each muscle has been proposed [10]. The medial and lateral recti are the easiest of the extraocular muscles to identify and measure by ultrasound. A maximum width of 4 mm for the medial rectus is the author's accepted norm.

Care should be taken when assessing the thickness of the superior rectus as it is often impossible to separate it from levator palpebrae and this may result in an apparently enlarged muscle.

Typical appearances of dysthyroid eye disease are shown in Fig. 24.21. Severe thickening of the muscles at the orbital apex may cause optic nerve compression and visual loss. Treatment by surgical decompression or radiotherapy is helpful in these cases but more precise imaging by CT or MRI is required.

Myositis of a rectus muscle may also cause localized enlargement; however, the eye is usually painful and the clinical history is more typical of an acute process. In myositis there is enlargement of the entire muscle and tendon insertion whereas in dysthyroid states it is only the central muscle belly that is enlarged.

PSEUDOTUMOUR

This is an inflammatory condition affecting one or both orbits and of varying severity. It often presents with proptosis due to a retrobulbar mass (Fig. 24.22). It may be indistinguishable on ultrasound from other pathologies such as lymphoma and biopsy is required for the diagnosis.

Pseudotumour may mimic thyroid eye disease by causing enlargement of one or more extraocular muscles.

In cases of pseudotumour with no mass effect the inflammation may be detected from the presence of fluid lying immediately posterior to the globe extending along the optic nerve. The fluid lies within Tenon's space and in typical examples exhibits the 'T-sign' (Fig. 24.23).

Table 24.2 Causes of proptosis

Unilateral	Bilateral
Thyroid eye disease	Thyroid eye disease
Inflammatory	Inflammatory
mucoceles	pseudotumour
pseudotumour	Tumours
cellulitis	optic nerves
cavernous sinus thrombosis	Pseudoexophthalmos
Tumours	severe myopia
primary/secondary	Congenital macrophthalmos
lymphoma	
Vascular	
aneurysm	
varicosities	
Cysts	
dermoids/epidermoids	

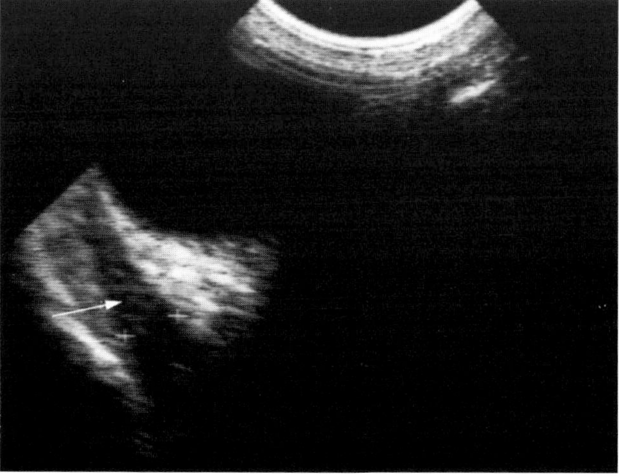

Fig. 24.21 Ultrasound of orbit—dysthyroid eye disease. Note the thickened nedial rectus muscle (arrow).

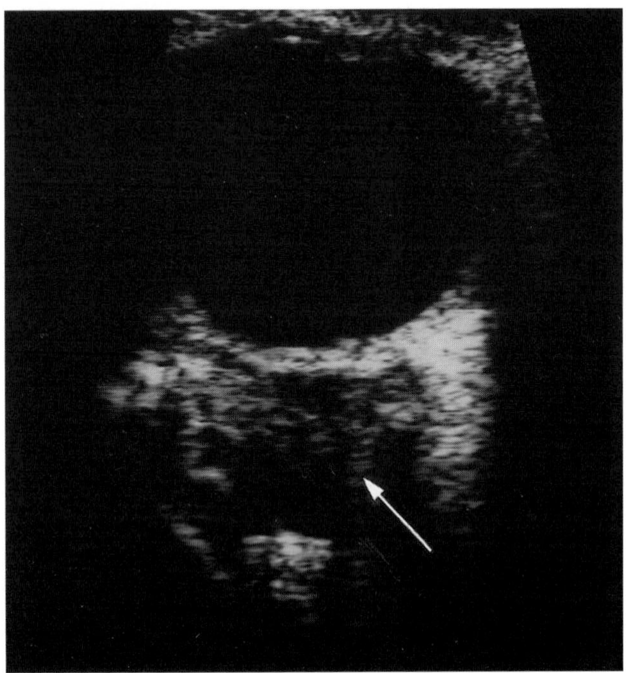

Fig. 24.22 Pseudotumour. Low reflectivity retrobulbar mass (arrow).

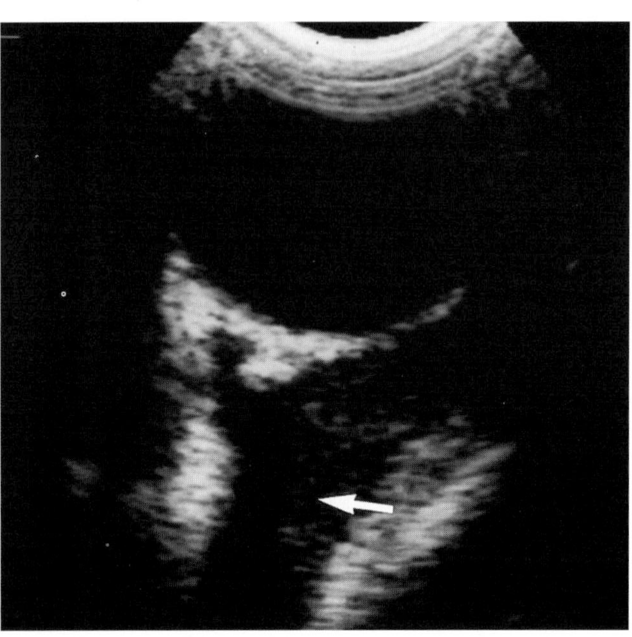

Fig. 24.24 Lymphoma. Large area of reduced reflectivity extending to the orbital apex paralleling the rectus muscle (arrow).

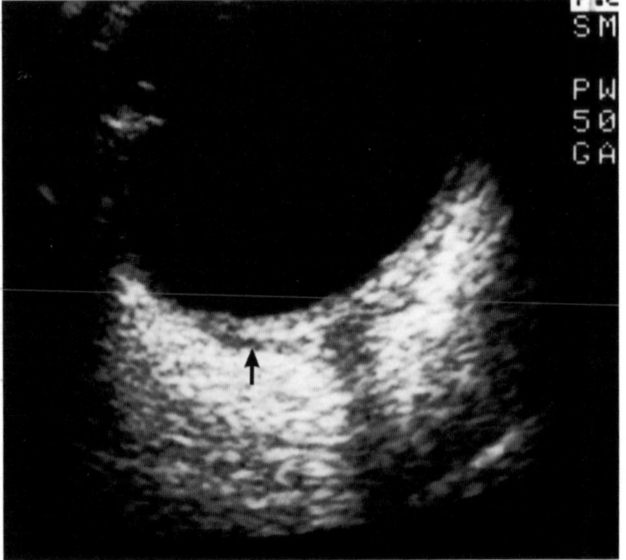

Fig. 24.23 Pseudotumour. 'T-sign' due to inflammatory fluid within Tenon's space (arrow).

Orbital tumours

Primary tumours may arise from any of the structures in the orbit but are usually related to the optic nerve or are part of a more widespread disease process such as lymphoma. The orbit is a recognized but unusual site for a metastasis, breast carcinoma being the most common primary tumour.

Orbital tumours are conveniently classified as intraconal and extraconal according to their location. These relate to the muscle cone formed by the four rectus muscles. The position of a mass within the orbit may be difficult to define with certainty by ultrasound and involvement at the orbital apex impossible to assess.

Intraconal lesions include optic nerve gliomas which are commonest in children, meningiomas, and neural sheath tumours such as schwannoma. Cavernous haemangioma is a benign slow growing tumour usually presenting in middle-aged female patients. They are well-defined masses and lie clearly within the muscle cone. They can be readily identified within the retrobulbar fat; however, they have typical signal characteristics on MRI which facilitates the diagnosis.

Lymphomas often present with proptosis but their appearance in the orbit is variable. They may be seen as a focal hypoechoic mass, or as a more diffuse process involving the muscles and orbital wall (Fig. 24.24). Additional imaging is required to assess any intracranial extension.

Lacrimal gland tumours characteristically displace the eye downwards and medially. Larger tumours can be identified by ultrasound, but their full extent must be assessed by CT or MRI.

Vascular anomalies such as varices are an uncommon

cause of proptosis but ultrasound may be able to establish a vascular aetiology with the aid of CFD.

Biometry

This is a technique for precisely assessing the dimensions of the globe, particularly the axial length and the curvature. These values enable appropriate intraocular lenses to be inserted after cataract removal. It is routinely performed in ophthalmic departments with dedicated equipment and is not usually practised by radiologists. Details regarding the technique can be found in the more specialized ophthalmic ultrasound textbooks [11,12].

Colour flow imaging of the orbit

G.M. BAXTER

Although B-mode ultrasound had been used successfully for many years in the delineation of normal and pathological anatomy within the orbit, Doppler ultrasound which has largely been confined to the examination of larger vessels in the body including the carotid arteries, cardiac and abdominal vessels, has only recently been employed. As the resolution of the orbital vasculature is below that of real-time ultrasound, study of these vessels has been impossible. With the introduction of colour Doppler technology it is now possible to visualize these vessels and obtain Doppler spectral waveforms from them [13–15]. Although the technique remains in its infancy, it provides an opportunity to investigate a wide variety of disorders affecting vascular perfusion.

Many techniques have been used to study orbital blood flow although some, such as labelled and unlabelled microspheres, are restricted to animal models [16,17], whilst others, i.e. laser Doppler velocimetry [18,19], are limited to studying the retinal circulation and blue field entoptic techniques [20] to the macular circulation. Other techniques that measure perfusion pressure in the retinal and ciliary arteries rely on orbital compression techniques by the induction of pressure on the globe [21]. These methods thus require abnormal physiological circumstances and as such may influence vascular flow itself. Colour Doppler ultrasound thus obviates many of these problems because it neither involves the addition of pharmacological agents nor abnormal globe pressure and can be used to examine orbital blood vessels that are not amenable to other methods of investigation (Fig. 24.25).

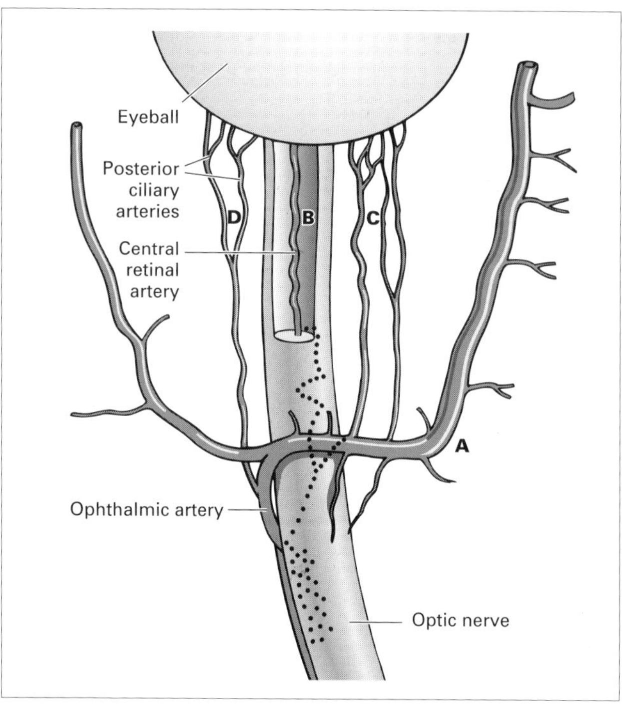

Fig. 24.25 Diagram of the orbital arterial vasculature. The largest vessel in the orbit, the ophthalmic artery, courses across the orbit and continues as a large nasal branch. It is along this nasal aspect of the orbit (A) that the artery is routinely interrogated by colour Doppler imaging. The CRA and CRV are normally visualized in their intraneural portion of the optic nerve (B) approximately 5 mm posterior to the choroid whilst the multiple small, tortuous arteries on either side of the optic nerve head, the posterior ciliary vessels, are visualized and examined with Doppler ultrasound in their nasal (C) and temporal (D) positions.

Technique

Patients can be scanned in either the supine, sitting or standing position although the author prefers the former as the examination is technically easier. All scanning is performed using a 7.5 MHz probe, either a sector/vector or linear array transducer. Contact jelly is placed onto the closed eyelid and the probe is applied with the minimum amount of pressure possible. Although scanning is performed in both transverse and longitudinal axes the transverse axis is the most informative and convenient plane. All vessels can be visualized in this plane and only on occasion is the longitudinal axis of additional benefit. It is necessary, however, to vary the position of the eye by asking the patient to look either to the right or left. This has the effect of changing the angle that the retro-orbital vessels subtend with the interrogating probe, and can result in improvement of the angle between probe and vessel.

All vessels are first localized using the colour flow facility and then by placing the Doppler spectral gate over the vessel, more specific quantitative velocity information is acquired (Fig. 24.26). The size of the Doppler gate has varied in published studies from as small as 0.2 mm [22] to 5 mm and some have also suggested using different gate sizes for different vessels. Standardization of gate size is important and the author and others prefer the use of a

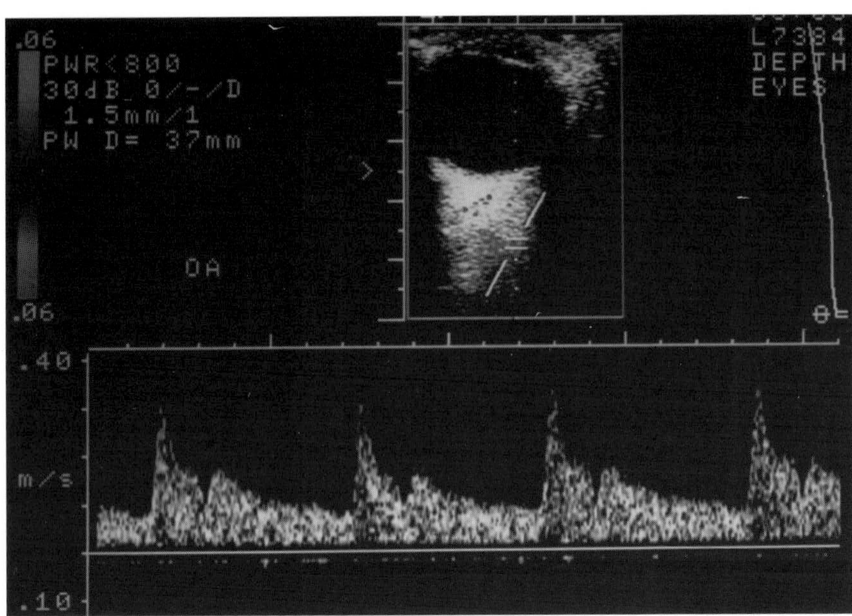

Fig. 24.26 Colour Doppler imaging of a normal Doppler waveform from the ophthalmic artery. Note the well-defined mid diastolic notch typical of the ophthalmic artery.

standard gate size of 1.5 mm as this is likely to represent an accurate velocity profile.

Routine colour Doppler examination of the eye takes approximately 5–10 min. Good technique is important in order to reduce ultrasonic exposure levels to a minimum. Some patients experience difficulty in keeping the eye still enough to allow optimal examination; however, these cases are exceptional.

Orbital vasculature

As many of these vessels are extremely tortuous attention to detail is important so that flow direction, accurate angle correction and subsequent velocity readings can be taken. Standard Doppler measurements include the peak systolic velocity, end-diastolic velocity and resistive index (RI).

The main arterial branch of the orbit is the ophthalmic artery, the first branch of the internal carotid artery. This vessel runs obliquely across the orbit from the infratemporal to a supranasal position. As the largest artery it can be interrogated by spectral analysis at any point along its path. It occupies a very constant position along the nasal wall (Fig. 24.27) and interrogation of this part of the vessel not only allows comparison of velocities between examinations but also makes a favourable Doppler angle with the probe [23].

The central retinal artery (CRA) and vein (CRV) lie side by side just posterior to the optic nerve head. By convention the CRA is colour coded in red and the vein in blue (Fig. 24.28). The small tortuous vessels on either side of the optic nerve head are the posterior ciliary vessels. These

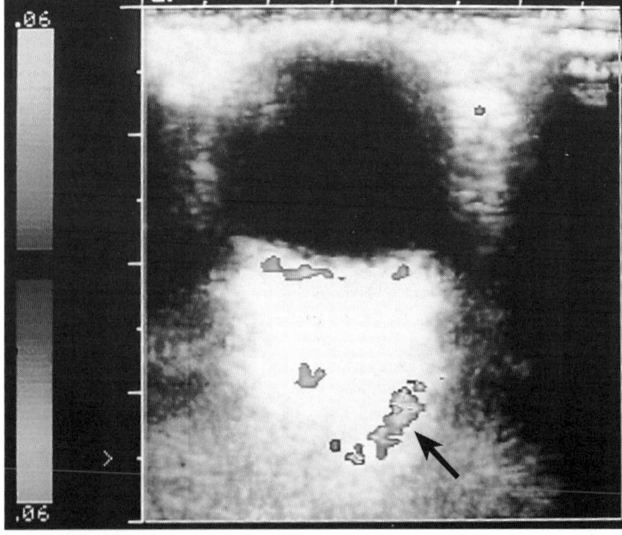

Fig. 24.27 Colour Doppler image of the ophthalmic artery. The ophthalmic artery crosses the optic nerve in the posterior aspect of the orbit and gives a large nasal branch (arrow) which occupies a constant anatomical position and as such is suitable for Doppler analysis. For colour, see Plate 24.27 (between pp. 308 and 309).

vessels can be extremely difficult to image as they tend to appear momentarily on the colour flow image, presumably due to a combination of their small size and tortuosity.

The superior ophthalmic vein (SOV) can be visualized in 85–96% of cases and the inferior ophthalmic vein has been visualized in 60% but quantitative data have not yet

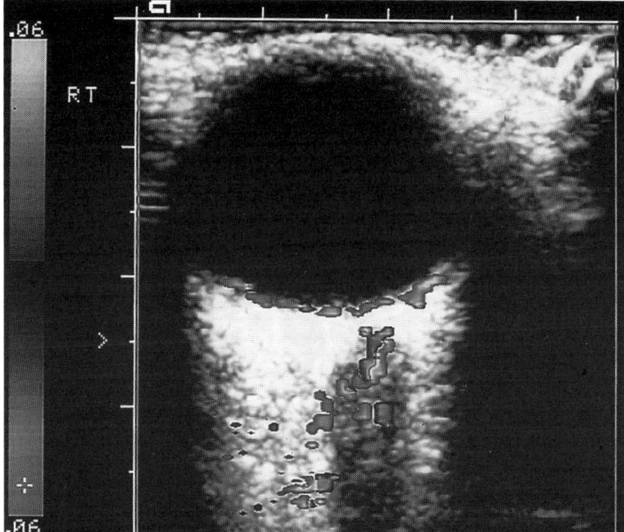

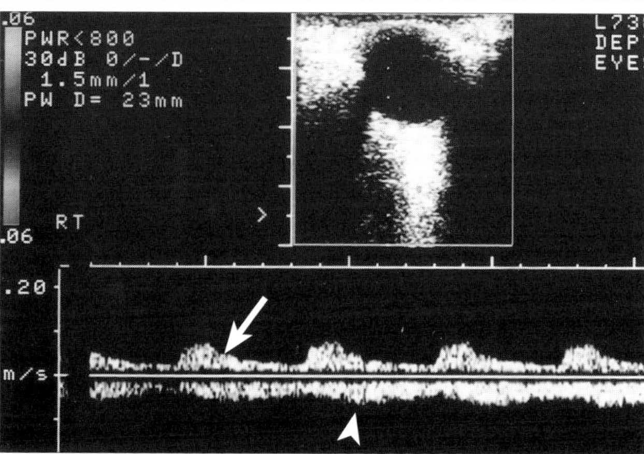

Fig. 24.28 (a) Colour flow image just posterior to the choroid demonstrating flow within both the CRV and CRA. Flow within the artery is towards the probe, whilst flow in the vein is in the opposite direction. Both these vessels lie within the intraneural portion of the optic nerve head. (b) Typical Doppler waveforms of both these vessels are shown. The arterial waveform has both systolic and diastolic components (arrow) whilst the venous waveform is more phasic (arrowhead). For colour, see Plate 24.28 (between pp.308 and 309).

been published [24,25]. Similarly, the author has experienced difficulty in visualizing the SOV in all normal individuals and has found a large variation in velocity readings. Its non-visualization should therefore not necessarily be regarded as pathological. Finally, there remains the vortex veins of which there are usually four, situated in the upper and lower quadrants behind the choroid. Although these have been visualized in normal control groups it is felt once again their absence should not necessarily be regarded as pathological.

Safety

There has been recent concern of potentially tissue-damaging energy being used at diagnostic levels. Tissue damage can be produced via two main pathways, either by a temperature increase, and thus tissue heating effects, or by tissue cavitation. The maximum transfer of energy occurs during spectral analysis and it is important that only short traces of waveforms are obtained to minimize the energy absorption by the delicate structures of the eye.

The degree of damage also depends upon the duration of exposure to the ultrasound beam. Colour Doppler imaging speeds the localization of the orbital vessels, and with good technique thereby shortens the exposure and dwell time of the Doppler examination. An awareness of these potential tissue damaging effects is essential especially in such a critical organ.

Normal velocity profiles and reproducibility

Although the ophthalmic artery, CRA and CRV, posterior ciliary arteries, vortex veins and SOV can all be detected and Doppler analysis performed, only waveforms from the CRA, CRV and ophthalmic artery have been reliably detected in the major series reported [22,26] (Table 24.3). Although spectral analysis can be performed on the posterior ciliary vessels the variability in velocity readings is marked and the author therefore feels that comments on their presence or absence are as useful as quantitative measurements (Table 24.4).

Age-related changes in the blood velocity measurements occur. A significant reduction in blood velocities from the ophthalmic artery with increasing age has been recorded [26,27] (Fig. 24.29) and this may reflect a reduction in the peripheral perfusion of the patient. An age-related increase in RI in the CRA may reflect an increase in peripheral resistance of the retina whilst an increase in the RI within the CRV is difficult to explain fully. These relatively small changes, however, are unlikely to influence results significantly.

In addition to age-related changes, postural effects also influence the spectral waveform within these vessels although these does not achieve statistical significance. Using the supine scanning position as standard on serial scans negates any small postural-related velocity changes.

Arterial disease

The flow of blood within the multiple vessels at the optic nerve head produces a very complex colour Doppler pattern. This conglomerate of vessels is due to a combination of the CRV and CRA with the posterior ciliary circulation, on either side (Fig. 24.30).

Table 24.3 Normal control velocity measurements—mean and (standard deviation): ophthalmic artery, CRA and CRV

Measurement	Ultrasound machine	No. of patients	Ophthalmic artery	CRA	CRV
Peak systolic velocity (cm s^{-1})	Acuson 128	83	35.0 (11.2)	10.2 (2.8)	5.7 (1.4)
	QAD 1	40	31.4 (4.2)	10.3 (2.1)	2.9 (0.73)
	ATL/Acuson	72	31.6 (9.0)	9.5 (3.1)	5.7 (1.5)
End-diastolic velocity	Acuson 128		8.6 (3.8)	3.1 (1.1)	3.8 (0.8)
	QAD 1		8.3 (3.9)	2.6 (1.2)	—
	ATL/Acuson		8.2 (3.7)	3.1 (1.6)	4.0 (1.0)
RI	Acuson 128		74.0 (8.2)	69.3 (7.7)	32.4 (9.7)

Table 24.4 Intra- and interobserver variation of the orbital vessels

		Coefficient of variation of repeated measurements (%)	
Vessel	Measurement	Intraobserver	Interobserver
Ophthalmic artery	Peak systolic velocity	6.5	8.2
	End-diastolic velocity	11.0	25.5
	RI	4.8	6.2
CRA	Peak systolic velocity	12.2	19.3
	End-diastolic velocity	20.0	25.0
	RI	6.4	6.3
Posterior ciliary artery (nasal)	Peak systolic velocity	29.8	
	End-diastolic velocity	22.2	
	RI	13.6	
Posterior ciliary artery (temporal)	Peak systolic velocity	36.6	
	End-diastolic velocity	38.8	
	RI	10.0	
CRV	Peak systolic velocity	13.6	20.3
	End-diastolic velocity	12.2	22.0
	RI	9.0	22.7

CRA occlusion

Although this diagnosis can be made with colour flow imaging in the acute situation, there being no detectable colour flow within the CRA at the optic nerve head (Fig. 24.31), this diagnosis can be easily made clinically and therefore colour Doppler has no role in the diagnosis or management of CRA occlusion.

Anterior ischaemic optic neuropathy

Anterior ischaemic optic neuropathy (AION) classically arises when there is occlusion of the posterior ciliary vessels; it is a cause of acute visual loss. It can be due to an arteritic process the most common being giant cell arteritis (GCA) or a non-arteritic process. In GCA the ophthalmic artery and CRA may also be involved reflecting a more diffuse vascular involvement in keeping with the systemic nature of the disease. It can be associated with local or systemic symptoms including jaw claudication, scalp tenderness, headache, malaise and a raised erythrocyte sedimentation rate (ESR). Clinical suspicion is normally confirmed by temporal artery biopsy and treatment is usually with oral steroids with frequent monitoring of the ESR and visual recovery.

Although quantification of flow within these vessels is difficult documentation of their presence or absence would appear from early pilot studies to be related to the clinical course and indeed may also reflect the severity of disease. In addition it would appear that the vascular changes are not simply confined to the posterior ciliary vessels but that changes in ophthalmic artery flow and the central artery are also detectable, not only in the clinically affected eye but also within the asymptomatic fellow eye [28]. This would certainly seem logical in view of the diffuse nature of many arteritic processes. Indeed it has

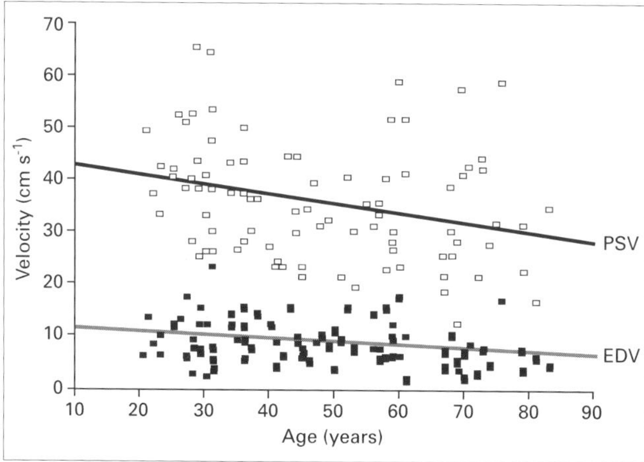

Fig. 24.29 Graph of the peak systolic velocity (PSV) and end-diastolic velocity (EDV) within the ophthalmic artery and their variation with age. A significant reduction is present in both these measurements with age (P, 0.003). This reduction is relatively small and is unlikely to influence results significantly when dealing with pathological processes.

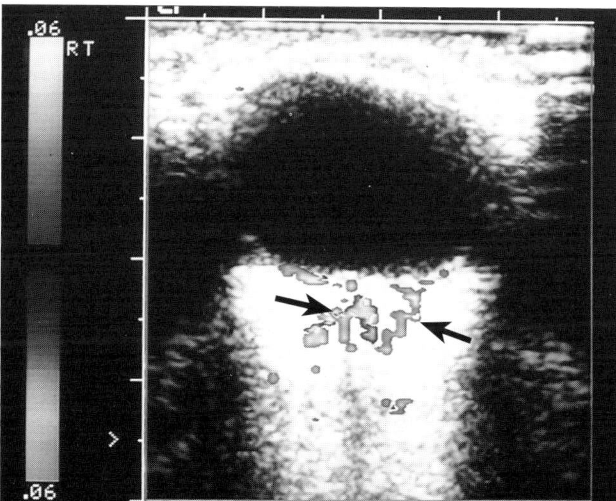

Fig. 24.30 Colour flow image of the vessels at and around the optic nerve head. The CRA and CRV are seen centrally within the optic nerve head whilst the peripapillary vessels on either side are the posterior ciliary arteries (arrows). These latter vessels appear as short flashes of colour flow and although seen during a dynamic examination are difficult to capture on still film. For colour, see Plate 24.30 (between pp. 308 and 309).

recently been demonstrated that the greater number of vessels involved and a reduction in ophthalmic artery velocity is associated with a poorer visual prognosis although these results are based upon very small numbers of patients [28].

Temporal monitoring of such vasculitic processes may

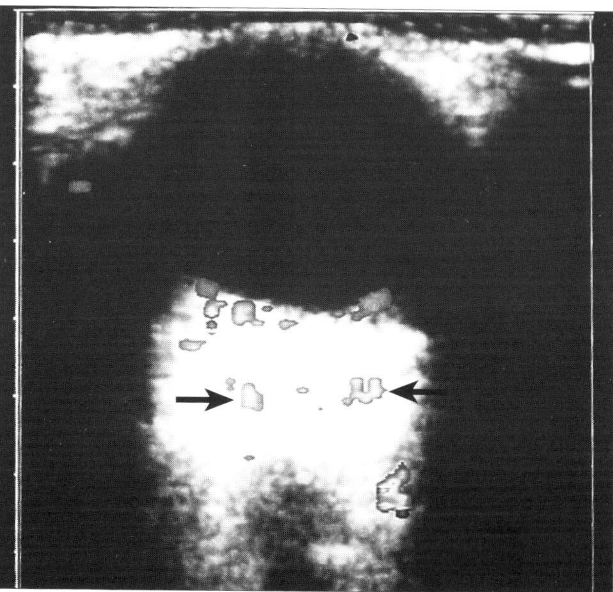

Fig. 24.31 Colour Doppler image just behind the choroid demonstrating complete absence of the CRA with maintenance of the posterior ciliary vessels on either side of the optic nerve (arrows). This patient presented clinically with an acute CRA occlusion which was confirmed on fluorescein angiography, the ultrasound scan being performed within 24 h of presentation. (Reproduced with permission from *Eye* (1993), **7**, 74–79.) For colour, see Plate 24.31 (between pp. 308 and 309).

also be useful. Indeed in one patient, serial Doppler studies demonstrated absent ophthalmic artery blood flow in a recurrent acute episode of AION resulting in blindness despite apparent control of the disease by corticosteroid therapy and a normal ESR. A subsequent increase in immunosuppression was followed by clinical improvement and reperfusion of the ophthalmic artery on colour Doppler imaging [29] (Fig. 24.32).

Significant increases in blood velocity in the ophthalmic artery and CRA, accompanied by a decrease in the vascular resistance within the posterior ciliary arteries following surgical optic nerve sheath decompression [30] in a small group of patients with progressive AION, also demonstrates the potential of monitoring such procedures with this technique. However, these clearly represent very early forays into the field and more detailed controlled studies are required before this technique can be adopted clinically.

Vein occlusion

Central retinal vein occlusion (CRVO) affects the end artery retinal circulation, by obstruction of its outflow at the level of or posterior to the lamina cribrosa. The degree

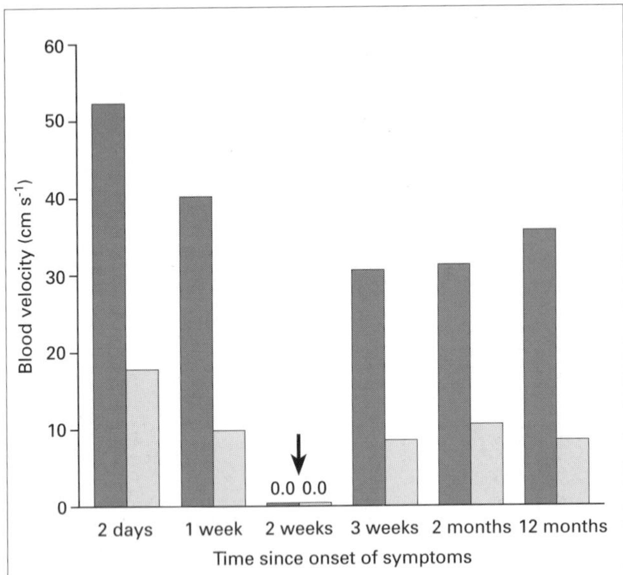

Fig. 24.32 Histogram of a patient with GCA demonstrating the variations in peak systolic (■) and end-diastolic (□) velocity in the ophthalmic artery with disease progression and remission. Interestingly when the disease was clinically in remission and the ESR was at its lowest, this patient suffered complete blindness in one eye. Colour Doppler ultrasound performed at that time (arrow) showed absent flow within the ophthalmic artery. Repeat Doppler examination 1 week later demonstrated return of vascularity, this corresponding with clinical improvement in vision. (Reproduced with permission from the *British Journal of Ophthalmology* (1992), **76**, 690–691.)

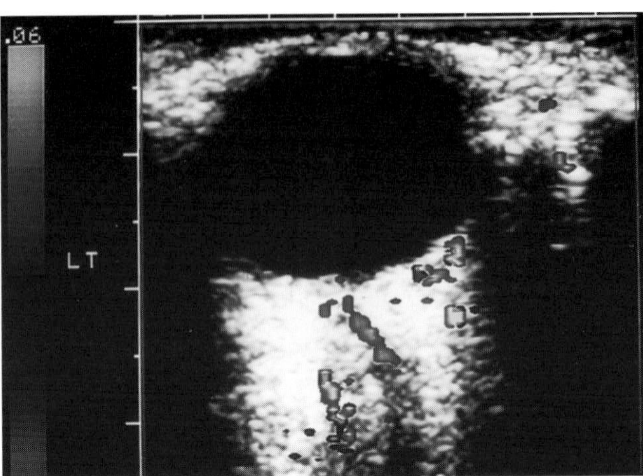

Fig. 24.33 Colour flow image of a patient with ischaemic CRVO. The CRA is still visualized; however, the CRV is absent as it is occluded. The venous signal was absent on both colour flow and Doppler analysis. For colour, see Plate 24.33 (between pp. 308 and 309).

of visual loss depends on many factors which include the speed of onset, degree of occlusion and the ability to form collateral vessels. Although there are many predisposing factors in this condition, e.g. diabetes, hypertension and increased blood viscosity, most cases are idiopathic [31,32].

The diagnosis can be made clinically; however, classification of the severity of the occlusion into ischaemic or non-ischaemic forms is of prognostic significance, the former having the worse prognosis, these patients being at risk of developing the complications of rubeosis iridis and neovascular glaucoma [33–35] both of which result in further visual deterioration. Classification of severity depends upon capillary non-perfusion on fluoroscein angiography. Unfortunately, this test may be uninterpretable in up to one-third of patients within the first 3 months of the onset of symptoms [36] and this is one area where colour flow imaging may prove to be useful.

A pilot study comparing 20 CRVO patients with a control group of 20 volunteers has shown a significant reduction in the maximum and minimum venous velocities from the CRV in the affected CRVO eye when compared to both the fellow eye and an age- and sex-matched control population. Furthermore, a more marked reduction was found in the ischaemic CRVO group compared with the non-ischaemic group [37] (Fig. 24.33). A larger subsequent study confirmed these findings and also demonstrated the effectiveness of colour Doppler in the prediction of iris neovascularization. Indeed, a minimum venous velocity in the CRV of $<3\,\mathrm{cm\,s^{-1}}$ within 3 months of onset had a sensitivity of 75% and a specificity of 86% in predicting this complication [38], which compares extremely favourably with alternative tests many of which are more invasive and subjective. Thus, colour Doppler may be helpful in a clinical setting facilitating the decision as to whether the patient should or should not receive pre-emptive laser therapy.

Tumours

Several series of patients with intraocular tumours have been published using colour Doppler ultrasound [39–41]. Tumour circulation can be visualized in almost all cases of choroidal malignant melanomas (Fig. 24.34). In those few patients in whom no tumour circulation was detectable, all had raised intraocular pressure from secondary glaucoma and may have secondary tumour necrosis from cessation of tumour blood supply. In addition, the author's experience would suggest that tumour circulation is very difficult to detect in very small raised choroidal lesions.

Temporal studies following radiotherapy have also been performed. Initially an increase in blood flow velocity was detected in the first few days following therapy with subsequent reduction from predosage levels. In fact, of 19 out of 20 cases described by Wolff-Kormann a reduc-

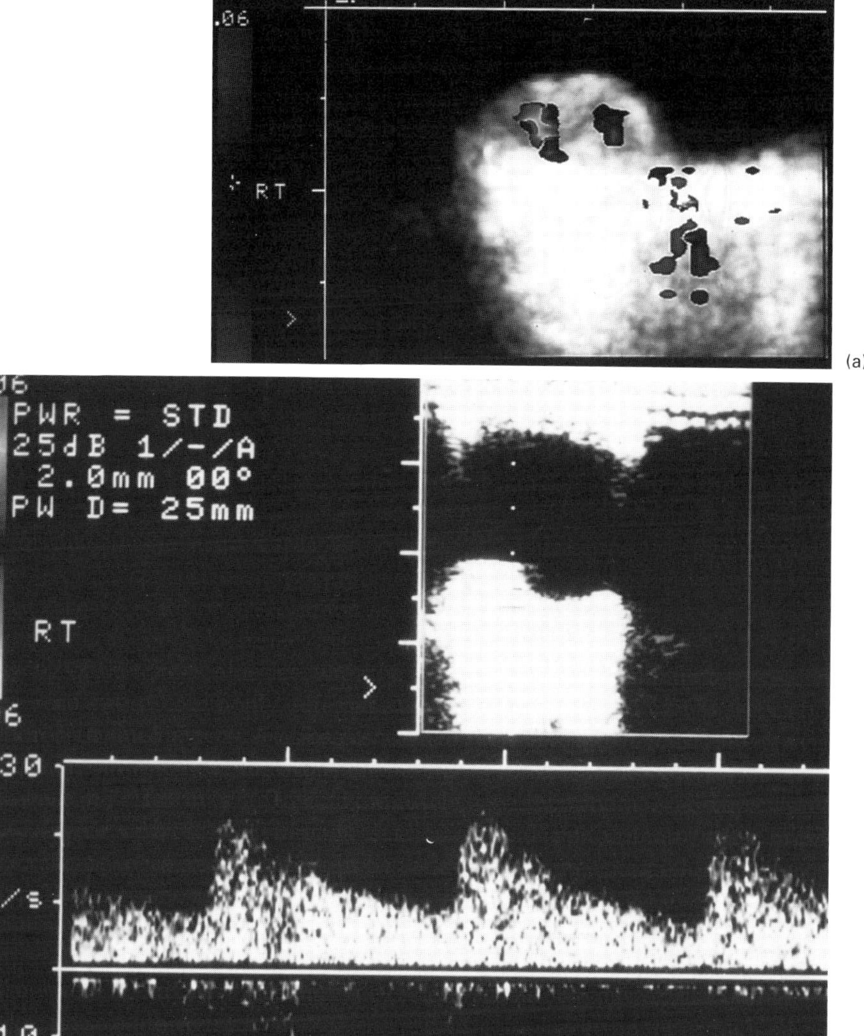

Fig. 24.34 (a) Colour flow image of a malignant melanoma demonstrating intratumoral flow. (b) This can be quantified using spectral analysis and velocity and Doppler indices measured in the usual manner. For colour, see Plate 24.34 (between pp. 308 and 309).

tion in blood velocity was detected prior to tumour regression by conventional grey-scale ultrasound. Interestingly, increased velocity was noted within the tumour mass in one patient and tumour recurrence subsequently developed [40].

Other intraocular tumours including choroidal haemangiomas (Fig. 24.35) and metastatic lesions also have pathological circulations, the former possessing reportedly higher velocities than the melanoma group. It remains unlikely that melanomas, haemangiomas and metastasis will be differentiated on Doppler analysis alone. Other lesions that potentially mimic malignant tumours such as age-related macular degeneration, choroidal osteoma and choroidal naevi have shown no detectable blood flow [42]. Colour flow imaging therefore may help in the differentation of some intraocular tumours and tumour-imitating lesions.

Drugs

Another potential growth area for this technique is in the study of pharmacological agents on retrobulbar haemodynamics. This technique is ideal for the task as it is safe, non-invasive and therefore accommodates repeated serial examinations. This potential has already been realized and a small study of 10 healthy volunteers following the administration of timolol 0.5% for 3 days has already been performed. Results of this trial perhaps indicate that timolol may have an effect on the retinal blood vessels themselves, indicating contrary to current opinion that sympathetic receptors are present in these vessels [23].

It would thus be possible to study the effects of many different types of β-blockers and other pharmacological agents to improve our understanding of how these drugs work.

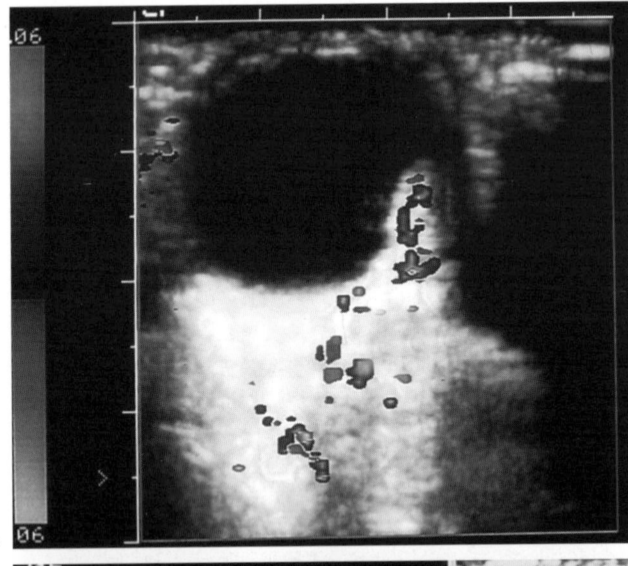

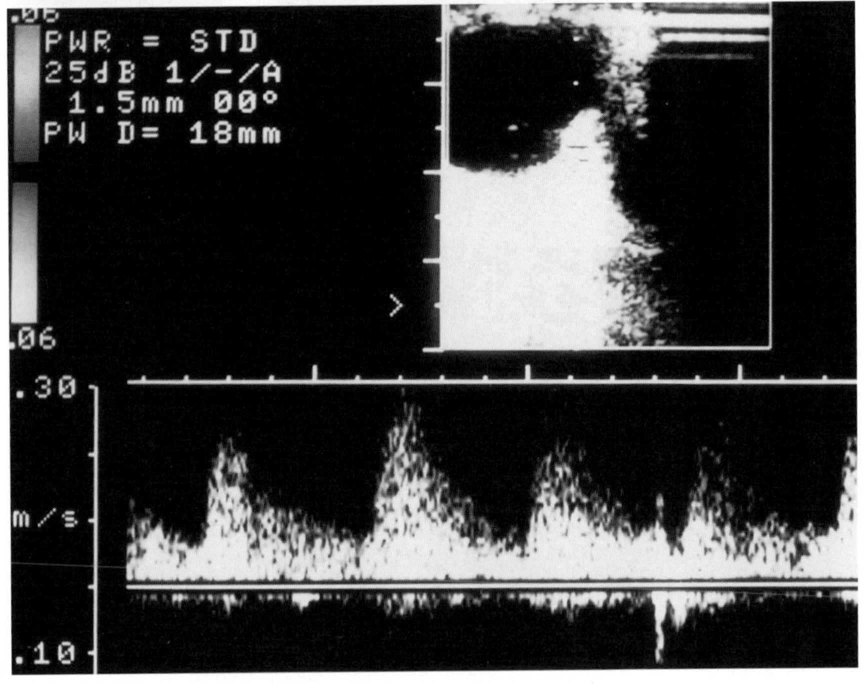

Fig. 24.35 (a) Colour flow image of a capillary haemangioma. Again flow within the mass is demonstrated using colour flow imaging whilst further analysis is possible using spectral Doppler (b). Although some differences have been demonstrated between capillary haemangiomas and malignant melanomas there is an overlap in Doppler measurements between the two groups and therefore they cannot be differentiated on Doppler analysis. For colour, see Plate 24.35 (between pp. 308 and 309).

Other vascular conditions affecting the eye

Carotid disease

Patients with major carotid vessel disease may also show flow abnormalities within the orbit [43]. In severe carotid stenosis and ocular ischaemic syndrome, the peak systolic velocities within the CRA and the posterior ciliary arteries are significantly reduced when compared with a control group. Of interest, in 12 out of 16 eyes examined, flow reversal was observed in the ophthalmic artery (Fig. 24.36) [44].

SOV occlusion

Absent flow within the SOV in association with dilated collateral venous channels have been described in this condition [45].

Caroticocavernous fistulae

In patients with caroticocavernous fistulae (CCF), dilated orbital veins, in particular, the SOV have been described. A pulsatile arterialized waveform from this vessel has also been noted on Doppler analysis and reversal of flow

Fig. 24.36 Doppler spectral analysis of the ophthalmic artery showing flow below the Doppler baseline, i.e. reverse flow. The peak systolic velocity was markedly increased and this was thought to be due to a stenotic lesion within the ophthalmic artery. Flow within the CRA was, however, still normal. Flow reversal within the ophthalmic artery is most commonly secondary to severe internal carotid artery stenoses or occlusions.

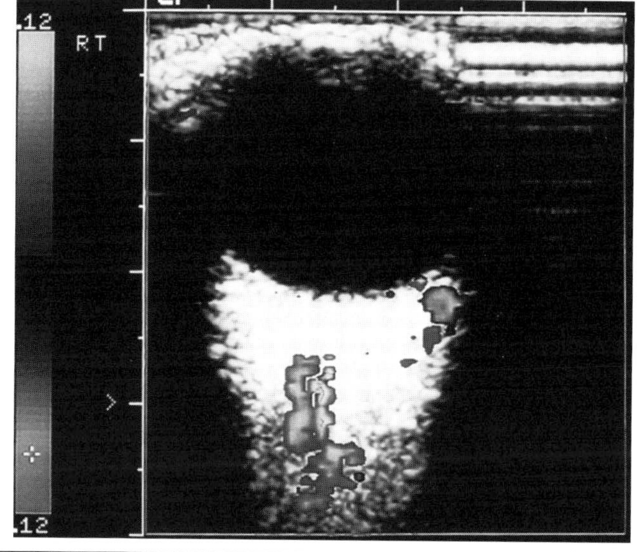

(a)

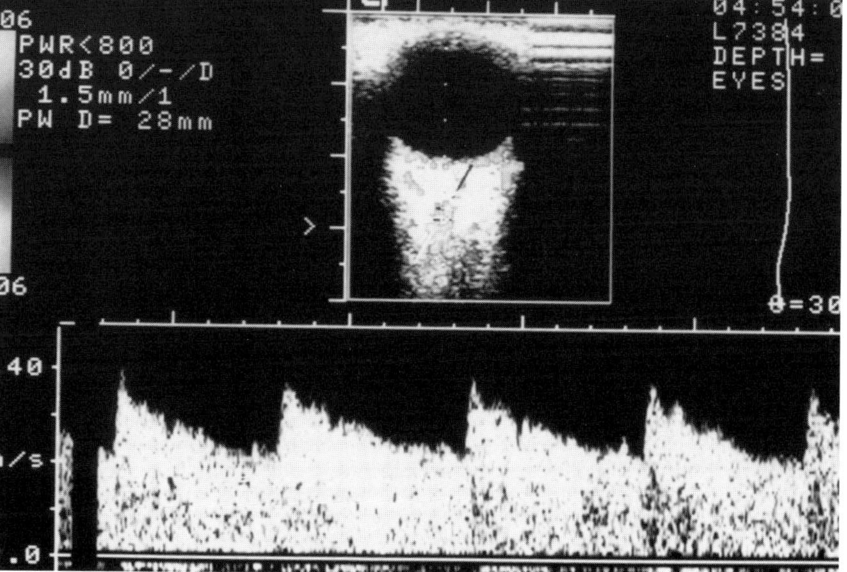

(b)

Fig. 24.37 (a) Colour flow image of a patient with a CCF showing marked enlargement of the ophthalmic artery. (b) Doppler analysis of the ophthalmic artery shows marked increase in diastolic flow with a consequent reduction in RI. For colour, see Plate 24.37 (between pp. 308 and 309).

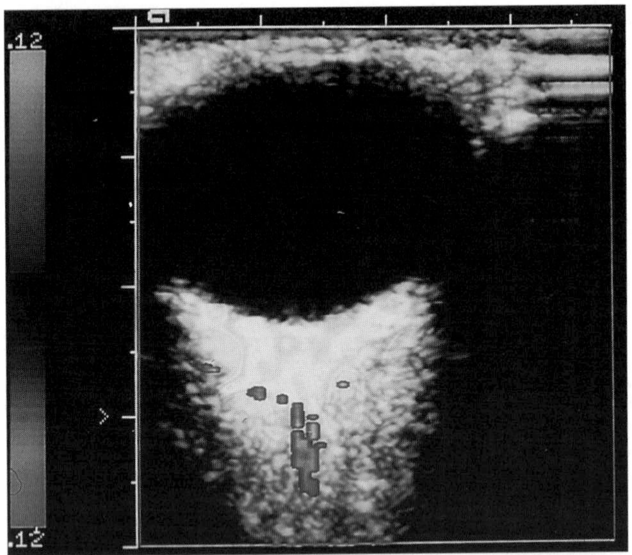

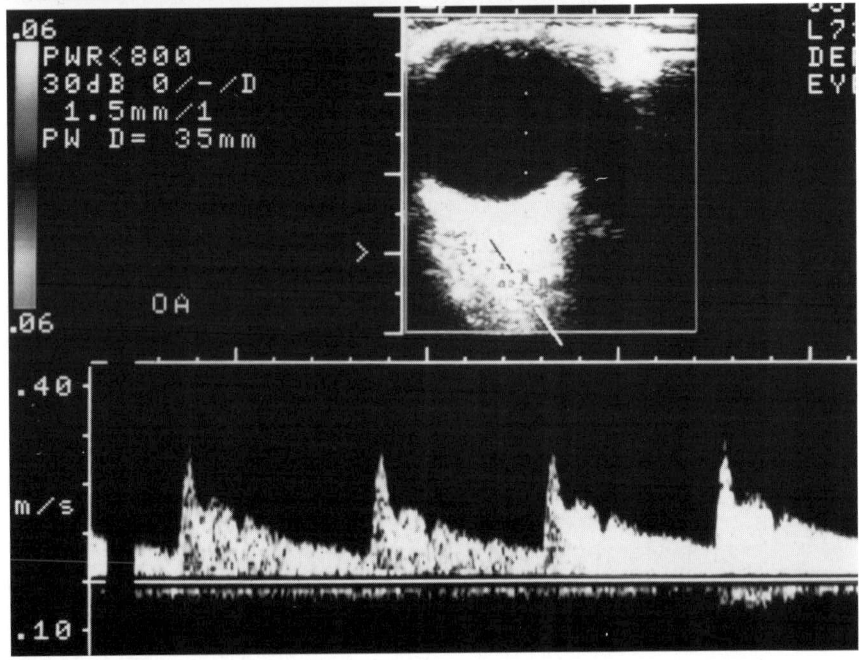

Fig. 24.38 (a) The opposite eye of the same patient as in Fig. 24.37 showing a normal appearance on colour flow imaging of the ophthalmic artery. (b) Similarly the Doppler spectrum of the ophthalmic artery is normal with significantly less diastolic flow when compared with Fig. 24.37b. For colour, see Plate 24.38 (between pp. 308 and 309).

direction has also been observed. Restoration from an arterialized waveform to a normal venous pattern within the SOV following embolization is also possible [46].

Orbital hypervascularity is also striking in some cases of CCF (Figs 24.37, 24.38).

Other vascular anomalies

Orbital arteriovenous malformations have also been demonstrated using colour Doppler imaging and low resistance arterial flow observed [25]. Flow has also been detected in orbital varices especially during the Valsalva manoeuvre as the vessel fills and empties [47].

References

1 Fielding, J.A. (1987) Ultrasound imaging of the eye through the closed lid using a non-dedicated scanner. *Clinical Radiology* **38**, 131–135.

2 Coleman, D.J., Smith, M.E. (1983) Pattern recognition of ocular tumours. Proceedings of symposium on medical and surgical diseases of the retina and vitreous. *Transactions of the New Orleans Academy of Ophthalmology* **22**, 272–290.

3 Fielding, J.A. (1996) Ocular ultrasound. *Clinical Radiology* **51**, 533–544.

4 Byrne, S.F., Green, R.L. (1992) Intraocular tumours. In: *Ultrasound of the Eye and Orbit*. CV Mosby, St Louis, pp. 133–213.

5 Shields, J.A. (1989) Tumours of the uveal tract. In: Tasman, W., Jaeger, E.A. (eds) *Clinical Ophthalmology*, Vol. 67. JB Lippincott, Philadelphia, pp. 1–13.

6 Char, D.H. (1980) Current concepts in retinoblastoma *Annals of Ophthalmology* **12**, 792–804.

7 Davidorf, F.H., Lang, J.R. (1975) The natural history of malignant melanoma of the choroid: small vs large tumors. *Transactions of the American Academy of Ophthalmology and Otolaryngology* **79**, 310–320.

8 Shammas, H.F., Blodi, F.C. (1977) Prognostic factors in choroidal and ciliary body melanomas. *Archives of Ophthalmology* **95**, 63–69.

9 Given-Wilson, R., Pope, R.M., Michell, M.J. *et al.* (1989) The use of real-time ultrasound in Graves' ophthalmopathy: a comparison with computed tomography. *British Journal Radiology* **62**, 705–709.

10 Demer, J.L., Kerman, M.D. (1994) Comparison of standardised echography with magnetic resonance imaging to measure extraocular muscle size. *American Journal of Ophthalmology* **118**, 351–361.

11 Byrne, S.F., Green, R.L. (1992) Axial eye length measurements. In: *Ultrasound of the Eye and Orbit*. CV Mosby St Louis, pp. 215–242.

12 Shammas, H.J. (1984) *Atlas of Ophthalmic Ultrasonography and Biometry*. CV Mosby, St Louis.

13 Berger, R.W., Guthoff, R., Helmke, K., Winkler, P., Draeger, J. (1989) Dopplersonographische Befunde der Arteria und Vena centrali retinae. *Fortschritte der Ophthalmologie* **86**, 334–336.

14 Canning, C.R., Restori, M. (1988) Doppler ultrasound studies of the ophthalmic artery. *Eye* **2**, 92–95.

15 Canning, C.R., Restori, M. (1988) Doppler ultrasound of orbital vessels. *Australian and New Zealand Journal of Ophthalmology* **16**, 229–233.

16 Alm, A. (1980) The effect of topical l-epinephrine on regional ocular blood flow in monkeys. *Investigations in Ophthalmology and Visual Science* **19**, 487.

17 Capriolo, J., Miller, J.M. (1988) Measurement of optic nerve blood flow with iodoantipyrene: limitations caused by diffusion from the choroid. *Experimental Eye Research* **47**, 641.

18 Riva, C.E., Grunwald, G.E., Sinclair, S.H., Petrig, B.L. (1985) Blood velocity and volumetric flow in human retinal vessels. *Investigations in Ophthalmology and Visual Science* **26**, 1124.

19 Robinson, F., Riva, C.E., Grunwald, J.E., Petrig, B.L., Sinclair, S.H. (1986) Retinal blood flow autoregulation in response to an acute increase in blood pressure. *Investigations in Ophthalmology and Visual Science* **27**, 722.

20 Sinclair, S.H., Azar-Cavanagh, M., Soper, K.A., Tuma, R.F., Mayrovitz, H.N. (1989) Investigation of the source of blue field entoptic phenomenon. *Investigations in Ophthalmology and Visual Science* **30**, 722.

21 Ulrich, W.P., Ulrich, C. (1985) Oculo-oscillo-dynamography: a diagnostic procedure for recording ocular pulses and measuring retinal and ciliary artery blood pressures. *Ophthalmic Research* **17**, 308.

22 Lieb, W.E., Cohen, S.M., Merton, D.A., Shields, J.A., Mitchell, D.G., Goldberg, B.B. (1991) Color Doppler imaging of the eye and orbit: technique and normal vascular anatomy. *Archives of Ophthalmology* **109**, 527–531.

23 Baxter, G.M., Williamson, T.W., McKillop, G., Dutton, G.N. (1992) Color Doppler ultrasound of orbital and optic nerve blood flow: effects of posture and timolol 0.5%. *Investigative Ophthalmology and Visual Science* **33**, 604–610.

24 Berges, O. (1992) Colour Doppler flow imaging of the orbital veins. *Acta Ophthalmologica* **204**, 55–58.

25 Erickson, S.J., Hendrix, L.E., Massaro, B.M., *et al.* (1989) Color Doppler flow imaging of the normal and abnormal orbit. *Radiology* **173**, 511–516.

26 Guthoff, R.F., Berger, R.W., Winkler, P., Helmke, K., Chumbley, L.C. (1991) Doppler ultrasonography of the ophthalmic and central retinal vessels. *Archives of Ophthalmology* **109**, 532–536.

27 Michelson, G., Gierth, K., Priem, R, Laumer, R. (1990) Blood velocity in the ophthalmic artery in normal subjects and patients with endophthalmitis. *Investigations in Ophthalmology and Visual Science* **31**, 1919–1923.

28 Ghanchi, F., Williamson, T.H., Lim, C.S., Butt, Z., Baxter, G.M., McKillop G., O'Brien, C. (1996) Colour Doppler imaging in giant cell (temporal) arteritis: serial examination and comparison with nonarteritic anterior ischaemic optic neuropathy. *Eye* **10**, 459–464.

29 Williamson, T.H., Baxter, G.M., Paul, R., Dutton, G.N. (1992) Colour Doppler ultrasound in the management of a case of cranial arteritis. *British Journal of Ophthalmology* **76**, 690–691.

30 Flaharty, P.M., Sergott, R.C., Lieb, W., Bosley, T.M., Savino, P.J. (1993) Optic nerve sheath decompression may improve blood flow in anterior ischemic optic neuropathy. *Ophthalmology* **100**, 297–305.

31 Appiah, A.P., Trempe, C.L. (1989) Risk factors associated with branch versus central retinal vein occlusion. *Annals of Ophthalmology* **21**, 153–155.

32 Cole, M.D., Dodson, P.M., Hendlers, S. (1989) Medical conditions underlying retinal vein occlusion in patients with glaucoma or ocular hypertension. *British Journal of Ophthalmology* **73**, 693–698.

33 Quinlan, P.M., Elman, M.J., Bhatt, A.K., Mardesich, P., Enger, C. (1990) The natural course of central retinal vein occlusion. *American Journal of Ophthalmology* **110**, 118–123.

34 Sinclair, S.H., Gagourdas, E.S. (1979) Prognosis for rubeosis iridis following central retinal vein occlusion. *British Journal of Ophthalmology* **63**, 735–743.

35 Hayreh, S.S., Rojas, P., Podhajsky, P., Montague, P., Woolson, R.F. (1983) Ocular neovascularisation with retinal vascular occlusion. III. Incidence of ocular neovascularisation with retinal vein occlusion. *Ophthalmology* **90**, 488–506.

36 Hayreh, S.S., Klugman, M.R., Beri, M., Kimura, A.E., Podhajsky, P. (1990) Differentiation of ischemic from non ischemic central retinal vein occlusion during the early acute phase. *Graefes Archives of Clinical Experimental Ophthalmology* **228**, 201–207.

37 Baxter, G.M., Williamson, T.H. (1993) Color flow imaging in central retinal vein occlusion: a new diagnostic technique? *Radiology* **187**, 847–850.

38 Williamson, T.H., Baxter, G.M. (1994) Central retinal vein occlusion, an investigation by colour Doppler imaging: blood velocity characteristics and prediction of iris neovascularisation. *Ophthalmology* **101**, 1362–1372.

39 Guthoff, R.F., Berger, R.W., Winkler, P., Helmke, K., Chumbley, L.C. (1991) Doppler ultrasonography of malignant melanomas of the uvea. *Archives of Ophthalmology* **109**, 537–541.

40 Wolff-Kormann, P.G., Kormann, B.A., Riedel, K.G., *et al.* (1992) Quantitative color Doppler imaging in untreated and irradiated choroidal melanoma. *Investigations in Ophthalmology and Visual Science* **33**, 1928–1933.

41 Lieb, W.E., Shields, J.A., Cohen, S.M., *et al.* (1990) Color Doppler

imaging in the management of intraocular tumors. *Ophthalmology* **97**, 1660–1664.
42 Wolff-Kormann, P.G., Kormann, B.A., Hasenfratz, G.C., Spengel, F.A. (1992) Duplex and color Doppler ultrasound in the differential diagnosis of choroidal tumours. *Acta Ophthalmologica* **204**, 66–70.
43 Ho, A.C., Lieb, W.E., Flaharty, P.M., *et al.* (1992) Color Doppler imaging of the ocular ischemic syndrome. *Ophthalmology* **99**, 1453–1462.
44 Lieb, W.E., Flaharty, P.M., Sergott, R.C., *et al.* (1991) Color Doppler imaging provides accurate assessment of orbital blood flow in occlusive carotid artery disease. *Ophthalmology* **98**, 548–552.
45 Flaharty, P.M., Phillips, W., Sergott, R.C., *et al.* (1991) Color Doppler imaging of superior ophthalmic vein thrombosis. *Archives of Ophthalmology* **109**, 582–583.
46 Flaherty, P.M., Lieb, W.E., Sergott, R.C., Bosley, T.M., Savino, P.J. (1991) Color Doppler imaging. A new non invasive technique to diagnose and monitor carotid cavernous sinus fistulas. *Archives of Ophthalmology* **109**, 522–526.
47 Lieb, W.E., Merton, D.A., Shields, J.A., Cohen, S.M., Mitchell, D.D., Goldberg, B.B. (1990) Colour Doppler imaging in the demonstration of an orbital varix. *British Journal of Ophthalmology* **74**, 305–308.

Part 5
Abdomen

Chapter 25: The liver

H. Meire & P. Farrant

Anatomy

Segmental anatomy

Historically the liver has been divided into four lobes: right, left, caudate and quadrate. Although these have some anatomical relevance they have been replaced by a system of numbered segments. The anatomical definition and boundaries of these segments are determined by the branching vascular structures within the liver (Fig. 25.1) and the system reflects relatively recent developments in surgical resections. The anatomical sites of the segments is given in Table 25.1.

It is necessary for sonographers to be fully conversant with this segmental anatomy as ultrasound has a significant role in determining the resectability of focal lesions.

Venous vascular anatomy

PORTAL VEIN

The portal vein enters the liver as a single vessel but divides almost immediately. The right portal vein continues laterally into the right lobe but the left branch passes to the left at a right angle to the parent vessel. The left branch normally divides into two main divisions supplying segments 2 and 3.

HEPATIC VEINS

There are normally three main hepatic veins—right, middle and left—all of which normally drain directly into the vena cava just before it passes through the diaphragm. The left and middle veins may fuse before entering the inferior vena cava (IVC). Smaller veins drain the caudate lobe (segment 1) and are not normally seen in most patients. The anatomy of the hepatic veins is very variable, especially those within the right lobe where there may be two or more veins replacing the normal single vein. In addition separate supernumerary veins are common draining segment 6 and entering the IVC several centimetres inferior to the diaphragm.

Liver shape and normal variants

The shape of the liver is relatively similar in the majority of patients, the left lobe being markedly smaller than the right. The inferior edge of the left lobe normally has a sharp margin with an angle of less than 45° (Fig. 25.2). The inferior surface of the left lobe is usually concave. The superoinferior diameter of the left lobe is, however, extremely variable ranging from 3 to 10 cm in different subjects.

The right lobe of the liver normally also has a sharp inferior margin with an angle of less than 90° (Fig. 25.3), the superoinferior diameter is also variable.

In a minority of subjects there is a lateral and inferior extension of the right lobe referred to as a Reidel's lobe, though it is not a true lobe. This lobe may extend down as far as the right iliac fossa and give a false clinical impression of hepatomegaly. Patients with a Reidel's lobe frequently have a small left lobe. Examination of the vessels within a suspected Reidel's lobe may help to confirm its nature as prominent portal and hepatic vein trunks can be seen passing down into the lobe in the long axis of the patient, quite unlike the anatomy of the vessels in an enlarged right lobe.

Normal appearances

The display of the parenchymal echo pattern in a normal liver varies considerably with different makes of scanner and different transducer frequencies. It is important, therefore, for every ultrasound user to become familiar with the characteristics of the image produced by their own equipment.

The echo pattern should be fairly homogeneous, except for the portal and hepatic vein branches. The mean echo amplitude should be slightly greater than that of the cortex of the adjacent normal right kidney. The portal vein branches normally have highly reflective walls which can

Table 25.1 Segmental liver anatomy

Segment number	Anatomical site
1	Caudate lobe
2	Left superior
3	Left inferior
4	Left medial
5	Right anterior inferior
6	Right posterior inferior
7	Right posterior superior
8	Right anterior superior

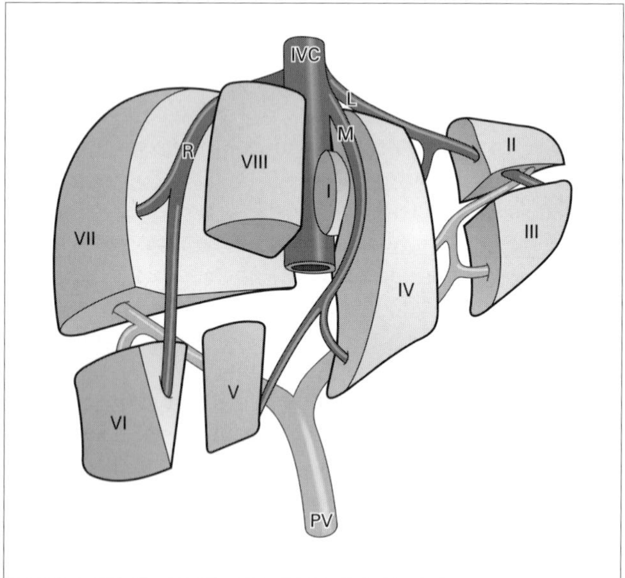

Fig. 25.1 Segmental liver anatomy showing the vascular boundaries of the major liver segments (see also Table 25.1). IVC, inferior vena cava; R, M, L, right, middle and left hepatic veins; PV, portal vein.

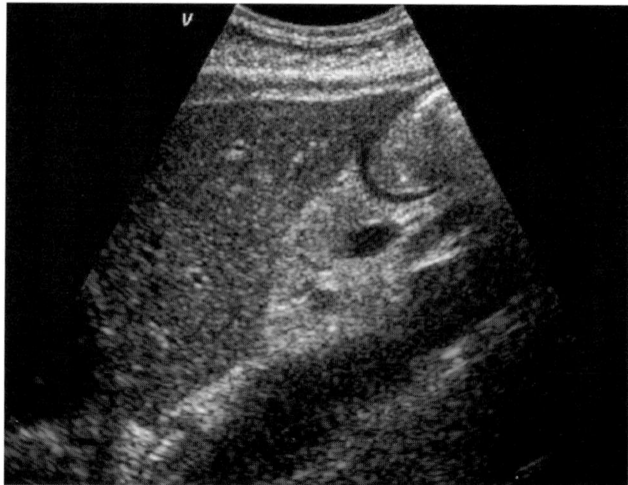

Fig. 25.2 Normal left lobe of liver. The inferior margin of the left lobe is sharp with an angle of less than 45°.

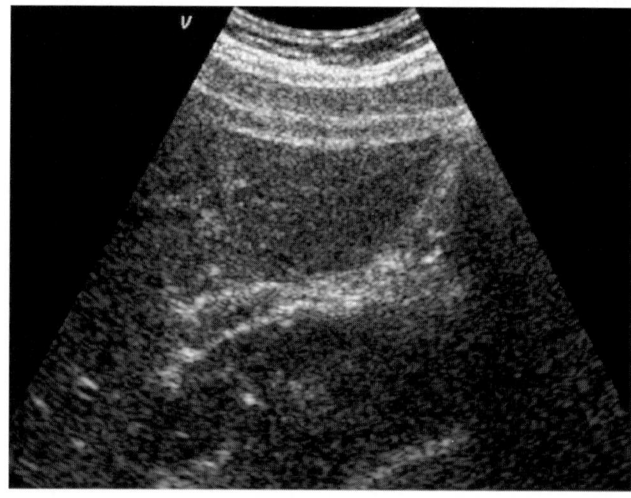

Fig. 25.3 Normal right lobe of liver. The inferior margin is sharp but the angle is between 45 and 90°.

be clearly distinguished from the adjacent parenchyma (Fig. 25.4). Indeed, the reflectivity of these vessel walls is a useful internal reference for the reflectivity of the liver parenchyma. The hepatic veins walls are not normally seen on ultrasound and these vessels thus appear merely as gaps in the liver parenchyma. The only exception to this rule occurs when an hepatic vein wall lies at right angles to the insonating beam, giving rise to specular reflection and a strong wall echo.

Assessment of liver size

Because of the variability in the size and proportions of the lobes no one measurement of the liver permits unequivocal identification of hepatomegaly. However, if the magnitude of the inferior angles is increased beyond the normal range or if the inferior margin of the left lobe is convex, hepatomegaly can be assumed. In many patients the relationship between the right lobe of the liver and the right kidney is also helpful. An anterior longitudinal scan of the right kidney through the right lobe of the liver normally shows the liver in contact with no more than two-thirds of the length of the kidney (see Fig. 25.4). When the liver is enlarged the area of contact is significantly increased.

In many patients with chronic liver disease there may be a complex combination of lobar or segmental hypertrophy and atrophy such that the liver shape is markedly

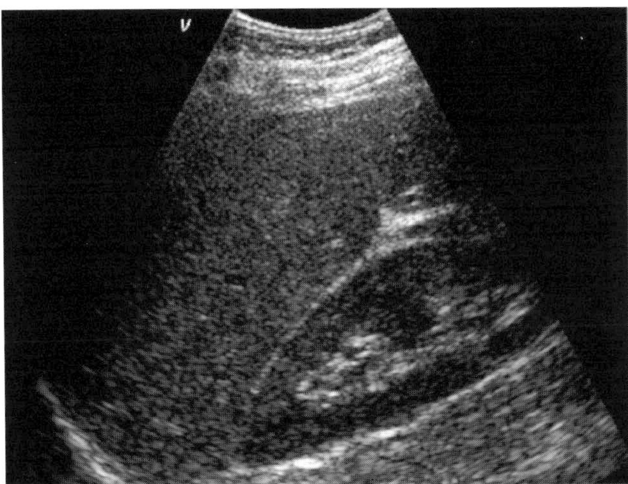

Fig. 25.4 Relationship of liver and right kidney. The normal right lobe is in contact with up to two-thirds of the length of the right kidney. The reflectivity of the liver parenchyma is slightly greater than that of the renal cortex at the same depth. The portal vein walls are clearly identifiable against the lower reflectivity parenchymal echo pattern.

altered [1]. One of the common sequelae of chronic liver disease is atrophy of the right lobe with enlargement of the left or caudate lobes. Caudate lobe size can be judged on transverse scans of the upper abdomen showing the left lobe anterior to the caudate lobe [2]. The anteroposterior diameter of the caudate lobe in this view should be no more than 50% of that of the left lobe, or the width of the caudate lobe should be no more than half of the width of the adjacent right lobe (Fig. 25.5).

Scanning technique

Preparation of the patient

No patient preparation is necessary for imaging of the liver. However, as most examinations of the liver will include assessment of the biliary tree and gallbladder it is wise routinely to fast all patients for hepatobiliary ultrasound. In addition, the utility of Doppler blood flow studies in the assessment of chronic liver disease is becoming more widely accepted and it is necessary to fast the patient prior to a Doppler study in order to interpret the portal vein findings.

Scanning guidelines

As a general principle it is useful for each department to develop guidelines for examination of the liver to ensure that a complete examination is performed. Failure to follow guidelines may lead to significant omissions in an examination, especially if the operator is diverted by some interesting or unusual finding before completing the examination. The following is the protocol used in the authors' department and has been evolved over a period of many years.

Patients are initially examined in the supine position, the first scans being obtained in a longitudinal plane to the left of the midline in the hypochondrium. If the patient is able to co-operate scans are obtained during short periods of suspended inspiration to optimize imaging of the left lobe. After finding the left lobe the examination is extended as far as possible to the left to assess the lateral extent of the left lobe and then imaging continues in the longitudinal plane moving to the right until access is impaired by the right costal margin. Oblique subcostal and transverse scans during suspended inspiration may be helpful in obtaining good views of the liver in many patients but will fail in those who cannot co-operate or who have a small liver or low costal margin. The majority of imaging of the right lobe is obtained via intercostal scans during neutral respiration. The right lobe is interrogated through a series of intercostal spaces on the right, angling the transducer to interrogate as large a volume of the liver as possible through each intercostal space.

Using the above protocol it is likely that about 90% of the liver volume is imaged. It is probably never possible to image 100% of the liver.

If imaging via the intercostal spaces is unsatisfactory the right lobe can sometimes be seen better with the patient in the left lateral decubitus position and the transducer placed either longitudinally or obliquely in the right subcostal space, during suspended inspiration if possible. This view is also extremely helpful in improving imaging of the gallbladder, common bile duct and pancreas as the right lobe of the liver tends to fall medially giving an excellent window to these structures.

Doppler studies

The splenic vein, superior mesenteric vein and extrahepatic portal vein should be accessed by appropriate subcostal scans, although obtaining an adequate beam–vessel angle from this approach may be difficult [3]. The distal extrahepatic and the intrahepatic portal system are best examined via a right lateral intercostal approach such that the portal vein is passing almost directly towards the transducer thus giving an optimal beam–vessel angle (Fig. 25.6). Measurements of mean portal vein flow velocity should be obtained using a range gate which is large enough to encompass the full width of the vessel (see Fig. 25.6) and, if respiratory excursion is not excessive, tracings should be obtained during quiet respiration. If it is neces-

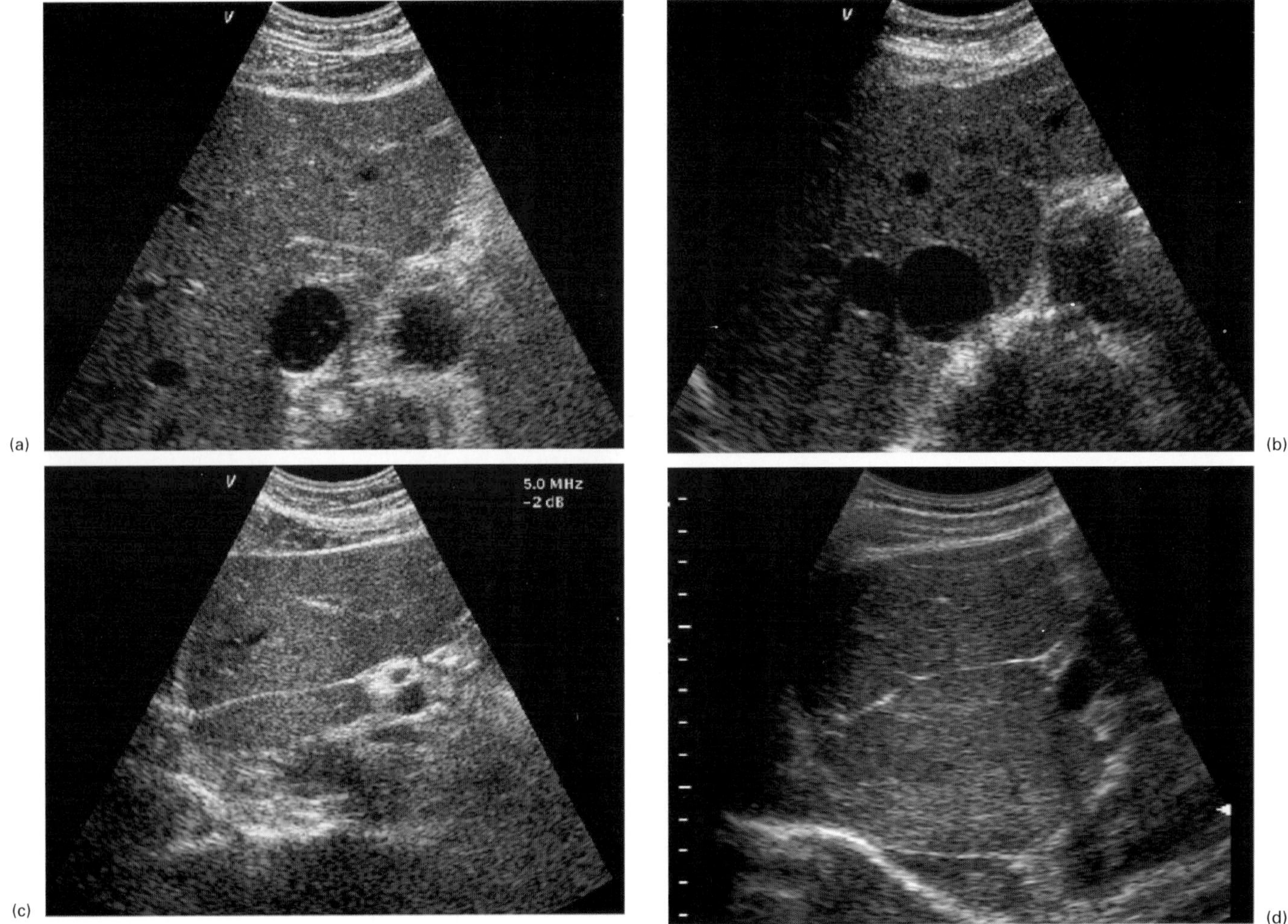

Fig. 25.5 Assessment of caudate lobe size. (a) Transverse scan of a normal caudate lobe. The anteroposterior diameter is less than half of the anteroposterior diameter of the left lobe anterior to the caudate. (b) Enlarged caudate lobe. The anteroposterior diameter of the caudate is now equal to the left lobe. (c) Longitudinal scan of a normal caudate lobe. (d) Longitudinal scan of an enlarged caudate lobe with an anteroposterior diameter greater than that of the left lobe.

sary to suspend respiration in order to obtain adequate traces the patient should be asked to hold their breath after only a small inspiration and the trace should be obtained as quickly as possible. Use of deep and prolonged inspiration may reduce the portal vein flow velocity.

Assessment of hepatic vein pulsatility is normally confined to the right hepatic vein [4,5] and this is also best imaged via a relatively posterior lateral intercostal scan (Fig. 25.7). Doppler tracings are obtained during quiet respiration or, if necessary, during suspended shallow inspiration. It is seldom necessary to obtain Doppler tracings from the left and middle hepatic veins, if their patency is being questioned this can usually be confirmed using colour Doppler imaging with a conventional anterior approach.

Benign focal liver disease

Cysts

Developmental cysts of the liver are relatively common [6,7] and are diagnosed with increasing frequency in older patients. They are often multiple, several may be grouped together, they may be partially or completely septated and often have lobulated shapes (Fig. 25.8). They are probably never of any clinical relevance. These simple cysts are virtually never seen in paediatric and young adult patients. Any liver cysts detected in these younger patients arise from and may communicate with the bile ducts, are usually single and are often lobulated but seldom sep-

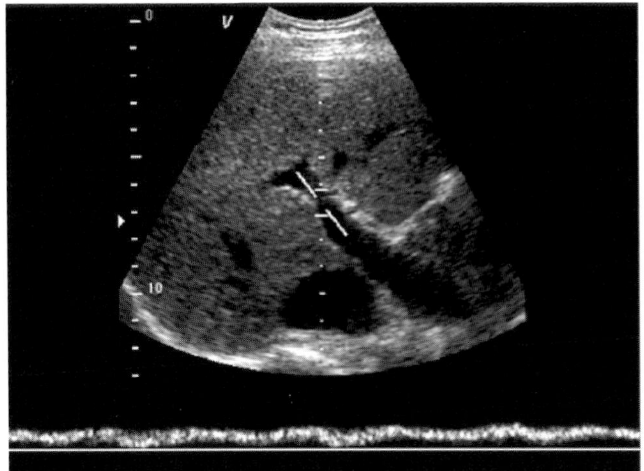

Fig. 25.6 Portal vein Doppler study. The portal vein is approached via a right lateral intercostal scan and the sample volume is adjusted to match the vessel width.

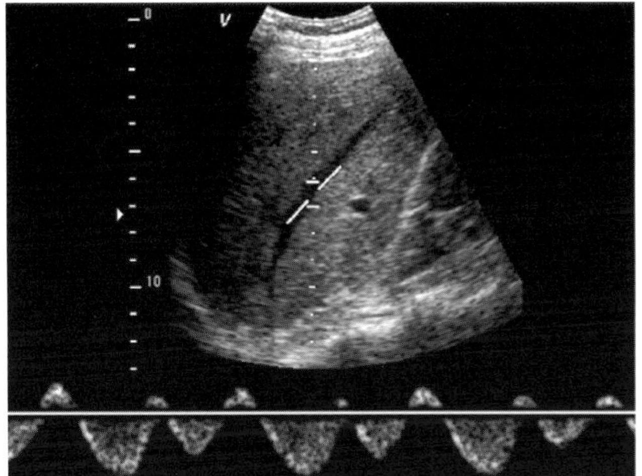

Fig. 25.7 Right hepatic vein Doppler study. The approach is similar to that for the portal vein. The normal waveform is biphasic with two periods of flow reversal during the cardiac cycle.

tated. They may be associated with other biliary anomalies. The presence of multiple intrahepatic cysts in a child or young adult is likely to be due to Caroli's disease [8,9].

True polycystic liver disease, although hereditary in origin, is normally only manifest in middle to late adult life and is characterized by the presence of numerous cysts with widely varying sizes and shapes [6] (Fig. 25.9). It may be associated with polycystic renal disease. The presence of multiple similar sized cysts within the liver is more likely to be due to hydatid disease in which a cyst has ruptured and given rise to many daughter cysts, all of the same age and size (Fig. 25.10). However, the appearance of

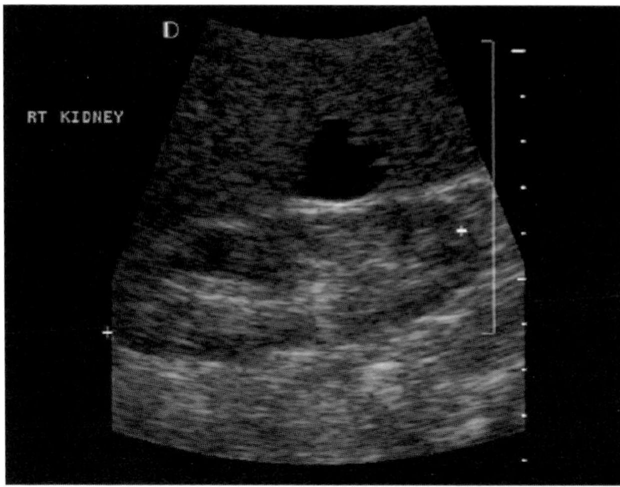

Fig. 25.8 Simple liver cyst. This cyst was an incidental finding in the right lobe of the liver. It shows the characteristic lobulated outline.

hydatid disease of the liver is extremely variable [10,11] ranging from single simple cysts to multiple cysts and apparently solid lesions, rarely with an onion skin layering appearance (Fig. 25.11) which is almost pathognomonic of this condition. Long-standing hydatid cysts may show mural calcification and may contain mobile dependent debris.

A rare form of cystic disease of the liver is the biliary cystadenoma. This normally benign tumour comprises both solid and cystic components and is often very complex in structure, similar to an ovarian cystadenoma. The lesion is always single, may recur after incomplete resection and may be frankly malignant.

Liver abscess

Pyogenic liver abscesses may occur at any site within the liver, though the large majority are posteriorly within the right lobe. In the early stage of evolution of an abscess ultrasound reveals an ill-defined area of reduced reflectivity [12]. As the abscess matures central necrosis gives rise to a cavitating lesion with a thick and irregular wall (Fig. 25.12). Cavitation may give rise to a multiloculated abscess and indeed many liver abscesses may be multifocal, particularly if secondary to portal pyaemia. It is important to interrogate the entire liver for the presence of gas within the portal system and to confirm patency of the portal vein.

Amoebic liver abscesses usually occur only in patients who have recently visited areas of the world where *Entamoeba histolytica* is endemic. Most patients give a history of amoebic dysentery some weeks or months prior to presentation. Amoebic abscesses are normally fairly mature by

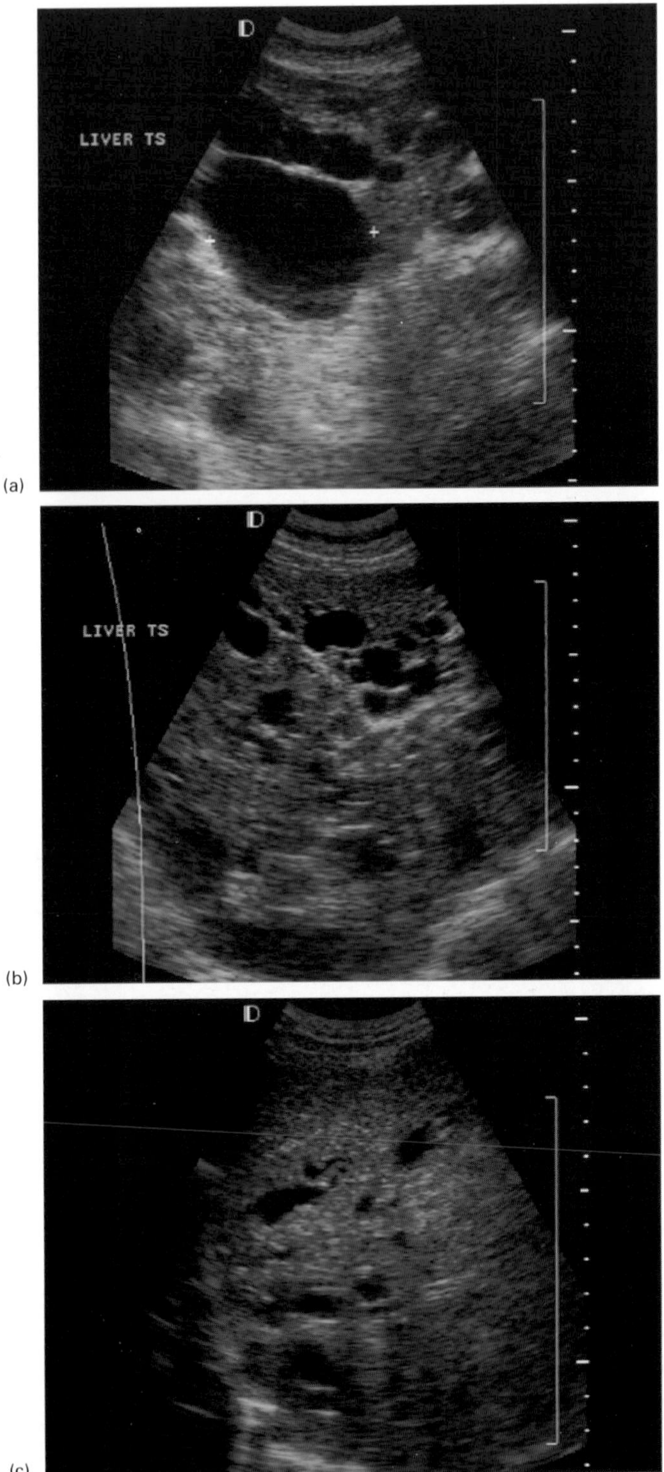

Fig. 25.9 Polycystic liver disease. (a) A single large and several small cysts are seen within the left lobe of the liver. (b) Right lobe of the same patient as in (a). Numerous small irregular shaped and varying sized cysts are present. (c) A further patient with irregular cystic spaces in the liver. In this case these are due to Caroli's disease of the biliary system. Biliary contrast studies may be necessary to differentiate this condition from polycystic liver disease.

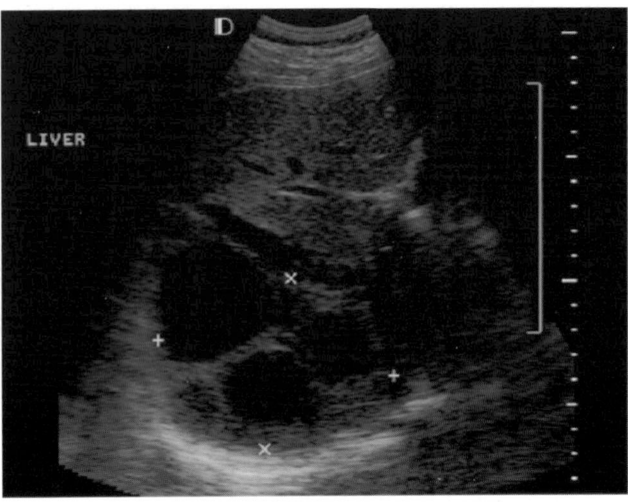

Fig. 25.10 Hydatid disease. Three similar-sized daughter cysts are seen posteriorly in the right lobe. The remainder of the liver is normal.

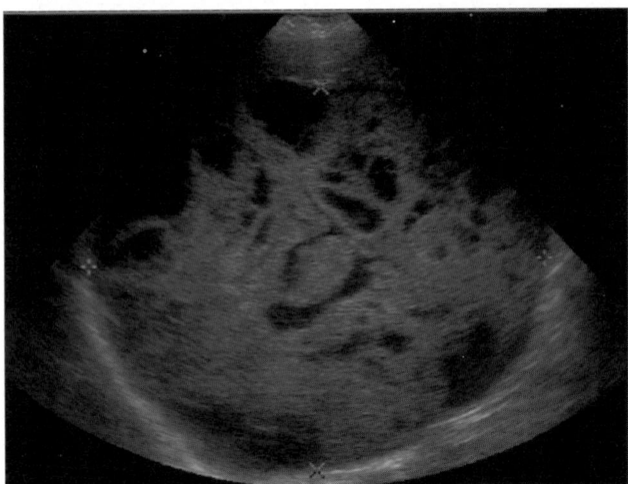

Fig. 25.11 Hydatid disease. This large hydatid cyst is filled with multiple small irregular cysts and alveolar material giving a false appearance of a mostly solid lesion. The distal acoustic accentuation helps to differentiate the lesion from a soft tissue mass.

the time the patient is investigated and they therefore appear as clearly defined thin-walled lesions [13] (Fig. 25.13). The pus is often moderately to highly reflective and uniform in appearance [14] and may give the false impression of a solid lesion, though there is invariably marked distal acoustic accentuation to confirm the true fluid nature of the pus.

Fungal granulomas of the liver occur rarely, usually in immunocompromised patients. Many are not detected with ultrasound but they may appear as small lesions, approximately 1 cm in diameter, with reduced reflectivity

(a)

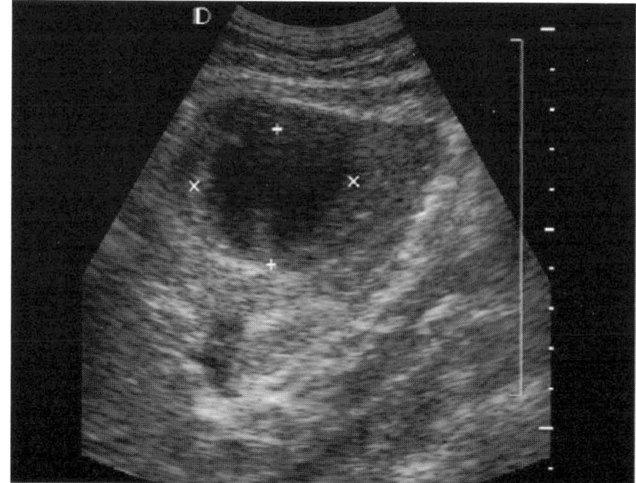

(b)

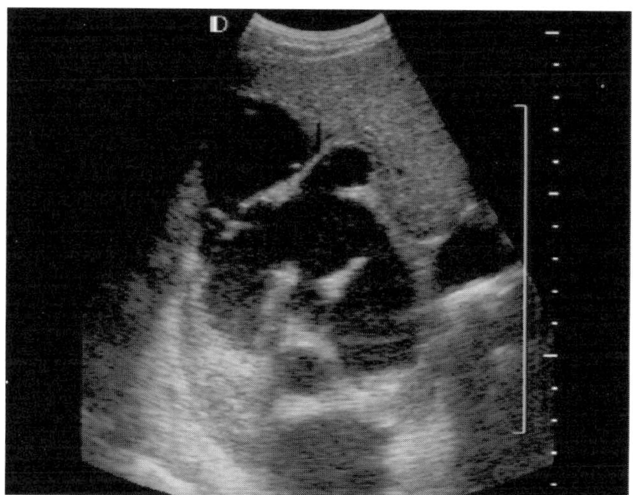

Fig. 25.12 Liver abscess. (a) A maturing liver abscess with a thick wall and irregular ill-defined cavity. (b) A relatively long-standing abscess with a thick wall and multiple septations. This must be differentiated from hydatid disease and multicystic metastasis.

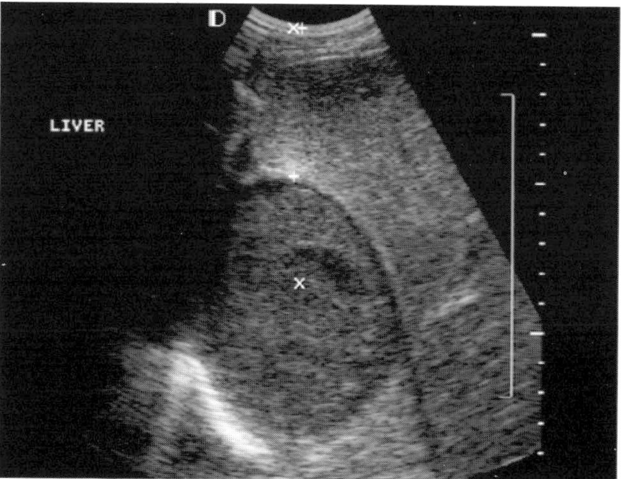

Fig. 25.13 Amoebic abscess. The abscess is very clearly defined and contains uniform highly reflective material but exhibits marked distal acoustic accentuation confirming its fluid-filled nature.

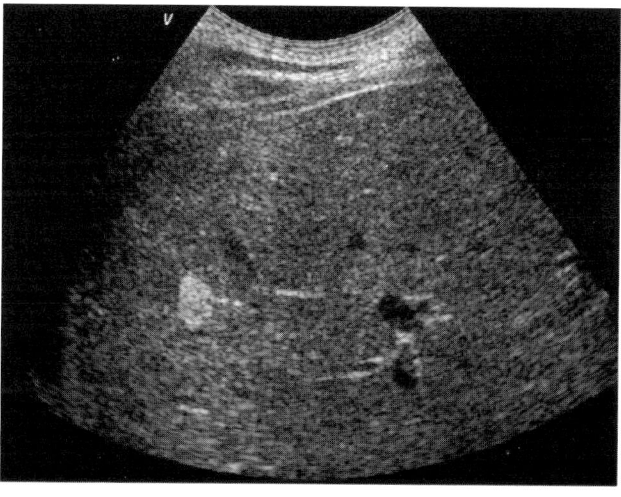

Fig. 25.14 Liver haemangioma. Typical appearance of a small haemangioma. It is clearly defined and uniformly highly reflective with no distal accentuation or shadowing.

and a central highly reflective nidus [15,16], probably a small vessel. In these patients similar lesions may also be seen in the spleen.

Solid lesions

HAEMANGIOMAS

Cavernous haemangiomas are the commonest benign liver tumour and are said to be present in 10% of the population on postmortem examination. Consequently, on ultrasound examination, they are almost always incidental findings and need to be differentiated from other liver tumours. Haemangiomas less than 5 cm in diameter are almost always highly reflective [17] with clearly defined lobulated outlines and occasionally containing small irregular echo-free areas (Fig. 25.14). Careful examination reveals close proximity to the wall of a major vessel and many lesions are also subcapsular. They are often multiple. Lesions greater than 5 cm in diameter have rather more variable echo patterns and are frequently heterogeneous with larger areas of reduced reflectivity [18], possibly indicating haemorrhage or necrosis.

The subcapsular lesions may give rise to localized liver pain, especially if they have undergone necrosis or haemorrhage and rarely haemangiomas may spontaneously rupture and give rise to a haemoperitoneum. In the appropriate clinical context the ultrasound examination should therefore be extended to search for free intraperitoneal fluid. The blood flow in haemangiomas is exceedingly slow and Doppler studies are therefore of no value in this condition as the red cell velocities cannot be detected.

HAEMANGIOENDOTHELIOMA

Haemangioendotheliomas present in the neonatal period, usually with hepatomegaly and occasionally as a cause for high output cardiac failure. On ultrasound imaging the lesions appear as multiple clearly defined spherical masses of lower reflectivity than the normal liver [19] (Fig. 25.15). Colour Doppler studies show them to be highly vascular and there is usually increase in the size of the hepatic artery with greatly increased flow velocity, often much greater than $100\,\mathrm{cm\,s^{-1}}$. Patients with these lesions are often treated by hepatic artery embolization or ligation. Although the clinical results of this are usually satisfactory postoperative Doppler studies always show continuing patency of the intrahepatic arterial tree with continuing high flow [20]. However, with the passage of time, the flow progressively spontaneously reduces and the lesions slowly reduce in size and may partially calcify. The liver is usually normal in appearance by the age of about 3 years, very rarely residual abnormalities may persist into adult life.

FOCAL NODULAR HYPERPLASIA

This strange condition is much less common than haemangioma and is again often an incidental finding. The characteristic feature of a central stellate scar so clearly seen on computed tomography (CT) scanning is seldom obvious on ultrasound examination [21,22] and the lesion therefore presents as an ill-defined mass, often of the same or similar reflectivity to the adjacent liver. There are no ultrasound characteristics which permit an accurate ultrasound diagnosis.

ADENOMA

Liver adenomas are rare benign tumours and are almost always single. The ultrasound features are variable [23], the lesion usually appearing as a clearly defined area with altered echo pattern and displacement of adjacent vessels. The reflectivity is variable and there are no specific ultrasound characteristics for this lesion.

Both focal nodular hyperplasia and liver adenoma may give rise to spontaneous intraperitoneal haemorrhage and their presence should thus always be sought in the appropriate clinical context.

FOCAL FATTY CHANGE

Although not a true lesion focal fatty change and focal fatty sparing masquerade as focal liver lesions [24,25]. Fatty change appears as an irregular often very angular shaped area of increased reflectivity against a background of normal liver echo pattern whilst focal sparing is again irregular in shape, often anterior to the porta hepatis [26], and is seen as an area of normal reflectivity against a background of increased parenchymal reflectivity secondary to generalized fatty change (Fig. 25.16). Both conditions

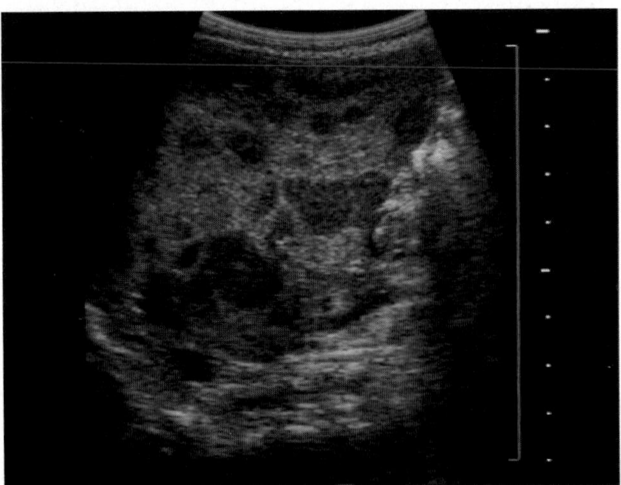

Fig. 25.15 Haemangioendothelioma. The typical appearance with multiple, irregular sized, clearly defined echo-poor lesions throughout the liver.

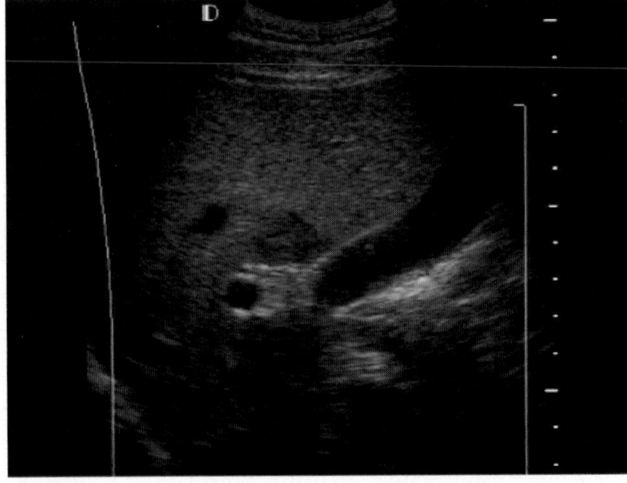

Fig. 25.16 Focal fatty sparing. The liver is uniformly increased in reflectivity but there is a 15 mm diameter area of lower reflectivity anterior to the porta hepatis due to focal fatty sparing.

occur as temporary manifestations of an evolving liver disorder and may therefore be expected to alter in size and appearance over a period of weeks or months. CT scanning may be necessary to confirm the diagnosis.

FOCAL CALCIFICATIONS

Isolated small foci of calcification within the liver are not uncommon as incidental findings. It is often not possible to be certain of their nature and origins. If the lesions are close to the portal tracts the possibility of intrahepatic biliary calculi should be considered but the majority of lesions are probably due to infarcted haemangiomas or parasitic infestations. These lesions are therefore almost always the tombstones of previous pathology and are thus not of any current clinical relevance.

Liver trauma

Although the liver may be damaged by bullets, knives and other sharp objects by far the most common cause of liver injury is blunt abdominal trauma, often not of sufficient severity to raise suspicion of liver injury. If the injury is relatively mild the liver capsule remains intact and the initial ultrasound finding is usually an irregular intrahepatic fluid-filled space. These haematomas often increase in size over a period of several days, either by continued bleeding or as a result of osmosis of fluid into the lesion. Thus the haematoma will normally become more clearly defined and spherical in shape. Late rupture of the capsule may occur, or may be the cause of rapid post-trauma collapse and shock after more severe trauma. In this situation the disruption of the liver may be difficult or impossible to identify, but free blood will be noted in the peritoneal cavity.

Fresh haematomas are relatively echo-poor but fill with echoes after a few days as fibrin fibres form. Later these may undergo lysis, with consequent loss of reflectivity, but alternatively may progress to organized thrombus with increase in reflectivity. Despite often quite severe compression of the underlying liver uncomplicated haematomas, with an intact liver capsule, require no active treatment and can be monitored by ultrasound. They may increase in size for a period of a few weeks and may take several months to resolve completely.

Malignant liver tumours

Hepatocellular carcinoma

Hepatocellular carcinoma (HCC) is the commonest primary malignant liver tumour. The majority arise against a background of chronic liver disease [27] and carry a very poor prognosis. The fibrolamellar variant tends to occur in younger patients without known liver disease, is often large at the time of presentation, and carries a rather better prognosis.

The ultrasound appearances of HCC are extremely variable. The lesions may be single or multiple, clearly defined or ill defined and of increased, decreased or variable reflectivity (Fig. 25.17). There are thus no characteristic ultrasound features and the diagnosis must be determined by the detection of one or more focal lesions against a background of known chronic liver disease, usually with elevation of the serum α-fetoprotein (AFP) level. Care must be taken not to confuse prominent regenerative nodules with HCC as most patients at risk for HCC will also have multiple regenerative nodules throughout the liver. Differentiation may be aided by studying the vascularity of the lesions as regenerative nodules are not hypervascular whereas many HCCs are more vascular than other liver tumours and colour Doppler and power Doppler studies can be used to demonstrate this feature [28]. It is possible that the new ultrasound contrast agents may also be helpful in differentiating HCCs from other tumours [29].

Direct invasion of the liver vessels is said to occur in up to 25% of HCCs [30]. This most commonly occurs into the portal vein and may extend throughout the portal system with expansion of the vessels on imaging. Even when the vessels are expanded the tumour does not occlude the vessel and colour flow imaging may be useful to confirm this and to show tumour vessels within the intraluminal mass [31], thus permitting an accurate diagnosis to be made. Metastases rarely invade vessels.

Ultrasound has been shown to have a valuable role in the treatment of HCC, primarily as a guidance tool for alcohol injection, laser and cryo treatment and follow-up of response to these therapies.

Hepatoblastoma

This malignant tumour virtually only occurs in paediatric patients and may be present at birth. The tumour is usually solitary and may show rapid increase in size and rapid spread throughout the liver. The overall reflectivity of the lesion tends to be similar to or a little greater than that of the normal liver [32] and the diagnosis may be difficult to make, although there is usually a mass effect with displacement of adjacent vessels (Fig. 25.18). These tumours occasionally contain a range of mesenchymal elements, including bone and cartilage, and may exhibit amorphous areas of calcification. There are no specific ultrasound characteristics but the presence of a liver tumour in a child is more likely to be due to hepatoblastoma than any other diagnosis.

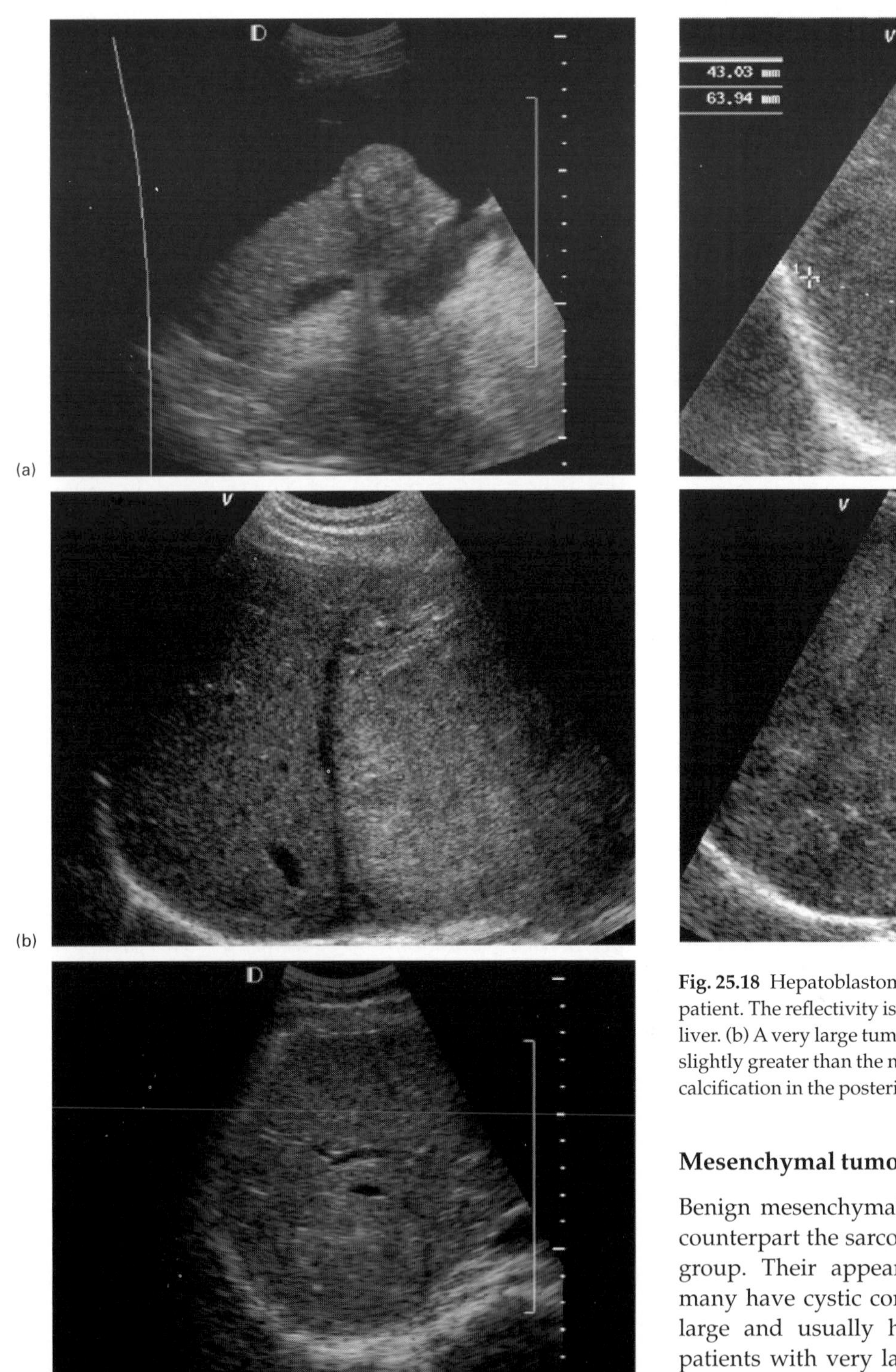

Fig. 25.17 Hepatocellular carcinoma. (a) A small heterogeneous lesion in a patient with ascites. The lesion also exhibits moderate distal acoustic shadowing. (b) A very large hepatoma with greater reflectivity and less attenuation than the adjacent liver. (c) An isoechoic 5 cm lesion is present posteriorly within this right lobe. The lesion shows less attenuation than the adjacent liver.

Fig. 25.18 Hepatoblastoma. (a) A 4×6 cm tumour in a neonatal patient. The reflectivity is similar to that of the overlying normal liver. (b) A very large tumour in a small child. The reflectivity is slightly greater than the normal liver and there is possibly multifocal calcification in the posterior part of the tumour.

Mesenchymal tumours

Benign mesenchymal hamartomas, and their malignant counterpart the sarcoma, may occur in the paediatric age group. Their appearances are extremely variable but many have cystic components. The lesions may be very large and usually have a clearly defined margin. In patients with very large lesions the compressed normal liver may be very difficult to identify with ultrasound and CT or magnetic resonance imaging (MRI) may be necessary to give a true picture of the whole anatomy.

Metastases

Metastases are the commonest liver tumours and exhibit a wide variety of ultrasound appearances. Although most

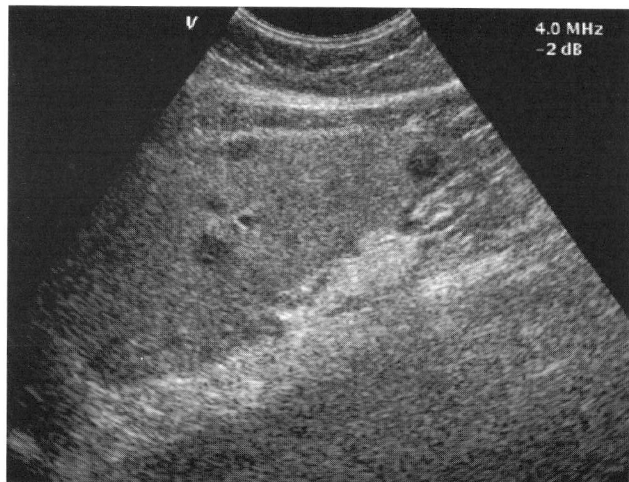

Fig. 25.19 Poorly reflective metastases. Multiple clearly defined lesions of lower reflectivity than the liver are present in this patient with carcinoma of the breast.

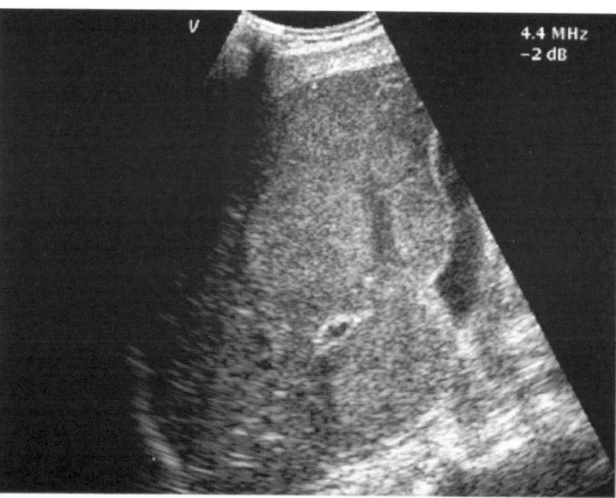

Fig. 25.20 Highly reflective metastases. Three large clearly defined and moderately highly reflective lesions are present in this patient with carcinoma of the colon.

liver metastases from carcinoma of the breast or bronchus are poorly reflective (Fig. 25.19) and metastases from carcinoma of the colon are highly reflective (Fig. 25.20), the ultrasound features of metastases never permit an accurate prediction for the site of origin. However, metastases from carcinoma of the breast are almost always multiple and small and may give rise to a moth-eaten appearance of the liver. Conversely, metastases from the colon tend to be single or few in number and may become very large. When the lesions are few the segmental anatomy of the lesions should be determined in order to assist the surgeon in consideration of their resectability.

Large metastases may outgrow their blood supply and undergo central necrosis sometimes giving an appearance not unlike a liver abscess. Rarely necrotic metastases may become infected. It is therefore important to be aware of this possibility and to consider biopsy of the wall of the lesion as well as aspirating its contents when undertaking a diagnostic tap for a suspected liver abscess.

Rarely metastases may exhibit a gross morphology similar to the primary lesion. Thus metastases from carcinoma of the ovary may show multi-cystic change and cysts or clearly defined fluid-filled spaces may also occur in metastases from colon, kidney, stomach, oesophagus and other mucus-secreting tumours.

Differential diagnosis of liver metastases

There are seldom any ultrasound features which assist in the differential diagnosis of poorly reflective liver lesions. However, if the lesions are highly reflective the presence or absence of excessive through transmission or attenuation should be observed. The majority of haemangiomas show normal or excessive transmission and may show distal acoustic accentuation. Conversely, metastases from carcinoma of the colon are often more attenuating than adjacent liver with consequent distal shadowing. Occasionally there may be frank calcification within the tumour giving rise to very strong shadowing. Lymphoma involvement of the liver usually gives rise to clearly defined, spherical, poorly reflective lesions, though there are no specific features that permit their differentiation from other echo-poor metastases.

If lesions are re-examined over an interval of 2–3 months the majority of metastases will show little change. If there has been rapid tumour growth the possibility of HCC should be considered.

In all cases where the diagnosis is uncertain ultrasound is invaluable to assist with guided biopsy. Even if the lesion is thought to be a possible haemangioma, biopsy is generally safe so long as the needle is passed through some normal liver before entering the tumour. It is of course wise to check the patient's coagulation status prior to all liver biopsies.

Diffuse liver disease

Ultrasound is essentially an anatomical imaging technique and its role in the diagnosis of diffuse liver disease is therefore rather limited. In patients thought to have diffuse liver disease ultrasound may be helpful in judging the size and shape of the liver. The liver outline should be

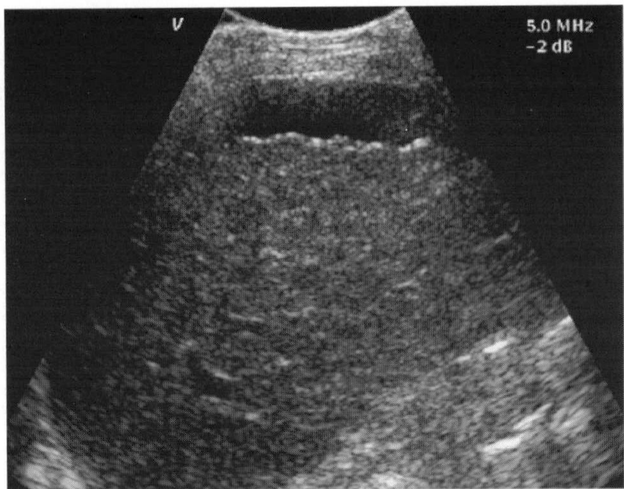

Fig. 25.21 Nodular regeneration of the liver. The parenchymal echo pattern is finely heterogeneous with multiple small nodules but these are most easily seen on the surface outlined by the ascites.

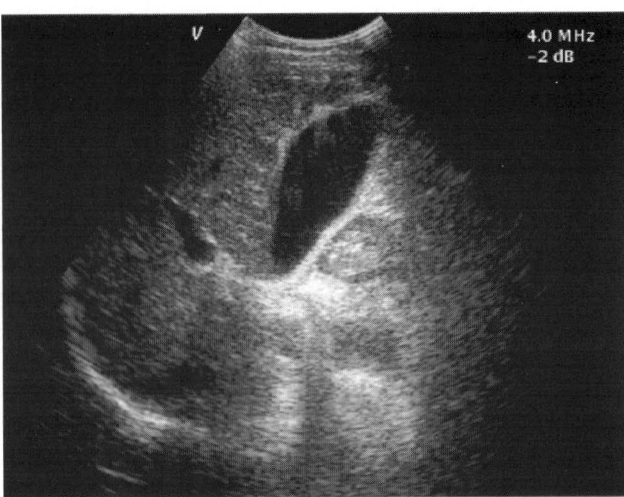

Fig. 25.22 Liver nodularity. This patient has cirrhosis with nodular regeneration. The outline of the nodules is best seen adjacent to the anterior wall of the gallbladder.

assessed to determine whether or not there is any evidence of nodularity. This is most easily achieved in the presence of ascites (Fig. 25.21). If no ascites is present the surface of the liver adjacent to the gallbladder and the right kidney should be assessed (Fig. 25.22) and it may also be helpful to inspect the margins of the major hepatic veins to see whether or not there is gross evidence of nodularity.

The liver echo pattern in diffuse liver disease is variable and many subjective changes have been reported in the literature but these unfortunately vary according to the make of equipment in use. There is, however, uniform agreement that an increase in liver fat content gives rise to an increase in reflectivity [33,34] (See Fig. 25.16) whilst acute inflammatory changes may cause a reduction in reflectivity. Mild to moderate cirrhosis without fatty change does not give any identifiable changes within the liver [33,34] though, of course, it may be associated with both fatty change and regenerative nodules. Acute hepatic inflammation, due to acute hepatitis and other insults such as some drugs, may be associated with a reduction in liver reflectivity with even the smallest portal radicals standing out clearly against the dark parenchyma.

Alcoholic liver disease is generally associated with enlargement of the liver and an increase in both reflectivity and attenuation [35] (Fig. 25.23). If the disorder is acute there may be rapid evolution in both the degree and distribution of the fatty change.

In patients with primary biliary cirrhosis the liver may appear normal in both size and echo pattern, even if the disease is sufficiently severe to threaten the patient's survival. However, in advanced cases it is usually possible to detect some nodularity and in many cases enlarged lymph nodes may be seen in the region of the hepatoduodenal ligament [36,37].

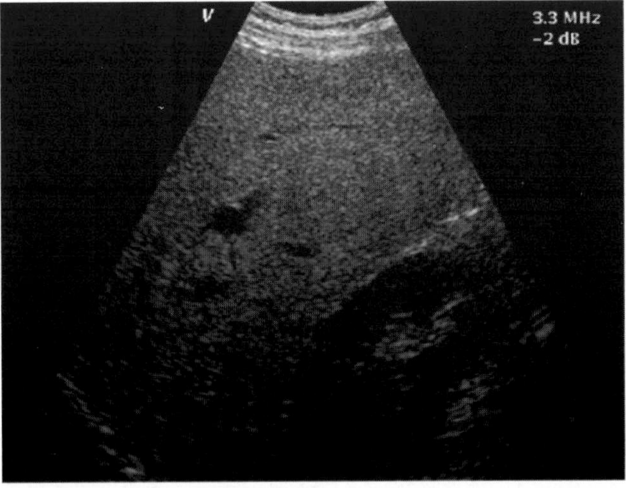

Fig. 25.23 Alcoholic liver disease. There is an increase in both reflectivity and attenuation. The liver is markedly brighter than the adjacent kidney and the deeper regions of the liver are poorly seen owing to increased attenuation.

The liver disease secondary to cystic fibrosis often has a characteristic appearance with the development of large nodules, typically 2–3 cm in diameter, with or without increased reflectivity due to fatty change. However, as the underlying diagnosis is almost always known in advance this feature is seldom of prospective diagnostic value.

Portal hypertension

Ultrasound imaging and Doppler studies are valuable both for the initial diagnosis and the management of portal hypertension. Imaging should be directed towards detection of portosystemic shunts, including the umbilical vein, gastro-oesophageal varices and spontaneous splenorenal shunts [38].

The umbilical vein passes from the left branch of the portal vein inferiorly and anteriorly along the undersurface of the liver to reach the anterior abdominal wall just below the liver edge (Fig. 25.24). Normally it cannot be detected by ultrasound but if it is recanalized and dilated it can be seen by both imaging and colour Doppler studies. When patent it gives absolute confirmation of portal hypertension [39,40] and is associated with normal or high flow velocity in the main portal vein, though there may be simultaneous reversed flow in the more peripheral branches of the right and left portal vein as these too drain towards the umbilical vein. The umbilical vein probably recanalizes in up to 50% of patients with portal hypertension.

The presence of gastro-oesophageal varices can be implied by the finding of tortuous venous channels superior to the splenic vein and by thickening of the lesser omentum.

Spontaneous splenorenal shunts only occur in about 15% of patients with portal hypertension. They are haemodynamically more efficient that all other spontaneous portosystemic shunts effectively decompressing the portal system and giving a high level of protection from gastro-oesophageal varix formation. Flow in the main portal vein and splenic vein is almost always reversed. These shunts are seen as a collection of 2–3 cm diameter vascular channels between the splenic hilum and the hilum of the left kidney (Fig. 25.25). Colour flow imaging confirms their vascular nature. When present they are confirmation of the presence of portal hypertension.

A further non-specific sign of portal hypertension is thickening of the gallbladder wall [41] but the same appearance may also be seen in any patient with acute or chronic liver disease.

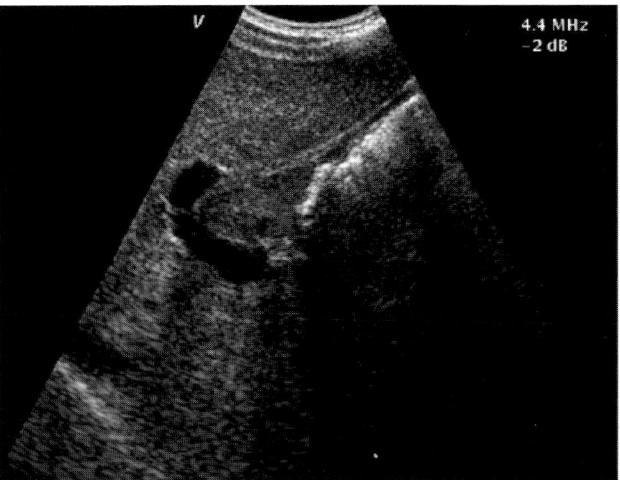

(a)

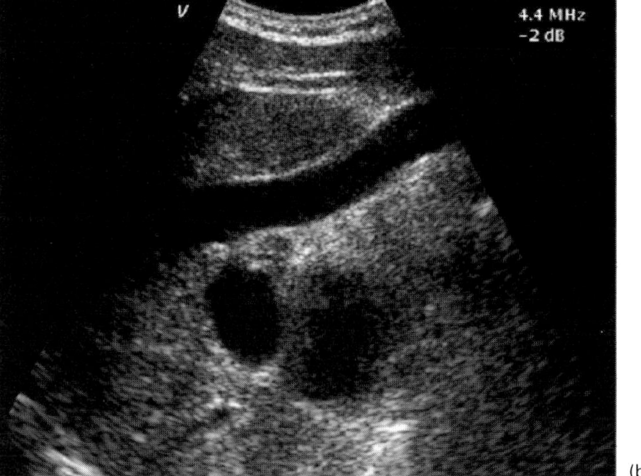

(b)

Fig. 25.24 Umbilical vein. (a) A normal obliterated umbilical vein can be seen in this patient passing anteriorly and inferiorly from the left portal vein. (b) A very large recanalized umbilical vein in which there was high velocity hepatofugal flow in this patient with portal hypertension.

Measurement of spleen size

Measurement of spleen size is an integral component of assessment of chronic liver disease and portal hypertension, though it must be remembered that a normal-sized spleen does not exclude portal hypertension [42].

The spleen should normally be measured during quiet respiration along the length of a left intercostal space with the patient supine. Care must be taken to identify both the inferior splenic tip and the superomedial extremity of the spleen simultaneously. Failure to do this will lead to undermeasurement of the spleen. Occasionally a small inspiration may help to bring the spleen into view but deep inspiration must be avoided as it will bring the lung down into the lateral costophrenic recess and obscure the spleen completely. Similarly turning the patient onto their right side may ease access to the spleen but the spleen may fall medially and become difficult or impossible to see. It must be remembered that as the spleen enlarges its tip migrates towards the right iliac fossa, not down the left flank.

In adults the size of a normal spleen varies with both body size and race. In an average white adult it should not have a length of greater than about 12.5 cm whilst in

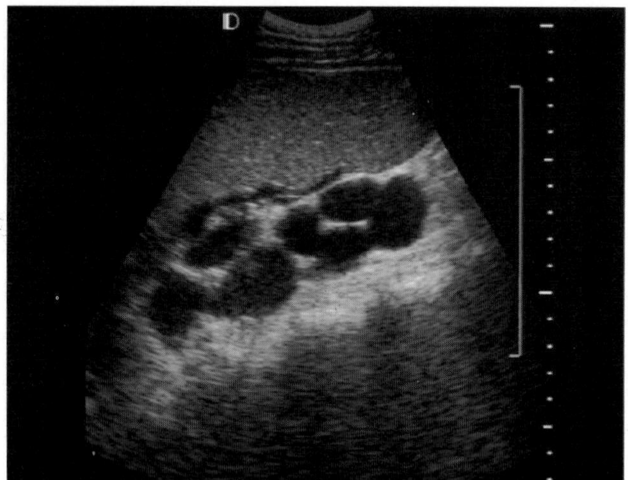

Fig. 25.25 Spontaneous splenorenal shunts. These large serpiginous venous channels close to the splenic hilum are typical of spontaneous splenorenal shunts.

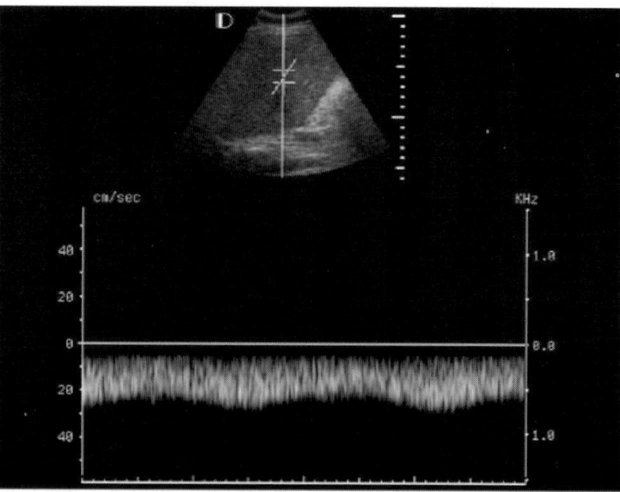

Fig. 25.26 Abnormal hepatic vein waveform. The blood flow waveform in this patient's hepatic vein is markedly damped due to diffuse liver disease. Compare with Fig. 25.7.

patients of African origin it may be no more than 8–9 cm in length.

Budd–Chiari syndrome

This syndrome is caused by occlusion of the major hepatic veins. It may be partial or complete. In those cases which present early it may be possible to see poorly reflective thrombus filling the hepatic veins. In more chronic cases the liver becomes enlarged and irregular in shape with patchy alteration in echo pattern. The underlying occlusion of the hepatic veins may not be immediately obvious in such a distorted liver and the diagnosis must therefore always be borne in mind and an active search made with colour Doppler for the hepatic veins. In complete cases there is usually reversal of flow in the portal vein early in the disease but this may revert to normal as intrahepatic channels open up from the hepatic veins to the subcapsular veins. Conversely, as the disease becomes chronic cirrhosis usually occurs and portal flow may reverse once again.

Doppler ultrasound in liver disease

The intra- and extrahepatic portal venous system, hepatic artery and major hepatic veins are all amenable to imaging and flow assessment with Doppler ultrasound. The clinical utility of hepatic vein measurements remains to be proven, though it has been shown that the pulsatility of the waveform in the right hepatic vein is reduced in many forms of acute and chronic liver disease [5,43] (Fig. 25.26), and it may be of some value in assessing the prognosis of some of these patients [44].

Examination of the hepatic artery is similarly of limited value, although its role has been shown to be crucial in monitoring young children with biliary atresia [45] and in the postoperative assessment of liver transplant subjects.

The main role for Doppler ultrasound in the diagnosis of liver disease is in the assessment of the patency of the portal vein and the characteristics of the flow within it.

PORTAL VENOUS SYSTEM

Investigation of the portal system should include identification of the splenic vein, superior mesenteric vein, both the extrahepatic and intrahepatic portal venous system, paraportal and portosystemic shunts.

The patency and direction of blood flow within the components of the portal system can be confirmed by colour Doppler examination and this is often all that is required in the diagnosis and assessment of liver disease (Fig. 25.27). However, particularly in pretransplant assessment patients, measurement of the time averaged mean portal vein flow velocity may be clinically valuable. If the flow is found to be unusually slow, irrespective of direction, the patient is at increased risk for spontaneous portal thrombosis and it is imperative to reassess the portal vein patency prior to transplantation.

The value of portal vein velocity measurement in the assessment of portal hypertension remains controversial, though it does have many protagonists. If the flow velocity is significantly decreased there is a high chance for portal hypertension being present but normal or high velocities may be present in some patients with portal hypertension.

Some patients with long-standing portal hypertension

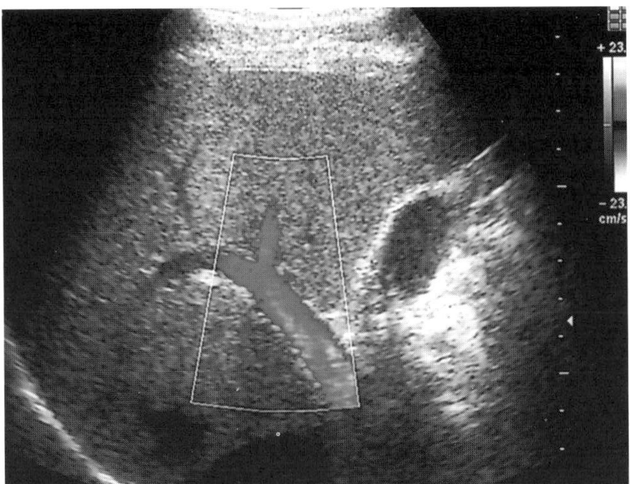

Fig. 25.27 Colour Doppler of the portal vein. Portal vein patency and flow direction is readily confirmed by a right lateral intercostal colour Doppler study. For colour, see Plate 25.27 (between pp. 308 and 309).

exhibit dilatation of the portal vein. The combination of this with reduced velocity has given rise to development of the 'congestion index' which may be more sensitive for the diagnosis of portal hypertension than portal vein diameter or flow velocity alone [46]. However, a normal congestion index does not exclude portal hypertension.

The published range of values for normal portal vein flow velocity is extremely wide [47]. This is partly due to a range of different measurement methods, including instantaneous peak, mean peak, computed time averaged mean and corrected mean values. In addition there is no uniformity of calibration between different makes of ultrasound equipment. It is therefore clear that any institution wishing to evaluate portal flow velocity in their patients must first establish their own normal range for the type of velocity measurement they prefer on the type of equipment available to them.

PORTAL VEIN OCCLUSION

The diagnosis of occlusion of the portal vein is surprisingly often overlooked. Recent thrombosis may be missed on imaging as the fresh thrombus has only minimally increased reflectivity. If the occlusion is of long standing there may be a partial recanalization, collateral formation or cavernous transformation (Fig. 25.28). In all of these a relatively large and apparently normal venous channel may be present and may masquerade to the unwary as a normal portal vein. However, careful examination with both imaging and Doppler should reveal the presence of

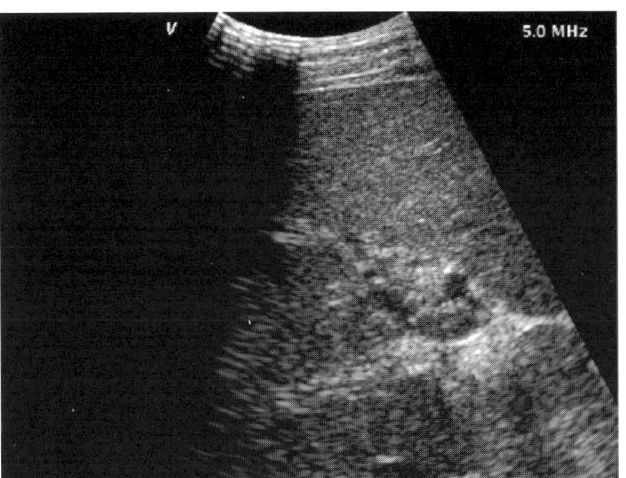

(a)

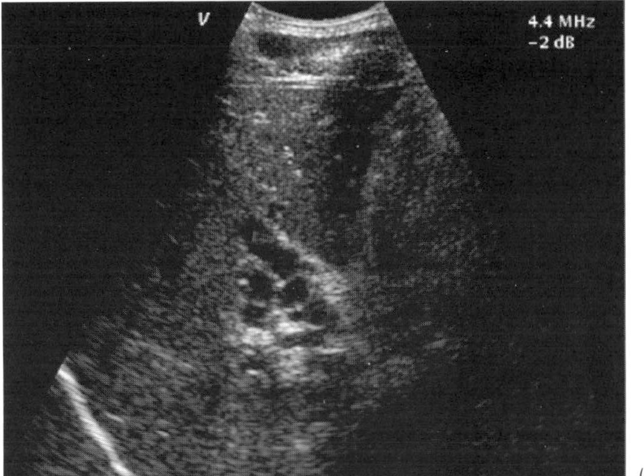

(b)

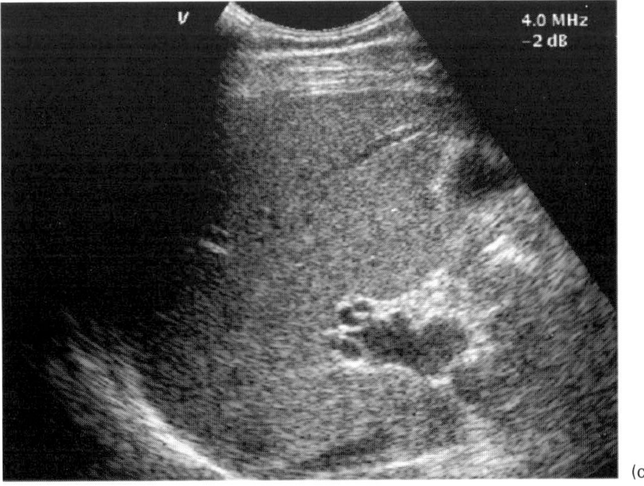

(c)

Fig. 25.28 Portal vein occlusion. (a) There is thrombus within the intrahepatic portal vein. (b) Cavernous transformation of the portal vein with multiple irregular collateral channels. (c) Cavernous transformation with a single large channel which may masquerade as a normal portal vein, though its shape and anatomy are clearly abnormal.

highly reflective material at the site of the occluded portal vein, or in any residual organized thrombus, whilst the collateral vessels are normally multiple and do not follow the same anatomical course as a normal portal vein. If the patency of the portal vein is under question it is important also to examine the splenic and superior mesenteric veins for patency as they may be required for possible shunt surgery.

IATROGENIC PORTOSYSTEMIC SHUNTS

A wide range of shunts has been devised including mesocaval, splenorenal, mesoatrial and transjugular intrahepatic portosystemic stent shunt (TIPS). Ultrasound assessment of shunt patency is frequently requested and is often difficult or impossible. An essential prerequisite is knowledge of both the direction and velocity of flow in the main portal vein prior to the shunt procedure. If preoperative forward flow changes to reverse flow postoperatively this is strong circumstantial evidence of shunt patency. Any subsequent change in flow direction implies shunt occlusion. Direct imaging of mesocaval shunts is frequently unsuccessful as the shunts are usually well below the splenic vein/superior mesenteric vein confluence and are thus obscured by overlying bowel. However, right lateral coronal scanning of the IVC may show the site of flow into the IVC if the shunt is patent. Care must be taken not to mistake a left renal vein for a mesocaval shunt. Patency of a splenorenal shunt requires prior knowledge of the flow direction within the splenic vein. Generally this will be forward prior to the shunt and reversed after successful shunting. If the shunt occludes, flow within the splenic vein may cease or may revert to forward in direction.

Careful scanning with a high frequency transducer will almost always permit direct visualization of a mesoatrial shunt as it passes anterior to the left lobe of the liver. The shunts are usually fashioned from a woven corrugated Teflon graft giving rise to the characteristic convoluted appearance of the graft material. These shunts are usually used as a temporary measure to decompress the liver after acute hepatic vein thrombosis and generally have a shorter life expectancy than other shunts.

TIPS are generally expanding metal shunts placed between the middle hepatic vein and portal vein. They are easily identified on grey-scale imaging and colour Doppler studies will usually easily confirm their patency. However, it is important to undertake a spectral Doppler study also in order to measure the peak flow velocity. If this is less than 50 $cm\,s^{-1}$ the shunt is at increased risk of occlusion [48], though Jalan *et al.* have found Doppler ultrasound of less value than portography [49].

Liver transplantation

Preoperative assessment

Ultrasound plays an important role in the preoperative assessment of patients being considered for liver transplantation. The two most important observations are continuing patency of the portal vein and the presence or absence of focal lesions which may indicate the development of HCC. As mentioned above low portal vein flow velocity may precede portal vein thrombosis and thus serial monitoring of flow velocity is important in the transplant candidate.

If focal lesions are discovered on ultrasound both the size and number of tumours should be assessed and ultrasound-guided biopsy should be considered to confirm the diagnosis. The cure rate of liver transplantation for HCC is reduced if large or numerous tumours are present. If more than three lesions are present and if any lesion is greater than about 4 cm in diameter the chances of success are so limited that transplantation is probably unjustified.

The spleen size should also be carefully measured prior to transplantation as a baseline value for post-transplant monitoring.

Ultrasound scanning with Doppler studies is also valuable during the evaluation of living related donors. In this context ultrasound is used to exclude fatty change and to exclude incidental benign lesions and major anomalies of the extrahepatic and intrahepatic vascular anatomy.

Peroperative scanning

Peroperative imaging may be helpful in confirming the number, site and size of liver tumours. Occasionally this may reveal the possibility of hepatic resection rather than transplantation as the preferred treatment choice whilst the detection of multicentric HCC usually mediates against transplantation.

If a donor liver is too large for the recipient, an on-table reduction procedure is necessary and ultrasound may have a role in helping the surgeon to determine the plane through which the liver can be divided, possibly to be split between two recipients.

Doppler studies may be helpful in confirming adequate flow after completion of the vascular anastomoses and before closure of the patient's abdomen.

Postoperative management

The postoperative role of ultrasound varies according to the time since transplantation and the surgical aspects of the transplant. In the immediate post-transplant period ultrasound is directed towards confirming vascular patency and detection of fluid collections which might indicate either a biliary or vascular leak. It is also important to assess the parenchymal echo pattern throughout the graft as preservation injury or postoperative occlusion of a major vessel or branch may give rise to localized irregular areas of reduced reflectivity indicating hepatic necrosis.

Portal vein patency can be confirmed with colour Doppler studies. The flow profile beyond the anastomosis is almost always disturbed and thus spectral Doppler studies are of little value.

Confirmation of hepatic arterial patency should include both the main hepatic artery and right and left intrahepatic branches. Again patency can be confirmed with colour Doppler, though this may be difficult as the peak flow velocities present within the adjacent portal vein may exceed the arterial velocity. High resolution colour flow imaging is therefore essential and the display velocity range should be manipulated to optimize differentiation between the arterial and portal flows. Once arterial patency has been confirmed on colour flow it is important to acquire spectral Doppler traces in order to study the flow velocity waveform. A wide range of velocity waveforms may be seen in the post-transplant patient [50] (Fig. 25.29). Low or absent diastolic flow is often observed but this seems to be of no clinical relevance and usually reverts to a more normal low resistance waveform within a week or two. However, the presence of a damped or tardus–parvus waveform (Fig. 25.30) in the intrahepatic branches indicates the likely presence of an anastomotic narrowing or arterial clamp injury [51] and indicates the need for immediate arteriography.

It has been stated that assessment of the hepatic vein waveform pulsatility may be a very sensitive and specific indicator of the onset of rejection [52]. However, the authors' experiences and those of Kok *et al.* [53] do not support this view.

The range of surgical variations in liver transplantation continues to expand and includes standard orthotopic transplant, cut-down livers (usually grafting segments 2 and 3, but occasionally other segments, including use of the right lobe) living related donation (usually segments 2 and 3) and auxiliary grafting where the left or right lobe only are replaced, leaving part of the recipient's own liver *in situ*. The postoperative vascular anatomy varies greatly with these different options and details of this must be known by the sonographer prior to examination of the patient [54]. All the anatomical variations cannot be discussed in the space available in this chapter. However, the most important postoperative features to be examined remain vascular patency, bile duct size and detection and

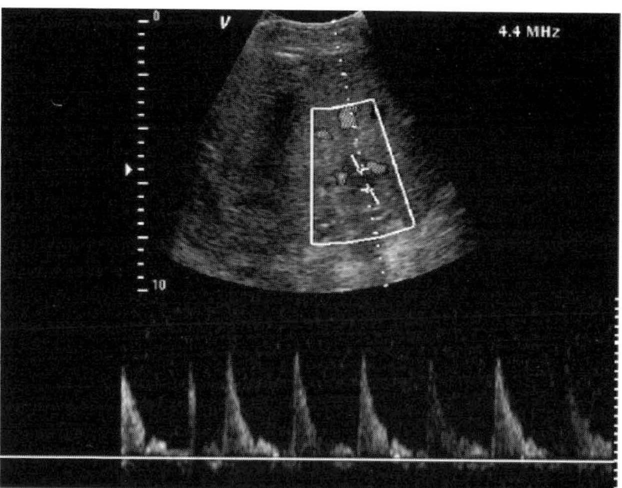

(a)

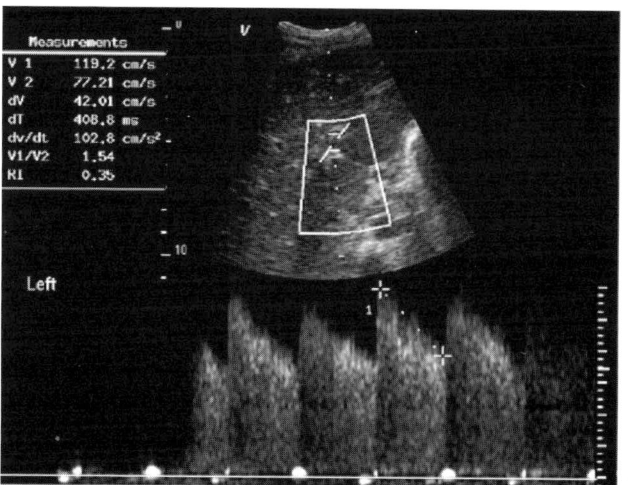

(b)

Fig. 25.29 Post-transplantation hepatic artery Doppler. These two figures show widely varying postoperative waveforms which did not correlate with any significant pathology and both patients made good postoperative recoveries.

monitoring of fluid collections, especially those related to the cut surface of a reduced graft.

The role of ultrasound in the later monitoring of hepatic transplantation again includes assessment of vascular patency, flow patterns, bile duct diameters and spleen size. Complications with the portal anastomosis are extremely unusual but arterial occlusion has been reported in up to 3% of adult recipients [55] and 25% of paediatric patients [56]; though recent improvements in surgical techniques have probably reduced these figures. The finding of a tardus–parvus waveform more than 1 month after transplantation is most likely to be due to arterial occlusion with collateral formation.

Assessment of the intrahepatic bile duct diameter is important to diagnose or exclude the development of

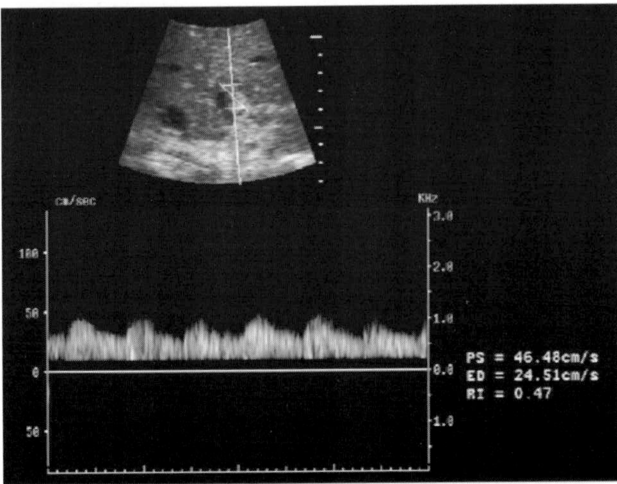

Fig. 25.30 Tardus–parvus hepatic artery waveform. The intrahepatic artery shows the typical waveform from an artery supplied by collateral vessels.

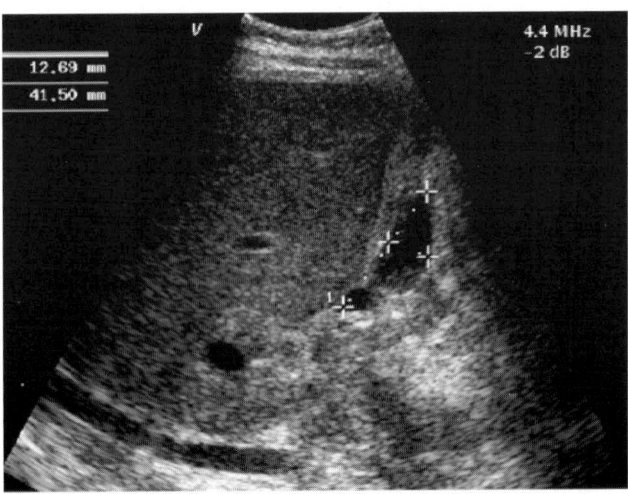

Fig. 25.31 Normal post-transplant periportal collection. This small subhepatic fluid collection is typical of that commonly seen in the post-transplant patient.

biliary stenoses. Late stenosis of the bile duct may occur at the anastomosis as a result of postsurgical fibrosis but can also occur close to the junction of the left and right hepatic ducts as a consequence of arterial deprivation. It is therefore important to examine the hepatic arterial tree in any patient found to have intrahepatic duct dilatation after transplantation.

Measurements of spleen size are an important corollary to assessment of portal vein flow. In patients with preoperative splenomegaly a reduction in spleen size by 1–2 cm can be expected in the first few post-transplant weeks. Thereafter the spleen should remain constant in size and any subsequent significant increase may indicate either portal vein stenosis or recurrence of chronic liver disease.

MANAGEMENT OF FLUID COLLECTIONS

Postoperative fluid collections are extremely common in these patients and the large majority are of little clinical relevance. There is almost always a perivascular haematoma at the porta hepatis within the first week (Fig. 25.31) but this should not exceed 3–4 cm in diameter and usually resolves rapidly. Lens-shaped subcapsular haematomas are also relatively common, particularly anteriorly on the left lobe and laterally on the right lobe. The aetiology is uncertain but they are probably related to handling of the liver. They can usually be differentiated from extrahepatic fluid collections by virtue of the fact that they indent the liver parenchyma. Subcapsular haematomas normally stabilize in size within the first week and virtually never require any intervention.

Leaks from the biliary anastomosis generally give rise to subhepatic fluid collections which are variable in size, shape and appearance. Although the bile is often echo-free during the first few days after a leak it usually subsequently fills with echoes which are often gravity dependent and thus make it impossible to differentiate bile from blood or pus. Serial monitoring of any doubtful fluid collections to assess changes in size is an integral component of their ultrasound evaluation. Those which are increasing rapidly in size, which may be causing vascular or ductal compression or which may be associated with sepsis probably deserve aspiration under ultrasound guidance. However, in the authors' experience, less than 10% of post-transplant fluid collections require any intervention [57].

Conclusion

Ultrasound imaging and Doppler studies continue to play a major role in the diagnosis and evaluation of patients with known or suspected liver disease. The advent of ultrasound echo-enhancing agents (contrast agents) may well expand this role by facilitating the acquisition of Doppler data and enhancing the evaluation of tumour vascularity [29,58]. Differential or dynamic tissue enhancement studies are currently under evaluation and may yield diagnostically useful information concerning the dynamics of liver parenchymal perfusion.

References

1 Ham, J.M. (1990) Lobar and segmental atrophy of the liver. *World Journal of Surgery* **14**, 457–462.

2 Giorgio, A., Amoroso, P., Lettieri, G., *et al.* (1986) Cirrhosis: value of caudate to right lobe ratio in diagnosis with US. *Radiology* **161**, 443.

3 Meire, H.B., Farrant, P. (1993) Liver transplants. In: Meire, H.B., Cosgrove, D.O., Dewbury, K.C. (eds) *Clinical Ultrasound—a Comprehensive Text*, vol. I. Churchill Livingstone, Edinburgh, p. 329.

4 Coulden, R.A., Lomas, D.J., Farman, P., Britton, P.D. (1992) Doppler ultrasound of the hepatic veins: normal appearances. *Clinical Radiology* **45**, 223–227.

5 Farrant, P., Meire, H.B. (1997) Hepatic vein pulsatility assessment on spectral Doppler ultrasound. *British Journal of Radiology* **70**, 829–832.

6 Weaver, R.M. Jr, Goldstein, H.M., Green, B., Perkins, C. (1978) Gray scale ultrasonographic evaluation of hepatic cystic disease. *American Journal of Roentgenology* **130**, 849–852.

7 Forbes, A., Murray-Lyon, I.M. (1991) Cystic disease of the liver and biliary tract. *Gut* (suppl.) S116–S122.

8 Tandon, R.K., Grewal, H., Anand, A.C., Vashisht, S. (1990) Caroli's syndrome: a heterogeneous entity. *American Journal of Gastroenterology* **85**, 170–173.

9 Guntz, P., Coppo, B., Lorimier, G., *et al.* (1991) Single-lobe Caroli's disease. Anatomoclinical aspects. Diagnostic and therapeutic procedure. Apropos of three personal cases and 101 cases in the literature. *Journal de Chirurgie (Paris)* **128**, 167–181.

10 Lewell, D.B., McCorkell, S.J. (1985) Hepatic echinococcal cysts: sonographic appearance and classification. *Radiology* **155**, 773.

11 Suwan, Z. (1995) Sonographic findings in hydatid disease of the liver: comparison with other imaging methods. *Annals of Tropical Medicine and Parasitology* **89**, 261–269.

12 Terrier, F., Becker, C.D., Triller, J.K. (1983) Morphologic aspects of hepatic abscesses at computed tomography and ultrasound. *Acta Radiologica Diagnostica* **24**, 129.

13 Ralls, P.W., Colletti, P.M., Quinn, M.F., Halls, J. (1982) Sonographic findings in hepatic amoebic abscess. *Radiology* **145**, 123.

14 Dalrymple, R.B., Fataar, S., Goodman, A., *et al.* (1982) Hyperechoic amoebic liver abscess: an unusual ultrasonic appearance. *Clinical Radiology* **33**, 541.

15 Maxwell, A.J., Mamtora, H. (1988) Fungal liver abscesses in acute leukaemia—a report of two cases. *Clinical Radiology* **39**, 197–201.

16 Mills, P., Saverymuttu, S., Fallowfield, M., Nussey, S., *et al.* (1990) Ultrasound in the diagnosis of granulomatous liver disease. *Clinical Radiology* **41**, 113–115.

17 Mirk, P., Rubaltelli, L., Bazzocchi, M., *et al.* (1982) Ultrasonographic patterns in hepatic haemangiomas. *Journal of Clinical Ultrasound* **10**, 373.

18 Moody, A.R., Wilson, S.R. (1993) Atypical hepatic hemangioma: a suggestive sonographic morphology. *Radiology* **188**, 413–417.

19 Dicks-Mireaux, C. (1993) The paediatric liver. In: Meire, H.B., Cosgrove, D.O., Dewbury, K.C. (eds) *Clinical Ultrasound—a Comprehensive Text*, vol. I. Churchill Livingstone, Edinburgh, p. 447.

20 Hazebroek, F.W., Tibboel, D., Robben, S.G., *et al.* (1995) Hepatic artery ligation for hepatic vascular tumors with arteriovenous and arterioportal venous shunts in the newborn: successful management of two cases and review of the literature. *Journal of Pediatric Surgery* **30**, 1127–1130.

21 Welch, T.J., Sheedy, P.F., Johnson, C.M., *et al.* (1985) Focal nodular hyperplasia and hepatic adenoma: comparison of angiography, CT, ultrasound and scintigraphy. *Radiology* **156**, 593.

22 Di Stasi, M., Caturelli, E., De Sio, I., *et al.* (1996) Natural history of focal nodular hyperplasia of the liver: an ultrasound study. *Journal of Clinical Ultrasound* **24**, 345–350.

23 Sandler, M.A., Petrocelli, R.D., Marks, D.S., Lopez, R. (1980) Ultrasonic features and radionuclide correlation in liver cell adenoma and focal nodular hyperplasia. *Radiology* **135**, 393.

24 Yates, C.K., Streight, R.A. (1986) Focal fatty infiltration of the liver simulating metastatic disease. *Radiology* **159**, 83.

25 Kawashima, A., Suehiro, S., Murayama, S., Russell, M.J. (1986) Focal fatty infiltration of the liver mimicking a tumour: sonographic and CT features. *Journal of Computer Assisted Tomography* **10**, 329.

26 Kissin, C.M., Bellamy, E.A., Cosgrove, D.O., *et al.* (1986) Focal sparing in fatty infiltration of the liver. *British Journal of Radiology* **59**, 25–28.

27 Shinagawa, T., Ohto, M., Kimura K., *et al.* (1984) Diagnosis and clinical features of small hepatocellular carcinoma with emphasis on the utility of real time ultrasonography. A study in 51 patients. *Gastroenterology* **86**, 495–502.

28 Hosoki, T., Mitomo, M., Chor, S., *et al.* (1997) Visualisation of tumor vessels in hepatocellular carcinoma. Power Doppler compared with color Doppler and angiography. *Acta Radiologica* **38**, 422–427.

29 Tanaka, S., Kitamra, T., Yoshioka, F., *et al.* (1995) Effectiveness of galactose-based intravenous contrast medium on color Doppler sonography of deeply located hepatocellular carcinoma. *Ultrasound in Medicine and Biology* **21**, 157–160.

30 Sugiura, N., Ohto, M., Kimura, K., *et al.* (1986) Imaging diagnosis of portal vein tumour thrombosis and its pathophysiology in hepatocellular carcinoma. *Japan Journal of Gastroenterology* **83**, 2151–2160.

31 Dodd, G.D. IIIrd, Memel, D.S., Baron, R.L., *et al.* (1995) Portal vein thrombosis in patients with cirrhosis: does sonographic detection of intrathrombus flow allow differentiation of benign and malignant thrombus. *American Journal of Roentgenology* **165**, 573–577.

32 de Campo, M., de Campo, J.F. (1988) Ultrasound of primary hepatic tumours in childhood. *Pediatric Radiology* **19**, 19–24.

33 Saverymuttu, S.H., Joseph, A.E., Maxwell, J.D. (1986) Ultrasound scanning in the detection of hepatic fibrosis and steatosis. *British Medical Journal* **292**, 13–15.

34 Joseph, A.E.A., Saverymuttu, S.H., Al-Sam, S., *et al.* (1991) Comparison of liver histology with ultrasonography in assessing diffuse parenchymal liver disease. *Clinical Radiology* **43**, 26–31.

35 Richard, P., Bonniaud, P., Barthelemy, C., *et al.* (1985) Value of ultrasonography in the diagnosis of cirrhoses. Prospective study of 128 patients. *Journal de Radiologie* **66**, 503–506.

36 Lyttkens, K., Prytz, H., Forsberg, L., *et al.* (1992) Ultrasound, hepatic lymph nodes and primary biliary cirrhosis. *Journal of Hepatology* **15**, 136–139.

37 Eustace, S., Buff, B., Kane, R., *et al.* (1995) The prevalence and clinical significance of lymphadenopathy in primary biliary cirrhosis. *Clinical Radiology* **50**, 396–399.

38 Gibson, P.R., Gibson, R.N., Donlan, J.D., *et al.* (1991) Duplex Doppler ultrasound of the ligamentum teres and portal vein: a clinically useful adjunct in the evaluation of patients with known or suspected chronic liver disease or portal hypertension. *Journal of Gastroenterology and Hepatology* **6**, 61–65.

39 Aagaard, J., Jensen, L.I., Sorensen, T.I.A., *et al.* (1982) Recanalised umbilical vein in portal hypertension. *American Journal of Roentgenology* **139**, 1107.

40 Mostbeck, G.H., Wittich, G.R., Herold, C., *et al.* (1989) Hemodynamic significance of the paraumbilical vein in portal hypertension: assessment with duplex ultrasound. *Radiology* **170**, 339.

41 Saverymuttu, S.H., Grammatopoulos, A., Meanock, C.I., *et al.* (1990) Gallbladder wall thickening (congestive cholecystopathy) in chronic liver disease: a sign of portal hypertension. *British Journal of Radiology* **63**, 922–925.

42 Gibson, P.R., Gibson, R.N., Ditchfield, M.R., Donlan, J.D. (1990) Splenomegaly—an insensitive sign of portal hypertension. *Australia and New Zealand Journal of Medicine* **20**, 771–774.

43 Arda, K., Ofelli, M., Calikoglu, U., *et al.* (1997) Hepatic vein Doppler waveform changes in early stage (Child–Pugh A) chronic parenchymal liver disease. *Journal of Clinical Ultrasound* **25**, 15–19.

44 Ohta, M., Hashizume, M., Kawanaka, H., *et al.* (1995) Prognostic significance of hepatic vein waveform by Doppler ultrasonography in cirrhotic patients with portal hypertension. *American Journal of Gastroenterology* **90**, 1853–1857.

45 Broide, E., Farrant, P., Reid, F., *et al.* (1997) Hepatic artery resistance index can predict early death in children with biliary atresia. *Liver Transplantation Surgery* **3**, 1–8.

46 Moriyasu, F., Ban, N., Nishida, O., *et al.* (1985) 'Congestion index' of the portal vein. *American Journal of Roentgenology* **146**, 735.

47 Bolondi, L., Gaiani, S., Barbara, L. (1993) The portal venous system. In: Meire, H.B., Cosgrove, D.O., Dewbury, K.C. (eds) *Clinical Ultrasound—a Comprehensive Text*, vol. I. Churchill Livingstone, Edinburgh, pp. 320–321.

48 Feldstein, V.A., Patel, M.D., LaBerge, J.M. (1996) Transjugular intrahepatic portosystemic shunts: accuracy of Doppler US in determination of patency and detection of stenoses. *Radiology* **201**, 141–147.

49 Jalan, R., Stanley, A.J., Redhead, D.N., Hayes, P.C. (1997) Shunt insufficiency after transjugular intrahepatic portosystemic stent-shunt: the whens, whys, hows and what should we do about it? *Clinical Radiology* **52**, 329–331.

50 Longley, D.G., Skolnick, M.L., Sheahan, D.G. (1988) Acute allograft rejection in liver transplant recipients: lack of correlation with loss of hepatic artery diastolic flow. *Radiology* **169**, 417–420.

51 Nghiem, H.V., Tran, K., Winter, T.C. IIIrd, *et al.* (1996) Imaging of complications in liver transplantation. *Radiographics* **16**, 825–840.

52 Britton, P.D., Lomas, D.J., Coulden, R.A., *et al.* (1992) The role of hepatic vein Doppler in diagnosing acute rejection following paediatric liver transplantation. *Clinical Radiology* **45**, 228–232.

53 Kok, T., Haagsma, E.B., Klompmaker, I.J., *et al.* (1996) Doppler ultrasound of the hepatic artery and vein performed daily in the first 2 weeks after orthotopic liver transplantation. Useful for the diagnosis of acute rejection? *Investigative Radiology* **31**, 173–179.

54 Someda, H., Moriyasu, F., Fujimoto, M., *et al.* (1995) Vascular complications in living related liver transplantation detected with intraoperative and postoperative Doppler US. *Journal of Hepatology* **22**, 623–632.

55 Wozeney, P., Zajko, A.B., Bron, K.M. (1986) Vascular complications after liver transplantation: a 5-year experience. *American Journal of Roentgenology* **147**, 657–663.

56 McDiarmid, S.V., Hall, T.R., Grant, E.G., *et al.* (1991) Failure of duplex sonography to diagnose hepatic artery thrombosis in a high risk group of pediatric liver transplant recipients. *Journal of Pediatric Surgery* **26**, 710–713.

57 Raby, N., Meire, H.B., Forbes, A., Williams, R. (1988) The role of ultrasound screening in management after liver transplantation. *Clinical Radiology* **39**, 507–510.

58 Ernst, H., Hahn, E.G., Balzer, T., *et al.* (1996) Colour Doppler ultrasound of liver lesions: signal enhancement after intravenous injection of the ultrasound contrast agent Levovist. *Journal of Clinical Ultrasound* **24**, 31–35.

Chapter 26: The biliary tree and pancreas

K.M. Carroll

Anatomy and normal appearance

Bile is secreted by hepatocytes into biliary canaliculi which converge to form intrahepatic biliary ducts. The intrahepatic bile ducts lie in the portal triads with branches of the portal vein and hepatic artery. The cystic duct joins the gallbladder to the common hepatic duct to form the common bile duct. It is not usually possible on ultrasonography to identify the level of insertion of the cystic duct and the term 'common duct' is generally used for both the common hepatic and common bile ducts. The intrahepatic ducts up to segmental level are not seen on ultrasound but the right and left hepatic ducts may be seen near the porta hepatis, measuring up to 2mm. The normal common duct measures up to 6mm but increases in size with advancing age [1]. At the porta hepatis the right hepatic artery crosses between the portal vein and the common duct and may resemble a filling defect in the duct. This is a tubular structure and colour Doppler imaging readily demonstrates its arterial nature (Fig. 26.1). The common bile duct passes down towards the pancreas, anterior to the portal vein and lateral to the hepatic artery in the free edge of the lesser omentum. The distal common duct then passes behind the duodenal bulb to lie in a groove on the posterior aspect of the pancreas, sometimes encircled by pancreatic tissue, before entering the medial aspect of the second part of the duodenum at the ampulla of Vater with the pancreatic duct. The gallbladder usually lies in a fossa along the inferior margin of the liver. The cystic duct may have a spiral configuration.

The pancreas lies in the retroperitoneum in the upper abdomen. The head is the bulkiest portion of the gland and lies in the concavity of the C loop of the duodenum. The neck, body and tail extend to the left and slightly superiorly towards the splenic hilum. The splenic vein lies posterior to the pancreas for most of its length and is a useful anatomical landmark for identifying the pancreas. On transaxial section the splenic vein has a 'tadpole' configuration with the head on the right due to confluence with the superior mesenteic vein forming the portal vein (Fig. 26.2). The uncinate process lies inferiorly, posterior to the superior mesenteric artery and vein. The pancreas varies in size. The maximum anteroposterior diameter of the head of the pancreas is 2.5–3.0cm and the tail 2cm. The pancreas is normally homogeneous in echogenicity on ultrasound. However, in a significant number of subjects, the uncinate process and part of the pancreatic head, derived from the ventral pancreas, are relatively echo-poor due to lower fat content, which may lead to false positive diagnosis of an hypoechoic lesion.

Ultrasound of the gallbladder, biliary tree and pancreas is performed after an overnight fast in supine and right anterior oblique positions. Left decubitus and erect positions may also be helpful. The normal gallbladder is seen as an ovoid structure containing anechoic bile. The wall thickness is less than 3mm [2]. The gallbladder may be folded (Fig. 26.3) or may contain a prominent incomplete septum, described as a 'Phrygian cap'. The normal transverse diameter measures up to 4cm (but may be up to 5cm in short gallbladders) and the length is 7–10cm. Ultrasound with measurement of gallbladder volume before and after a fatty meal or cholecystokinin may demonstrate patency of the cystic duct [3,4]. After a fatty meal there is normally a reduction in the diameter of the common duct. Enlargement indicates obstruction [5,6].

The pancreas may be difficult to visualize because of overlying gastric and bowel gas. Visualization may be improved by using the liver as an acoustic window and by scanning with the patient erect. Using an oral fluid load to create an acoustic window in the stomach and proximal duodenum may help, especially in visualization of the tail, which is usually the most difficult part of the pancreas to demonstrate. The normal pancreatic duct measures up to 2mm and can be seen in most subjects with good quality scanners (Fig. 26.4) [7]. The duct is easiest to see in the body. The side branches are not visualized in the normal gland.

Pancreas divisum results from failure of fusion of the embryological ventral and dorsal ducts and is controversially associated with an increased risk of pancreatitis [8]. This diagnosis is most commonly made at endoscopic retrograde cholangiopancreatography (ERCP) but the

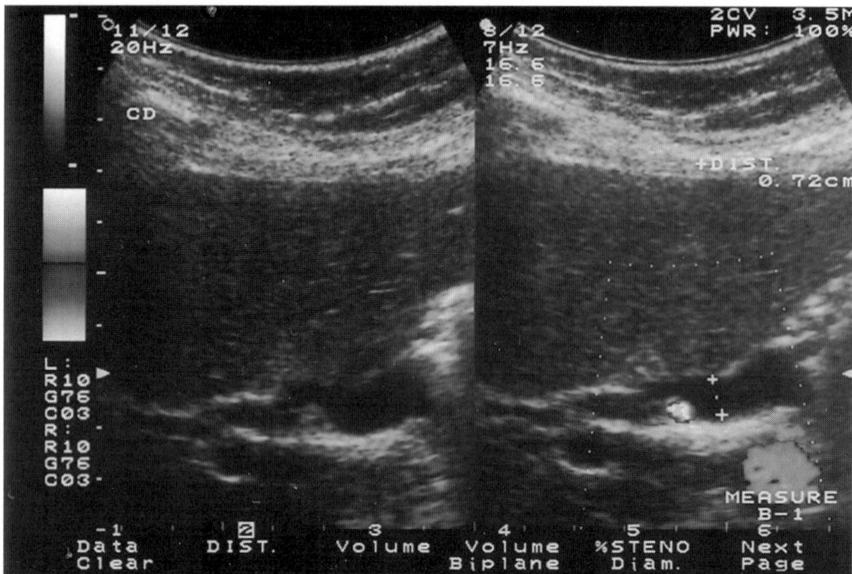

Fig. 26.1 Normal anatomy at the porta hepatis. Right hepatic artery crossing between the portal vein (posteriorly) and a slightly dilated common duct (7 mm) might be mistaken for a filling defect in the duct but this is a tubular structure on scanning along its length. Colour Doppler imaging (on the right) demonstrates arterial pulsation in the right hepatic artery. For colour, see Plate 26.1 (between pp. 308 and 309).

(a)

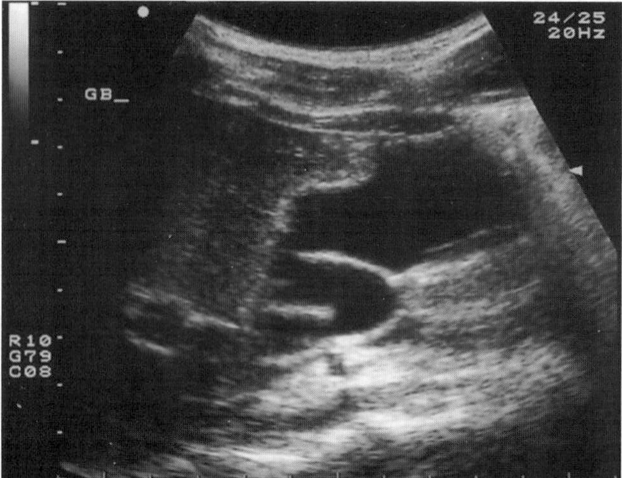

(b)

Fig. 26.2 (a,b) Prominent folds in gallbladder. Such folds may lead to false positive diagnosis of intraluminal filling defects such as stones or polyps.

separate pancreatic ducts may sometimes be visible on ultrasound. Annular pancreas is a congenital anomaly resulting from the pancreas encircling the duodenum, usually the second part. About half will present early with duodenal obstruction. In children and adults with a later presentation, the ring may be incomplete. Pancreatic tissue may be seen encircling the duodenum.

Recent developments in ultrasound of the biliary tree and pancreas include the use of endoscopic, endoluminal, laparoscopic and intraoperative ultrasound which allow high frequency contact imaging. Endoscopic ultrasound provides detailed images of structures close to the lumen of the stomach and duodenum. This technique is comparable to cholangiography in evaluation of the common bile duct for stones with a negative predictive value of 97% for common duct stones [9]. Pancreatic diseases can be accurately characterized and targeted biopsy can be performed [10,11]. This technique is expensive, difficult to use and available in only a small number of centres. Micro-ultrasound probes with frequencies up to 30 MHz. are used for intraductal imaging [e.g. 12]. Laparoscopic ultrasound is very sensitive for common duct stone detection [e.g. 13]. Endoscopic and intraoperative ultrasound are described in more detail in Chapter 27.

Evaluation of acute right upper quadrant pain

Ultrasound is the initial imaging modality of choice in acute right upper quadrant (RUQ) pain and this is one of

(a)

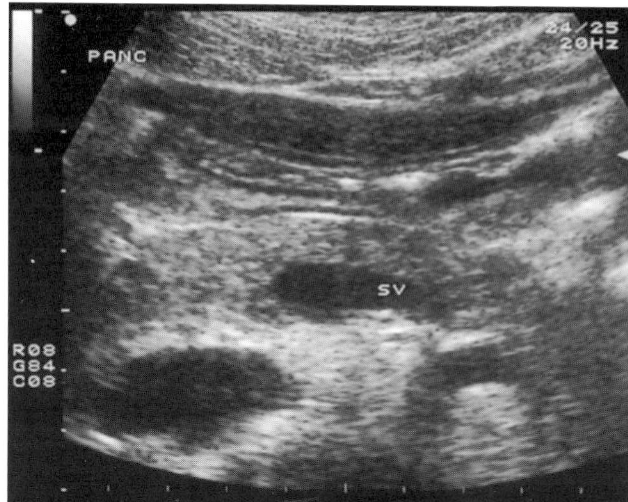

(b)

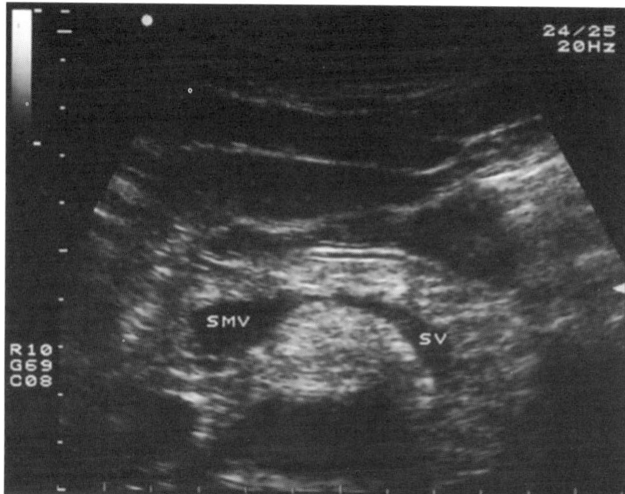

Fig. 26.3 Normal pancreas. (a) Transverse view showing body of pancreas anterior to the splenic vein (SV). (b) Transverse view in a different patient with a SV on the left and the confluence with the superior mesenteric vein (SMV) forming the portal vein on the right like the head of a tadpole.

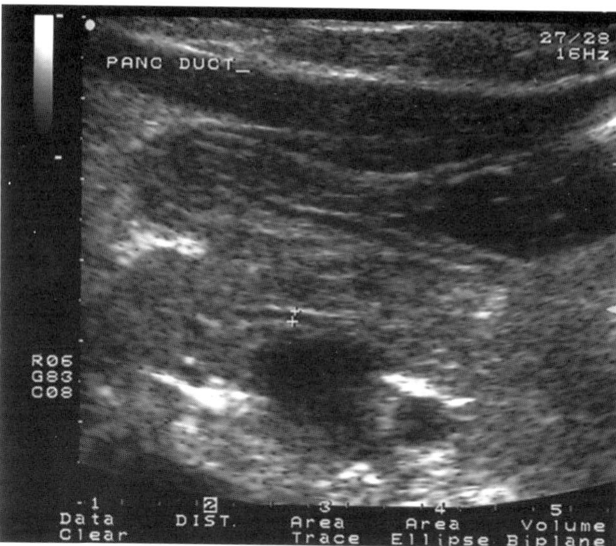

Fig. 26.4 Transverse view of a normal pancreas showing a normal pancreatic duct (1.2 mm).

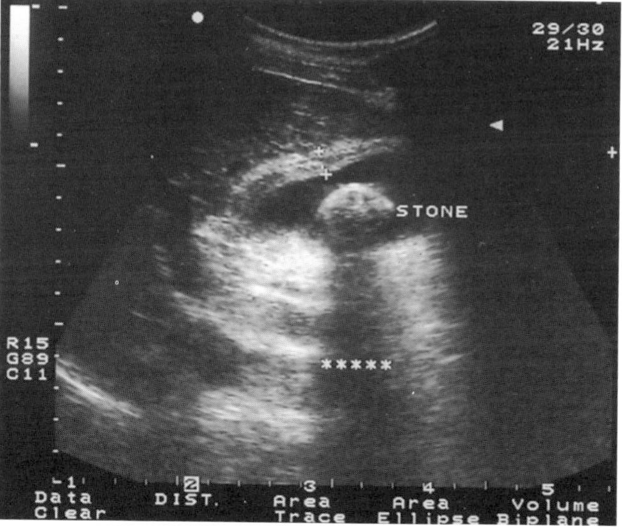

Fig. 26.5 Gallstone and cholecystitis. Oblique view of gallbladder showing typical appearance of a gallstone as an echogenic filling defect with acoustic shadowing (*****). The stone was mobile on changing the patient's position. The gallbladder wall is thickened and oedematous at 8 mm consistent with cholecystitis.

the commonest indications for ultrasound referral. Lesions of the gallbladder are a common cause of RUQ pain. Ultrasound may also demonstrate other sources of pain.

Gallstones

About 10% of the population develop gallstones but most are asymptomatic [14,15]. About three-quarters of gallstones contain cholesterol and the rest are pigment stones. Gallstones are commonly detected in patients being scanned for other reasons. Patients become symptomatic at around 2% per annum with an overall risk at 20 years of 18%. Patients are unlikely to become symptomatic after 20 years of asymptomatic gallstones [16]. The clinical syndromes associated with symptomatic gallstones include biliary colic, cholecystitis, gallstone ileus and pancreatitis.

The typical appearance of a gallstone on ultrasound is a mobile, highly reflective intraluminal structure which casts a clean sharp acoustic shadow (Figs 26.5, 26.6). Ultrasound is very sensitive in the detection of gallbladder

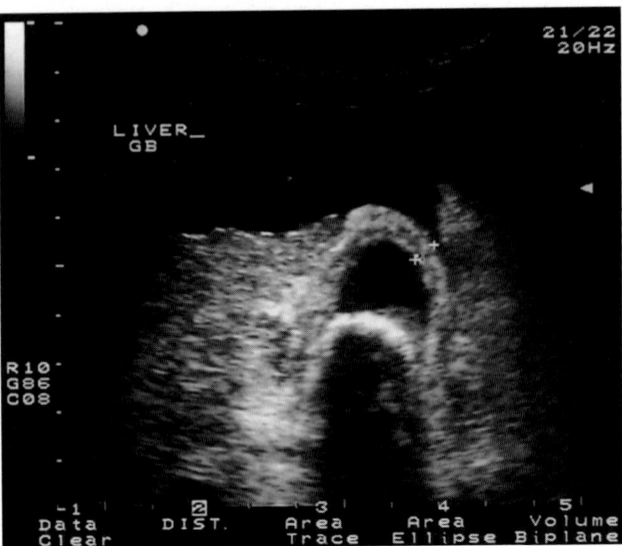

Fig. 26.6 Gallbladder wall thickening in cirrhosis. Note the nodular outline of the cirrhotic liver, the ascites and the gallstone in the gallbladder. There is thickening of the gallbladder wall (5 mm) which may be found in cirrhosis without any inflammation in the gallbladder.

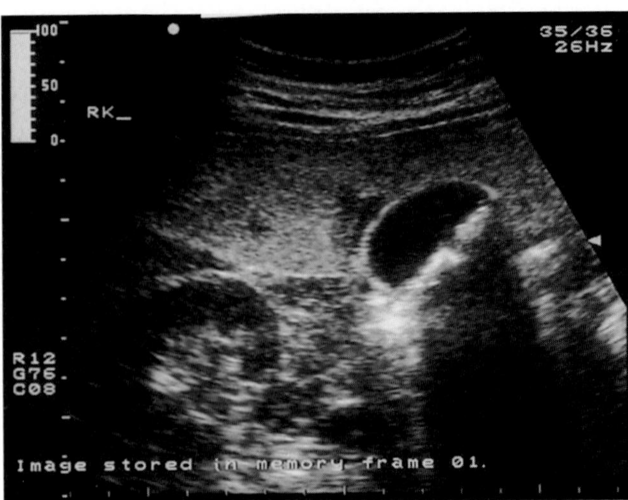

Fig. 26.7 Layering of multiple gallstones. Transverse oblique view of gallbladder with dependent layering of multiple mobile gallstones and distal acoustic shadowing. The liver is diffusely echogenic apart from a focal area adjacent to the gallbladder which is a common site for focal fatty sparing.

stones. Scanning the patient in multiple positions is important to demonstrate the mobility of the stones as other lesions may cause fixed filling defects in the gallbladder and stones may become more apparent in a different position. Occasionally shadowing from bowel gas in the duodenum adjacent to the gallbladder may cause problems, but this shadowing is less well defined and 'dirty' due to reverberation artefacts. Changing the patient's position may redistribute the bowel gas. Small stones may clump together on changing the patient's position giving a better acoustic shadow (Fig. 26.7). Image quality is optimized by using as high a frequency as possible and by setting the focal zone of the ultrasound beam at the level of the gallbladder. Contracted gallbladders are difficult to evaluate for gallstones. If the patient has not been fasted it may be worth repeating the examination after an adequate overnight fast. The gallbladder may be chronically contracted as a result of chronic inflammation and fibrosis. The finding of a contracted gallbladder in a genuinely fasted patient is a good indicator of pathology [17]. Other filling defects in the gallbladder include sludge, polyps and tumour. Sludge is mobile, gravity dependent, non-shadowing and can form mass-like tumefactive sludge or sludgeballs. Sludge formation usually results from bile stasis and may be due to prolonged fasting, often in an intensive care setting, total parenteral nutrition, gastrointestinal surgery or pathological biliary obstruction. Biliary sludge usually resolves if the underlying problem is removed and normal diet reintroduced. Echogenic bile may result from pus or blood in the biliary tree and may be seen in infection or post-trauma (often iatrogenic).

Prior to the availability of ultrasound, oral cholecystography was the standard imaging investigation for gallstones. Gallstones are seen as mobile filling defects in the contrast excreted by the liver and concentrated by the gallbladder. Failure of opacification of the gallbladder is seen with an obstructed gallbladder, but there are many other reasons for this finding, including failure of the patient to take the contrast medium tablets the night before the examination, vomiting and diarrhoea, malabsorption and failure of the hepatocytes to excrete the contrast into the biliary system. Oral cholecystography is still occasionally performed if it is not possible to obtain good quality ultrasound images or in cases where the clinical index of suspicion is high for gallstones but none are seen on ultrasound. Plain abdominal radiography is only 10–15% sensitive for gallstones as only those stones with a significant amount of calcium are detected. Computed tomography (CT) is approximately 80% sensitive for gallstones.

BILIARY COLIC

Biliary colic is caused by a gallstone temporarily obstructing the neck of the gallbladder or the cystic duct. The patient usually complains of RUQ or epigastric pain lasting for several hours. The term colic is a misnomer as the pain is usually steady rather than colicky but there may be periodic exacerbations. Tenderness to palpation is unusual on clinical examination and on scanning over the gallbladder. The gallstone may be seen impacted in the neck. Small stones obstructing the cystic duct may be more difficult to visualize. The natural history of most episodes of biliary colic is for the stone to disimpact spontaneously and for the pain to resolve. However, in some cases the stone may remain impacted for more than 6 h resulting in cholecystitis or may pass into the common bile duct and may result in obstruction of the common bile duct and/or pancreatic duct.

CHOLECYSTITIS

Most patients who develop cholecystitis will have a history of biliary colic, although they may not have sought medical attention. If obstruction of the cystic duct or gallbladder neck persists, an episode of biliary colic may become acute cholecystitis. The classical clinical features of acute cholecystitis are pain lasting more than 6 h, usually in the RUQ but possibly radiating to the right shoulder, the right side of the chest, the interscapular area or the epigastrium, jaundice, fever, chills, nausea and vomiting. On clinical examination, there is usually tenderness and guarding in the RUQ with a positive Murphy's sign (the patient stops inspiration when asked to inspire as the tender gallbladder comes into contact with the examiner's hand in the subcostal area of the RUQ).

Ultrasound is usually the initial imaging investigation in patients with suspected cholecystitis and may demonstrate an alternative cause for the pain in about one-third of patients and most patients with RUQ pain do not have acute cholecystitis [18]. Ultrasound provides information about the size and number of gallstones, the gallbladder wall, pericholecystic fluid, presence of common duct stones and the appearance of the liver and pancreas. This information is not available from cholescintigraphy.

Ultrasound features of acute cholecystitis (see Fig. 26.5) include:

1 gallstones, possibly impacted in gallbladder neck or cystic duct;
2 gallbladder wall oedema and thickening >3 mm;
3 maximal tenderness on scanning over the gallbladder;
4 distended gallbladder, round or oval shape, >5 cm in diameter; and
5 pericholecystic fluid.

Severe acute cholecystitis may lead to necrosis and gangrene of the gallbladder with perforation. The presence of pericholecystic fluid suggests more advanced changes. A focal collection adjacent to the gallbladder wall may indicate localized perforation. CT is helpful in problem solving in these more severe cases of cholecystitis. A gallbladder defect may not be seen on ultrasound but gallbladder wall bulging can be seen and may represent presumptive evidence of perforation, as CT frequently shows the bulge to be the site of the perforation [19]. The sonographic Murphy's sign may be negative or indeterminate in patients who are unresponsive or medicated, in cases where the gallbladder is deep and in gallbladder wall necrosis [20]. In emphysematous cholecystitis there is acoustic shadowing from air in the lumen and wall in addition to the stones and this complication is more commonly found in patients with diabetes mellitus.

Laparoscopic cholecystectomy has replaced open surgery in many centres. Preoperative ultrasound is helpful in planning surgery and in deciding whether more invasive investigation such as ERCP is required. Complicated cholecystitis, e.g. perforation or possible tumour, is an indication for open surgery. Ultrasound features which may predict difficulty during laparoscopic surgery are controversial but may include small, contracted or poorly functioning gallbladder. Complications of cholecystectomy include bile leak or obstruction. Early ultrasound looking for possible fluid collections or biliary dilatation is important when patients present a few days after surgery with symptoms of RUQ pain or discomfort, jaundice, fever or abdominal distension. Possible intervention in the form of ERCP and stenting or percutaneous drainage of collections may be indicated.

ACALCULOUS CHOLECYSTITIS

Acalculous cholecystitis accounts for 5–10% of patients with acute cholecystitis. It is usually found in patients in intensive care settings after major surgery, serious trauma, extensive burns, prolonged hypotension or parenteral nutrition or in the generally debilitated. The absence of stones and the inability to elicit tenderness on scanning over the gallbladder make the diagnosis difficult to make [21]. The presence of gallbladder wall thickening and distension indicates the diagnosis but there are many other causes of gallbladder wall thickening (Table 26.1). There may be sludge in the gallbladder (Fig. 26.8). Gangrene and perforation are more common than in calculous cholecystitis. Cholecystokinin-induced contraction of an unobstructed gallbladder excludes the diagnosis [22]. Nuclear medicine ^{99m}Tc-labelled iminodiacetic acid (IDA) scintigraphy shows no activity in the gallbladder in cases of cholecystitis. Percutaneous aspiration of bile may be performed at the patient's bedside under ultrasound guidance.

CHRONIC CHOLECYSTITIS AND ADENOMYOMATOSIS

Chronic inflammation in the gallbladder may lead to

Table 26.1 Causes of gallbladder wall thickening

Inflammatory disease of the gallbladder
Cholecystitis, acute and chronic (see Fig. 26.5)
Sclerosing cholangitis
AIDS
Crohn's disease
Non-inflammatory gallbladder disease
Adenomyomatosis (see Fig. 26.9)
Carcinoma
Leukaemia
Myeloma
Liver disease
Cirrhosis (see Fig. 26.6)
Hepatitis
Hypoalbuminaemia
Portal hypertension
Varices, especially if portal vein thrombosis
Other causes of gallbladder oedema
Heart and renal failure
Lymphatic obstruction
Pancreatitis
Physiological
Contraction as normal response to a meal

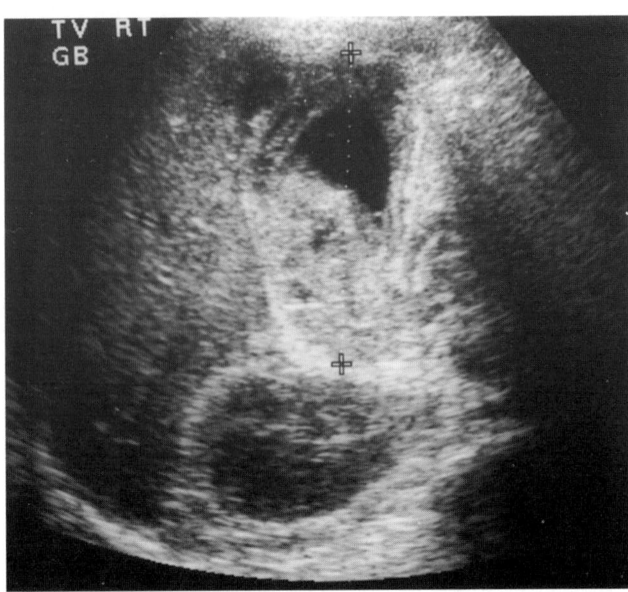

Fig. 26.8 Acalculous cholecystitis. Patient in intensive care unit after major surgery with distended (9 cm long) thick-walled (1.1 cm) gallbladder containing a lot of mass-like sludge but no calculi.

adenomatous hyperplasia which may be diffuse, localized or segmental. The epithelium extends between muscle bundles with formation of Aschoff–Rokitansky sinuses which may extend beyond the serosa of the gallbladder. Chronic cholecystitis is usually associated with gallstones. Adenomatous hyperplasia is also found in adenomyomatosis in the absence of gallstones or inflammation.

On ultrasound there is diffuse or segmental gallbladder wall thickening with intramural diverticula which may contain anechoic (bile) or echogenic (concretions) foci (Fig. 26.9). The diverticula extend for variable depth into the wall. Bile concretions in the Aschoff–Rokitansky sinuses may give a 'diamond ring' appearance [23,24].

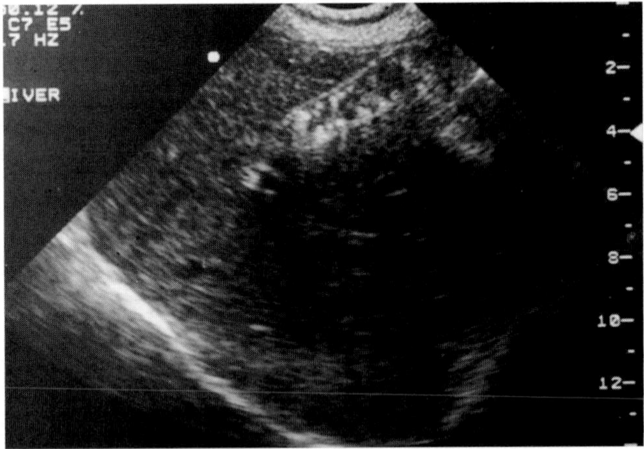

Fig. 26.9 Adenomyomatosis. Transverse view of liver and gallbladder showing multiple reflective foci in the gallbladder wall due to concretions in Aschoff–Rokitansky sinuses. No gallstones were seen. Similar features may be seen in chronic cholecystitis associated with gallstones and inflammation. On oral cholecystography there was filling of the sinuses with contrast.

Other gallbladder pathology

CHOLESTEROLOSIS (STRAWBERRY GALLBLADDER)

Cholesterolosis is a non-inflammatory process resulting from deposition of lipids in the mucosa of the gallbladder with tiny surface nodules not seen on ultrasound. Larger polypoid cholesterol deposits may be seen as single or multiple, non-mobile, small echogenic foci [25].

GALLBLADDER POLYPS

Pseudopolyps may be seen as small intraluminal echogenic structures with no acoustic shadowing in inflammation (cholecystitis), cholesterolosis and adenomyomatosis. True adenomatous polyps are sessile or papillary, and 10% are multiple. These polyps may be premalignant especially if larger. Polyps may cause intermittent obstruction of the cystic duct [26]. Gallbladder polyps are seen as fixed, non-shadowing, soft tissue masses projecting into the gallbladder lumen on ultrasound (Fig. 26.10). Polyps may be found in the gallbladder in Peutz–Jegher syndrome [27].

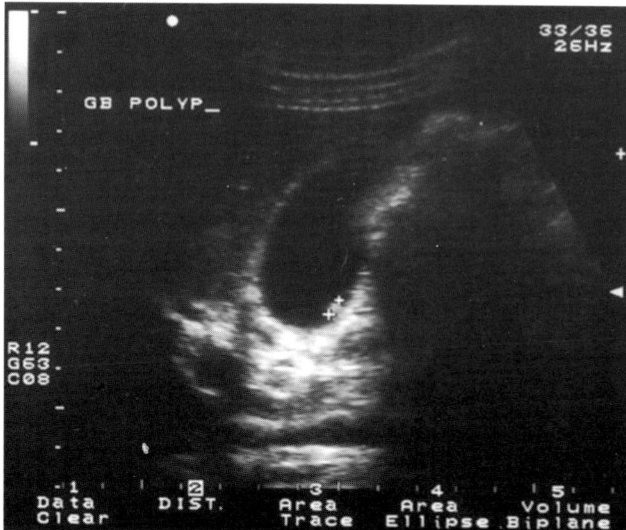

Fig. 26.10 Gallbladder polyp. Oblique view of gallbladder shows small non-shadowing filling defect in the gallbladder which did not move when the patient changed position.

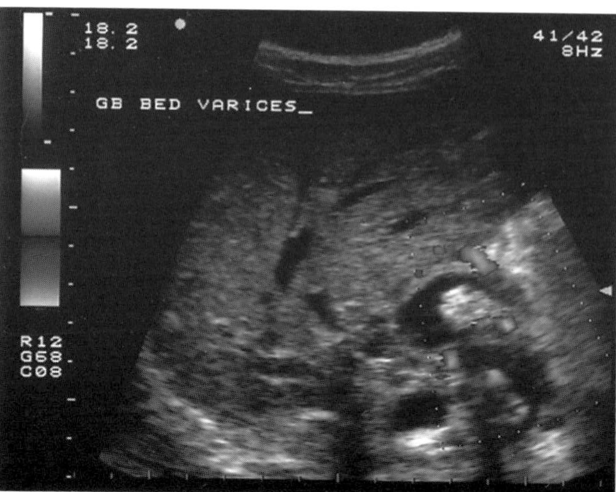

Fig. 26.11 Gallbladder varices. Multiple serpiginous anechoic channels were seen around the gallbladder in this patient with portal vein thrombosis. Colour Doppler imaging shows flow within these venous collaterals. For colour, see Plate 26.11 (between pp. 308 and 309).

GALLBLADDER CARCINOMA

Gallbladder carcinoma is most commonly found in elderly female patients and is an aggressive malignancy. Patients may be asymptomatic or present with anorexia, nausea and vomiting. There is a strong association with gallstones and chronic cholecystitis. Liver invasion and infiltration of the biliary tree results in jaundice. At ultrasound gallstones are seen in 80–90%. There may be irregularity of the gallbladder wall. Calcification of the gallbladder wall is seen in 'porcelain gallbladder' which is associated with an increased incidence of gallbladder carcinoma (20–25%) and cholangiocarcinoma (10%) [28]. Gallbladder carcinoma may be infiltrating or fungating in type. Metastases to the gallbladder are unusual but on ultrasound may manifest as asymmetrical wall thickening or polypoid intraluminal mass.

GALLBLADDER VARICES

Varices in the gallbladder bed are common in patients with portal vein thrombosis. The venous collaterals are seen as tortuous, serpentine, anechoic structures 3–8 mm in size with venous flow on colour and spectral Doppler (Fig. 26.11) [29].

Evaluation of obstructive jaundice

Ultrasound is the screening modality of choice for evaluating the biliary tree in patients with jaundice or suspected biliary obstruction. Ultrasound is readily available, fast, safe and not dependent on liver function. The main clinical questions are as follows.

1 Are the bile ducts dilated?
2 What is the level of obstruction?
3 What is the cause of obstruction?

Ultrasound signs of biliary obstruction

Intrahepatic ducts are not usually seen. When dilated they are visible as tubular structures in the liver running with portal vein branches. When scanned in short axis, the duct and portal vein are described as having a 'double-barrelled shotgun' appearance (Fig. 26.12) [30]. When seen along long axis, the dilated duct and accompanying portal vein are described as 'parallel-channel sign' (Fig. 26.12) [31]. Other descriptions of dilated intrahepatic ducts include 'too many tubes' [32] and in diffuse fatty infiltration 'the stilette sign' where the outer walls of the ducts merge with bright liver [33]. The common duct is dilated if more than 6 mm in diameter (Fig. 26.13; see Fig. 26.15).

Ultrasound is more than 90% accurate in discriminating 'medical' versus 'surgical' jaundice. The sensitivity of ultrasound for biliary dilatation is 68–99% and the specificity is 75–100% [34]. Ultrasound correctly identified the level of obstruction in 71–92% of cases and the cause of obstruction in 50–71% [35,36]. The success rates are variable, depending on the patient population, equipment, operators and the effort made to get optimal quality

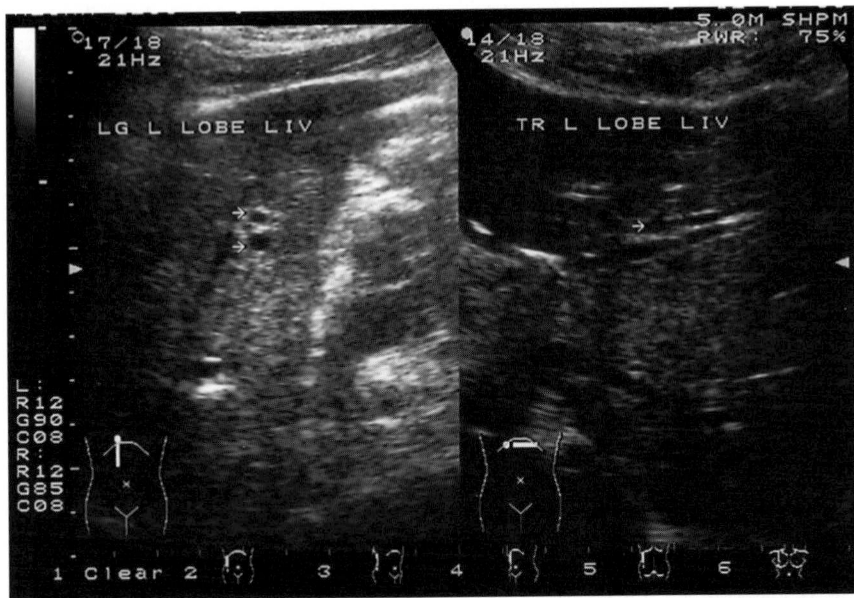

Fig. 26.12 Dilated intrahepatic ducts in patient with carcinoma of head of pancreas. The left image is a longitudinal view along the short axis of the duct and portal vein radicle resembling a 'double-barrelled shotgun'. The transverse view along the long axis of the duct and accompanying portal vein shows 'parallel tubes'. Same examination as Fig. 26.20 (dilated pancreatic duct).

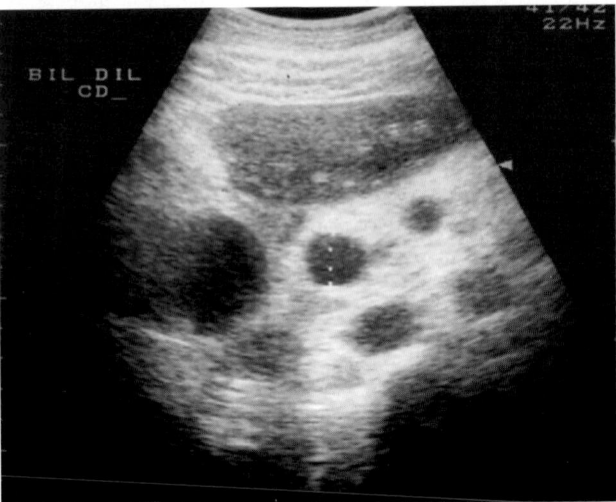

Fig. 26.13 Dilated common bile duct. Transverse view of pancreatic head with slightly dilated distal common bile duct (8 mm).

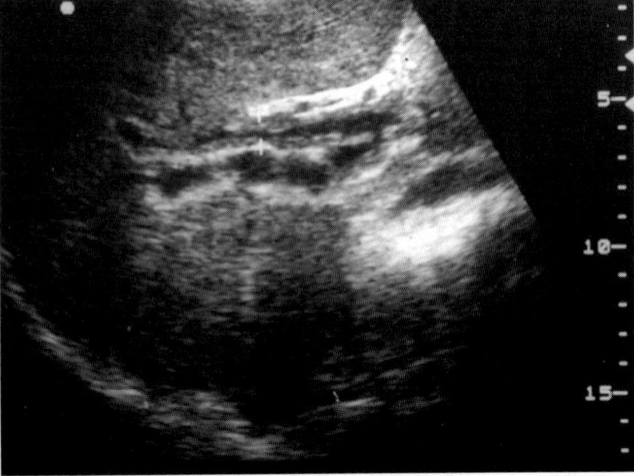

Fig. 26.14 Primary sclerosing cholangitis. Longitudinal view along the common duct showing the characteristic mural thickening of PSC. The duct lumen is irregular but not dilated.

imaging. The site and cause of obstruction guide the choice of further imaging and possible therapeutic intervention. In patients with proximal obstruction, percutaneous transhepatic cholangiography (PTC) is indicated, while in distal duct obstruction, ERCP is indicated. Both of these procedures have therapeutic options with biliary drainage or stenting. Magnetic resonance cholangiopancreatography (MRCP) is now gaining acceptance as a non-invasive modality which may aid in planning intervention. MRCP is also useful when ERCP is not possible [37].

Biliary obstruction in the absence of dilatation is uncommon but may be found in the very early stages of obstruction (e.g. bile duct injury or surgical clip placed erroneously over common hepatic duct at cholecystectomy). Repeat scanning will demonstrate the proximal dilatation. In some circumstances the obstructed ducts do not dilate. This may be due to abnormality in the ducts (e.g. fibrosis in sclerosing cholangitis) (Fig. 26.14) or surrounding tissues (e.g. encasement of duct by tumour).

Causes of biliary obstruction

Bile duct obstruction may result from intraluminal filling

defects such as stones, stricture due to trauma, especially surgery, inflammation or neoplasm or extrinsic compression. Most cases of obstruction occur at the level of the distal common bile duct.

CHOLEDOCHOLITHIASIS

Common duct stones are found in up to 15% of patients with stones in the gallbladder. Stones are seen as curvilinear reflective structures in the lumen of the common duct with an acoustic shadow (Fig. 26.15). Stones in the common duct cause obstructive jaundice and cholangitis which is classically associated with Charcot's triad; biliary colic, jaundice and swinging fever. However, one or more of these features may be absent. The sensitivity of early ultrasound was poor for diagnosing stones in the common duct but with better quality equipment, sensitivities of up to 75–80% have been reported [38]. The difficulties encountered in attempting to demonstrate stones in the common duct include overlying gas which may be minimized by scanning the patient after a fast or by filling the proximal duodenum with fluid. Stones are harder to demonstrate in non-dilated ducts or when the stone fills the lumen of the duct (Fig. 26.16). Stones in the common duct, especially distally, may not cast an acoustic shadow. Gas in the bile ducts causes ringdown artefact rather than a sharp clean acoustic shadow of a stone (Fig. 26.17). The commonest cause of pneumobilia is now iatrogenic, usually postsphincterotomy or stenting at ERCP or post-choledochojejunostomy. Visualization of the common duct is optimized by careful attention to equipment and technique and by scanning in different planes and patient positions.

Common bile duct dilatation after cholecystectomy is more common after common duct exploration, cholangitis or previous obstruction [39]. Occasionally a large stone in the neck of the gallbladder or cystic duct or cystic duct remnant may compress the common hepatic duct resulting in proximal biliary dilatation (Mirizzi's syndrome). Mirizzi's syndrome may be associated with a low insertion of the cystic duct into the common duct. Further investigation by CT or cholangiography may be required [40,41].

CHOLANGITIS

Cholangitis may be associated with calculi (see above). Primary sclerosing cholangitis (PSC) may be found in association with inflammatory bowel disease, especially ulcerative colitis, and may precede the onset of the bowel changes. It is characterized by recurrent episodes of cholangitis and strictures and beading of the ducts. The characteristic ultrasound feature of PSC is mural thickening of the common duct (see Fig. 26.14) [42]. The major limitation of ultrasound in PSC is the inability to exclude intrahepatic duct disease. There is an increased incidence of cholangiocarcinoma, which may be suggested on ultrasound by the presence of non-segmental intrahepatic duct dilatation or a mass [43]. There may also be features of cirrhosis and portal hypertension.

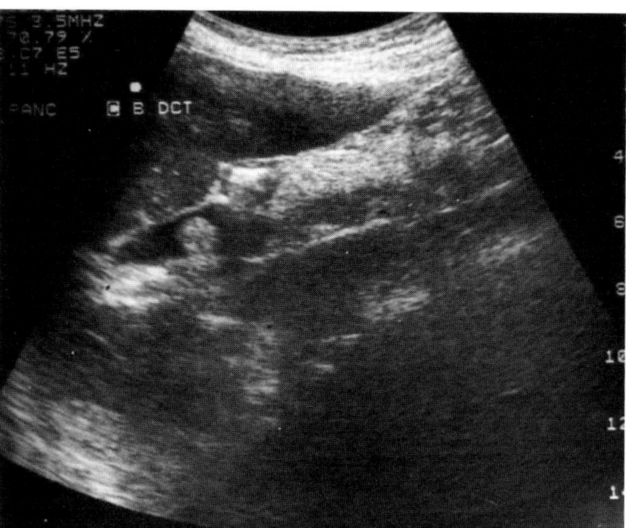

Fig. 26.15 Dilated common bile duct with calculus. Oblique view along the dilated common bile duct showing echogenic filling defect due to a calculus (1.4 cm) with little distal acoustic shadowing.

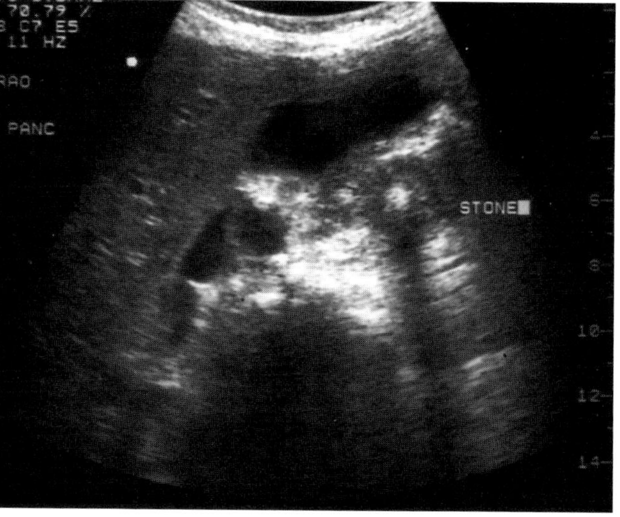

Fig. 26.16 Gallstone with acoustic shadowing filling the distal common bile duct. Dilated intrahepatic ducts are seen in the liver. The image quality is suboptimal due to overlying bowel gas.

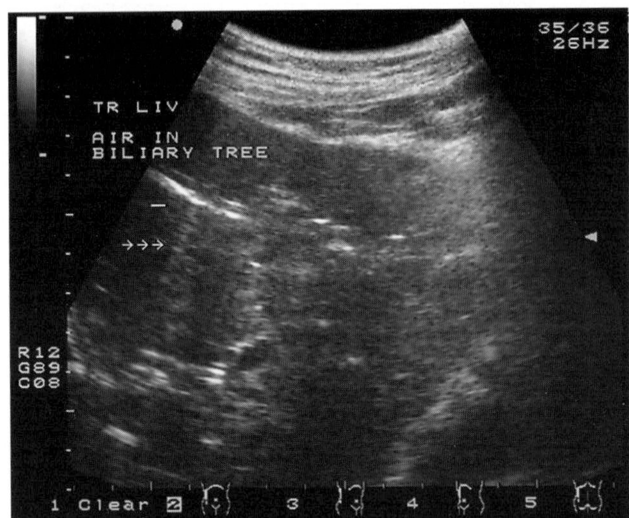

(a)

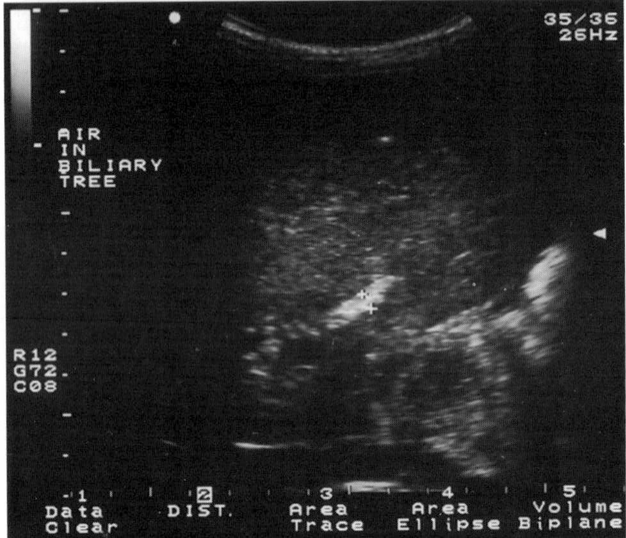

(b)

Fig. 26.17 Pneumobilia. (a) Air in intrahepatic bile ducts (dash) secondary to a sphincterotomy. There is ringdown artefact (arrows) from the pneumobilia rather than the clean acoustic shadowing beyond a stone. Dilated pancreatic duct. (b) Transverse view through left hepatic duct (4 mm) showing mild dilatation and pneumobilia.

Acquired immune deficiency syndrome (AIDS) related cholangitis or AIDS-related sclerosing cholangitis may involve the gallbladder and biliary tree in a focal or diffuse way. Characteristically there is mural thickening with stricture in the distal common duct with relatively mild proximal dilatation [44]. The commonest organisms involved are cytomegalovirus (CMV) and *Cryptosporidium*.

Clonorchis sinensis (Chinese liver fluke) is associated with cholangiohepatitis. Occasionally the flukes may be seen as filling defects on cholangiography or as echogenic foci in bile duct or rarely in the gallbladder [45]. *Ascaris* (roundworms) in the adult stage usually live in the proximal intestine but may enter the bile ducts at the ampulla. Adult worms are typically more than 10 cm in length and 3–6 mm in diameter and can be seen as tubular structures in the extrahepatic duct [46] and rarely in the gallbladder [47].

BILE DUCT NEOPLASMS

Benign tumours of the bile ducts are rare. Papilloma and adenoma appearing on ultrasound are seen as solid non-shadowing intraluminal masses. Primary bile duct carcinoma is unusual in the intrahepatic ducts and the most common intrahepatic biliary tumour is cystadenoma. Cystadenoma may be seen as a large multiloculated cystic mass with mural nodules, usually in young or middle-aged women. Calcification may be seen in the soft tissue components [48,49].

Cholangiocarcinoma is the commonest malignant tumour of bile ducts. The bile ducts are dilated down to the point of obstruction. It may be possible to detect a mass (usually poorly reflective). Larger masses are ill defined and heterogeneous. Cholangiocarcinoma at the confluence of the right and left hepatic ducts (Klatskin tumours) results in dilated intrahepatic bile ducts but normal extrahepatic ducts. If the biliary obstruction is long standing there may be parenchymal atrophy. Ultrasound diagnosis of cholangiocarcinoma has a high predictive value and may aid in mapping tumour site [50]. Percutaneous biopsy under ultrasound or CT guidance may yield a histological diagnosis but samples may be difficult to obtain due to fibrous tissue in the tumour. In the absence of a visible mass it may be worth taking a biopsy from the transition point, which is the expected site of the tumour. Cholangiocarcinoma is increased in incidence in PSC and may be multifocal.

OTHER NEOPLASMS

Other tumours obstructing bile ducts include intrahepatic tumours, lymphadenopathy at porta hepatis which may be seen as several discrete masses and masses arising from the head of the pancreas or ampulla. The head of the pancreas may be enlarged by tumour or infiltration. Chronic pancreatitis may cause fibrous stricturing of the common duct indistinguishable from malignancy. On ultrasound carcinoma is seen as hypoechoic solid mass with proximal common duct dilatation (see below). The presence of common duct dilatation with a normal head of pancreas may suggest ampullary carcinoma. The diagnosis can be made at endoscopy.

Table 26.2 Classification of choledochal cysts [51,52]

Type	Relative prevalence	Features
I	Most common type 68–90%	Ia: cystic dilatation of the common bile duct Ib: focal segmental dilatation of the common bile duct Ic: fusiform dilatation
II	2%	Choledochal diverticulum
III	Least frequent	Choledochocele
IV	19–26%	IVa: multiple intra- and extrahepatic cysts IVb: multiple extrahepatic cysts only
V		Caroli's disease: intrahepatic cysts only may be associated with renal cystic disease and hepatic fibrosis

Table 26.3 Causes of pancreatitis

Alcohol	Increasing in incidence
Gallstones	>60% in UK
Trauma	
Viral	Including mumps
Familial	Family history, prominent calcification
Hypercalcaemia	
ERCP	
Biopsy	
Drugs	Including immunosuppressants such as azathioprine
Hyperlipidaemia	
Pancreas divisum	Controversial
Scorpion bite	Always remembered by students!

CHOLEDOCHAL CYSTS

Choledochal cyst is a rare congenital abnormality, predominantly in Asian females (female to male ratio is 3 to 1), characterized by cystic dilatation of the extra- and/or intrahepatic biliary tree. Choledochal cysts are classified according to the pattern of dilatation and the anatomical level of bile duct involvement (Table 26.2). The cysts in Caroli's disease are intrahepatic only and this has been classified by some authors as part of the spectrum of choledochal cysts [51,52]. Caroli's disease may be associated with congenital hepatic fibrosis, renal tubular ectasia or other cystic renal disease.

On ultrasound, choledochal cysts are seen as large cystic masses separate from the gallbladder. A dilated common hepatic or common bile duct may be seen entering directly into the cystic mass or the cystic mass may be due to dilatation of the duct itself. The cyst may contain calculi. Continuity between cyst and biliary tree must be seen to make the diagnosis and this may require cholescintigraphy as the communication may not be definite on ultrasound. Choledochal cysts may be complicated by biliary obstruction, recurrent bacterial cholangitis, and biliary tumours, typically cholangiocarcinoma involving the cyst but there is also an increased incidence in the gallbladder and the rest of biliary tree. The risk of malignancy is 50% by age 50 years [53]. A drainage procedure is inadequate; surgical treatment and complete cyst excision and hepatico jejunostomy is recommended especially in types I, II and IV [52,53]. The biliary obstruction and cholangitis may cause progressive changes of biliary cirrhosis and portal hypertension.

Pancreatitis

Acute pancreatitis is characterized by inflammatory changes in and around the pancreas with activation of pancreatic enzymes. It can be a difficult diagnosis to make and be very difficult to manage clinically. The classical presentation is upper abdominal pain radiating to the back, but there may be no pain even in severe cases. There is usually nausea and vomiting. Laboratory investigations show elevated amylase and lipase and there may be leucocytosis and hypocalcaemia. Gallstones and alcohol account for over three-quarters of cases. Biliary sludge or microscopic calculi may play a part in many of the other cases [54–56] (Table 26.3). Pancreatitis is a well-recognized complication of ERCP. About three-quarters of cases of acute pancreatitis are mild and self-limiting (acute interstitial pancreatitis). Severe pancreatitis may result in irreversible destruction of pancreatic tissue and multiorgan failure (Table 26.4).

Ultrasound is the most sensitive modality in the detection of gallstones and biliary dilatation. Good quality ultrasound will demonstrate common duct stones in up to 75% of cases [57]. The use of water to distend the stomach and duodenum and scanning in erect and semi-erect positions improves the chances of visualization of common duct stones. The pancreas and upper abdomen may appear normal on ultrasound in mild cases. In more severe cases the abnormalities range from hypoechoic focal areas of swelling to a diffuse hypoechoic, swollen, ill-defined pancreas. Increased pancreatic echogenicity is

Table 26.4 Complications of acute pancreatitis

Biliary obstruction (? cause and effect relationship)
Obstruction of bowel
Renal obstruction or non-obstructive failure
Vascular occlusion and pseudoaneurysm formation
Pseudocyst formation
Adult respiratory distress syndrome
Hypovolaemic shock
Disseminated intravascular coagulation
Pancreatic necrosis and abscess
Myocardial depression
Subcutaneous fat necrosis
Metabolic acidosis
Hypocalcaemia

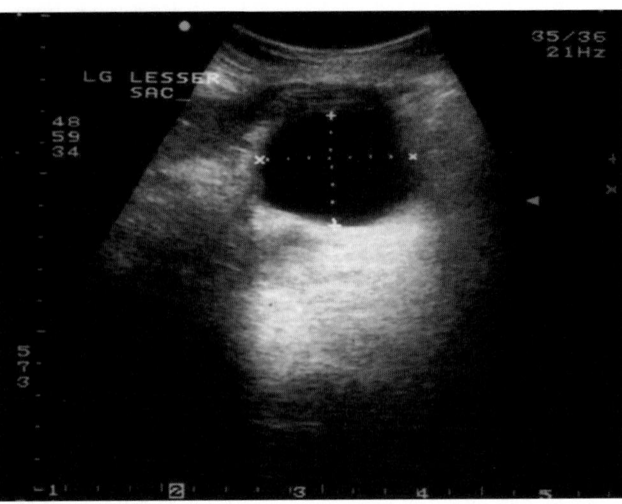

Fig. 26.18 Pancreatitis: pseudocyst in lesser sac. Longitudinal view of a well-defined fluid collection in the lesser sac of the peritoneum with distal acoustic enhancement. Pseudocysts usually 'mature' in about 6 weeks and usually do not resolve spontaneously after this time.

occasionally seen in haemorrhage or fat saponification. CT is better than ultrasound at demonstrating surrounding tissues.

Fluid collection

Peripancreatic fluid collections are common in pancreatitis. Most of the collections are in the lesser sac of the peritoneum but the pararenal spaces and transverse mesocolon are also common sites. The spread of inflammatory exudate along perivascular spaces is characteristic of acute pancreatitis [58]. Pseudocysts are contained collections of pancreatic secretions and debris without an epithelial lining and may be found in the pancreas or anywhere else in the abdomen or pelvis but most commonly in the lesser sac of the peritoneum. Even mild episodes of pancreatitis may be complicated by pseudocysts. Pseudocysts may also result from blunt trauma or from tumour (see below). On ultrasound pseudocysts are seen as smooth-walled fluid collections with layering of debris and posterior enhancement (Fig. 26.18). There may be secondary infection of the pseudocysts. Pseudocysts may drain spontaneously into stomach or bowel. Most collections resolve within a few weeks but at about 6 weeks pseudocysts are mature and rarely resolve spontaneously thereafter [59–61]. A drainage procedure is usually indicated for mature pseudocysts, either surgically or percutaneously under ultrasound or CT guidance. The volume of fluid drained depends on whether there is communication between the pseudocyst and the pancreatic ducts. Persisting communication may require surgical treatment.

The early diagnosis of pancreatic abscess is important in reducing morbidity and mortality. CT is preferred to ultrasound in detecting pancreatic abscesses. Fever may be present in pancreatitis even without sepsis, but high fever should prompt a search for a focus of sepsis [62]. The ultrasound and CT appearances are non-specific but imaging-guided aspiration of suspicious fluid collections may yield diagnostic fluid or pus. Colour Doppler imaging can demonstrate flow in pseudoaneurysms due to enzymatic digestion of vessel walls (Fig. 26.19). The aneurysms, most commonly of the splenic artery, take 2–3 weeks to develop. Other vascular complications of pancreatitis include occlusion of the splenic, portal and superior mesenteric veins.

Chronic pancreatitis

Chronic pancreatitis is characterized by parenchymal scarring and fibrosis, strictures of the main and branch ducts, intrapancreatic cavities, intraductal protein plugs and calculi and focal necrotic areas. This condition may result from recurrent acute or subacute episodes of pancreatitis and is commonly associated with alcohol. Patients may complain of constant epigastric pain radiating to the back. Complications of chronic pancreatitis include pseudocyst formation, biliary or duodenal obstruction and portal vein thrombosis. On ultrasound the pancreas is often atrophied with an irregular border and dilatation of the pancreatic duct (>2 mm). Calculi may be seen in the main pancreatic duct or branch ducts. There may be focal gland enlargement, usually in the head which may be difficult to distinguish from carcinoma. The presence of calcification in the focal mass indicates pan-

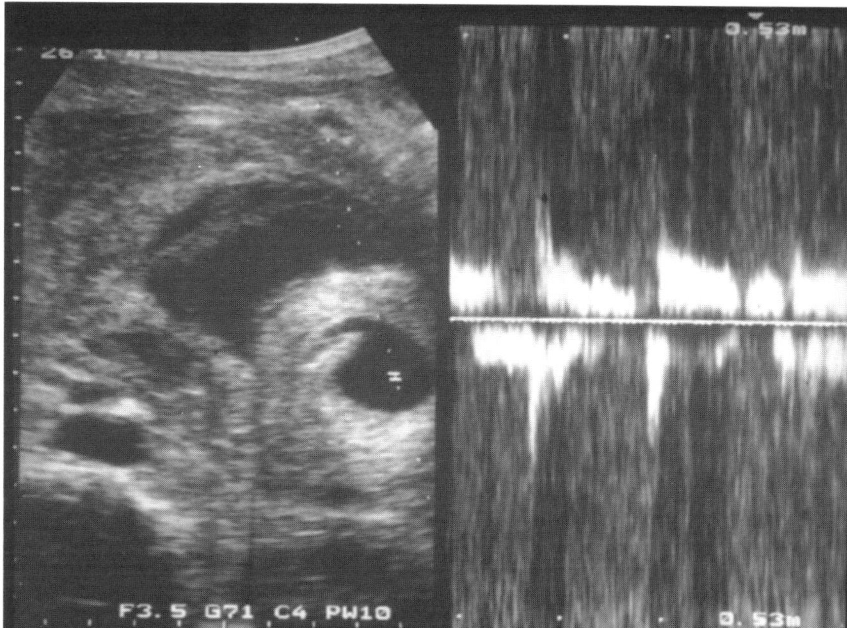

Fig. 26.19 Pseudoaneurysm of splenic artery complicating pancreatitis. Ultrasound showing 2.5 cm low echogenicity structure in the left upper quadrant with spectral Doppler trace demonstrating the vascular nature of this structure. (Courtesy of Dr P.J. Guest.)

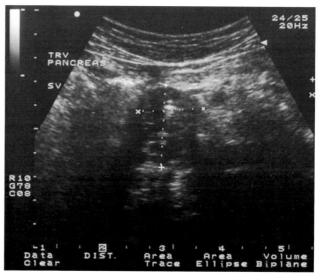

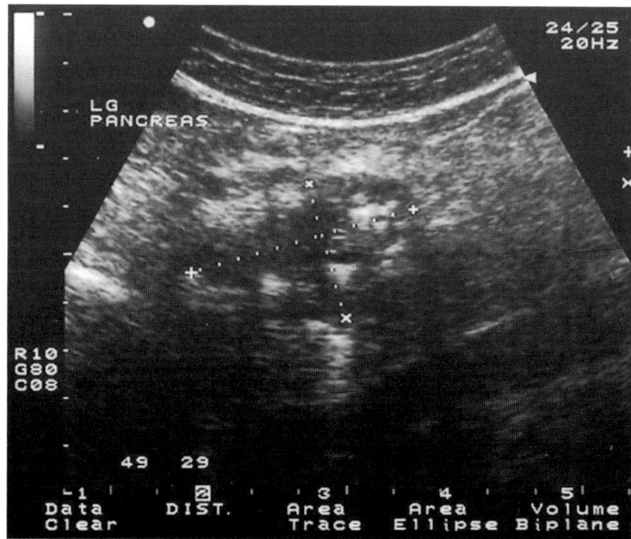

(a) (b)

Fig. 26.20 Pancreatic mass in chronic pancreatitis. (a) Longitudinal and (b) transverse views of head and uncinate process of pancreas with hypoechoic mass containing focal areas of calcification. The patient had a history of episodes of pancreatitis. Differentiating masses in chronic pancreatitis from tumour can be difficult.

creatitis but tumour may develop in patients with chronic pancreatitis (Fig. 26.20). Duct dilatation may be found in both carcinoma and chronic pancreatitis. Biopsy may be required. Positron emission tomography (PET) scanning with ^{18}F-labelled fluorodeoxyglucose (FDG) may prove useful in differentiating carcinoma from pancreatitis [63].

Pancreatic tumours

Pancreatic carcinoma is a common gastrointestinal cancer which is increasing in incidence. Most pancreatic malignancies are ductal adenocarcinomas and most are found in the head and body of the pancreas. Islet cell tumours are often associated with production of excessive hormone with characteristic clinical syndromes. Other uncommon pancreatic tumours include giant cell, adenosquamous, mucinous, acinar, microadenocarcinoma or cystandenocarcinoma. Rare tumours include pancreatoblastoma, papillary cystic and anaplastic carcinomas and tumours

(a)

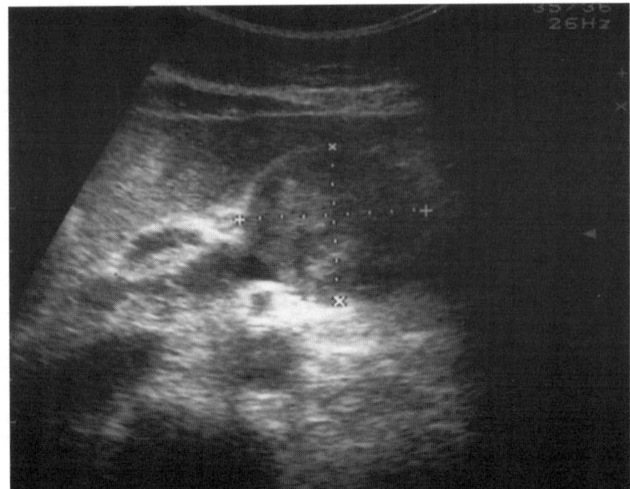

(b)

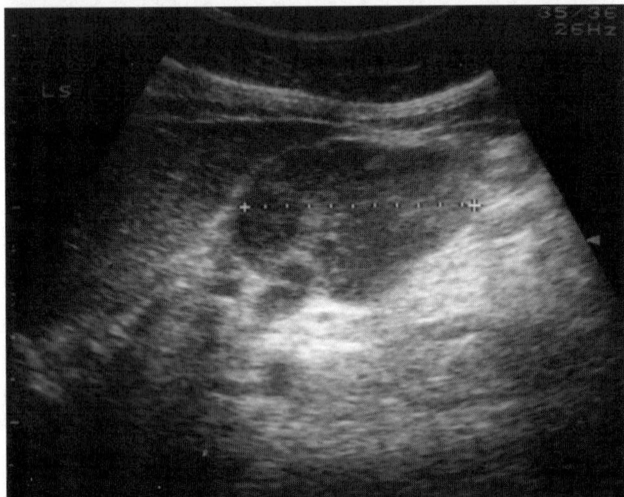

Fig. 26.21 Pancreatic carcinoma. Transverse (a) and longitudinal (b) views of the pancreas showing a large mass in the body compressing the splenic vein. Tumours that do not obstruct the bile ducts present later.

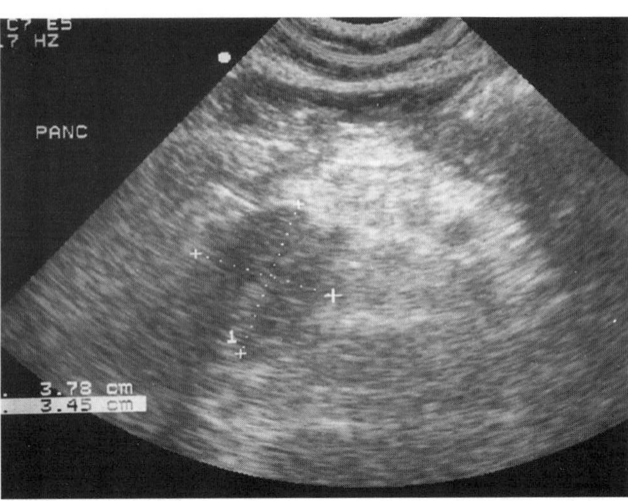

Fig. 26.22 Pancreatic head mass. Transverse view of head of pancreas showing 3.78 × 3.45 cm hypoechoic mass in head of pancreas.

of connective tissue origin. These unusual tumours are mostly similar in appearance to the common ductal adenocarcinoma. Ductectatic tumours are characterized by dilated mucin-filled pancreatic branch ducts usually in the uncinate process and head. Mucin-hypersecreting carcinoma usually has more extensive ductal dilatation. Metastases to the pancreas are rarely clinically significant but have been well documented in autopsy series. Breast, lung, colon, stomach and melanoma are the commonest primary sites. Lymphoma may rarely involve the pancreas but is potentially treatable [64].

Pancreatic carcinoma commonly presents with painless jaundice due to obstruction of the common bile duct in elderly patients. There may also be weight loss, nausea, vomiting and abdominal pain. The gallbladder may be palpable and enlarged on ultrasound. The prognosis for patients with pancreatic carcinoma is very poor and surgery offers the only hope of cure. However, only 10–20% of patients are suitable for attempted curative resection. Curative resection is not possible in the presence of extrapancreatic spread, vascular invasion and large masses. Even with apparently resectable tumours, the prognosis is poor. Ultrasound and CT may help in confirming inoperability of a tumour. Resectability is much more difficult to predict and many patients are found to be unresectable at laparotomy. Stenting or surgical bypass may give symptomatic relief. Ultrasound is routinely the first imaging modality in the investigation of obstructive jaundice or suspected pancreatic cancer [65,66]. Ultrasound has very good spatial and contrast resolution in the pancreas but inconsistent visualization of the entire pancreas is a major problem, even with the best technique. CT consistently demonstrates the entire pancreas. However, some pancreatic masses may be demonstrated on ultrasound but not on CT. Ultrasound may also distinguish peripancreatic nodes from pancreatic parenchyma.

Pancreatic carcinoma is usually seen on ultrasound as a focal irregular hypo- or isoechoic mass with distal attenuation (Figs 26.21, 26.22). The dilated common bile duct may be seen down to the obstructing mass. The pancreatic duct may also be dilated (Fig. 26.23) ('double-duct sign'). A chronically obstructed pancreatic duct may be elongated and tortuous. There may be invasion of adjacent structures. Venous encasement and invasion more fre-

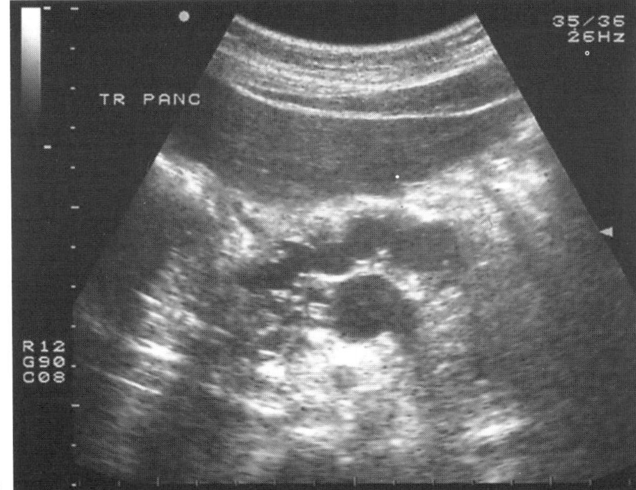

(a)

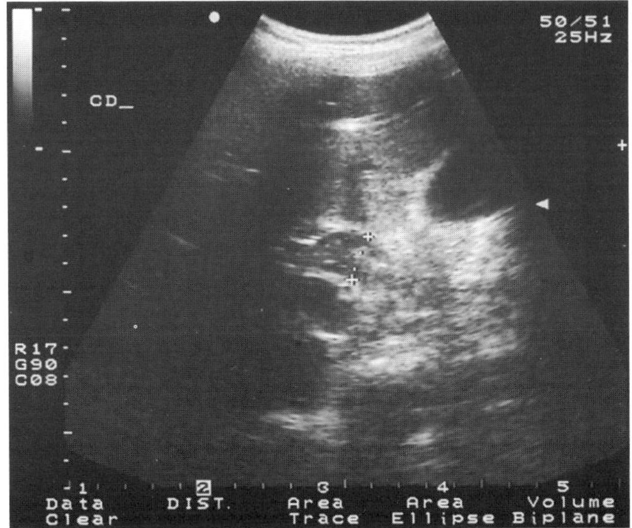

(b)

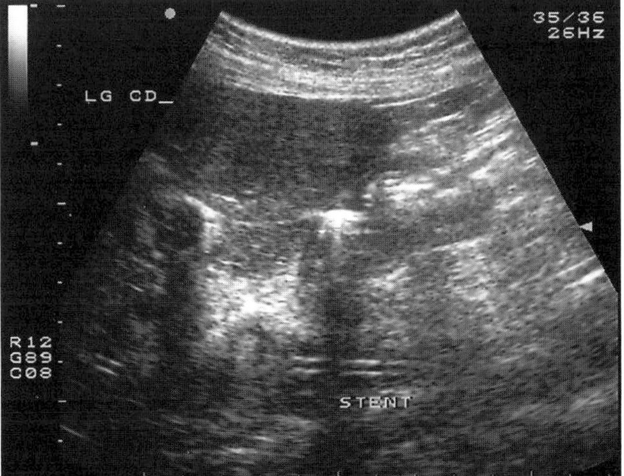

(c)

Fig. 26.23 Dilated tortuous pancreatic duct and dilated common bile duct with debris and indwelling stent. (a) Transverse view of pancreas with tortuous dilated main pancreatic duct and parenchymal atrophy due to long-standing obstruction by tumour in the pancreatic head (same examination as Fig. 26.12). (b) Dilated common duct (16 mm) containing debris poststenting proximal to the tumour. (c) Stent in common duct distal to (b).

quently precludes surgical resection for cure than arterial encasement.

Colour Doppler imaging may show evidence of compression with high velocity jets and turbulence. Characteristic low impedance Doppler signals due to tumour neovascularity have been described [67]. There may be metastatic spread to lymph nodes around the pancreas or to the liver. Obstruction of the pancreatic duct occasionally results in pseudocyst formation. Non-obstructing tumours present later.

Many pancreatic tumours are diagnosed from clinical, laboratory and imaging findings without histological proof. If surgery is not being performed and confirmation of the diagnosis is sought, then a fine-needle aspirate (FNA) or a core biopsy may be obtained percutaneously under ultrasound or CT guidance [68].

Cystic pancreatic tumours

Cystic pancreatic neoplasms are relatively uncommon [69]. Serous (microcystic) carcinoma is almost always benign. These tumours are commoner in females and in the elderly. There are multiple small cysts, most less than 2 cm. There may be a central stellate scar and about half of the tumours calcify. On ultrasound, there is increased echogenicity of those parts of the tumour with tiny cysts. Larger cysts are hypoechoic. The central stellate scar may be visible.

Mucinous cystic pancreatic neoplasms are commoner in women and are made up of larger cysts. Most are found in the tail or body. These tumours are very difficult to separate into benign and malignant groups, even histologically. All of these tumours should be surgically removed if possible as complete resection is curative and these

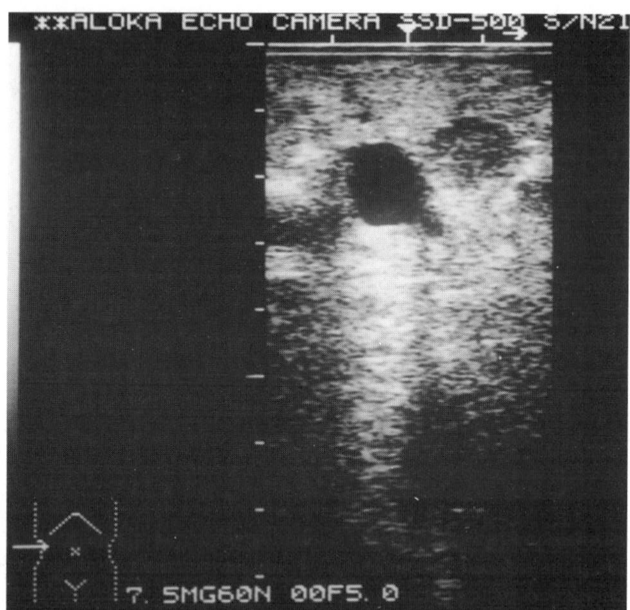

Fig. 26.24 Intraoperative ultrasound showing transverse view of a small (1 cm) hypoechoic islet cell tumour to the left of the superior mesenteric vein that was not demonstrable on transabdominal ultrasound or CT. (Courtesy of Dr J.F. Olliff.)

tumours have a better prognosis than ductal adenocarcinoma. Calcification is seen in about 20%. On ultrasound the cystic masses are usually septated and of variable size. The septations are variable in number, thickness and outline. The differential diagnosis of these cystic pancreatic neoplasms includes pseudocyst, abscess or hydatid disease and other rare cystic pancreatic neoplasms such as papillary cystic tumour, cystic metastases or cystic islet cell tumour.

Islet cell tumours

Endocrine tumours of the pancreas arise from islet cells, most commonly insulinoma and gastrinoma. Other rare islet cell tumours include glucagonoma, somatostatinoma, vasoactive intestinal peptidoma (VIPoma), carcinoid and phaeochromocytoma. Insulinoma is usually benign. Patients present with hypoglycaemic episodes due to excess secretion of insulin. Other islet cell tumours tend to be malignant. Gastrinomas are frequently malignant (60%), multiple, small and outside of the pancreas. Islet cell tumours are a feature of multiple endocrine neoplasia syndromes. These tumours are difficult to locate on imaging. Routine transabdominal ultrasound is relatively insensitive but endoscopic or intraoperative ultrasound are more sensitive [70]. On ultrasound islet cell tumours are generally small, well-defined, round or ovoid hypoechoic lesions (Fig. 26.24). Other imaging modalities which may be useful in imaging islet cell tumours include CT, magnetic resonance imaging, ERCP and angiography with venous sampling.

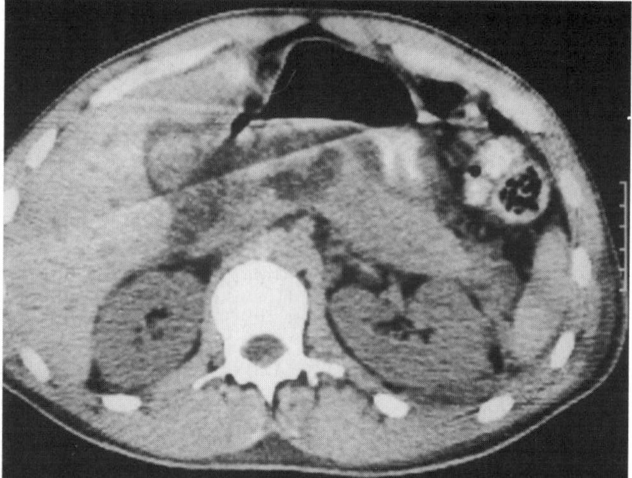

(a)

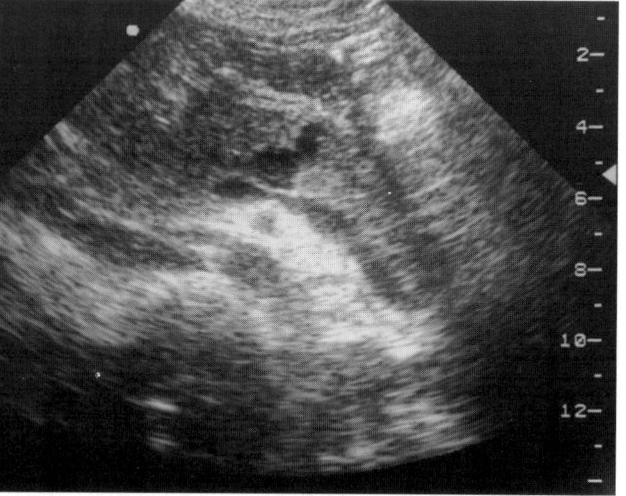

(b)

Fig. 26.25 Pancreatic transection. (a) Axial CT scan through the pancreas without intravenous contrast showing low attenuation band in pancreas at the site of transection. The pancreas is fixed in the retroperitoneum and this injury usually results from blunt trauma, e.g. high velocity road traffic collisions. (b) Ultrasound at the same level within the pancreas showing low echogenicity band at the site of the transection. (Courtesy of Dr P.J. Guest.)

Acinar cell carcinoma

Acinar cell carcinoma of the pancreas is a rare aggressive tumour which has a distinct clinical presentation and imaging appearance from the more common ductal adenocarcinoma. Biliary obstruction and jaundice are

(a)

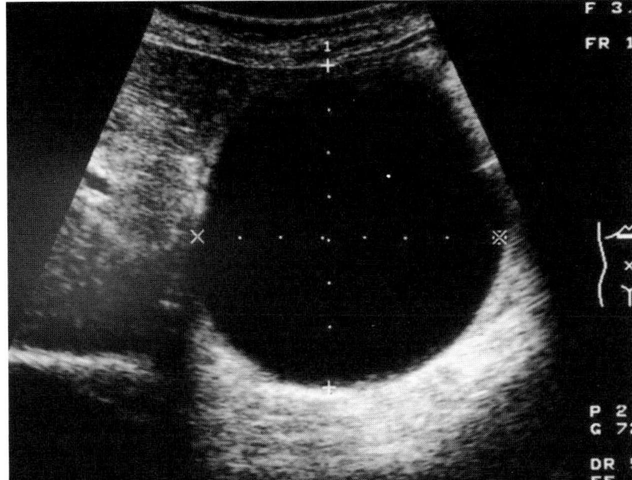

(b)

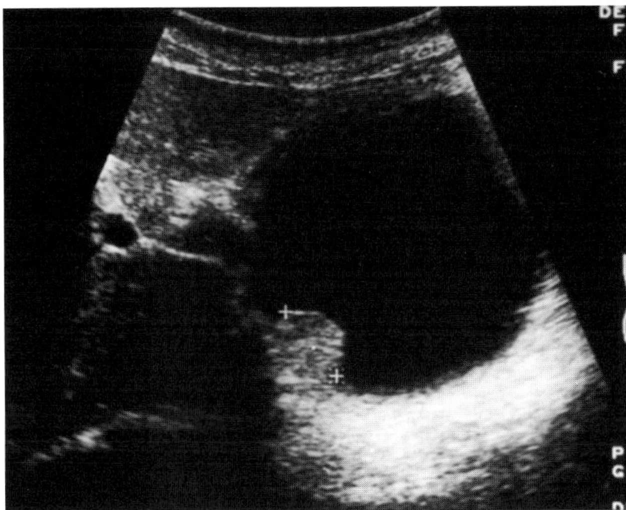

Fig. 26.26 Post-traumatic pseudocyst of the pancreas. (a) Transverse view of the pancreas showing large (7.4 × 7.3 cm) well-defined fluid containing structure in a teenager complicating blunt trauma to the pancreas as a result of an assault. (b) There is a nodule of soft tissue posteriorly within the pseudocyst.

uncommon. There may be disseminated fat necrosis due to lipase production and secretion by the tumour. [71]. The tumours are usually large at presentation and are well defined with a thin capsule and necrotic areas on ultrasound and CT [72]. Large non-functioning islet cell tumours may have a similar appearance.

Pancreatic trauma

Trauma to the pancreas, including blunt injury, may result in pancreatic duct injury, transection (Fig. 26.25) and pseudocyst formation (Fig. 26.26).

References

1 Wu, C.C., Ho, Y.H., Chen, C.Y. (1984) Effect of aging on common bile duct diameter: a realtime sonographic study. *Journal of Clinical Ultrasound* **12**, 473.

2 Engel, J.M., Deitch, E.A., Sikkema, W. (1979) Gallbladder wall thickness: sonographic accuracy and relation to disease. *American Journal of Roentgenology* **134**, 907–909.

3 Bellamy, P.R., Hicks, A. (1988) Assessment of gallbladder function by ultrasound; implications for dissolution therapy. *Clinical Radiology* **39**, 511–512.

4 Hopman, W.P.M., Rosenbusch, G., Jansen, J.B.M.J., de Jong, A.J.L., Lamers, C.B.H.W. (1985) Gallbladder contraction: effects of fatty meals and cholecystokinin. *Radiology* **157**, 37–39.

5 Wilson, S.A., Gosink, B.B., van Sonnenberg, E. (1986) Unchanged size of a dilated common bile duct after a fatty meal: results and significance. *Radiology* **160**, 29–31.

6 Darweesh, R.M.A., Dodds, W.J., Hogan, W.J., *et al.* (1988) Fatty meal sonography for evaluating patients with suspected partial common duct obstruction. *American Journal of Roentgenology* **158**, 63–68.

7 Bryan, P.J. (1982) Appearance of normal pancreatic duct. *Journal of Clinical Ultrasound* **10**, 63–66.

8 Cotton, P.B. (1980) Congenital anomaly of pancreas divisum as a cause of obstructive pain and jaundice. *Gut* **21**, 105.

9 Palazzo, L., Girrolet, P.P., Salmeron, M., *et al.* (1995) Value of endoscopic ultrasound in the diagnosis of common bile duct stones: comparison with surgical exploration and ERCP. *Gastrointestinal Endoscopy* **42**, 225–231.

10 Muller, M.F., Meyenberger, C., Bertschinger, P., Schaer, R., Marincek, B. (1994) Pancreatic tumours: evaluation with endoscopic US, CT, and MR imaging. *Radiology* **190**, 745–751.

11 Chang, K.J., Albers, C.G., Erickson, R.A., Butler, J.A., Wuerker, R.B., Lin, F. (1994) Endoscopic ultrasound-guided fine needle aspiration of pancreatic carcinoma. *American Journal of Gastroenterology* **89**, 263–266.

12 Furukawa, T., Tsukamoto, Y., Naitoh, Y., Hirooka, Y., Hayakawa, T. (1994) Differential diagnosis between benign and malignant localized stenosis of the main pancreatic duct by intraductal ultrasound of the pancreas. *American Journal of Gastroenterology* **89**, 2038–2041.

13 Stieggman, G.V., Soper, N.J., Filipi, C.J., McIntyre, R.C., Culley, M.P., Cordova, J.F. (1995) Laparoscopic ultrasonography as compared with static or dynamic cholangiography at laparoscopic cholecystectomy: a prospective multicentre trial. *Surgical Endoscopy—Ultrasound and Interventional Techniques* **9**, 1269–1273.

14 Barbara, L. (1984) Epidemiology of gallstone disease: the 'Sirmione study'. In: Capocaccia, L., Ricci, G., Angelico, F., Angelico, M., Attili, A.F. (eds) *Epidemiology and Prevention of Gallstone disease*. MTP Press, Lancaster, pp. 23–25.

15 Laing, F.C. (1987) Ultrasonography of gallbladder and biliary tree. In: Sarti, D.A. (ed.) *Diagnostic US: Text and Cases*, 2nd edn. Year Book, Chicago, pp. 142–153.

16 Gracie, W.A., Ransohoff, D.F. (1982) The natural history of silent gallstones: the silent gallstone is not a myth. *New England Journal of Medicine* **307**, 798–800.

17 Harbin, W.P., Ferrucci, J.T., Wittenberg, J., Kirkpatrick, R.H. (1979) Non-visualized gallbladder by cholecystosonography. *American Journal of Roentgenology* **132**, 727–728.

18 Laing, F.C., Federle, M.P., Jeffrey, R.B., Brown, T.W. (1981) Ultrasonic evaluation of patients with acute right upper quadrant pain. *Radiology* **140**, 449–455.
19 Kim, P.N., Lee, K.S., Kim, I.Y., Bae, W.K., Lee, B.H. (1994) Gallbladder perforation: comparison of US findings with CT. *Abdominal Imaging* **19**, 239–242.
20 Simeone, J.F., Brink, J.A., Mueller, P.R., *et al.* (1989) The sonographic diagnosis of acute gangrenous cholecystitis: importance of the Murphy sign. *American Journal of Roentgenology* **152**, 289–290.
21 Deitch, E.A., Engel, J.M. (1981) Acute acalculous cholecystitis: an ultrasonic diagnosis. *American Journal of Surgery* **142**, 290–292.
22 Mirvis, S.E., Vainright, J.R., Nelson, A.W., *et al.* (1986) The diagnosis of acute acalculous cholecystitis; a comparison of sonography, scintigraphy, and CT. *American Journal of Roentgenology* **147**, 1171–1175.
23 Raghavendra, B.N., Subramanyam, B.R., Balthazar, E.J., Horii, S.C., Megibow, A.J., Hilton, S. (1983) Sonography of adenomyomatosis of the gallbladder: radiologic–pathologic correlation. *Radiology* **146**, 747–752.
24 Fowler, R.C., Reid, W.A. (1988) Ultrasound diagnosis of adenomyomatosis of the gallbladder: ultrasonic and pathological correlation. *Clinical Radiology* **39**, 402–406.
25 Price, R.J., Stewart, E.T., Foley, W.D., Dodds, W.J. (1982) Sonography of polypoid cholesterolosis. *American Journal of Roentgenology* **139**, 1197.
26 Niv, Y., Kosakov, K., Shcolnik, B. (1986) Fragile papilloma (papillary adenoma) of the gallbladder. A cause of recurrent biliary colic. *Gastroenterology* **91**, 999–1001.
27 Foster, D.R., Foster, D.B.E. (1980) Gallbladder polyps in Peutz–Jegher's syndrome. *Postgraduate Medical Journal* **56**, 373–376.
28 Kane, R.A., Jacobs, R., Katz, J., Costello, P. (1984) Porcelain gallbladder: ultrasound and CT appearence. *Radiology* **152**, 137–141.
29 Ghawla, Y., Dilawari, J.B., Katariya, S. (1994) Gallbladder varices in portal vein thrombosis. *American Journal of Roentgenology* **162**, 643–645.
30 Weill, F., Eisencher, A., Zetlner, F. (1978) Ultrasonic study of the normal and dilated biliary tree: shotgun sign. *Radiology* **127**, 221.
31 Conrad, M.R., Landay, M.J., Jones, J.O. (1978) Sonographic 'parallel channel' sign of biliary tree enlargement in mild to moderate obstructive jaundice. *American Journal of Roentgenology* **130**, 279.
32 Laing, F.C., London, L.A., Filly, R.A. (1978) Ultrasonographic identification of dilated intrahepatic bile ducts and their differentiation from portal venous structures. *Journal of Clinical Ultrasound* **6**, 90.
33 Ingram, C., Joseph, A.E.A. (1989) The stilette sign: the appearance of dilated ducts in the fatty liver. *Clinical Radiology* **40**, 257–258.
34 Zeman, R.K., Burrel, M.L. (1987) Biliary obstruction: general principles. In: Zeman, R.K., Burrel, M.L. (eds) *Gallbladder and Bile Duct Imaging: A Clinical Radiologic Approach.* Churchill Livingstone, New York, pp. 385–469.
35 Laing, F.C., Jeffrey, R.B. Jr, Wing, V.W. (1986) Biliary dilatation: defining the level and cause by realtime US. *Radiology* **160**, 9–42.
36 Blackbourne, L.H., Earnhardt, R.C., Sistrom, C.L., Abbitt, P., Jones, I.G. (1994) The sensitivity and role of ultrasound in the evaluation of biliary obstruction. *American Surgeon* **60**, 683–690.
37 Soto, J.A., Yucel, E.K., Barish, M.A., Chuttani, R., Ferucci, J.T. (1996) MR cholangiopancreatography after unsuccessful or incomplete ERCP. *Radiology* **199**, 91–98.
38 Dong, B., Chen, M. (1987) Improved sonographic visualization of choledocholithiasis. *Journal of Clinical Ultrasound* **15**, 185–190.
39 Bucceri, A.M., Brogna, A., Ferrara, B.R. (1994) Common bile duct caliber following cholecystectomy: a two-year sonographic survey. *Abdominal Imaging* **19**, 251–252.
40 Jackson, V.P., Lappas, J.C. (1984) Sonography of the Mirizzi syndrome. *Journal of Ultrasound Medicine* **3**, 281–283.
41 Becker, C.D., Hassler, H., Terrier, F. (1984) Preoperative diagnosis of the Mirizzi syndrome: limitations of sonography and computed tomography. *American Journal of Roentgenology* **143**, 591–596.
42 Carroll, B.A., Oppenheimer, D.A. (1982) Sclerosing cholangitis: sonographic demonstration of bile duct wall thickening. *American Journal of Roentgenology* **139**, 1016–1018.
43 Majoie, C.B., Smits, N.J., Phoa, S.S., Reeders, J.W., Jansen, P.I. (1995) Primary sclerosing cholangitis: sonographic findings. *Abdominal Imaging* **20**, 109–112.
44 McCarthy, M., Choudhri, A.H., Helbert, M., *et al.* (1989) Radiological features of AIDS related cholangitis. *Clinical Radiology* **40**, 582–585.
45 Morikawa, P., Ischida, H., Niizawa, M., Komatsu, M., Arakawa, H., Masamune, O. (1988) Sonographic features of biliary clonorchiasis. *Journal of Clinical Ultrasound* **16**, 655–658.
46 Schulman, A., Loxton, A.J., Heydenrych, J.J., *et al.* (1982) Sonographic diagnosis of biliary ascariasis. *American Journal of Roentgenology* **139**, 485–489.
47 Filice, C., Marchi, L., Meloni, C., Patruno, S.F., Capellini, R., Bruno, R. (1995) Ultrasound in the diagnosis of gallbladder ascariasis. *Abdominal Imaging* **20**, 320–322.
48 Choi, B.I., Lim, J.H., Han, M.C., *et al.* (1989) Biliary cystadenoma and cystadenocarcinoma: CT and sonographic findings. *Radiology* **171**, 57–61.
49 Korobkin, M., Stephens, D.H., Lee, J.K.T., *et al.* (1989) Biliary cystadenoma and cystadenocarcinoma: CT and sonographic findings. *American Journal of Roentgenology* **153**, 507–511.
50 Garber, S.J., Donald, J.J., Lees, W.R. (1993) Cholangiocarcinoma: ultrasound features and correlation of tumor position with survival. *Abdominal Imaging* **18**, 66–69.
51 Todani, T., Watanabe, Y., Narusve, M., Tabuchi, K., Okajima, K. (1977) Congenital bile duct cysts: classification, operative procedures and review of 37 cases including cancer arising from choledochal cyst. *American Journal of Surgery* **134**, 263–269.
52 Savader, S.J., Benenati, J.F., Venbrux, A.C., *et al.* (1991) Choledochal cysts: classification and cholangiographic appearance. *American Journal of Roentgenology* **156**, 321–327.
53 Chijiiwa, K., Koga, A. (1993) Surgical management and long-term follow-up of patients with choledochal cysts. *American Journal of Surgery* **165**, 238–242.
54 Acosta, J.M., Ledesma, C.L. (1974) Gallstone migration as a cause of acute pancreatitis. *New England Journal of Medicine* **290**, 484–487.
55 Lee, S.P., Nicholls, J.F., Park, H.Z. (1992) Biliary sludge as a cause of acute pancreatitis. *New England Journal of Medicine* **326**, 589–593.
56 Ros, E., Navarro, S., Bru, C., *et al.* (1991) Occult microlithiasis in 'idiopathic' acute pancreatitis: prevention of relapses by cholecystectomy or ursodeoxycholic acid treatment. *Gastroenterology* **101**, 1701–1709.

57 Laing, F.C., Jeffrey, R.B., Wing, V.W. (1984) Improved visualisation of choledocholithiasis by sonography. *American Journal of Roentgenology* **143**, 949–952.
58 Jeffrey, R.B., Laing, F.C., Wing, V.W. (1986) Extrapancreatic spread of acute pancreatitis: new observations with real-time US. *Radiology* **159**, 707–711.
59 Hill, M.C., Barkin, J., Isikoff, M.B., Silverstein, W., Keilser, M. (1982) Acute pancreatitis: clinical vs. CT findings. *American Journal of Roentgenology* **139**, 263–269.
60 Sarti, D.A. (1977) Rapid development and spontaneous regression of pancreatic pseudocysts documented by US. *Radiology* **125**, 789–793.
61 Bradley, E.L., Clements, L.J. (1976) Spontaneous resolution of pancreatic pseudocyst: implications for timing operative intervention. *American Journal of Surgery* **129**, 23–28.
62 Marshall, J.B. (1993) Acute pancreatitis. *Archives of Internal Medicine* **153**, 1185–1191.
63 Bares, R., Klever, P., Hauptmann, S., *et al.* (1994) F-18 Fluorodeoxyglucose PET *in vivo* evaluation of pancreatic glucose metabolism for detection of pancreatic glucose metabolism for detection of pancreatic cancer. *Radiology* **192**, 79–86.
64 Pasanen, P.A., Eskelinen, M., Vornanen, M., Partanen, K. (1993) Pancreatic lymphoma. *Annales Chirurgie et Gynaecologiae* **82**, 207–209.
65 Campbell, J.P., Wilson, S.R. (1988) Pancreatic neoplasms: how useful is evaluation with ultrasonography? *Radiology* **167**, 341–344.
66 Nghiem, H.V., Freeny, P.C. (1994) Radiologic staging of pancreatic carcinoma. *Radiology Clinics of North America* **32**, 71–79.
67 Taylor, K.J.W., Ramos, I., Carter, D., Morse, S.S., Dhower, D., Fortune, K. (1988) Correlation of Doppler ultrasound tumor signals with neovascular morphological findings. *Radiology* **166**, 57–62.
68 Hall-Craggs, M.A., Lees, W.R. (1986) Fine needle aspiration biopsy: pancreatic and biliary tumors. *American Journal of Roentgenology* **147**, 399–403.
69 Grieshop, N.A., Wiebke, E.A., Kratzer, S.S., Madura, J.A. (1994) Cystic neoplasms of the pancreas. *American Surgeon* **60**, 509–514.
70 Glover, J.R., Shorvon, P.J., Lees, W.R. (1992) Endoscopic ultrasound for localization of islet cell tumours. *Gut* **33**, 108–110.
71 Radin, D.R., Colletti, P.M., Forrester, D.M., *et al.* (1986) Pancreatic acinar cell carcinoma with subcutaneous and intra-osseous fat necrosis. *Radiology* **158**, 67–68.
72 Lim, J.H., Chung, K.B., Cho, O.K., *et al.* (1990) Acinar cell carcinoma of pancreas. Ultrasonography and CT findings. *Clinical Imaging* **14**, 301–304.

Chapter 27: Endoluminal ultrasound of the upper gastrointestinal tract

D.A. Nicholson

Endoscopic ultrasound (EUS) is the adopted term for the technique which enables endoluminal ultrasound to be performed using a specially designed endoscope with a fixed piezoelectric transducer. It is now over 10 years since initial reports described the use of this technique in patients and its use in clinical practice in Europe, the Far East and the USA has been steadily increasing over this period. The technique has been described as the most significant advance in gastrointestinal endoscopy during the last decade, providing structural information about the gastrointestinal tract and tissues immediately surrounding it. Advances in instrumentation are on-going and there are now several types of instrument available; axial and sagittal imaging transducers (radial and linear array scanners), colour Doppler sagittal probes, and miniaturized catheter probes for use through the biopsy channel of conventional endoscopes.

The main advantage of EUS in imaging the upper gastrointestinal tract and adjacent organs is that the transducer proximity to the tissues under investigation allows relatively high ultrasound frequencies to be used, with a consequent improvement in spacial resolution. Some of the information obtained by EUS is not available by any other imaging modality. The commonly available instruments operate at frequencies ranging from 5 to 20 MHz.

This chapter covers the technique of EUS and describes the EUS appearances of common pathology. Indications for EUS in the upper gastrointestinal tract include the following.

1 Staging of malignancy—oesophageal/gastric cancer and lymphoma.

2 Follow-up of malignant disease—assessment of recurrence.

3 Evaluation of submucosal lesions.

4 Diagnosis and follow-up of oesophageal varices.

5 Evaluation of the pancreas, particularly for the assessment of small pancreatic cancers, neuroendocrine tumours and chronic pancreatitis.

6 Assessment of bile duct strictures and staging of cholangiocarcinoma.

Anatomy of gastrointestinal tract wall

Using transducer frequencies of between 7.5 and 12 MHz resolution is improved so that the intestinal mucosa (Fig. 27.1) can be visualized as a five (or occasionally seven) layer structure with alternating echogenic and echo-poor bands [1]. EUS is the only available modality that routinely provides such images of the structure of the wall of the intestinal tract. The actual histological correlation of the various bands seen on the ultrasonographic image has been a matter of debate for some years with some authors claiming a close relationship between the sonographic layers and the anatomical/histological layers of the gut wall. More recently, however, it has been shown that the various sonographic layers cannot be related directly to histological layers in a simplistic manner (Fig. 27.2) [2,3]. The first hyperechoic layer corresponds to the superficial surface of the gut mucosa. The deep part of the mucosa and adjacent muscularis mucosa form a hypoechoic layer. The submucosa which histologically contains a large number of vessels and fat is equivalent to the third hyperechoic layer. There is good correlation between the width of the fourth band and the varying amount of muscle in the muscularis propria, which varies with anatomical site (Fig. 27.3). The fifth hyperechoic layer corresponds to the interface between the serosa/adventitia, and surrounding tissues/organs.

Technique

Although EUS combines visual endoscopy and ultrasonography it is not possible to perform both aspects of the technique simultaneously. Endoscopy requires air distension for visualization of the mucosa whereas ultrasound examination requires direct contact with the mucosa, ideally in a collapsed or fluid-filled viscus.

Endoscopic ultrasound is performed following pharyngeal anaesthesia and intravenous sedation as the endoscopes are of relatively large calibre (approximately 13 mm diameter). Although the endoscopic procedure is performed as for conventional upper endoscopy, it is techni-

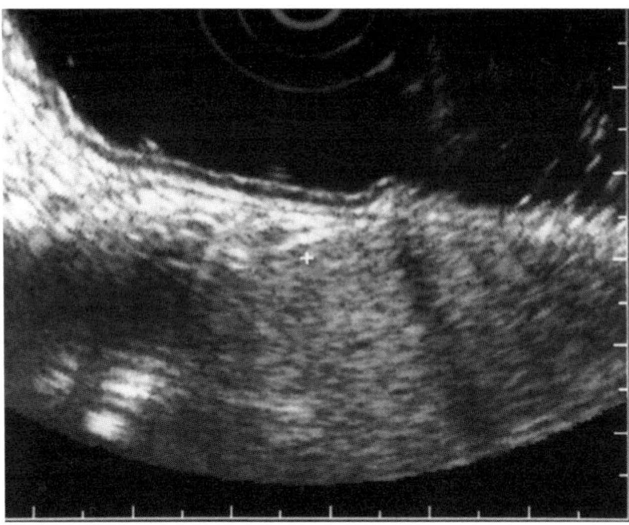

Fig. 27.1 Ultrasound of water-filled gastric body. This demonstrates the normal five layer appearance to the intestinal wall. Compare with Fig. 27.2.

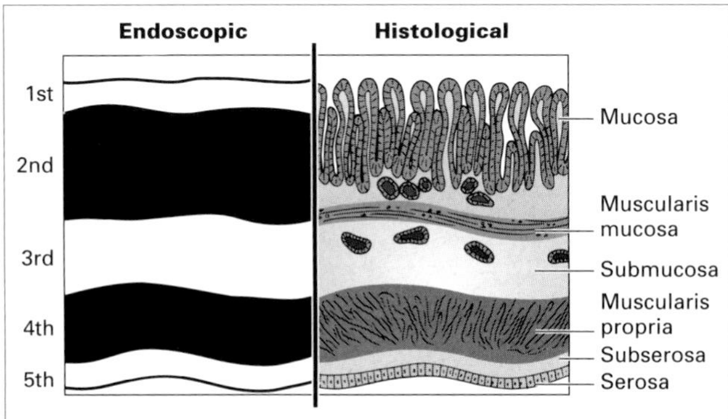

Fig. 27.2 Endoscopic layers compared with histological layers. The second and fourth layers appear hypoechoic. Note that the thickness of the fourth layer is equivalent to the thickness and distribution of the muscularis propria.

cally more difficult to perform as the endoscopic image is obliquely orientated and because the housing of the probe at the end of the endoscope causes a longer rigid segment. In order to fully utilize EUS it is therefore essential that the operator is trained in both endoscopy and EUS interpretation or that there is good collaboration between the endoscopist and radiologist as the technique bridges both disciplines.

The patient is initially examined in the left decubitus position with the endoscope passed into the second part of the duodenum. Negotiation of the pylorus and first part of the duodenum may prove difficult due to the rigid distal portion of the endoscope, which measures 4 cm in length. More often than not the focus of interest has been

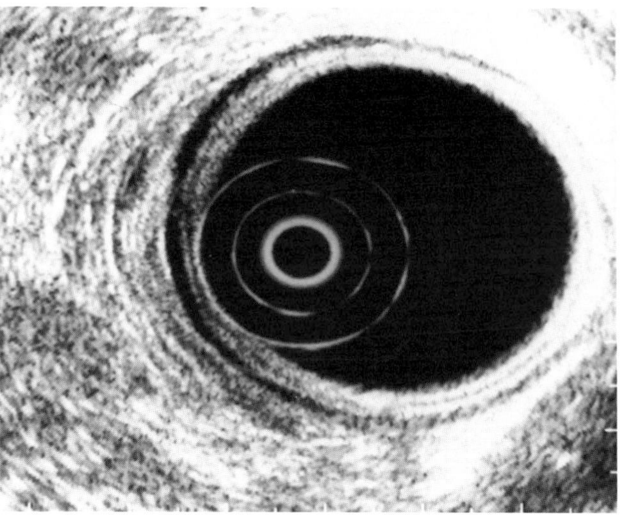

Fig. 27.3 Endoscopic ultrasound of a normal gastric antrum. The balloon is distending the antrum. Note the difference in thickness of the endoscopic layers particularly the muscularis propria compared to Fig. 27.1.

identified previously by other investigations, e.g. oesophageal or gastric cancer, submucosal tumour, pancreatic or biliary disease. Once the endoscope is in an appropriate position as much air as possible is aspirated in order to optimize ultrasonic visualization. The endoscopic image is therefore lost and the orientation of the endoscope is subsequently adjusted according to the ultrasonic image. The endoscope is withdrawn through the duodenum and stomach in a staged pullback technique as described by Caletti *et al.* [4] Acoustic coupling between the transducer and the stomach mucosa is achieved by the use of either a water-filled balloon surrounding the transducer head (see Fig. 27.3) or organ distension by the installation of water (see Fig. 27.1), or a combination of both. The water-filled technique is most appropriate for examination of the stomach and duodenum and particularly for the evaluation of mucosal lesions or extraluminal structures such as the pancreas and biliary tree (see Fig. 27.3). During the procedure the patient position can be changed in order to shift the water in the stomach to lie adjacent to the surface to be examined. In the oesophagus the water-filled balloon technique is most appropriate as good circumferential contact can be achieved [5]. For complete examination of the pancreas and biliary tree the endoscope needs to the introduced into the second part of the duodenum (Figs 27.4–27.6). Visualization of the head of the pancreas and distal bile duct is initially obtained by withdrawing the endoscope and later the rest of the bile duct and hepatoduodenal ligament may be seen by partly intussuscepting the duodenal cap into the gastric antrum. The body and tail of the pancreas (Fig. 27.7) can be visual-

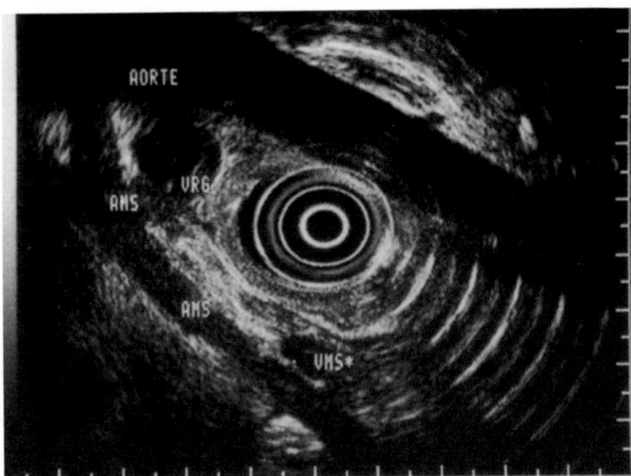

Fig. 27.4 The transducer is in the second part of the duodenum. This allows good visualization of the superior mesenteric artery (AMS), left renal vein (VRG), right renal artery, inferior vena cava and superior mesenteric vein (VMS). (Courtesy of Dr Laurent Pallazzo, Paris.)

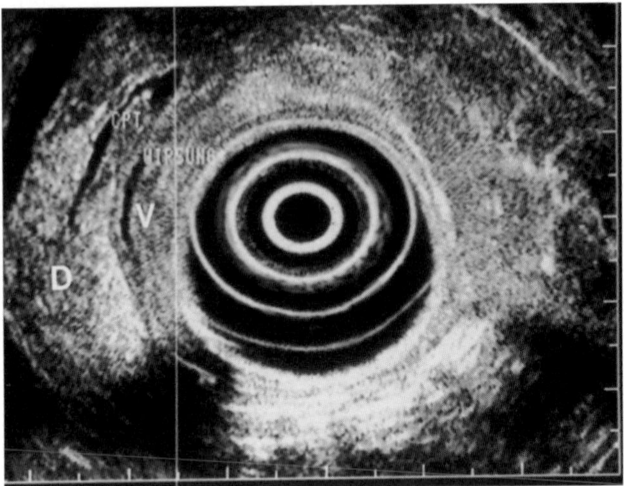

Fig. 27.5 The transducer is in the second part of the duodenum. The duct of Wirsung can be identified in the ventral pancreas as well as the main pancreatic duct (CPT). D, dorsal pancreas; V, ventral pancreas.

ized by maintaining contact with the posterior wall of the stomach and slowly withdrawing the scope into the fundus [6].

The most commonly used endoscope (Olympus EU-M3 system) produces a 360° radial image in a transverse plane perpendicular to the shaft of the endoscope. The transducer can be switched between 7.5 and 12 MHz allowing a depth of field of either 4 or 8 cm, respectively. Most current endoscope have an instrument channel to allow fine-needle aspiration or biopsy under direct ultrasound guidance.

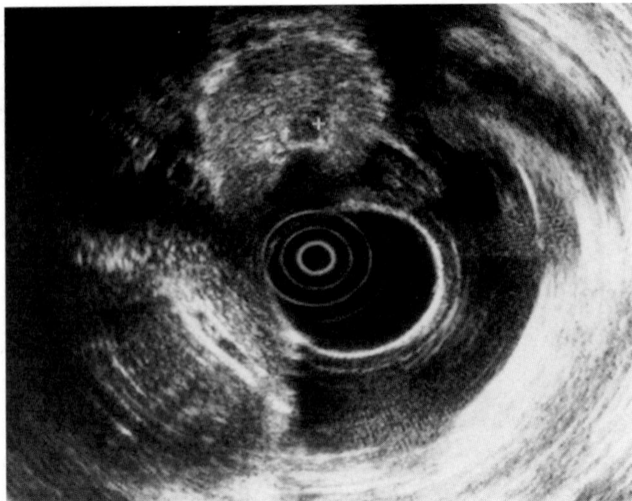

Fig. 27.6 The transducer again is in the second part of the duodenum. This gives excellent visualization of the head of the pancreas. Lying within the head of the pancreas there is a small 7 mm hypoechoic lesion which is well defined (crosses). This was later confirmed on angiography and following resection to be an insulinoma.

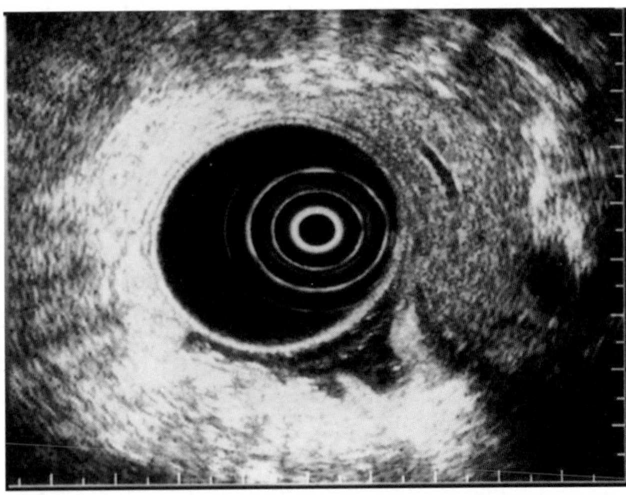

Fig. 27.7 The remaining body and tail of the pancreas is visualized through the posterior wall of the stomach. In this example the transducer is lying in the fundus of the stomach making visualization of the tail of the pancreas and normal pancreatic duct possible.

Clinical uses of EUS

Assessment of malignancies

Endoscopic ultrasound is valuable in assessing various malignancies for several reasons. Principally it is the only imaging modality that can attempt to stage tumours according to current TNM classification (T, primary tumour; N, regional lymph node metastasis; M, remote metastasis) [7]. EUS provides useful information about tumour growth patterns which can facilitate the classification of early and advanced cancer and is therefore complementary to both endoscopy and biopsy. The information gleaned can be valuable for assessing prognosis and will impact on tumour therapy determining surgical and non-surgical options. EUS may also have a role in evaluation and surveillance of patients with inoperable carcinomas and in assessing the response to chemotherapy and radiotherapy [8].

TUMOUR STAGING

There is now increasing evidence that EUS has the ability to diagnose and stage tumours of the upper gastrointestinal tract accurately. The standard convention for assessing tumour extent, nodal involvement and distant metastatic lesions is the TNM classification. The T staging is based on the tumour penetration of the normal histological layers which EUS is uniquely equipped to assess. The main limitation is the difficulty in distinguishing peritumoral inflammation and true tumour which appear similar and may therefore lead to overstaging [9,10]. Despite these limitations of EUS concordance with the histology of surgically resected tumours is approximately 90%. Because of the spacial resolution achieved by EUS, the technique is also very sensitive for demonstrating very small lymph nodes. As with other techniques it may prove difficult distinguishing benign from malignant disease. However, EUS allows estimation of not only the size but also the shape and internal architecture of nodes which improves overall nodal staging to an accuracy of 75–90%, with a specificity of 50–70%.

Full staging of metastases (M staging) is not possible with EUS because of its limited depth of penetration/visualization, which is related to the high frequencies used. The role of EUS should therefore be limited to patients who have potentially resectable/curable disease after exclusion of metastatic disease with conventional imaging of the liver and lungs with ultrasound, computed tomography (CT) or magnetic resonance imaging (MRI).

Oesophageal cancer

To date EUS has had the greatest impact on the staging of oesophageal cancer (Fig. 27.8–27.10) and thereby assisting in the treatment of choice for individual patients. Various studies have shown accuracies of 82–86% for T staging and 70–86% for N staging of tumours which is vastly superior to other modalities such as CT [11–13]. However, a difference in 'prediction of resectability' has also been documented when assessing different histological types of tumour specifically adenocarcinomas and squamous cell carcinoma of the oesophagus. This has occurred because of the difficulty in assessing microscopic infiltration in squamous cell carcinoma [14]. In addition because of the late presentation and obstructive nature of oesophageal malignancy problems have arisen in negoti-

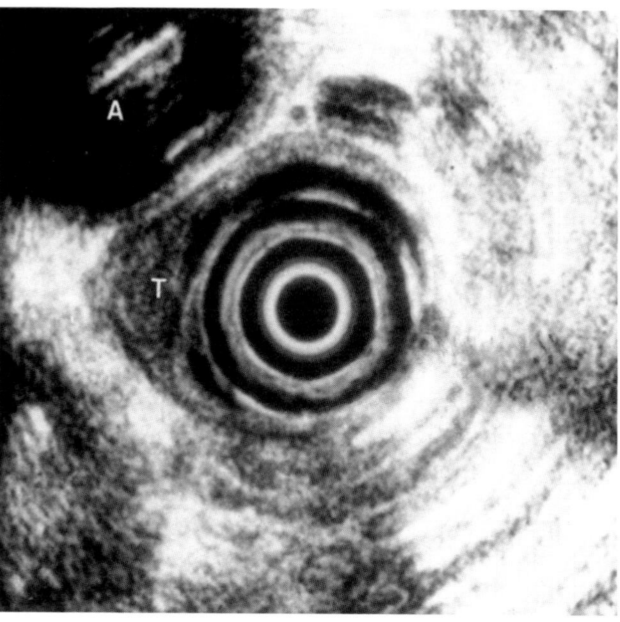

Fig. 27.8 Small cancer of the middle third of the oesophagus. The tumour (T) is disrupting the fourth hypoechoic layer with invasion of the perioesophageal fat (T3 cancer). A fat plane between the tumour and the aorta (A) is still evident.

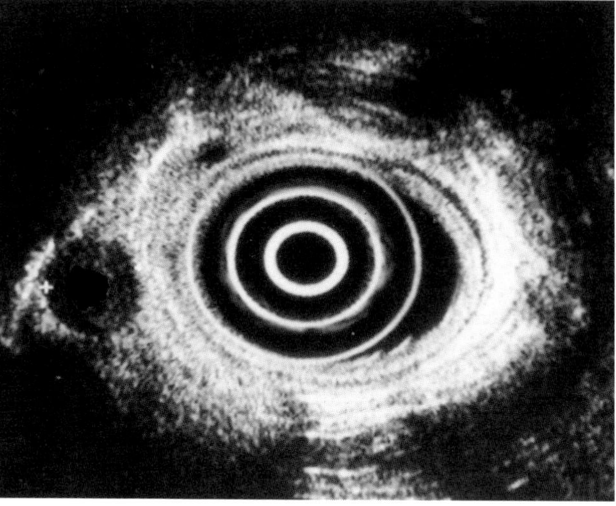

Fig. 27.9 Small rounded well-defined hypoechoic lymph node situated between the left wall of the oesophagus and the aorta. Although only 7 mm in diameter this node has the typical features of metastatic involvement.

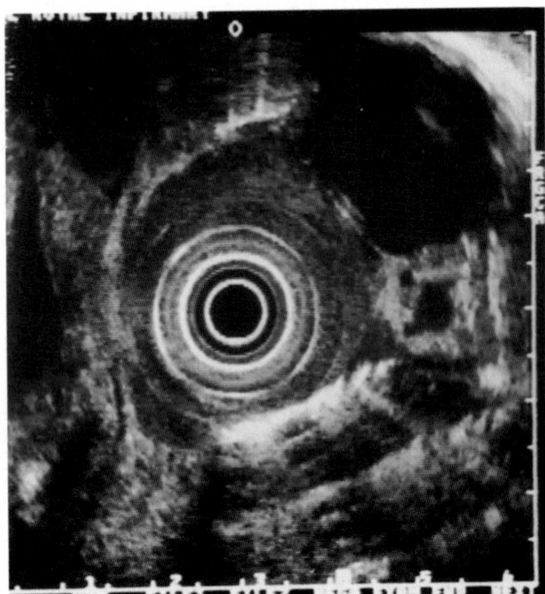

Fig. 27.10 Extensive oesophageal cancer spreading circumferentially penetrating and disrupting all the usual visible layers. The tumour is also seen to be inseparable from the aorta with loss of the fat plane indicating aortic invasion at this site.

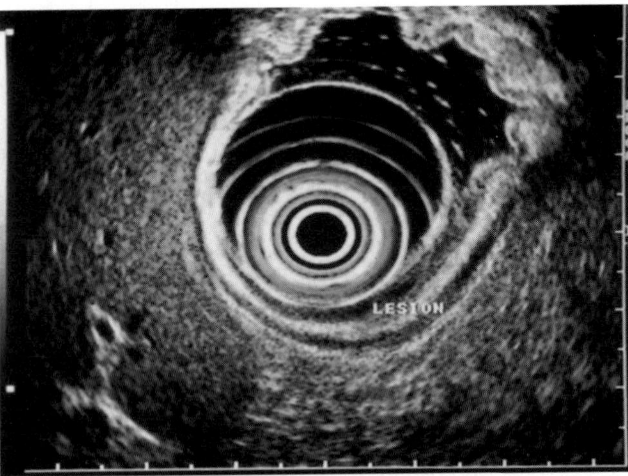

Fig. 27.11 Small lesser curve gastric ulcer on biopsy showed adenocarcinoma. This staging EUS shows a very small tumour limited to the superficial two layers of the gastric wall. The third hyperechoic layer is still intact with no evidence of invasion. This lesion corresponds to a T1 cancer.

ating tight strictures with the large calibre endoscope/transducer. This has resulted in incomplete staging of tumours which has been reported in up to 50% of cases in some series. The use of mini-probes in such situations has been suggested as a possible solution in these circumstances. As well as staging of oesophageal cancer the role of EUS in evaluating non-operative tumours is also being explored as new approaches to the treatment of tumours with chemotherapy and/or radiotherapy as adjuvunct treatments with surgery are developed [15]. EUS may therefore have a role in monitoring/tumour response assessment. The role of EUS in the assessment of premalignant conditions such as Barrett's oesophagus is still to be determined but is another potential for this modality. Tumour characteristics of oesophageal cancer are illustrated in Figs 27.8–27.10.

Gastric cancer

Endoscopy and barium radiology remain the primary diagnostic methods in detecting gastric cancer; however, studies from Japan, where early gastric cancer is seen relatively commonly, have shown EUS to be of great value in staging small malignancies.

Early gastric carcinoma most often appears as an irregular hypoechoic intraluminal tumour with no distinguishing features from a benign ulcer [16], whereas advanced tumours show intramural extension infiltrating the deep layers [17]. The accuracy of differentiating between early and advanced gastric cancer has been impressive (greater than 95%; Fig. 27.11), although confusion between peritumoral inflammation and fibrous tissue and true tumour has led to a degree of over staging. Infiltration of the muscularis propria confers a T2 stage lesion. Overall EUS accurately determines the depth of gastric cancer invasion in around 80% of cases, slightly lower than for oesophageal cancer, however, EUS has a good accuracy of approximately 95% in predicting resectability [18].

Endoscopic ultrasound has also been shown to be valuable in the assessment of patients with linitis plastica or gastric fold thickening. Such appearances may be due to hypertrophic gastritis or scirrhous carcinoma which has a tendency to spread in the submucosa producing a marked desmoplastic response (Fig. 27.12). Scirrhous carcinoma accounts for approximately 10% of gastric cancer causing a marked fibrotic response in the submucosa and muscularis propria in the typical 'leather bottle' stomach—linitis plastica. Preservation of the mucosa can make endoscopic diagnosis difficult. On EUS there is preservation of the normal five layer structure with thickening of the third and fourth sonographic layers by irregular hypoechoic tissue [19]. This contrasts with hypertrophic gastritis where there is usually only thickening of the superficial second layer (Fig. 27.13).

Pancreatic cancer

The complicated anatomy of the pancreas renders the diagnostic and therapeutic approaches to it difficult. The

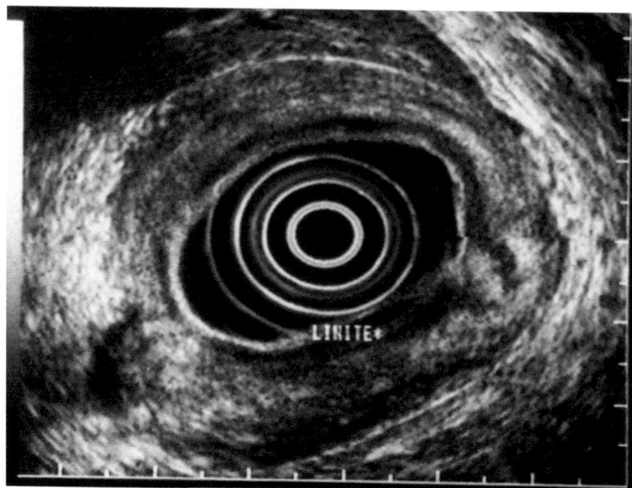

Fig. 27.12 Circumferential adenocarcinoma of the body of the stomach. There is predominantly thickening of the third and fourth layers of the gastric wall corresponding to the typical appearances of linitis plastica. (Courtesy of Dr Laurent Pallazzo, Paris.)

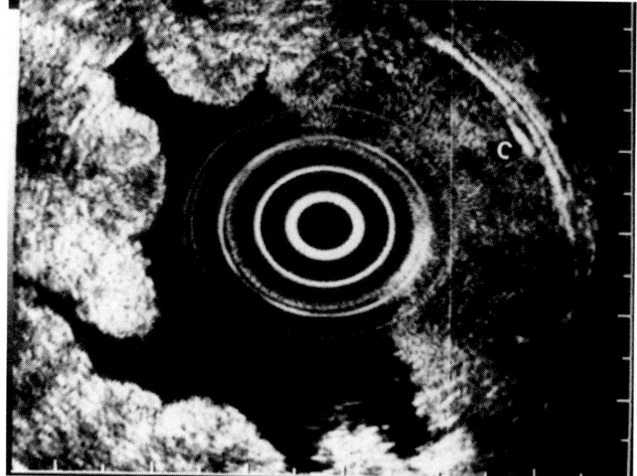

Fig. 27.13 Ménétrier's disease. There is thickening of the superficial layers of the gastric mucosa with preservation of the deep layers. A small cyst (C) measuring 3 mm in diameter is evident in the depth of the mucosal thickening.

organ lies deep in the retroperitoneum covered by a variety of solid and gas-filled organs. In the last decade ultrasound, CT and endoscopic retrograde cholangiopancreatography (ERCP) have significantly improved the diagnosis of small tumours; however, all these techniques have limitations. Since many pancreatic tumours are advanced at the time of clinical presentation standard imaging (ultrasound, CT, ERCP) is all that is required; however, early detection and accurate staging of small pancreatic tumours (<3 cm) is still a problem, and in this

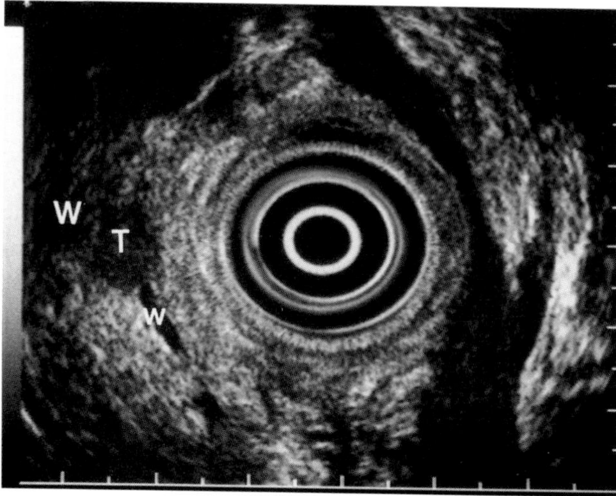

Fig. 27.14 Typical appearance of a small pancreatic cancer. There is a 9 mm hypoechoic lesion lying in the body of the pancreas (T). The main pancreatic duct (W) can be visualized and shows dilatation proximal to the small tumour.

group EUS may provide valuable staging information. With the close proximation of the endoscope to the gland through the posterior wall of the stomach there is no intervening bowel gas. This with the use of high frequency ultrasound has allowed improved accuracy of tumour detection and staging. For the detection of masses in the pancreas, EUS has been proved to be more sensitive than ultrasound, CT, MRI and ERCP. Its superiority is especially evident when dealing with small tumours less than 3 cm in diameter [20].

Detection. Pancreatic cancer usually appears as a hypoechoic lesion which is distinct from the normal surrounding pancreatic parenchyma (Fig. 27.14). Small tumours are usually roundish whereas larger tumours have a nodular contour and appear more heterogeneous due to necrosis. The contour of the tumour is dependent on both the degree of infiltration and the amount of peritumoral inflammation. Problems have been encountered in differentiating small tumours from inflammatory masses in pancreatitis. In contrast to pancreatic cancer, pseudotumours observed in chronic pancreatitis normally have a mottled pattern with an irregular edge which varies depending on the degree of surrounding inflammation (Fig. 27.15). However, general criteria must be sought to differentiate between inflammatory and malignant masses (enlarged lymph nodes, vascular involvement, liver metastases).

Staging. As with other tumours the prognosis and treatment of pancreatic cancer depends on the stage of tumour

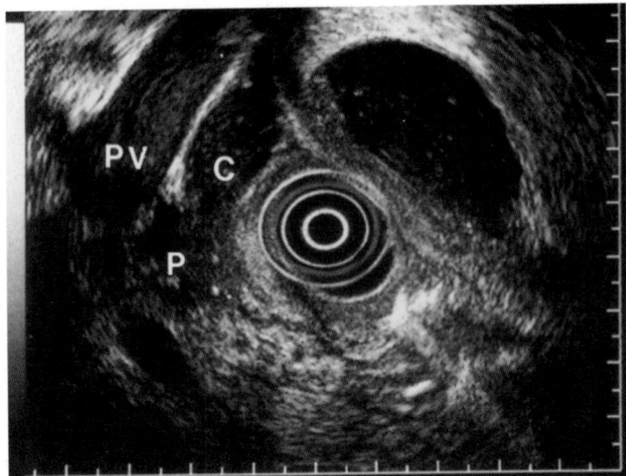

Fig. 27.15 Patient with chronic pancreatitis. A pseudotumour (P) is seen at the level of the head of the pancreas. There is gross dilatation of the proximal pancreatic duct (C) and thrombosis of the portal vein (PV).(Courtesy of Dr Laurent Pallazzo, Paris.)

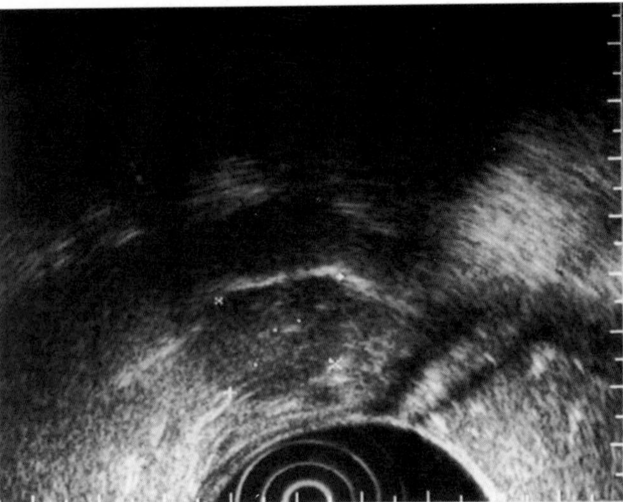

Fig. 27.16 Small 2 cm insulinoma located in the tail of the pancreas. The lesion has a typical well-circumscribed border and appears hypoechoic.

infiltration. EUS gives detailed information about the tumour and adjacent structures. However, as will other pathologies, it has limited value in assessing distant metastases. Tumour staging by EUS has been shown to be accurate in 88–92% and in determining correctly invasion into major vessels in 80% [21,22]. Again, the accuracy of EUS in nodal staging has been relatively disappointing varying from 50 to 80% in various reports. Nevertheless this compares favourably with other modalities such as CT [23].

At present EUS is the most accurate method of imaging pancreatic cancer especially when the lesions are small. Though accuracies of 90% have been achieved, differentiation between cancer and pseudotumours is a problem. With new advances in scope technology and the ability to biopsy under direct endoscopic visualization, some of these problems should be overcome in the future.

Pancreatic islet cell tumours. Islet cell tumours like all endocrine tumours are rare, mostly benign and difficult to diagnose because of their small size. They commonly become clinically apparent because of their severe hormonal secretions. Despite aggressive preoperative localization using ultrasound, CT, angiography and portal venous sampling about 40% of all pancreatic adenomas usually escape detection. Angiography has been reported as the most sensitive modality but false negatives are frequent with small nodules. Selective pancreatic venous sampling is the specific technique but is invasive, difficult to perform and does not provide accurate tumour localization. Several studies have shown improved detection rates for islet cell tumours using EUS [24,25]. Islet cell tumours are generally well circumscribed and hypoechoic in comparison with the normal pancreatic parenchyma (Fig. 27.16). The internal echo pattern is usually homogeneous; however, in malignant lesions irregular central echogenic areas may be identified. The advantage of detecting such tumour preoperatively is that this greatly reduces the extent of surgical mobilization required at operation and in the size of the resected specimen.

Clinicopathological studies have shown that the clarity of the margin of tumours is related to the degree of surrounding inflammation. When a carcinoma obstructs the pancreas there is secondary pancreatitis; this leads to fibrosis which in turn creates a more blurred margin. In comparison islet cell tumours cause little secondary fibrosis and therefore are generally well defined. In pancreatic pseudotumours an indistinct margin is seen around the entire circumference due to the inflammatory changes. The internal structure of small pancreatic mass lesions varies depending on the histology. The majority of malignancies are hypoechoic with irregular central echogenic tissue whereas islet cell tumours are usually homogeneously hypoechoic.

Cholangiocarcinoma (extrahepatic bile duct cancer)

These lesions usually present with jaundice, abdominal pain, pruritis and weight loss. Accurate preoperative staging is essential because the extent of tumour may be difficult to assess at surgery due to the anatomical location and the fibrotic response to such tumours. Cholangiocarcinoma appears as hypoechoic, inhomogeneous, intraductal or transductal tissue which may be surrounded by

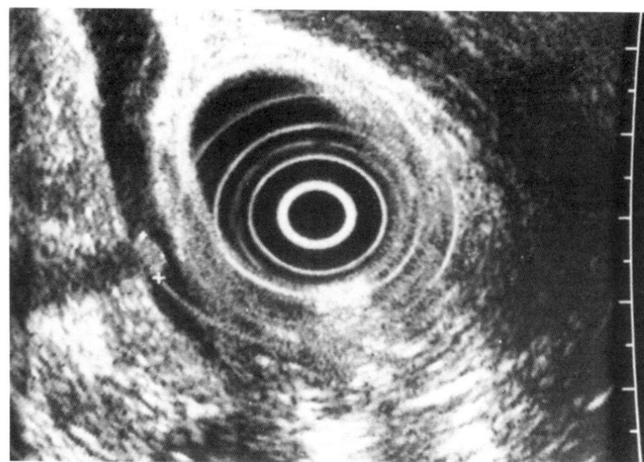

Fig. 27.17 Patient presented with obstructive jaundice. Duct dilatation was identified both at ultrasound and CT although no cause was established. EUS demonstrates a small 4 mm calculus (crosses) in the lower common bile duct causing the duct dilatation.

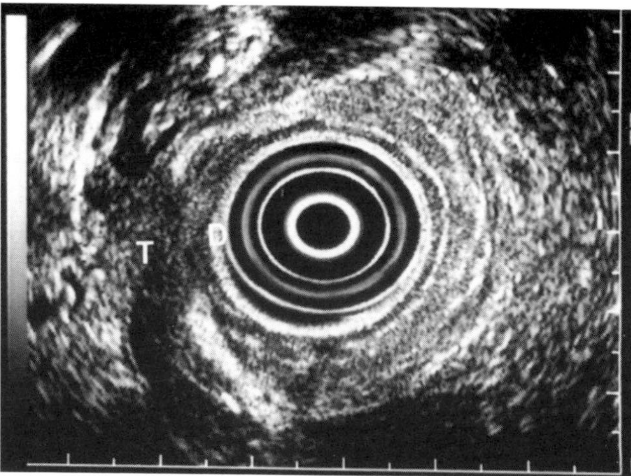

Fig. 27.19 Cholangiocarcinoma (T) on the upper portion of the common bile duct. The tumour is seen to be causing invasion of the adjacent duodenal wall (D), staging the tumour as a T3 lesion.

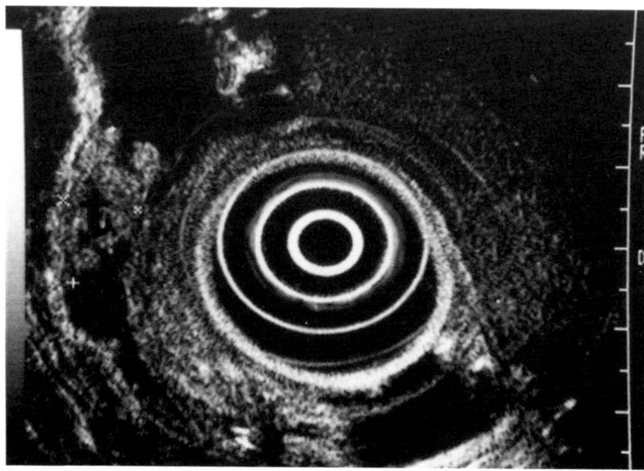

Fig. 27.18 Intraductal polypoid tumour measuring 15 mm in diameter located in the mid portion of the common bile duct. Note no acoustic shadowing is seen from the tumour (t). The prestenotic dilatation of the common bile duct is obvious.

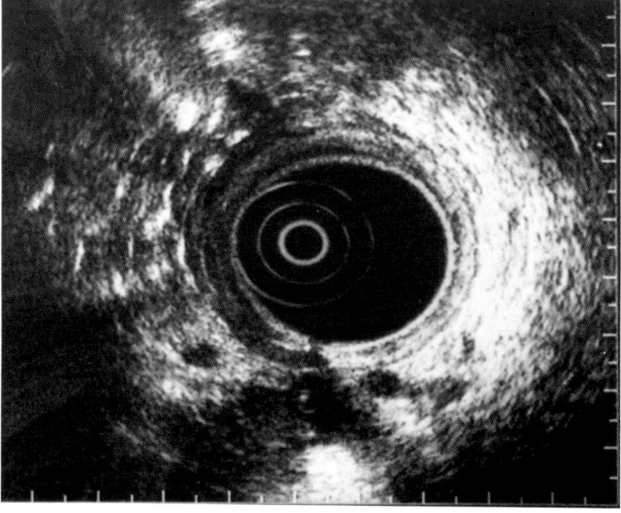

Fig. 27.20 Normal gastrojejunal anastomosis showing only three endosonographic layers (12 to 6 o'clock on the right). The left side of the anastomosis shows a hypoechoic rim of tissue measuring up to 10 mm in diameter in keeping with a gastric cancer recurrence.

a rim of echogenic material representing the associated fibrosis (Figs 27.17–27.19). Prestenotic dilatation of the bile duct is usually seen and readily identified at EUS. The accuracy of EUS in diagnosing cholangiocarcinoma has been reported as approximately 85% and again it appears as a very promising technique in assessing extent of tumour infiltration and local lymph node metastases [26].

Anastomotic recurrence

Another clinical problem is the diagnosis of local or submucosal tumour recurrence following surgical anastomoses in patients with oesophageal or gastric cancer. EUS can detect postoperative recurrence of carcinoma on the serosal surface of an anastomosis [27] with a sensitivity of 95% and a specificity of 80%. The false positive rate of 20% occurs as fibrosis will often distort the layers in an eccentric fashion, hence biopsy is needed to confirm the tissue type. Following surgical anastomoses as few as three sonographic layers may be identified (Fig. 27.20). Recurrent tumour is identified as nodularity or irregular hypoechoic thickening to greater than 7 mm which may be localized or circumferential in the region of the anastomosis (see Fig. 27.20). Furthermore, abnormal local lymph nodes may be identified.

Lymph node assessment

As with other imaging modalities micrometastases in normal-sized lymph nodes cannot be visualized using EUS, and the differentiation of enlarged inflammatory nodes from malignant nodes is also a problem. Nevertheless EUS has proved more accurate than other modalities in the assessment of local nodes in both oesophageal and gastric cancer with quoted accuracies of 50 to 80%. EUS has the ability to identify normal-sized nodes which often appear elliptical in shape. In comparison malignant nodes appear well defined, round and hypoechoic with a similar echogenicity to the primary tumour (see Fig. 27.9) [28,29]. Limited beam of penetration prevents EUS being an effective way of evaluating distant metastases.

Gastric lymphoma

As with submucosal tumours gastric lymphoma is a difficult endoscopic diagnosis as the appearances can mimic gastric carcinoma. A definitive diagnosis is essential for assessing prognosis and allowing appropriate management. In addition, early gastric lymphoma often occurs with an intact mucosa and biopsies are often inconclusive. EUS has the ability to define the extent of gastric lymphoma even when the tumour is covered with normal mucosa. On EUS lymphoma shows some characteristics which may help distinguish it from carcinoma. In primary gastric non-Hodgkin's lymphoma three different EUS patterns have been described, a polypoid pattern with protrusion into the gastric lumen, ulceration with a localized hypoechoic thickening of the gastric wall causing complete disruption of the normal five layer pattern and ulceration with diffuse underlying hypoechoic infiltration with longitudinal extension [30]. Such infiltration is characteristic of lymphoma is usually confined to the second and third sonographic layers but may involve the whole thickness of the gut wall (Fig. 27.21) [31].

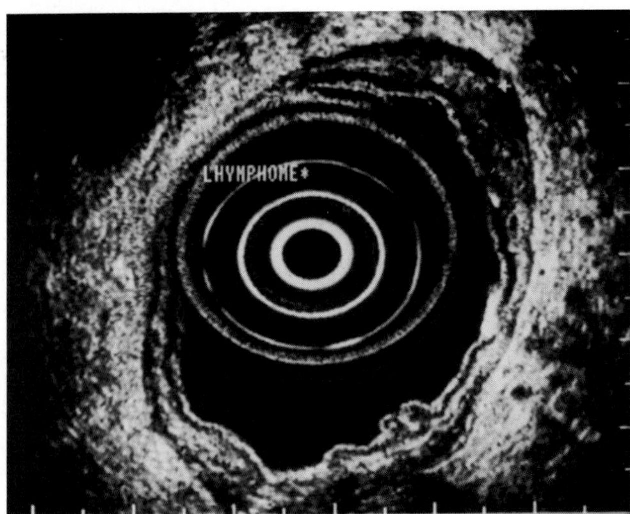

Fig. 27.21 Infiltrating lymphoma of the gastric fundus. The muscularis mucosa is actually preserved and the tumour is seen to extend longitudinally in this case affecting mainly the third layer. (Courtesy of Dr Laurent Pallazzo, Paris.)

Gastric submucosal lesions

The most widely reported European use of EUS in the stomach has been the evaluation of gastric submucosal lesions which have to be differentiated from extraluminal compression caused by adjacent normal or pathological organs. Several studies have shown EUS is able to characterize lesions in over 95% of cases, even when lesions measure less than 5 mm in size [32]. Submucosal lesions can be a diagnostic problem as small lesions often cause no mucosal ulceration and endoscopic biopsies are often negative.

Leiomyomas are the most common lesion identified and appear as round hypoechoic masses with smooth margins that are continuous with the fourth hypoechoic layer (muscularis propria) [33]. Malignant transformation to leiomyoblastomas or leiomyosarcomas can occur and should be considered in any lesion over 3 cm in size, or which has cystic foci within it which are due to necrosis or has an irregular outer margin [33,35]. However, malignant changes are possible in benign appearing lesions and biopsy is recommended in most circumstances [35].

Gastric varices appear as linear, hypoechoic structures with smooth outer margins (Fig. 27.22). Pancreatic rests are seen as well-circumscribed submucosal lesions of varying echogenicity with central cystic or tubular structures corresponding to duct systems. They tend to arise from the innermost three sonographic layers. Gastric lipomas are identified as compressible hyperechoic well-defined lesions generally arising from the third echogenic layer (Fig. 27.23). As well as intrinsic wall lesions EUS can accurately differentiate compression by adjacent organs, cysts and masses. Such pathologies compress the wall; however, the normal five layer structure is maintained.

Although a definitive histological diagnosis cannot be achieved by EUS the technique demonstrates whether the lesion is cystic, solid or vascular and by accurately defining its layer of origin frequently infers a diagnosis. Appropriate therapeutic decisions, however, can only be made on the basis of histology. Using the echo endoscopes

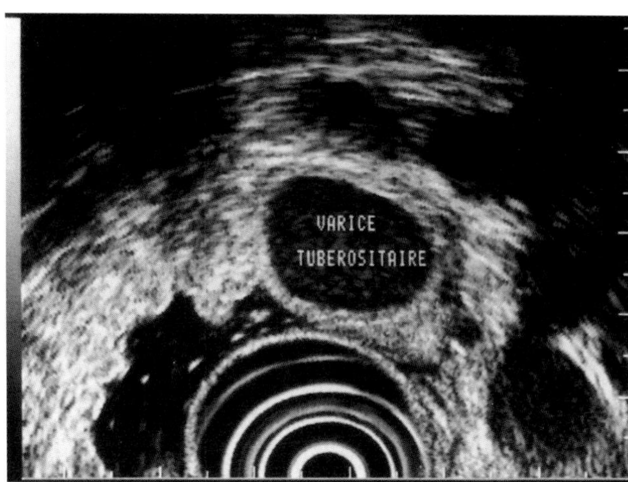

Fig. 27.22 Endoscopy revealed an extrinsic mass with no mucosal abnormality. EUS revealed the cause as gastric varices as shown by this image. (Courtesy of Dr Laurent Pallazzo, Paris.)

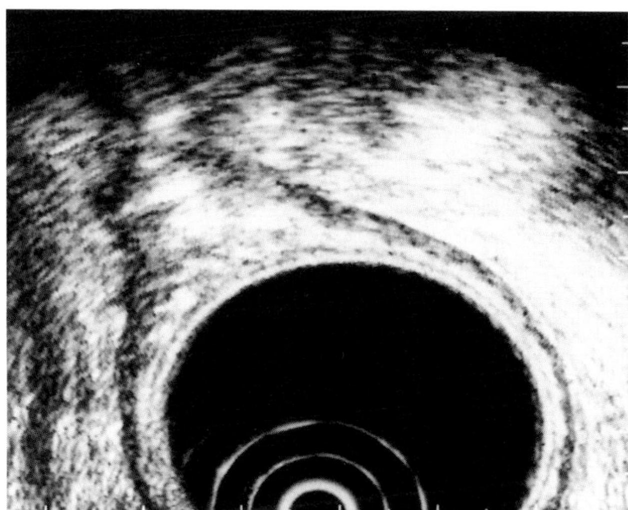

Fig. 27.23 Another submucosal lesion with no abnormality of the stomach mucosa. EUS demonstrates a compressible, hyperechoic submucosal lesion arising from the third layer consistent with a benign gastric lipoma.

biopsy channel samples can be taken from such lesions under direct ultrasound guidance. This technique allows small benign gastric tumours to be followed up without the need for more aggressive procedures such as partial gastrectomy.

Conclusion

EUS has been shown to be a safe and accurate technique in the investigation of a variety of upper gastrointestinal pathologies. It improves the local staging of carcinomas, and can provide useful information in the assessment of pathologies such as submucosal masses, pancreatic and biliary lesions. Although EUS is more accurate than other imaging modalities there are limitations to the technique such as differentiating inflammatory changes from tumour, assessing regional lymph nodes and its inability to assess distant/liver metastases. It is accurate in determining the depth of tumour invasion and therefore has the potential to be used in the TNM classification of cancer staging. With experience it can be a valuable technique for staging of oesophageal and gastric malignancies which can aid patient management. At present EUS is expensive as the only proven equipment is dedicated to its use. Hopefully the cost of EUS will fall; this is most likely to be achieved by the ability to interface endoscopic probes with existing ultrasonographic display units. In addition the technique is invasive and requires a combination of endoscopic and ultrasound skills which are seldom found in a single individual. Despite this the applications of the technique are diverse and will no doubt increase in the future as different types of scope and the ability to perform therapeutic procedures through scope channels widens. EUS is a valuable tool in pretreatment staging of many cancers, and with the development of new techniques of endoscopic resection or minimally invasive surgical techniques EUS may have a role in the assessment of many tumours. However, further studies are needed to show that the information obtained by the technique is cost-effective and will translate into changes in patient management and improved outcome.

References

1 Kimmey, M.B., Martin, R.W., Haggitt, R.C., *et al.* (1989) Histological correlates of gastrointestinal endoscopic ultrasound images. *Gastroenterology* **96**, 411.

2 Aibe, T., Fuji, T., Okita, K., Takemoto, K. (1986) A fundamental study of normal layer structure of the gastrointestinal wall visualised by endoscopic ultrasonography. *Scandinavian Journal of Gastroenterology* **21** (suppl. 123), 6–15.

3 Tio, T.L., Tygat, G.N.J. (1986) Endoscopic ultrasonography of normal and pathologic upper gastrointestinal wall structure. Comparison of studies *in vivo* and *in vivo* with histology. *Scandinavian Journal of Gastroenterology* **21** (suppl. 123), 6–15.

4 Caletti, G., Bolindi, L., Barbara, L. (1988) Instrumentation and scanning techniques. In: Kawai, K. (ed.) *Endoscopic Ultrasonography in Gastroenterology*. Igaku-shoin, New York, pp. 1–17.

5 Caletti, G.C., Bolondi, L., Lorena, Z., *et al.* (1986) Technique of endoscopic ultrasonography investigations: esophagus, stomach and duodenum. *Scandinavian Journal of Gastroenterology* **21** (suppl. 123), 1–5.

6 Lightdale, C.J. (1992) Normal endosonographic anatomy of the

esophagus and stomach. *Gastrointestinal Endoscopy* **38**(2), 193–194.
7 Ziegler, K., Sanft, C., Zeitz, M., *et al.* (1991) Evaluation of endosonography in TN staging of esophageal cancer. *Gut* **32**, 16–20.
8 Nousbaum, J.B., Robaszkiewicz, M., Cauvin, J.M., Calament, G., Gouerou, H. (1992) Endosonography can detect residual tumour infiltration after medical treatment of oesophageal cancer in the absence of endoscopic lesions. *Gut* **11**, 1459–1461.
9 Rice, T.W., Boyce, G.A., Sivak, M.V. (1991) Esophageal ultrasound and the preoperative staging of carcinoma of the esophagus. *Journal of Thoracic Cardiovascular Surgery* **101**, 536–544.
10 Tio, T.L., Schouwink, M.H., Cikot, R.J., *et al.* (1989) Preoperative TMN classification of gastric carcinoma by endoscopy in comparison with the pathological TNM system: a retrospective study. *Hepato-Gastroenterology* **36**, 51–56.
11 Vilgrain, V., Mompoint, D., Palazzo, L., *et al.* (1990) Staging of esophageal carcinoma: comparison of results with endoscopic sonography and CT. *American Journal of Roentgenology* **155**, 277–281.
12 Tio, T.L., Coene, P.P.L.O., Schouwink, M.H., *et al.* (1989) Esophagogastric carcinoma: preoperative TNM classification with endosonography. *Radiology* **173**, 11–17.
13 Grimm, H., Binmoeller, K.F., Hamper, K., *et al.* (1993) Endosonography for preoperative locoregional staging of oesophageal and gastric cancer. *Endoscopy* **25**(3), 224–230.
14 Dittler, H.J., Siewert, J.R. (1993) Role of endoscopic ultrasonography in oesophageal carcinoma. *Endoscopy* **2**, 156–161.
15 O'Reilly, S., Forestiere, A. (1994) New approaches to treating oesophageal cancer. *British Medical Journal* **308**, 1249–1250.
16 Rosch, T., Classen, M. (1991) Endoscopic ultrasonography. In: Cotton, P.B., Tygot, G.N.J., Williams, C.B. (eds) *Gastrointestinal Endoscopy*. London, Current Science, pp. 66–82.
17 Okai, T., Yamakawa, D., Matsuda, N., *et al.* (1991) Analysis of gastric carcinoma growth by endoscopic ultrasonography *Endoscopy* **23**, 121–125.
18 Dittler, H.J., Siewert, J.R. (1993) Role of endoscopic ultrasonography in gastric carcinoma. *Endoscopy* **25**, 162–166.
19 Fujishima, H., Misawa, T., Chijiwa, Y., *et al.* (1991) Scirrhous carcinoma of the stomach versus hypertrophic gastritis: findings at endoscopic US. *Radiology* **181**, 197–200.
20 Rosch, T., Lorenz, R., Braig, C., *et al.* (1991) Endoscopic ultrasound in pancreatic tumour diagnosis. *Gastrointestinal Endoscopy* **3**, 347–352.
21 Grimm, H., Mayedo, A., Soehendra, N. (1990) Endoluminal ultrasound for the diagnosis and staging of pancreatic cancer. *Baillière's Clinical Gastroenterology* **4**, 869–888.
22 Palazzo, L., Roseau, G., Gayet, B., *et al.* (1993) Endoscopic ultrasonography in the diagnosis and staging of pancreatic adenocarcinoma. *Endoscopy* **25**, 143–150.
23 Rosch, T., Lorenz, R., Braig, C., *et al.* (1991) Endoscopic ultrasound in pancreatic tumour diagnosis. *Gastrointestinal Endoscopy* **37**, 345–352.
24 Yamanda, M., Komoto, E., Naito, Y., Tsukamoto, Y., Mitake, M. (1991) Endoscopic ultrasonography in the diagnosis of pancreatic islet cell tumours. *Journal of Ultrasound Medicine* **10**, 271–276.
25 Glover, J.R., Shorvon, P.J., Lees, W.R. (1992) Endoscopic ultrasound for localisation of islet cell tumours. *Gut* **1**, 108–110.
26 Tio, T., Cheung, J., Wijers, O., Sars, P., Tygat, G. (1991) Endosonographic TNM staging of extra hepatic bile duct cancer. *Gastroenterology* **100**, 1351–1361.
27 Lightdale, C., Botet, J., Kelsen, D., Turnbull, A., Brennan, M. (1989) Diagnosis of recurrent upper gastrointestinal cancer at surgical anastomosis by endoscopic ultrasound. *Gastrointestinal Endoscopy* **35**, 407–412.
28 Akahoshi, K., Misawa, T., Fujishima, H., *et al.* (1991) Preoperative evaluation of gastric cancer by endoscopic ultrasound. *Gut* **32**, 479–482.
29 Botet, J., Lightdale, C., Zauber, A., *et al.* (1991) Preoperative staging of gastric cancer: comparison of endoscopic US and dynamic CT. *Radiology* **181**, 426–432.
30 Boyce, G.A., Sivac, M.V., Rosch, T., *et al.* (1991) Evaluation of submucosal upper gastrointestinal tract lesions by endoscopic ultrasound. *Gastrointestinal Endoscopy* **37**, 449–454.
31 Caletti, G., Ferrari, A., Brocchi, E., *et al.* (1993) Accuracy of endoscopic ultrasonography in the diagnosis and staging of gastric cancer and lymphoma. *Surgery* **113**, 14–27.
32 Caletti, G.C., Zani, L., Bolondi, L., *et al.* (1989) Endoscopic ultrasonography in the diagnosis of gastric submucosal tumour. *Gastrointestinal Endoscopy* **35**, 413–418.
33 Yasuda, K., Nakajima, M., Yoshida, S., *et al.* (1989) The diagnosis of submucosal tumours of the stomach by endoscopic ultrasonography. *Gastrointestinal Endoscopy* **3**, 10–15.
34 Tio, T.L., Tygatt, G.N.J., Den Hartog Jager, F.C.A. (1990) Endoscopic ultrasonography for the evaluation of smooth muscle tumours in the upper gastrointestinal tract; an experience with 42 cases. *Gastrointestinal Endoscopy* **36**, 342–350.
35 Caletti, G.C., Brocchi, E., Ferrari, A., *et al.* (1991) Guillotine needle biopsy as a supplement to endosonography on the diagnosis of gastric submucosal tumours. *Endoscopy* **23**, 251–254.

Chapter 28: Endoluminal ultrasound of the lower gastrointestinal tract

C.I. Bartram

Intraluminal endosonography of the gastrointestinal tract was performed first by Wild and Reid [1] in the mid-1950s. Rectal endosonography (RES) for cancer staging did not become a practical reality until the 1980s, when transducers with sufficient resolution to identify the bowel wall layers became available. Endosonography of the anal canal (AES), where the water-filled balloon system for rectal examination is replaced by a hard cone [2], is a more recent development that has proved valuable in the investigation of sphincter disorders.

RES

Tumour staging, which has been the main application for RES, requires high anatomical resolution to relate the depth of tumour penetration to bowel wall layer. The initial experience was with 5 MHz transducers [3], but the value of higher frequency probes of 7 MHz or greater was soon recognized [4,5]. Unfortunately, in spite of good results, the general impact of RES on clinical management has been limited, and it has not become a routine procedure prior to rectal cancer surgery. To quote one authority [6], RES 'remains the preserve of a minority of enthusiasts'. Lack of available expertise may have prevented more widespread acceptance of the technique, which does has specific indications in rectal disease, and should be available as part of the range of imaging techniques required by modern coloproctology.

Technique

Most rigid rectal probes are designed for prostatic examination, and have a water-filled balloon system for acoustic coupling. Only B & K Medical [7], Kretz-technik and Aloka [8] have probes designed specifically for rectal examination. B & K Medical has a mechanically rotated 7 or 10 MHz transducer mounted on a probe 24 cm in length, which may be inserted through a short 20 cm sigmoidoscope (Fig. 28.1) to allow examination of lesions higher than 12 cm in the rectum, i.e. above the main rectal fold. Aloka also manufacture a 7.5 MHz mechanically rotating probe, which is shorter. Both give a 360° radial cross-sectional image. The Kretz-technik probe is 22 mm in diameter, may be inserted through a sigmoidoscope, and gives a radial 355° image. There is a wide selection of sector, longitudinal or endfire linear arrays, which although designed for prostatic examination may also be used for rectal wall studies. Endoscopic ultrasound systems are ideal for rectal scanning, as lesions at any level may be imaged.

Prior to examination the rectum must be cleared of faecal residue, by giving either full bowel preparation or a disposable enema. Patients are usually examined in the left lateral position. The balloon system should be cleared of any air bubble, deflated and inserted either through a sigmoidoscope or directly into the rectum. It is important to remember the posterior angulation of the distal rectum when inserting the instrument, and never to apply force when introducing a rigid probe.

The balloon should be slowly distended with about 50 ml of water, until there is good contact with the rectal wall. Greater distension may be required in the distal ampulla. If the sigmoidoscope has been used to insert the transducer high into the rectum, both will have to be pulled down together as the rectum is scanned, and the sigmoidoscope reinserted if the upper rectum has to be viewed again. With rotating endoprobes it is important to keep the probe at right angles to the rectal wall. Angled views of a lesion may give a false impression of its depth.

Anatomy

The rectal wall is described as a five-layered structure, with three hyperechoic and two intervening hypoechoic layers (Fig. 28.2). The sonographic appearance is a complex of reflections from tissue layers and interfaces between layers of differing acoustic impedance.

The first echogenic layer is an interface between water (and balloon) and superficial mucosa. Beneath this the relatively echo-poor deep mucosa (lamina propria) forms the second layer, which is hypoechoic. The mucosaris

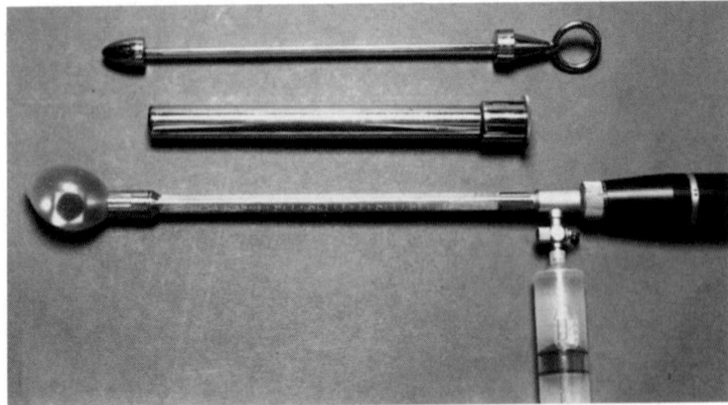

Fig. 28.1 The B & K Medical 1850 endoprobe with water-filled balloon system and short rectoscope.

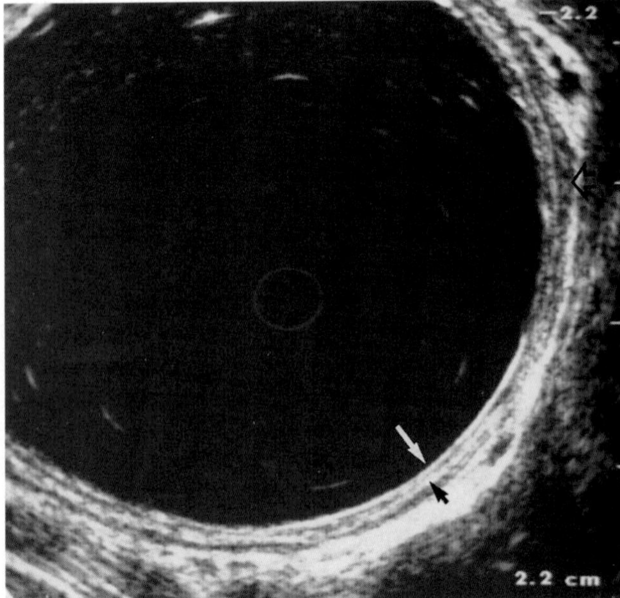

Fig. 28.2 Normal rectal wall anatomy. Bright interface reflection from inner mucosal surface (white arrow), and broad echogenic submucosa (black arrowhead) with outer adventitial reflection seen. Note the two intervening hypoechoic layers of the deep mucosa and muscularis propria. The latter is divided into an inner circular and outer longitudinal layer in part of the wall (open arrowhead). Some small perirectal veins are visible.

mucosae was considered to be part of this layer, but recent work [9] has indicated that there is a sufficient difference in acoustic impedance for an interface to be present between the lamina propria and the muscularis mucosae. As the muscularis is <0.1 mm thick, the interface reflection would be thicker than the tissue layer. This interface is not seen normally as it is lost within the next echogenic layer of the submucosa (Fig. 28.3). There is a further interface with the muscularis propria on the other side of the submucosa. This reflection will extend down into the muscularis, which is hypoechoic. The effect of these interface reflections is that the third echogenic layer contains two interfaces, and that the outer interface with the muscularis propria will make the layer appear thicker sonographically than it is histologically. The thickness of the interface reflection depends on the axial resolution of the transducer, which is typically about 0.25 mm [10]. The fourth layer (second outer hypoechoic layer) is hypoechoic and represents the muscularis propria, minus the interface reflection. The fifth layer is hyperechoic, and is due to an interface and the adventitial border. With high definition probes [11] (7.5 MHz linear or 12 MHz rotating), the muscle layer may be seen to be divided in two by a thin fascial reflection, separating the inner circular from the outer longitudinal muscle coat. The bowel wall then becomes a seven layer structure. These layers are summarized in Table 28.1.

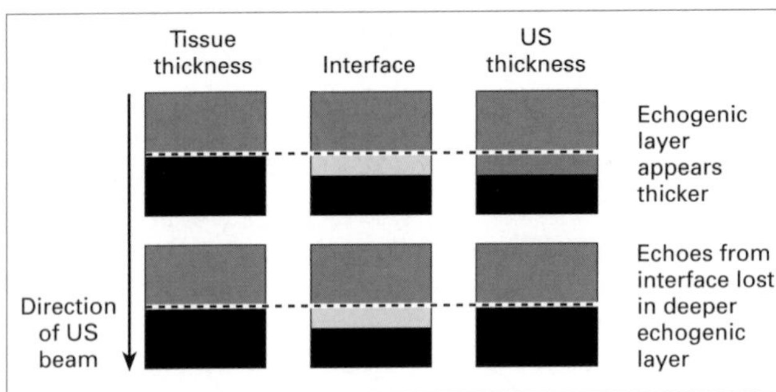

Fig. 28.3 Diagram to show the effect of an interface reflection on the apparent depth of the layer.

Table 28.1 Endosonography of the rectal wall

Acoustic layer	Histological layer	Interface	Echogenicity of layer
1	Water/mucosa	+	↑
2	Mucosa (lamina propria)	–	↓
3	Submucosa	+	↑
		+	
4	Muscularis propria	–	↓
5	Adventitia	+	↑

The perirectal fat is hyperechoic with a slightly heterogenous texture. The normal mesorectum contains eight to 20 lymph nodes about 3 mm in size. These are considered to be isoechoic with the perirectal fat and not seen routinely. The superior rectal artery divides at S3 into two branches passing down either side of the rectum. Branches of the middle and inferior rectal arteries are not usually visible. The venous plexus is very variable. Small veins running away from the rectal wall almost at right angles will be seen coursing in and out of view.

In the male the bladder, seminal vesicles, prostate, urethra and bulbourethral glands are anterior. The recto-vesical fascia of Denonvilliers separates the rectum from the prostate. In females the vagina, rectovaginal septum, urethra and Bartholin's glands are the main anterior relationships. The uterus, and sometimes the ovaries may be seen. Depending on how far the probe has been inserted and the depth of the pouch of Douglas, bowel loops may be present anterolaterally to the rectum.

Artefacts are common. Gas bubbles within the rectal balloon creat acoustic shadows. Solid faeces smeared on the balloon cast a broad acoustic shadow obscuring the rectal wall. Liquid faeces cause a more heterogeneous reflection between the balloon and rectal wall. Other artefacts include mirror image reflections from the balloon, which may produce very confusing pictures creating pseudomasses [12].

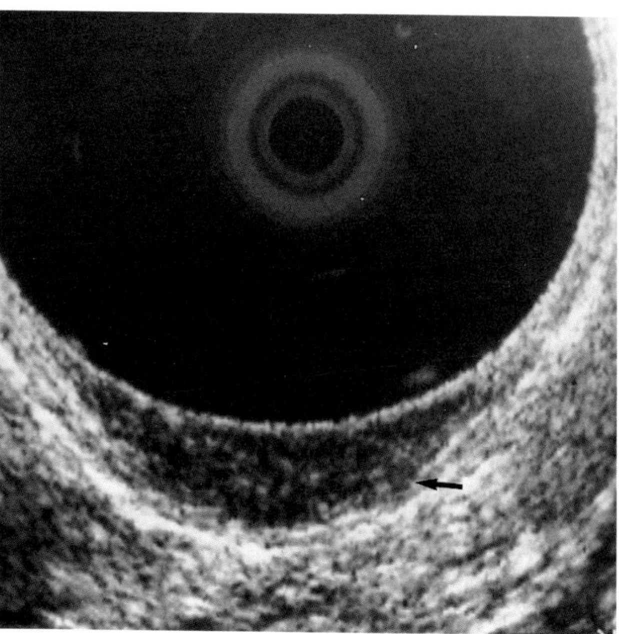

Fig. 28.4 T1 carcinoma. Small hypoechoic polypoid lesion is pressed into the bowel wall. The white line of the submucosa is mostly intact, but is breached in part (arrow) indicating invasion.

Staging of rectal cancer

The Dukes' classification [13] is based on detailed pathological examination of surgical specimens, and highlights two prognostic factors, depth of invasion and lymph node involvement. Depth of invasion is divided simply into tumours limited to the bowel wall (Dukes' A) and those that have spread into the perirectal fat (Dukes' B). Any lymph node involvement is defined as Dukes' C, irrespective of the depth of invasion.

The TNM [14] classification categorizes each component of tumour spread: depth of infiltration (T), lymph node involvement (N) and metastasis (M) separately. The T staging relates tumour infiltration to bowel wall layer. To signify that a tumour has been staged with endosonography, and not pathologically, a 'u' prefix has been suggested [15].

T STAGING

T1: the tumour has invaded the submucosa (Fig. 28.4). In the oesophagus and stomach, invasion of the lamina propria would define a cancer. In the colorectum the lymphatics are not thought to extend into the lamina propria, hence a lesion is not defined as a cancer until cells have penetrated the submucosa, and so have the potential for lymphatic spread. Cancer *in situ* is not an accepted term for colorectal tumours.

T2: the muscularis propria is involved, but tumour invasion is limited to this and the outer edge remains intact (Fig. 28.5).

T3: the tumour has penetrated through the rectal wall. In the early stages small pseudopodia of tumour extend into perirectal fat (Figs 28.6, 28.7). With more extensive spread bulky perirectal growth becomes obvious.

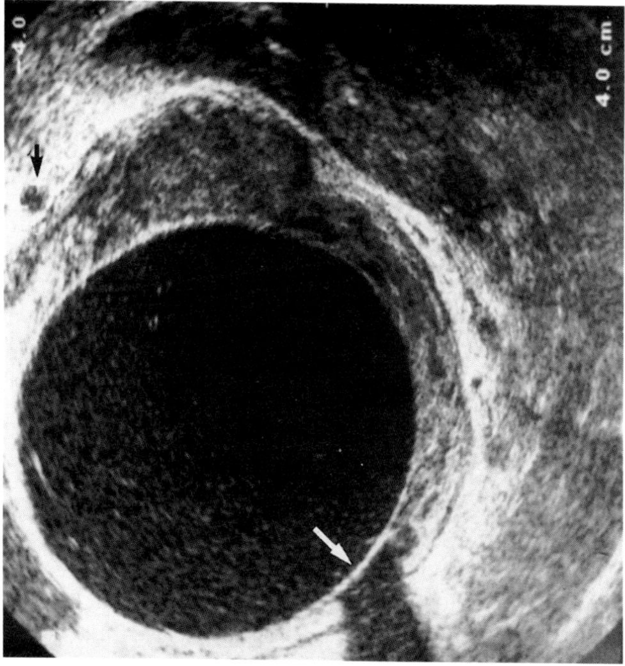

Fig. 28.5 T2 carcinoma. The muscularis propria is involved but the outer margin remains clearly defined. Note a small involved node (black arrow), preservation of the fascial plane to the prostate, and acoustic shadow (white arrow) from a pocket of gas outside the balloon.

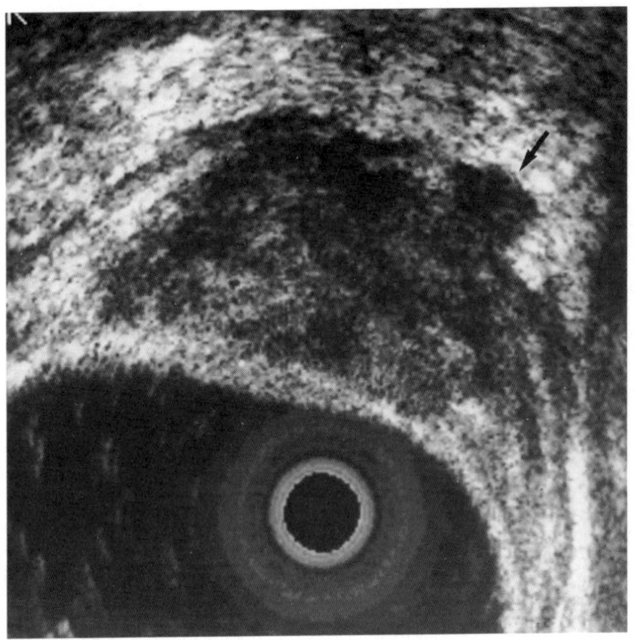

Fig. 28.6 T3 tumour. The lesion has clearly breached the muscularis propria with tumour growth into the perirectal fat (arrow).

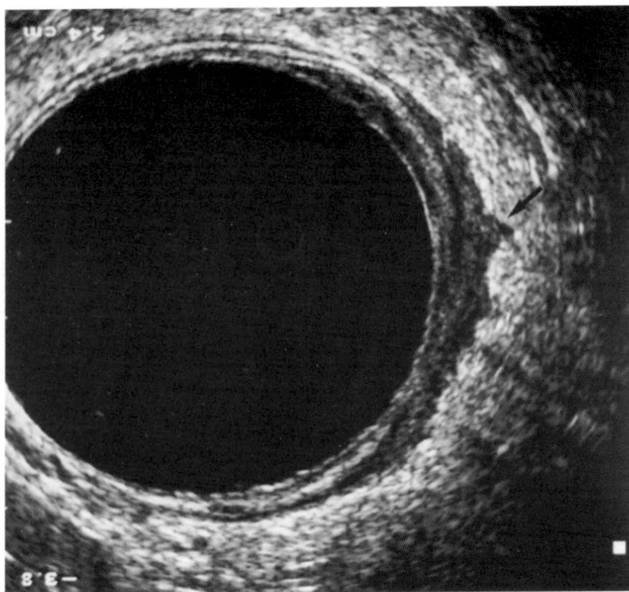

Fig. 28.7 T3 tumour. Small pseudopodia of tumour growth are seen extending outside the muscularis propria (arrow).

T4: invasion of surrounding structures, such as the vagina or prostate.

N STAGING

N0: no regional lymph node metastasis.
N1: one to three mesorectal lymph nodes involved.
N2: four or more nodes involved.

M STAGING

Metastatic involvement to liver, lung or bone.

Endosonography and TNM staging

The accuracy of sonographic T staging for tumour penetration is 81–93% [16]. There is a greater tendency to overstage (10.2%, 8.3%) rather than understage (0.8%, 5.3%) [17,18]. Technique is important, and a learning curve must be overcome. However, once mastered the main reason for understaging is minimal histological penetration. Tumour cell budding, with small peg-like projections into the perirectal fat, is the initial histological change in a T3 lesion. Minor tumour budding is below sonographic resolution. Conversely, overstaging is more common. This is due to an inflammatory cellular infiltrate associated creating a hypoechoic zone around the tumour. A recent paper suggests that this inflammatory zone is of lower echogenicity than tumour, and can be recognized sonographically. Once this is taken into account staging accuracy increases dramatically as T2 tumours are no longer overstaged as T3 [19].

Another cause for incorrect staging is failure to view the lesion at right angles to the wall. The balloon may be of relatively low compliance, but when distended with water will push any polypoid lesion into the wall (Fig. 28.8). With axial imaging, if the lesion is sectioned at an angle to the wall, geometric distortion may give an incorrect impression of the depth of penetration (Fig. 28.9). Lesions low in the rectal ampulla are difficult to view in the correct plane with rotating probes in a transverse section. In one series [17] 16.7% of tumours in the lower rectum were staged incorrectly, compared to only 6.3% in the mid and upper rectum. Linear probes do not have this disadvantage, as although the lesion may be acutely angled sagittally, it may be viewed perpendicular to the wall in the transverse plane. If it is not possible to traverse a stenotic lesion, a radial transducer will give an incomplete view. Forward viewing transducers may then be preferable to demonstrate the outer limits of the tumour.

The maximum thickness of the tumour should be recorded, as this indicates the extent of perirectal infiltration which is relevant to local recurrence. A good correlation between the sonographic and histological thickness has been demonstrated, again providing the tumour is viewed at right angles. With perirectal extension (T3) it is most important to exclude infiltration of adjacent structures (T4) such as the prostate or vagina. Supplementing endorectal with endovaginal scanning may help confirm

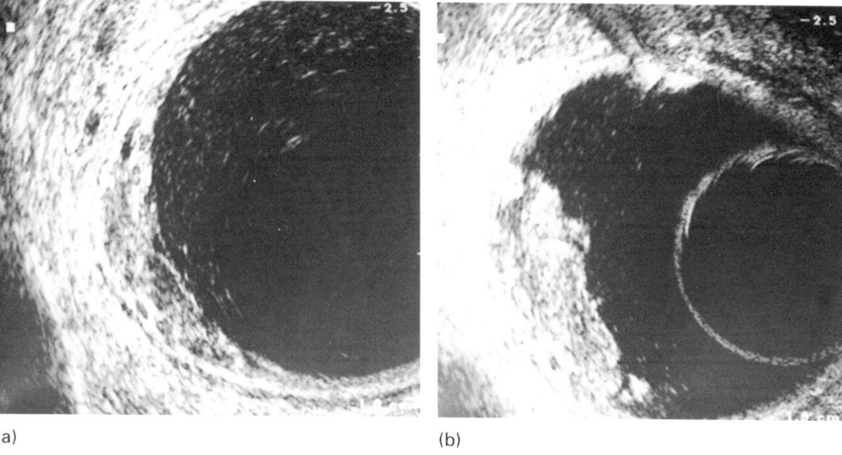

Fig. 28.8 Benign villous adenoma. (a) The balloon is intact, and has deformed the polyp, pressing it into the wall. (b) The balloon had burst and the rectum filled with water. The rectum is now circular, and the exophytic nature of the polyp visible.

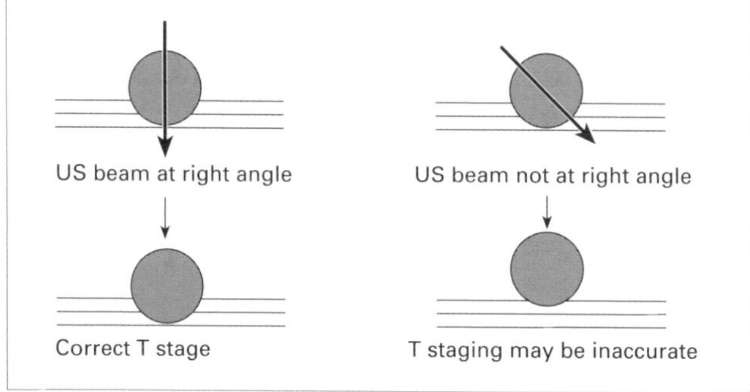

Fig. 28.9 Diagram to show that staging may be inaccurate if the lesion is not interrogated with the beam at right angles to the wall.

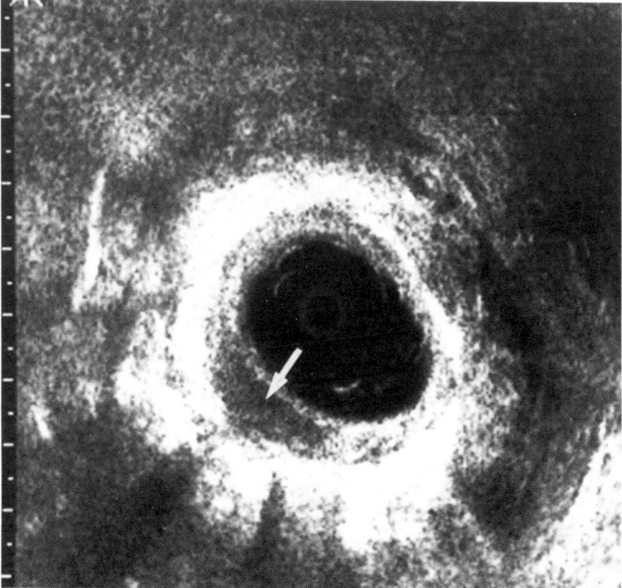

Fig. 28.10 Radiotherapy changes. The tumour is still visible (arrow), but the wall poorly defined and indistinct from the rather echogenic perirectal fat.

rectovaginal septal involvement. Radiotherapy complicates sonographic staging as oedema and fibrosis obliterate normal tissue planes (Fig. 28.10), and the tumour becomes less clearly demarcated. Reductions in staging accuracy from 86 to 47% [20], and from 63 to 53% [21] have been reported, so that endosonographic T staging after radiotherapy is not recommended.

Local recurrence

The incidence of local recurrence for rectal cancer is 5–20% after restorative anterior resection. This is due to inadequate clearance of tumour from the mesorectum. Tumour implantation at the anastomosis is rare. Sonographically the site of anastomosis is seen as a localized thickening of the muscularis and submucosal layers. Staples cause multiple short bright reflections. Recurrent cancer, as with primary disease, is hypoechoic. Any hypoechoic mass in the perirectal tissues or at the anastomosis must be considered a possible recurrence. The main differential diagnosis is a stitch line granuloma. These are situated at the anastomosis, usually visible sigmoidoscopically and present early in the postoperative period. Any lesion with an intraluminal component may be biopsied endoscopically. Extramucosal or perirectal lesions may also be biopsied under ultrasound guidance.

Alternatively, a suspicious lesion may be followed up with repeated scanning. Any increase in size indicates a recurrence. Early diagnosis with biopsy is advisable, as recurrent cancers are operable only in the early stages. Following resection for rectal carcinoma in 120 patients [22], 17 recurrences were detected by RES. Six were asymptomatic and surgery was possible in each, but in the 11 with symptomatic recurrence surgery was possible in only two. RES would seem a worthwhile part of follow-up, though it should be noted that there is a study where computed tomography (CT) was more accurate than RES in detecting recurrence [23].

Lymph node involvement

Lymph node involvement places a patient in Dukes' C category, and is associated with a significant reduction in 5-year survival.

Most studies have reported a 73–86% accuracy for detecting lymph node involvement (N1+). Often the only criterion used was that the node was visible on endosonography. Size [24] and echogenicity [25] are important factors. Involved nodes tend to be large and hypoechoic relative to perirectal fat. Reactive nodes may also be slightly enlarged, but relatively hyperechoic (Fig. 28.11). *In vitro* correlation [26] suggested that all nodes with a short axis of >9 mm were malignant, as were nodes with marked inhomogeneity or hypoechogenicity. Nodes exhibiting a hilar reflection were benign, but this sign is difficult to detect *in vivo*. Altogether no clear differentiation was possible in about 60% of the nodes examined. Nodes that are >7 mm in diameter, round not oval, and homogeneous rather than heterogeneous are more likely to be malignant than benign, although the positive predictive value of these criteria is only 55% [27].

Nodes are usually easy to distinguish from veins, which can be traced branching out from the rectal wall. Sometimes this is difficult and Doppler is then useful to differentiate vessel from node [28]. Following radiotherapy, lymph node (N) staging does not seem to be affected as much as staging of the primary tumour (T).

One of the main problems in node detection is the limited field examined by rigid probes. Beynon *et al.* [7] estimate that only about 40% of the nodes in the average resected specimen would have been viewed at endosonography. Node assessment remains unsatisfactory. If hypoechoic nodes are seen, lymph node involvement is likely, but if no node is detected it should not be assumed that the nodes are clear.

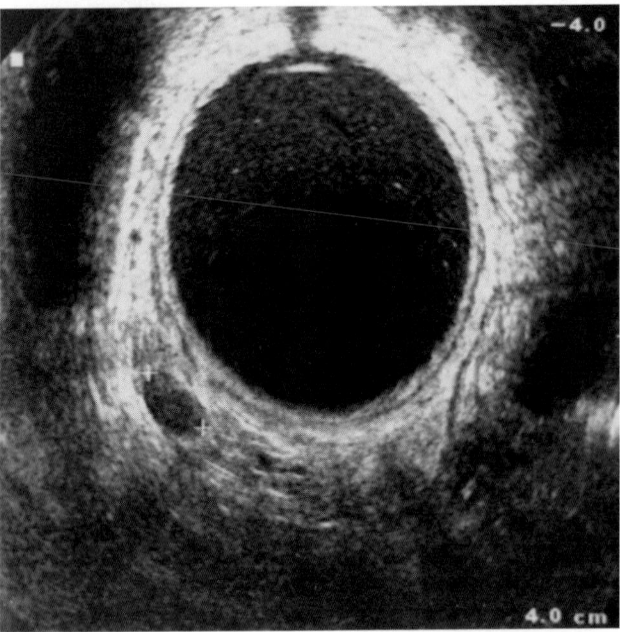

Fig. 28.11 Reactive lymph node measuring 9 mm. Note the small acoustic shadow from a gas bubble in the balloon.

RES compared to CT

Most of the literature suggests that RES is more accurate than digital [29] or CT [30] for staging rectal cancer, although with the latter it is possible that optimum techniques in each field have not been compared. CT is better at demonstrating the extent of a bulky tumour, and for showing iliac node involvement. RES has clear superiority in demonstrating early tumour infiltration of the bowel wall, and for demonstrating small mesorectal nodes. Continued development in transducer technology and the use of higher frequency transducers will improve definition, but how this will match other modalities, notably magnetic resonography with an endocoil remains to be evaluated.

The role of RES

In a review of the literature Solomon and McLeod [31] concluded that RES was reasonably accurate for determining tumour penetration ($\kappa = 0.85$), but only moderately so for lymph node involvement ($\kappa = 0.58$). The criterion for any radiological examination must be that it will alter clinical management. Most patients with rectal cancer undergo resection irrespective of any RES finding. The situations in which RES may affect management are as follows.

1 Small rectal cancers (<3 cm) that are clinically mobile and well differentiated are eligible for local excision. RES should be performed to assess such lesions. The absence of penetration of the muscularis propria (T2 stage) and nodal involvement provide supportive evidence that the tumour has not spread, and is suitable for local resection.

2 Malignant change in a villous adenoma may be difficult to detect clinically. RES is indicated prior to local excision to exclude unsuspected invasion of the wall.

3 Large tumours may seem fixed clinically just from inflammatory changes. RES will confirm invasion of local structures (T4 lesion). Should ablation with laser therapy be considered, it is important to know if the tumour is particularly thin at any one point, or closely related to the bladder.

4 RES is recommended in follow-up, particularly if the primary tumour was high grade and close to the resection margins.

5 RES may be used to examine a pararectal mass. Although a precise diagnosis may not be possible purely on the sonographic appearances, directed biopsy may be performed for histological confirmation.

AES

Anal endosonography may be technically simpler to perform than RES, but the anatomy is more complex to interpret. Balloon systems with rotating transducers are inappropriate within the anal canal, and must be replaced by a hard cone with parallel walls to avoid anatomical distortion (Fig. 28.12). Most work in this field has been performed with the B & K Medical 1850 rectal endoprobe (Sandtoften 9, Gentofote, Denmark), using either a 7 or more recently a 10 MHz transducer and a hard plastic cone of outer diameter 1.7 cm [32]. This gives a complete 360° cross-sectional image, that is ideal for assessing circular structures such as the sphincters. The bifocal multiplane rectal Kretz-technik (Zipf, Austria) transducer [33] is an alternative that gives a 355° cross-sectional image.

No patient preparation is required. The cone may be covered with a condom, and gelled on both sides for acoustic contact and lubrication. It may be more convenient to examine patients in the left lateral position, but females should be examined prone as the anterior perineal structures are more symmetric in this position [34]. The probe should be orientated so that anterior is uppermost at 12 o'clock on the screen. The axis of the probe should be kept in line with that of the anal canal to minimize distortion of the cross-sectional image of the sphincters (Fig. 28.13).

Normal anatomy

The anus has a basic four layer pattern. As the layers are thicker, there is less dependence on interface reflections than in the rectal wall.

The mucosa is lost within a major echo from an interface reflection from the outside of the cone. The subepithelial space does not have a complete muscularis mucosae, so that the term 'submucosa' is not used. The subepithelial tissues contain venous channels and extensive smooth muscle with an elastic component, derived from the longitudinal muscle, and are moderately echogenic. Vaginal endosonography [35] has shown that the undisturbed internal sphincter has an inner diameter of 6–8 mm (Fig. 28.14). The canal is sealed by the subepithelial tissues, par-

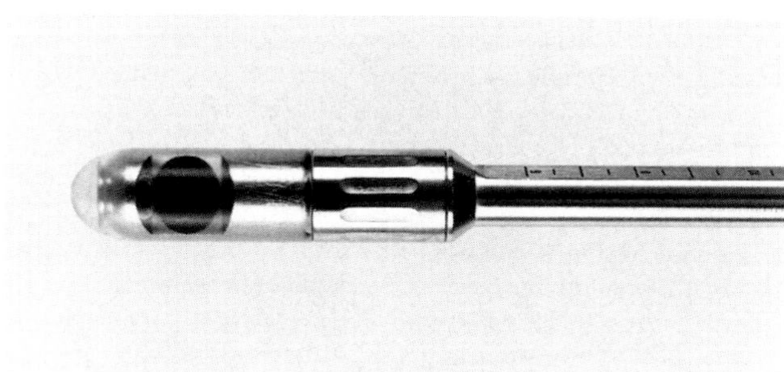

Fig. 28.12 The B & K Medical 1850 endoprobe with plastic cone 1.7 cm in outer diameter, filled with degassed water, for AES.

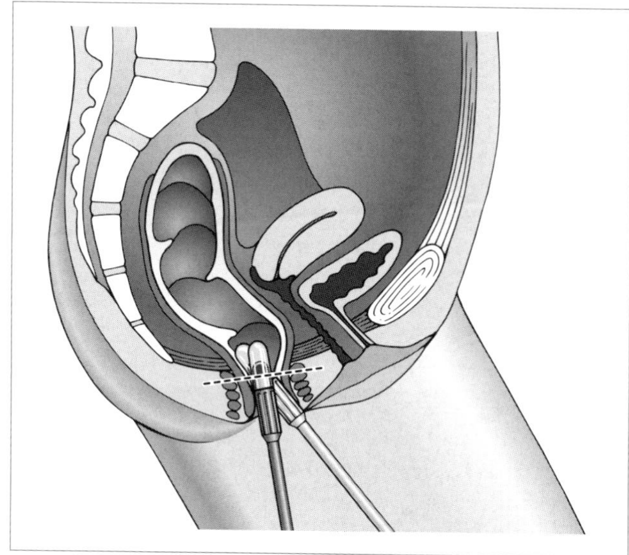

Fig. 28.13 Sagittal section of the pelvis to emphasize the importance of keeping the probe in the same axis as the canal in order to maintain an undistorted view of the sphincter anatomy.

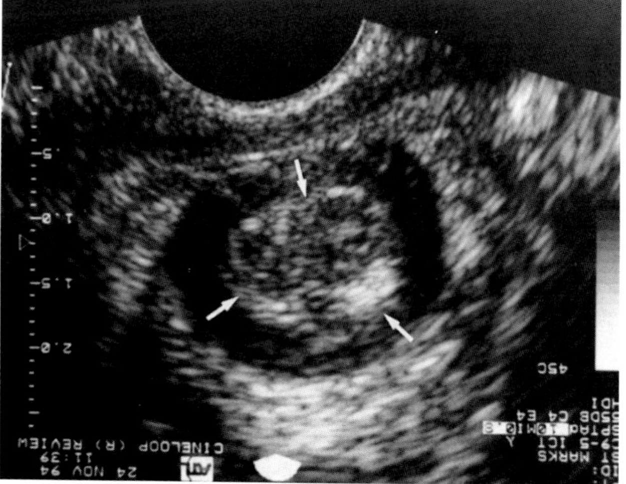

Fig. 28.14 View of the internal sphincter from the vagina. The inner diameter of the sphincter is about 10 mm. The internal sphincter appears thicker than at AES as it is not stretched by the probe. The anal cushions that seal off the canal are just visible (arrows).

ticularly by the anal cushions, which are three specialized enlargements in the proximal canal.

The internal sphincter is a condensation of the circular muscle of the rectum and is in continuity with this. It terminates at the lower border of the superficial external sphincter. It is about 2 mm thick, symmetric and hypoechoic. The longitudinal muscle surrounds the internal sphincter. This is an extension of the longitudinal muscle of the rectum, with some striated muscle from the levators and a major fibroelastic component derived from the pelvic floor fascia. It pierces the subcutaneous external sphincter to insert into the perianal skin, but also extends into the ischioanal fossae, perineum and subepithelial space. The longitudinal muscle is of intermediate echogenicity. Small hypoechoic bundles of smooth muscle may be seen within this layer. In males the longitudinal muscle becomes very echogenic at the level of the superficial external sphincter. Interface reflections may be visible between the longitudinal muscle and external sphincter, and demarcate the site of the intersphincteric plane.

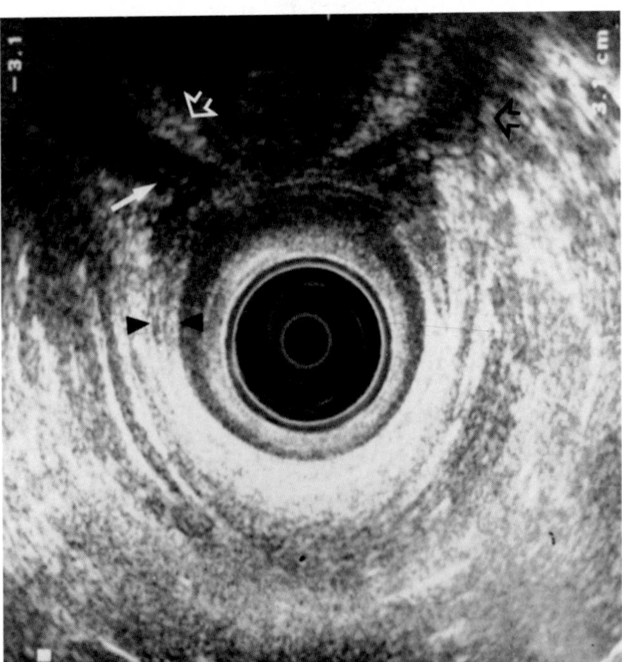

Fig. 28.15 High canal level in a female patient. The image is normally orientated with anterior uppermost. The puborectalis (black open arrowhead) is seen extending anteriorly to the pubic symphysis, and with the deep external sphincter forms a striated U-shaped sling around the canal. The longitudinal muscle is visible as a separate structure (black arrowheads) just outside the hypoechoic ring of the internal sphincter. Anteriorly the curve of the bulbospongiosus is visible (white open arrowhead). The triangular hypoechoic segment just posterior to this is the superficial transverse perineii muscle (white arrow).

The external sphincter is composed of striated muscle, and is a complex structure divided into three parts [36]. The deep layer is continuous with the puborectalis sling (Fig. 28.15). Although circular, its anterior aspect is not clearly defined sonographically in the female, as it is lost within amorphous reflections from the perineal body. The superficial external sphincter is elliptical, arising posteriorly from the sides of the anococcygeal ligament and decussating anteriorly within the perineal body (Fig. 28.16). The subcutaneous part lies below the level of the internal sphincter (Fig. 28.17) and is either conical in outline, pointing posteriorly to the anococcygeal ligament, or annular.

The acoustic texture of the external sphincter changes at different levels. The deep part is typical of striated muscle throughout the body, with a fine striated texture due to reflections from the supporting fascial stroma, and is indistinguishable from the puborectalis. The superficial

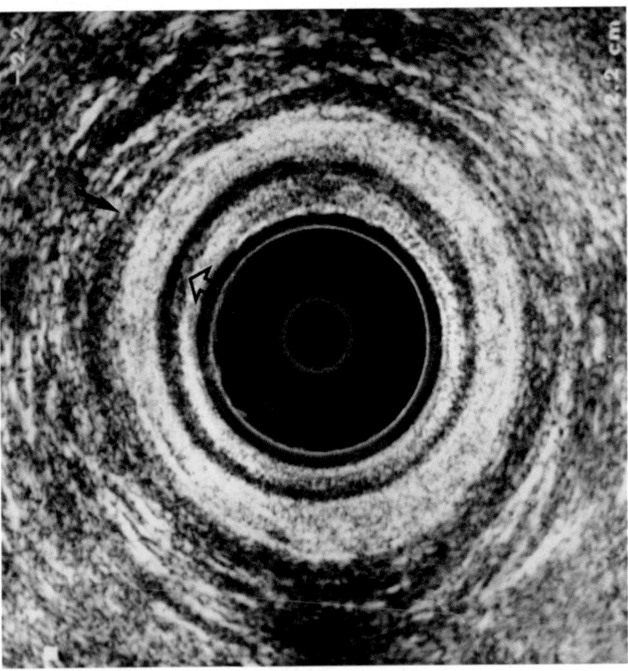

Fig. 28.16 Mid canal level in a male at a higher level of magnification. The internal sphincter is seen as a well-defined thin symmetric hypoechoic ring (arrowhead). Deep to this is the relatively hyperechoic subepithelium. Anteriorly at 12 o'clock there is a small hypoechoic space within the subepithelium representing a normal vascular channel. The cone creates two inner bright reflections. Outside the internal sphincter, is the broad hyperechoic layer of the longitudinal muscle. Outside this is the external sphincter (arrow), which is typically relatively hypoechoic in males at this level. Posteriorly the ill-defined shadow from the anococcygeal ligament is just visible. Posterolaterally around the external sphincter are ill-defined reflections from fat and fascia in the ischioanal fossae.

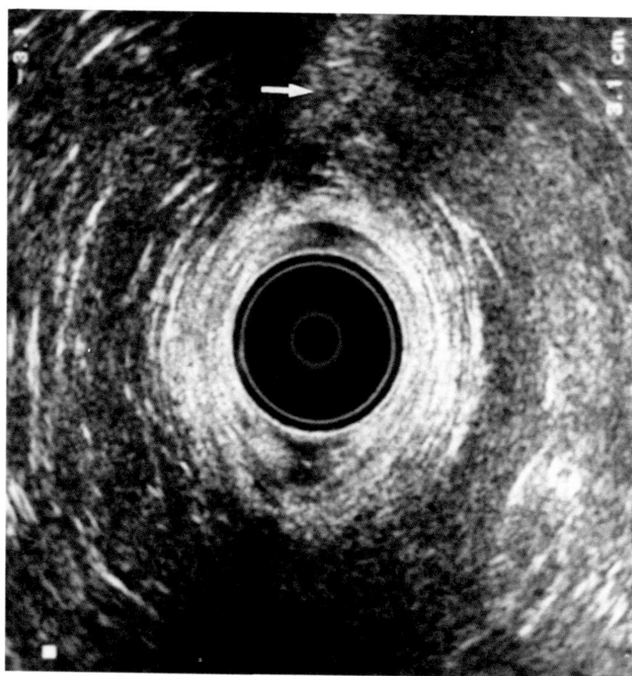

Fig. 28.17 Low canal level. This is below the termination of the internal sphincter. Note the striated texture of the subcutaneous part of the external sphincter which is penetrated by the longitudinal muscle as it sends fascial extensions into the perianal skin. Anteriorly a fascial extension (arrow) into the central point of the perineum is seen in a male.

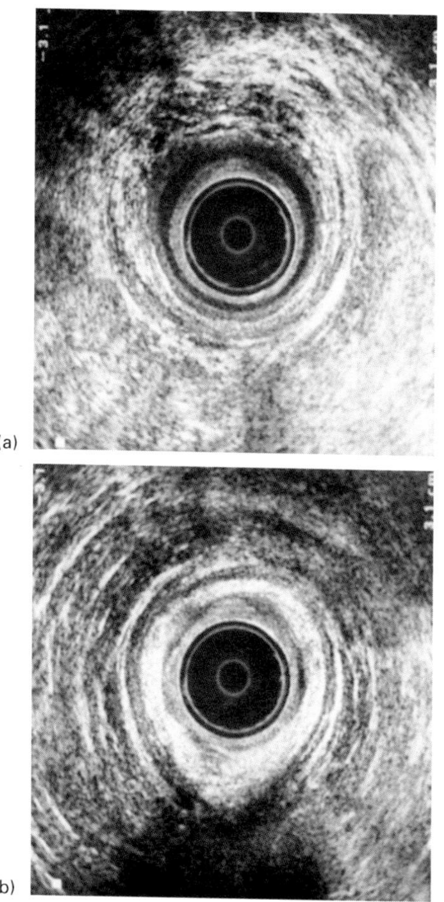

Fig. 28.18 (a) High and (b) mid canal levels in a male patient. Note the almost complete symmetry of the external sphincter and longitudinal muscle anterior at a high level.

part in males is hypoechoic without striation. In females the lower aspect of this part of the external sphincter may be similar, but the upper part tends to be striated. The subcutaneous part is sometimes echogenic, but often shows a striated pattern. The lower part of the superficial sphincter may overlap the subcutaneous component, forming an outer hypoechoic ring around the echogenic subcutaneous sphincter, below the level of the internal sphincter.

There is a gender difference in the external sphincter layout. In males the longitudinal muscle and the three divisions of the external sphincter are roughly symmetric, so that the sagittal and coronal arrangements are similar (Fig. 28.18). This is not so in females, where sonographically there seems to be a large defect anteriorly in the upper canal (Fig. 28.19). The external sphincter is shorter anteriorly than posteriorly. The deep and superficial fibres slope downwards as they run forwards to join the subcutaneous part to form a well-defined anterior muscle ring lower in the canal. Axial imaging in the upper canal gives the appearance of a defect, but as the probe is withdrawn down the canal, the sloping side walls of external sphincter can be seen coming together anteriorly to form an intact muscle ring.

Structures that may be recognized within the perineum are the bulbospongiosus around the vagina or base of the penis. The bulbospongiosus fuses with the superficial external sphincter. The superficial transverse perineii insert at this level from each side. Bartholin's glands in females and the bulbourethral glands in males are paired lobulated posterolateral to the bulbospongiosus, but are not visible unless abnormal. A reflection from the inner surface of the pubic bones may be seen anteriorly, with the ischiocavernous muscles visible on the side wall of the pelvis (Fig. 28.20). The fat in the ischioanal fossae has an irregular coarse texture with some striations. The striated pattern of the levators may be seen posterolaterally in some patients.

Internal sphincter

The sphincter becomes slightly thicker in old age. The exact ranges have yet to be established, but is probably

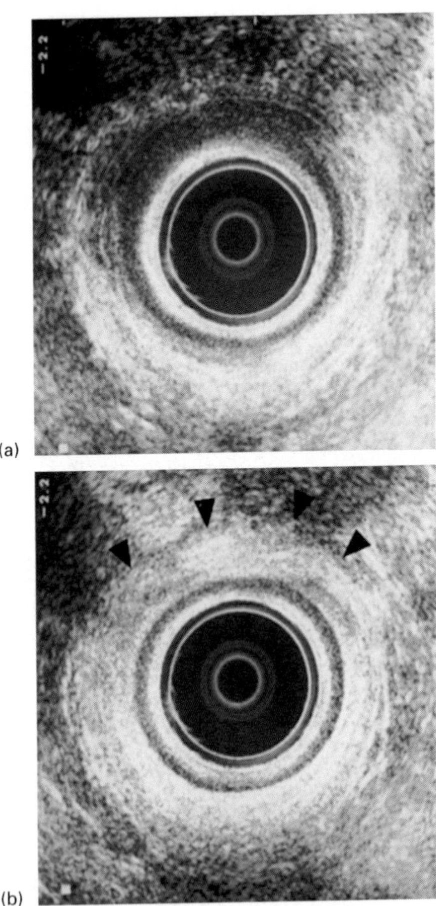

Fig. 28.19 High and mid canal levels in a female. (a) The high level is at the deep/superficial external sphincter level. Anteriorly the external sphincter is not defined, and appears cut off at between 10 and 2 o'clock. (b) As the probe is withdrawn slightly the intact anterior muscle ring (arrowheads) comes into view.

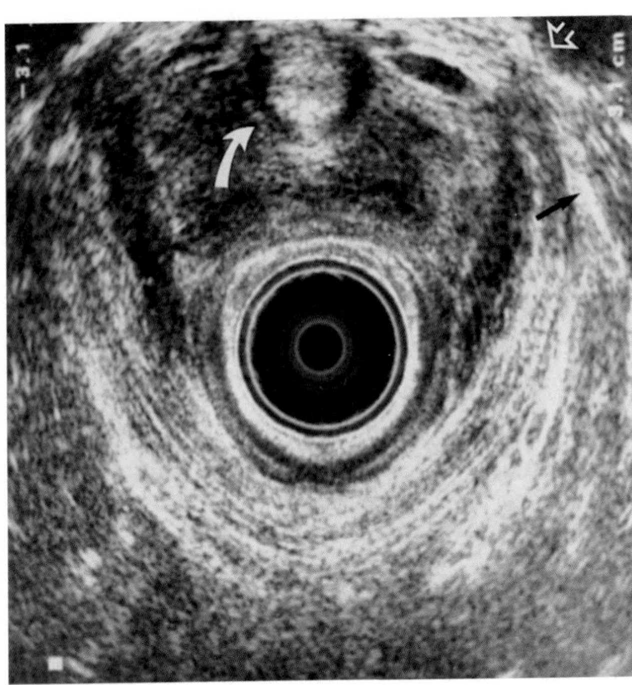

Fig. 28.20 High level in a female. The U-shaped striated sling of the puborectalis and deep external sphincter are seen around the canal. The internal sphincter is not clearly defined at this level, which is a common finding, and may be just due to a change in the orientation of the fibres. The puborectalis runs forward to the pubic symphysis (arrowhead). The obturator internus (black arrow) is seen on the lateral pelvic wall. The amorphous perivaginal tissues separate the canal from the urethra (curved white arrow).

about 1 mm in children, 1–2 mm in young adults, becoming 2–3 mm in those over 55 years old. This is mainly due to increased fibrous tissue content [37]. Any sphincter above 3.5 mm is abnormal whatever the age. Thick sphincters may be found with anal pain (Fig. 28.21) or the solitary rectal ulcer syndrome (Fig. 28.22). In the latter the subepithelial tissues are also prominent, producing a diagnostic complex [38]. Very thick sphincters of over 6 mm may be associated with a rare hereditary myopathy presenting with severe proctalgia fugax. A thin sphincter of less than 2 mm in an older patient may be due to internal sphincter degeneration and associated with passive faecal incontinence [39].

The ring of the internal sphincter should always be intact. There may be some variation in circumferential thickness at any one level, but any gross thinning or actual break in the ring is abnormal. Anal stretch procedures, often performed for fissure, may cause single or multiple tears [40] (Figs 28.23, 28.24). Fragmentation of the internal sphincter is characteristic of this sort of trauma (Fig. 28.25). An alternative treatment for fissure is sphincterotomy, where the distal third of the sphincter is divided. If the division is more extensive, there is the risk of precipitating incontinence (Fig. 28.26). This may happen inadvertently in females due to the shortness of the anal canal [41]. Haemorrhoidectomy should not involve the sphincter, but in patients who become incontinent following surgery, a localized defect may be found.

External sphincter

Rupture of the striated muscle fibres in the external sphincter muscle results in some separation at the site of the tear, the degree of separation depending on the linear extend of the tear, and how well the muscle fibres are supported by surrounding stroma. Initial haemorrhage becomes organized and heals with granulation tissue and fibrous repair.

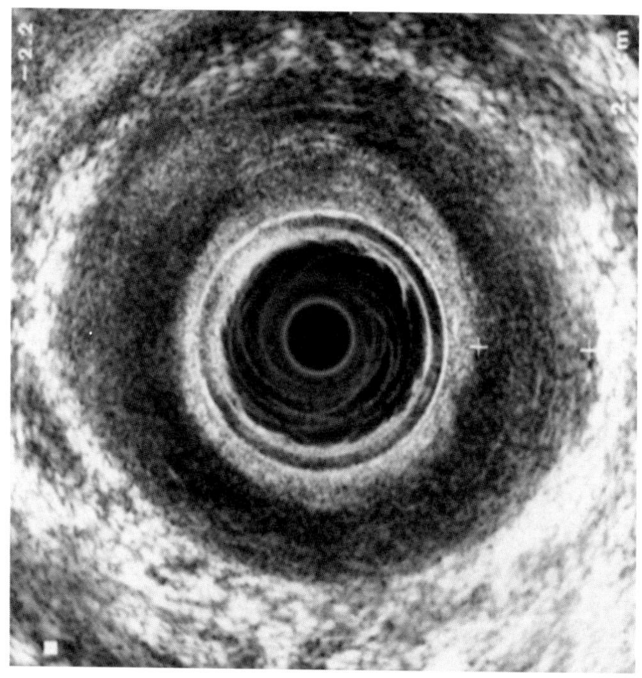

Fig. 28.21 Gross thickening of the internal sphincter (7.1 mm, between crosses) in a 74-year-old patient with a long-standing history of severe proctalgia fugax. This was familial with her mother and daughter affected, and is a rare case of hereditary internal sphincter myopathy.

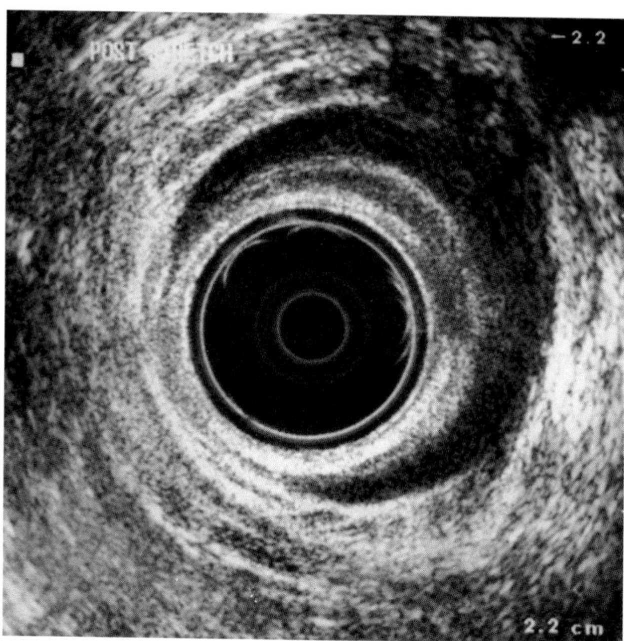

Fig. 28.23 Localized posterior break in the internal sphincter following an anal stretch for fissure.

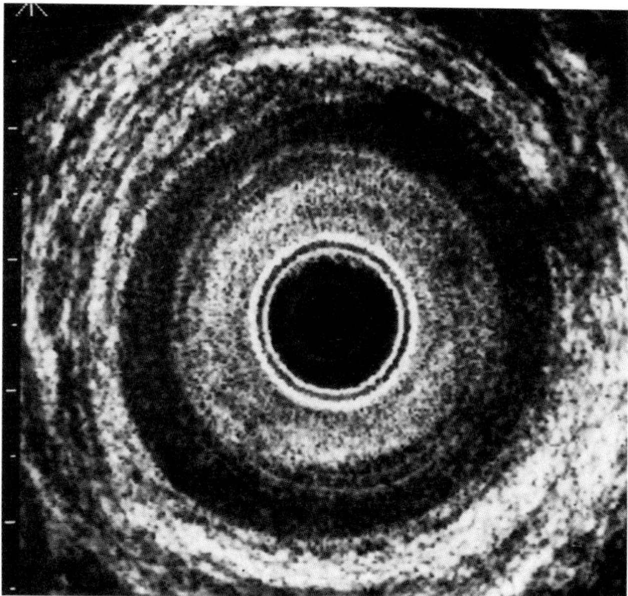

Fig. 28.22 Thickened internal sphincter (3.2 mm) and subepithelial tissues in a young male patient with rectal prolapse.

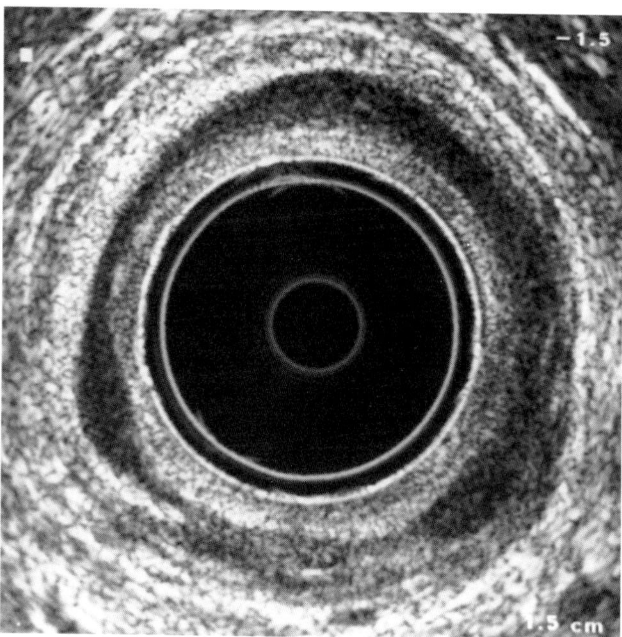

Fig. 28.24 Irregular thinning of the internal sphincter following an anal stretch.

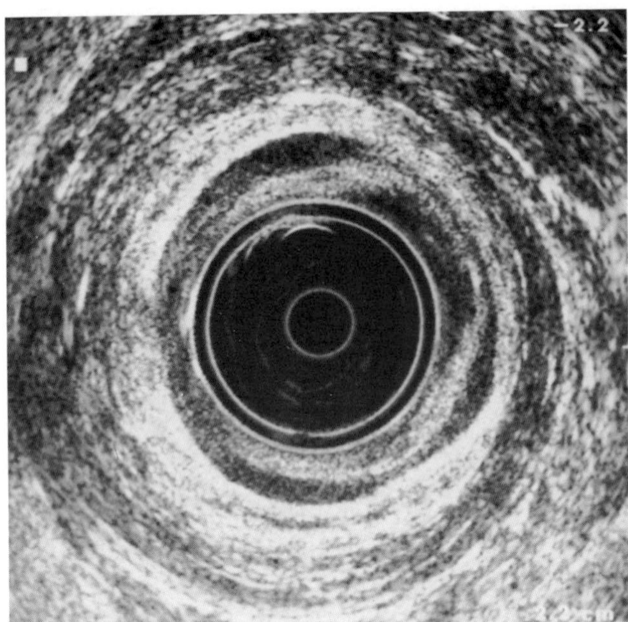

Fig. 28.25 Fragmentation of the internal sphincter after an anal stretch.

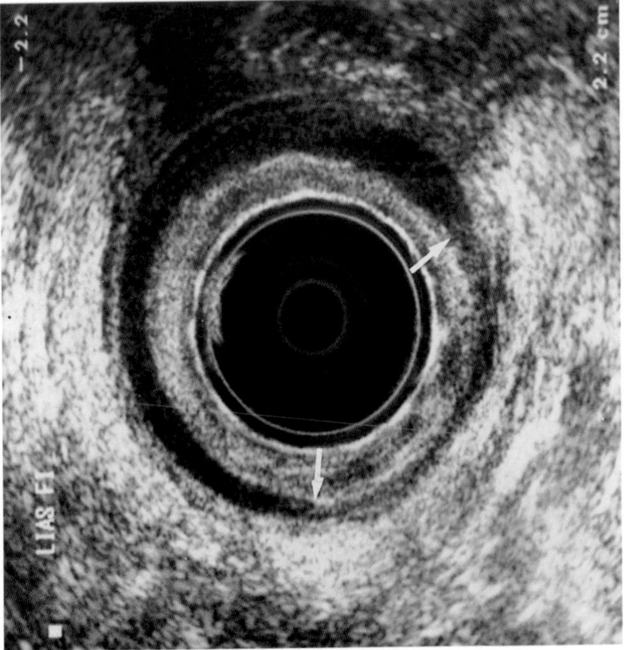

Fig. 28.26 Lateral sphincterotomy for fissure, extending high (arrows) into the canal in a female patient, and resulting in faecal incontinence.

Fibrous tissue is relatively homogeneous and only moderately echogenic. Tears are therefore seen as amorphous areas, usually less echogenic than the external sphincter and longitudinal muscle. The longitudinal muscle is often involved in external sphincter tears, especially when there is a defect in the internal sphincter (Fig. 28.27). Tears, or rather the remaining scars, may be referred to as 'defects'. This term originates from electromyograph studies, where the electrical activity of the muscle was mapped out by multiple needle insertions, with a scar shown as a segment of electrical inactivity, or defect in normal activity. Endosonography has been shown to be more accurate than digital examination, anal manometry or concentric needle electromyography in the detection of tears [42].

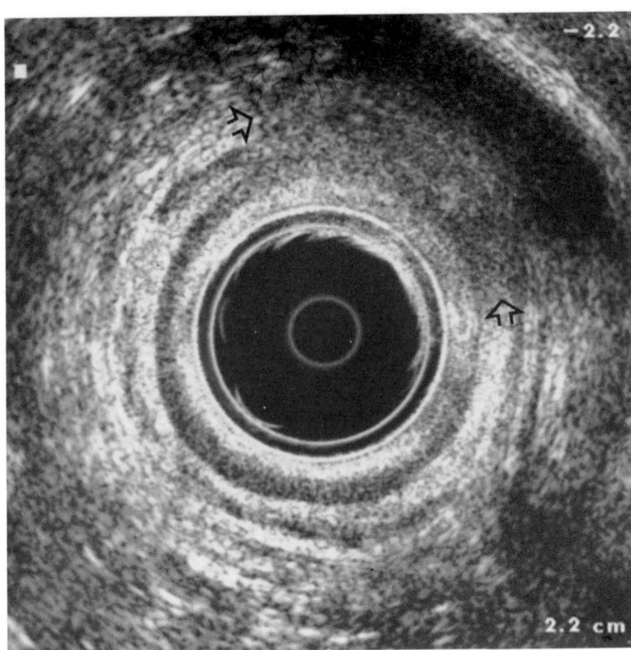

Fig. 28.27 An external sphincter tear (12–3 o'clock; arrowheads) due to obstetric trauma, with a relatively homogeneous hypoechoic pattern, also involving the longitudinal muscle and internal sphincter.

The external sphincter damage may be surgical, obstetric or traumatic in origin. Childbirth is the commonest cause, with 35% of first-time vaginal deliveries resulting in some sphincter damage [43] (Figs 28.28, 28.29). Forceps-assisted deliveries, particularly if rotational, are associated with the highest incidence of sphincter trauma [44].

Anal sepsis

About 25% of fistulas recur after surgery. This is attributed mainly to incomplete clearance of the fistula. A meticulous approach is needed to locate all tracks and abscesses to prevent recurrence. Any imaging method that could map out the full extent of sepsis preoperatively would be very helpful to recognize that a fistula was complex, and to plan the most appropriate surgical approach.

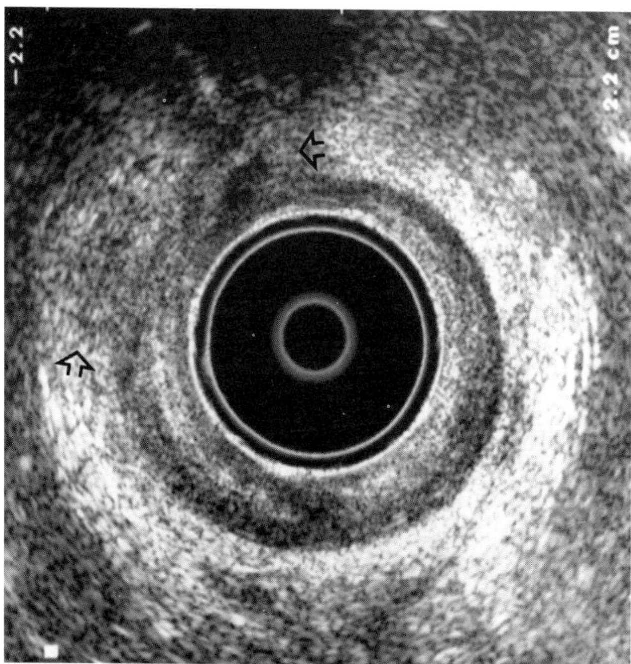

Fig. 28.28 Obstetric trauma with external sphincter tear (arrowheads). The tear is not so clearly defined as in Fig. 28.27. Between 9 and 10 o'clock there is patchy fibrosis in the sphincter, with a short segment of more normal-looking sphincter between 10 and 11 o'clock, leading to a well-defined scar between 11 and 12 o'clock. Note that the internal sphincter is also deficient between 9 and 12 o'clock.

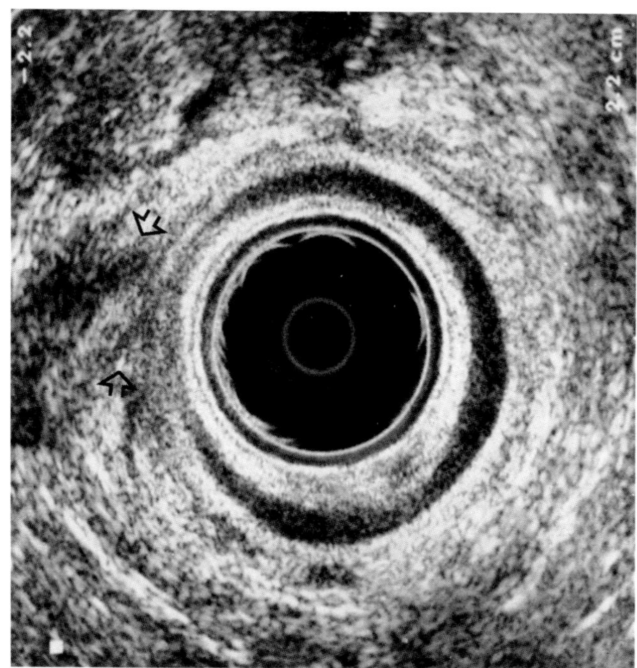

Fig. 28.29 A right lateral obstetric tear between 9 and 10 o'clock (arrowheads), with an associated defect in the internal sphincter.

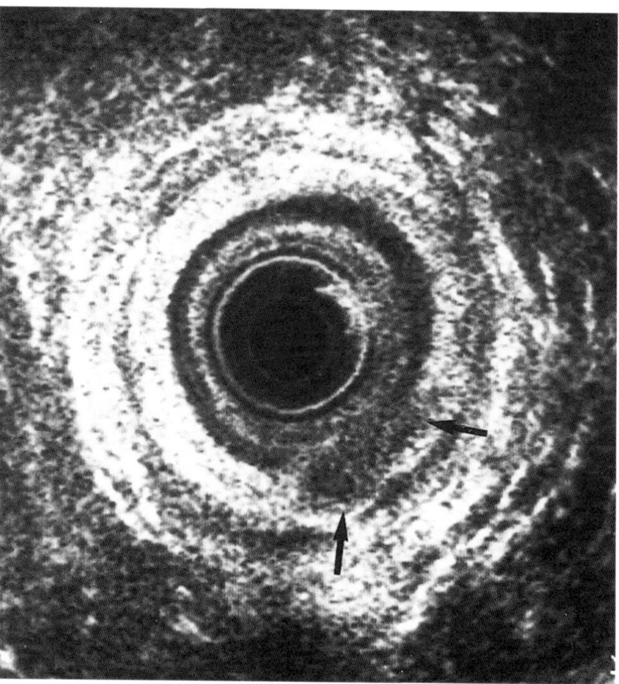

Fig. 28.30 Broad intersphincter track (arrows) running in the longitudinal muscle with a defect in the internal sphincter and internal opening at 6–7 o'clock.

Endosonography is capable of documenting sepsis within the sphincter [45]. The internal opening is inferred by the site where the primary track fuses with the internal sphincter (Fig. 28.30), as the actual track into the subepithelial tissues is seldom visible. A fistulous track presents as a hypoechoic band within the longitudinal muscle. Its extent and any branching may be traced throughout the length of the anal canal. Transsphincteric extension is present when irregular tracks are seen extending through the external sphincter (Fig. 28.31). Fluid collections are typically hypoechoic with increased through transmission. These may be difficult to palpate [46]. Small gas bubbles confirm an abscess. Small bright areas in tracks may represent pockets of gas, lumps of granulation tissue or foreign bodies (Fig. 28.32). Suprasphincteric tracks require changing to a balloon system for acoustic coupling in the rectal ampulla. Using the cone, examination is limited to sepsis within the canal. Following surgery scarring may be extensive, and a restriction in chronic cases is that it is difficult sonographically to distinguish fibrosis from residual infection.

Magnetic resonance imaging (MRI) is now the gold standard for imaging anal sepsis [47]. Fat suppression techniques highlight infected granulation tissue, and there is no difficulty in visualizing the extent of infection in any plane.

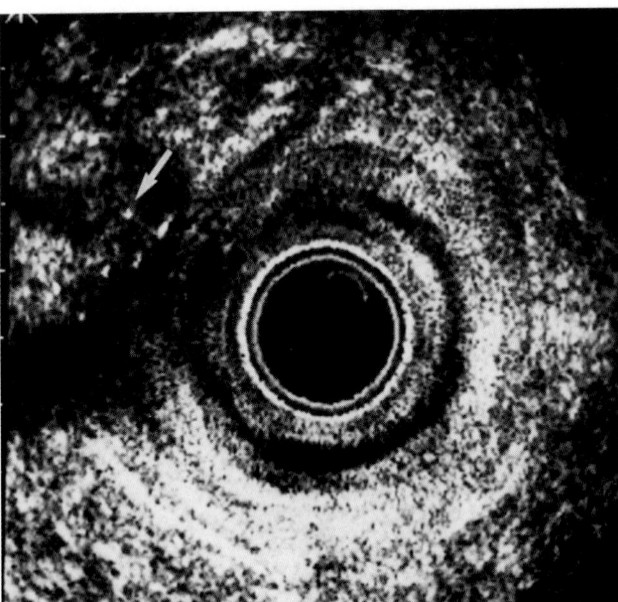

Fig. 28.31 Transsphincteric extension of an intersphincteric abscess with gas bubbles (arrow). Note the irregular permeation of the external sphincter.

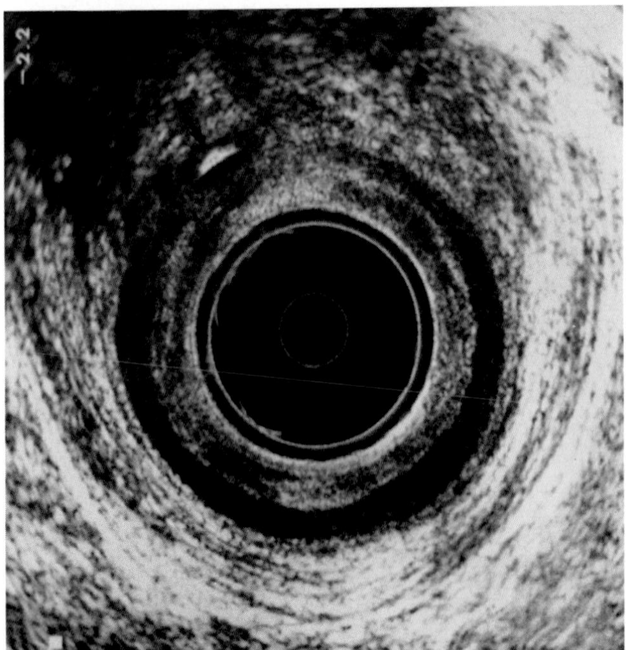

Fig. 28.32 Echogenic focus in an anterior track at 11 o'clock (arrow). This could be due to a gas bubble, granulation tissue or foreign body.

Table 28.2 Endosonographic equivalent of TNM classification of anal cancer

TNM classification for anal cancer
T1: tumour <2 cm in size
T2: >2 cm <5 cm in size
T3: >5 cm in maximum diameter
T4: any size with invasion adjacent structure
Endosonographic staging [48]
T1: confined to subepithelial tissues
T2: confined to sphincter muscles
T3: penetration of external sphincter
T4: invasion adjacent structure

Anal malignancy

In keeping with other gastrointestinal cancers, anal cancers are hypoechoic and their extent in relation to the sphincter may be mapped out using endosonography. The current TNM classification is based on the size of the tumour. An endosonographic equivalent [48] has been suggested (Table 28.2). Sonography may be helpful in screening for recurrence, which presents as a hypoechoic mass.

Indications for AES

1 Faecal incontinence [49]—to determine if there is any sphincter damage.
2 Anal pain—to see if the sphincter is abnormally thick.
3 Anal sepsis—may be helpful in complex cases, particularly for showing fluid collections, which are not always palpable.
4 Anal malignancy—staging small tumours and screening for recurrent disease.

References

1 Wild, J.J., Reid, J.M. (1956) Diagnostic use of ultrasound. *British Journal of Physical Medicine* **19**, 128–257.
2 Law, P.J., Bartram, C.I. (1989) Anal endosonography: technique and normal anatomy. *Gastrointestinal Radiology* **14**, 349–353.
3 Dragsted, J., Gammelgaard, J. (1985) Endoluminal ultrasonic scanning in the evaluation of rectal cancer: a preliminary report of 13 cases. *Gastrointestinal Radiology* **8**, 367–369.
4 Hildrebrandt, U., Feifel, G., Schwarz, H.P., Scherr, O. (1985) Endorectal ultrasound: instrumentation and clinical aspects. *International Journal of Colorectal Disease* **1**, 203–207.
5 Beynon, J. (1989) An evaluation of the role of rectal endosonography in rectal cancer. *Annals of the Royal College of Surgeons of England* **71**, 131–139.
6 Mortensen, N.J. McC. (1992) Rectal and anal endosonography. *Gut* **33**, 148–149.
7 Beynon, J., Feifel, G., Hildebrandt, U., Mortensen, N.J. McC. (1991) *An Atlas of Rectal Endosonography*. Springer-Verlag, London.

8 Detry, R.J., Kartheuser, A., Kestens, P.J. (1993) Endorectal ultrasonography for staging rectal tumours: technique and contribution to treatment. *World Journal of Surgery* **17**, 271–276.

9 Ødegaard, S., Kimmey, M.B. (1994) Location of the muscularis mucosae on high frequency gastrointestinal ultrasound images. *European Journal of Ultrasound* **1**, 39–50.

10 Kimmey, M.B., Martin, R.W., Haggitt, R.C., Wang, K.Y., Franklin, D.W., Silverstein, F.E. (1989) Histological correlates of gastrointestinal endoscopic ultrasound images. *Gastroenterology* **96**, 433–441.

11 Konishi, F., Ugajai, H., Ito, K., Hanazawa, K. (1990) Endorectal ultrasonography with a 7.5 MHz linear array scanner for the assessment of invasion of rectal cancer. *International Journal of Colorectal Disease* **5**, 15–20.

12 Hulsmans, F.J.H., Castelijns, J.A., Reeders, J.W.A.J., Tygat, G.N.J. (1995) Review of artifacts associated with transrectal ultrasound: understanding, recognition, and prevention of misintepretation. *Journal of Clinical Ultrasound* **23**, 483–494.

13 Dukes, C.E., Bussey, H.J.R. (1958) The spread of rectal cancer and its effect on prognosis. *British Journal of Cancer* **12**, 309–320.

14 Sobin, L.H., Wittekind, C. (eds) (1997) *TNM Classification of Malignant Tumours*, 5th edn. John Wiley, New York.

15 Hildebrandt, U., Feifel, G. (1985) Pre-operative staging of rectal cancer by intrarectal ultrasound. *Diseases of the Colon Rectum* **28**, 42–46.

16 Bartram, C.I., Beynon, J. (1994) Endosonographic staging of rectal cancer. In: Freeny, P.C., Stevenson, G.W. (eds) *Alimentary Tract Roentgenology*. Mosby-Year Book, St Louis, pp. 813–823.

17 Herzog, U., von Flue, M., Tondelli, P., Schuippisser, J.P. (1993) How accurate is endorectal ultrasound in the preoperative staging of rectal cancer? *Diseases of the Colon and Rectum* **36**, 127–134.

18 Katsura, Y., Yamada, K., Ishizawa, T., Yoshinaka, H., Shimazu, H. (1992) Endorectal ultrasonography for the assessment of wall invasion and lymph node metastasis in rectal cancer. *Diseases of the Colon and Rectum* **35**, 362–368.

19 Maier, A.G., Barton, P.P., Neuhold, N.R., Herbst, F., Teleky, B.K., Lechner, G.L. (1997) Peritumoral tissue reaction at transrectal US as a possible cause of overstaging in rectal cancer: histopathologic correlation. *Radiology* **203**, 785–789.

20 Napoleon, B., Pujol, B., Berger, F., Valette, P.J., Gerard, J.P., Souquet, J.C. (1991) Accuracy of endosonography in the staging of rectal cancer treated by radiotherapy. *British Journal of Surgery* **78**, 785–788.

21 Fleshman, J.W., Myerson, R.J., Fry, R.D., Kodner, I.J. (1992) Accuracy of transrectal ultrasound in predicting pathologic stage of rectal cancer before and after preoperative radiation therapy. *Diseases of the Colon and Rectum* **35**, 823–829.

22 Mascagni, D., Corbellini, L., Urciuoli, P., Matteo di, G. (1989) Endoluminal ultrasound for early detection of local recurrence of rectal cancer. *British Journal of Surgery* **76**, 1176–1180.

23 Romano, G., Esercizio, L., Santangelo, M., Vallone, G., Santangelo, M.L. (1993) Impact of computed tomography vs intrarectal ultrasound on the diagnosis, resectability, and prognosis of local recurrent rectal cancer. *Diseases of the Colon and Rectum* **36**, 261–265.

24 Beynon, J., Mortensen, N.J. McC, Foy, D.M.A., Channer, J.L., Rigby, H., Virjee, J. (1989) Preoperative assessment of mesorectal lymph node involvement in rectal cancer. *British Journal of Surgery* **76**, 276–279.

25 Hildebrandt, U., Klein, T., Feifel, G., Schwarz, H.-P., Koch, B., Schmidtt, R.M. (1990) Endosonography of pararectal lymph nodes: *in vitro* and *in vivo* evaluation. *Diseases of the Colon and Rectum* **33**, 863–868.

26 Hulsmans, F.-H., Bosma, A., Mulder, P.J.J., Reeders, J.W.A., Tygat, G.N.J. (1992) Perirectal lymph nodes in rectal cancer: *in vitro* correlation of sonographic parameters and histopathologic findings. *Radiology* **184**, 553–556.

27 Rafaelsen, S.R., Kronborg, O., Fenger, C. (1992) Echo pattern of lymph nodes in colorectal cancer: in *in vitro* study. *British Journal of Radiology* **65**, 218–220.

28 Lindmark, G., Elvin, A., Påhlman, L., Glimelius, B. (1992) The value of endosonography in preoperative staging of rectal cancer. *International Journal of Colorectal Disease* **7**, 162–166.

29 Rafaelsen, S.R., Kronberg, O., Fenger, C. (1994) Digital examination and transrectal ultrasonography in staging of rectal cancer. *Acta Radiologica* **35**, 300–304.

30 Goldman, S., Arvidsson, H., Norming, U., Lagerstedt, U., Magnusson, I., Frisell, J. (1991) Transrectal ultrasound and computed tomography in preoperative staging of lower rectal adenocarcinoma. *Gastrointestinal Radiology* **16**, 259–263.

31 Solomon, M.J., McLeod, R.S. (1993) Endoluminal transrectal ultrasonography: accuracy, reliability, and validity. *Diseases of the Colon and Rectum* **36**, 200–205.

32 Bartram, C.I., Frudinger, A. (1997) *A Handbook of Anal Endosonography*. Wrightson Biomedical Publishing, Petersfield, UK.

33 Schafer, A., Enck, P., Heyer, T., Gantke, B., Frieling, T., Lubke, H.J. (1994) Endosonography of the anal sphincters: incontinent and continent patients and healthy controls. *Zeitschrift fur Gastroenterologie* **32**, 328–331.

34 Frudinger, A., Bartram, C.I., Halligan, S., Kamm, M. (1998) Examination techniques for endosonography of the anal canal. *Abdominal Imaging* **23**, 301–303.

35 Sultan, A.H., Loder, P.B., Bartram, C.I., Kamm, M.A., Hudson, C.N. (1994) Vaginal endosonography: new approach to image the undisturbed anal sphincter. *Diseases of the Colon and Rectum* **37**, 1296–1299.

36 Sultan, A.H., Kamm, M.A., Hudson, C.N., Nicholls, R.J., Bartram, C.I. (1994) Endosonography of the anal sphincters: normal anatomy and comparison with manometry. *Clinical Radiology* **49**, 368–374.

37 Burnett, S.J.D., Bartram, C.I. (1991) Endosonographic variations in the normal internal anal sphincter. *International Journal of Colorectal Disease* **6**, 2–4.

38 Halligan, S., Sultan, A., Rottenburg, G., Bartram, C. (1995) Endosonography of the anal sphincters in solitary rectal ulcer syndrome. *International Journal of Colorectal Diseases* **10**, 79–82.

39 Vaizey, C.J., Kamm, M.A., Bartram, C.I. (1997) Primary degeneration of the internal anal sphincter as a cause of passive faecal incontinence. *Lancet* **349**, 612–615.

40 Nielsen, M.B., Rasmussen, O.Ø., Pedersen, J.F., Christiansen, J. (1993) Risk of sphincter damage and anal incontinence after anal dilatation for fissure-in-ano. An endosonographic study. *Diseases of the Colon and Rectum* **36**, 677–680.

41 Sultan, A.H., Kamm, M.A., Nicholls, R.J., Bartram, C.I. (1994) Prospective study of the extent of internal anal sphincter division during lateral sphincterotomy. *Diseases of the Colon and Rectum* **37**, 1031–1033.

42 Sultan, A.H., Kamm, M.A., Talbot, I.C., Nicholls, R.J.,

Bartram, C.I. (1994) Anal endosonography for identifying external sphincter defects confirmed histologically. *British Journal of Surgery* **81**, 463–465.

43 Sultan, A.H., Kamm, M.A., Hudson, C.N., Thomas, J.M., Bartram, C.I. (1993) Anal sphincter disruption during vaginal delivery. *New England Journal of Medicine* **329**, 1905–1911.

44 Sultan, A.H., Kamm, M.A., Bartram, C.I., Hudson, C.N. (1993) Anal sphincter trauma during instrumental delivery. *International Journal of Gynecology and Obstetrics* **43**, 263–270.

45 Choen, S., Burnett, S., Bartram, C.I., Nicholls, R.J. (1991) Comparison between anal endosonography and digital examination in the evaluation of anal fistulae. *British Journal of Surgery* **78**, 445–447.

46 Deen, K.I., Williams, J.G., Hutchinson, R., Keighley, M.R.B., Kumar, D. (1994) Fistulas in anoendoanal ultrasonographic assessment assists decision making for surgery. *Gut* **35**, 391–394.

47 Barker, P.G., Lunniss, P.J., Armstrong, P., Reznek, R.H., Cottam, K., Phillips, R.K. (1994) Magnetic resonance imaging of fistula-in-ano: technique, interpretation and accuracy. *Clinical Radiology* **49**, 7–13.

48 Goldman, S., Norming, U., Svensson, C., Glimelius, B. (1991) Transanorectal ultrasonography in the staging of anal epidermoid carcinoma. *International Journal of Colorectal Disease* **6**, 152–157.

49 Bartram, C.I., Sultan, A.H. (1995) Anal endosonography in faecal incontinence. *Gut* **37**, 4–6.

Chapter 29: General principles of biopsy and drainage

H.C. Irving

Interventional ultrasound

'Interventional ultrasound' is the term that has come to be applied to the use of ultrasound for the guidance of needles into patients for diagnostic and/or therapeutic purposes. Diagnostic uses include biopsy of solid masses or organs and aspiration of fluid-containing lesions or collections. Therapeutic procedures encompass drainage of both fluid-containing masses, such as cysts and abscesses, and organ systems such as the biliary and urinary tracts, as well as the insertion of needles into tumours for the instillation of therapeutic agents.

In many instances, 'interventional ultrasound' has become an integral part of 'interventional radiology' in that a procedure will commence by using ultrasound to guide a needle into position so that a guide-wire can be introduced and the procedure then continues using radiological or other imaging methods. Portable ultrasound machines are essential and may be taken into X-ray screening rooms, computed tomography (CT) or magnetic resonance imaging (MRI) scanning suites, and into operating theatres. Renal, hepatobiliary, vascular and many other imaging-guided interventions are some of the many techniques that are reliant on ultrasound for their initial stages.

Needle guidance

Purpose-built needle-guide devices for ultrasound probes are available from most manufacturers of ultrasound equipment. Whilst some have designed ultrasound transducer housings with an integral biopsy channel, these are expensive, lack versatility and are difficult to sterilize. Such problems are overcome by using needle-guide attachments which clip or screw on to conventional ultrasound transducers. Designs vary, but there are several essential features. The construction should be rigid to ensure that the needle pathway will be consistent and metal is therefore preferable to plastic. There must be a mechanism for varying the size of the needle channel (spring loading or a choice of inserts with different calibre lumens), so that needles of different outer diameters can be used for the various applications and will always fit snugly through the channel. It must be possible to release the needle from the guide rapidly during a procedure, and the guide should be capable of easy detachment from the probe to allow for sterilization between cases. Sterility can be achieved by placing the ultrasound transducer within a sterile cover over which the sterile needle-guide can then be placed and fixed to the transducer housing. Finally, since the optimum needle entry point may be close to ribs or other bony protuberances, the ideal systems will have as small a scan probe head as possible in order to permit adequate transducer–skin contact and to allow the needle entry site to be as close as possible to the entry portal of the ultrasound beam (Fig. 29.1).

Once the needle-guide is attached to the transducer housing, the needle pathway can be programmed into the ultrasound machine so that it will appear as a line superimposed on the ultrasound image (Fig. 29.2). If the design constraints referred to above are met, then it becomes possible to guide needles to small deep targets with considerable precision (Fig. 29.3).

Needle visualization

With needle-guide systems as described above, needle visualization is restricted to the bright echo emanating from the tip of the needle and this is adequate for most clinical purposes (Fig. 29.4). The gain settings should be adjusted so that there is maximum contrast between the needle-tip echo and the surrounding tissues, and thus it is usually easier to see the needle tip as it passes through fluid as opposed to solid tissue. The amplitude of the needle-tip echo varies with the construction of the needle and there have been attempts to increase reflectivity by using a roughened surface coating and by the incorporation of an air-containing notch near to the needle tip. The cutting action of some types of core biopsy needles, particularly those operated by a spring loaded gun, generate a cluster of echoes within the tissues as the core is ensnared within the device. This is a useful aid to the operator who

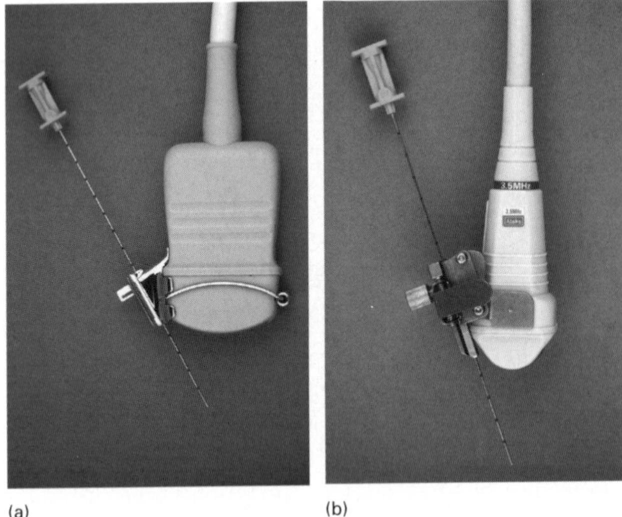

(a) (b)

Fig. 29.1 (a) A sector array probe with clip-on needle-guide. (b) A small headed sector array probe with screw-on needle guide.

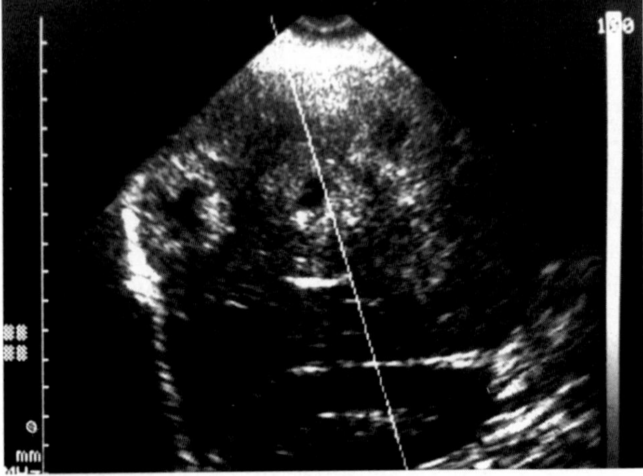

Fig. 29.2 The needle-guide device has been directed at one of the liver metastases and the dotted line indicates the intended needle path.

can then be confident as to the precise origin of the biopsy sample (Fig. 29.5).

Free hand techniques

In routine clinical practice, there will be many occasions when the target is either sufficiently large or superficial to permit a free hand approach to the puncture procedure. The proposed needle entry site is simply marked on the skin after careful ultrasound scanning has been performed for localization and characterization of the target, assessment of the proposed needle pathway, measure-

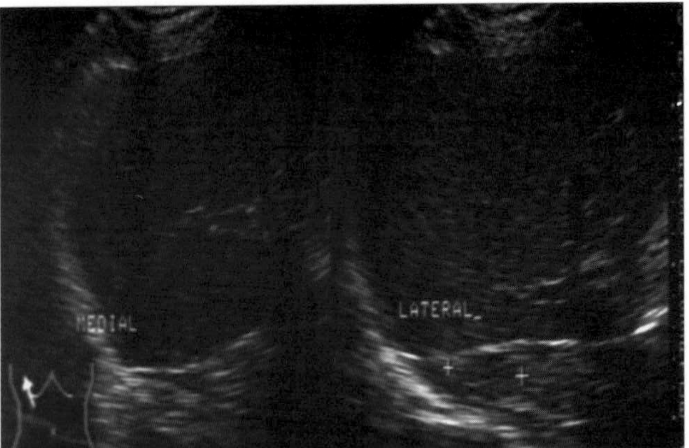

(a)

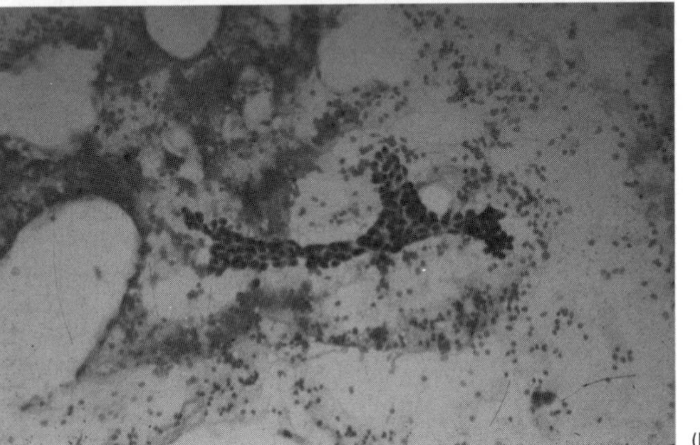

(b)

Fig. 29.3 (a) Sagittal and transverse scans through an enlarged right adrenal gland in a patient with a primary bronchial carcinoma. (b) The fine-needle aspiration cytology sample from the adrenal gland shows a cluster of malignant cells confirming a metastatic deposit. For colour, see Plate 29.3 (between pp. 308 and 309).

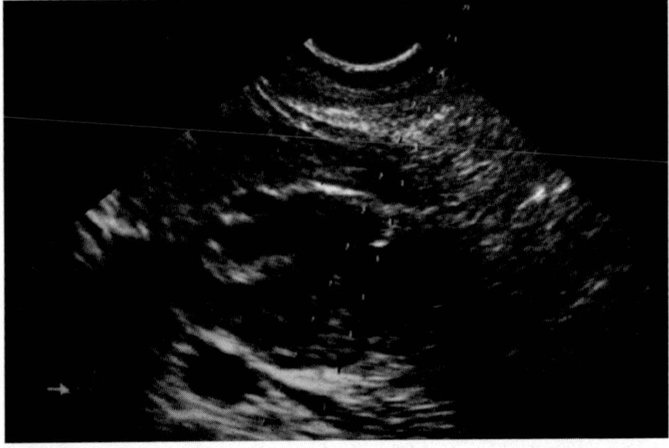

Fig. 29.4 Transverse scan showing the needle tip approaching a mass in the tail of the pancreas. 18-gauge core biopsy confirmed pancreatic carcinoma.

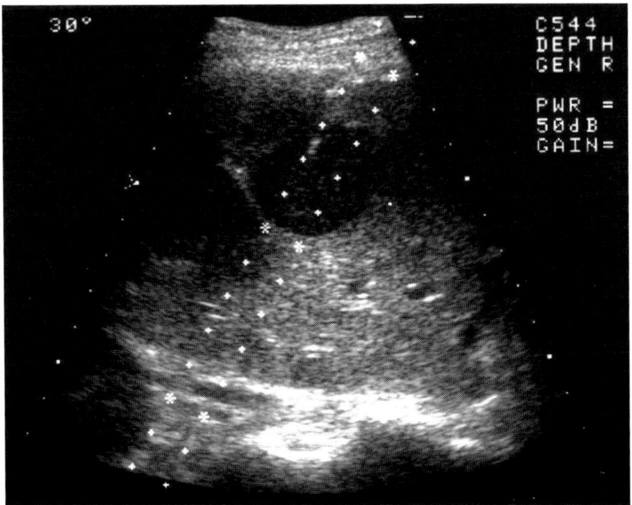

Fig. 29.5 One of the multiple liver metastases has been biopsied and a linear track of echoes has been generated by the cutting action of the spring loaded core biopsy needle.

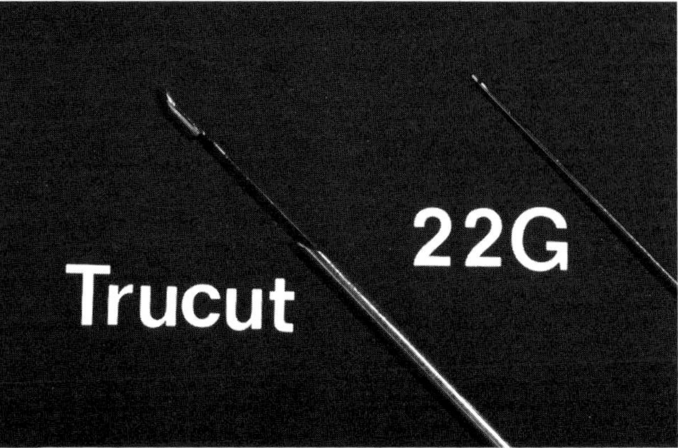

Fig. 29.6 Biopsy needles: 14-gauge 'Trucut' for core biopsy, and 22-gauge fine needle for aspiration biopsy.

ment of the correct depth for needle insertion and demonstration of the effect of respiratory motion. Free hand punctures should be performed with the minimum of needle angulation since accuracy of placement rapidly diminishes as angulation away from a true vertical or horizontal approach increases. In this way free hand needle guidance following ultrasound localization can be a quick and effective method for aspiration and drainage of fluid collections such as pleural effusions and ascites, as well as for biopsy of large superficial structures, although small and deep targets are not amenable to this technique.

Indirect needle guidance

Indirect needle guidance is a compromise technique by which real-time ultrasound is used to monitor a free hand puncture without a needle-guide attachment. The needle is introduced into the patient close to the ultrasound probe and, with practice, the needle tip can be visualized passing through the tissues towards the target. The advantage of this method is freedom from the constraints of a rigid needle-guide confering greater versatility of approach and opportunity for modification of angulation along the needle pathway. The problems concern the difficulty of locating the needle tip and the ease with which the tip is lost from direct visualization during needle manipulations. However, even when the needle tip itself is not seen, movement of the tissues around the needle tip may give the operator an appreciation of the course of the needle. This method of needle guidance is used most commonly when lesions are relatively superficial such as in breast biopsies.

Biopsies

Pathological examination of a sample of tissue from a solid organ or tumour is often required for diagnosis, and suitable tissue samples can be rapidly and atraumatically collected via ultrasound-guided needle biopsy. The pathological information to be derived from the biopsy will influence the size and nature of tissue sample needed and will be a major factor in determining the type and size of biopsy needle to be used.

Fine-needle aspiration biopsies

Certain tumours and inflammatory conditions may be diagnosed from a cytological examiantion in which a small cluster of cells has been aspirated into the lumen of a fine gauge needle. Such a sample can be obtained by using a 22-gauge (or finer) needle (outer diameter 0.72 mm) (Fig. 29.6) and these fine needles can be introduced into most sites in the body without fear of damaging either the target organ or intervening structures such as bowel, and the risk of haemorrhage is minimal. Once the needle tip has been placed within the target, cells are encouraged to enter the needle lumen by the application of suction at the same time as mechanical disruption is caused by 'jiggling' the needle tip back and forth. The suction pressure is then released, the needle withdrawn and the aspirate is expelled from the needle lumen. The sample is prepared for cytological examination according to the instructions of the local cytologist—some pathologists prefer an immediate smear onto microscope slides with half the slides sprayed with fixative and half air-dried, while others prefer the aspirate to be placed in cytological culture fluid so that the smears can be made later in the laboratory. The interpretation (and hence the ultimate value) of fine-needle aspiration biopsies is critically dependent upon the expertise of the cytologist who is usually able to decide if the cells are from a malignant or benign (including inflammatory) process, and may also be able to type certain tumours (see Fig. 29.3).

Core (large needle) biopsies

Larger cores of tissue are required if a histological diagnosis is needed, when the arrangement of the cells and the tissue architecture can be studied. The needles for core biopsies are more traumatic than fine needles and most have a cutting edge to facilitate detachment of the tissue core from its surroundings (see Fig. 29.6). For ultrasound-guided core biopsies, automatic triggering of the biopsy needle via a spring loaded 'gun' is preferable so that the ultrasound probe can be held in one hand and the biopsy gun in the other. As the needle tip is seen to approach the target, the biopsy mechanism can then be automatically triggered by pressing a small button with the thumb or finger of the hand which is holding the gun. The inner notched obturator is fired into the lesion and the outer cutting sheath rapidly follows—within a split second. These devices dramatically reduce the time taken for the biopsy and reliably produce excellent quality cores of tissue. As mentioned above, the motion of the cutting action generates a 'core' of highly reflective echoes in the tissues so that the operator can immediately be aware of the exact site of origin of the biopsy (see Fig. 29.5) [1,2].

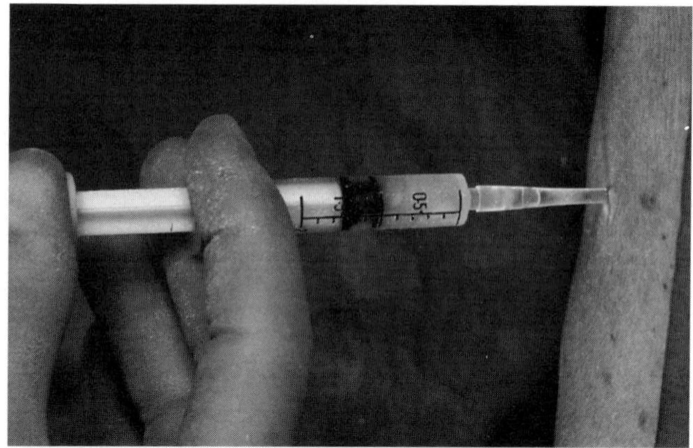
(a)

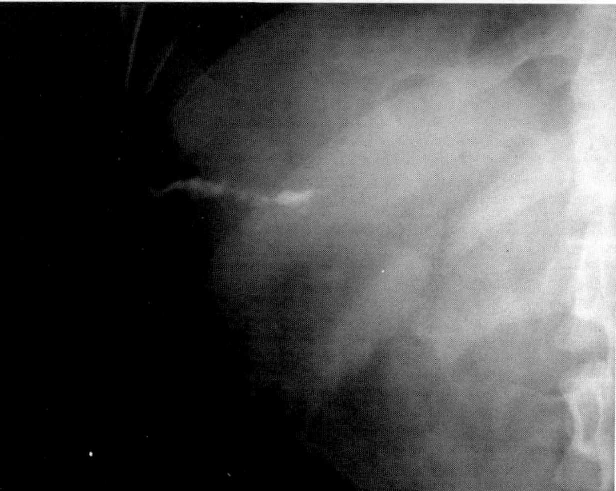
(b)

Fig. 29.7 (a) The plugging material is injected through the outer sheath following the biopsy. (b) Radiograph to show the needle track plugged with gelfoam (Sterispon) soaked in contrast medium for demonstration purposes only.

Plugged biopsies

Percutaneous liver biopsies from patients with impaired blood coagulation may carry an unacceptably high risk of intraperitoneal haemorrhage when a core biopsy is needed for definitive diagnosis of the underlying liver disease. In such patients, with a prolonged prothrombin time or low platelet count, the biopsy may be safely performed following ultrasound localization by introducing the biopsy needle through an outer sheath so that the track may be 'plugged' with particulate matter as soon as the core biopsy has been obtained and the biopsy needle removed. Pledget of gelfoam (Sterispon) or other inert material (e.g. Lyostypt) which have been rendered pliable by soaking in sterile saline solution can thus form an effective mechanical barrier and so greatly reduce the risk of bleeding (Fig. 29.7) [3].

Complications of biopsy

Fine-needle aspiration biopsy is virtually free from complications [4] and there are thus hardly any contraindications. With such small needle diameters, haemorrhage and perforation are insignificant complications, and even vascular tumours, such as capillary haemangiomas of the liver, can be safely biopsied—as long as the needle pathway traverses normal liver tissue prior to entering the tumour [5]. However, it is prudent to avoid puncturing distended gallbladders which may leak if they are not then decompressed with a drainage catheter and phaeochromocytomas which may produce a hypertensive crisis if traumatized [6]. Tumour seeding along the needle track has been reported following fine-needle biopsy, but cumulative experience shows that this is an extremely rare phenomenon and is probably avoidable by restricting the number of needle passes through the tumour [7,8].

The larger size of core biopsy needle mitigates for more cautious use. These needles cannot be passed through bowel or other viscera without consideration of the risks of perforation or haemorrhage. It is therefore necessary to check blood coagulation before embarking upon a percutaneous core biopsy, and the needle pathway should be carefully planned. However, transgastric or transbowel passage of an 18-gauge (outer diameter 1.26 mm) needle carries very little risk of subsequent leakage of bowel content in the absence of bowel obstruction, and many radiologists (including the author) do not now regard such approaches as a contraindication to core biopsy [9].

Aspiration and drainage procedures

Ultrasonically guided punctures of fluid-containing lesions or structures may be for either diagnostic or therapeutic purposes.

Diagnostic tap

The ultrasound diagnosis of a simple (and hence benign) cyst, whether in liver, kidney or other viscus, requires the presence of an echo-free content, increased through transmission of sound, and smooth, clearly defined walls. If any of these diagnostic criteria are in doubt, or if the clinical features are worrying, then the diagnosis can be confirmed by aspirating fluid from the cyst for pathological examination. Using a 22- or 20-gauge needle (outer diameters 0.72 or 0.90 mm), the suspected cyst can be aspirated without risk, and this can be done as an outpatient procedure. Cyst fluid should be sent for cytological examination, and depending upon the particular circumstances, microbiological studies, estimation of tumour markers or biochemical tests may be relevant. The presence of blood in the aspirate should raise the index of suspicion for malignancy so that even in the absence of positive cytology further investigations such as CT or MRI may be indicated.

Similarly, with the aid of ultrasound guidance, even very small fluid collections within body compartments (e.g. pleural effusions of intraperitoneal fluid) may be needled and samples obtained for pathological examination.

Therapeutic aspiration and drainages

Simple cysts invariably reaccumulate after aspiration, although it may take weeks or months for their original volume to be regained. Aspiration of cysts that are symptomatic by virtue of their size and/or pressure effects upon adjacent organs will afford temporary relief. Repeated aspirations can be performed and may be an acceptable form of treatment—especially in the elderly. If a more permanent ablation of the cyst is required, a sclerosant such as absolute ethanol can be instilled. This is usually performed by inserting a fine bore catheter into the cyst under ultrasound guidance, aspirating the cyst to dryness, and instilling the sclerosant which is left in contact with the cyst lining for approximately 30 min before finally aspirating to dryness and removing the catheter [10]. Therapeutic drainage of pleural effusions and ascites are now commonly performed procedures in departments with an oncology referral practice, and can be safely and quickly accomplished via the insertion of a catheter under ultrasound guidance, either using a one-stage catheter over needle system or a three-stage catheter over guide-wire procedure.

Aspiration and drainage of abscesses

Abscesses often present with the clinical features of fever and tenderness, but may sometimes only be suspected on the ultrasound evidence of debris within a fluid collection or ill-defined margins of a mass. Occasionally none of these clues is present and the diagnosis is only apparent after the aspiration of pus (Fig. 29.8). Experience has shown that enough pus for diagnostic purposes can usually be aspirated through a 22-gauge needle, but a larger calibre needle or catheter will be needed for therapeutic benefit.

The management of intra-abdominal abscesses has been revolutionized by the use of ultrasound for early diagnosis and minimally invasive therapy (via ultrasound-guided drainage). Despite much scepticism (largely on the part of surgeons), it has been established that effective control of the suppurative process can be gained with the use of relatively narrow bore 'radiological' drains that can be inserted under either ultrasound or CT guidance [11–13].

In some circumstances, it is now accepted that insertion of a drain may be omitted and simple aspiration of pus in combination with systemic antibiotic therapy will suffice. This form of therapy has been particularly successful in the treatment of pyogenic liver abscesses [14] when there is a good blood supply to the tissues around the abscesses, ensuring access of antibiotics to the focus of infection.

However, the majority of intra-abdominal abscesses do require drainage and a variety of specially designed catheters are available for this purpose. The essential principle is that a sheathed needle is inserted into the abscess under imaging guidance, a guide-wire is passed through

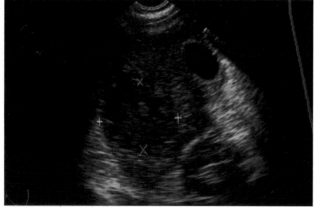

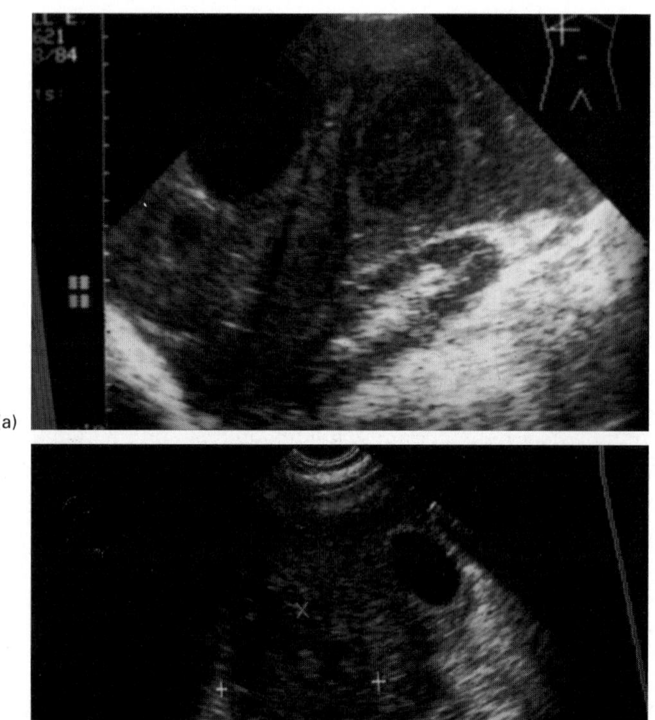

Fig. 29.8 (a) Sagittal scan through the right lobe of the liver showing two pyogenic abscesses at different stages of evolution. (b) Transverse scan through the right lobe of liver in which there is an abscess (crosses) which appears 'solid' in the early stages of its natural history. This was treated by aspiration rather than drainage.

the sheath, the track is dilated and a catheter is then passed over the guide-wire into the abscess cavity (Fig. 29.9). All purpose drainage catheters with wide side-holes are available in 8 or 12 F sizes and will suffice for most purposes, although larger bore catheters and sump drains (with an air inlet to aid effective drainage) are available for abscesses with particularly thick contents.

Subsequent management of the patient depends upon the clinical course. All patients should be treated with appropriate antibiotics and many abscesses will cease to drain within 24–48 h when the catheter can be removed. If there is continuing drainage, then further imaging by ultrasound, CT or sinography will be required in order to search for other pockets of pus and/or fistulas.

Important practical tips regarding abscess drainage include the following.

1 Give antibiotic cover.

2 Aspirate the abscess to dryness in the ultrasound department.

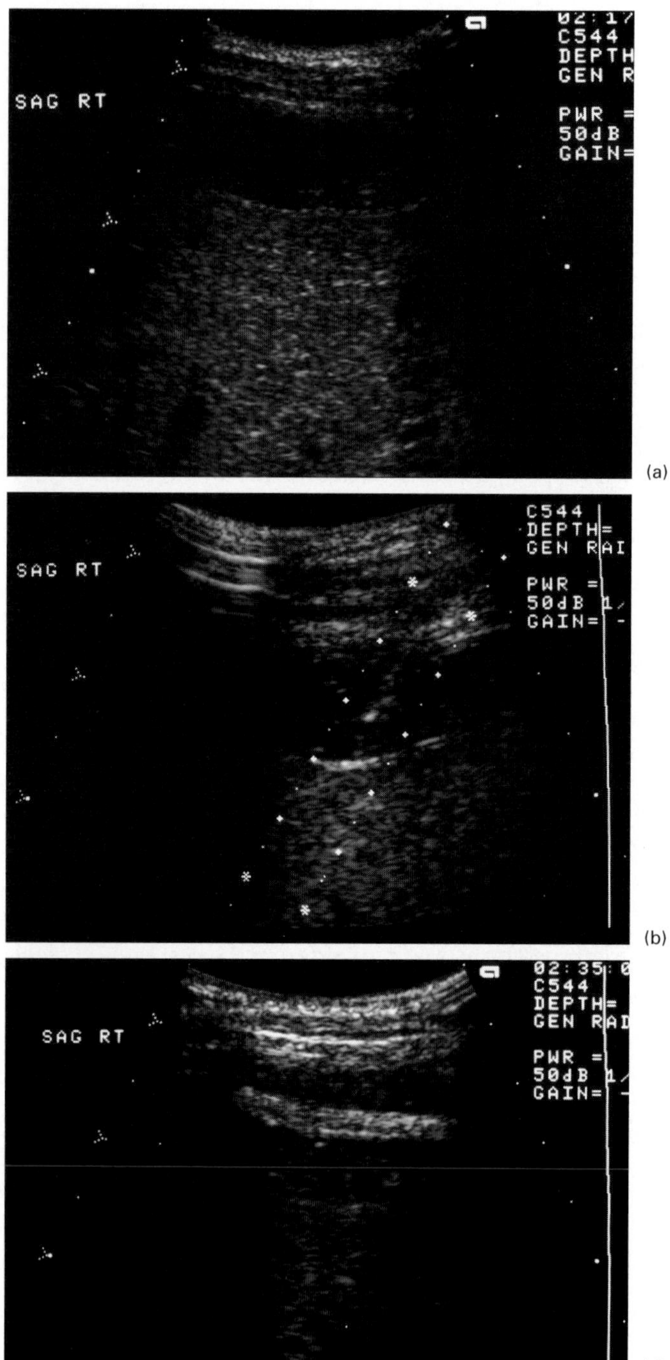

Fig. 29.9 (a) Coronal scan showing a right subphrenic abscess. (b) The tip of a sheathed needle is seen within the abscess. (c) A drainage catheter has been introduced into the abscess which has been aspirated to dryness.

3 Remove all taps from the drainage system (the lumen of the tap is often narrower than the internal diameter of the drainage catheter).

4 Avoid transpleural punctures (for subphrenic, hepatic or splenic abscesses).

5 Avoid transbowel punctures if possible (but the transgastric approach for pancreatic abscess is fine).
6 Flushing the catheter rarely helps and may lead to dislodgement.
7 Investigate continued drainage.
8 Do not place drains in uninfected haematomas (aspirate for culture first).
9 Failure to respond may be due to undrained collections, fistulous connections or underlying necrotic tumour.

Using these methods, the results of percutaneous abscess drainage are impressive. For example, it has been shown that the mortality rate from pyogenic liver abscesses has been reduced from almost 50% to zero, due to earlier diagnosis and effective treatment via ultrasound-guided drainage [15]. However, most large centres find it difficult to reproduce the high cure rate reported in the early papers on the subject [11,12] as the case mix has changed over the years. We are now faced with many patients who develop septic conditions secondary to some form of immunosuppression, e.g. transplant recipients, acquired immune deficiency syndrome, and so on, and it has become more difficult to render these patients free of sepsis [16]. Another problematic group are oncology patients receiving chemotherapy, who are not only immunosuppressed, but may also have large volumes of ischaemic and necrotic tumour which act as a nidus for infection.

Drainage of viscera

Interventional uroradiology relies heavily on the use of ultrasound to guide needles into the urinary tract so that guide-wires, catheters, stents and large bore sheaths can be introduced into pelvicalyceal systems, ureters and the bladder. Percutaneous nephrostomy of both native and transplanted kidneys is performed by ultrasound-guided puncture of the pelvicalyceal system either by a catheter over needle system or by a sheathed needle with subsequent introduction of a guide-wire over which a catheter can be passed. Drainage of an obstructed urinary tract can thus be performed quickly and safely using just ultrasound for guidance, but additional X-ray fluoroscopy is needed for diagnostic nephrostogram or antegrade stent insertion [17].

There is less dependence on ultrasound for biliary tract catheterization procedures when most radiologists are content to use X-ray screening. However, ultrasound-guided puncture of the gallbladder for drainage of empyema can prove life-saving in elderly patients who are unfit for acute surgery [18,19].

Other fluid-containing anatomical structures which are the target of ultrasonically guided puncture include the pancreatic duct for percutaneous pancreatic ductography,

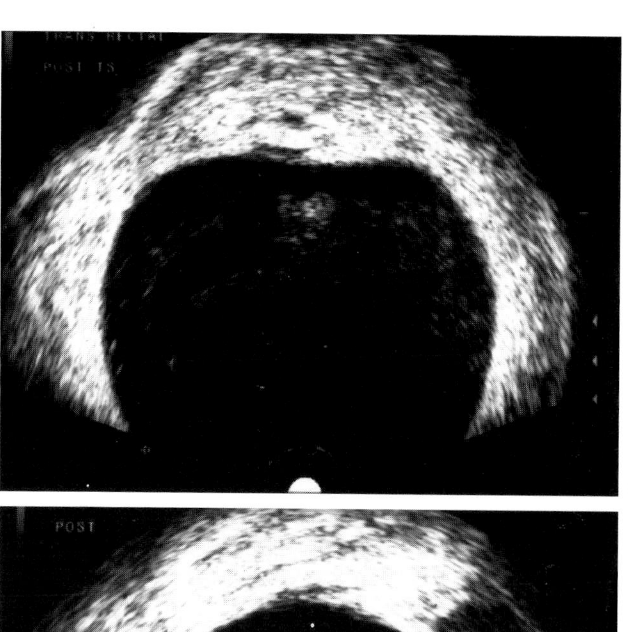
(a)

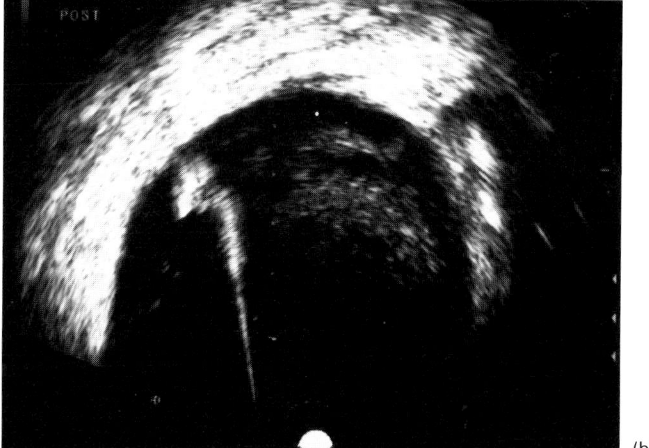

(b)

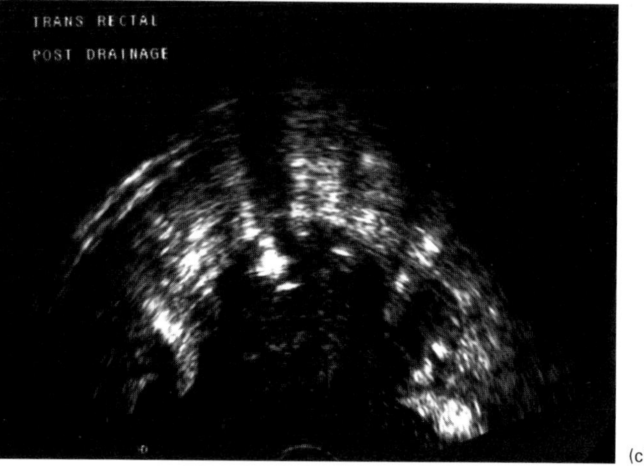

(c)

Fig. 29.10 (a) Transrectal scan shows a deep pelvic (diverticular) abscess. (b) A needle has been introduced into the abscess. (c) The abscess has been aspirated.

the stomach for percutaneous feeding gastrostomy and percutaneous pancreatic cystogastrostomy [20,21], various systemic arteries and veins for percutaneous placement of intravascular catheters [22,23] and even targeted nerve blocks for pain relief [24].

Percutaneous tumour ablation

Percutaneous ethanol injection has been used to treat hepatocellular carcinomas with encouraging survival rates [25,26], liver metastases for palliative purposes and is of proven value in reducing hormone output from parathyroid adenomas and functioning thyroid nodules [27–29]. Indeed, there is much current activity in exploring the potential for using ultrasound to guide various physical agents capable of local tissue destruction, e.g. radioactive seeds [30,31], laser fibres, microwave transducers, hypothermic probes, and so on, into tumours for therapeutic purposes.

Conclusion

Interventional ultrasound is a rapidly expanding field. Advances in technology have led to improved imaging, more accurate diagnosis and better visualization of needles. The increasing portability of ultrasound equipment means that procedures can be performed on sick patients at the bedside or in the intensive care unit. Progress in the wider field of interventional radiology has resulted in improved needle and catheter design, and to the increasing acceptance of, and demand for, guided interventional procedures.

Other applications of interventional ultrasound include needle guidance by intracavitary probes (transrectal, transvaginal, transgastric, etc.) for biopsies, aspirations and drainages (Fig. 29.10) [32–34], and by intraoperative probes for liver, pancreatic and other visceral punctures.

There can be no doubt that the ingenuity and inventiveness of ultrasonologists worldwide will ensure continuing expansion of this exciting and rewarding field.

References

1 Lindgren, P.G. (1982) Percutaneous needle biopsy. A new technique. *Acta Radiologica. Diagnosis* **23**, 653–656.
2 Ubhi, C.S., Irving, H.C., Guillou, P.J., Giles, G.R. (1987) A new technique for renal allograft biopsy. *British Journal of Radiology* **60**, 599–600.
3 Riley, S.A., Ellis, W.R., Irving, H.C., Lintott, D.J., Axon, A.T.R., Losowsky, M.S. (1984) Percutaneous liver biopsy with plugging of needle track: a safe method for use in patients with impaired coagulation *Lancet* **ii**, 436.
4 Smith, E.H. (1991) Complications of percutaneous abdominal fine-needle biopsy. *Radiology* **178**, 253–258.
5 Solbiati, L., Livraghi, T., De Pra, L., Ierace, T., Masciadri, N., Ravetto, C. (1983) Fine-needle biopsy of hepatic haemangioma with sonographic guidance. *American Journal of Roentgenology* **144**, 471–474.
6 Casola, G., Nicolet, V., van Sonnenberg, E., *et al.* (1986) Unsuspected phaeochromocytoma: risk of blood pressure alterations during percutaneous adrenal biopsy. *Radiology* **159**, 733–735.
7 Ferucci, J.T., Wittenberg, J., Margolies, M.N., Carey, R.W. (1979) Malignant seeding of the tract after thin-needle aspiration biopsy. *Radiology* **130**, 345–346.
8 Smith, F.P., Macdonald, J.S., Schein, P.S., Ornitz, R.D. (1980) Cutaneous seeding of pancreatic cancer by skinny-needle aspiration biopsy. *Archives of Internal Medicine* **140**, 855.
9 Watkinson, A.F., Adam, A. (1994) Complications of abdominal and retroperitoneal biopsy. *Seminars in Interventional Radiology* **2**, 254–266.
10 Bean, W.J. (1981) Renal cysts: treatment with alcohol. *Radiology* **138**, 329–331.
11 Van Sonnenberg, E., Mueller, P.R., Ferucci, J.T. (1984) Percutaneous drainage of 250 abdominal abscesses and fluid collections. 1. Results, failures and complications. *Radiology* **151**, 337–341.
12 Gronvall, S., Gammelgaard, J., Haubek, A., Holm, H.H. (1982) Drainage of abdominal abscesses guided by sonography. *American Journal of Roentgenology* **138**, 527–529.
13 Mueller, P.R., Van Sonnenberg, E., Ferucci, J.T. (1984) Percutaneous drainage of 250 abdominal abscesses and fluid collections. 2. Procedural concepts. *Radiology* **151**, 343–347.
14 Berger, L.A., Osborne, D.R. (1982) Treatment of pyogenic liver abscesses by percutaneous needle aspiration. *Lancet* **i**, 132–134.
15 Farges, O., Leese, T., Bismuth, H. (1988) Pyogenic liver abscess: an improvement in prognosis. *British Journal of Surgery* **75**, 862–865.
16 Lambiase, R.G., Deyoe, L., Cronan, J.J., Dorfman, G.S. (1992) Percutaneous drainage of 335 consecutive abscesses: results of primary drainage with 1-year follow-up *Radiology* **184**, 167–179.
17 Irving, H.C., Arthur, R.J., Thomas, D.F.M. (1987) Percutaneous nephrostomy in paediatrics. *Clinical Radiology* **38**, 245–249.
18 Stafford Johnson, D., Mueller, P.R., Varghese, J., Lee, M.J. (1996) Percutaneous cholecystostomy: a review. *Journal of Interventional Radiology* **11**, 1–8.
19 Boland, G.W., Lee, M.J., Leung, J., *et al.* (1994) Percutaneous cholecystostomy in critically ill patients: early response and final outcome in 82 patients. *American Journal of Roentgenology* **162**, 339–342.
20 Hancke, S., Henriksen, W.F. (1985) Percutaneous pancreatic cystogastrostomy guided by ultrasound scanning and gastroscopy. *British Journal of Surgery* **72**, 916–917.
21 Sacks, B., Greenberg, J.J., Porter, H.D., *et al.* (1989) An internalised double-J catheter for percutaneous transgastric cystogastrostomy. *American Journal of Roentgenology* **152**, 523–526.
22 Machi, J., Takeda, J., Kakegawa, T. (1987) Safe jugular and subclavian venipuncture under ultrasonographic guidance. *American Journal of Surgery* **153**, 321–323.
23 Nolsøe, C., Nielsen, L., Karstrup, S., Lauritsen, L. (1989) Ultrasonically guided subclavian vein catheterisation. *Acta Radiologica* **30**, 108–109.
24 Das, K.M., Chapman, A.H. (1992) Sonographically guided coeliac plexus block. *Clinical Radiology* **45**, 401–403.

25 Livraghi, T., Festi, D., Monti, F., Salmi, A., Vettori, C. (1986) US-guided percutaneous alcohol injection of hepatic and abdominal tumours. *Radiology* **161**, 309–312.

26 Ebara, M., Ohto, M., Sugiura, N., *et al.* (1990) Percutaneous ethanol injection for the treatment of small hepatocellular carcinoma. Study of 95 patients. *Gastroenterology* **5**, 616–618.

27 Solbiati, L., Gigrande, A., De Pra, L., *et al.* (1985) Percutaneous ethanol injection of parathyroid tumours under US guidance: treatment for secondary hyperparathyroidism. *Radiology* **155**, 607–610.

28 Karstrup, S., Holm, H.H., Torp-Pedersen, S., Hegedus, L. (1987) Ultrasonically guided percutaneous inactivation of parathyroid tumours. *British Journal of Radiology* **60**, 667–670.

29 Karstrup, S., Transbøl, I., Holm, H.H., Glenthøj, A., Hegedüs, L. (1989) Ultrasound-guided chemical parathyroidectomy in patients with primary hyperparathyroidism: a prospective study. *British Journal of Radiology* **62**, 1037–1042.

30 Holm, H.H., Strøyer, I., Hansen, H., Stadil, F. (1981) Ultrasonically guided percutaneous interstitial implantation of iodine 125 seeds in cancer therapy. *British Journal of Radiology* **54**, 665–670.

31 Holm, H.H., Juul, N., Pedersen, J.F., Hansen, H., Strøyer, I. (1983) Transperineal ^{125}I seed implantation in prostatic cancer guided by transrectal ultrasonography. *Journal of Urology* **130**, 283–286.

32 Nosher, J.L., Winchman, H.K., Needell, G.S. (1987) Transvaginal pelvic abscess drainage with US guidance. *Radiology* **165**, 872–873.

33 Carmody, E., Thurston, W., Yeung, E., *et al.* (1993) Transrectal drainage of deep pelvic collections. *Journal of Canadian Association of Radiologists* **44**, 429–433.

34 van Sonnenberg, E., A'Agostino, H.B., Casola, G., *et al.* (1991) US-guided transvaginal drainage of pelvic abscesses and fluid collections. *Radiology* **181**, 53–56.

Chapter 30: The kidneys

P.L.P. Allan & S.A. Moussa

Anatomy

The kidneys are retroperitoneal organs lying in the paravertebral fossae. The superoinferior axes are orientated with the lower ends lying more anteriorly and laterally than the upper ends; in addition, the mediolateral axes lie at approximately 45° to the coronal plane so that the anterior surfaces face anterolaterally and the posterior surfaces face posteromedially. The hilum of the right kidney usually lies about 1.5 cm lower than the left hilum; the exact level of the kidneys, however, varies with respiration as both kidneys move down with inspiration, the amount of movement is normally less than 2.5 cm.

The kidneys are surrounded by perirenal fat, which is separated from the anterior and posterior pararenal spaces by the anterior and posterior renal fascia. The fascia layers and peritoneal spaces are not normally visible on ultrasound but they may affect the appearances and spread of fluid or inflammatory processes in and around the kidneys.

In the adult the normal kidneys are usually between 10 and 12 cm in length but can range from 7 cm up to 14 cm in individuals with normal renal function [1]. The size of the kidneys increases steadily from birth; after the first year, this is at a rate of approximately 5 mm for each 10 cm increase in height, or about 2–3 mm year^{-1}.

The kidney is surrounded and contained by a thin capsule, the cortex forms the outer component of the renal parenchyma and surrounds the more centrally placed medullary pyramids. These are arranged around the central renal sinus which contains the main blood vessels and collecting system surrounded by fat. The renal pelvis is usually contained mainly within the renal substance but it can project out of the kidney to a variable extent.

The renal vessels divide into segmental branches which lie in front and behind the renal pelvis at the hilum. These segmental branches divide into interlobar branches, which run out towards the periphery between the lobules; finally, the interlobular branches divide and form the arcuate vessels which run across the bases of adjacent medullary pyramids, parallel to the capsule.

Technique

Access

Ultrasonic examination of the kidneys begins with the patient supine. The right kidney is examined from an anterolateral or lateral approach, using the liver as an acoustic window. The kidney is examined initially in the longitudinal plane and then in the transverse plane. It is important to check both planes as peripheral lesions may be missed by a cursory examination in the longitudinal plane only. In addition to assessing the shape, size and echogenicity of the kidney, some attention should be paid to the perirenal areas and the movement of the kidney relative to the liver and other adjacent structures during respiration as some processes, such as inflammation, may affect motion; furthermore, examination at different phases of respiration may allow visualization of portions of the kidney which are partially obscured. If the right kidney cannot be visualized adequately from an anterolateral approach, then further access should be sought through more posterior scan planes.

The left kidney is more difficult to see clearly as the spleen does not normally provide as big an acoustic window as the right lobe of the liver. It is best approached from a lateral or posterolateral scan plane with the patient lying in a left anterior oblique position. Once again, alteration of renal position in different phases of respiration may improve visualization. If this approach is unsuccessful imaging may be achieved by turning the patient prone, or into the right decubitus position with a pillow under the hip and the left arm raised over the head in order to open up the intercostal and subcostal spaces.

Small, chronically diseased kidneys may be difficult to distinguish from surrounding tissues, especially on the left. Careful observation during quiet respiration may allow distinction of the kidney moving in perirenal tissues.

Measuring the size of the kidneys

One of the common indications for ultrasound examinations of the kidneys is the request for an assessment of their size. The simplest measurement is renal length; this is found by scanning the kidney along its long, craniocaudal axis and measuring the longest length found. Care must be taken as, due to the ellipsoidal shape of the organ, it is easy to measure an incorrect, short dimension, despite seeing an apparently satisfactory renal outline. However, with care and attention, measurements which are reproducible to within 10% can be achieved [2]. Although renal lengths between people may vary, the lengths of an individual's kidneys do not normally vary by more than a centimetre.

The renal volume can also be estimated using ultrasound. Various methods for estimating the volume of the kidneys have been proposed but the most straightforward is the use of a modified formula for an ellipsoid: length × transverse diameter × anteroposterior diameter × 0.5 [3]. The normal values for adult kidneys are also variable but are typically 145 cm^3 on the left and 135 cm^3 on the right [1]. It should be noted that renal size normally increases during pregnancy, the length by approximately 7 mm and the volume by about 80–90 cm^3 between the 12th and 36th weeks [4].

Some estimate of renal parenchymal thickness can be made. Again this can be very variable, especially in the elderly, but a value of less than 12–15 mm is suggestive of significant parenchymal loss [5].

Biopsy and fine-needle aspiration of the kidneys

Real-time ultrasound allows accurate placing of needles in the kidney in order to retrieve material for cytology (fine needle aspiration or FNA) or histology (biopsy). For FNA the most direct safe route between the skin and the lesion is chosen; with the patient in an appropriate position, a 20- or 22-gauge needle is directed, under ultrasound control, into the area of interest. It is desirable to avoid adjacent structures such as the colon or spleen, and care should be taken not to produce a pneumothorax when aspirating upper pole lesions. Occasionally it may be necessary to approach right-sided lesions through the liver and care must be taken not to tear or damage this organ.

Biopsy is usually undertaken with the patient lying prone and a pillow under the stomach to compress the kidneys posteriorly. Either kidney can be sampled, depending on various factors including the symptoms, ease of access, the presence of cysts or collecting system dilatation. An 18-gauge needle normally provides adequate diagnostic material with three to four passes and samples are sent for light microscopy, electron microscopy and immunofluorescence [6]. Careful thought should be given to the necessity of aspiration or biopsy of solid renal lesions as most of these will require surgical removal and there is a small, but real, risk of needle track seeding of tumour which will adversely affect the prognosis, this is less likely with smaller needles.

Normal appearances

Parenchyma

The three main components of the kidney which can be identified on ultrasound are the cortex, the medullary pyramids and the renal sinus (Fig. 30.1). The outer margin of the cortex is well defined due to the presence of the renal capsule but the inner margin is more irregular due to the medullary pyramids and renal sinus.

The echogenicity of the cortex used to be described as less than that of adjacent liver but modern equipment and signal processing make this distinction less valid and normal cortex may be equal to, or slightly more echogenic than, the liver. In the neonate the renal cortex is generally more echogenic than in the adult due to the different, more complex histological structure found at this stage of renal development. Echogenicity which is significantly greater than that of the liver in an adult or older child is, however, an indicator of parenchymal disease.

The medullary pyramids have a lower echogenicity than the cortex and appear as darker, round or triangular areas uniformly arranged in the deeper part of the parenchyma around, and distinct from, the renal sinus [7]. Some pathological processes accentuate this corticomedullary differentiation, whilst others make it less distinct. In some subjects the interlobular and arcuate arteries may be distinguished as echogenic foci adjacent to the

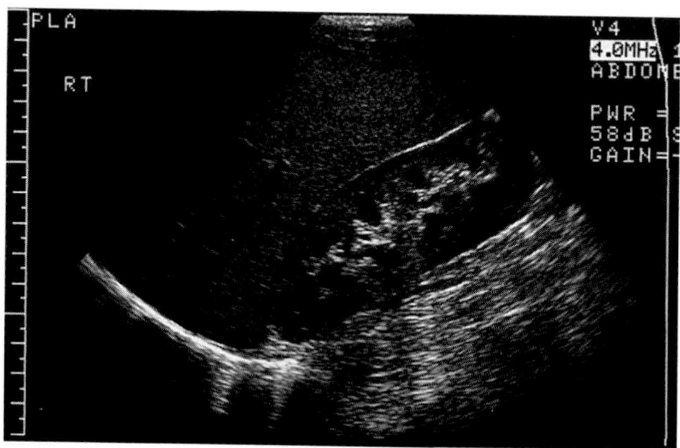

Fig. 30.1 Longitudinal view of normal right kidney.

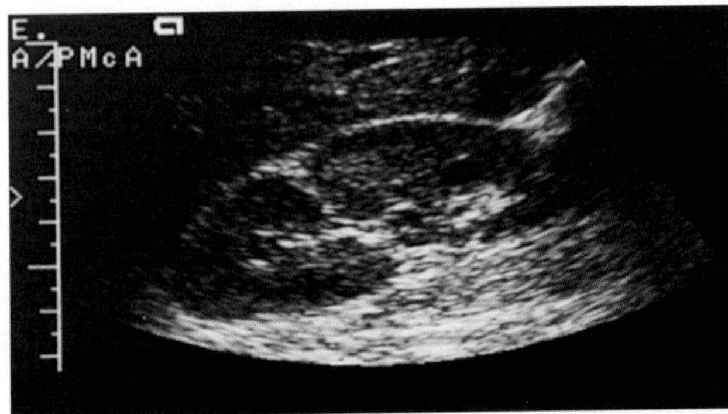

Fig. 30.2 The 'junctional line'.

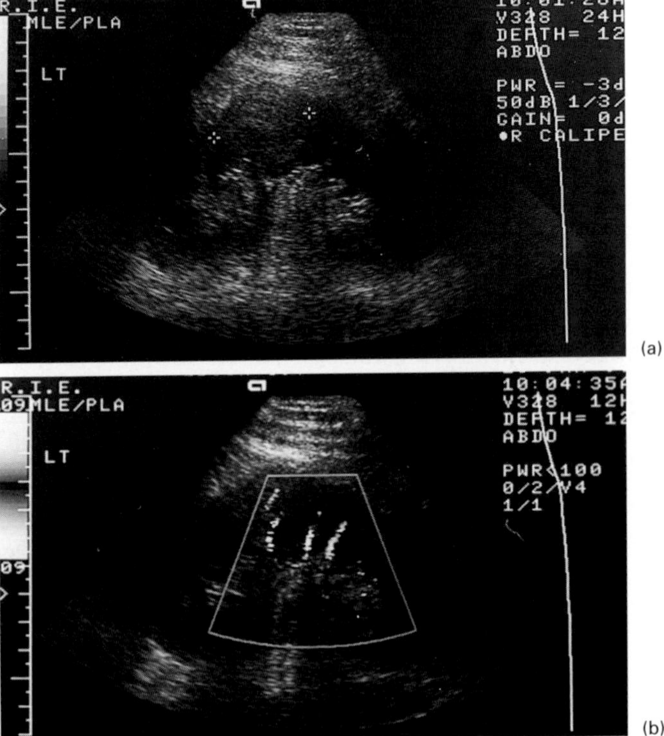

Fig. 30.3 (a) A splenic hump. (b) Colour Doppler shows normally disposed vessels.

medullary pyramids, their vascular nature can be confirmed using Doppler.

A thin echogenic line is sometimes seen running from the anteromedial cortex to the hilum (Fig. 30.2). This has been called the junctional parenchymal defect and was thought to represent a plane of fusion between two 'renunculi' which joined together to form the kidney but more detailed studies suggest that this appearance is due simply to an extension of sinus fat into the parenchyma when the sinus is lying in a deep position [8]. The main importance of this appearance is that it should not be mistaken for cortical scarring.

The renal sinus and collecting system

The renal sinus is made up of the collecting system, the renal arteries, the renal veins and fat; it is seen as an echogenic region due to the fat around the vessels and collecting system. The amount of fat can vary, tending to increase in some circumstances such as obesity and steroid therapy. There is also a relative increase in the size of the central echo complex with age, this is due to a degree of atrophy of the parenchyma, rather than an increase in the amount of sinus adipose tissue [1].

The main vessels can be distinguished as they pass through the sinus. In some individuals, especially children, the relative prominence of the larger vessels may suggest a degree of dilatation of the collecting system; this can be excluded using colour Doppler.

The collecting system is not usually visible in normal subjects but may be seen if there is a diuresis, especially if the bladder is full for a pelvic ultrasound examination. Part of the renal pelvis may lie outside the kidney to a variable degree; if this is a significant portion then it may be mistaken for a parapelvic cyst if it is not recognized. In pregnancy the collecting systems can dilate significantly, particularly on the right. This is thought to be due to a combination of circumstances: a degree of obstruction produced by the enlarging uterus, hormonal changes resulting in decreased smooth muscle tone and increased renal blood flow [9].

Humps, lobulations and columns of Bertin

The renal parenchymal margin is normally a smooth, curved shape but some normal variations should be recognized and not mistaken for pathological changes. Fetal lobulation produces irregularity of the parenchyma which may be mistaken for cortical scarring. The distinguishing feature of fetal lobulation is that the indentations of the cortex lie between the medullary pyramids, whereas in scarring they lie adjacent to them and there is an associated loss of parenchymal thickness [7].

The spleen is related closely to the left kidney and pressure from it on the developing kidney may result in the formation of a 'splenic hump'. This can mimic a tumour but careful scanning will show an extension of the sinus echoes into the 'hump' and the parenchymal thickness is seen not to be increased. Colour or power Doppler show a normal distribution of vessels (Fig. 30.3).

The columns, or septa, of Bertin are produced by the fusion of adjacent portions of cortex as the fetal lobules fuse. Normally they do not stand out but occasionally they may be unduly prominent, to the extent that

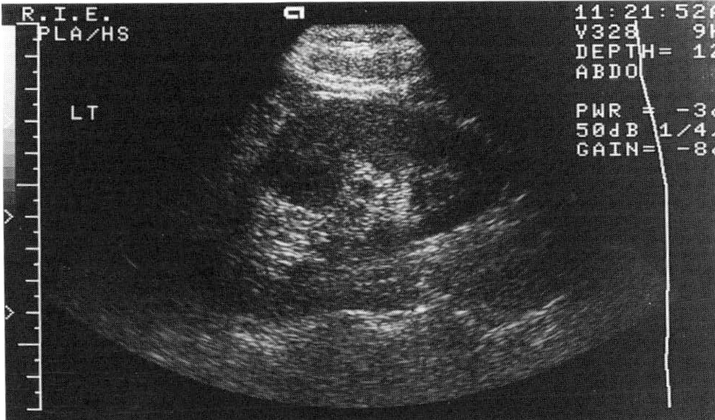

Fig. 30.4 A prominent column of Bertin.

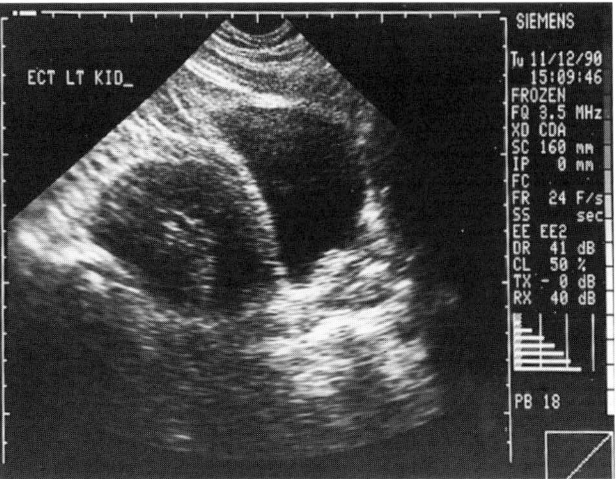

Fig. 30.5 Part of an ectopic left kidney, lying above a partly filled bladder.

they simulate a tumour (Fig. 30.4). Careful examination will show that the parenchymal surface is not distorted by the 'mass' and that the echogenicity is the same as adjacent cortex; echoes from the sinus may be seen enveloping the septum [10].

Congenital abnormalities

Agenesis and hypoplasia

The distinction between hypoplasia and atrophy can be difficult to make. Many 'congenital' hypoplastic kidneys are the result of damage sustained during fetal life rather than following birth. The size of the renal vessels may give a clue as vessels which are relatively large in relation to the kidney suggest atrophy rather than hypoplasia; similarly, parenchymal scarring and dilatation of the collecting system indicate previous pathological problems.

Agenesis is relatively common, being found in 1 in 100 autopsies although detected clinically in only about 1 in 1500 patients [11]; it is found more commonly on the left side. A loop of colon may lie in the empty renal fossa and mimic the appearance of a kidney if it is not recognized—a 'pseudokidney'; this may also be seen following nephrectomy. Compensatory hypertrophy of the opposite kidney is seen in patients with agenesis; if this is not present then an ectopic kidney should be sought.

Ectopic locations

Ectopic kidneys are also more common on the left side and may be found anywhere between the renal fossa and pelvis (Fig. 30.5). They may be recognized by their renal structure but pelvic kidneys may be more difficult to define as they can develop with unusual shapes. The ectopic kidney may lie on the contralateral side of the abdomen, in which case it is nearly always fused to the other kidney—crossed, fused renal ectopia.

Horseshoe kidneys

Horseshoe kidney is found in 1 in 425 autopsies and is the commonest fusion abnormality of the urinary tract [12]. The two kidneys are joined by a band, or isthmus, of tissue between their lower poles which can vary from a thin, fibrous band to a full-thickness mass of parenchyma. On ultrasound the long axes of the kidneys are seen to be orientated in a more vertical angle, with the lower poles lying more medially than usual and the kidneys may have a distinctive inverted triangular or pyramidal shape [13]. The isthmus may be seen as it crosses in front of the aorta if it is of sufficient bulk and not obscured by bowel gas (Fig. 30.6). The collecting systems of the kidneys are orientated in a more sagittal plane than normal.

Duplex systems

Duplex systems may be identified on ultrasound if there is sufficient splitting of the intrarenal collecting system for the two components to be recognized. The renal sinus echoes are split into two sections by a bridge of parenchymal tissue (Fig. 30.7) but the two ureters cannot normally be identified unless one, or both, is dilated.

Nephroptosis

The degree of vertical movement of the kidneys is normally less than 2.5 cm but more marked degrees of movement are sometimes seen [14]. The significance of nephroptosis in relation to symptoms is still a matter of discussion; medial movement may be of more clinical relevance than vertical motion. Vertical movement can be

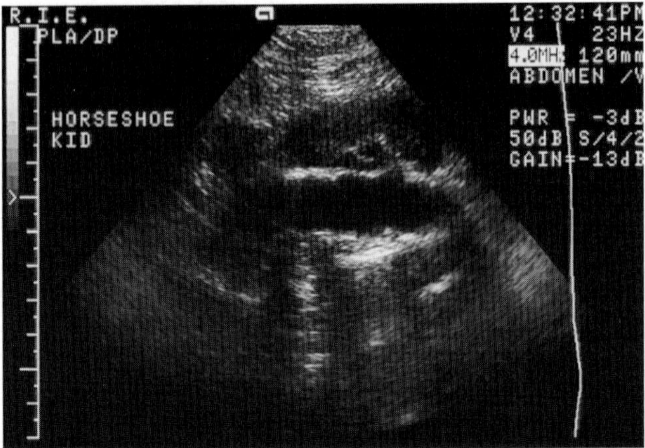

(a)

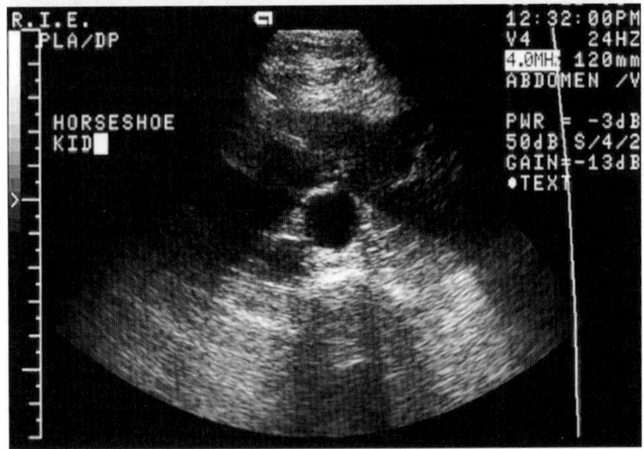

(b)

Fig. 30.6 (a) Longitudinal view of a horseshoe kidney lying in front of the aorta. (b) Transverse view of the same kidney.

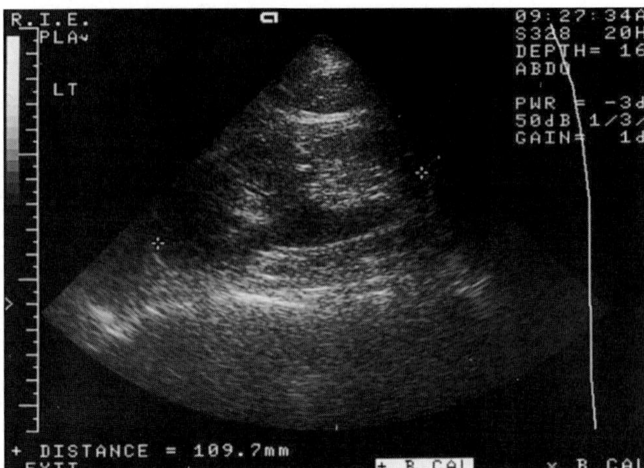

Fig. 30.7 A duplex collecting system showing the sinus echo split by a bridge of parenchyma.

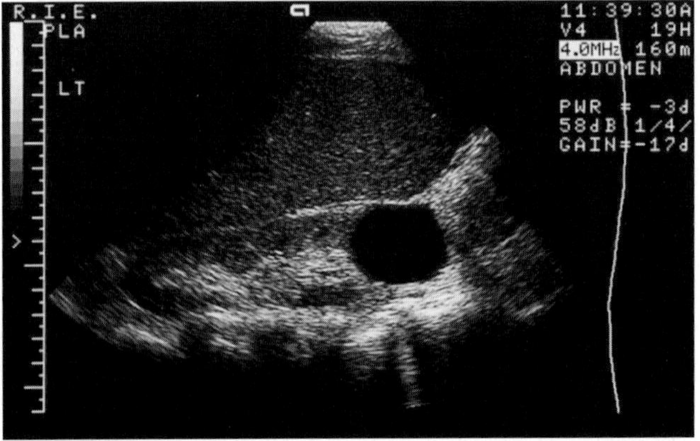

Fig. 30.8 A simple renal cyst at the lower pole of the left kidney in a patient with splenomegaly.

assessed by scanning in the prone and erect positions and relating the kidney to a fixed bony landmark, such as the 12th rib, or the lumbar transverse processes. Medial movement can be assessed by scanning in the supine and decubitus positions and relating the position of the kidney to the spine or the aorta.

Renal cysts

Several classifications of renal cystic lesions have been proposed. The main practical diagnostic problem in assessing renal cysts with ultrasound is to separate those which are simple and benign, which can be left alone, from those which are not simple and require further investigation or surgery. Bosniak has proposed four categories of cysts [15]: (a) uncomplicated, benign, simple cysts; (b) minimally complicated cysts, which have only one or two features that cause concern; (c) lesions which are more complex, in which malignancy cannot be excluded; and (d) lesions which are clearly malignant.

Simple renal cysts

These are common findings on abdominal ultrasound examinations; prevalence and size increase with age. They are usually incidental findings but may be symptomatic if they produce obstruction, become infected or develop a haemorrhage. The criteria for diagnosis of a simple cyst on ultrasound are well defined: they should be anechoic, have sharply marginated, smooth walls, with good through sound transmission giving distal acoustic enhancement (Fig. 30.8) [15]. Providing all these criteria are met then a simple renal cyst can be diagnosed with a high degree of accuracy. The presence of a single thin septum, or a minor indentation of the wall by an adjacent vessel, do not significantly affect the diagnosis of a simple cyst. However, multiple septae, or obvious thickenings and irregularities of the wall must be treated with suspicion. Cysts arising near the renal pelvis may sometimes simulate a dilated collecting system and careful scanning is required to make the distinction.

Complicated cysts

Infection or haemorrhage can lead to changes in the appearance of cysts with the presence of internal echoes, calcification in the wall and solid components due to pus or blood clot. In these circumstances distinction from a tumour can be difficult or impossible and further imaging is required. Diagnostic cyst puncture may also be helpful but the interpretation of the findings must be treated with care [15]. Hydatid cysts can be found in the kidneys and the appearance may be non-specific. However, the presence of daughter cysts within the cyst, together with calcification in the wall may give a clue to the true nature of the lesion.

Occasionally a cystic lesion is due to neoplasia. Necrosis and degeneration can result in a cystic lesion but the irregularity of the margins and internal echoes will usually indicate that it is not a simple cyst. Cystadenocarcinomas may be unilocular or multilocular, these are cystic lesions with areas of solid tumour lying between the cystic areas and their complex nature is usually apparent [16]. The development of carcinoma in simple cysts is very uncommon.

Polycystic kidney disease

INFANTILE POLYCYSTIC KIDNEY DISEASE (AUTOSOMAL RECESSIVE)

The kidneys are enlarged, with increased echogenicity and loss of corticomedullary differentiation. Tiny cysts (<5 mm) may be identified and dilated tubules distinguished amongst them [17]. An hypoechoic rim may be discerned around the margin of the kidney which is thought to represent residual renal cortex.

AUTOSOMAL DOMINANT POLYCYSTIC KIDNEY DISEASE

This presents clinically in adult life, usually after the third decade; although cysts can be detected earlier in teenagers, children and neonates. There have also been reports of cysts being detected *in utero*. By the time of clinical presentation the kidneys show the typical changes of enlargement, multiple cysts of variable size, no visible residual renal cortex and the renal sinus is not distinguished (Fig. 30.9). Screening of relatives may show earlier stages of the disease with variable numbers of cysts and varying degrees of renal enlargement; in younger patients the presence of cysts, with at least two in one kidney is strongly suggestive of autosomal dominant polycystic kidney disease [18]. Some 30–50% of patients do not have a relevant family history.

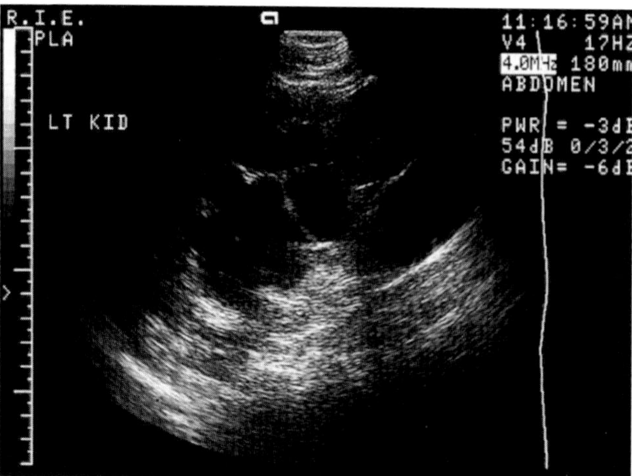

Fig. 30.9 Autosomal dominant polycystic kidney disease.

Hepatic cysts are seen in approximately 50% of patients; pancreatic cysts and splenic cysts may also be seen in a small proportion of patients. Cystic changes are occasionally seen in other organs such as the testis and ovary.

The cysts in autosomal dominant polycystic kidney disease can become infected or bleed. Ultrasonic examination may show echoes within a cyst but distinguishing a single complicated cyst in these patients can be extremely difficult.

Other congenital cysts

MULTICYSTIC DYSPLASTIC KIDNEY

The typical form of this condition is the result of ureteric atresia in early fetal life. It presents as a mass in the abdomen of the child, occasionally it may be discovered in adulthood. On ultrasound the kidney is replaced by a mass of multiple cysts of variable size. The condition is usually unilateral but the contralateral kidney may sometimes show an anomaly, usually ureteropelvic obstruction. A second form of the disorder is known as the hydronephrotic form of the condition in which dilatation of the collecting system may be distinguished amongst the cysts as the condition results from incomplete ureteric obstruction occurring later in fetal life [19]. Affected kidneys atrophy with age and, in the adult, may appear small and atrophic; calcification may develop in the cyst walls.

MEDULLARY CYSTIC DISEASE

This presents in children or young adults, usually with signs of renal failure. The kidneys are small, echogenic and there are small cysts present, especially in the medulla [20]. The condition is also referred to as juvenile nephronophthisis.

MISCELLANEOUS RENAL CYSTS

Various conditions are associated with cysts in the kidneys. These include Conradi's disease, Zellweger's syndrome (cerebrohepatorenal syndrome), orofaciodigital syndrome, Laurence–Moon–Biedl syndrome, Jeune's syndrome, tuberose sclerosis, glomerulocystic renal disease and some of the trisomies.

Acquired cystic disease of the kidneys

Acquired cystic disease of the kidney is seen in patients with end-stage renal failure, or who are on dialysis. The changes are more marked with increasing duration of haemodialysis but are also seen in continuous ambulatory peritoneal dialysis patients [21]. Multiple small cysts and adenomas develop in the native kidneys of these patients and can be identified with ultrasound (Fig. 30.10), although distinction between small cysts and adenomas may not be possible. In addition there is a small risk of carcinoma developing and this should be considered in any dialysis patient who develops renal pain or haemorrhage in relation to their native kidneys. There is some evidence that a successful transplant will lead to reversal of these changes.

Renal tumours

Benign

ANGIOMYOLIPOMA

Angiomyolipomas are hamartomatous lesions which contain varying amounts of fat, smooth muscle and blood vessels; there is an association with tuberose sclerosis, particularly if they are multiple. Their appearance on ultrasound varies, depending on the relative amounts of the component tissues, and the presence of haemorrhage, necrosis or calcification; if there is sufficient fat present then the typical, well-defined, echogenic lesion is seen (Fig. 30.11). However, a spectrum of appearances may be seen making diagnosis on ultrasound in these circumstances difficult [22]. The typical echogenic appearance is suggestive but not diagnostic as, rarely, a carcinoma can have a similar echogenicity. Computed tomography (CT) is of value in confirming the presence of fat within the lesion, although very occasionally larger adenocarcinomas and oncocytomas can contain areas of fat due to the inclusion of sinus fat by the expanding tumour.

ONCOCYTOMA

Oncocytomas are solid tumours of the kidney which are pathologically distinctive due to their granular, eosinophilic cytoplasm packed with mitochondria. They can grow to a large size and may be locally invasive but very rarely metastasize. It may be difficult to distinguish them from carcinoma on ultrasound but the identification of a central, stellate or 'spoke-wheel' arrangement of hypoechoic or low attenuation bands on ultrasound or CT,

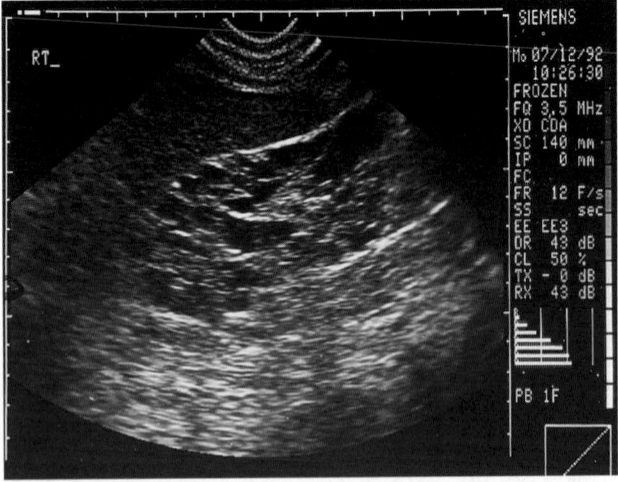

Fig. 30.10 Acquired cystic disease of the kidney, multiple small cysts throughout the kidney.

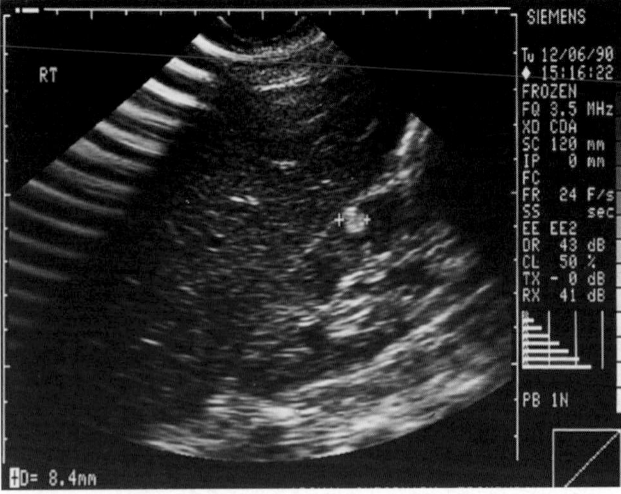

Fig. 30.11 A small angiomyolipoma in the cortex of a kidney.

particularly in larger tumours, provides a clue to their nature [23].

ADENOMA

Benign adenomas are relatively common findings at autopsy and are being detected more frequently in life by improved imaging techniques such as ultrasound and CT. They are also associated with acquired cystic disease of the kidney. It is not possible to distinguish benign from malignant lesions on imaging on the grounds of size or characteristics and histological distinction is also often impossible [24].

Malignant

ADENOCARCINOMA

This is the commonest malignant neoplasm of the kidneys. They are usually solid, isoechoic or relatively hypoechoic lesions arising from the cortex (Fig. 30.12); however, hyperechoic and cystic appearances may also be seen. Smaller lesions tend to have a uniform internal structure but larger lesions may undergo necrotic or haemorrhagic changes which result in inhomogeneity of the lesion [25]. Some lesions have a significant cystic component and, in a few cases, distinction from simple cysts may be difficult; any irregularity or thickening of a cyst margin, or solid components in the wall should arouse suspicion of malignancy (Fig. 30.13). Tumours will distort the renal outline if they are large enough but some small tumours may not produce any distinct disruption of the renal shape. The margins of the lesion are often well defined in smaller lesions but in larger masses they may be indistinct, both in relation to any residual renal tissue and to perirenal fat. Calcification may be detected within the lesion in a small number of cases.

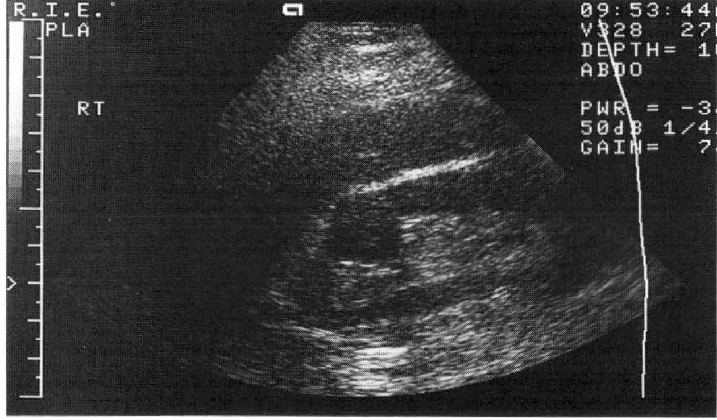

Fig. 30.12 Carcinoma of the kidney in the upper pole.

Lesions vary in size at the time of detection: some are very large by the time symptoms appear and investigations are commenced; others declare themselves earlier, when they are still relatively small; some are detected as an incidental finding during examinations for other disorders. The size of the lesion has no relevance to the likelihood of malignancy; solid lesions less than 3 cm are sometimes considered to be 'adenomas' with low malignant potential but this is a false distinction and all solid renal lesions which are not obviously an angiomyolipoma, metastasis or lymphoma deposit should be considered as potential carcinomas and treated accordingly [24].

Some 70% of renal tumours are sufficiently vascular for abnormal blood flow signals to be detected by Doppler [26]. The signals obtained are of high peak frequency (>2.5 kHz), and broad spectrum. Inflammatory masses may also show similar characteristics, therefore Doppler findings are useful but not diagnostic indicators of the likelihood of malignancy.

Renal carcinomas can spread to the renal vein and thence to the inferior vena cava. Tumour thrombus may be seen in the veins and as this progresses the vein becomes swollen and filled by the tumour within it. This can extend into the inferior vena cava and sometimes up to the right atrium. Colour Doppler makes the diagnosis of venous involvement more straightforward. Tumours may also spread to perirenal tissues and structures; this may be apparent on the image but fixation of the kidney on respiration may be a sign of local invasion. Spread to the liver and to the hilar and para-aortic lymph nodes can occur and should be sought on ultrasound, although this is less sensitive than CT for the detection of nodal disease and perirenal spread.

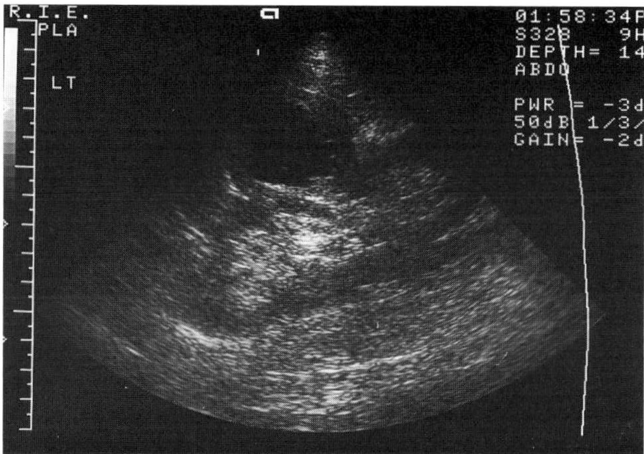

Fig. 30.13 A cystic neoplasm showing an irregular, thickened wall and some low level echoes within the 'cyst'.

WILMS' TUMOUR

This is the commonest abdominal tumour in neonates and children, presenting as an abdominal mass, which may be large. Ultrasound shows a solid renal mass, which has an even echogenicity with small cysts within the mass corresponding to areas of cystic degeneration [27].

Multilocular cystic nephroma is a benign tumour which is found in children and, very rarely, in adults. It is considered by some authors to be a benign form of Wilms' tumour, but this is not accepted universally. There are no specific features to distinguish it from other multicystic lesions on ultrasound [28].

TRANSITIONAL CELL CARCINOMA

These may be recognized as masses within the collecting system (Fig. 30.14), especially if this is dilated; solid masses within the renal sinus echoes will also suggest this diagnosis [29]. Larger lesions are indistinguishable from other renal tumours. Very rarely small transitional cell tumours may mimic renal calculi due to relatively large amounts of keratin within them.

LYMPHOMA

Primary lymphoma of the kidney is rare; secondary involvement, usually by non-Hodgkin's lymphoma, can occur. Deposits are usually focal, multiple and hypoechoic [24]; diffuse infiltration of the parenchyma and renal sinus is also seen and this may be associated with general enlargement of the kidneys.

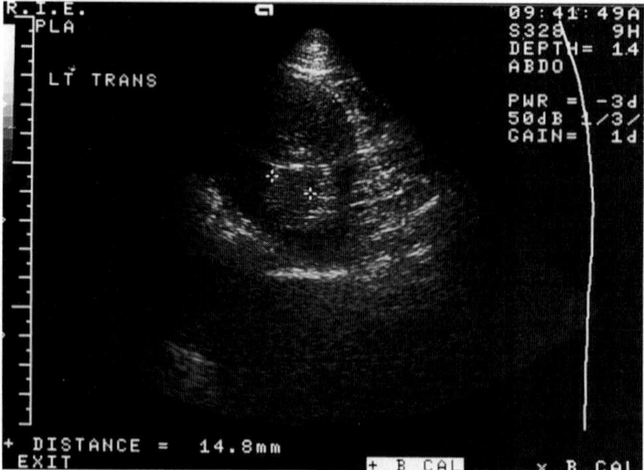

Fig. 30.14 Transverse view of a kidney showing an ill-defined 1.4 cm transitional cell carcinoma.

OTHER MALIGNANT TUMOURS

Secondary deposits are seen on occasion. There are no particular diagnostic features but the clinical situation may suggest the diagnosis if there is a known primary tumour. Rarely a solitary metastasis may be found in the kidney and aspiration/biopsy will be required to ascertain its nature.

Primary sarcomas are rare tumours of the kidney and have no specific features which allow differentiation from other solid renal malignancies.

Trauma

Kidneys can suffer trauma in various situations: blunt, crushing injuries are the most common, occurring in sports injuries, falls, car accidents, assaults, and so on; penetrating injuries from knife wounds or bullets; and deceleration injuries from car accidents. Iatrogenic trauma from percutaneous procedures must also be considered as a cause of renal injury.

Trauma from blunt injury is classified according to the degree of trauma: parenchymal contusion and subcapsular haematoma; capsular laceration; deep laceration which communicates with the collecting system; and shattered or fractured kidney. In addition vascular and pedicle injuries can occur ranging from intimal dissection and haematoma to complete avulsion of the vessels and ureter [30].

Penetrating injuries can damage the parenchyma, capsule, vessels and collecting system leading to haematomas and urine collections, arteriovenous fistulae or vascular interruption. Bullet wounds will also produce a degree of more diffuse blast injury, depending on the velocity of the projectile. Most iatrogenic damage to the kidney results from penetrating injuries—biopsies, nephrostomies and stent placement can all damage the organ.

Imaging of patients with suspected renal trauma who do not require immediate surgery has been centred around intravenous urography, which provides information on function as well as structure, and CT with contrast enhancement, which images the kidneys and other abdominal organs, as well as providing information on tissue perfusion and renal function. Ultrasound, together with Doppler, will provide information on the renal parenchyma, perirenal collections and blood flow; it will also allow some assessment of other abdominal organs; it is generally more available than CT but may be limited by bowel gas or patient immobility. Ultrasound can be used for initial assessment of patients with renal trauma and is also of value in the follow-up of patients and confirming the resolution of collections [30,31].

Contusions are seen as focal areas of altered echogenicity in the parenchyma with an intact capsule; they are usually of predominantly lower echogenicity at first but show increased echogenicity with time after the injury. Subcapsular collections are crescentic in shape and the line of the renal capsule is not broken, although it may be displaced a little and there is compression of the underlying parenchyma. Capsular lacerations are usually associated with perirenal collections, the capsular laceration may, or may not be positively identified. Fragmented kidneys show separation of the component parts with haematoma and urine between and around them [31], ultrasound is unable to distinguish between blood and urine collections. Vascular occlusion as a result of vessel transection or intimal dissection and thrombosis will be detected if Doppler is used to assess arterial and venous circulation in the parenchyma or fragments. However, lesser degrees of intimal dissection which do not result in occlusion may be missed.

Penetrating injuries can produce perirenal collections but also arteriovenous fistulae and pseudoaneurysms, Doppler ultrasound is of value in the diagnosis and follow-up of these as it will demonstrate changes in the arterial and venous waveforms in the relevant vessels and colour Doppler may show the associated tissue bruit [32].

Dilatation and obstruction

Ultrasound is very sensitive at detecting dilatation of the renal collecting system and, in the appropriate clinical situation this allows a diagnosis of obstruction to be made. However, distinction between obstructed and non-obstructed kidneys may be difficult as the presence of dilatation does not always equate with obstruction [33]. A further problem in a small group of patients is that there may be significant obstruction with only minimal dilatation. Causes of dilatation without obstruction include pregnancy, postobstructive dilatation, chronic reflux, ileal loop diversions, and may be seen in normal patients with a full bladder undergoing diuresis—such as those having pelvic ultrasound examinations. Obstruction without marked dilatation may be seen in some cases of acute obstruction and in cases of retroperitoneal fibrosis.

Appearances

The diagnosis of dilatation is made by demonstrating the anechoic calyces and collecting system in the central part of the kidney (Fig. 30.15). A dilated collected system is recognized by the fact that the various components are seen to be in continuity. Focal dilatation of part of the collecting system may be seen in patients with duplex systems, usually the upper moiety is affected; or in cases where

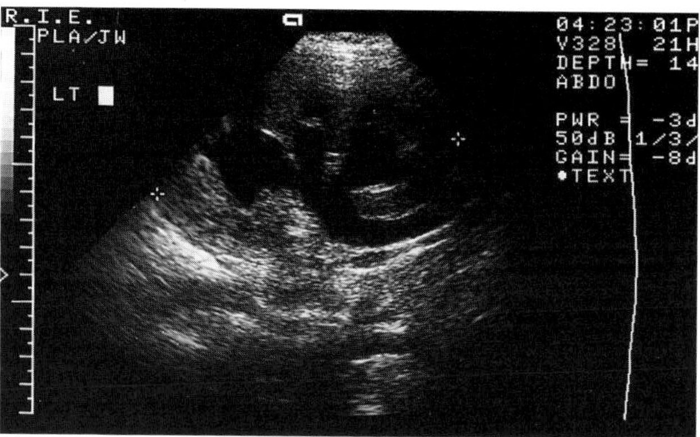

Fig. 30.15 The dilated collecting system and upper ureter in a patient with ureteric obstruction.

tumours, calculi or strictures have obstructed only part of the collecting system. Papillary necrosis and reflux may also result in dilatation of only part of the collecting system.

The main diagnostic problem is in distinguishing dilatation from central renal cysts; in these cases the cystic areas will not be in continuity and regions of normal renal sinus echoes may be seen. Minor degrees of dilatation may be simulated by prominent central vessels in some patients and colour Doppler allows rapid recognition of the vascular nature of these. The presence of echoes in a dilated collecting system suggests the presence of pyonephrosis or haemorrhage. Large staghorn calculi can obscure the dilated collecting system and lead to dilatation being overlooked if they are not recognized.

The parenchyma appears normal in acute obstruction, although renal size generally may be a little increased; in a small number of cases of acute obstruction the parenchyma may show a minor degree of thinning due to the high intrarenal pressure but returns to normal on relief of the obstruction. Cortical atrophy occurs with long-standing obstruction and in severe chronic cases no significant remaining cortex may be seen around the large dilated collecting system.

Once a diagnosis of obstruction has been reached a search should be made to try and identify the level and cause of the obstruction. Careful scanning of the retroperitoneal region may show a dilated ureter adjacent to the aorta or inferior vena cava. Large masses, such as lymph nodes, may be seen but ureteric calculi and small areas of retroperitoneal fibrosis are not usually identified. The ureter cannot usually be visualized as it passes into the pelvis due to overlying bowel gas but a dilated distal ureter may be seen behind a full bladder and a calculus, or other cause of obstruction identified. Pelvic and bladder tumours producing obstruction, or evidence of bladder outflow obstruction may also be seen.

Doppler ultrasound and obstruction

Doppler ultrasound is of value in reaching a diagnosis of obstruction in difficult cases as the resistance index is increased in the affected kidney: a resistance index greater than 0.7, or more than 0.1 higher than the other kidney, is strongly suggestive of obstruction [34]. However, the sequence of events in relation to blood flow following acute severe obstruction is complex and care should be taken in the interpretation of the resistance index in acute obstruction of less than 4–6 h, in young children and in the presence of diffuse renal disease, as it may be misleading in these cases.

Calculi and lithotripsy

Intrarenal calculi are seen well on ultrasound in many cases but small (<2 mm) stones and papillary stones can be missed in a third of cases [35,36]. Calculi are seen as echogenic foci which cast an acoustic shadow (Fig. 30.16), although the shadow may not be seen with tiny calculi [37]; conversely, large staghorn calculi can be overlooked in some cases as the acoustic shadowing may be less intense than expected. Ultrasound is also relatively poor at detecting the number of small calculi, or localizing them precisely within the calyces or parenchyma; plain radiographs of the renal areas are more accurate for assessing the size and number of renal stones.

Ureteric calculi are difficult to see with ultrasound. The larger part of the ureter is obscured by overlying bowel gas but calculi may be seen in the lower ureter behind the bladder, or in the upper ureter if there is dilatation. However, ultrasound and plain films together provide a sensitive technique for assessing patients with possible renal colic and some reports suggest that they provide an alternative to intravenous urogram in these patients [38]; however, others are less enthusiastic [39].

With the advent of lithotripsy for urinary tract calculi, ultrasound has gained an important role in the diagnosis, treatment and follow-up of patient presenting for stone management.

Lithotripsy

Lithotripsy is the disintegration of calculi using shock waves. These can be applied directly onto the stone, e.g. during percutaneous nephrolithotomy, or extracorporeally, e.g. extracorporeal shock wave lithotripsy (ESWL).

In ESWL the shock waves are generated by one of three mechanisms:

1 piezoelectric;
2 electrohydraulic; or
3 electromagnetic.

The early lithotriptors used one localization modality either ultrasound or fluoroscopy to focus the shock wave onto the stone. Modern lithotriptors operate dual localization systems [40,41].

The majority of renal and upper ureteric calculi as well as calculi at the vesicoureteric junction (VUJ) can be easily visualized with ultrasound (Figs 30.17, 30.18). Those in the mid ureter generally require fluoroscopic localization.

Very small calculi <2 mm in diameter particularly when associated with other echogenic structures such as scars, arcuate arteries or a bright parenchyma can be difficult to visualize with ultrasound. Difficulties can also arise in the presence of renal cysts adjacent to the calyces harbouring the calculus or when the collecting system is very dilated.

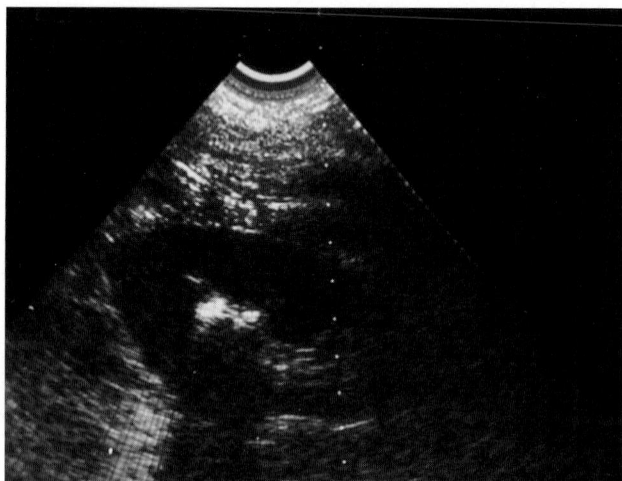

Fig. 30.16 Calculi in upper pole calyx casting acoustic shadow.

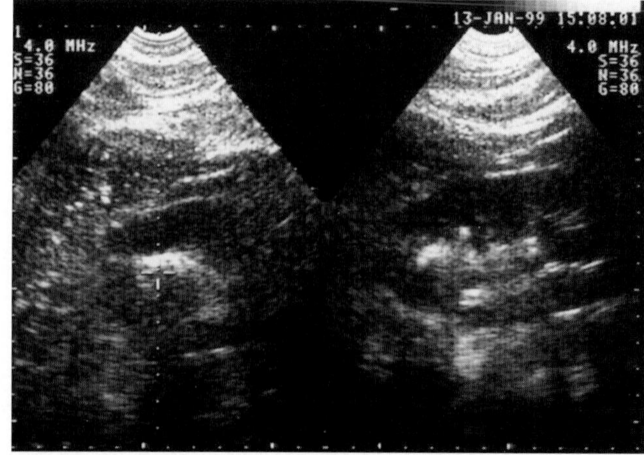

Fig. 30.17 Calculi in upper calyx targeted during ESWL.

(a)

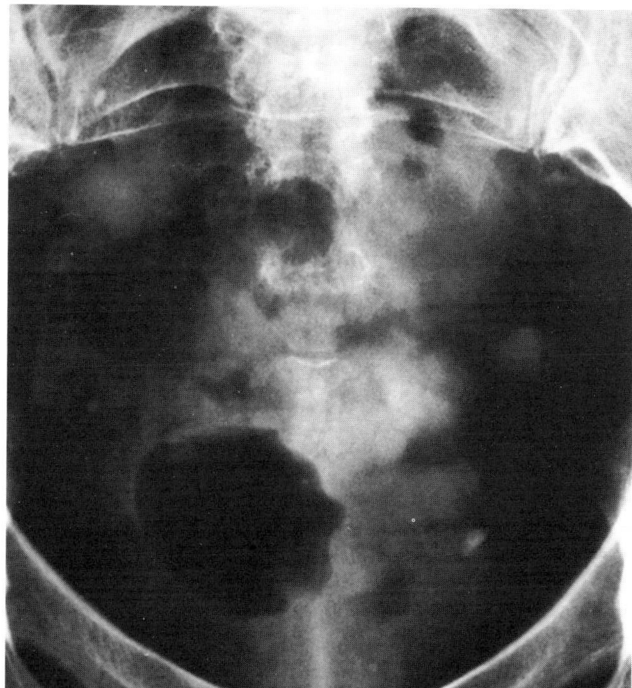

(b)

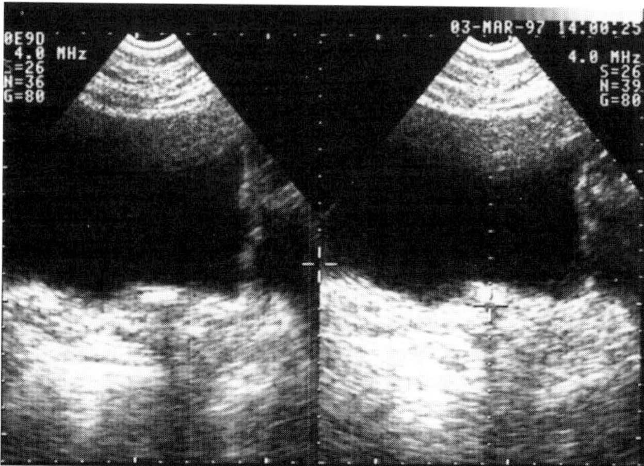

Fig. 30.18 (a) Radiograph showing calculus in lower left ureter at VUJ. (b) Calculus at left VUJ targeted during ESWL.

Not all renal calculi are suitable for lithotripsy. This depends on the size of the calculus, the location of the calculus within the collecting system or ureter and the configuration of the collecting system which should allow free drainage after fragmentation. The intravenous urogram remains an important modality to confirm the position of the calculi within the collecting system and to exclude any abnormalities which may impede clearance of the fragments after treatment.

Patients with residual fragments in the ureter or after ureteric instrumentation should be followed up by plain radiography and ultrasound. Absence of upper tract dilatation or resolution of previously documented hydronephrosis is often a good indication for continuing conservative management.

Medullary sponge kidney is an abnormality in which there is dilatation of the distal collecting tubules in the pyramids. Tiny calculi may form in these dilated segments and these may be seen on ultrasound as small echogenic foci in the region of the papillae [42].

Vesicoureteric reflux

Vesicoureteric reflux is associated with renal parenchymal scarring and dilatation of the collecting system. Ultrasound can identify scarring when the changes are marked but it is less good at detecting minor or moderate changes, which are best detected using isotope techniques [43]. Similarly it will not detect minor degrees of reflux which are better seen with micturating cystography or isotopes.

'Medical' diseases of the kidneys

Many disease processes affect the kidneys and result in varying degrees of impairment of renal function. The appearances of the kidneys on ultrasound will vary depending on the nature of the disorder and whether it is acute or chronic. However, the sonographic appearances are non-specific and rarely allow a particular disease process to be identified on ultrasound alone [44–46]. In acute disorders the kidneys are often normal in size but may be enlarged; the cortical echogenicity can be normal, increased or sometimes decreased; the medullary pyramids can be normal in appearance, more prominent, indistinct or enlarged; the collecting system may be normal or more prominent. In chronic disorders there is generally a decrease in renal size as the disease progresses and renal cortical scarring may be seen but these changes can be variable and do not correlate particularly with the deterioration in renal function, or the underlying pathology.

Doppler ultrasound findings may also be abnormal. Normal renal waveforms have a resistance index of less than 0.7 but many parenchymal disorders will cause an increase in this, particularly those with a predominantly vascular involvement. However, the changes are not sufficiently specific to allow distinction between various types of renal disease.

Ultrasound is useful in the assessment of patients with impaired renal function as it allows the exclusion of obstruction as the cause of the renal impairment and the information it provides on the size and appearance of the kidneys does help in the overall assessment of the diagnosis and the prospects for recovery. Many causes of impaired renal function can only be diagnosed by renal biopsy and ultrasound provides an excellent means of directing biopsy needles under real-time control.

Glomerulonephritis

This term covers a group of disorders which affect mainly the glomeruli; there are a variety of causes and pathological findings but ultrasound shows no particular features which allow distinction between them. In many cases the appearances of the kidneys are within normal limits but they may show a variety of abnormal changes in acute and chronic disease. In acute disease the kidneys may be increased in size and show increased cortical echogenicity with some loss of definition of corticomedullary differentiation (Fig. 30.19). In chronic disease the kidneys are reduced in size and cortical thickness, cortical echogenicity is often increased.

Acute pyelonephritis and renal infections

In most cases of acute pyelonephritis the kidneys appear normal. In more severe cases, the most common finding is enlargement of the kidneys with a decrease in cortical echogenicity, these changes can be diffuse or patchy in distribution. An underlying anatomical abnormality, or obstruction, may be identified in a small number of cases [47,48]. Thickening of the margins of the pelvicalyceal system may occur but is a non-specific finding. These changes usually resolve completely with appropriate antibiotic therapy; diffuse loss of cortical parenchyma may be seen after severe infections but focal scarring is rare in adults, although it may be seen in young children.

FOCAL BACTERIAL NEPHRITIS (LOBAR NEPHRONIA)

Focal changes may be seen in patients with renal infection; these may represent focal areas of infection, or focal changes in a kidney during resolution of more diffuse changes. Ultrasound shows a focal area of reduced echogenicity within the renal parenchyma, although increased echogenicity is occasionally seen if haemorrhage has occurred; swelling of the parenchyma may be seen but this is not a constant feature. These changes may resolve on antibiotic treatment, or progress to frank abscess formation [49].

RENAL ABSCESS

These may result from local renal pathology, or embolic spread from elsewhere. Typically they appear as an hypoechoic area in the renal parenchyma, which show a variable degree of echogenicity, but also shows good through sound transmission consistent with its liquid nature [50]. Abscesses also occur in the perirenal and pararenal areas and can be identified using ultrasound but some of these can be quite complex and CT provides a better assessment of their full extent. Ultrasound can be used to guide drainage procedures.

PYONEPHROSIS

If an obstructed collecting system becomes infected then it fills with debris and pus, this will show as echoes within the collecting system and fluid–fluid levels may be seen as layers; gas may be seen in the collecting system in cases of infection with gas-forming organisms: these appearances should alert the sonographer to the diagnosis, particularly if the patient is a diabetic, or is toxic (Fig. 30.20). Ultrasound may fail to show any internal echoes in the collecting system in some cases and patients with staghorn calculi can also present difficulties in making a diagnosis of pyonephrosis; blood in a sterile hydronephrosis can lead to a false positive diagnosis [51].

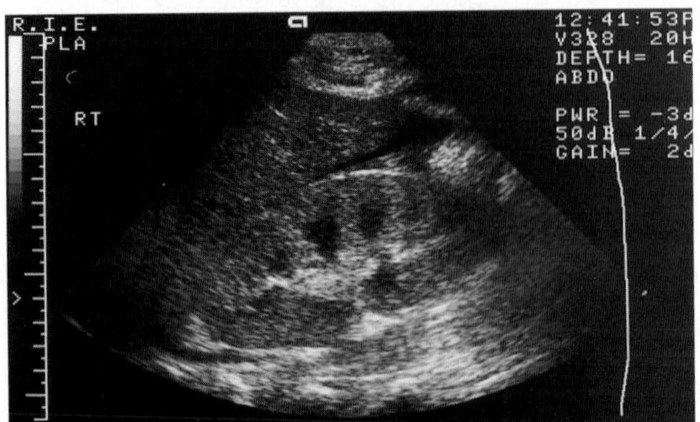

Fig. 30.19 A large, echogenic kidney in a patient with acute glomerulonephritis.

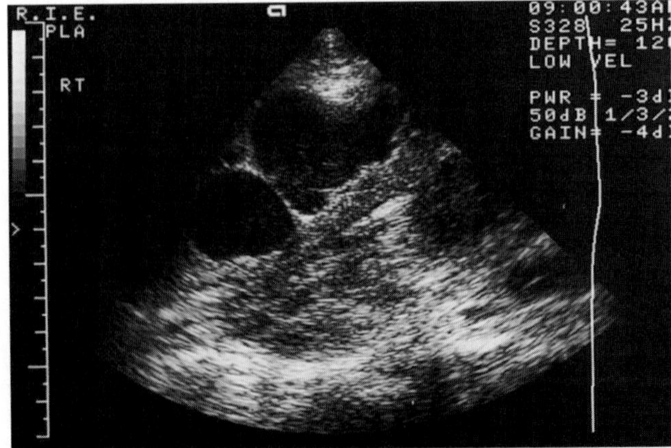

Fig. 30.20 Chronic obstruction with low level echoes in the collecting system compatible with pyonephrosis.

If the diagnosis is suspected then diagnostic aspiration should be performed with a view to proceeding to drainage if necessary.

XANTHOGRANULOMATOUS PYELONEPHRITIS

This condition occurs with chronic obstruction of all or part of the collecting system. Histologically the renal tissue is replaced by chronic inflammatory tissue and the changes may be focal or generalized; fibrosis of the collecting system occurs which reduces or abolishes dilatation of the calyces and pelvis. The affected kidney, or part of a kidney, is enlarged and the normal parenchymal anatomy is replaced by areas of predominantly hypoechoic, heterogeneity. The collecting system may not be visible, or may contain multiple echoes which make it difficult to define; associated calculi may be seen but can be difficult to distinguish amid the general distortion of normal appearances. If there is doubt about the diagnosis FNA may confirm the nature of the changes.

TUBERCULOSIS

Tubercle usually affects the kidneys from the lungs but may not become apparent clinically for up to 20 years after the pulmonary episode. The early stages affect the papillae and calyces and are not apparent on ultrasound. In more advanced disease the renal parenchyma is abnormal with focal and infiltrative changes of mixed echogenicity being present; debris-filled cavities, dilated calyces and calcification may be seen, and in severe cases there is complete replacement of the renal parenchyma [52]. Tuberculosis also affects the ureters, producing multiple strictures which result in hydronephrosis of the collecting system; these changes may affect individual calyces, producing focal caliectasis.

HYDATID DISEASE

Hydatid disease affects the kidneys only rarely. The appearances of the cysts are similar to those more commonly seen in the liver: daughter cysts, detached membranes, thickened capsule and hydatid sand may all be seen.

Acute tubular necrosis

This is the most common cause of acute renal failure in hospital patients, it is usually the result of renal ischaemia but other factors are often associated with its development. These include sepsis, drugs, dehydration, radiographic contrast agents and haemoglobinuria/myoglobinuria. The most common finding on ultrasound is a normal renal appearance and the main reason for examining patients is to exclude obstruction as a cause of the renal failure. In some patients generalized enlargement of the kidneys may be seen and the pyramids may be large and prominent; the corticomedullary differentiation is usually preserved. Other patients may show an increase in cortical echogenicity, particularly if nephrotoxic agents are responsible for the acute renal failure [53,54].

Doppler ultrasound may be of value in the assessment of some patients with acute renal failure as the resistive index is significantly higher in most patients with acute tubular necrosis than in patients with a prerenal cause for their failure [55].

Acute interstitial nephritis is another cause of acute renal failure which, clinically, may be similar to acute tubular necrosis. However, on ultrasound there may be a marked increase in cortical echogenicity and this finding in a patient with acute renal failure suggests acute interstitial nephritis as a cause [56].

Acute cortical necrosis

This is a rare type of acute renal failure which is associated with shock, postpartum haemorrhage, burns, sepsis and myocardial infarction [57]. The parenchyma shows patchy areas of increased echogenicity with loss of the normal corticomedullary differentiation but there may be an hypoechoic subcapsular rim around the kidney which represents tissue perfused by capsular vessels (Fig. 30.21). Calcification may appear in this junctional region within a few days in some cases.

Renal papillary necrosis

Renal papillary necrosis may result from several disorders including analgesic abuse, diabetes, sickle cell trait/disease, obstruction, reflux, vasculitis and infantile diar-

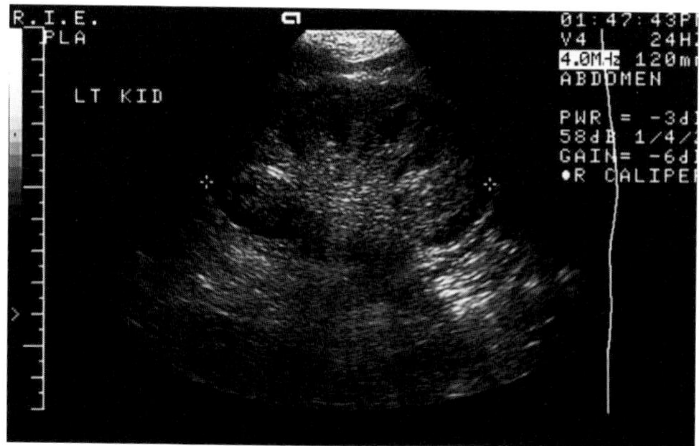

Fig. 30.21 Acute cortical necrosis showing increased cortical echogenicity with a subcapsular region of lower echogenicity.

rhoea. Early changes are best seen with urography but if calcification or sloughing of the papillae occur then these changes will be seen on ultrasound. Sloughed papillae result in small fluid-filled spaces at the periphery of the collecting system, whereas calcified papillae may mimic calculi in the calyces or in the pelvis and ureter if they have sloughed and are producing obstruction [58,59].

Diabetes

No specific changes are seen in the kidneys of patients with diabetic nephropathy. In the early stages an increase in renal size may be apparent if serial examinations are performed; this is a reflection of the increased glomerular filtration rate which occurs at this time [60]. As the disease progresses the kidneys decrease in size and can be indistinguishable from other causes of end-stage renal disease. Doppler ultrasound is non-specific, the resistive index being normal in early disease and raised in the later stages.

Table 30.1 Causes of increased parenchymal echogenicity

Medullary
Calcification
renal tubular acidosis
hypercalcaemia and hypercalciuria
frusemide therapy in children
medullary sponge kidney
dystrophic calcification after acute tubular necrosis
renal papillary necrosis
Hyperoxaluria
Hyperuricaemia
Medullary fibrosis
Cortical
Calcification
renal cortical necrosis
oxalosis
chronic glomerulonephritis
Acute glomerulonephritis
Acute amyloid
Acute interstitial nephritis
Acute cortical necrosis

Amyloid

Amyloid is a complex disorder in which an abnormal fibrillar protein is laid down in the extracellular tissues of many organs, various patterns of deposition can occur and the kidneys are most commonly involved in the systemic forms of amyloid. In the acute stages the kidneys may be enlarged with a patchy increase in cortical echogenicity but in chronic disease they shrink and the appearances are indistinguishable from other causes of chronic renal failure [61,62].

Acquired immunodeficiency syndrome

There are no specific changes in the kidneys. A variety of pathological processes can affect the kidneys in these patients: the glomeruli, tubules and interstitial tissues can all be affected [63] and the sonographic appearances reflect these changes. In the majority of patients the kidneys appear normal in size and appearance but enlargement may be a feature and a patchy, or diffuse increase in cortical echogenicity may be seen. Focal lesions due to infection or neoplastic lesions, including lymphoma, have been reported and hydronephrosis may result from ureteric obstruction by tumour or fungal balls [64,65].

Nephrocalcinosis

Several disorders result in the deposition of calcium in the medulla and, rarely, the cortex of the kidneys. When present, this calcification produces increased echogenicity of the affected region, there may not be significant acoustic shadowing as the individual foci are often smaller than the beam width. Causes of nephrocalcinosis are given in Table 30.1.

Bright medullary pyramids are seen in a variety of disorders in children; this is often due to nephrocalcinosis but may be seen in patients with other disorders which result in medullary fibrosis, the deposition of urates or proteins in the medulla [66]. In neonates a transient echogenicity, seen in the first few days of life, has been described in babies without any evidence of significant renal impairment [67].

Chronic renal disease and end-stage kidneys

In chronic renal disease the functioning renal tissue is lost and replaced with fibrosis (Fig. 30.22). The kidneys tend to become smaller in size with loss of parenchymal thickness. There are no specific features which allow the aetiology of the chronic renal failure to be identified on ultrasound except for cases of adult polycystic kidney disease. The degree of shrinkage can be quite variable and is not related to the nature of the underlying disease process.

Patients on dialysis may develop acquired cystic disease of the kidney. In these patients there is proliferation of tissues in the kidney which results in multiple small cysts forming, the development of adenomas and, rarely, the development of carcinomas. Occasionally these changes may be seen in patients with severe renal failure

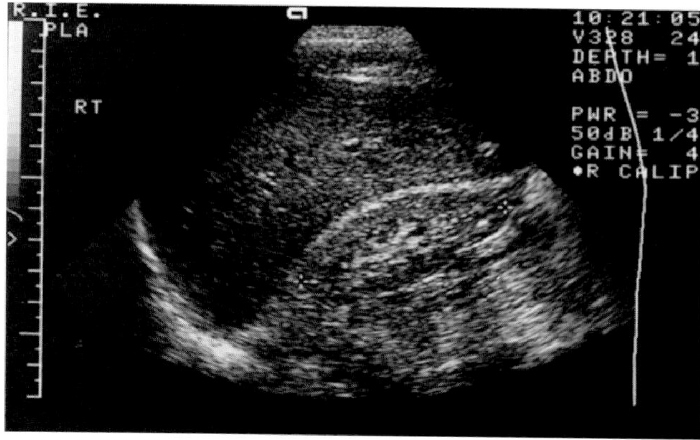

Fig. 30.22 A small bright kidney in a patient with end-stage renal disease.

but who are not yet on dialysis [68]. On ultrasound the kidneys show a variable number of hypoechoic and cystic areas corresponding to the adenomas and cysts, in severe cases the kidneys are enlarged and may be difficult to distinguish from adult polycystic kidneys. Interestingly these changes can regress if the patient undergoes a successful renal transplant [69]. Renal carcinoma should be considered if patients develop pain or haematuria in relation to their native kidneys.

Complications affecting haemodialysis access shunts can be assessed using colour Doppler: thrombosis, stenosis and aneurysms can be diagnosed [70] and an approximate assessment of volume flow in the supplying artery can be obtained; although it is recognized that volume flow calculations are associated with several sources of error, it is still possible to separate shunt volumes into broad categories of low (<400 ml min^{-1}), satisfactory (400–1000 ml min^{-1}) and high flow (>1000 ml min^{-1}).

Complications associated with continuous ambulatory peritoneal dialysis can be seen with ultrasound. Loculated or infected collections of fluid, leakage of fluid around the catheter insertion and other problems can all be assessed. In a few patients thickened omentum due to chronic sclerosing peritonitis may be seen [71].

Miscellaneous disorders

Many other diseases affect the kidneys directly, or indirectly but the appearances of the kidneys are generally non-specific. Connective tissue disorders may produce a renal vasculitis, and drug therapy for the disorder, or secondary amyloid, may affect the kidneys.

Haemolytic–uraemic syndrome in children is of interest as it has been shown that the return of diastolic flow on Doppler ultrasound is a predictor of returning renal function over the next 24–48 h [72].

Vascular abnormalities

Acute arterial insufficiency

Acute occlusion of a renal artery may produce surprisingly little change in the general appearance of the kidney; there may a slight increase in size due to oedema and a thin subcapsular rim of hypoechoic parenchyma may be seen in some patients representing oedematous tissue supplied by capsular collaterals. Over a period of time the affected kidney slowly shrinks in size [73]. Occlusion of a segmental artery produces local swelling in the acute stage, followed by cortical scarring as contraction and fibrosis take place.

Colour Doppler or power Doppler make the diagnosis of acute arterial occlusion more straightforward, providing the system is set up appropriately then the failure to demonstrate arterial flow in the renal sinus or parenchyma is strongly suggestive of arterial occlusion.

Renal artery stenosis

This is usually the result of atheroma or fibromuscular hyperplasia but occasionally aneurysms, emboli or arteritis may be the cause; in about 5% of patients with hypertension recognition and correction of a stenosis can improve or abolish the increase in blood pressure. Careful examination of the abdominal aorta from anterior and coronal approaches may allow visualization of the proximal renal arteries, usually about the level of the superior mesenteric artery; the right is easier to demonstrate as it may be identified passing behind the inferior vena cava. Once located the vessels can be examined with spectral Doppler and abnormally high shifts or velocities detected [74,75]. Unfortunately there can be problems with locating the vessels, determining their alignment for accurate angle correction and locating accessory arteries, which may be responsible for the hypertension. If accurate angle correction is not possible then a ratio of >3.5 between the shifts in the renal artery and adjacent abdominal aorta has been shown to be a good indication of significant stenosis [76].

An alternative approach is to assess the waveform in the intrarenal arteries; these are accessible in nearly every case and a decrease in the rate of systolic acceleration (<3 m s^{-2}), or an increase in acceleration time (>0.12) resulting in a damped waveform (Fig. 30.23), correlate well with severe (>70%) stenosis [77]. However, lesser degrees of stenosis are not detected reliably and accessory arteries may still be missed.

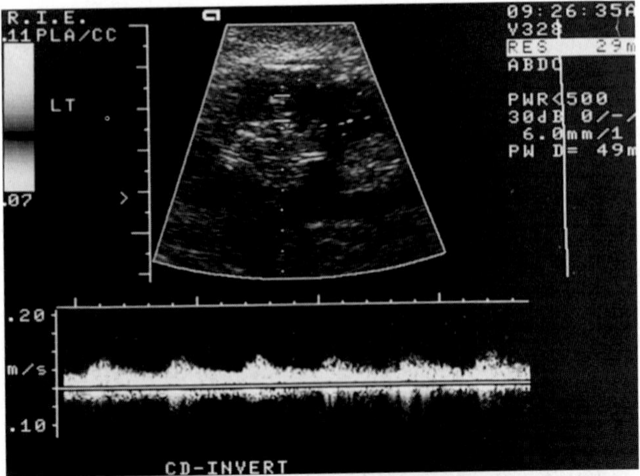

(a)

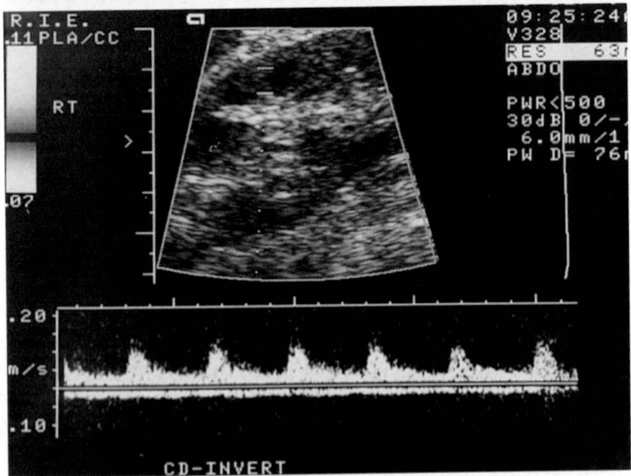

(b)

Fig. 30.23 (a) A damped intrarenal waveform in the left kidney consistent with renal artery stenosis; the normal side in the same patient. (b) A normal waveform on the right side.

Venous thrombosis

Bilateral renal vein thrombosis is rare in adults but may be seen in infants, particularly if they have been severely dehydrated. In adults unilateral, or segmental vein thrombosis usually occurs on a background of underlying renal disease, rather than spontaneously; although severe dehydration, trauma, steroids and oral contraceptives may be associated with it in a few cases; tumours of the kidney may extend into the renal vein and produce thrombosis [78].

In acute thrombosis the kidney is swollen and generally hypoechoic; anechoic areas may be seen within the parenchyma, corresponding to areas of infarction. After 1–2 weeks the affected kidney starts to shrink in size, if resolution of the thrombosis has not occurred and over several weeks becomes small and echogenic [79,80]. Segmental vein thrombosis produces similar but localized changes and, in the acute phase, is difficult to distinguish from other causes of focal, hypoechoic swelling of the parenchyma. The renal vein may appear swollen and low level echoes may be seen in it but fresh thrombus can be anechoic and difficult to visualize; Doppler and colour Doppler are of value in confirming the absence of flow in the main renal veins; flow in the renal artery shows absent, or reversed diastolic flow. Thrombosis may be complete or only partial and this should be remembered when performing Doppler examinations as a partial thrombosis may be overlooked. The artery on the affected side will show absent or reversed diastolic flow.

Arteriovenous fistula

This can occur spontaneously but is usually seen following penetrating trauma, including renal biopsy. The diagnosis may be suggested on colour Doppler by the presence of a visible tissue 'bruit' at the site of the fistula. Spectral Doppler may be used to assess the area of the fistula. It is also useful to examine the segmental arteries and veins in the area as, in the presence of a significant fistula, there will be decreased pulsatility (increased diastolic flow) in the artery supplying the fistula and flow in the veins draining the fistula will be abnormally fast and pulsatile. The fistula can be followed on Doppler as some will close spontaneously, others will remain static and some will deteriorate.

References

1 Emammian, S.A., Nielsen, M.B., Pedersen, J.F., Ytte, L. (1993) Kidney dimensions at sonography: correlation with age, sex and habitus in 665 adult volunteers. *American Journal of Roentgenology* **160**, 83–86.

2 Sargent, M.A., Wilson, B.P. (1992) Observer variability in the sonographic measurement of renal length in childhood. *Clinical Radiology* **46**, 344–347.

3 Hricak, H., Lieto, R.P. (1983) Sonographic determination of renal volume. *Radiology* **148**, 311–312.

4 Cietak, K.A., Newton, J.R. (1985) Serial, quantitative maternal nephrosonography in pregnancy. *British Journal of Radiology* **58**, 405–413.

5 Rodger, S.D., Beale, A.M., Catell, W.R., Webb, J.A.W. (1994) What is the value of measuring renal parenchymal thickness before renal biopsy? *Clinical Radiology* **49**, 45–49.

6 Cozens, N., Murchison, J., Allan, P.L., Winney, R.J. (1992) Comparison of 18G renal biopsy with conventional 14G technique. *British Journal of Radiology* **65**, 594–597.

7 Marchal, G., Verbeken, E., Oyen, R., Moerman, F., Baert, A.L., Lauweryns, J. (1986) Ultrasound of the normal kidney: a sonographic, anatomic and histologic correlation. *Ultrasound in Medicine and Biology* **12**, 999–1009.

8 Dalla Palma, L., Bazzocchi, M., Cressa, C., Tomasini, G. (1990) Radiological anatomy of the kidney revisited. *British Journal of Radiology* **63**, 680–690.

9 Cietak, K.A., Newton, J.R. (1985) Serial qualitative maternal nephrosonography in pregnancy. *British Journal of Radiology* **58**, 399–404.

10 Mahoney, B.S., Brooke-Jeffrey, R., Laing, F.C. (1983) Septa of Bertin: a sonographic pseudotumour. *Journal of Clinical Ultrasound* **11**, 317–319.

11 Mascatello, V., Lebowitz, R.L. (1976) Malposition of the colon in left renal agenesis and ectopia. *Radiology* **120**, 371–376.

12 Pitts, W.R. Jr, Maecke, E.C. (1975) Horseshoe kidney: a 40-year experience. *Journal of Urology* **113**, 743–746.

13 Bannerjee, B., Brett, I. (1991) Ultrasound diagnosis of horseshoe kidney. *British Journal of Radiology* **64**, 898–900.

14 Morgan, R.A., Dubbins, P.A. (1992) Pancreatic and renal mobility. *Clinical Radiology* **45**, 88–91.

15 Bosniak, M.A. (1986) The current radiological approach to renal cysts. *Radiology* **158**, 1–10.

16 Hartman, D.S., Davis, C.J., Johns, T., Goldman, S.M. (1986) Cystic renal carcinoma. *Urology* **28**, 145–153.

17 Hayden, C.J., Swischuk, L.E. (1990) Renal cystic disease. *Seminars in US, CT and MRI* **12**, 361–373.

18 Ravine, D., Gibson, R.N., Walker, R.G., Sheffield, L.J., Kincaid-Smith, P., Danks, D.M. (1994) Evaluation of sonographic criteria for autosomal dominant polycystic kidney disease. *Lancet* **343**, 824–827.

19 Felson, B., Cussen, L.J. (1975) The hydronephrotic type of unilateral congenital multicystic disease of the kidney. *Seminars in Roentgenology* **10**, 125–131.

20 Garel, L.A., Habib, R., Apariente, D., *et al.* (1984) Juvenile nephronophthisis: sonographic appearance in children with severe uraemia. *Radiology* **151**, 93–96.

21 Thompson, B.J., Jenkins, D.A.S., Allan, P.L., *et al.* (1986) Acquired cystic disease of the kidney: an indication for renal transplantation? *British Medical Journal* **293**, 1209–1210.

22 Hartman, D.S., Goldman, S.M., Friedman, A.C., Davis, C.J., Madewell, J.E., Sherman, J.L. (1981) Angiomyolipoma: ultrasonic–pathologic correlation. *Radiology* **139**, 451–458.

23 Borgstein, R.L., Moran, B., Davison, L.M. (1991) Characteristic ultrasonographic appearance of a large renal oncocytoma. *Clinical Radiology* **43**, 426–428.

24 Bosniak, M.A. (1991) The small (<3.0 cm) renal parenchymal tumour: detection, diagnosis and controversies. *Radiology* **179**, 307–317.

25 Yamashita, Y., Takahashi, M., Watanabe, O., *et al.* (1992) Small renal cell carcinoma: pathologic and radiologic correlation. *Radiology* **184**, 493–498.

26 Kier, R., Taylor, K.J.W., Feyock, A.L., Ramos, I.M. (1990) Renal masses: characteristation with Doppler ultrasound. *Radiology* **176**, 703–707.

27 Hartman, D.S., Sanders, R.C. (1982) Wilms' tumor versus neuroblastoma: usefulness of ultrasound in differentiation. *Journal of Ultrasound in Medicine* **1**, 117–122.

28 Dalla Palma, L., Pozzi-Mucelli, F., di Donna, A., Pozzi-Mucelli, R.S. (1990) Cystic renal tumours: US and CT findings. *Urological Radiology* **12**, 67–73.

29 Leder, R.A., Reed Dunnick, N. (1990) Transitional cell carcinoma of the pelvicalices and ureter. *American Journal of Roentgenology* **155**, 713–722.

30 Pollack, H.M., Wein, A.J. (1989) Imaging of renal trauma. *Radiology* **172**, 297–308.

31 Furtschegger, A., Egender, G., Jakse, G. (1988) The value of sonography in the diagnosis and follow-up of patients with blunt renal trauma. *British Journal of Radiology* **62**, 110–116.

32 Middleton, W.D., Kellman, G.M., Melson, G.L., Madrazo, B.L. (1989) Postbiopsy renal transplant arteriovenous fistulas: colour Doppler US characteristics. *Radiology* **171**, 253–257.

33 Amis, E.S., Cronan, J.J., Pfister, R.C., Yoder, I.C. (1982) Ultrasonic inaccuracies in diagnosing renal obstruction. *Urology* **19**, 101–105.

34 Platt, J.F., Rubin, J.M., Ellis, J.H. (1993) Acute renal obstruction: evaluation with intrarenal duplex Doppler and conventional ultrasound. *Radiology* **186**, 685–686.

35 Vrtiska, T.J., Hattery, P.R., King, B.F., *et al.* (1992) Role of ultrasound in medical management of patients with renal stone disease. *Urological Radiology* **14**, 131–138.

36 Middleton, W.D., Dodds, W.J., Lawson, T.L., Foley, W.D. (1988) Renal calculi: sensitivity for detection with ultrasound. *Radiology* **167**, 239–244.

37 King, W., Kimme-Smith, C., Winner, J. (1985) Renal stone shadowing: an investigation of contributing factors. *Radiology* **154**, 191–196.

38 Dalla Palma, L., Stacul, F., Bazzochi, M., Pagnan, L., Festini, G., Marega, D. (1993) Ultrasonography and plain film versus intravenous urography in ureteric colic. *Clinical Radiology* **47**, 333–336.

39 Laing, F.C., Jeffrey, R.B., Wing, V.W. (1985) Ultrasound versus excretory urography in acute flank pain. *Radiology* **144**, 613–616.

40 Martin, X., Mestas, J.L., Cathignol, D., Margonan, J., Dubenard, J.M. (1986) Ultrasound stone localisation for ESWL. *British Journal of Urology* **58**, 349–352.

41 Geschwend, J., Miller, K., Hautmann, R. (1993) Combined ultrasound and roentgen localisation in ESWL. initial clinical experience. *Urologe-Ausgabe A* **32**, 141–144.

42 Tayoda, K., Miyamoto, Y., Ida, M., Tada, S., Utsunomiya, M. (1989) Hyperechoic medulla of the kidneys. *Radiology* **173**, 431–434.

43 Tasker, A.D., Lindsell, D.R., Moncrieff, M. (1993) Can ultrasound reliably detect renal scarring in children with urinary tract infection? *Clinical Radiology* **47**, 177–179.

44 Hricak, H., Cruz, C., Romanski, R., *et al.* (1982) Renal parenchymal disease: sonographic–histologic correlation. *Radiology* **144**, 141–147.

45 Rosenfield, A.T., Siegel, N.J. (1981) Renal parenchymal disease. Histopathologic–sonographic correlation. *American Journal of Roentgenology* **137**, 793–798.

46 Huntington, D.K., Hill, S.C., Hill, M.C. (1991) Sonographic manifestations of medical renal disease. *Seminars in US, CT and MRI* **12**, 290–307.

47 Johnson, J.R., Vincent, L.M., Wang, K., Roberts, P.L., Stamm, W.E. (1992) Renal ultrasonic correlates of acute pyelonephritis. *Clinical Infectious Diseases* **14**, 15–22.

48 Neal, D.E., Steele, R., Sloane, B. (1990) Ultrasonography in the differentiation of complicated and uncomplicated acute pyelonephritis. *American Journal of Kidney Disease* **16**, 478–480.

49 McInstry, C.S. (1985) Acute lobar nephronia. *British Journal of Radiology* **58**, 1217–1219.

50 Goldman, S.M., Fishman, E.K. (1991) Upper urinary tract infection: the current role of CT, ultrasound and MRI. *Seminars in US, CT and MRI* **12**, 335–360.

51 Jeffrey, R.B., Laing, F.C., Wing, V.W., Hoddick, W. (1985)

Sensitivity of sonography in pyonephrosis: a re-evaluation. *American Journal of Roentgenology* **144**, 71–73.
52 Premkumar, A., Lattimer, J., Newhouse, J.H. (1987) CT and sonography of advanced urinary tract tuberculosis. *American Journal of Roentgenology* **148**, 65–69.
53 Rosenfield, A.T., Zeman, R.K., Cicchetti, D.V., Siegel, N.J. (1985) Experimental acute tubular necrosis: US appearance. *Radiology* **157**, 771–774.
54 Nomura, G., Kinoshita, E., Yamagata, Y., Koga, N. (1984) Usefulness of renal ultrasonography for the assessment of severity and course of acute tubular necrosis. *Journal of Clinical Ultrasound* **12**, 135–139.
55 Platt, J.F., Rubin, J.M., Ellis, J.H. (1991) Acute renal failure: possible role of duplex Doppler US in distinction between acute pre-renal failure and acute tubular necrosis. *Radiology* **179**, 419–423.
56 Gross, H.H., Hricak, H., Filly, R.A. (1984) Ultrasonography in patients with acute renal failure. In: Resnick, M.I., Sanders, R.C. (eds) *Ultrasound in Urology*, 2nd, edn. Williams & Wilkins, Baltimore, p. 156.
57 Sefczek, R.J., Beckman, I., Lupetin, A.R., Dash, N. (1984) Sonography of acute cortical necrosis. *American Journal of Roentgenology* **142**, 553–554.
58 Hoffman, J.C., Schnerr, M.J., Koenigsberg, M. (1982) Demonstration of renal papillary necrosis by sonography. *Radiology* **45**, 785–787.
59 Cheung, H., Chan, P.S.F., Metriweli, C. (1992) Echogenic necrotic renal papillae simulating calculi: case report. *Clinical Radiology* **46**, 61–62.
60 Segel, M.C., Leehy, J.W., Slasky, B.S. (1984) Diabetes mellitus: the predominant cause of bilateral renal enlargement. *Radiology* **153**, 341–342.
61 Ekelund, L. (1977) Radiographic findings in amyloidosis. *American Journal of Roentgenology* **129**, 851–853.
62 Subramanyam, B.R. (1981) Renal amyloidosis in juvenile and rheumatoid arthritis: sonographic features. *American Journal of Roentgenology* **136**, 411–412.
63 Bourgoignie, J.J., Meneses, R., Ortiz, C., Joffe, D., Pardo, V. (1988) The clinical spectrum of renal disease associated with human immunodeficiency virus. *American Journal of Kidney Disease* **12**, 131–137.
64 Kay, C.J. (1992) Renal diseases in patients with AIDS: sonographic findings. *American Journal of Roentgenology* **159**, 551–554.
65 Miller, F.H., Parikh, S., Gore, R.M., Nemcek, A.A. Jr, Fitzgerald, S.W., Vogelzang, R.L. (1993) Renal manifestations of AIDS. *Radiographics* **13**, 587–596.
66 Jequier, S., Kaplan, B.S. (1991) Echogenic renal pyramids in children. *Journal of Clinical Ultrasound* **19**, 85–92.
67 Riebel, T.W., Abraham, K., Wartner, R., Muller, R. (1993) Transient renal medullary hyperechogenicity in ultrasound studies of neonates: is it a normal phenomenon and what are the causes? *Journal of Clinical Ultrasound* **21**, 25–31.
68 Mikisch, O., Bommer, J., Bachman, S., Waldkerr, R., Mann, J.F.E., Ritz, E. (1984) Multicystic transformation of the kidneys in chronic renal failure. *Nephron* **38**, 93–99.
69 Ishikawa, I., Yuri, T., Kitada, H., Shinoda, A. (1983) Regression of acquired cystic disease of the kidney after successful renal transplantation. *American Journal of Nephrology* **3**, 310–314.
70 Middleton, W.D., Picus, D.D., Marx, M.V., Melsen, G.L. (1989) Color Doppler sonography of hemodialysis vascular access: comparison with angiography. *American Journal of Roentgenology* **152**, 633–639.
71 Holland, P. (1990) Sclerosing encapsulated peritonitis in chronic ambulatory dialysis. *Clinical Radiology* **41**, 19–23.
72 Patriquin, H.B., O'Regan, S., Robitaille, P., Paltiel, H. (1989) Hemolytic-uremic syndrome: intrarenal arterial Doppler patterns as a useful guide to therapy. *Radiology* **172**, 625–628.
73 Spies, J.B., Hricak, H., Slemmer, T. (1984) Sonographic evaluation of experimental acute renal artery occlusion in dogs. *American Journal of Roentgenology* **142**, 341–346.
74 Robertson, R., Murphy, A., Dubbins, P.A. (1988) Renal artery stenosis: the use of duplex ultrasound as a screening technique. *British Journal of Radiology* **61**, 196–201.
75 Greene, E.R., Avasthi, P.S., Hodges, J.W. (1987) Noninvasive Doppler assessment of renal artery strenosis and hemodynamics. *Journal of Clinical Ultrasound* **15**, 653–659.
76 Kohler, T.R., Zierler, R.E., Martin, R.L., *et al.* (1986) Noninvasive diagnosis of renal artery stenosis by ultrasonic duplex scanning. *Journal of Vascular Surgery* **4**, 450–456.
77 Kliewer, M.A., Tupler, R.H., Carroll, B.A., *et al.* (1993) Renal artery stenosis: analysis of Doppler waveform parameters and tardus–parvus pattern. *Radiology* **189**, 779–787.
78 Clark, R.A., Wyatt, G.M., Colley, D.P. (1979) Renal vein thrombosis: an underdiagnosed complication of multiple renal abnormalities. *Radiology* **132**, 43–50.
79 Hricak, H. (1981) Sonographic manifestation of renal vein thrombosis: experimental study. *Investigative Radiology* **16**, 30–35.
80 Rosenfield, A.T., Zeman, R.K., Cronan, J.J., Taylor, K.W.T. (1980) Ultrasound in clinical and experimental renal vein thrombosis. *Radiology* **137**, 735–741.

Chapter 31: Renal transplantation

R.S.C. Rodger & G.M. Baxter

There has been a steady increase in the number of new patients with end-stage renal disease who are accepted for renal replacement therapy in the developed world [1]. With the improvement in dialysis techniques and renal transplantation such treatment now offers a good outlook for many elderly patients and those with significant comorbidity such as diabetics [2]. As a result the total number of patients receiving renal replacement continues to rise dramatically and is unlikely to plateau before the early part of the next century (Fig. 31.1).

For the majority of patients with end-stage renal disease, transplantation is the optimum long-term treatment and the major limitation to its use is the shortage of suitable donor kidneys [3]. The improvement in outcome following renal transplantation over the last decade is generally attributed to better donor to recipient matching [4] and more potent immunosuppressive drugs particularly cyclosporin [5]. The 1- and 5-year graft survival in Europe is now 77–82% and 57–64%, respectively [6] and in order to achieve and improve upon these results early recognition and prompt treatment of a variety of complications is needed.

Ultrasound has proved to be a valuable non-invasive aid over many years following renal transplantation. This chapter reviews its application and highlights the value of the latest techniques in current practice.

Indications/contraindications

Renal transplantation should be considered for all patients with chronic renal failure severe enough to warrant dialysis treatment. Patients may be unsuitable because of the dangers of surgery (e.g. severe cardiac disease), the hazards of immunosuppression (e.g. pre-existing infection or malignancy) or the risk of disease recurrence (e.g. oxalosis or active vasculitis).

Donor supply

The use of cadaveric and live related donors for organ transplantation is widely accepted throughout the world. In most developed countries the majority of renal transplantation is carried out using kidneys from brain dead ventilated organ donors whilst in developing countries live donor transplantation predominates. Although there are minor differences in surgical technique and recipient outcome (see below) there is little need for distinction between the two as far as management of the recipient is concerned.

Histocompatibility testing

The presence of donor-specific antibodies detected by the lymphocyte cross-match test, is a contraindication to transplantation because of the likelihood of developing hyperacute rejection. Graft acceptance following renal transplantation, in patients with a negative lymphocyte cross-match test, is thought to depend upon the degree of matching between donor and recipient of the human lymphocytic antigens (HLA). For example, the 5-year graft survival rate was 17% better in patients who received HLA B and DR matched rather than mismatched kidneys in one study [7].

Preoperative management

Renal transplantation should be carried out within 24 h or at the most 48 h of organ retrieval. This should allow sufficient time to select a suitable recipient and prepare him or her for theatre. The recipient should be screened for infection, their cardiorespiratory reserve assessed and additional dialysis given where needed to correct fluid overload or hyperkalaemia.

Immunosuppressive regimens

A wide variety of maintenance immunosuppressive regimens are used to prevent rejection. Most incorporate cyclosporin with or without steroids and/or azathioprine. Monoclonal or polyclonal antibody therapy (OKT3, antithymocyte globulin, antilymphocyte globulin) may be used in the first 7–14 days particularly if cyclosporin is

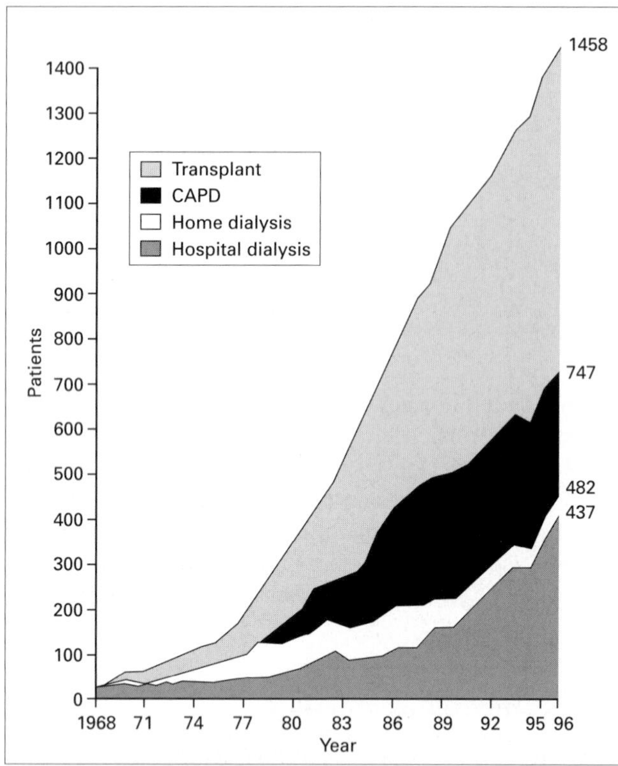

Fig. 31.1 Number of patients receiving renal replacement therapy and other treatments in the west of Scotland 1968–96. CAPD, continuous, ambulatory peritoneal dialysis.

withheld or if the recipient is considered to be at increased risk of rejection. Newer immunosuppressive drugs such as tacrolimus and mycophenolate are currently the subject of clinical trials and may become standard treatment in the future [8,9].

Treatment of established acute rejection is usually with high dose oral or intravenous corticosteroids or in more severe or resistant cases immunodepletion by antibody therapy or tacrolimus. There is no effective treatment for hyperacute or chronic rejection.

Surgery

The retroperitoneal and iliac approach and placement has been the standard technique for many years. The donor renal artery and a patch of donor aorta is usually anastomosed end to side to the external iliac artery. In live related transplantation the donor renal artery does not have an aortic patch and is anastomosed end to end with the internal iliac artery. For patients receiving a third transplant where both iliac fossae have been used an intraperitoneal approach to the iliac vessels is often undertaken. The vesicoureteric anastomosis is performed by attaching the shortened donor ureter end to side to the dome of the bladder.

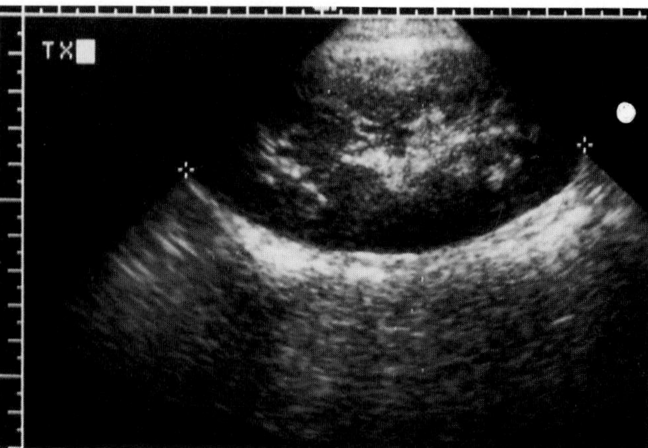

Fig. 31.2 Grey-scale image of a normal transplant kidney. The renal parenchyma is well visualized and easily differentiated from the echogenic renal sinus fat.

Ultrasound appearances of the normal transplant kidney

B-mode

The transplant kidney is easily visualized within either iliac fossa lying usually within a few centimetres of the skin surface. Its orientation is rather variable and dependent upon the surgical technique; however, with the appropriate scanning technique a conventional longitudinal and transverse axis view can usually be obtained. As the kidney orientation is variable, if biopsy is being considered then the biopsy site should be marked on the skin surface to avoid confusion.

Scanning can be performed with a selection of probes; however, the best overall assessment is usually with a vector probe operating at 4 or 3 MHz. Linear array transducers can also be utilized and whilst both 7 and 5 MHz probes give excellent near-field resolution their field of view and tissue penetration are restricted, limiting their use. The use of a 4 MHz probe not only allows an overall grey-scale assessment of the kidney but is better suited to detect peritransplant collections and the iliac and transplant vasculature.

Morphologically the renal transplant is very similar in appearance to the native kidney and many of the subtle differences are attributable to improved resolution from its superficial position. As in the normal kidney there is a well-defined renal parenchyma peripherally with a bright echogenic renal sinus centrally (Fig. 31.2). In distinction to the native kidney the renal pyramids are more commonly visualized within the transplant—these are often hypoechoic relative to the parenchyma. Confusion with dilated minor calyces should not arise as the pyramids bear a constant relationship to the medulla and are regularly spaced with no communication between them.

Minor calyces and the renal pelvis are sometimes visualized within a 'normal' transplant kidney. This is not uncommon in the early post-transplant period when oedema at the vesicoureteric anastomosis may cause some proximal dilatation. As this oedema subsides, the dilatation may resolve but in some it remains. Assuming renal function is normal this can simply be documented so as not to cause confusion at subsequent scans.

The transplant vessels can also be visualized at the renal hilum—these should not be confused with a dilated renal pelvis, and vice versa—and can easily be distinguished by the use of colour or power Doppler. The iliac vessels can also normally be identified but further interrogation with spectral Doppler is required for quantitative information. Finally, the bladder should be routinely visualized—it is normally well defined and echo-free. The presence of more solid echoes may delineate haemorrhage or infection in the appropriate clinical setting.

Colour Doppler

Colour Doppler allows a global assessment of the intrarenal vasculature (Fig. 31.3) and a more specific examination of the transplant artery, vein and iliac vessels, if required. As at many other sites the technique is similar, i.e. identify an intrarenal vessel, normally an interlobar vessel with colour or power Doppler, place the spectral gate over the vessel and obtain a tracing. The waveforms of these vessels are almost identical to that of the native kidney and other low resistance vascular beds and has been previously described as having a ski slope appearance (Fig. 31.4). Normally end-diastolic flow is approximately one-third to one-half the amplitude of peak systole and it is a reduction in the end-diastolic flow that reflects disease during the early post-transplant period. A single, isolated examination is, however, of little benefit and patients must have serial studies. These are often performed every second day following transplantation until the kidney is functioning satisfactorily.

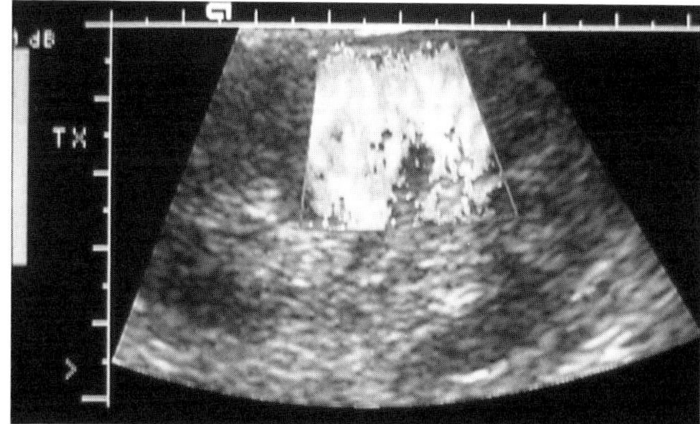

Fig. 31.3 Power Doppler image of a normal transplant kidney. The intrarenal vasculature is well visualized with flow demonstrated as far as the cortical margin. Good colour flow visualization allows accurate placement of the spectral gate to obtain spectral Doppler waveforms and reduces examination time to a minimum. For colour, see Plate 31.3 (between pp. 308 and 309).

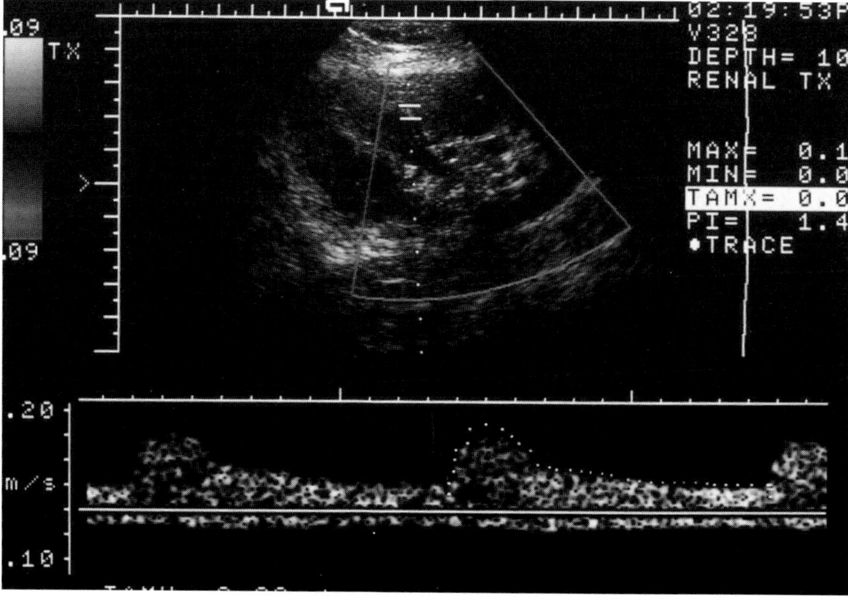

Fig. 31.4 Normal Doppler waveform from an interlobar artery. The systolic peak rises sharply with a generalized reduction in velocity throughout diastole. This has been termed the 'ski slope' appearance. The end-diastolic velocity is approximately one-third or greater that of the peak systolic velocity. For colour, see Plate 31.4 (between pp. 308 and 309).

Many different indices have been used in an attempt to quantify 'flow' within the kidney. These include pulsatility index (PI), resistive index (RI), systolic/diastolic ratio (SDR) and diastolic/systolic ratio (DSR). The two commonest employed measurements are PI and RI. Examination of the transplant artery is a technically difficult study due to the tortuosity of the transplant vessel. A Doppler angle of <65° is mandatory and this can, on occasion, be difficult to achieve. A wide range of normal peak systolic velocities have been quoted ranging from 1.0 to 2.5 $m\,s^{-1}$ which may reflect the difficulty of the technique [10–12]—it is probably more important that each individual centre has a cut-off value and that this has been documented against angiography. The renal vein is normally easily visualized and whilst no specific reference velocity values exist, the presence or absence of flow is clearly of paramount importance in the early postoperative period. The iliac artery and vein should also be identified at each examination—this allows differentiation of the iliac from renal vessels and also excludes a local lesion within the iliac artery which may have an adverse effect on transplant function.

Early complications

Acute tubular necrosis

Acute tubular necrosis (ATN) is common following cadaveric renal transplantation, 10–50% of patients requiring to be dialysed in the postoperative period. Delayed graft function, which is rare following live related transplantation, is principally related to factors in the donor and donor kidney especially warm ischaemic time. In those patients requiring to be dialysed recovery of renal function from ATN usually occurs 1–2 weeks after transplantation but may be delayed for up to 3 months.

Rejection

The classification of the histological changes of renal allograft rejection has been the subject of an International Working Party [13]. This group has published an agreed standardization of criteria for diagnosis which have become widely adopted. Renal biopsy remains the gold standard for diagnosing suspected rejection against which all other investigations must be judged. When carried out in experienced hands it is generally very safe and complications such as bleeding requiring blood transfusion or pain requiring opiate analgesia occur in less than 5% of cases [14]. Fine-needle aspiration of renal allografts is almost free of complications and can be repeated frequently. However, its diagnostic value has not proved to be as reliable as conventional biopsy samples.

Acute rejection occurs in up to 40% of patients in the early postoperative period with a peak incidence between 1 and 3 weeks. When promptly recognized it is usually reversed by treatment with high dose steroids or antibody therapy. However, its occurrence is an adverse long-term prognostic factor [15]. Rejection should be excluded in any patient with deteriorating renal function for which the principle differential diagnoses are obstruction, cyclosporin nephrotoxicity and ascending infection. It is usually asymptomatic but may be accompanied by graft tenderness, flu-like symptoms and a pyrexia. As it is often asymptomatic the diagnosis is particularly difficult in patients with non-functioning grafts.

Ultrasound in delayed function

Enthusiasm for ultrasound in the assessment of delayed function of the transplant has varied since the 1980s and the literature has been both confusing and contradictory; inhomogeneous study populations, lack of definable end-points and differing diagnostic criteria have all contributed to this. The initial expectation of being able to differentiate ATN from rejection on Doppler criteria has not been realized and led to disappointment in many centres. Currently the true role of Doppler ultrasound is in the monitoring of patients with delayed function.

B-mode

Many varied grey-scale findings have been described in acute rejection [16] ranging from a reduction in corticomedullary differentiation, reduction in renal sinus echoes, both increased and reduced renal pyramid echoes, increased cortical reflectivity, and so on. In general these findings occur late, well after the onset of acute rejection and either revert or remain static even after successful treatment. They are such arbitrary and inconstant findings, that they are of limited use.

Increases in renal length [17] and cross-sectional area [18] of the kidney during rejection but not ATN have been noted. These measurements, however, have never been adopted routinely and may perhaps be worthy of reassessment. However, full accurate measurement of renal length is difficult since the full length of the kidney can be difficult to judge on a single image using vector/sector probes.

Colour Doppler

This is routinely used by many centres in early post-transplant assessment. An overall assessment is possible using colour flow imaging and flow can often be visualized as far as the cortical margin. However, to avoid subjective assessment quantitative analysis with spectral Doppler is necessary. Serial measurements are mandatory as an isolated value is of little benefit. Patients with delayed non-function may be scanned daily or three times per week until function recovers. Although the initial Doppler studies suggested that ATN and acute rejection could be distinguished [19,20] it is now generally accepted that this level of differentiation is not possible [21,22]. However, serial measurements of PI or RI (Fig. 31.5) in conjunction with the clinical and biochemical findings can be used to monitor the transplant and can influence the decision as to when to proceed to biopsy. A PI of < 1.5 or RI < 0.7 can be regarded as normal whilst a PI > 1.8 or RI > 0.9 is regarded as pathological. Although both ATN and acute rejection can give rise to increases in PI and RI, acute rejection is more likely with higher values. Indeed complete absence or reverse diastolic flow is in the majority of cases due to acute rejection. Once the diagnosis has been confirmed histologically Doppler can then be used to monitor the response to treatment.

The introduction of power imaging has resulted in improved sensitivity in the detection of flow. It has been postulated that this may result in a better overall assessment of the transplant renal vasculature and identify areas of infarction within the kidney. As yet there have been no formalized studies to assess this or to measure its clinical impact. Some interesting recent work has looked at the use of acceleration time in the post-transplant period and has concluded that a short acceleration time on day 1 following transplantation is associated with a longer duration of delayed function. Persistently short acceleration times of <90 ms at day 5 were associated with a high risk of rejection and this was more sensitive than conventional RI measurements [23]. These results, however, remain to be substantiated by other studies.

Thrombosis

Arterial thrombosis is a rare and often initially asymptomatic early complication following renal transplantation. Typically it is discovered in the early postoperative period by routine isotope renography or Doppler ultrasound examination in a patient with a non-functioning graft. Predisposing factors include multiple renal arteries, young paediatric donor kidneys and atherosclerosis in the donor kidney or recipient. Arterial thrombosis is usually irreversible and causes infarction necessitating graft nephrectomy. In kidneys with multiple arteries, where only one vessel has thrombosed, segmental infarction occurs and satisfactory long-term renal function can still occur.

The ultrasonic appearances of an arterial occlusion are striking in that there is complete absence of flow in both the intrarenal vessels and the transplant renal artery on colour flow and Doppler analysis, occasionally leading the sonographer to question whether the appropriate settings have been used. A similar marked reduction in intrarenal colour flow may also occur secondary to hyperacute rejection or renal vein thrombosis; however, in these latter two conditions the transplant artery is usually patent but exhibits reverse diastolic flow [24]. Trauma may also lead to major arterial thrombosis although this usually occurs outwith the early postoperative period.

Venous thrombosis is more common and causes acute pain and swelling of the graft associated with an abrupt reduction in urine output. Typically this occurs in patients with non-functioning grafts 3–8 days postoperatively [25]. Strategies to reduce this complication include avoidance of cyclosporin in patients with delayed graft function and the use of subcutaneous heparin or aspirin, although the benefits of these manoeuvres have not been proven by controlled clinical trials. Clinicians should have a low threshold for suspecting incipient venous thrombosis, which can be confirmed by Doppler ultrasound examination as rapid diagnosis and intervention may salvage the graft, although unfortunately nephrectomy is required in most cases.

The diagnosis is suggested by typical Doppler ultrasound findings. Ultrasonic criteria include a dilated transplant vein containing thrombus, visible thrombus within the major intrarenal veins, absent venous flow on colour flow imaging both intrarenal and within the transplant vein and reverse diastolic flow within the intrarenal and main transplant artery, [26,27] (Fig. 31.6). Reverse diastolic flow may also occur in cases of severe acute rejection. A low amplitude rounded intrarenal arterial waveform similar to a 'parvus–tardus' waveform has also been described in incomplete renal vein thrombosis where residual venous flow persists; however, very few cases have been described and it is not clear if the prognosis is improved in this subgroup [28].

Obstruction

Obstruction occurring in the immediate postoperative period is usually due to clot in the ureter or bladder and may be relieved by simple bladder irrigation. Haematuria usually resolves within 72 h of transplantation and obstruction thereafter is most likely due to stenosis of the distal ureter or external compression from a lymphocele. Where a lymphocele is present it should be drained externally or intraperitoneally and reaccumulation may be prevented by installation of a sclerosant. In cases of ureteric stenosis a nephrostomy catheter should be inserted to allow recovery of renal function and later a nephrostogram performed to delineate the site of obstruction. Thereafter reoperation is usually required although some

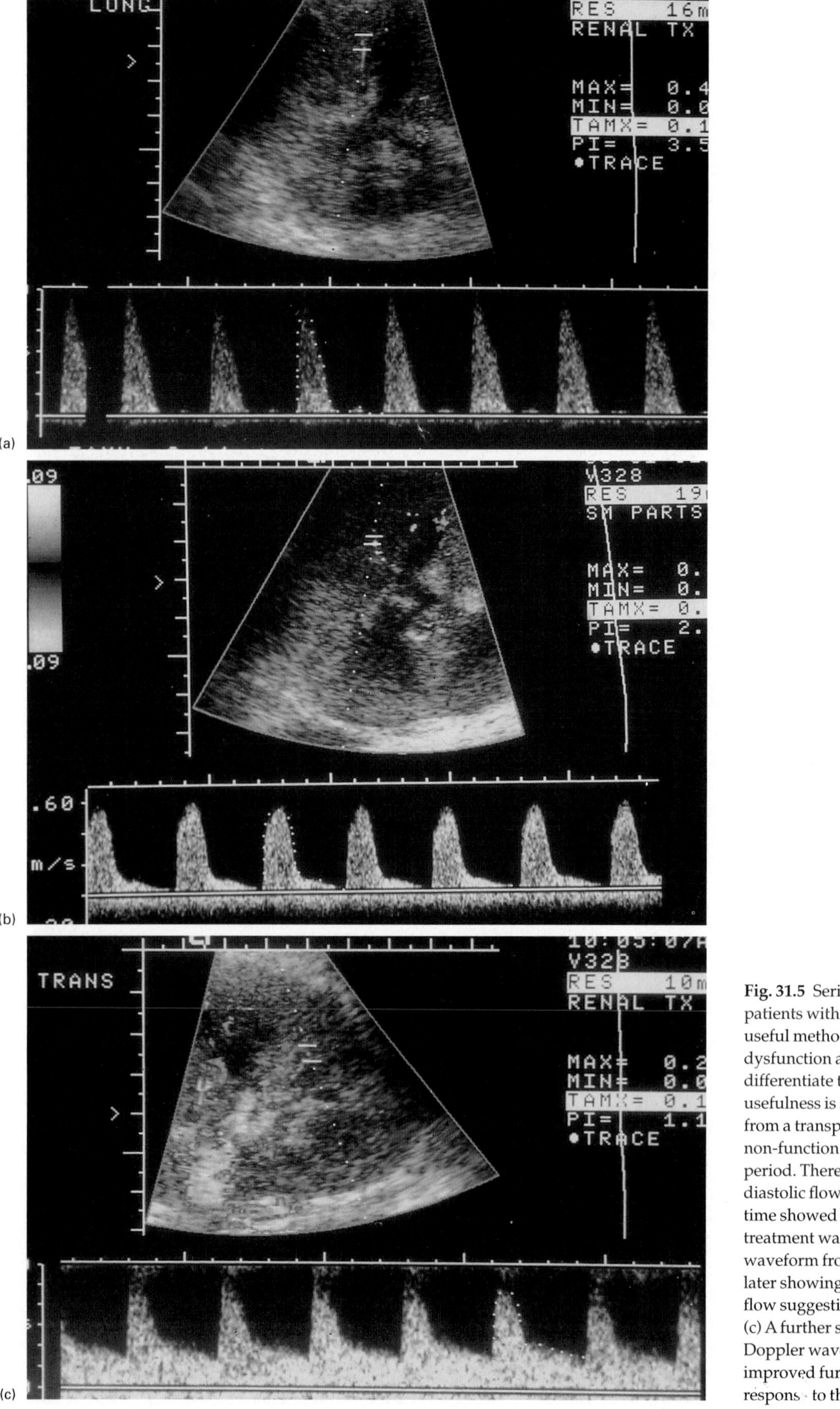

Fig. 31.5 Serial Doppler examination in patients with primary non-function is a useful method of monitoring graft dysfunction although clearly it cannot differentiate the causes. An example of its usefulness is shown. (a) Spectral waveform from a transplant patient with primary non-function in the early postoperative period. There is almost complete loss of diastolic flow. A biopsy performed at this time showed acute rejection. Appropriate treatment was begun. (b) Spectral waveform from the same patient 2 days later showing an improvement in diastolic flow suggestive of a response to therapy. (c) A further scan 2 days later and the Doppler waveform has dramatically improved further, reflecting an excellent response to therapy.

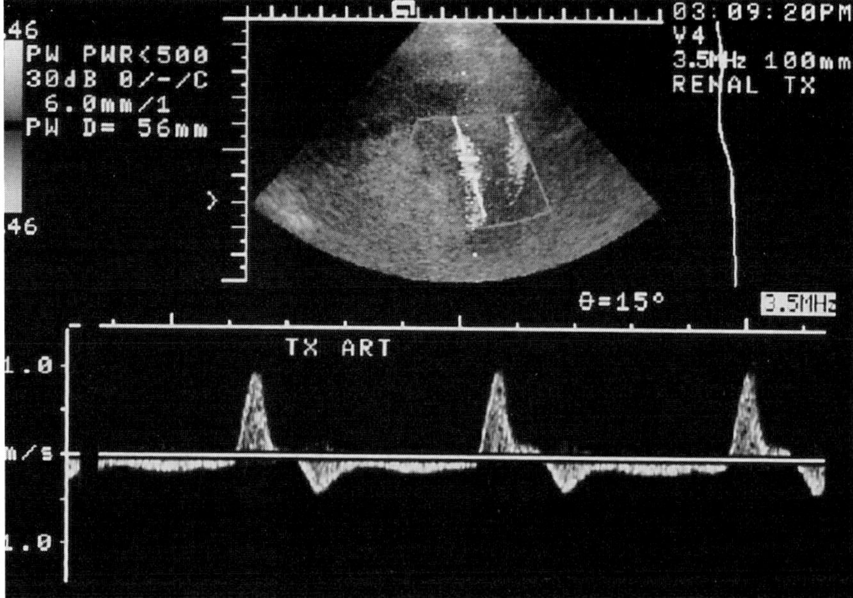

Fig. 31.6 A Doppler waveform from the transplant renal artery in a patient 4 days postoperatively with a sudden onset of anuria and graft tenderness. The waveform shows reverse diastolic flow this also being observed in the intrarenal arteries. The renal vein could not be visualized and was presumably occluded by thrombus. The overall appearances are consistent with renal vein thrombosis. Despite urgent surgical exploration, nephrectomy was performed.

(a) 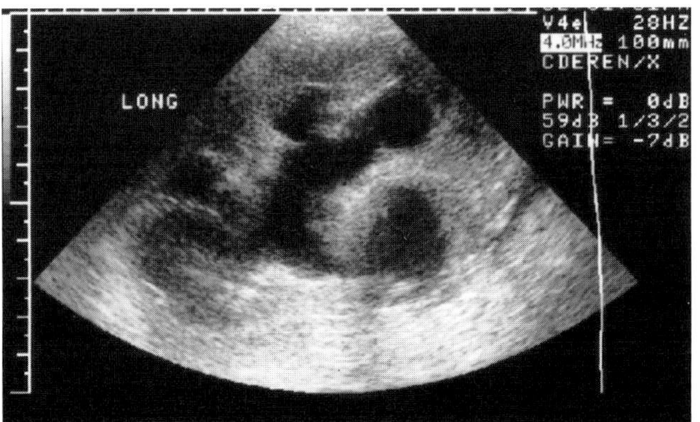

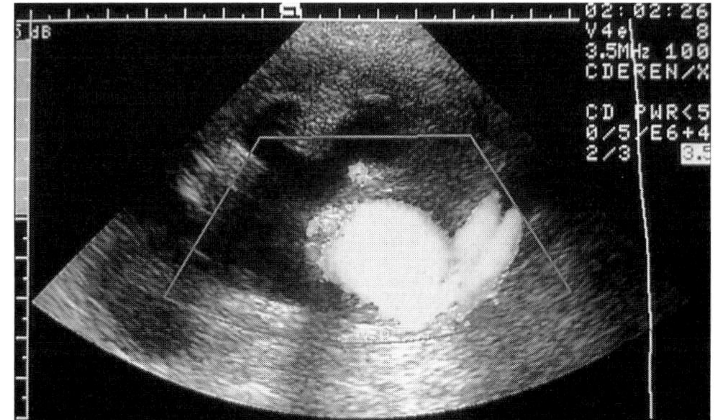 (b)

Fig. 31.7 (a) Real-time image of a transplant kidney with fairly typical features of hydronephrosis, i.e. the renal sinus is opened up by the dilated minor and major calyces and renal pelvis. There is, however, a separate less well-circumscribed cystic area with a thick margin to it. (b) Power Doppler image of the iliac vessel showing flow within the focal cystic area at the iliac artery consistent with a pseudoaneurysm. Hydronephrosis noted as in (a). For colour, see Plate 31.7 (between pp. 308 and 309).

cases can be treated by percutaneous transluminal ureteroplasty [29].

Hydronephrosis is easily identified using ultrasound (Fig. 31.7) and can be easily monitored. Its significance should be related to renal function. Occasionally a trial of nephrostomy drainage will be required to clarify its relevance. It should be remembered that a significant hydronephrosis may account for an elevated PI or RI ratio in the early post-transplant period.

Haemorrhage

Postoperative bleeding may be exacerbated by the use of aspirin or anticoagulants and may arise from the transplanted kidney or the wound. The resulting haematoma is readily detected by ultrasound and the bleeding is usually self-limiting. Occasionally re-exploration is required to identify the bleeding point and evacuate the associated haematoma. Rarely catastrophic haemorrhage can occur due to rupture of the vascular anastomosis requiring emergency surgical intervention. This is most likely where there is a severe deep wound infection.

Urinary leak

This complication has been described in up to 6% of renal transplant recipients [30]. It occurs due to disruption of the vesicoureteric anastomosis or necrosis of the distal ureter. It is heralded by increasing abdominal pain, a reduction in urine output and sometimes the appearance of urine through the wound. Ultrasound may reveal a new pelvic or perinephric collection, a cystogram may demonstrate leakage directly from the bladder and isotope renography is often helpful. Exploration may still be required even when these investigations are inconclusive and once identified the defect needs to be repaired surgically.

Ultrasonic appearance of post-transplant collections

Post-transplant collections including lymphocele, abscess, haematoma and urinoma can all be identified with ultrasound. Features such as more solid echoes or multiple septations may, in conjunction with the clinical findings, help to distinguish the different types of collection (Fig. 31.8).

Cyclosporin toxicity

Although cyclosporin has proved to be a major advance in organ transplantation, its nephrotoxicity remains a distinct disadvantage. The drug produces a reversible renal vasoconstriction acutely and may cause chronic interstitial fibrosis [31] thus it may attenuate recovery from ATN and cause irreversible deterioration in functioning grafts.

The diagnosis of cyclosporin nephrotoxicity is notoriously difficult particularly in non-functioning grafts and in this situation many clinicians prefer to avoid its use. Trough cyclosporin levels and renal biopsy are the traditional but imperfect aids to diagnosis. Some have advocated the measurement of intrarenal pressure to differentiate nephrotoxicity from rejection [32] but this test has not been widely adopted.

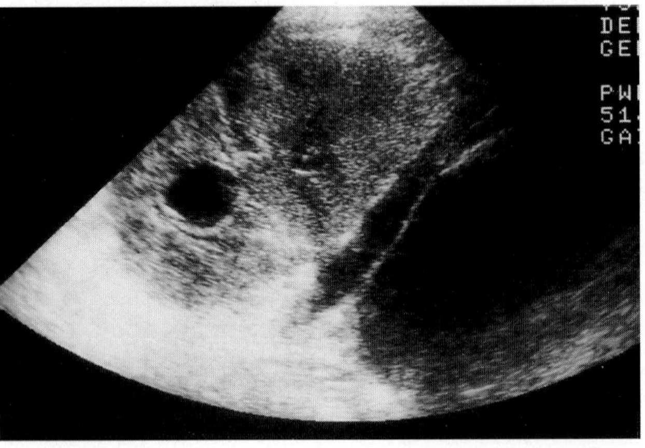

Fig. 31.8 Image through the transplant kidney and iliac vessels demonstrating a large cystic collection lying posterior to both. This was drained percutaneously and was found to be a lymphocele.

Ultrasound also is generally of little help. The effect of cyclosporin toxicity upon renal waveforms is variable. It generally does not produce any visible effect on the Doppler parameters but occasionally can cause a reduction in diastolic flow [21].

Infection

Patients in the early postoperative period are susceptible to bacterial infections in the chest, wound and urinary tract. Wound infections are usually due to *Staphylococcus aureus* and are particularly likely in patients requiring reoperation. Urinary infections are predisposed to by the presence of a urinary catheter and vesicoureteric reflux into the transplant. They may cause bacteraemia and be associated with a deterioration in renal function. As previously stated this may produce symptoms and signs difficult to distinguish from rejection and occasionally the diagnosis of pyelonephritis is made following a transplant biopsy for suspected rejection.

Ultrasound has little or no role in this diagnosis, however. The presence of infection may elevate the PI or RI ratio leading to biopsy for suspected rejection or ATN.

Late renal complications

Obstruction

Chronic ischaemia may cause stenosis of the transplant ureter and progressive hydronephrosis. This usually follows an insidious course and deterioration in renal function is a late event. Routine ultrasound screening can therefore detect this process before severe renal damage occurs.

Transplant artery stenosis

This has been described in up to 10% of renal transplant recipients [33] and may contribute to hypertension and cause progressive renal impairment particularly following the introduction of angiotensin-converting enzyme inhibitor therapy. Unfortunately the natural history of transplant renal artery stenosis is unknown and this makes clinical decisions about intervention difficult. It is more likely to occur in patients in whom the donor kidney vessels are atherosclerotic and where a small paediatric kidney is given to an adult. Most centres use arteriography to confirm the diagnosis as the literature is confusing concerning the most appropriate screening investigation. Captopril renography, ultrasound and magnetic resonance imaging (MRI) scanning all have their advocates [34–36]. In the authors' centre Doppler ultrasound has been found to be both a highly sensitive and specific test

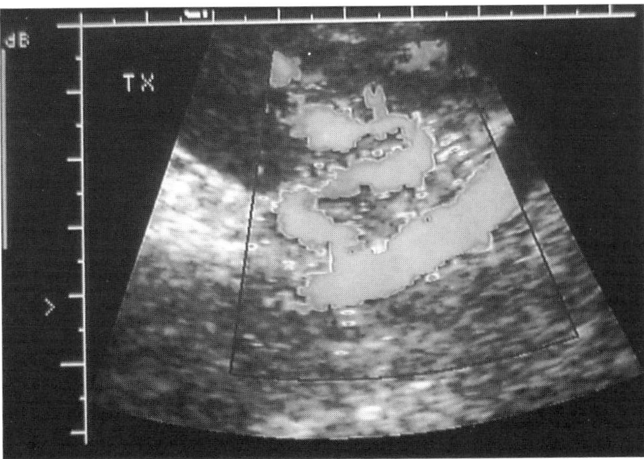

Fig. 31.9 Power Doppler scan of the transplant renal artery. The marked vessel tortuosity can be easily appreciated, this being a very common finding. Clearly, good visualization of this vessel is required to allow accurate Doppler vessel angle correction when interrogating it for suspected renal artery stenosis. For colour, see Plate 31.9 (between pp. 308 and 309).

for the detection of transplant artery stenosis [35]. Patients are initially screened with ultrasound and if percutaneous intervention is being considered then angiography will be performed.

Colour Doppler examination for transplant artery stenosis is fraught with difficulty and full of pitfalls, mainly because of the tortuous course of the transplant artery (Fig. 31.9). As a result the artery is difficult to visualize throughout its length and therefore angle correction is difficult. In addition, it may be difficult to distinguish between a stenosis and an area of tortuosity in the vessel since the velocity of blood flow will be increased in both cases. The iliac artery should also be routinely examined as a proximal stenosing lesion can also be responsible for a reduction in renal function.

Widely differing diagnostic criteria for renal artery stenosis have been described [10–12]. Classically, a significant stenosis results in an increased peak systolic velocity at the site of stenosis and a dampening of the waveforms downstream, i.e. in the intrarenal vessels (Fig. 31.10). Most stenoses occur at or close to the surgical anastomoses and can be initially suspected when using colour Doppler by identifying a focal area of aliasing within the artery on medium to high pulse repetition frequency (PRF) setting. Quantification using spectral Doppler is required and the authors have found a peak systolic velocity cut-off value of $2.5\,m\,s^{-1}$ to be accurate and reproducible for the diagnosis of stenosis [37].

Turbulence, areas of reverse flow and spectral broadening may also occur close to the stenotic area and are secondary phenomena. The authors have not found the downstream parvus and tardus effects, currently being evaluated in the native kidney, to be as useful in the transplant kidney when good visualization of the artery is obtained [37]. Doppler ultrasound is also useful to detect restenosis following angioplasty or renal artery stenting. Branch stenoses, which are of uncertain clinical significance, are uncommon. Detection with ultrasound and indeed angiography is difficult.

Arteriovenous fistula

Arteriovenous fistulae usually occur secondary to a previous transplant biopsy with an estimated incidence of 1–2%. One recent study noted a rate of 10%; however, all but one resolved completely [38]. Whilst they often give rise to very spectacular appearances on colour flow ultrasound they are usually of little clinical significance. It has been postulated that they cause both hypertension and renal impairment but if this is true it is rare. At the authors' centre, intervention is generally not contemplated unless the fistula is bleeding or increasing in size as the risks of embolization are thought to outweigh any potential benefits.

Ultrasonic appearances include a focal pool of colour flow representing both arterial and venous high flow states (Fig. 31.11). This can easily be differentiated from an area of 'well-perfused' kidney by increasing the PRF to a level at which the normal intrarenal vessels would not be expected to be visualized. At such high levels the only visible areas of colour flow are pathological, i.e. fistulae. On spectral analysis the peak velocities within the feeding artery are either normal or increased in comparison with similar-sized vessels elsewhere within the kidney and the PI and RI ratios are normal or reduced [39] due to a direct communication between the artery and a low resistance venous bed. Venous flow may be normal or turbulent in up to 33% and a large draining vein may be visible on colour flow (Fig. 31.12).

Cyclosporin toxicity

Chronic cyclosporin nephrotoxicity may lead to progressive graft dysfunction. Although typical histological changes such as tubular microcalcification and interstitial striped or patchy fibrosis have been described; in practice, it is often difficult to distinguish this from chronic rejection. A therapeutic trial of a reduction in cyclosporin dosage or conversion to another immunosuppressive drug such as azathioprine may need to be considered. Where this has been tried a small but significant number of patients will have reversible graft dysfunction due to cyclosporin damage.

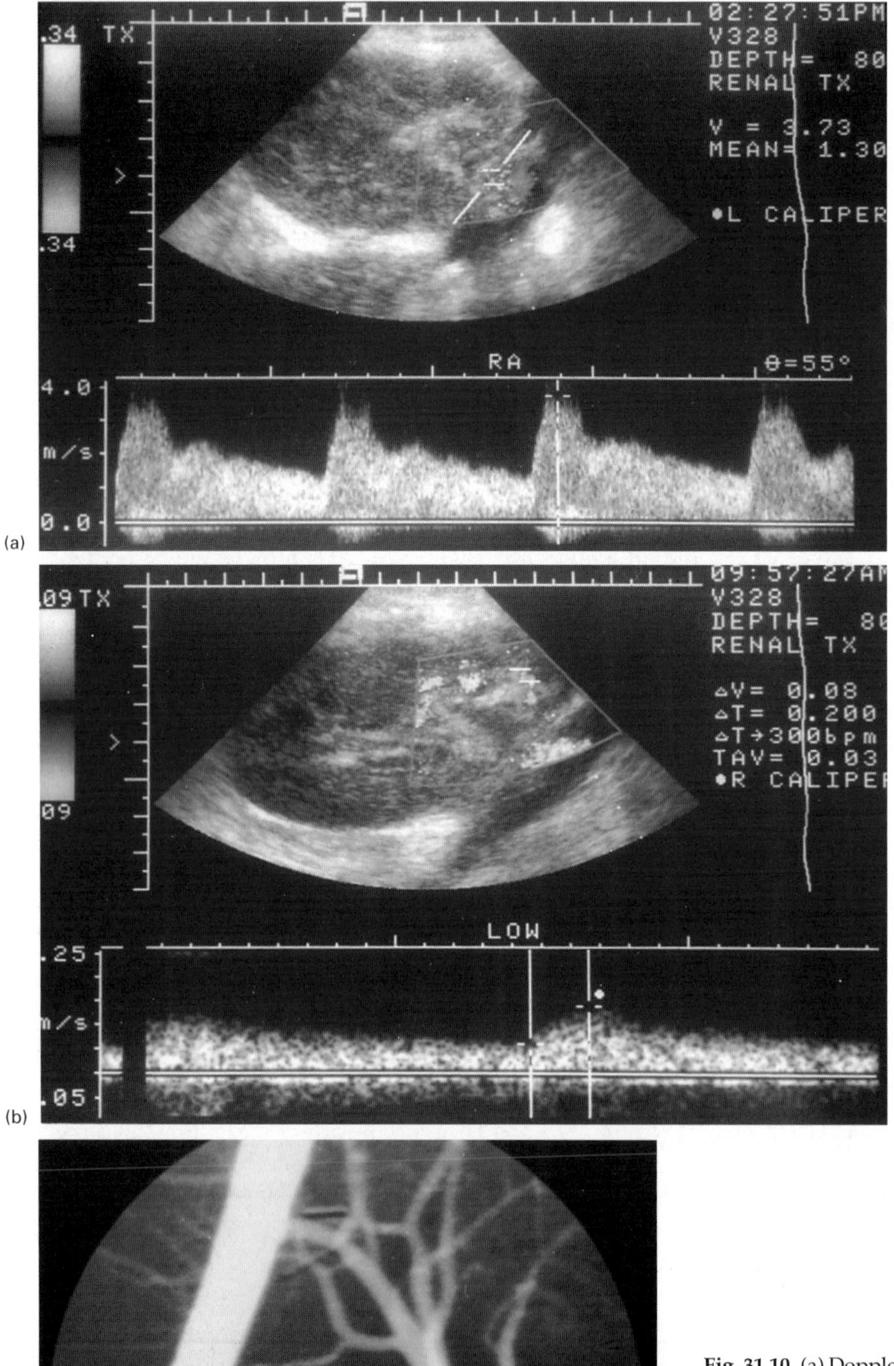

Fig. 31.10 (a) Doppler waveform in a patient with suspected transplant artery stenosis showing a markedly elevated peak systolic velocity of 3.73 m s^{-1} at the origin of the transplant artery and spectral broadening consistent with a transplant artery stenosis. (b) Spectral waveform in the same patient from an interlobar artery demonstrating the parvus–tardus effect with dampening and rounding of the waveform reflective of a more proximal stenosing lesion. The acceleration time is markedly prolonged at 0.20 s (normal <0.07 s). (c) Digital subtraction angiogram demonstrating back to back high grade renal artery stenoses just distal to the origin of the vessel, consistent with the Doppler findings.

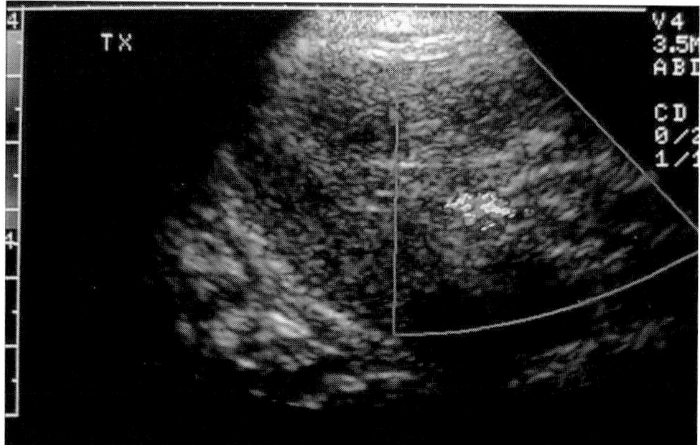

Fig. 31.11 Colour flow image of a transplant kidney with a small focal flow abnormality towards one pole. The colour velocity scale (PRF) was increased to a level where normal intrarenal flow could not be visualized. This area is clearly an abnormal area of high flow representative of an arteriovenous fistula. For colour, see Plate 31.11 (between pp. 308 and 309).

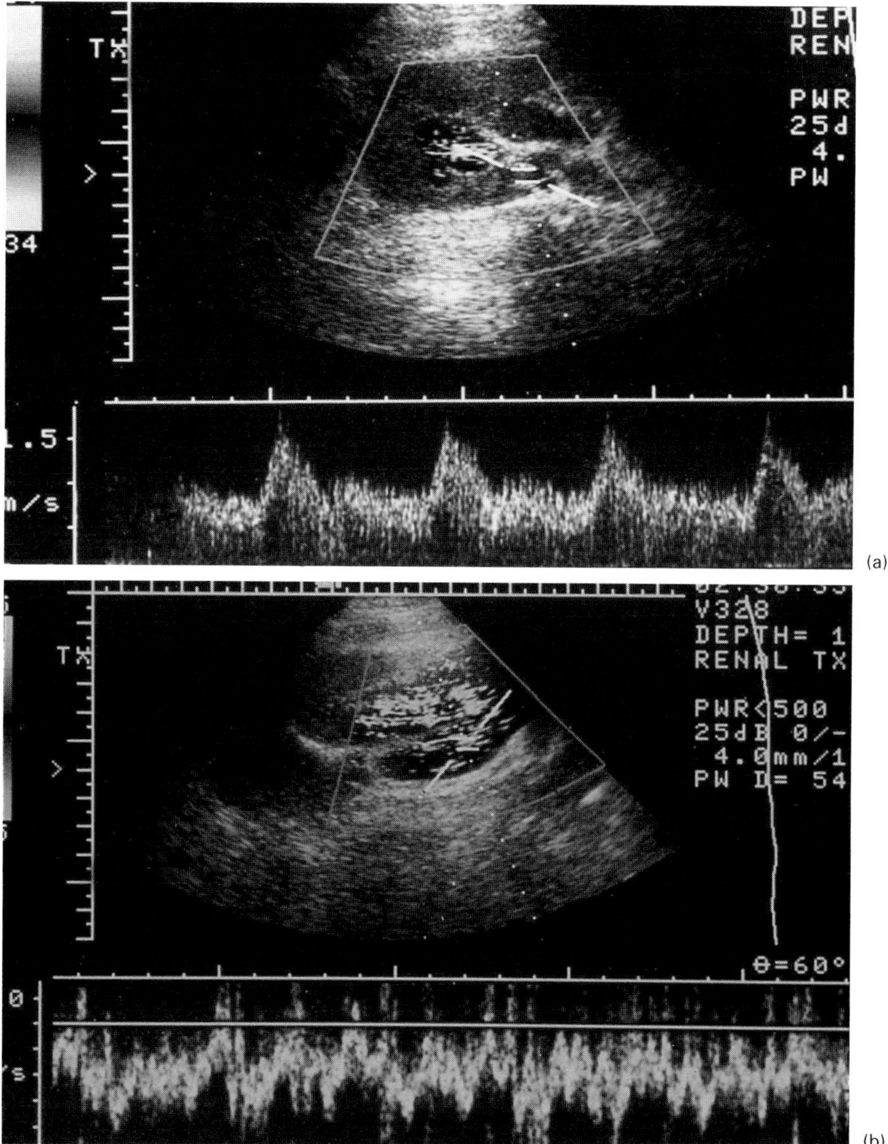

Fig. 31.12 (a) Doppler waveform from a patient with an arteriovenous fistula showing the typical appearances of a feeding arterial vessel. The diastolic flow relative to the systolic is increased, this being reflected in a low PI. Spectral broadening and turbulent flow are also present. (b) Turbulent flow is noted in the draining vein in the same patient.

Rejection

Acute rejection is an unusual late complication following transplantation. When it occurs, the question of non-compliance with immunosuppressive therapy should be raised. Diagnosis and treatment of acute rejection in this setting are as described above.

Chronic rejection has been defined as a gradual deterioration in graft function starting at least 3 months post-transplant in association with characteristic biopsy appearances such as fibrous intimal thickening with interstitial fibrosis and tubular atrophy. Numerous studies have shown that previous acute rejection is the most consistent risk factor for the subsequent development of chronic rejection. Unfortunately, there is no effective treatment for chronic rejection and so currently efforts are being directed towards the prevention of acute rejection in the hope that this will reduce the incidence of chronic rejection.

Ultrasound has no significant role in chronic rejection. Whilst the kidney may reduce in size, or the echogenicity may increase and the number of intrarenal vessels reduce in number, these findings are of little prognostic significance.

Urinary infection

Asymptomatic bacteriuria is common in long-term renal transplant recipients and generally carries a good prognosis. Symptomatic urinary infections are also relatively common and are occasionally severe enough to cause pyelonephritis, bacteraemia and a temporary deterioration in renal function. Patients suffering repeated infection should be investigated to look for a structural abnormality such as calculi, obstruction or severe reflux. Rarely repeated severe infection may lead to malakoplakia.

De novo glomerulonephritis and recurrent disease

Most forms of glomerulonephritis can cause disease recurrence in the transplanted kidney. Fortunately early recurrence is rare and it remains an unusual cause of graft failure. Recurrent disease can be detected in long-term renal transplant recipients with diabetes, amyloidosis and cystinosis but again this is usually an incidental finding. However, patients with active vasculitis and those with oxalosis are considerably more at risk of damaging their grafts at an early stage with recurrent disease and careful consideration needs to be given before transplanting such patients [40].

Ultrasound has little specific role except for excluding treatable causes of reduced function such as hydronephrosis, and so on.

Late non-renal complications

Successful renal transplant recipients suffer considerable morbidity and have an increased mortality due to cardiovascular disease and an increased susceptibility to developing infections and malignancy. Renal transplantation is associated with a number of risk factors for cardiovascular disease such as hypertension, left ventricular hypertrophy and abnormal lipid profiles but as yet the efforts to reduce these risk factors has not been associated with any improvement in survival. In contrast the risk of death from infection following renal transplantation has reduced considerably in each decade principally due to a reduction in the overall level of immunosuppression but also because of an increased awareness of the type of infections which can occur and better specific therapy for these diseases. The incidence of neoplasia also relates to the overall level of immunosuppression. Skin and cervical cancer and non-Hodgkin's lymphomas are the most common malignancies encountered and careful supervision of the transplant population should allow early detection and the best prognosis for these disorders [41].

Conclusion

In conclusion, colour Doppler ultrasound is the main imaging technique in the assessment of the renal transplant. It has both a role in the early transplant period in the sequential monitoring of graft dysfunction and in the delineation of peritransplant and local transplant collections, some of which can be treated under ultrasound guidance. In addition, it is also useful in the diagnosis of more chronic vascular complications including transplant artery stenosis and arteriovenous fistulae although it is of little use in the diagnosis of chronic rejection.

References

1 Valderrabano, F., Jones, E.H.P., Mallick, N.P. (1995) Report on the management of renal failure in Europe XXIV, 1993. *Nephrology, Dialysis and Transplantation* **10** (suppl. 51), 1–25.

2 Charra, B., Calemerd, E., Ruffet, M., *et al.* (1992) Survival as an index of the adequacy of dialysis. *Kidney International* **41**, 1286–1291.

3 Gore, S.M., Cable, D.J., Holland, A.J. (1992) Organ donation from intensive care units in England and Wales—two year confidential audit of deaths in intensive care. *British Medical Journal* **304**, 349–355.

4 Takemoto, S., Terasaki, P.I., Cecka, J.M., Chong, Y.W., Gjertson, D.W. (1992) Survival of nationally shared HLA-matched kidney transplants from cadaveric donors. *New England Journal of Medicine* **327**, 834–839.

5 The Canadian Multicentre Transplant Study Group (1986) A randomised clinical trial of cyclosporin in cadaveric renal

transplantation: analysis at three years. *New England Journal of Medicine* **314**, 1219–1220.
6 Berthoux, F.C., Jones, E.H.P., Mehls, O., Valderrabano, F. (1996) Transplantation report: report on management of renal failure in Europe, XXV, 1994. *Nephrology, Dialysis and Transplantation* **11** (suppl. 1), 37–40.
7 Opelz, G. (1985) Correlation of HLA matching with kidney graft survival in patients with or without cyclosporine treatment. *Transplantation* **40**, 240–243.
8 Vincenti, F., Laskow, D.A., Neylan, J.F., Mendez, R., Matas, A.J. (1996) One year follow up of an open label trial of FK506 for primary kidney transplantation. *Transplantation* **61**, 1576–1581.
9 European Mycophenolate Mofetil Cooperative Study Group (1995) Placebo controlled study of mycophenolate mofetil combined with cyclosporin and corticosteroids for prevention of acute rejection. *Lancet* **345**, 1321–1325.
10 Duda, S.H., Erley, C.M., Wakat, J.P., *et al.* (1993) Post-transplant renal artery stenosis—outpatient intraarterial DSA versus color aided duplex Doppler sonography. *European Journal of Radiology* **16**, 95–101.
11 Snider, J.F., Hunter, D.W., Moradian, G.P., Castaneda-Zuniga, W.R., Letourneau, J.G. (1989) Transplant renal artery stenosis: evaluation with duplex sonography. *Radiology* **172**, 1027–1030.
12 Taylor, K.J.W., Morse, S.S., Rigsby, C.M., Bia, M., Schiff, M. (1987) Vascular complications in renal allografts: detection with duplex Doppler US. *Radiology* **162**, 31–38.
13 Solez, K., Anderson, R.A., Benediktsson, H., *et al.* (1993) International standardisation of criteria for the histologic diagnosis of renal allograft rejection: the Banff working classification of kidney transplant pathology. *Kidney International* **44**, 411–422.
14 Wilczek, H.E. (1990) Percutaneous needle biopsy of the renal allograft. *Transplantation* **50**, 790–797.
15 Pirsch, J.D., Ploeg, R.J., Gange, S., *et al.* (1996) Determinants of graft survival after renal transplantation. *Transplantation* **61**, 1581–1585.
16 Cochlin, D.L.L., Wake, A., Salaman, J.R., Griffin, P.J.A. (1988) Ultrasound changes in the transplant kidney. *Clinical Radiology* **39**, 373–376.
17 Pozniak, M.A., Kelcz, F., D'Alessandro, A., Oberley, T., Stratta, R. (1992) Sonography of renal transplants in dogs: the effect of acute tubular necrosis, cyclosporin nephrotoxicity and acute rejection on resistive index and renal length. *American Journal of Radiology* **158**, 791–797.
18 Parvin, S.D., Rees, Y., Veitch, P.S., *et al.* (1986) Objective measurement by ultrasound to distinguish cyclosporin a toxicity from rejection. *British Journal of Surgery* **73**, 1009–1011.
19 Rifkin, M.D., Needleman, L., Pasto, M.E., *et al.* (1987) Evaluation of renal transplant rejection by duplex Doppler examination: value of the resistive index. *American Journal of Radiology* **148**, 759–762.
20 Rigsby, C.M., Taylor, K.J.W., Weltin, G., *et al.* (1986) Renal allografts in acute rejection: evaluation using duplex sonography. *Radiology* **158**, 375–378.
21 Genkins, S.M., Sanfilippo, F.P., Carroll, B.A. (1989) Duplex doppler sonography of renal transplants: lack of sensitivity and specificity in establishing pathologic diagnosis. *American Journal of Radiology* **152**, 535–539.
22 Kelzc, F., Pozniak, M.A., Pirsch, J.D., Oberly, T.D. (1990) Pyramidal appearance and resistive index: insensitive and nonspecific indicators of acute renal transplant rejection. *American Journal of Radiology* **155**, 531–535.
23 Merkus, J.W.S., Hoitsma, A.J., van Asten, W.N.J.C., Koene, R.A., Scotnicki, S.H. (1994) Doppler spectrum analysis to diagnose rejection during post transplant acute renal failure. *Transplantation* **58**, 570–576.
24 Kaveggia, L.P., Perella, R.R., Grant, E.G., *et al.* (1990) Duplex doppler sonography in renal allografts: the significance of reversed flow in diastole. *American Journal of Roentgenology* **155**, 295–298.
25 Penny, M.J., Nankivell, B.J., Disney, A.P.S., Blyth, K., Chapman, J.R. (1994) Renal graft thrombosis: a survey of 134 consecutive cases. *Transplantation* **58**, 565–569.
26 Baxter, G.M., Morley, P., Dall, B. (1991) Acute renal vein thrombosis in renal allografts: new Doppler ultrasonic findings. *Clinical Radiology* **43**, 125–127.
27 Reuther, G., Wanjura, D., Bauer, H. (1989) Acute renal vein thrombosis in renal allografts: detection with duplex Doppler ultrasound. *Radiology* **170**, 557–558.
28 MacLennan, A.C., Baxter, G.M., Harden, P., Rowe, P.A. (1995) Renal transplant vein occlusion; an early diagnostic sign? *Clinical Radiology* **50**, 251–253.
29 Benoit, G., Alexandre, L., Monkarezel, M., *et al.* (1993) Percutaneous antegrade dilatation of ureteral strictures in kidney transplants. *Journal of Urology* **150**, 37–39.
30 Nargund, V.H., Cranston, D. (1996) Urological complications after renal transplantation. *Transplantation Reviews* **10**, 24–33.
31 Myers, B.D., Sibley, R., Newton, L., *et al.* (1988) The long term course of cyclosporin associated chronic nephropathy. *Kidney International* **33**, 590–600.
32 Salamen, J.R., Griffen, P.J.A. (1983) Fine needle intrarenal manometry: a new test for rejection in cyclosporin treated recipients of kidney transplants. *Lancet* **ii**, 709–711.
33 Gray, D.W.R. (1994) Graft renal artery stenosis in the transplanted kidney. *Transplantation Reviews* **8**, 15–21.
34 Erley, C.M., Duda, S.H., Wakat, J.P., *et al.* (1992) Non invasive procedures for diagnosis of renovascular hypertension in renal transplant recipients and prospective analysis. *Transplantation* **54**, 863–867.
35 Baxter, G.M., Ireland, H., Moss, J.G., *et al.* (1995) Colour Doppler ultrasound in renal transplant artery stenosis: which Doppler index? *Clinical Radiology* **50**, 618–622.
36 Gedroye, W.M., Negus, R., al Kautoubi, A., *et al.* (1992) Magnetic resonance angiography of renal transplants. *Lancet* **339**, 789–791.
37 Baxter, G.M., Ireland, H., Moss, M.G., *et al.* (1995) Colour Doppler ultrasound in renal transplant artery stenosis; which Doppler index? *Clinical Radiology* **50**, 618–622.
38 Merkus, J.W.S., Zeebregts, C.J.A.M., Hoitsma, A.J., van Asten, W.N.J.C., Koene, R.A.P., Skotnicki, S.H. (1993) High incidence of arteriovenous fistula after biopsy of kidney allografts. *British Journal of Surgery* **80**, 310–312.
39 Renowden, S.A., Blethyn, J., Cochlin, D.I. (1992) Duplex and color flow sonography in the diagnosis of post biopsy arteriovenous fistulae in the transplant kidney. *Clinical Radiology* **45**, 233–237.
40 Matthew, T.H. (1991) Recurrent disease after transplantation. *Transplantation Reviews* **5**, 31–45.
41 Penn, I. (1986) Cancer is a complication of severe immunosuppression. *Surgery in Gynaecology and Obstetrics* **162**, 603–610.

Part 6
Pelvis

Chapter 32: The lower urinary tract and prostate

S.A. Moussa

Anatomy

Bladder

The urinary bladder lies in the mid line extraperitoneally within the bony pelvis. It is bounded anteriorly by the symphysis pubis but rises above it when filled, and by the obturator internus muscles and umbilical ligaments laterally, giving it its characteristic quadrangular shape in the transverse plane. Together with the prostate it is anchored to the urogenital diaphragm inferiorly. The rectum lies immediately behind it in the male. In the female the uterus and vagina are interposed between the bladder and urethra anteriorly and the rectum posteriorly.

The bladder vault is mobile allowing it to expand on filling, with the peritoneum loosely attached to it anteriorly but more firmly attached posteriorly [1].

The ureters are inserted into the bladder base posteriorly and have a short intramural segment traversing the bladder musculature.

Prostate

The prostate is a cone-shaped or inverted pyramid formed of glandular and fibromuscular tissue. It surrounds the beginning of the male urethra, lying behind the inferior border of the symphysis pubis and anterior to the rectal ampulla.

It is surrounded anteriorly by loose adipose tissue and venous plexus and is anchored to the pubic bone from its superior aspect by the puboprostatic ligaments. Laterally the fibrous sheath consists of fibrous tissue and venous plexus with a pair of neurovascular bundles on each side. Posteriorly the fibrous sheath is avascular [2]. Initial anatomical studies by McNeal suggested a zonal concept of the prostate anatomy [3], with concentric zones surrounding the proximal urethra [4] having anatomical, functional and pathological significance.

The prostatic urethra can be used as an anatomical landmark dividing the glands into an anterior fibromusculature portion and a posterior glandular portion. The prostatic urethra itself is divided into a proximal segment from the bladder neck to the verumontanum and a distal segment from the verumontanum to the external sphincter at the apex of the gland. The two segments form an obtuse angle (approximately 145°) at the verumontanum. The posterior glandular portion consists of three concentric zones. The transitional zone (TZ; approximately 5% of glandular tissue) surrounds the lateral aspect of the proximal urethral segments about the level of the verumontanum. The central zone (CZ; approximately 25% of glandular tissue) is wedged posteriorly between the seminal vesicle and ejaculatory ducts and posterior aspect of the proximal urethral segment. The peripheral zone (PZ; approximately 70% of glandular tissue) forms the remainder of the posterior glandular tissue (Fig. 32.1).

Seminal vesicles

The seminal vesicles which are formed by lateral outpouchings from the vas deferens are relatively symmetrical structures lying behind the bladder base obliquely. They are slightly lobulated (Fig. 32.2) and taper medially towards the mid line, joining the vas from either side to form the ejaculatory ducts. These in turn traverse the prostate and enter the prostatic urethra at the verumontanum.

Urethra

The urethra is a tubular structure, short in the female (2.5–4 cm) and longer and more complex in the male (7.5–20 cm).

The male urethra is divided mainly into two parts. The posterior urethra consisting of a proximal prostatic segment surrounded by the prostate and the membranous urethra extending from the external sphincter at the apex of the prostate to the urogenital diaphragm. The anterior urethra commences at the urogenital diaphragm swinging ventrally inferior to the symphysis pubis then running along the penile shaft. Its proximal portion is dilated (bulbar segment). The remaining penile segment is

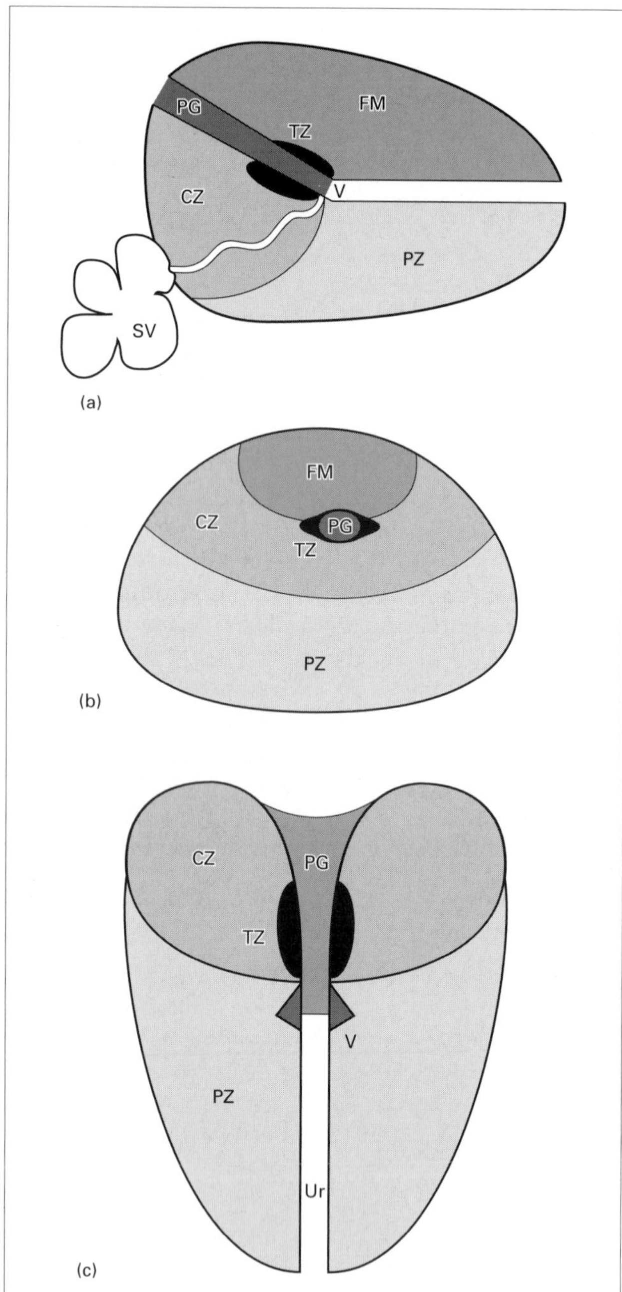

Fig. 32.1 Schematic representation of the zonal concept of prostate anatomy. (a) Mid line sagittal section. (b) Transverse section just above level of verumontanum. (c) Coronal section. CZ, central zone; FM, fibromuscular tissue; PG, periurethral glands; PZ, peripheral zone; SV, seminal vesicle; TZ, transition zone; Ur, urethra; V, verumontanum. (Redrawn from Rifkind, 1988 [15].)

uniform in size measuring approximately 6 mm in diameter. It is surrounded by the corpus spongiosum. The very distal segment in the glans penis is slightly dilated forming the fossa navicularis.

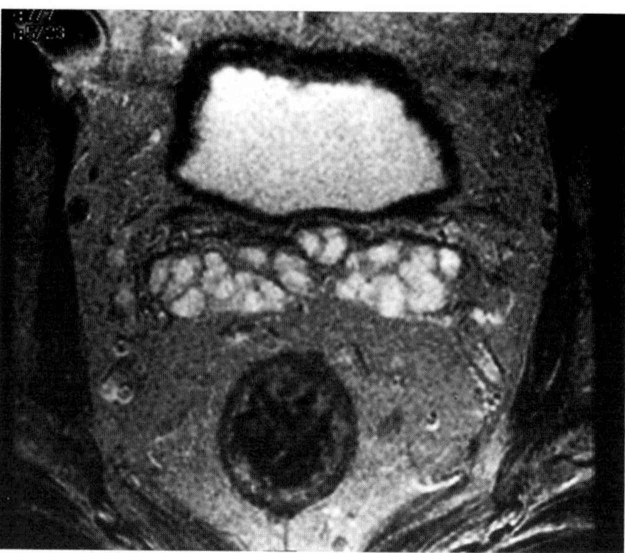

Fig. 32.2 Seminal vesicles: T_2-weighted magnetic resonance imaging image showing the symmetrically lobulated seminal vesicles lying behind the bladder base.

The female urethra is short extending from the bladder neck to the external urinary meatus. It lies behind the symphysis pubis and is closely related to the anterior wall of the vagina [5,6].

Techniques and instruments

Ultrasound imaging of the lower urinary tract is now a well-established and widely used technique to assess the bladder and female pelvic organs as well as the prostate, seminal vesicles and urethra. Recent advances in probe technology allow examinations of these areas to be carried out using different approaches; transabdominal (suprapubic), transurethral (endoluminal), transrectal (TRUS), transvaginal and transperineal.

Bladder

TRANSABDOMINAL (SUPRAPUBIC)

A full bladder is an obvious requirement for this examination. The patient is scanned in a supine position, using conventional 3.5–5 MHz, sector or curvilinear probes. When filled, the bladder gives an ideal window to scan deeper pelvic organs particularly in the female and also allows good visualization of the bladder neck, prostate and seminal vesicles in the male. However, a more detailed evaluation of the morphology of these structures is better achieved using the transrectal approach.

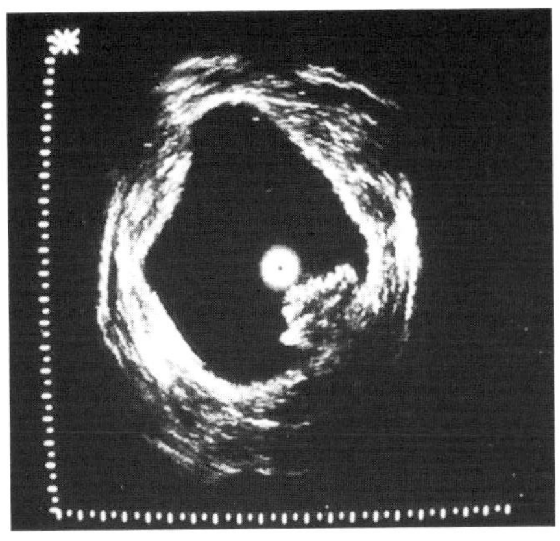
(a)

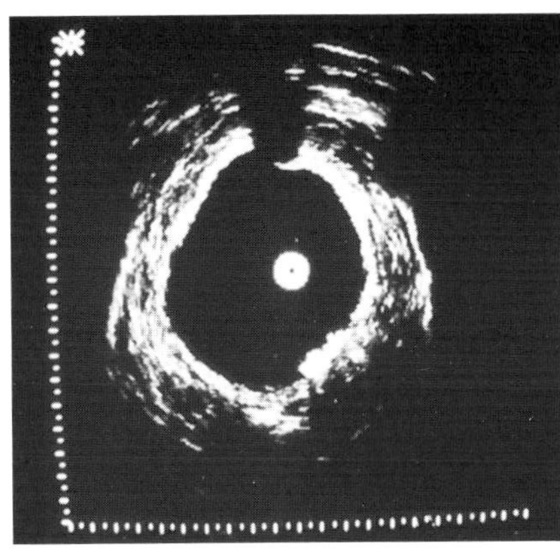
(b)

Fig. 32.3 Transurethral (endoluminal) bladder ultrasound. (a) Tumour arising from posterolateral wall of the bladder. (b) Appearances after resection.

TRANSURETHRAL (ENDOLUMINAL)

This imaging technique was introduced in the early 1970s (Fig. 32.3) [7]. Although this technique is not widely used in the UK it is still in use in specialized units mainly by urologists. The technique requires the necessary skills and training for cystoscopy and is carried out using a circumferential scanner (7–10 MHz) with a 90° side viewing transducer introduced through a 24 Ch cystoscope sheath. This allows detailed scanning of the bladder mucosa and musculature. The bladder neck and bladder vault represent relative blind spots and scanners with different angled transducers are used to visualize these areas [8]. Scanning of the bladder using this approach is usually carried out in conjunction with cystoscopy and when available it is particularly useful when poor vision due to bleeding makes cystoscopic examination inadequate as well as in conjunction with new laser-based transurethral resection of bladder tumours.

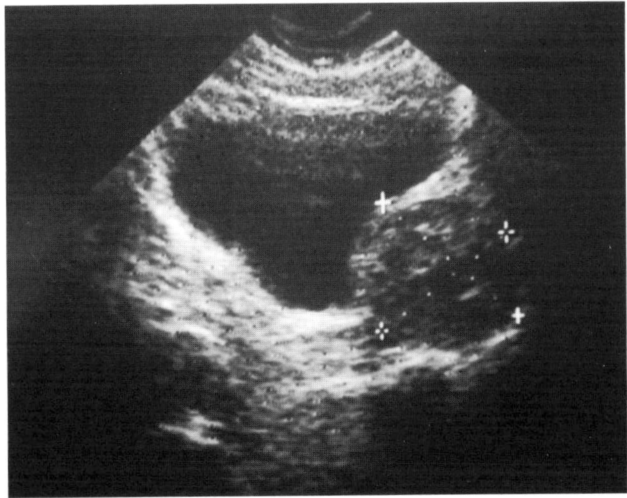

Fig. 32.4 Enlarged prostate indenting the bladder base (sagittal view).

Prostate and seminal vesicles

TRANSABDOMINAL

During conventional transabdominal scanning of the full bladder, the bladder neck, prostate and seminal vesicles can be visualized and a large prostate indenting the bladder base can be evaluated and its volume measured (Fig. 32.4). Large abscesses or cystic lesions deep to the bladder base can also be visualized to some extent; however, the detailed zonal anatomy of the prostate and surrounding structures and any smaller focal lesions will not be easily seen.

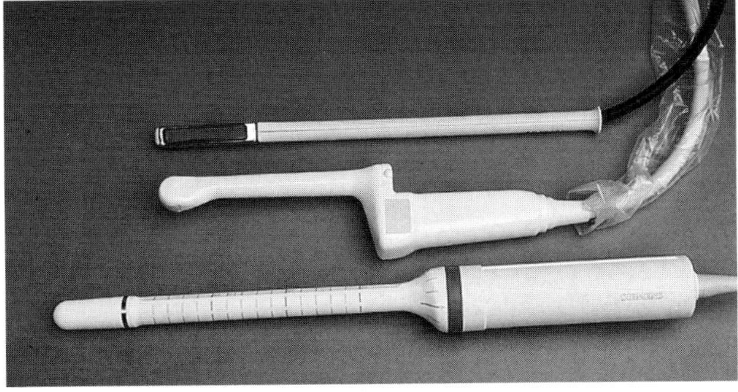

Fig. 32.5 Some of the single and multiplane probes available for transrectal scanning.

TRANSRECTAL ULTRASOUND (TRUS)

A large number of dedicated transrectal probes are now available (Fig. 32.5). These vary in frequency from 5 to 7.5 MHz. Multi-frequency probes are now standard with the majority of ultrasound equipment. Probes can be single plane, sector, linear or curvilinear allowing scanning of the prostate in the transverse or sagittal planes.

These scans, however, require physical rotation during the examination to scan into perpendicular planes. Biplane and multiplane probes are now also widely available with more modern probes allowing simultaneous scanning in both transverse and sagittal planes viewed on a split screen. Probes are routinely covered using general purpose or specifically designed condoms. Some probes are equipped with a water-filled balloon acting as a stand-off and allowing the whole of the prostate to be visualized in a wider image field. Care should be taken to clean the probe adequately between examinations by following the manufacturer's guidelines or local infection control policies.

The patient is usually scanned in the left lateral position and apart from a relatively filled bladder no specific preparation is required. When examining the prostate the gland should be scanned in both axial (transverse) and sagittal planes. The seminal vesicles are easily seen behind the bladder base mainly in the axial plane, slight angling of the probe allows scanning of these structures through their longitudinal axis. The lower ureters and intramural segments are often clearly seen along the same plane entering the superior aspect of the trigone (Fig. 32.6).

TRANSPERINEAL

In rare circumstances transperineal scanning can be used to visualize the prostate when the transrectal route is not available following abdominoperineal resection of the rectum or in the presence of severe anal strictures. Imaging of the prostate using this route is relatively poor. This technique, however, can be useful in carrying out ultrasound-guided biopsies of the prostate in these circumstances.

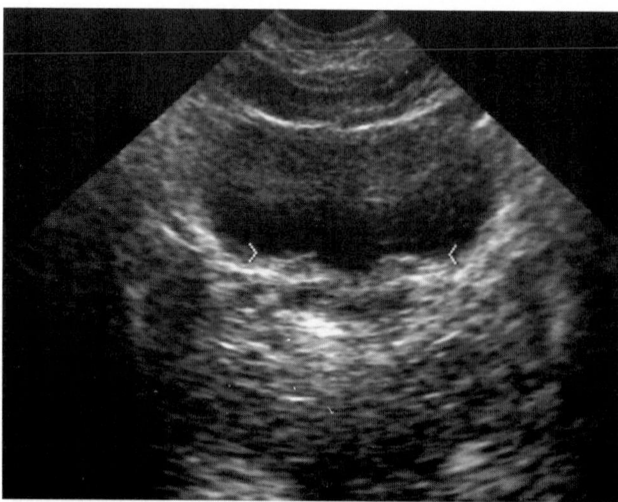

Fig. 32.6 Intramural segment of distal ureters (arrowheads) seen on transabdominal scanning.

Urethra

TRANSRECTAL

The bladder neck and prostatic urethra can easily be imaged in the sagittal plane using the transrectal route. If bladder voiding can be achieved with the rectal probe *in situ* clear images of the bladder neck, prostatic urethra, verumontanum and external sphincter can be obtained (Fig. 32.7) and functional studies carried out and recorded on video (ultrasound videourethrography [8]).

TRANSVAGINAL

In females dedicated transvaginal probes (sector or curvilinear), similar in design to the single plane transrectal probes and interchangeable, are used to visualize the bladder neck and distal ureters as well as the short female urethra and any distended urethral lesions.

Penile urethra

Ultrasound scanning of the penile and bulbar urethra can be carried out using a small part linear probe 6–7.5 MHz which can be applied to the dorsal or ventral aspect of the penis. The urethra is distended with sterile water or saline using standard urethrographic technique. Alternatively, the urethra can be filled by asking the patient to compress the urethra firmly at the glans during micturition (Fig.

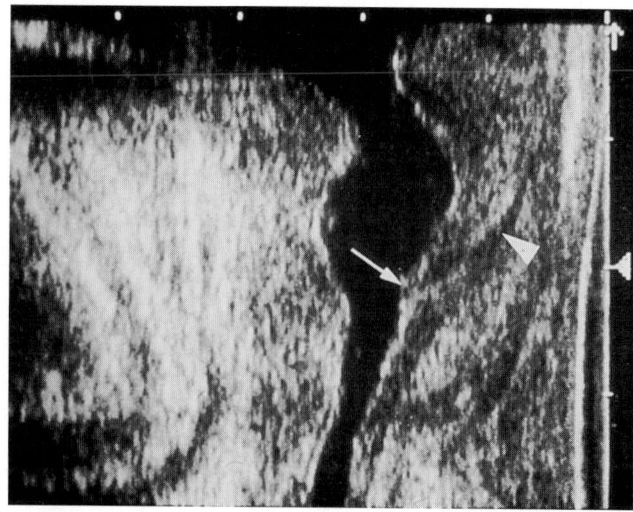

Fig. 32.7 Transrectal ultrasound during voiding, demonstrating open bladder neck and prostatic urethra, verumontanum (arrow) and ejaculatory ducts (arrowhead).

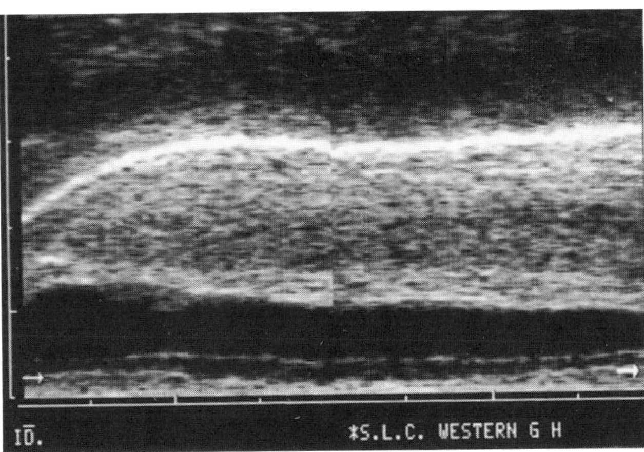

Fig. 32.8 Normal penile urethra using linear array probe applied to the ventral aspect of the penis.

32.8). This avoids the need for catheterization and greatly reduces the duration of the examination [9].

Normal appearances

BLADDER

The normal full urinary bladder is triangular or ellipsoid in shape in the mid line sagittal plane but has a more quadrangular outline within the bony pelvis in the transverse plane, becoming more rounded as the bladder vault rises upward outside the true pelvis. The bladder wall is relatively echogenic and well demarcated, and although the wall thickness varies with the degree of bladder filling, this should not exceed 5 mm in a well-distended bladder. The anterior wall of the bladder is often less well defined due to reverberation artefacts.

A small indentation in the inferior aspect of the bladder represents the bladder neck. This is more easily seen in males where the prostate indicates its exact position. The prostate and seminal vesicles are seen in relation to the inferior and posterior aspect of the bladder behind the trigone. The ureteric orifices can often be identified as slight localized thickening of the bladder mucosa on either side of the mid line at the level of the seminal vesicles. Urinary jets into the bladder are often clearly seen during the examination as a result of ureteric peristalsis (Fig. 32.9). These jets can be depicted more easily with the higher sensitivity of colour flow Doppler [10].

Bladder volume assessment

Bladder volume measurement is based on mathematical formulae for measuring ellipsoid shapes. Two methods are widely used [11,12].

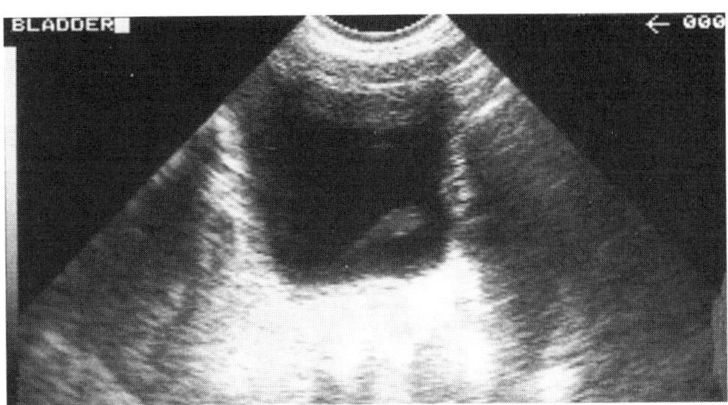

Fig. 32.9 Transverse view of the bladder: ureteric jet from right ureter.

ELLIPSOID METHOD

The bladder is imaged in both transverse and sagittal mid line planes. The images are stored or viewed simultaneously on a split screen. The volume is calculated using the prolate ellipsoid formula

$$V = L \times H \times W \times c$$

where L represents the length of the bladder and H the height (both of these measurements are best taken on the sagittal image); W represents the width or transverse diameter; and c represents a constant $\pi/6$ or approximately 0.53.

The same formula is used to measure the volume of the prostate gland.

THE PLANIMETRIC METHOD

This is a more accurate but time-consuming method. The volume is calculated by determining the surface area of a number of successive parallel images taken at equal intervals through the organs. This required an accurate stepping unit allowing only movement in equidistant steps (e.g. 5 mm). In each image the bladder is outlined using the trackerball. Using the surface areas measured and the spacing between the steps allows relatively accurate estimation of the volume.

The majority of ultrasound machines are now equipped with software packages for volume estimation (Fig. 32.10) as well as dedicated urological packages for estimation of residual volume after voiding, prostate volume and if prostate-specific artigen (PSA) values are known, other calculations such as PSA densities can be carried out automatically. These softwares also include facilities for on-screen reporting (Fig. 32.11).

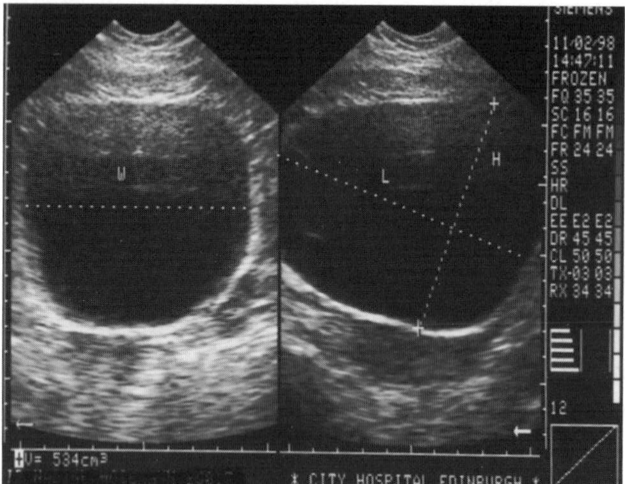

Fig. 32.10 Bladder volume measurements. H, height; L, length; W, width.

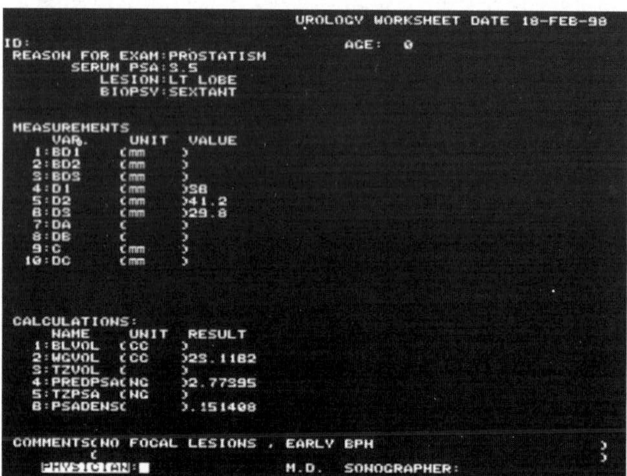

Fig. 32.11 Example of on-screen worksheet for measurement recording and reporting.

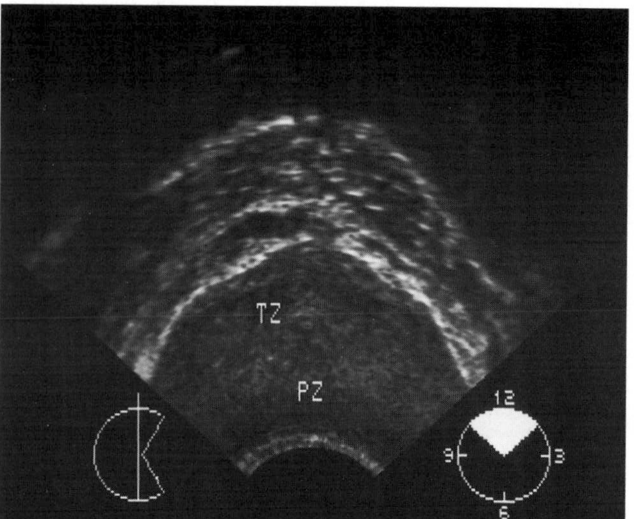

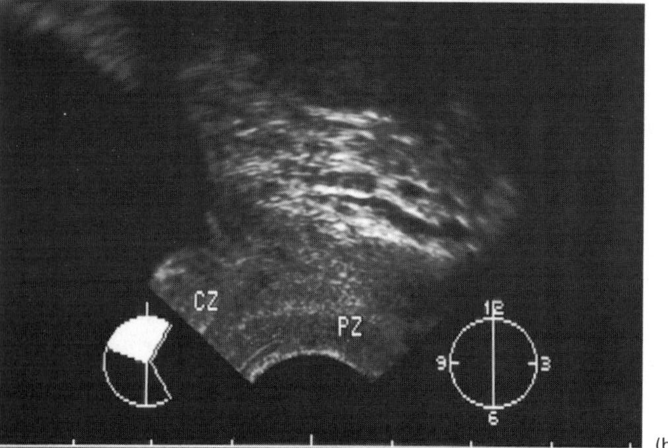

Fig. 32.12 Normal appearances of the prostate on transrectal scanning. (a) Transverse view. (b) Sagittal mid line view. CZ, central zone; PZ, peripheral zone; TZ, transitional zone.

Prostate and seminal vesicles

Viewed through the bladder during transabdominal scanning, the prostate is seen as a rounded relatively hypoechoic homogeneous structure situated caudal to the bladder neck. Estimation of the size of the gland can be obtained from these views but evaluation of the glandular architecture is poor. The seminal vesicles are seen as a pair of elongated structures just above the prostate lying behind the bladder neck and bladder trigone. They also appear hypoechoic and homogeneous [13].

On transrectal ultrasound the appearances of the prostate vary depending on the plane of scanning and the level within the gland. Much of the zonal anatomy described by McNeal [3] can be visualized [14].

In the transverse plane starting at the apex of the prostate, the urethra is centrally situated surrounded laterally and posteriorly by the PZ which is homogeneously stippled. This increases in size as scanning progresses proximally into the gland up to the level of the verumontanum (Fig. 32.12a). Anteriorly the fibromuscular stroma forms a small hypoechoic zone.

At the level of the verumontanum which appears as a small hypoechoic structure in the posterior aspect of the urethra, TZ material is recognized on either side of the urethra. This is surrounded posteriorly by a small CZ with the PZ which is slightly more echogenic forming the rest of the gland posteriorly and laterally.

As scanning progresses proximally, the urethra is seen more anteriorly and is surrounded posteriorly by a larger CZ which is in turn surrounded by the PZ forming the base of the gland.

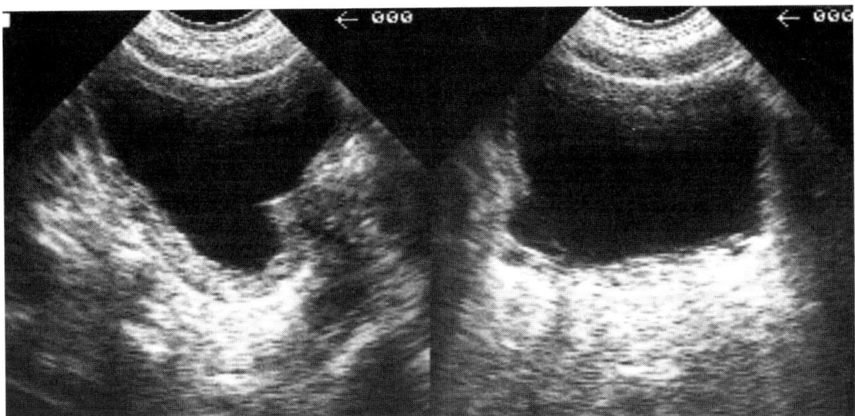

Fig. 32.13 Sagittal and transverse views of the bladder with gross thickening and trabeculation of the wall secondary to outflow obstruction due to benign prostatic hypertrophy.

At a higher level, a thick echogenic fat plane separates the trigone from the base of the prostate and the medial aspect of the seminal vesicles.

The seminal vesicles appear as relatively symmetrical paired structures, slightly lobulated mostly homogeneous in echo texture. Their convoluted tubular structure, however, is often recognizable. They overlap in the mid line with the ampullary segments of the vas joining their medial aspect to form the ejaculatory ducts.

In the longitudinal (sagittal) mid line plane (Fig. 32.12b), the bladder neck and empty prostatic urethra are recognizable. The urethra angles at the verumontanum. The PZ and CZ cannot be easily separated but the course of the ejaculatory duct can often be seen as a thin hypoechoic or hyperechoic line running obliquely towards the verumontanum.

In the lateral sagittal plane, the 'lateral lobes' are ovoid in shape and consist mainly of the PZs.

The small amount of fat separating the seminal vesicles and base of the prostate form the prostatic–seminal vesicles angle [15]. This is often acute but can vary; however, it should be symmetrical in the same individual.

Disorders of the bladder

Bladder outflow obstruction

Videocystometrography remains the definitive examination to assess the function of the lower urinary tract. However, this examination is invasive, time-consuming and carries a small risk of complications such as infection.

Using ultrasound estimation of the bladder volume before and after voiding to assess the bladder residual volume combined with uroflowmetry often provides sufficient information as to the nature of the outflow obstruction and can negate the need for formal urodynamic studies [16].

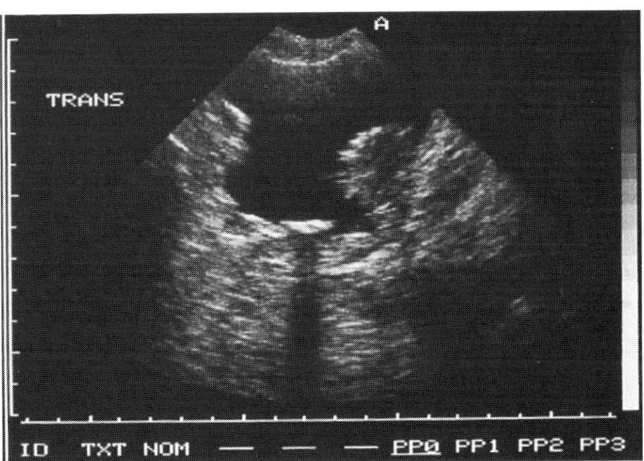

Fig. 32.14 Tumour arising from left lateral wall of the bladder. Echogenic stone with distinct acoustic shadowing resting on posterior wall.

Measuring the bladder volume before voiding ensures the presence of sufficient volume of at least more than 200 cm^3 needed to achieve an adequate flow study. In some patients with chronic outflow obstruction, the bladder may be overdistended. Thickening of the bladder wall and the presence of trabeculations is indicative of the long-standing nature of the condition (Fig. 32.13).

Bladder calculi are usually seen in association with outflow obstruction or bladder disfunction (e.g. neurogenic). Like renal calculi they are strongly echogenic with distinct acoustic shadowing (Fig. 32.14). Most calculi originate from the upper tracts.

Clots and other debris resulting from infection, haemorrhage from the upper tract or following endoscopic surgery (transurethral resection of the prostate or tumour resection) presents as mobile relatively hyperechoic structures within the bladder lumen but without the characteristic shadowing of calculi (Fig. 32.15).

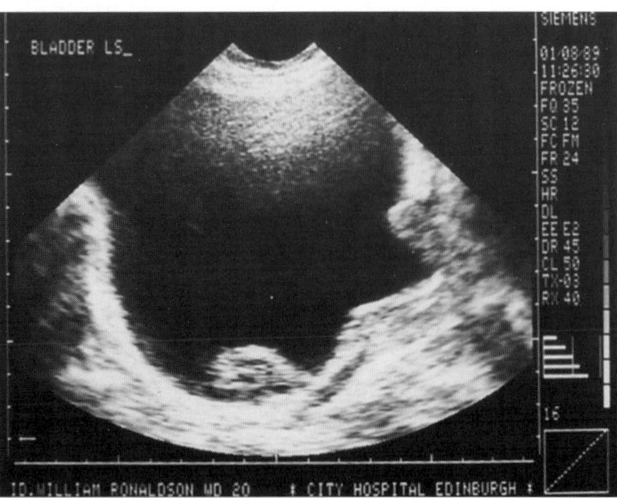

Fig. 32.15 Sagittal view of the bladder in the early postoperative period following transurethral reaction of the prostate: large defect at bladder neck and echogenic clot resting on posterior bladder wall.

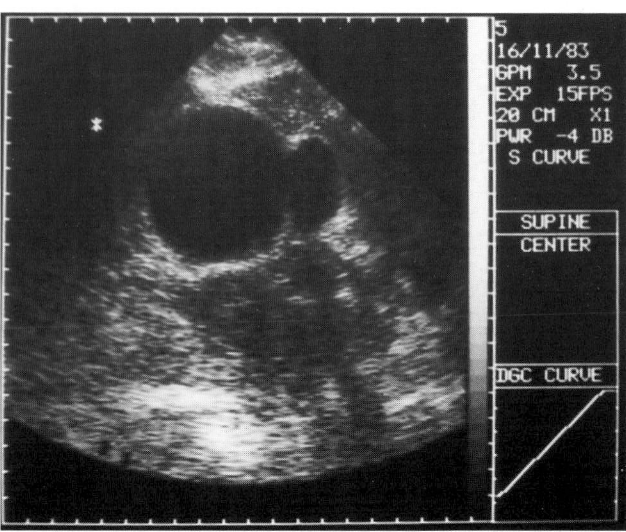

Fig. 32.16 Bladder diverticulum.

Bladder diverticula are also often seen in association with the above conditions although they are rarely congenital (Fig. 32.16). They usually arise from the posterior and lateral aspect of the bladder wall or in a paraureteral location. They appear as sonolucent masses varying in size. The opening onto the diverticulum is often identified and they may increase in size during voiding. If the opening cannot be seen they can be mistaken for extrinsic pelvic cystic lesions such as ovarian cysts, haematoma or lymphocele. Stones, blood clots or neoplastic lesions will occasionally be seen within these structures.

Benign prostatic hypertrophy

Although the degree of prostatic enlargement can be correlated with a degree of outflow obstruction, this correlation is rather poor. The configuration as well as the size of the prostate can be evaluated by transabdominal or transrectal ultrasonography. This helps to define the relationship of the bladder neck to the prostate, enlargement of the median lobe and displacement of the posterior urethra. These factors may assist the urologist in the choice of different available treatment modalities.

Bladder neck dyssynergia

This is a common condition causing bladder outflow obstruction in young men often undiagnosed. It can be complicated at later stages by the development of benign prostatic hypertrophy. Transrectal ultrasonography shows a hypoechoic region around the bladder neck as well as characteristic trapping of fluid in the prostatic urethra and intraprostatic reflux on interruption of micturition. Periurethral ductal calculi are also seen [17].

Cystitis

Inflammation of the bladder is a common finding. The changes are often too subtle and non-specific for ultrasound evaluation. Although the pathogenesis is often unknown, predisposing conditions such as diabetes, immunosuppression or depression, or local factors such as obstruction, calculi or the presence of indwelling catheters may be responsible for persistence or recurrence of cystitis.

INFECTIOUS CYSTITIS

Bacterial

The most common pathogens are *Escherichia coli* and other organisms originating from the intestine. Acute cystitis gives rise to little morphological changes except in the very severe cases where the bladder wall is irregular with thickening of the mucosa [18].

Chronic forms of cystitis may present as small focal bullous hypoechoic lesions due to bullous mucosal oedema. This should be distinguished from cystitis cystica and cystitis glandularis.

Tuberculosis of the bladder

Relatively rare it is always secondary to lesions in the upper tract and much less frequently as extension from the prostate. Ultrasonography reveals diffuse bladder wall thickening with reduced bladder capacity. Filling tumour-like defects (vesical tuberculoma) may be seen on rare occasions. When bladder wall fibrosis occurs, the bladder may become deformed and asymmetrical. These changes affect the trigone, the areas adjacent to the ureteric orifices and are associated with the presence of hydronephrosis.

Fungal cystitis

Immunosuppression and diabetes are predisposing factors. Debris and clusters of fungal masses are present in the bladder lumen [19].

Schistosomiasis

Parasitic infection (*Schistosoma haematobium*) endemic in the Middle East and Africa. Changes are due to deposition of ova in the submucosal plexuses mainly in the region of the trigone and lower ureter but may be more extensive. This leads to mucosal thickening and later calcification seen as extended linear hyperechogenicity of the bladder wall. Rarely tumour-like granulomas may also form. As a result of associated squamous metaplasia, patients with schistosomiasis have a higher incidence of squamous cell carcinoma [20].

Chronic non-infectious cystitis

Apart from the characteristic finding of small cystic filling defects of cystitis cystica [21] most other forms of chronic cystitis such as cystitis glandularis [22], amyloidosis, drug-induced cystitis and radiation cystitis generally present on sonography with marked thickening of the bladder wall which may be focal or diffuse. Neoplastic-like mass formation makes differentiation from tumours difficult. As with other forms of cystitis as well as bladder pathology in general, the cystoscopy and biopsies are usually required to reach a definitive diagnosis.

Bladder neoplasms

Tumours of the urothelium constitute approximately 95% of bladder neoplasms. Other parts of the urinary tract lined with transitional cell epithelium can also be affected by similar tumours but the bladder is by far the commonest site [23] (Fig. 32.17).

Non-epithelial tumours involving the bladder musculature such as leiomyosarcomas and rhabdomyosarcomas are relatively rare and present as smooth mural defects. These may ulcerate simulating an invasive transitional cell tumour. Other lesions such as pleochromocytomas and lymphoma can primarily involve the bladder wall [24].

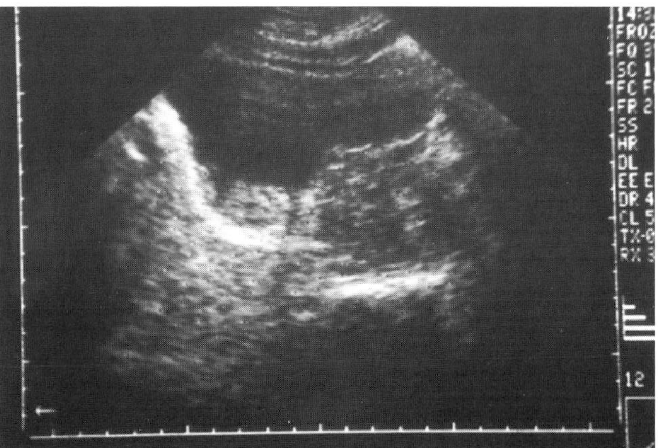
(a)

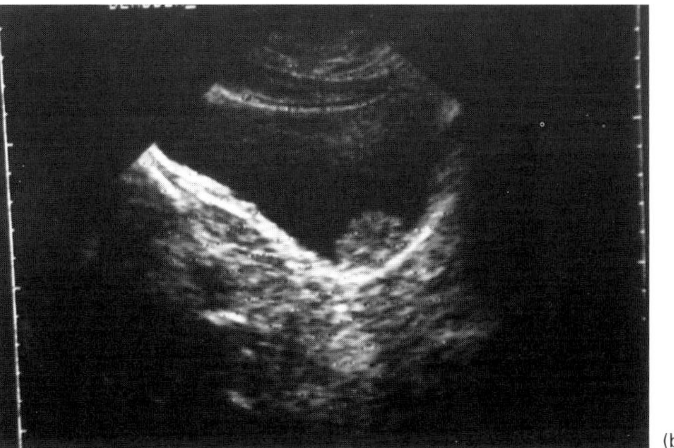
(b)

Fig. 32.17 Bladder neoplasm. (a) Small tumour mass arising from posterior wall of bladder. (b) The prostate is also enlarged.

Secondary bladder tumours represent slightly more than 1% of all neoplastic bladder lesions (Fig. 32.18). The most frequent metastatic lesions encountered are malignant melanomas but other tumours also involve the bladder via haematogenous or intraperitoneal spread. More commonly, however, the bladder is involved by direct extension of tumours arising from other adjacent pelvic structures (prostate, colon or cervix).

Urothelial bladder tumours

Of the epithelial tumours approximately 25% are transitional cell carcinomas, 4% are squamous cell carcinomas and 1% adenocarcinomas. These cannot be differentiated on imaging. Cystoscopy and biopsies are required for definitive diagnosis. Squamous cell carcinoma is more often found in patients with a history of chronic or recurrent urinary tract infection, stones or schistosomiasis. Adenocarcinomas arising in the dome of the bladder must be considered urachal in origin [25].

Transitional cell carcinoma

This is the second commonest urological tumour following carcinoma of the prostate. It occurs more commonly in men, the male to female ratio is 3–4 to 1. These tumours are relatively rare under the age of 40 years. The prognosis depends on the grade and stage of the tumour at diagnosis. The early stages (Ta and T2) show a 3-year survival of 53–90%, while with later stages (T3 and T4) this drops down to between 15 and 27%. Equally there is a high recurrence rate in the more undifferentiated higher grade tumours [26].

The majority of patients present with gross haematuria. Cystoscopy is the main definitive diagnostic modality. The role of the intravenous urogram in patient evaluation remains controversial but there is a general consensus regarding its value in detecting upper tract lesions which may affect the overall management of the patient [27].

Sonographically bladder transitional cell carcinomas are easily seen as well-demarcated slightly echogenic lesions projecting into the bladder lumen. However, difficulties arise with small lesions less than 5 mm in size which are not easily detected [28]. Lesions arising on the anterior wall of the bladder may also be difficult to visualize but this is less of a problem with more modern equipment. With extensive bladder tumours there is irregular and diffuse bladder wall thickening. Calcific encrustation are also often seen on the surface of the tumour (Fig. 32.19). Conventional ultrasound is also considered less accurate than other imaging modalities such as magnetic resonance imaging in assessing the degree of invasion through the bladder wall [29,30].

Despite these limitations, recent studies indicate that periodic ultrasound examinations combined with urine cytology can be an alternative to regular check cystoscopy in the follow-up of patient with superficial bladder tumours [31]. A similar policy has also been recently advocated for the investigation of patients presenting with asymptomatic microscopic haematuria.

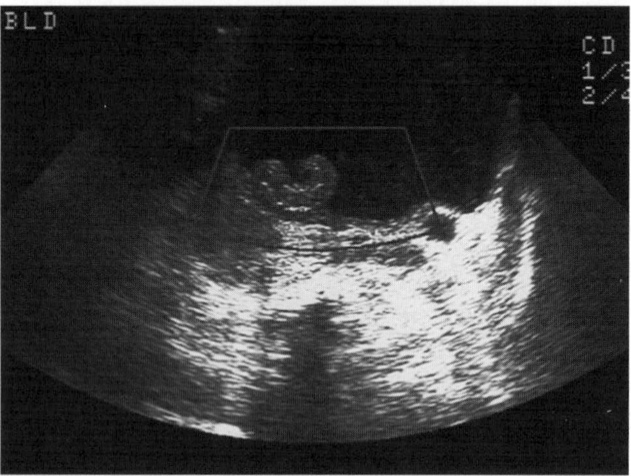

Fig. 32.18 Vascular lesion arising from bladder wall near the right vesicoureteric junction; very rare metastasis from gastric carcinoma.

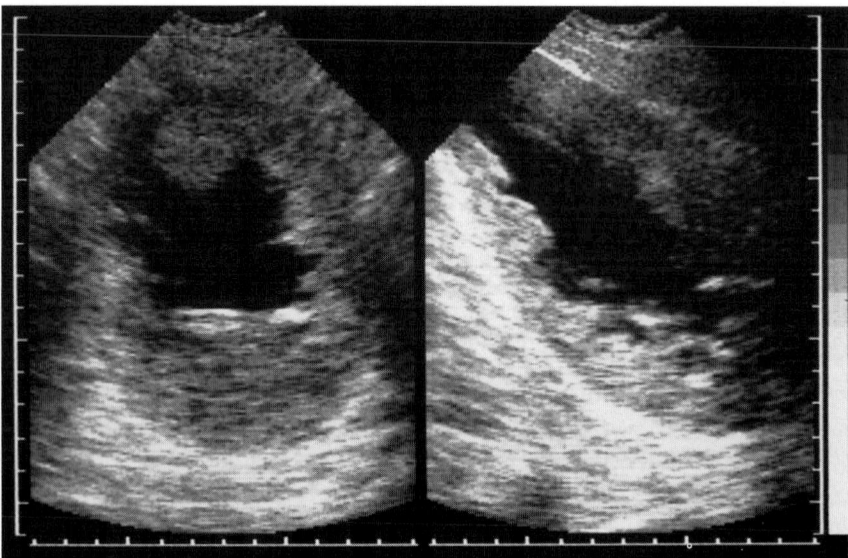

Fig. 32.19 Extensive bladder transitional cell carcinoma. Note irregular bladder mucosal thickening and echogenic encrustation.

Disorders of the prostate

Benign prostatic hypertrophy

The prostate usually increases in size with advancing age. Changes occur between the ages of 45–60 years and are rare below the age of 40 years. Occasionally the prostate may atrophy; however, enlargement is more common and has been estimated to affect up to 90% of the adult male population [32].

The exact pathogenesis is unclear and is characterized by the formation of nodules or adenomas invariably involving the TZ and periurethral glands [33]. These adenomas may enlarge to a massive size or there may be diffuse enlargement of the TZ.

The clinical manifestations may vary but their severity is not always related to the absolute size of the gland. Patients may present with irritative symptoms such as urinary frequency, nocturia or sensation of incomplete voiding, or obstructive symptoms including retention which may be acute or chronic, poor urinary stream, difficulty in initiating voiding and incomplete voiding with varying degrees of postmicturition bladder residue.

Sonographically, on conventional suprapubic scanning the enlarged prostate presents as a relatively homogeneous structure indenting the bladder base particularly when changes involve the middle portion of the gland posteriorly (median lobe) causing anterior displacement of the bladder neck and impingement on the proximal urethra. Focal lesions and zonal changes are, however, more clearly defined on transrectal scanning. Early changes include diffuse enlargement of the TZ with reduced echogenicity or discrete nodules (Figs 32.20, 32.21). These may enlarge symmetrically causing exaggeration of the Eiffel Tower configuration of the urethra at the level of the verumontanum. Asymmetrical enlargement may cause distortion of the prostatic outline (capsule) mimicking malignant infiltration (Fig. 32.22). The enlarging adenomas may show cystic changes and are associated with foci of calcification (calculi) or hyperechoic foci representing corpora amylacea (Fig. 32.23). These changes give rise to a heterogeneous echo pattern.

The enlargement of the adenomas and TZ causes posterior and lateral compression of the PZ and CZ which become relatively hyperechoic. Compression can be considerable. The compressed tissues are separated from the hypertrophied adenomatous tissues by a sharp demarcation identified as the 'surgical capsules' [34,35].

Transrectal ultrasound of the benign prostate is often carried out to assess the size of the gland (using the same prolate ellipsoid formula used for bladder volume estimation) as well as any impingement on the bladder neck. This may assist in the choice of treatment modality.

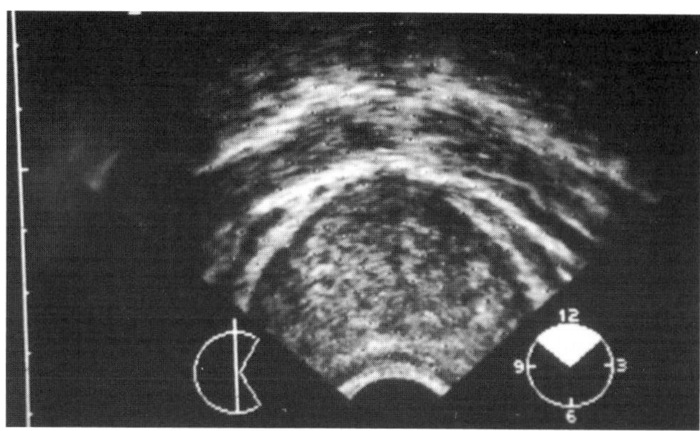

Fig. 32.20 Moderate benign prostatic hypertrophy: diffuse enlargement of the TZ.

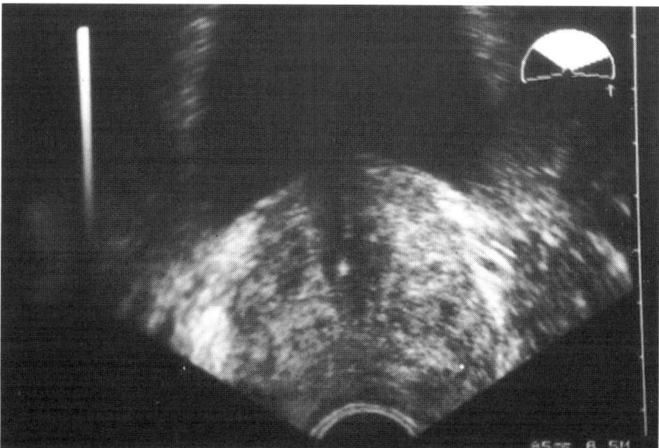

Fig. 32.21 Benign prostatic hypertrophy: gross enlargement of the TZ with heterogeneous nodularity.

Although transurethral resection of the prostate remains the most widely used technique in patients requiring intervention, other treatments including drug therapy and various forms of heat treatment are now also widely available. Patients scanned after transurethral resection of the prostate usually show re-expansion of the compressed tissue and a characteristic defect at the bladder neck and proximal urethra is seen (Fig. 32.24). This is much smaller than the amount of tissue resected even when the study is carried out in the immediate postoperative period to investigate clot retention [36]. The prostate may undergo recurrent hyperplastic growth.

Inflammatory disorders

Prostatitis is a common problem. Unfortunately, diagnostic assessment may be problematic with non-specific sonographic findings in the majority of cases. These include a hypoechoic rim surrounding the gland, a

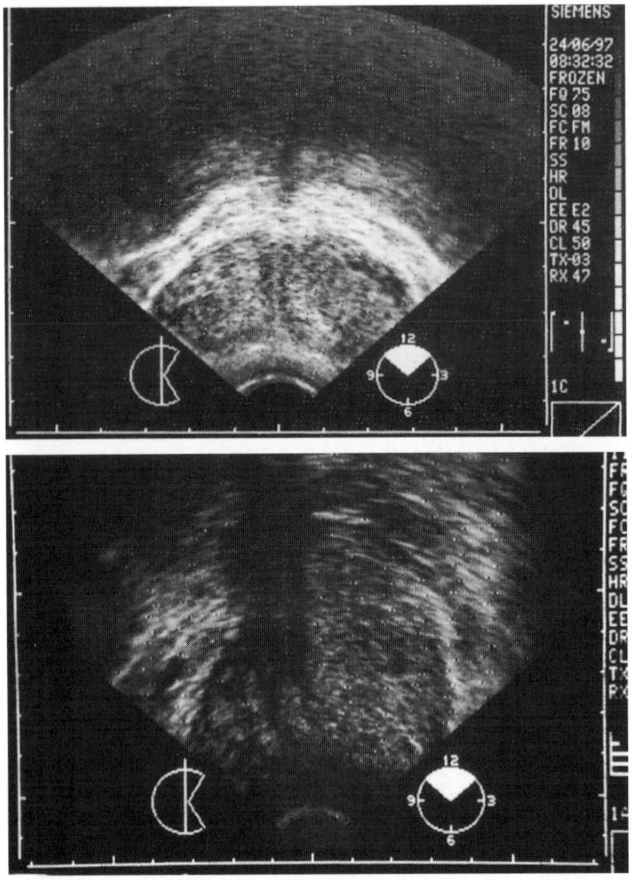

Fig. 32.22 Benign prostatic hypertrophy. (a) Symmetrical enlargement of TZ adenomas. (b) Asymmetrical enlargement of the adenomas.

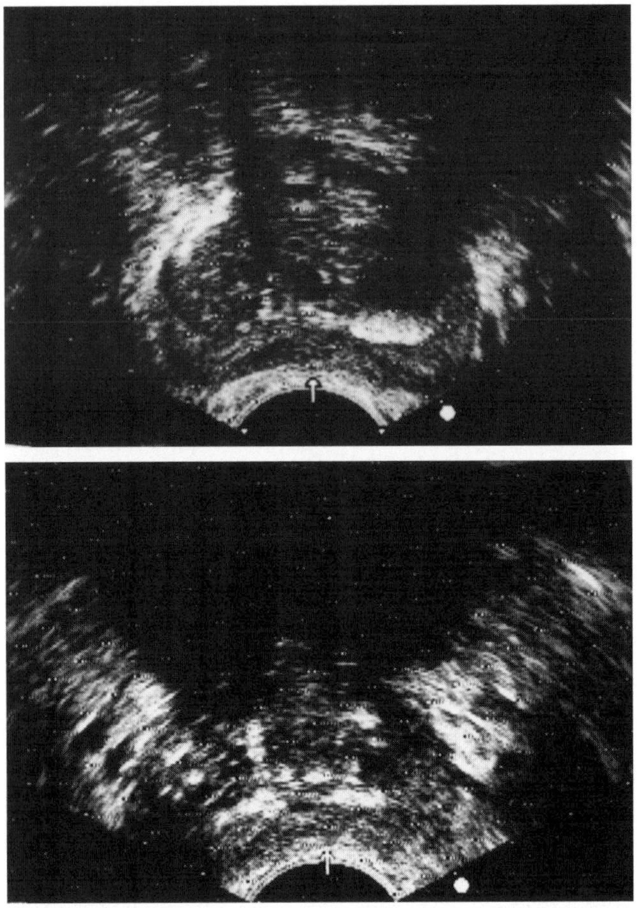

Fig. 32.23 Benign prostatic hypertrophy. (a) Calcification at the level of the 'surgical capsule' on the left side. (b) Multiple echogenic foci without acoustic shadowing representing corpora amylacea.

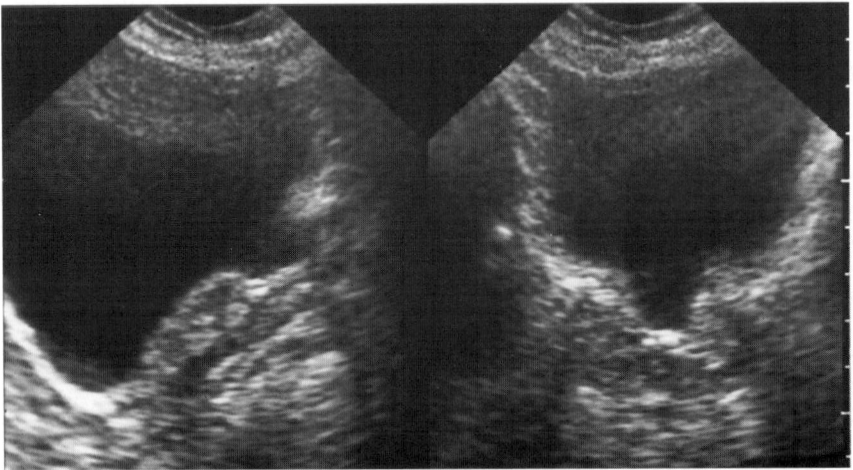

Fig. 32.24 Post-transurethral reaction of the prostate: typical defect in the bladder neck and proximal prostatic urethra.

sonolucent halo around the periurethral tissue and reduced echogenicity within the peripheral zone (Fig. 32.25). These changes have been described by Griffiths *et al.* as indicative of acute prostatitis [37]. Difficulties in diagnosis also arise due to non-prostatic abnormalities causing pelviperineal pain (prostadenia) simulating prostatitis [38]. Diagnostic imaging is generally not warranted unless abscess formation or underlying malignancies is suspected.

ACUTE BACTERIAL PROSTATITIS

This commonly occurs in sexually active young males aged 20–40 years. The most frequent causative organism is *E. coli* but *Pseudomonas* and enterococci or mixed infection can also be found. Following transrectal procedures anaerobic organism (*Bacteroides* and clostridia) are usually responsible.

Patients present with local symptoms in the form of pelviperineal pain, pain on defaecation or micturition associated with tenderness on digital rectal examination (DRE). Systemic symptoms of infection may also be present particularly with abscess formation. Sonographically the non-specific changes previously described may be present unless complicated with abscess formation. The abscess may vary in size presenting as a well-circumscribed hypoechoic lesion with a thick hyperechoic rim (Fig. 32.26) or the appearances may be complex with cystic and solid components. The abscess can be diagnostically aspirated under ultrasound guidance preferably using a transperineal approach with instillation of a suitable antibiotic. Alternatively, transurethral drainage (often with transrectal ultrasound guidance) can be effective.

(a)

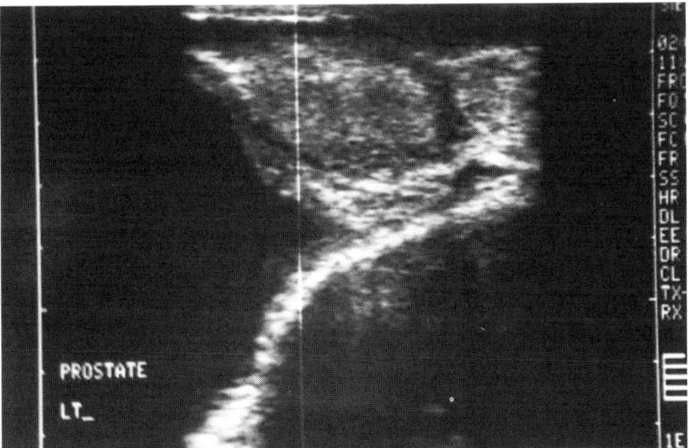

(b)

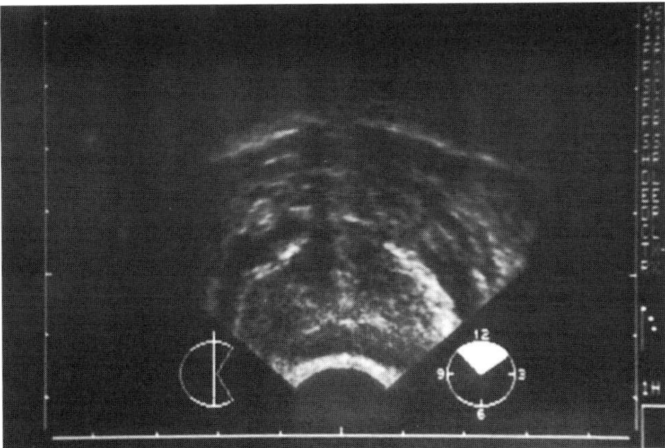

Fig. 32.25 Prostatitis. (a) Hypoechoic rim surrounding the lateral lobe (sagittal view). (b) Reduced echogenicity of the peripheral zone and dilated periprostatic veins.

CHRONIC BACTERIAL PROSTATITIS

This may or may not be preceded by acute prostatitis. Sonographically non-specific alteration in echo pattern may be seen but there are no pathognomonic ultrasound features. Prostatic calcification and calculi are suspected sequelae but these are also seen in patients with no clinical history of acute or chronic prostatitis. Some authors believe that the entire prostatovesicular complex is involved in chronic prostatitis [39].

GRANULOMATOUS PROSTATITIS

This is usually a histological diagnosis. The sonographic features are altered echogenicity of the PZ with scattered hypoechoic areas which may closely resemble malignant changes. Different pathological entities of granulomatous prostatitis are recognized [40].

1 Specific granulomatous prostatitis caused by tuberculosis, fungi, brucellosis or *Treponema pallidum*.
2 Non-specific granulomatous prostatitis accounts for at least 70% of granulomatous prostatitis. No causative agent is found.
3 Eosinophilic or allergic granulomatous prostatitis associated with peripheral eosinophilia, a history of asthma and mucocutaneous allergies [41].

NON-BACTERIAL PROSTATITIS

This is diagnosed when the prostatic fluid is purulent but no organisms are grown on culture. *Mycoplasma*, *Trichomonas* and *Chlamydia* may be the causative agents [42].

Prostate carcinoma

Carcinoma of the prostate is the second most common malignant neoplasm in men and currently the second most common cause of cancer deaths. At autopsy it is found in 12–50% of men over the age of 50 years. The incidence increases with age [43,44]. The aetiology is

(a)

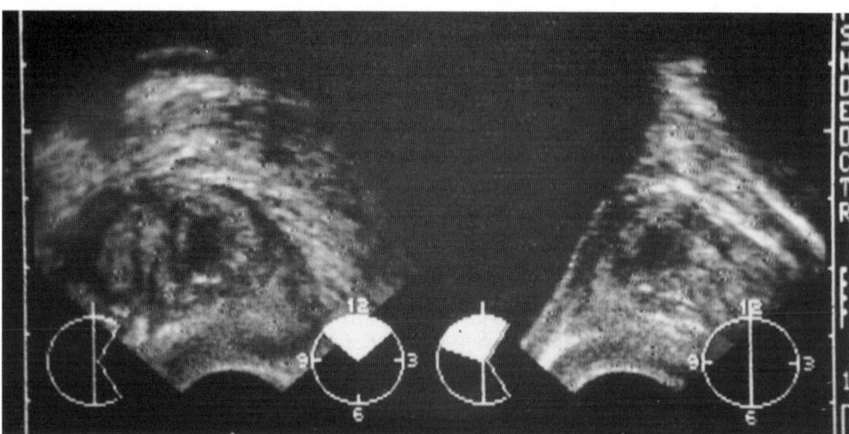

(b)

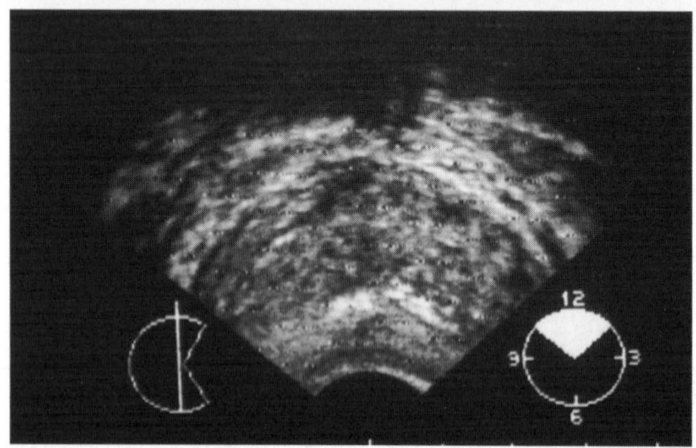

Fig. 32.26 Acute bacterial prostatitis: prostate abscess in the left lobe. (a) At presentation, note thick wall and sonolucent centre. (b) Complete resolution 1 month after ultrasound-guided transperineal aspiration.

unknown but risk factors include age, race, geographical location and a strong family history [45].

Patients may be asymptomatic or present with symptoms related to coexisting benign prostatic hypertrophy. Other symptoms such as bone pain may indicate metastatic spread.

With the PZ forming the greater part of the gland, 70% of tumours arise in this area. Of the remaining tumours 20% are found in the TZ and 10% in the CZ. The disease has an unpredictable course which causes controversy for diagnosis and treatment.

The TNM staging system is widely used where T0 represents a localized non-palpable tumour. T1 and T2 are intracapsular tumours. The tumour involving a larger proportion of the gland is T2 often causing some deformity of the gland but the capsule remains intact. T3 tumours extend beyond the capsule and T4 represents locally advanced tumours fixed to the wall of the pelvis or invading neighbouring structures [46].

Tumours are also graded histologically using the Gleason system [47] taking into consideration the degree of glandular differentiation and relationship of the glandular tissue to prostatic stroma as seen under low power magnification.

The diagnosis has traditionally relied on DRE for the palpation of abnormal nodules, asymmetry and focal induration. Unfortunately, DRE has a low sensitivity and specificity. Approximately 50% of palpable nodules are found to be benign and, furthermore, glands with extensive tumour may feel normal on DRE [48–50].

Recent advances in transrectal ultrasound imaging and biopsy techniques coupled with the wide use of serum PSA measurements [51] have combined to improve the detection rate of prostate cancers. The diagnostic triad of DRE, PSA and the appearances of the prostate on transrectal ultrasound, must be considered together [52].

Sonographically prostatic cancer is commonly seen as a hypoechoic lesion in the PZ (Fig. 32.27). However, this appearance is not specific; only about 40% of hypoechoic lesions are malignant [53]. Biopsies are required to establish the diagnosis. Hyperechoic lesions are rare. Tumours may be isoechoic, particularly those involving the TZ with pre-existing benign hypertrophy making identification of the tumour difficult. This adds to the value of systemic biopsies when focal lesions are not visualized.

Other features of tumour infiltration include loss of definition of the surgical capsule, distortion of the shape of the gland and loss of the normal smooth contour. Locally advanced tumours may show evidence of extracapsular extension usually involving a neurovascular bundle (Fig. 32.28). Obliteration of the seminal vesicle–prostate angle may indicate tumour infiltration of the seminal vesicle. Invasion of the ejaculatory duct can lead to unilateral seminal vesicle obstruction and distension.

TRANSRECTAL ULTRASOUND-GUIDED BIOPSIES

This is now a widely used technique in assessing patients with suspicious lesions detected on DRE or elevated PSA to detect early cancer or to confirm the histological diagnosis (Fig. 32.29). There is continuing controversy

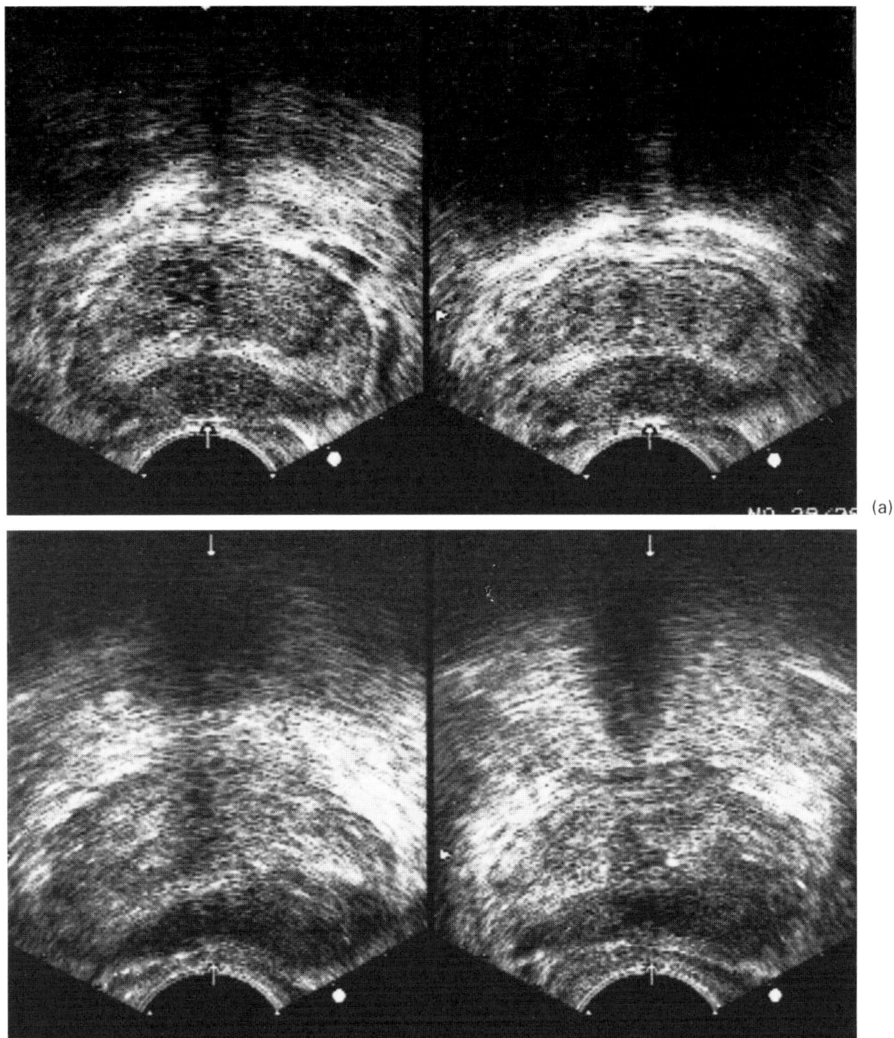

Fig. 32.27 Prostate cancer. (a) Hypoechoic peripheral lesion (two transverse views). There are also features of benign prostatic hypertrophy. (b) More extensive infiltration of the PZ. Tumour still confined to the gland.

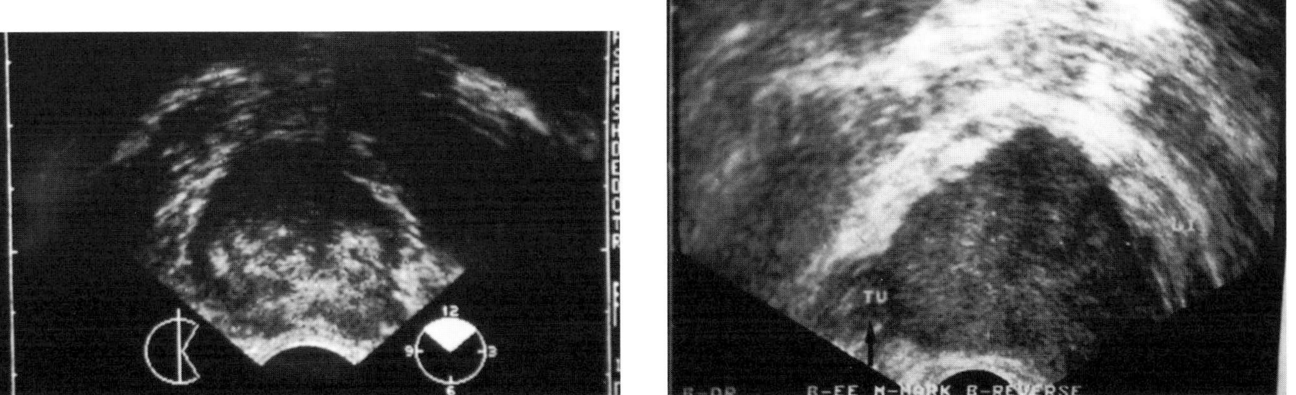

Fig. 32.28 Prostate cancer. (a) Extensive infiltration with loss of separation between the PZ and the TZ and irregular contour. (b) Tumour (TU) spread along neurovascular bundle.

(a)
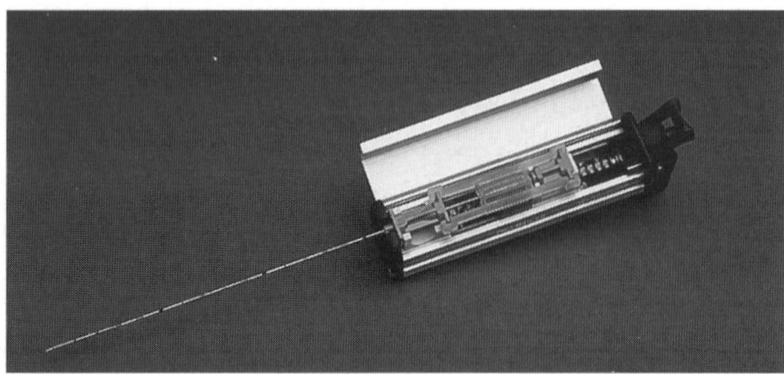

(b)
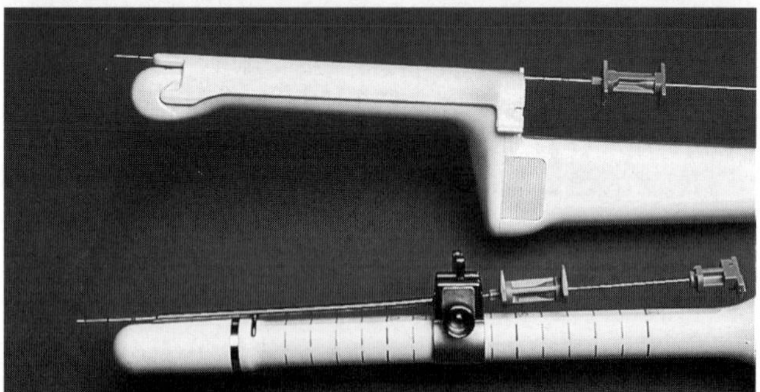

Fig. 32.29 Prostate biopsies. (a) Trucut needle (18 gauge) mounted in biopsy device. (b) Different biopsy attachments used for transrectal approach.

Table 32.1 Prostate specific antigen measurements. Commonly used PSA measurement: figures are those regarded as suspicious of malignancy

Serum PSA	<4 ng ml^{-1}
PSA velocity	<0.75 ng ml^{-1} per year
PSA density	<0.15 ng ml^{-1}

Table 32.2 Differences between transperineal and transrectal techniques

	Transperineal	Transrectal
Position	Lithotomy or lateral	Lateral
Anaesthesia	Local anaesthesia	None
Antibiotic cover	Not routine	Essential
Technique	Free hand	Biopsy attachment
	Sterile	Non-sterile
Probe	Linear	Sector or linear

regarding significant levels of PSA at which referral for biopsies should be made, as well as the significance of other PSA values such as PSA density, PSA velocity (Table 32.1) and the concept of predicted PSA levels [54–56].

Biopsies can be carried out using a transperineal or transrectal approach (Fig. 32.30). The differences between the two techniques is summarized in Table 32.2. No specific preparation is generally required except for a full bladder. Although routine checking of blood clotting is not necessary, patients are advised to stop all anticoagulant therapy a few days before the procedure. Routine sextant biopsies are recommended as well as biopsies of any suspicious lesions.

Transient haematuria, haemospermia and passage of blood per rectum often occurs after the procedure but major complications are rare [57]. These include urinary retention or more persistent bleeding in the immediate postoperative period. Infection and septicaemia are serious complications and should be prevented by appropriate antibiotic cover. The exact antibiotic regime will largely depend on local practices.

COLOUR DOPPLER IN PROSTATIC ULTRASOUND

Modern ultrasound equipment and transrectal probes have colour and pulsed Doppler capability. Some recent studies suggested various patterns of increased flow within areas of tumours. Focal increased PZ flow as well as diffuse increased flow in isoechoic areas were reported as being associated with a high likelihood of underlying cancer [58–60]. There is, however, considerable overlap in colour flow Doppler ultrasound patterns between prostate cancer and prostatitis. Some benign adenomas may also exhibit abnormal peripheral flow. These features have limited the benefit of colour flow ultrasound over conventional grey-scale ultrasound, particularly in the assessment of the PZ [61]. The role of colour Doppler therefore remains controversial. The wider availability and use of power Doppler in recent years remains to be assessed.

Disorders of the seminal vesicles

As well as routine imaging of the seminal vesicles during the assessment of inflammatory and malignant changes of the prostate, specific imaging of the seminal vesicles is often requested during the investigation of infertility or in patients presenting with haemospermia to evaluate the integrity of the distal seminal tract [62]. Congenital absence of one or both seminal vesicles may be associated with clinical absence of the vas deferens (Fig. 32.31). This can be recognized on ultrasound by failure to identify one or both seminal vesicles in their normal position behind the bladder base. Alternatively, unilateral or bilateral hypoplasia may be noted.

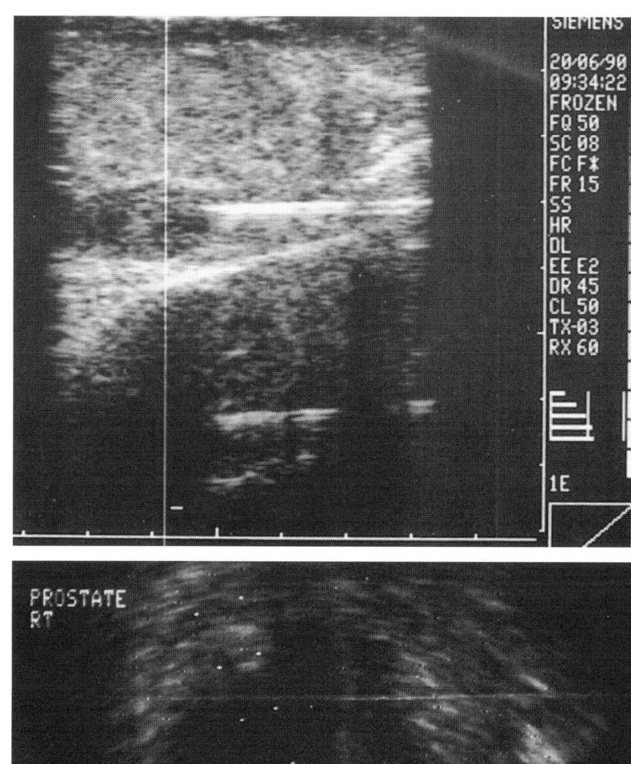

Fig. 32.30 Prostate biopsies. (a) Transperineal approach: needle and target clearly seen with transrectal linear array probe. (b) Transrectal approach: needle fired through lesion along biopsy guide (dots).

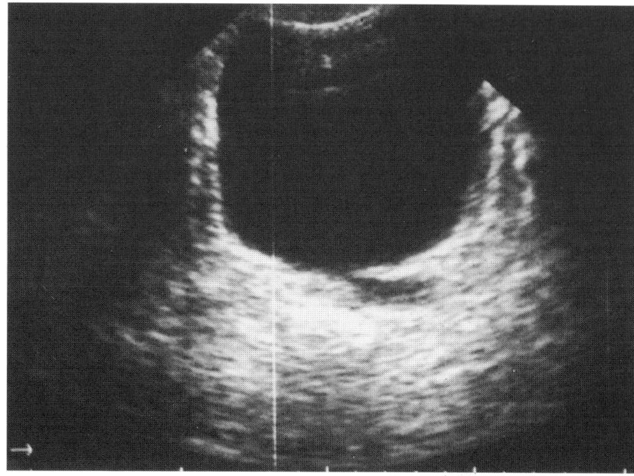

Fig. 32.31 Congenital absence of the right seminal vesicle.

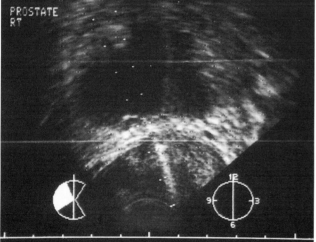

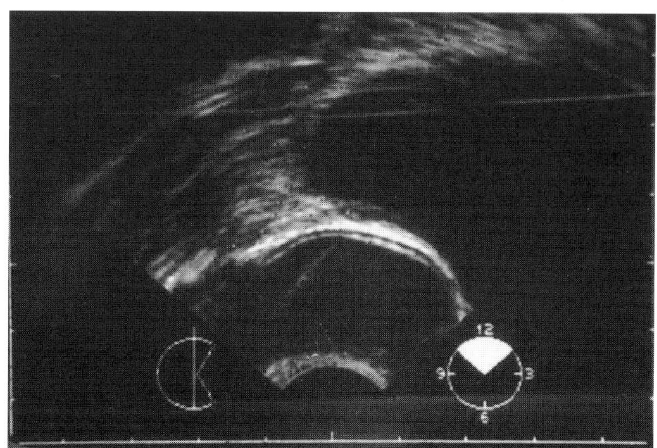

Fig. 32.32 Grossly distended right seminal vesicle with thin echogenic rim and septae.

Obstruction of the ejaculatory duct may lead to cystic dilatation of one or both seminal vesicles. Sonographically there is considerable enlargement of the seminal vesicle which is sonolucent with a distinct rim of tissue and occasional septae (Figs 32.32, 32.33). Transrectal ultrasound-guided puncture of the seminal vesicle for fluid aspiration or contrast studies (seminal vesiculography) to assess obstruction of the ejaculatory duct should be carried out using the transperineal approach [63] to avoid infective complications (Fig. 32.34). The same technique can also be used for the diagnostic aspiration in the rare event of abscess formation.

Ejaculatory duct cysts or Mullerian duct remnants generally present as a small mid line thin wall cyst situated within the posterior aspect of the prostate above the verumontanum (Fig. 32.35). Rare congenital communication between ejaculatory ducts, proximal vas and ectopic ureters have also been reported [64].

Primary tumour of the seminal vesicles are very rare. Direct spread particularly from the prostate is by far the commonest cause of malignancy in the seminal vesicles. Extension from other neighbouring tumours involving the bladder or rectum may also occur.

Disorders of the urethra

Diverticula

Diverticula are rare in males but more common in females. They may be congenital but are more often acquired due

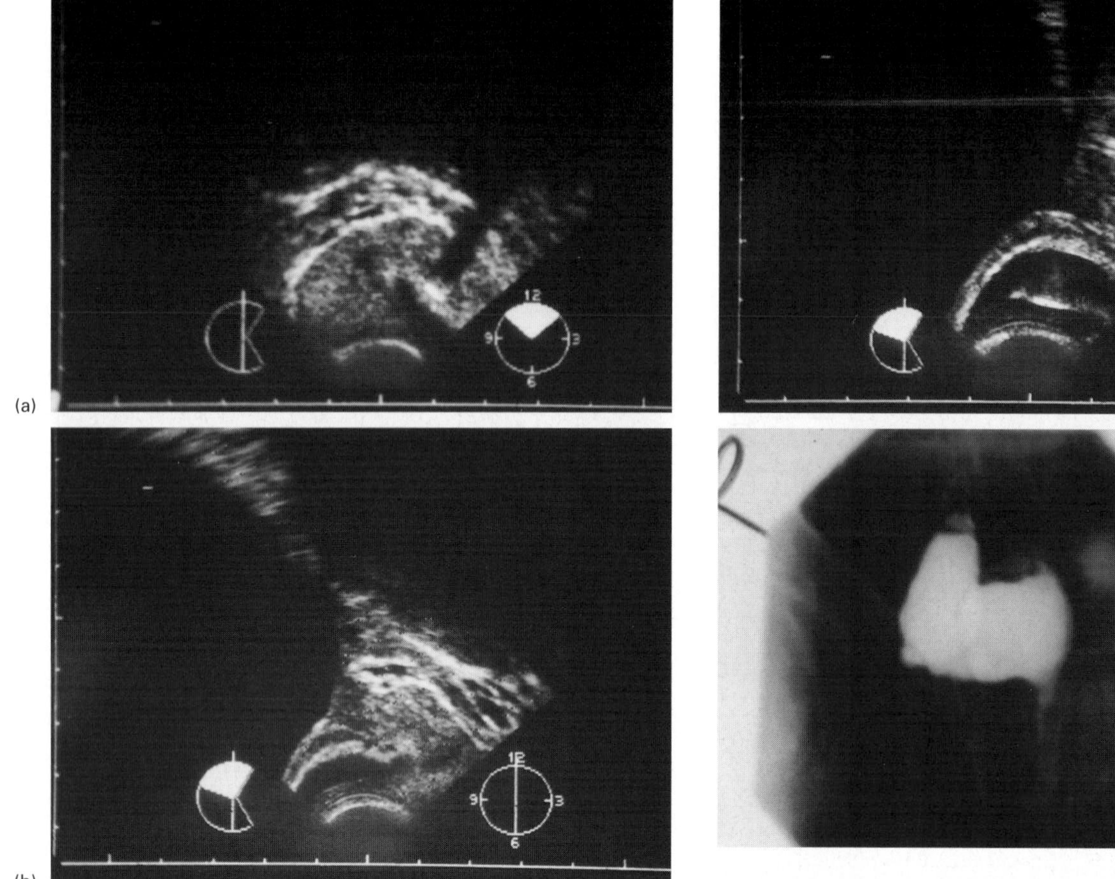

Fig. 32.33 (a) Transverse and (b) sagittal views of the obstructed dilated ejaculatory duct (sonolucent) pointing towards the verumontanum.

Fig. 32.34 Seminal vesiculography. (a) Transrectal ultrasound demonstrates distended right seminal vesicle with needle *in situ* inserted transperineally. (b) Contrast image of distended seminal vesicle.

to obstruction and secondary infection of the paraurethral glands. They may be an overlooked cause of frequency, dysuria, postvoiding dribbling, recurrent urinary tract infection and dyspareunia [65].

In females these are best imaged transvaginally and present characteristically as a small sonolucent fluid-filled structure near or adjacent to the urethra even when the urethra is empty and collapsed [66,67]. Communication with the urethra may not always be apparent.

Urethral strictures

The most common stricture affecting the anterior urethra in males is the result of infection (postgonococcal) which may have been inadequately treated. A stricture may also complicate trauma which may be retrogenic particularly following transurethral reaction of the prostate and indwelling catheters or fractures of the bony pelvis (straddle injury). These tend to affect the bulbar and

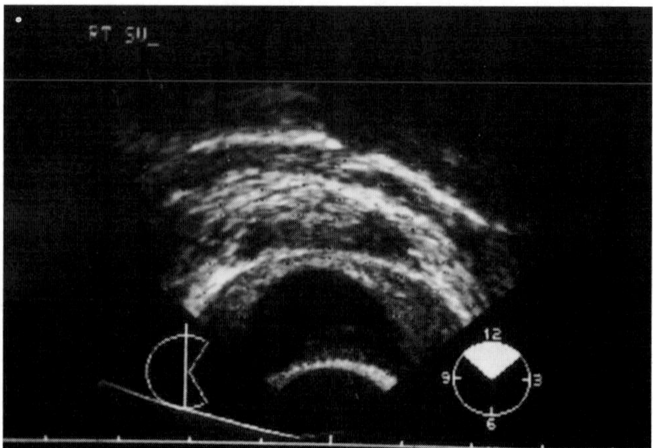

Fig. 32.35 Mullerian duct remnant; mid line cystic lesion.

membranous urethra and are more difficult to visualize on ultrasound.

As with conventional radiographic urethrography, strictures of the anterior urethra present sonographically as a focal narrowing of the lumen; in addition, the hyperechoic periurethral fibrosis can be evaluated [68].

Rare intraluminal filling defects due to granulomatous tissue or warts (condyloma accuminata) can be characterized with ultrasound [69].

References

1 Sandler, C.M., Phillips, J.M., Harris, J.D., Toombs, B.D. (1981) Radiology of the bladder and urethra in blunt pelvic trauma. *Radiology Clinics of North America* **19**, 995.

2 Williams, P.L., Warwick, R., Dyson, M., Bannister, L.H. (eds) (1989) Reproductive organs of the male. In: *Gray's Anatomy*, 37th edn. Churchhill Livingstone, Edinburgh, pp. 1424–1435.

3 McNeal, J.E. (1968) Regional morphology and pathology of the prostate. *American Journal of Clinical Pathology* **49**, 347–357.

4 Blacklock, N.J., Boushill, K. (1977) The zonal anatomy of the prostate in man and rhesus monkey. *Urology Research* **5**, 163–167.

5 Amis, Jr E.S., Newhouse, J.H. (1991) *Essentials of Uroradiology*. Little, Brown, Boston, pp. 335–349.

6 Rifkin, M.D. (1985) *Diagnostic Imaging of the Lower Genitourinary Tract*. Raven Press, New York, pp. 19–20.

7 Holm, H.H., Northeved, A. (1974) A transurethral ultrasonic scanner. *Journal of Urology* **111**, 238–241.

8 Nustrøm, H., Holm, H.H., Christensen, N.E.H., Movild, A.F., Nolsøc, C. (1991) 3-dimensional ultrasound based demonstration of the posterior urethra during voiding combined with urodynamics. *Scandinavian Journal of Urology and Nephrology* Suppl. 137, 125–129.

9 Beacroft, P.W.P., Berman, L.H. (1994) Sonography in evaluation of the male anterior urethra. *Clinical Radiology* **49**, 621–626.

10 Jequier, S., Palitl, H., Lafortune, M. (1990) Ureterovesical jets in infants and children. Duplex and colour Doppler ultrasound studies. *Radiology* **175**, 349–353.

11 Potson, G.L., Riddle, P.R. (1983) The accuracy of bladder volume with ultrasound. *British Journal of Urology* **55**, 361–363.

12 Geirsson, R. (1982) Ultrasound volume measurements comparing a prolate ellipsoid method with a parallel planimetric method against a known volume. *Journal of Clinical Ultrasound* **182**, 329–332.

13 Rifkin, M.D. (1985) *Diagnostic Imaging of the Lower Genitourinary Tract*. Raven Press, New York, p. 135.

14 Cochlin, D.L., Dubbins, P.A., Goldberg, B.B., Alexander, A.A. (1994) *Urogenital Ultrasound. A Text Atlas*. Martin Dunitz, London, pp. 273–280.

15 Rifkin, M.D. (1988) *Ultrasound of the Prostate*. Raven Press, New York, pp. 51–91.

16 Boothroyd, A.E., Dixon, P.J., Rickards, D. (1990) The ultrasound urodynamogram. *British Journal of Urology* **63**, 311–333.

17 Turner Warwick, R.T., Whitside, C.G. (1983) Symposium on clinical urodynamics. *Urology Clinics of North America* **6**, 1–25.

18 Gooding, G.A.W. (1986) Varied sonographic manifestations of cystitis. *Journal of Ultrasound Medicine* **5**, 61–63.

19 Gooding, G.A. (1989) Sonography of *Candida albicans* cystitis. *Journal of Ultrasound Medicine* **8**, 121–124.

20 Jorulf, H., Lindstedt, E. (1985) Urogenital schistosomiasis: CT evaluation. *Radiology* **157**, 745–749.

21 Goff, W.B. (1983) Cystitis cystica and cystitis glandularis: cause of bladder mass. *Journal of Computer Assisted Tomography* **7**, 347–349.

22 Kauzlaric, D., Barmeir, E., Campana, A. (1987) Diagnosis of cystitis glandularis. *Urologic Radiology* **9**, 50–52.

23 Bosniak, M.A., Siegelman, S.S., Evans, J.A. (1976) *The Adrenal, Retroperitoneum and Lower Urinary Tract: An Atlas of Tumour Radiology*. Year Book, Chicago, pp. 440–450.

24 Heiken, J.P., McClennan, B.L., Disantis, D.J. (1988) Non transitional cell tumours of the bladder. In: Taveras, J.M., Ferruci, J.T. (eds) *Radiology: Diagnosis and Imaging—Intervention*. Lippincott, Philadelphia.

25 Kwok-Lin, J.P., Zikman, J.N., Cockshott, W.P. (1980) Carcinoma of the urachus: the role of computerised tomography. *Radiology* **137**(3), 731–734.

26 Stacul, F. (1994) Early cancer of the urogenital tract: the bladder. In: Dalla Palma, L., Thomsen, H.S. (eds) *European Uroradiology 94*, pp. 188–190.

27 Yousen, D.M. (1988) Synchronous and metachronous transitional cell carcinoma of the urinary tract: Prevalence, incidence and radiographic detection. *Radiology* **167**, 613.

28 Brun, B., Gammelgaard, J., Christoffersen, J. (1984) Transabdominal dynamic ultrasonography in the detection of bladder tumours. *Journal of Urology* **132**, 19–20.

29 Wood, D.P. Jr. (1988) The role of magnetic resonance imaging with staging of bladder carcinoma. *Journal of Urology* **140**, 741.

30 Husband, J.E.S., Olliff, J.F.C., Williams, M.P. (1989) Bladder cancer: staging with CT and MR imaging. *Radiology* **173**, 435–440.

31 Berlac, P.A., Holm, H.H. (1992) Bladder tumour control by abdominal ultrasound and urine cytology. *Journal of Urology* **147**, 1510–1512.

32 Berry, S.J., Coffey, D.S., Walsh, P.C., Ewing, L.L. (1984) The development of human benign prostatic hyperplasia with age. *Journal of Urology* **132**, 474–479.

33 McNeal, J.E. (1978) Origin and evolution of benign prostatic enlargement. *Investigative Urology* **15**, 340–345.

34 Rifkin, M.D., Kurtz, A.B. (1986) Prostatic ultrasound. *Clinical Diagnostic Ultrasound* **18**, 195–227.

35 Watanabe, H., Igari, D., Tanahashi, Y., Harada, K., Saitoh, M. (1975) Transrectal ultrasonography of the prostate. *Journal of Urology* **114**, 734–740.

36 Rifkin, M.D. (1988) Post-transurethral resection: endorectal ultrasound. In: *Ultrasound of the Prostate*. Raven Press, New York, pp. 200–209.

37 Griffiths, G.J., Crooks, A.J.R., Roberts, E.E., Evans, K.T., Buck, A.C., Thomas, P.J. (1984) Ultrasonic appearances associated with prostatic inflammation: a preliminary study. *Clinical Radiology* **35**, 343–345.

38 Cochlin, D.L., Dubbins, P.A., Goldberg, B.B., Alexander, A.A. (1994) *Urogenital Ultrasound: A Text Atlas*. Martin Dunitz, London, p. 294.

39 Baert, L., Leonard, A., D'Hoedt, M., Vandeursen, R. (1987) Seminal vesiculography in chronic bacterial prostatitis. *Journal of Urology* **136**, 844.

40 Epstein, J.I., Hutchins, G.M. (1984) Granulomatous prostatitis: distinction among allergic, non specific and post-transurethral resection lesions. *Human Pathology* **15**, 818–822.

41 Towfighi, J., Sedeghee, S., Wheller, J.J. (1972) Granulomatous prostatitis with emphasis on the oesinophilic variety. *American Journal of Clinical Pathology* **58**, 630–641.
42 Doble, A., Thomas, B.J., Walker, M.M. (1989) The role of *Chlamydia trachomatis* in chronic and bacterial prostatitis; a study using ultrasound guided biopsy. *Journal of Urology* **141**, 332–333.
43 Andrew, G.S. (1949) Latent carcinoma of the prostate. *Journal of Clinical Pathology* **2**, 197.
44 Scardino, P.T. (1989) Early detection of prostatic cancer. *Urology Clinics of North America* **16**(4), 635–655.
45 Stamey, T.A., McNeal, J.E. (1992) Adenocarcinoma of the prostate. In: *Campbell's Urology*, vol. 2, 6th edn. WB Saunders, Philadelphia, pp. 1159–1215.
46 Clements, R., Griffiths, G.J., Feeling, W.B. (1992) Staging prostatic cancer. *Clinical Radiology* **46**, 225–231.
47 Gleason, D.F. and the Veterans Administration Cooperative Urological Research Group (1977) *Histological Grading and Clinical Staging of Prostatic Carcinoma*. Lea & Febiger, Philadelphia.
48 Chodak, G.W., Keller, P., Schoenberg, H.W. (1989) Assessment of screening for prostate cancer using digital rectal examination. *Journal of Urology* **141**, 1136–1138.
49 Jewett, H.J. (1956) Significance of the palpable prostatic nodule. *Journal of the American Medical Association* **160**, 838–839.
50 Daniels, G.F., McNeal, J.E., Stamey, T.A. (1992) Predictive value of contralateral biopsies in unilaterally palpable prostate cancer. *Journal of Urology* **147**, 870–874.
51 Parkes, C., Wald, N.J., Murphy, P. (1995) Prospective observational study to assess value of prostate specific antigen as screening test for prostate cancer. *British Medical Journal* **311**, 1340–1343.
52 Clements, R. (1996) The changing role of transrectal ultrasound in the diagnosis of prostate cancer. *Clinical Radiology* **51**, 671–676.
53 Lee, F., Torp-Pederson, S., Littrup, P.J. (1989) Hypoechoic lesions of the prostate: clinical relevance of size, digital rectal examination and prostate specific antigen. *Radiology* **170**, 29–32.
54 Carter, H.B., Pearson, J.D., Metter, J., *et al.* (1992) Longitudinal evaluation of prostatic specific antigen levels in men with and without prostate disease. *Journal of the American Medical Association* **267**, 2215–2220.
55 Clements, R., Etherington, R.J., Griffiths, G.J. (1992) Interrelation between measurement of serum PSA and transrectal ultrasound in the diagnosis of benign prostatic hypertroplasia and prostate cancer. *British Journal of Urology* **70**, 183–187.
56 Lee, F., Littrup, P.J., Loft Christenson, L., *et al.* (1992) Predicted prostate specific antigen results using transrectal ultrasound gland volume. *Cancer* **70**, 211–220.
57 Clements, R. (1994) Prostate biopsy: side effects and the influence of prostatic specific antigen. *Current Opinions in Urology* **4**, 85–88.
58 Rifkin, M.D., Sudakoff, G.S., Alexander, A.A. (1993) Prostate: techniques, results and potential applications of colour Doppler ultrasound scanning. *Radiology* **186**, 509–513.
59 Newman, J.S., Brea, R.L., Rubin, J.M. (1995) Prostate cancer: diagnosis with colour Doppler sonography with histologic correlation of each biopsy site. *Radiology* **195**, 86–90.
60 Kelly, I.M.G., Lees, W.R., Rickards, D. (1993) Prostate cancer and the role of colour Doppler ultrasound. *Radiology* **189**, 153–156.
61 Alexander, A.A. (1995) To colour Doppler image the prostate or not: that is the question. *Radiology* **195**, 11–13.
62 Carter, S.S., Shimohara, K., Lipshultz, L.I. (1989) Transrectal ultrasonography in disorders of the seminal vesicles and ejaculatory ducts. *Urology Clinics of North America* **16**, 773–790.
63 Holm, H.H., Gammelgaard, J. (1981) Ultrasonically guided precise needle placement in the prostate and seminal vesicles. *Journal of Urology* **125**, 385–387.
64 Negrin, D.A., Fernandez, F.A., Perales, C.L. (1989) Ectopic opening of the ureter into the ejaculatory duct. Use of ultrasound directed vesiculography in the diagnosis of this type of malformation. *Archivos Espanoles de Urologia* **42**, 925–927 (Spanish).
65 Oyen, R. (1994) Acquired urethral diverticula. In: Dalla Palma, L., Thomsen, H.S. (eds) *European Uroradiology 94*, p. 229.
66 Wexler, J.S., McGovern, T.B. (1980) Ultrasonography of the female urethral diverticula. *American Journal of Roentgenology* **134**, 737–740.
67 Baert, L., Willemen, P., Oyen, R. (1992) Endovaginal sonography: new diagnostic approach for urethral diverticula. *Journal of Urology* **147**, 464–466.
68 Merkle, W., Wagner, W.I. (1988) Sonography of the distal male urethra and new diagnostic procedure for urethral strictures. Results of a retrospective study. *Journal of Urology* **140**, 1409.
69 Gluck, C.D., Bundy, A.L., Fine, C., Laughlin, K.R., Ritchie, J.P. (1988) Sonographic urethrogram: comparison with roentgenographic technique in 22 patients. *Journal of Urology* **140**, 1404.

Chapter 33: The female pelvis

L.M. Macara & K.P. Hanretty

Donald laid the foundations for the clinical application of ultrasound almost 40 years ago [1]. Using the relatively crude equipment of that time the features which could most easily be recognized were those in which there was a fluid interface. Since pelvic tumours are commonly cystic, an enthusiasm for gynaecological ultrasound, though for a limited number of problems, developed. With the introduction of high resolution machinery and transvaginal probes, definition of tissues and organs has improved substantially such that ultrasound is now a significant diagnostic tool in gynaecological practice.

Examination technique

Both the transabdominal and transvaginal (endovaginal) approach can be utilized to examine the gynaecological patient. For reasons outlined below, a transabdominal examination should always precede any transvaginal examination. Direct contact, real-time ultrasound should be used for a transabdominal ultrasound examination. The bladder should be fully distended to displace bowel from the pelvis and provide a fluid interface over the anterior uterine wall. In the average adult a 5 or 3.5 MHz probe offers optimal penetration. Sensitivity and swept gain settings are critical and must be optimized to delineate the soft tissue in detail, particularly when examining the ovaries. Standard longitudinal and transverse views permit adequate inspection of the pelvic viscera. The uterus should be identified, its position determined (anteverted or retroverted) and the body of uterus viewed in its long axis. The entire uterine body should be examined to each lateral extremity before rotating at 90° to the long axis and systematically inspecting transverse images from cervix to uterine fundus. The adnexae are ideally inspected using a transverse view.

A transvaginal ultrasound examination should be performed while the bladder is empty and with the patient in a semi-lithotomy position. An overdistended bladder will displace the pelvic organs beyond the range of the transvaginal probe and causes undue patient discomfort. A 6 MHz probe provides optimal penetration and excellent image quality. The tip of the vaginal probe should be covered with transducer gel, then protected with a rubber covering such as a condom or surgical glove. Care should be taken to ensure that no air is trapped at the tip of the condom as this can cause significant artefact. The condom should then be lubricated externally with further gel prior to insertion. The probe should be cleaned between patients with one of the recommended solutions such as Spocidin or Cidex. It is important that adequate privacy and an appropriate chaperon are provided. Far too frequently little attention is given to these factors even though patient dissatisfaction with their care often centres around them.

Three standard views are used during a transvaginal scan (TVS): a sagittal (longitudinal), coronal (transverse) and semi-axial (transverse view directed anteriorly) view. The uterus should be identified in a sagittal plane initially to allow the entire long axis to be viewed before rotating 90° either clockwise or anticlockwise and inspecting the uterus from cervix to fundus (coronal and semi-axial views). The same direction of rotation should be used every time. With an acutely retroverted uterus the handle of the probe will be very anterior, near the symphysis pubis, with the transducer pointing to the rectum while with an acutely anteverted uterus, the transducer will point towards the symphysis pubis with the handle directed backwards until at times it touches the perineal area. Thereafter the adnexae may be inspected by directing the probe into the right and left vaginal fornix. The focal range of a transvaginal probe is limited to about 7–8 cm. For this reason an abdominal scan should always precede a TVS, even if the bladder is not full. This will exclude large masses and cysts and most pregnancies of 12 weeks gestation or more, all of which can be completely missed if only a transvaginal approach is used. In addition, valuable information on the position of the uterus can be obtained from the transabdominal scan allowing the angle of the transvaginal probe to be adjusted accordingly thus saving much embarrassment for the patient and doctor.

In many cases, particularly those presenting with a possible malignancy, the ultrasound examination should be extended to assess the renal tract for evidence of obstruction and the regional lymph nodes, the liver and the peritoneal cavity for evidence of tumour dissemination.

The uterus

Anatomy of the uterus

The uterus is a pear-shaped hollow fibromuscular organ that lies between the bladder and the rectum. It is thick walled with a narrow lumen lined by endometrium which is firmly attached to the underlying muscle, the myometrium. The lumen is continuous with the fallopian tubes superiorly and the cervical canal and vagina inferiorly (Fig. 33.1). In the majority of women (80%) the uterus lies anteverted and anteflexed to the vagina.

The uterine or fallopian tubes arise from the superior lateral aspects of the uterus, the isthmus, above the round and ovarian ligaments. They are approximately 10 cm in length, traverse laterally in the broad ligament to the pelvic side walls where they curve over the lateral aspect of the ovary, expanding into the fringed funnel-shaped infundibulum which opens into the peritoneal cavity.

The uterine fundus is covered in peritoneum except in its lower anterior portion where it is contiguous with the bladder. Posteriorly the peritoneum extends to cover the upper portion of the vagina. These peritoneal reflections form the uterovesicle pouch anteriorly, and the rectovaginal pouch of Douglas posteriorly. The uterus is supported by the cardinal and uterosacral ligaments inferiorly and the round ligaments superiorly.

The cervix of the uterus is cylindrical and is inserted into the upper anterior vaginal wall at an angle of almost 90°. In the adult, the cervix is approximately 2.5 cm in length.

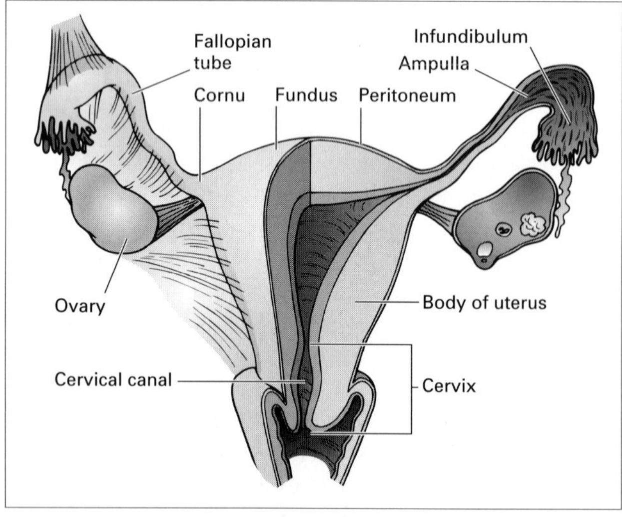

Fig. 33.1 The normal uterus is divided into three portions; the fundus, body and cervix as shown.

The vagina is a muscular tube measuring 12–13 cm in length in the adult. With the bladder empty its axis is towards the sacral promontory, and as the bladder fills its axis becomes more posterior.

In the non-pregnant adult the uterus measures approximately 8 cm in length (from fundus to lower pole of cervix). It does, however, show a large interperson variation (5–8 cm × 2–5 cm × 1.3–3 cm) with an upper limit of normal quoted at 9 × 5 × 3 cm. In the prepubertal uterus the body of the uterus is much smaller but the cervix is similar in size to that in the adult. After the menopause the uterus decreases rapidly in size so that by the age of 60 years, it will have reduced by 50%.

Ultrasound appearance of the normal uterus

The uterus is normally positioned behind the bladder, is smooth in outline and has a granular texture. Prior to the menarche the uterus has a more homogeneous appearance. Using a long axis image of the uterus, a central line of increased reflectivity from the endometrial interface, known as the 'mid line echo' will be seen. Measurements of endometrial thickness should be obtained using this long axis view and include both layers of the reflective endometrium. The endometrium changes in appearance (reflectivity) and thickness in conjunction with the menstrual cycle (Fig. 33.2).

During the proliferative phase of the menstrual cycle, endometrial thickness varies between 4 and 8 mm. Following ovulation, the endometrium thickens (8–14 mm), is more echogenic and is surrounded by a distinct hypoechoic layer which represents the inner layers of compact myometrium. Increasing thickness and reflectivity of the endometrium is associated with increasing levels of circulating oestrogens. During menstruation, the presence of blood in the lumen may produce a central sonolucent echo.

In the postmenopausal woman, the uterus is significantly smaller, and has a uniform echogenic pattern. The endometrial lining is extremely thin and is sometimes hard to differentiate from the underlying myometrial tissue (Fig. 33.3).

Intrauterine contraceptive device

Changes in the endometrium and cavity must be differentiated from the strongly reflective echo of the intrauterine contraceptive device (IUCD). Ultrasound may be employed to check the position of the IUCD postinsertion, to localize the IUCD if the coil threads are not visible, or

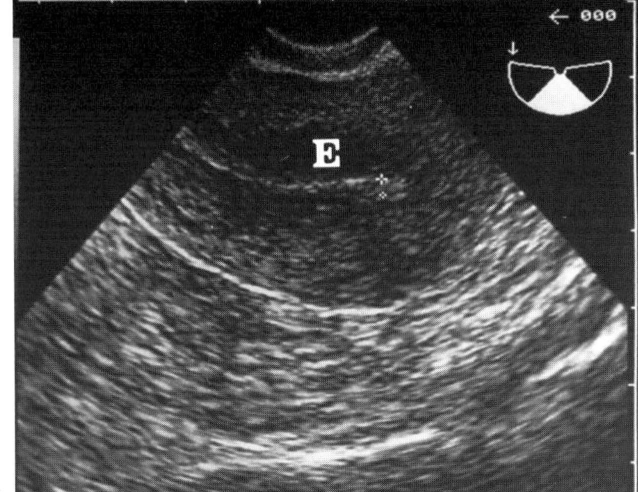

(a)

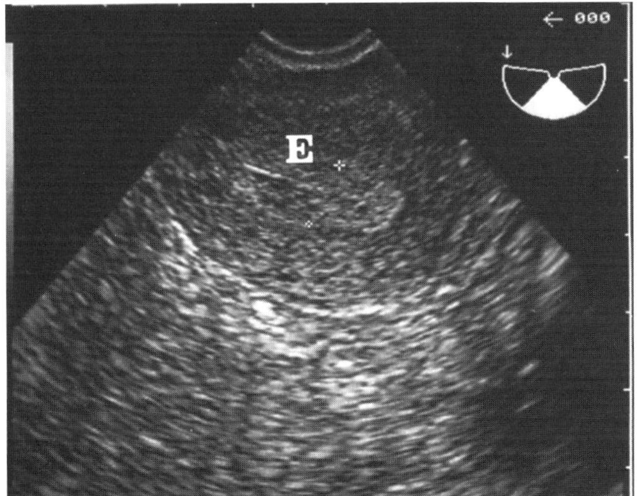

(b)

Fig. 33.2 (a) Transvaginal scan of a normal uterus during the first half of the menstrual cycle demonstrating a thin poorly reflective endometrium (E). (b) TVS of a normal uterus during the second half of the menstrual cycle in which the endometrium (E) is thicker and more echogenic.

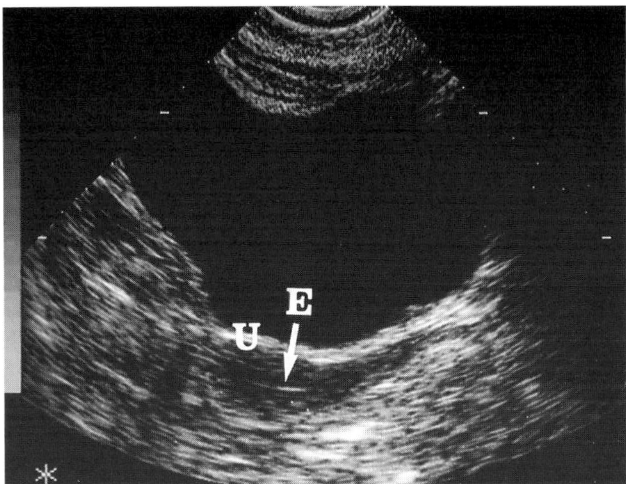

Fig. 33.3 Transabdominal image of a postmenopausal uterus in long section showing a small uterus (U) and a very thin endometrial layer (E).

visualize the IUCD when pregnancy ensues. There are a wide range of devices available. The majority of these give highly reflective linear echoes on a longitudinal scan, but newer hormonal-based IUCDs have proved difficult to visualize by ultrasound as they contain no copper elements (Fig. 33.4).

Congenital uterine anomalies

Imperfect fusion of the Mullerian tract during fetal life produces a wide spectrum of abnormalities ranging from uterus didelphys, in which the uterus, cervix and vagina are duplicated to rudimentary nodules in which the uterine body is not formed. The most common anomalies seen are the variants of a 'double or bicornuate uterus' (Fig. 33.5) and these are frequently asymptomatic. As there is an association with renal abnormalities [2] the renal tract should be carefully examined in the presence of a uterine anomaly. The ultrasound appearance of the uterus will vary depending on the abnormality present. Anomalies are often more easily detected during the puerperium when the uterus is enlarged. Diagnosing the presence of incomplete uterine septae is difficult. Contrast TVS using echogenic media or saline may prove useful in the future, permitting delineation of the uterine cavity more clearly. The introduction of the operating hysteroscope has led to minimally invasive resection of these septae. Uterine abnormalities of this type may be found in up to 20% of women with recurrent spontaneous abortions [3].

Evaluating the postmenopausal endometrium

In patients with postmenopausal bleeding, further investigation is indicated to exclude underlying endometrial pathology, particularly endometrial carcinoma. Previously, both transabdominal [4] and transvaginal sonography [5,6] have been used to evaluate the endometrium, but since transvaginal ultrasonography permits high resolution imaging, the endometrial–myometrial interface is more clearly visualized with TVS. Even in cases of morbid obesity, when there is a particular risk of endometrial cancer, reasonable images can be obtained as the ultrasound echoes do not require to pass through the abdominal adipose layer. The entire endometrium should be examined in a longitudinal plane of the uterus and the

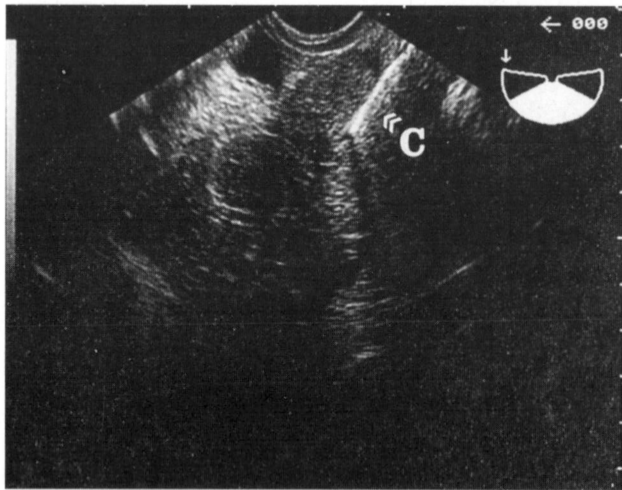

(a)

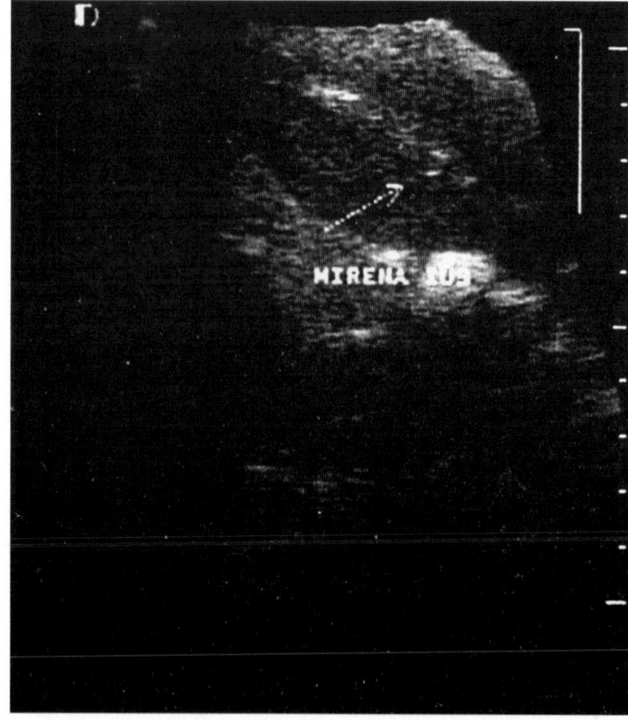

(b)

Fig. 33.4 (a) Transvaginal scan of a normal uterus with a copper-containing echogenic IUCD (C) *in situ*. (b) In contrast a TVS of a normal uterus containing a hormone-based (Mirena) IUCD. There is little reflection from the IUCD itself thus making it very difficult to distinguish with confidence from the surrounding endometrium.

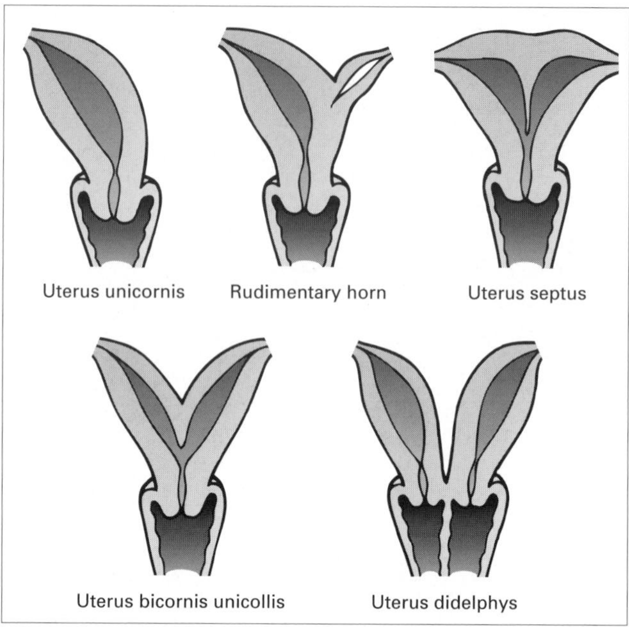

Fig. 33.5 Uterine malformations. When only one Mullerian duct develops uterus unicornis ensues with only one fallopian tube, a single uterine body and vagina. When the second Mullerian duct is present in a rudimentary form, a rudimentary uterine horn is formed. This contains functioning endometrium. If the canal connecting the horn is not patent a haematometra will develop. Both Mullerian ducts may form and fuse externally but the cavity may be partly or completely divided by a mid line septum—uterus septus or uterus bicornis unicollis. There is usually normal menstruation but there may be an increased incidence of miscarriage, preterm labour and malpresentations such as breech during pregnancy. Complete lack of fusion of the Mullerian ducts results in a double uterus and double vagina—uterus didelphys.

thickest area of endometrium identified. Most studies have measured from the outer highly reflective border of the endometrium on one side to the outer reflective border of endometrium on the other side, thus including any distension of the endometrial cavity (Fig. 33.6). This technique identifies any patients with endometrial pathology, such as polyps, and not only patients with endometrial carcinoma. The low amplitude 'halo' around the endometrium, which should be intact is not included in this measurement. Nasri *et al.*, however, have deducted any intracavity fluid from their endometrial measurements [5], to increase the specificity of endometrial thickness measurement. These studies are relatively small at present and until larger studies are available, it would seem prudent to use total endometrial thickness measurements, including any fluid with the endometrial cavity.

Isolated cases of endometrial carcinoma have been reported where the endometrial thickness is <4 mm [7] but in the large Nordic trial and others [5,6] no carcinoma was 'thinner' than 5 mm. Using this 4 mm cut-off level, the sensitivity of vaginal ultrasound for any endometrial pathology was 96% with a specificity of 68%. Increasing the cut-off level to 5 mm improved the specificity but obviously reduced the sensitivity of the technique. In postmenopausal women, not on hormone replacement

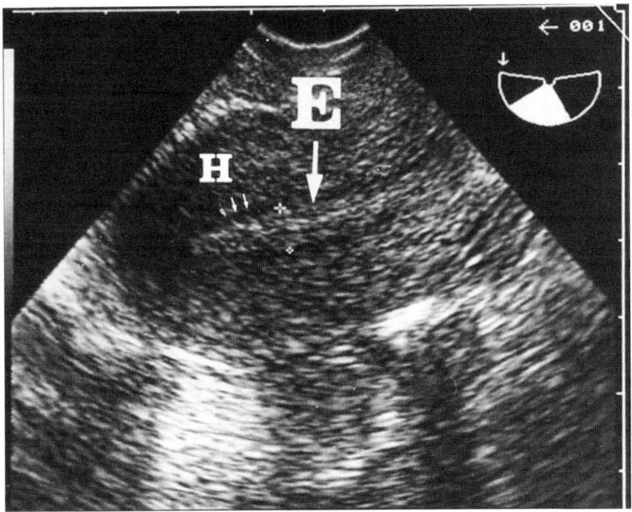

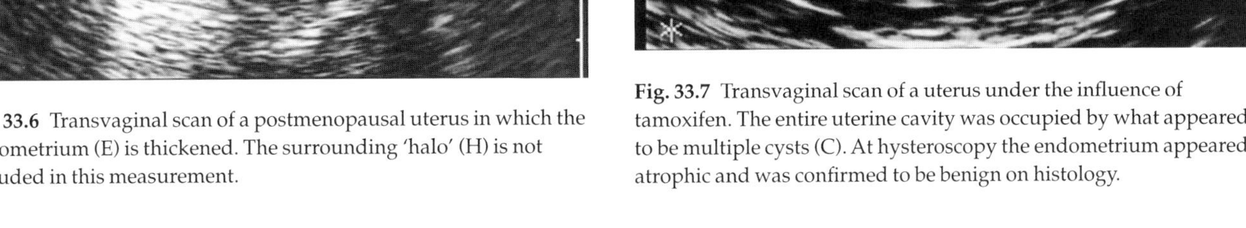

Fig. 33.6 Transvaginal scan of a postmenopausal uterus in which the endometrium (E) is thickened. The surrounding 'halo' (H) is not included in this measurement.

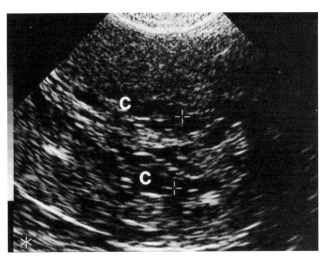

Fig. 33.7 Transvaginal scan of a uterus under the influence of tamoxifen. The entire uterine cavity was occupied by what appeared to be multiple cysts (C). At hysteroscopy the endometrium appeared atrophic and was confirmed to be benign on histology.

therapy (HRT), 'with an endometrial thickness of <4 mm, it would seem justified therefore to refrain from curettage' [6]. Outpatient methods of endometrial sampling accompanied by ultrasound assessment of endometrial thickness have some role in those not fit for anaesthesia but the gold standard for assessment, even though itself imperfect, remains examination under anaesthesia with hysteroscopy and curettage.

Women taking HRT, are more difficult to evaluate as the endometrium is stimulated by exogenous oestrogen. In the Nordic trial, women on HRT with a normal endometrium, had an endometrial thickness of 5.2 ± 3.1 mm. Those with endometrial pathology had measurements of 13.2 ± 8.6 mm [6]. Larger studies are required to define the normal appearance of the endometrium in women on each class of HRT, particularly with the introduction of new continuous combined 'no bleed' preparations. Until these studies are available, endometrial thickness measurements in this group of women should be interpreted cautiously.

Tamoxifen and the endometrium

Tamoxifen is a synthetic oestrogen antagonist, with partial agonist activity used in the treatment of breast cancer. Many of these women develop irregular or postmenopausal bleeding and are referred for evaluation.

Tamoxifen induces some striking ultrasound changes in the endometrium, particularly in the postmenopausal uterus; the endometrial thickness frequently measures more than 5 mm, suggestive of significant endometrial pathology in a postmenopausal woman. In addition, the endometrium may be hyperechoic and have multiple small cysts throughout (Fig. 33.7). Endometrial polyps are very common and may contribute to the thickened endometrial measurements. Though these polyps are almost always benign, it must be remembered that there is a sixfold excess of endometrial cancer in women on tamoxifen [8]. Doppler ultrasound has been applied to both uterine [9] and subendometrial/myometrial vessels [10] to discriminate between benign thickening and endometrial cancer in patients on tamoxifen treatment. However, it would appear that tamoxifen reduces vascular impedance in the uterus, mimicking the changes associated with endometrial cancer and Doppler is therefore of little diagnostic value. At hysteroscopy, most of these women will have atrophic endometrium or endometrial polyps but to date it is difficult to differentiate benign or hyperplastic/malignant disease in patients treated with tamoxifen by ultrasound appearances alone.

Uterine tumours

UTERINE LEIOMYOMA

These are the most common uterine tumours in women, noted in up to 20% of women between 25 and 55 years. They arise from uterine smooth muscle as single or multiple tumours and are commonly known as fibroids or myomas. The majority are within the uterine wall (intramural) though others may be found subserosal, submucosal or rarely cervical. Leiomyomas situated in the latter three positions may become pedunculated. There is an association with nulliparity, obesity and some ethnic origins such as those from sub-Saharan Africa. Oral contraceptive use appears to offer some protection. Postmenopausally fibroids become firmer and are often partially or wholly calcified.

Many women with fibroids are asymptomatic but most will present with infertility, heavy regular periods or pressure symptoms such as urinary frequency. Diagnosis of a pelvic mass is usually readily possible by clinical examination although difficulty may be encountered in the obese. Ultrasound examination, however, can distinguish if the mass is uterine or adnexal in origin.

On ultrasound leiomyomas are well-circumscribed, discrete round masses comprised of a mixed echo pattern. The moderately echogenic smooth muscle echos are interspersed with a variable amount of very echo-dense fibrous tissue. The exact sonographic appearance will obviously vary depending on the relative quantities of smooth muscle and connective tissue present (Fig. 33.8). As a result of the echo-dense fibrous tissue present, an area of 'fall-out' will often be noted behind the myomatous mass. Calcification may also be present and will be identified as highly reflective echoes, causing distal and at times complete shadowing. When leiomyomas degenerate, the centre of the myoma becomes liquefied and appears sonolucent, while the periphery becomes more echogenic. During pregnancy fibroids become less echogenic, perhaps as a result of the increased vascularity of the uterus at this time. The wide spectrum of acoustic features which are seen may cause diagnostic problems, particularly when the 'myoma' is pedunculated and in a subserous position. These atypical scans should always be interpreted with caution and the possibility of an ovarian tumour borne in mind.

In women with minimal symptoms, management of fibroids may be conservative. Those with symptoms who wish to retain fertility may be treated by myomectomy.

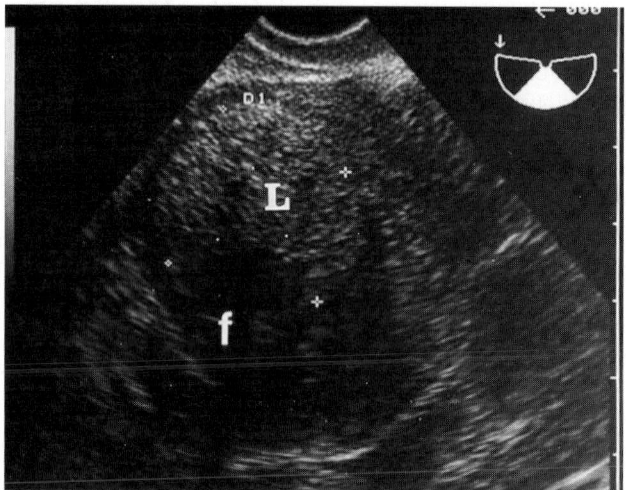

(a)

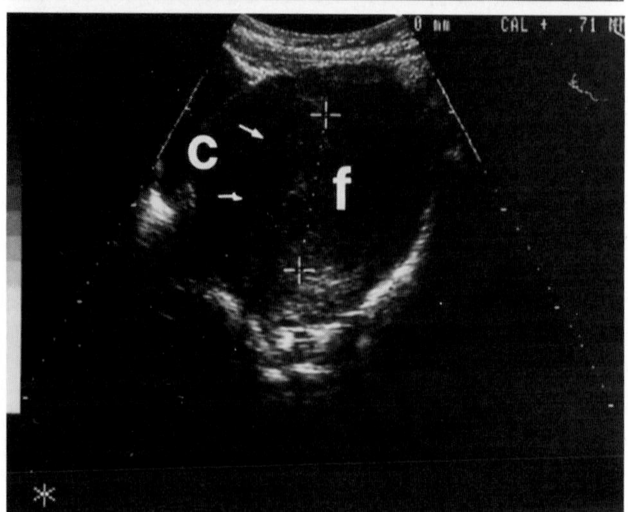

(c)

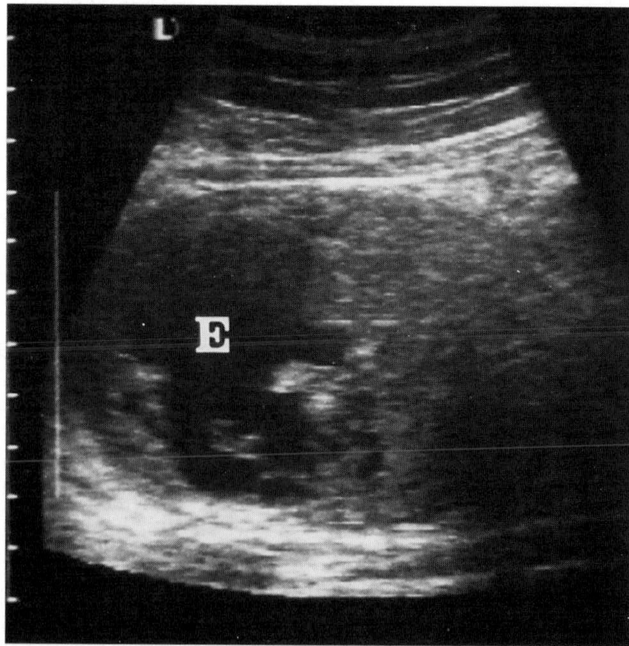

(b)

Fig. 33.8 The variable images seen with uterine leiomyomas. (a) A well-circumscribed intramural leiomyoma (L) with a mixed echo pattern. The dense tissue causing an area of 'fall-out' (f) just below the fibroid. (b) A pedunculated fibroid with an irregular echolucent area (e) in keeping with an area of liquefaction. Such an appearance may be very difficult to distinguish from a semi-solid ovarian mass. (c) Transabdominal image of an enlarged uterus containing a large intramural fibroid (f). The uterine cavity is displaced to the side (C).

The development of gonadotrophin analogues has provided a medical pretreatment which reduces the fibroid size (up to 50%) and may reduce blood loss at time of operation [11]. In women seeking to become pregnant medical treatment may have a short-term role. Unfortunately, prolonged treatment with analogue reduces bone density and may be unwise in women at risk for osteoporosis. Where medical treatment is being undertaken it seems likely that CA125 levels, which are elevated in the presence of fibroids, can be serially measured in combination with ultrasound assessment to give some indication of shrinkage [12]. Hysterectomy with conservation of the ovaries should be performed in women whose families are complete.

UTERINE SARCOMAS

Mesenchymal sarcomas of the uterus are rare, accounting for approximately 3% of all tumours of the body of uterus. They carry a very poor prognosis, irrespective of the size at initial presentation.

Leiomyosarcomas are the most frequently encountered uterine sarcoma. Up to two-thirds may occur in an existing leiomyoma. The uterus containing a single myoma which shows signs of growth should be viewed with caution. There are no specific ultrasound features which distinguish these malignant tumours from their benign counterpart (Fig. 33.9). Frequently they appear solid with lots of cystic spaces throughout giving rise to the term a 'dropped knitting' appearance. Ultrasound may be useful to monitor these patients postoperatively or following radiotherapy/chemotherapy. There is a very strong tendency to recur following removal, with blood-borne metastasis to lung, bone and liver.

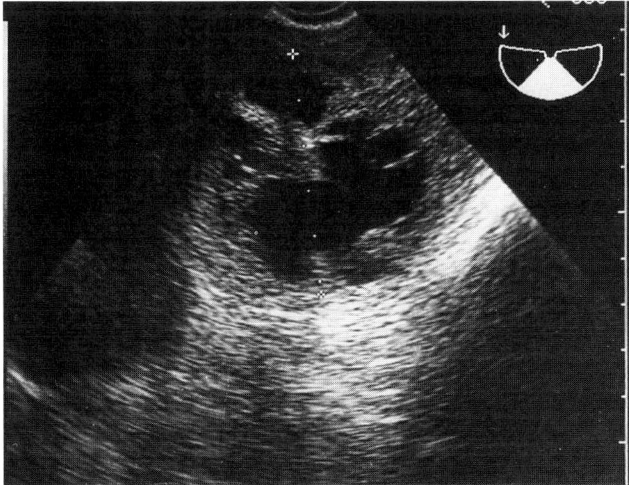

Fig. 33.9 A solitary fibroid in the posterior wall of the uterus with multiple irregular echolucent areas within it. Its appearance is not dissimilar from Fig. 33.8b but the 'cystic' areas are seen throughout the fibroid rather than in one isolated area. At the time of surgery this was confirmed to be a uterine leiomyosarcoma.

ENDOMETRIAL CANCER

Endometrial cancer, predominantly adenocarcinoma, is a disease of postmenopausal women. However, endometrial cancer may also be seen amongst women with polycystic ovarian syndrome (PCOS) because of the prolonged action of unopposed oestrogen. There is an association with endometrial hyperplasia and endometrial polyps. Endometrial cancers metastasize primarily by direct invasion and lymphatic spread. Haematogenous spread is usually a late feature. The prognosis of endometrial cancer is dependant on the clinical staging and pathological grading of the tumour. The International Federation of Gynecology and Obstetrics (FIGO) have recently revised the clinical staging [13] (Table 33.1).

The tumour usually develops in a localized portion of the endometrium. With further growth the uterine cavity becomes enlarged and filled with a firm, soft, often necrotic neoplasm. The ultrasound features of endometrial cancer reflect this. In its early stage, the only ultrasound evidence in the postmenopausal woman may be a thickened endometrium with a well-defined endometrial–myometrial interface. As described above, this always merits further investigation. Other features which should raise suspicion are breech of the endometrial 'halo', the presence of blood/debris in the uterine cavity and/or enlargement of the uterine body. Most endometrial tumours are echogenic, though less well-differentiated neoplasms may be hypoechoic (Fig. 33.10). TVS has been used to assess the depth of tumour invasion prior to surgery though the presence of leiomyomas in the

Table 33.1 The FIGO surgical staging of endometrial cancer (from 1989)

Stage	Features
Ia	Tumour limited to endometrium
Ib	Invasion < half of the myometrium
Ic	Invasion > half of the myometrium
IIa	Endocervical glandular involvement only
IIb	Cervical stromal invasion
IIIa	Tumour invades serosa and/or adnexae and/or positive peritoneal cytology
IIIb	Vaginal metastases
IIIc	Metastases to pelvic and/or para-aortic lymph nodes
IVa	Tumour invades bladder and/or bowel mucosa
IVb	Distant metastases including intra-abdominal and/or inguinal lymph node

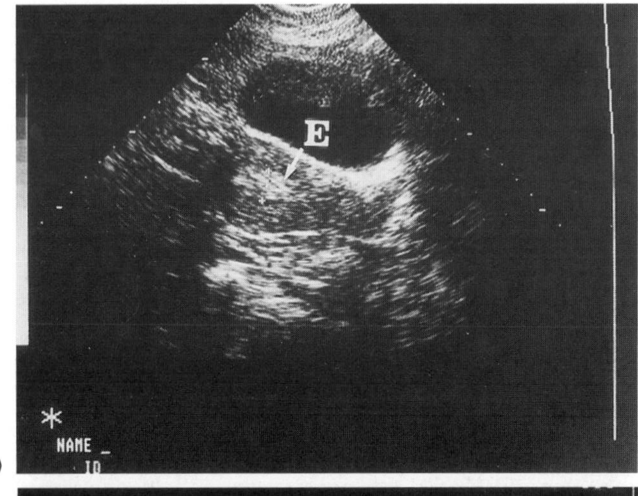

(a)

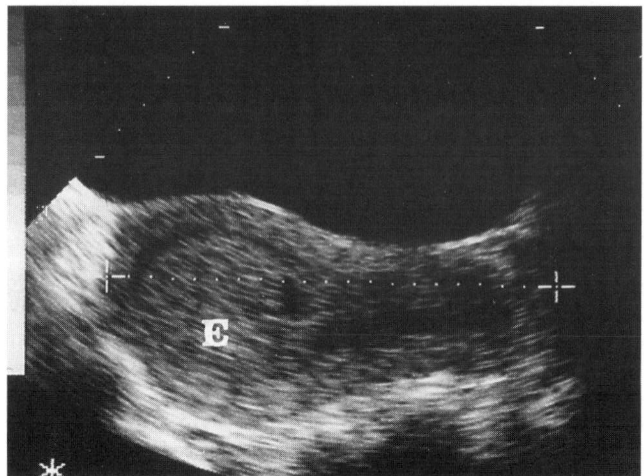

(b)

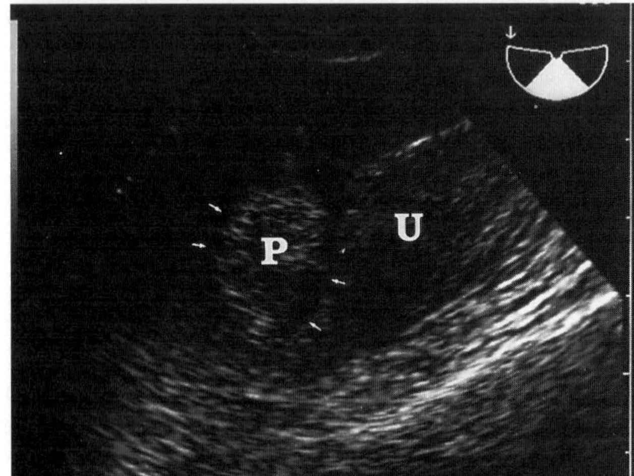

(c)

Fig. 33.10 (a) Transabdominal image of a small postmenopausal uterus. A dense echogenic area (E) measuring 10 mm is seen within the cavity. The 'halo' surrounding the endometrium has been breached at the lower pole. This was an early invasive endometrial cancer. (b) A transabdominal image of an endometrial cancer (E) arising from the posterior wall of the uterus. A small amount of blood is seen within the uterine cavity. The tumour is echogenic and was well differentiated on histology. (c) Transvaginal image of a uterus from a patient with persistent bleeding while on a 'no-bleed' HRT preparation. A hypoechoic polyp (P) is seen within the uterine cavity (U) surrounded by a rim of blood.

uterus may make this difficult. Ultrasound is poor at detecting invasion of local/distant lymph nodes. Transvaginal colour Doppler ultrasound has demonstrated that vascular impedance is lower in intratumoral, peritumoral and arcuate vessels associated with endometrial cancer than in vessels associated with normal endometrium [14–16]. These patients will almost always have other features such as a thickened endometrium to suggest the possibility of endometrial cancer.

Where there are ultrasound features to suggest endometrial pathology examination under anaesthesia with hysteroscopy and curettage should be performed. If carcinoma is identified the definitive treatment will be total abdominal hysterectomy with bilateral salpingo-oophorectomy (TAH/BSO). Staging is surgical (see Table 33.1). Radiotherapy may also be used postoperatively in those with more advanced disease (stage Ib or greater). For a proportion of women radiation alone may be used although this is not the ideal. Five-year survival rates of 75–80% might be expected for women with stage I disease, falling to 50% for stage II. One-third of women with stage III disease survive for 5 years but 85–90% of women presenting with stage IV disease succumb during the same period.

Ultrasound may also be useful in assessing patients following surgery and/or radiotherapy. Local recurrence usually occurs around the vaginal vault and will be seen as soft tissue swelling.

TROPHOBLASTIC DISEASE

Hydatidiform mole

Complete hydatidiform mole, in which there is no true fetal component, results from fertilization of an abnormal ovum. There are no maternal chromosomes in true moles and the genetic constitution results from duplication of a haploid sperm or from dispermy. In partial moles there are three sets of chromosomes, two being paternal and one maternal and a triploid fetus, is found. These pregnancies result in abortion, but in contrast with complete mole carry, no risk of subsequent choriocarcinoma. Complete moles often present with threatened abortion and classically are associated with the passage vaginally, of grape-like vesicles. Evacuation of the uterus is required following diagnosis. The risk of choriocarcinoma is difficult to establish but may be around 3%. Fortunately, human chorionic gonadotrophin (HCG) is produced by the abnormal trophoblast and acts as a highly effective marker in the management of trophoblast disease. Elevated HCG levels following molar pregnancy are an indication for further investigation and treatment.

On ultrasound examination the uterus is often larger than would be expected for the gestational age. In the case of a complete mole, no fetal parts can be identified. The uterus is filled with multiple cysts of varying size and reflectivity, though they are usually very small in diameter (Fig. 33.11). The ultrasound appearances of the uterus may be confused with hydropic degeneration of the placenta. Other differential diagnoses are blighted ovum and incomplete abortion. Histology and serial HCG estimations will establish the diagnosis. Postevacuation, HCG levels should fall. If they do not, ultrasound is useful to evaluate if the uterine cavity has been incompletely or completely evacuated. Theca lutein cysts are present in the ovary in about one-fifth of cases, as a result of the excessive HCG levels.

Pregnancy should be avoided for at least a year following molar pregnancy. Following each subsequent pregnancy urine or blood should be screened for HCG to exclude a further molar pregnancy. There is said to be a 2% risk of a second molar pregnancy. In the UK there is a well-established system for registering and monitoring trophoblast diseases and this is based in three centres, Dundee, Sheffield and Charring Cross Hospital in London.

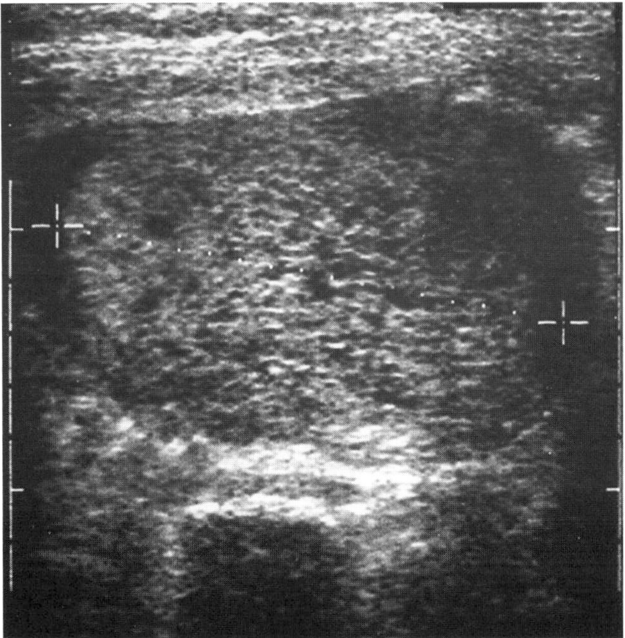

(a)

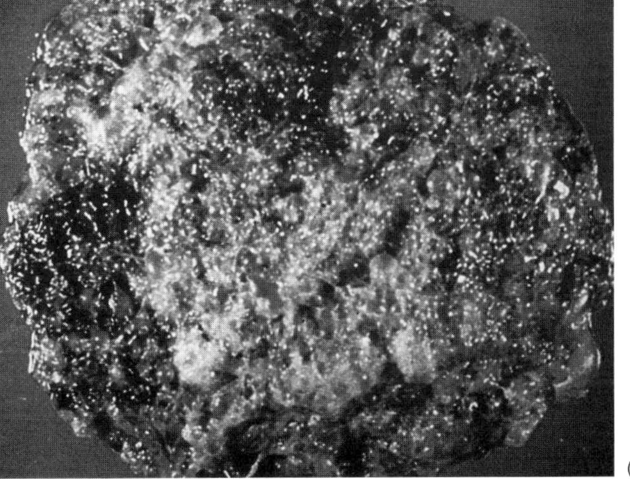

(b)

Fig. 33.11 (a) Tansabdominal image of a uterus at a 12-week 'booking' ultrasound scan. The uterus measuring 16 cm in length, is filled with multiple small cysts of varying size and density. (b) Pathology specimen of the tissue removed from the patient in (a), illustrating the grape-like vesicles which give rise to the ultrasound images.

Choriocarcinoma

Choriocarcinoma is an epithelial malignancy of trophoblastic cells. It invades the underlying myometrium, may involve local structures and invades vessels and lymphatics. It does not usually produce a large mass but has often metastasized to the lungs and bone by the time of diagnosis.

Fluid within the uterine cavity

The uterine cavity may be distended with pus (pyometra) or blood (haematometra) which will appear as an echolucent area within the uterine cavity. At times the cavity may be so distended that the endometrial echo may not be visible.

PYOMETRA

Pus collects within the uterine cavity as a result of blockage at the level of the cervix (e.g. from a cervical tumour) or at the lower uterus (e.g. following radiotherapy for a gynaecological malignancy). The pus may be sterile or frequently in the case of tumours be infective, from organisms such as coliforms or streptococci. The uterine cavity will appear grossly distended on ultrasound examination,

(a)

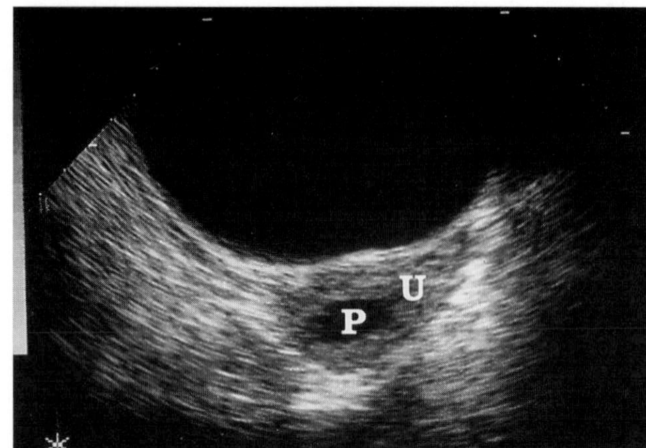

(b)

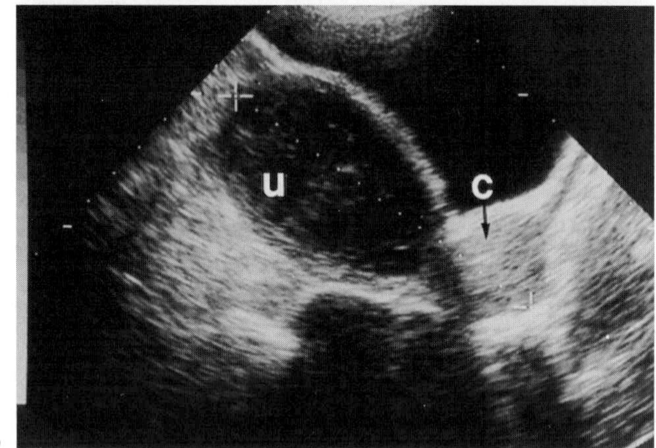

Fig. 33.12 (a) Transabdominal scan of a small perimenopausal uterus (U) filled with echolucent material (P). This was secondary to tuberculosis. (b) Transabdominal scan of a grossly enlarged postmenopausal uterus (u). The uterine cavity contains particulate, echogenic material. The cervix (c) is also enlarged. This pyometra was secondary to a cervical cancer.

with echolucent material, which at times may be particulate (Fig. 33.12). Dilatation of the cervix, usually under general anaesthesia, allows release of the pus. Further investigations are required to identify the underlying cause in every case.

HAEMATOMETRA

The uterine cavity may also be distended by blood secondary to obstruction at the level of the cervix or lower. Cervical obstruction may again be due to malignancy but more frequently is secondary to surgery involving the cervix, such as a Manchester-type pelvic floor repair or cone biopsy. The treatment for this problem is again dilatation of the cervix to allow free drainage of the menstrual blood. The ultrasound appearances are similar to those seen with pyometra (Fig. 33.13).

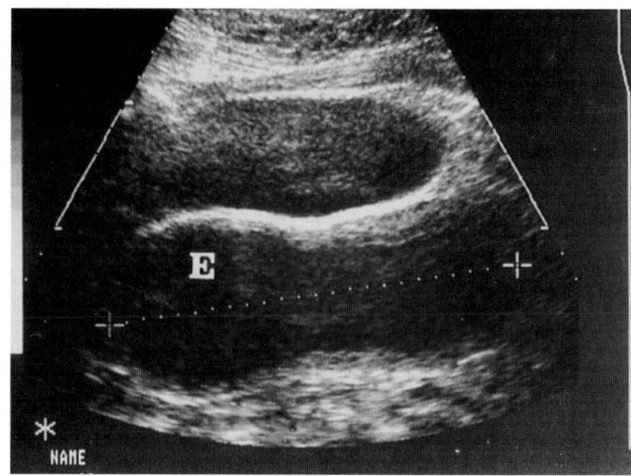

Fig. 33.13 Longitudinal transabdominal image of a uterus in which the uterine wall is very thin and the cavity distended with echolucent material (E). This haematometra was secondary to cervical stenosis following surgery.

Obstruction below the cervix, is caused by persistence of the hymenal membrane, resulting in distension of the vagina (haematocolpos) and uterus. Treatment is incision of the membrane.

Cervical cancer

Cervical cancer is associated with high parity, young age at first sexual intercourse, cigarette smoking and possibly viral infection. A number of subtypes of human papilloma virus have been implicated in cervical premalignancy (cervical intraepithelial neoplasia, CIN) and progression to invasive cancer is sufficiently frequently encountered to suggest an aetiological association. Cervical carcinoma is most commonly squamous epithelial disease and presents as intermenstrual, irregular or postcoital bleeding. The diagnosis is based upon clinical examination and histological assessment of cervical tissue. Once the diagnosis of cervical cancer is confirmed it is staged using the FIGO guidelines which is a clinical staging with the addition of cystoscopy and intravenous pyelography (Table 33.2). Ultrasound and computed tomography (CT) scanning may provide additional information but they do not alter clinical staging.

On ultrasound, the cervical canal may be seen to be enlarged or distorted by tumour. If blocked, a pyometra or haematometra may be present (see Fig. 33.13). Parametrial spread to the pelvic side wall may be demonstrated but requires optimal use of gain settings. Hydronephrosis or ureteric dilatation from tumour occlusion is readily identified. During or following treatment such imaging

Table 33.2 The FIGO staging classification for cervical cancer

Stage	Features
0	Preinvasive carcinoma (CIN)
I	Carcinoma confined to the cervix (corpus extension should be disregarded)
Ia	Preclinical carcinoma of cervix diagnosed only by microscopy; depth of invasion from the base of the epithelium should not be greater than 5 mm and horizontal spread must not exceed 7 mm
Ib	Lesions of greater dimensions than stage Ia whether seen clinically or not
II	Carcinoma extending beyond the cervix and involving the vagina (but not the lower third) and/or infiltrating the parametrium (but not reaching the pelvic side wall)
IIa	Carcinoma has involved the vagina
IIb	Carcinoma has infiltrated the parametrium
III	Carcinoma involving the lower third of the vagina and/or extending to the pelvic side wall
IIIa	Carcinoma involving the lower third of the vagina
IIIb	Carcinoma extending to the pelvic wall and/or hydronephrosis or non-functioning kidney due to ureterostenosis caused by tumour
IVa	Carcinoma involving the mucosa of the bladder or rectum and/or extending beyond the true pelvis
IVb	Spread to distant organs

may prove useful. Differentiating recurrent tumour from fibrosed tissue following treatment is difficult.

Management and prognosis of cervical cancer are dependent upon staging. Radiotherapy may be used for all stages of the disease although adjuvant chemotherapy before treatment of stage III and IV disease may improve outcome. For early stage disease, radical hysterectomy in which the uterus, fallopian tubes and upper half of vagina are removed along with pelvic lymphadenectomy, may be performed. The success rate is the same as for radiotherapy but it may have the advantage that ovarian function and vaginal stenosis may be avoided. For stage I disease the 5-year survival rate is between 85 and 90% regardless of treatment modality. Two-thirds of women with stage II disease will survive for 5 years but this will fall to one-third for stage III and around 10–15% for stage IV disease.

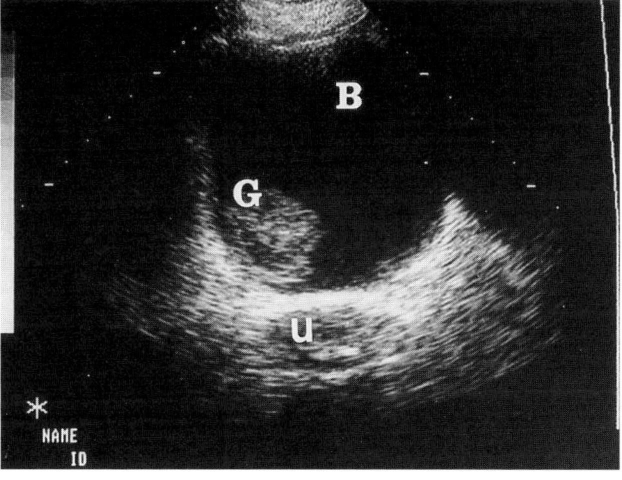

Fig. 33.14 Transabdominal scan in a postmenopausal woman with a full bladder (B) and a small uterus (U) behind. A frond-like growth (G) is seen to arise from the posterior bladder wall. This was confirmed to be a transitional cell carcinoma.

Bladder tumours

These tumours are surprisingly common in elderly women and it is therefore particularly wise to perform a transabdominal scan with a full bladder in all women presenting with supposed postmenopausal bleeding (Fig. 33.14). A proportion of women presenting with post-menopausal bleeding will in fact have had bleeding per urethra but assumed it to be per vaginam.

The ovary

Anatomy

The ovaries are found at the distal end of each fallopian tube and lie near the lateral pelvic side wall. The fimbriated end of the fallopian tube curves round the ovary, assisting the 'pick-up' of ova during ovulation. The lateral surface of each ovary lies in close apposition to the internal iliac artery on the pelvic side wall, near its root at the bifurcation of the common iliac artery. Each ovary is small with dimensions of 2.5–5 cm length, 1.5–3 cm breadth and 1–1.5 cm width. They are pearly white in appearance with a smooth, wrinkled surface.

During each menstrual cycle one or two follicles begin to enlarge, but one follicle soon becomes dominant and outgrows the others. By mid cycle, the follicle will be

18–30 mm in size. With ovulation, the follicle ruptures, releasing the ovum, which enters the fimbrial end of the fallopian tube.

Ultrasound appearance of the ovary

The ovaries can usually be detected by transabdominal scanning using the full bladder technique, though difficulty may be experienced in the obese patient. The internal iliac vessels which are posterolateral to the ovary serve as a useful landmark. During the reproductive years, ovaries can be clearly identified by the presence of 'follicles'. TVS is increasingly used for normal ovarian scans as a full bladder is not required and the close, high frequency probes ensure high resolution pictures of these small organs. Ovaries are identified on TVS laterally and slightly posterior to the uterus. The internal iliac vessels serve as further landmarks and ovarian follicles confirm the identity of the structures (Fig. 33.15).

Follicle measurements and tracking

Follicles can be pictured early in the menstrual cycle at 3–5 mm, particularly with TVS. With increasing follicle-stimulating hormone levels the follicles grow to 8–10 mm. In normal patients follicles are found in only one ovary in any given cycle. A dominant follicle will develop and reach a maximum diameter of 20–30 mm at the time of ovulation. Of circulating oestradiol 95% emanates from the growing follicle. Such assays can therefore be used to assess follicular growth during ovulation induction in the treatment of infertility. Once the ovum is expelled, there is bleeding into the collapsed follicle. This is seen as echogenic material within the area of the old follicle 1–5 days following ovulation. During the luteal phase, cystic enlargement of the corpus luteum may take place and can sometimes reach diameters of 30–100 mm. Sudden haemorrhage into an enlarged corpus luteum can mimic signs and symptoms of an ectopic pregnancy.

Polycystic ovarian syndrome

Polycystic ovaries may occur in up to 20% of the population [17–19]. Classically, these ovaries are enlarged, with an echo-dense central stroma and multiple small cysts (approximately 5 mm in diameter) located around the periphery of the ovary (Fig. 33.16). These features are more easily defined by TVS than with transabdominal ultrasound. When this finding of polycystic ovaries is found in association with reduced fertility, menstrual and endocrine irregularities the clinical entity is known as PCOS. Impaired fertility is usually due to anovulation and this can be treated using different ovulation induction techniques; the commonest of these are the antioestrogens of which clomiphene is the most widely used. For resistant cases treatment with exogenous gonadotrophins is required. These regimes are potentially dangerous and require careful patient selection. In particular, the development of follicles within the ovary must be carefully monitored to prevent ovarian hyperstimulation syndrome (OHS).

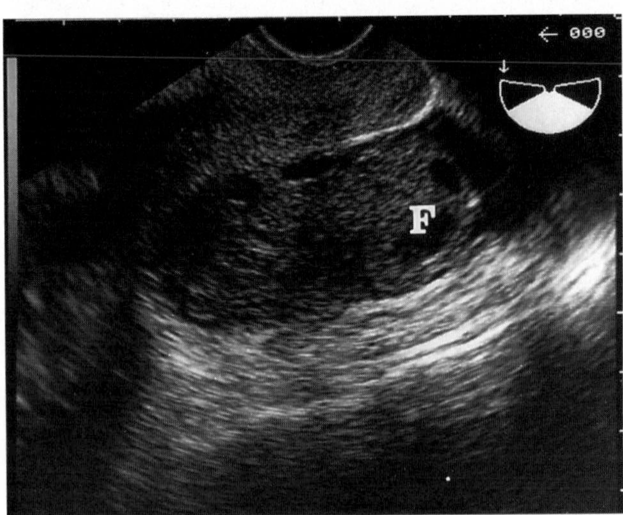

Fig. 33.15 Transvaginal scan of a normal ovary containing several small follicles (F).

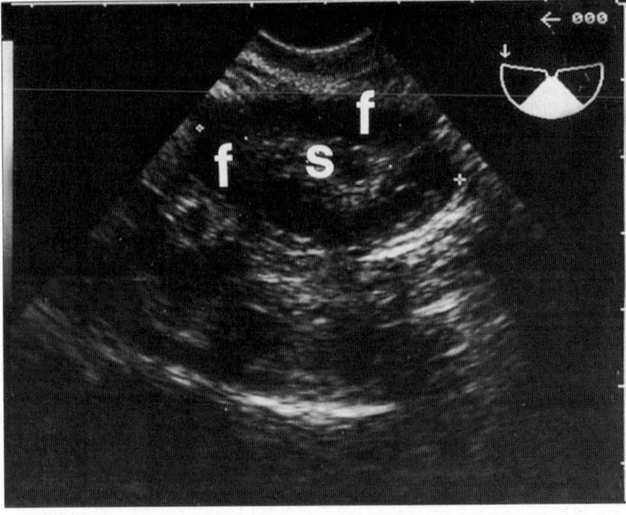

Fig. 33.16 Transvaginal scan of a polycystic ovary with dense ovarian stroma (S) and multiple small follicles (f) around the entire periphery.

Follicle tracking during ovarian stimulation

Transvaginal ultrasound is almost always employed for this. A baseline scan of each ovary should be completed and the presence of polycystic ovaries documented. Once treatment begins, the ovaries are examined on alternate days. In amenorrhoeic women preparing for *in vitro* fertilization (IVF), a small number of large follicles usually develops. Ideally, at least 10 mature follicles will form and reach a diameter of 18–20 mm. At this stage the follicles are aspirated to collect the ova. Serum oestradiols correlate well with follicular development.

An increasing number of women are seen for ovulation induction. These women may have endogenous oestrogens or polycystic ovaries and are at considerable risk of higher order (triplets or greater) pregnancy. This risk can be greatly reduced with adequate assessment of ovarian follicular growth. As for IVF cycles, ovarian scans are performed on alternate days to assess follicular growth. Smaller doses of gonadotrophins are usually required and frequently several follicles of varying size will be recruited. Ideally two or three follicles should reach a diameter of 18–20 mm, at which time HCG is administered to promote final follicular maturation and ovulation. Great care must be taken that the entire ovary is scanned to ensure that additional follicles have not also reached a 'mature' diameter, as once HCG is administered, potentially all follicles will ovulate (Fig. 33.17). Where four or five mature follicles are present the chances of a multiple pregnancy increase. In these circumstances, the cycle should be discontinued and HCG withheld. These patients are at risk of OHS. In this condition, which usually develops 1 week after ovulation has been induced with HCG, the ovaries become oedematous, multiple large cysts form and abdominal pain/swelling result. Severe cases can be life-threatening with the development of ascites, electrolyte imbalance, disseminated intravascular coagulation and pleural effusions. OHS can still occur in those patients who achieve a successful pregnancy. Spontaneous resolution will occur with supportive medical management. The ultrasound features of OHS reflect these clinical signs with large, bilateral multicystic ovaries and ascites.

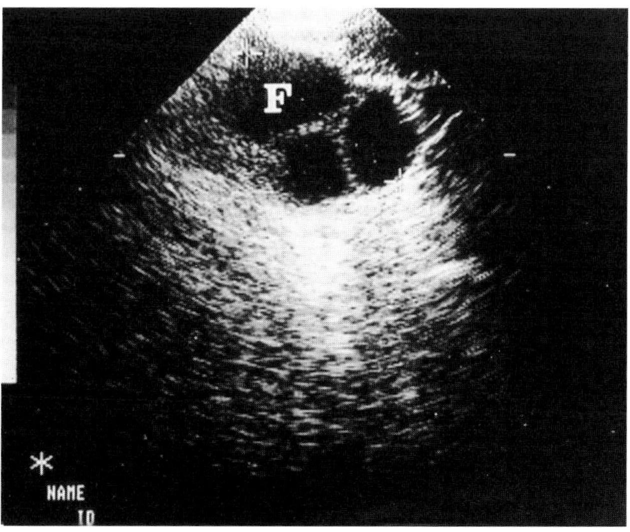

Fig. 33.17 Transvaginal scan of an ovary stimulated by exogenous gonadotrophins. Three large follicles (F) can be seen here, but on rotating the probe a further two large follicles were identified and the cycle therefore abandoned.

Ovarian masses

Ovarian cancer remains a difficult condition to identify in the early and potentially curable stages. It most commonly occurs in postmenopausal women who present with increasing abdominal girth, pain, anorexia or a palpable abdominal/pelvic mass. Recently, there has been increasing concern that younger women requiring ovarian stimulation for the treatment of infertility are at increased risk of ovarian cancer [20] and therefore the possibility of this diagnosis should be contemplated in any women presenting with an ovarian mass.

Although TVS affords excellent detail of the ovaries, as a result of the short focal range of TVS probes, ovarian masses greater than 10 cm or those outwith the true pelvis are best examined with transabdominal scanning.

CYSTIC AND SEMI-CYSTIC OVARIAN MASSES

Cystic adnexal masses are well-circumscribed, echolucent areas which contain no internal echoes (Fig. 33.18). In premenopausal women this is usually a 'physiological' cyst, formed from a graffian follicle or corpus luteum. These cysts are >3 cm in diameter and are surrounded by normal ovarian tissue. Corpus luteal cysts may have a thicker wall and contain some internal echoes due to bleeding into the cyst. Such cysts normally regress spontaneously. Larger physiological cysts which persist for more than three or four menstrual cycles may be drained during laparoscopy to prevent cyst accidents such as torsion occurring. With the introduction of ovarian cancer screening, it has been noted that up to 17% of the postmenopausal population may also have 'simple', small (3–4 cm) ovarian cysts [21]. Large cystic structures should always be scanned with a full and empty bladder as some may just be bladder alone or may be large bladder diverticuli. If necessary and there is any doubt, the patient should be catheterized.

Serous cystadenomas are benign tumours of epithelial origin. They are usually completely anechoic, unilocular

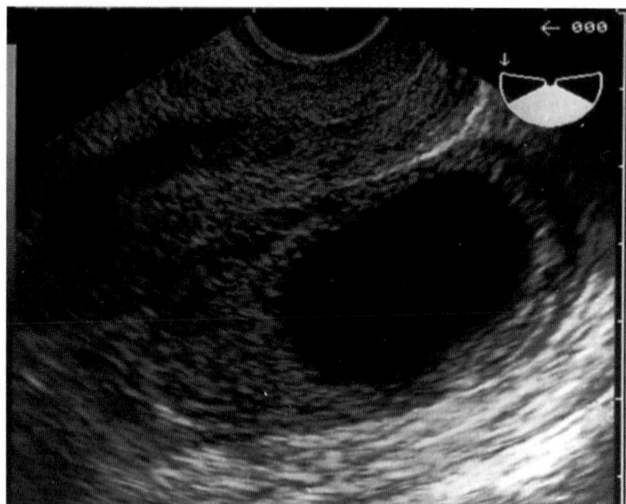

Fig. 33.18 Transvaginal scan of a single echolucent 'cyst' in an ovary. This disappeared after 2 months and was most likely a large corpus luteum cyst.

and have a regular, thin, smooth wall. They vary in size from 10 to 30 cm and occasionally may be bilateral. The malignant variant of this, the serous cystadenocarcinomas, account for 60% of all ovarian carcinomas. Malignancy is suggested by the presence of multiple loculations, irregular thickening of the cyst wall, ascites or papillary processes arising from the cyst wall (Fig. 33.19).

Mucinous cystadenomas are also of epithelial origin. They are commonly multiloculated with thin septae (Fig. 33.20) and have areas of irregular echoes within, due to the mucin they contain. It is difficult to differentiate benign and malignant mucinous cysts, though bilateral cysts are ominous. If they rupture, mucinous material fills the peritoneal cavity producing a variable echo pattern.

Teratomas (dermoid cysts) arise from germ cells and therefore contain a variety of adult epithelial tissue derivatives, including hair, bone and teeth. As a result, the ultrasound appearances vary considerably from primarily cystic lesions to dense echogenic solid masses (Fig. 33.21). Elements such as bone and teeth are very echogenic and often cast shadows, limiting the detail which can be obtained. These tumours are commonly unilateral but may be bilateral in young women especially. The presence of bilateral tumours must raise suspicion about possible malignancy. Malignant teratomas (dermoids) are usually solid or complex in appearance but may be very difficult to distinguish from the benign variant.

Endometriomas ('chocolate cysts') are found in women with endometriosis. Endometriosis describes the findings of tissue which is histologically similar to the endometrium but in another site. The condition affects

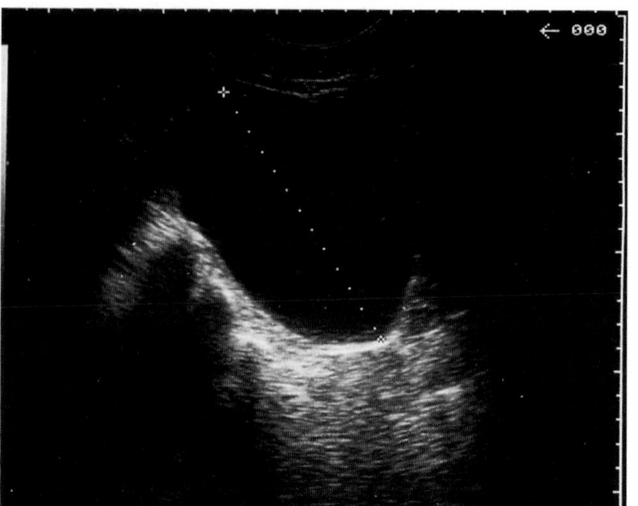

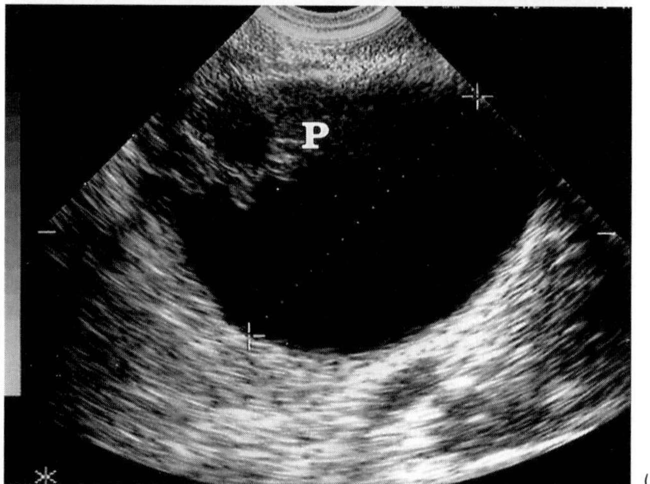

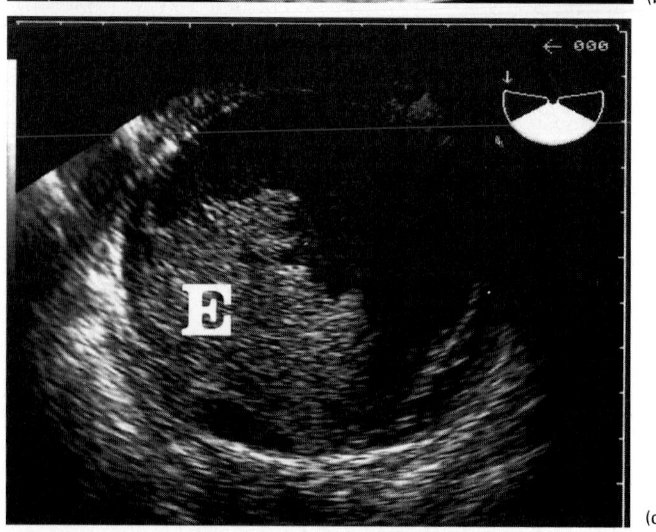

Fig. 33.19 (a) A simple unilocular serous cystadenoma. (b) Transabdominal image of a large unilateral ovarian cyst. Irregular protrusions (P) are seen to arise from one area. This was confirmed to be a serous cystadenocarcinoma. (c) Transabdominal image of an irregular semi-cystic, semi-solid mass (E) with a poorly defined border typical of a malignant adenocarcinoma.

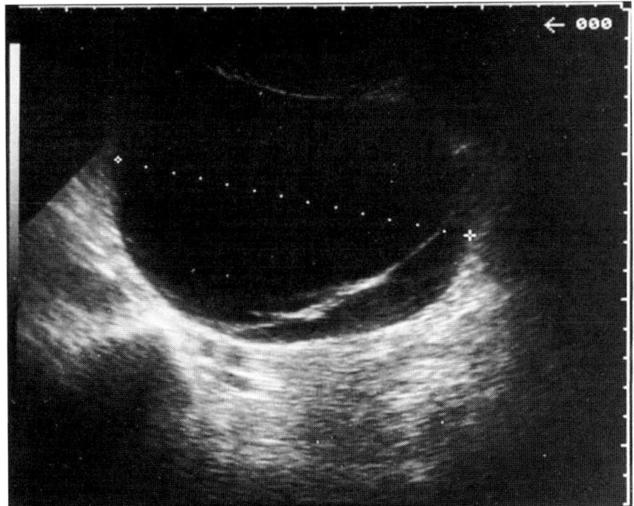

Fig. 33.20 A large unilocular cyst with internal septae and slightly particulate matter within it suggestive of mucinous cystadenoma.

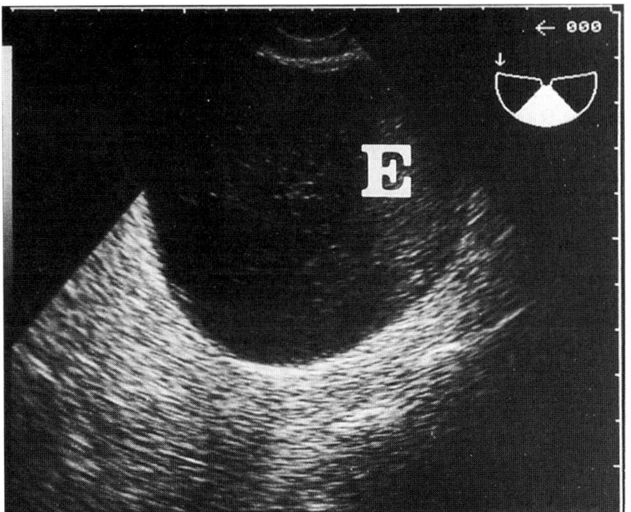

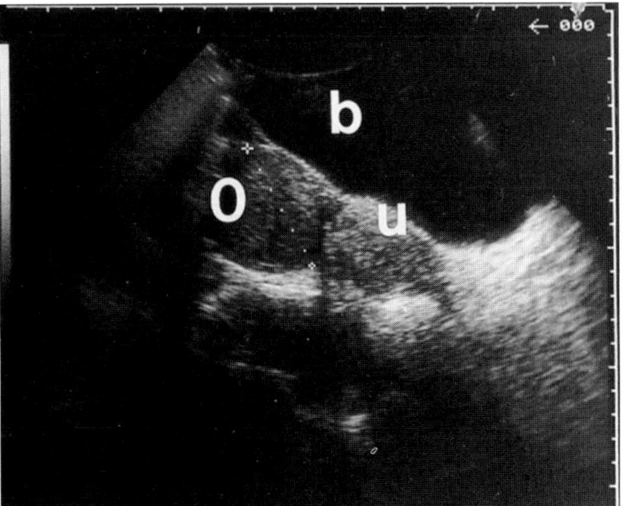

Fig. 33.21 (a) Transabdominal image of an ovarian cyst which contained particulate material and two echogenic areas within it (E), confirmed to be a dermoid cyst. (b) Transabdominal image of a solid unilateral ovarian mass which appears dense and echogenic. Pathology confirmed this to be a dermoid but the appearance could easily be mistaken for a leiomyosarcoma if care is not taken to identify the origin of the mass. b, Bladder; O, ovary; u, uterus.

women in the reproductive age group. The ectopic endometrium responds to both exogenous and endogenous oestrogen stimulation in a similar fashion to the uterine tissue. Such bleeding in the peritoneal cavity/ ovary may lead to the development of adhesions, and cause any further blood to collect, giving rise to blood cysts. These appear less regular than common ovarian cysts and usually demonstrate a mixed echo pattern on ultrasound reflecting the debris composed of blood clot they contain (Fig. 33.22). The appearances resemble those of dermoid cysts. The clinical presentation is often very helpful in establishing the most likely diagnosis.

SOLID OVARIAN MASSES

These tumours are rare and may be confused with a uterine fibroid (see Fig. 33.22). They appear irregular in shape and are echogenic. The two can usually be differentiated by TVS; a uterine fibroid will have the same texture as the uterus and will be connected to it. Imaging a normal ovary by TVS would suggest a uterine fibroid to be more likely. Some ovarian cysts in the semi-cystic category may also appear solid and should remain on the differential diagnosis of any solid adnexal mass. These include dermoids, thecomas, endometriomas and importantly Krukenberg tumours. Krukenberg tumours especially can be forgotten about by most sonographers. They are usually complex, solid and bilateral. There may be accompanying free abdominal or pelvic fluid present. When solid adnexal masses are detected, the liver and kidneys should be inspected for any signs of more widespread malignancy.

MANAGEMENT OF OVARIAN CYSTS

Ultrasound-guided aspiration of ovarian cysts has been advocated both in the acute presentation with pain [22] and also electively to avoid surgery. Unfortunately, false negative aspiration cytology is a real danger [23] and in one series cytological study was unsatisfactory in 18% of cases [24]. Ovarian cystectomy in cases of benign disease may be performed by laparotomy or minimal access techniques. The management of all ovarian cancer comprises TAH/BSO with infracolic omentectomy. The underlying principle of the surgical approach is to debulk as much

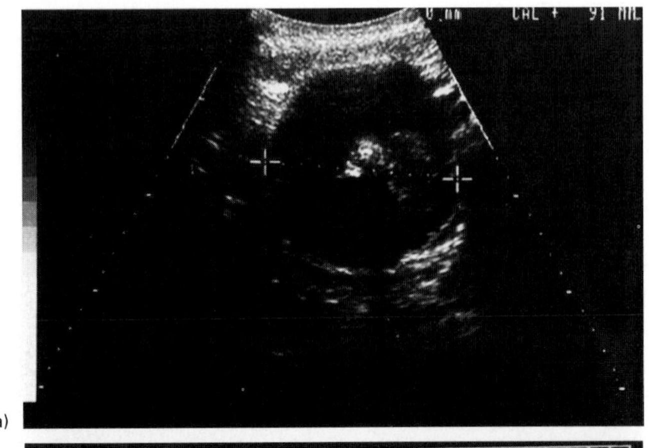
(a)

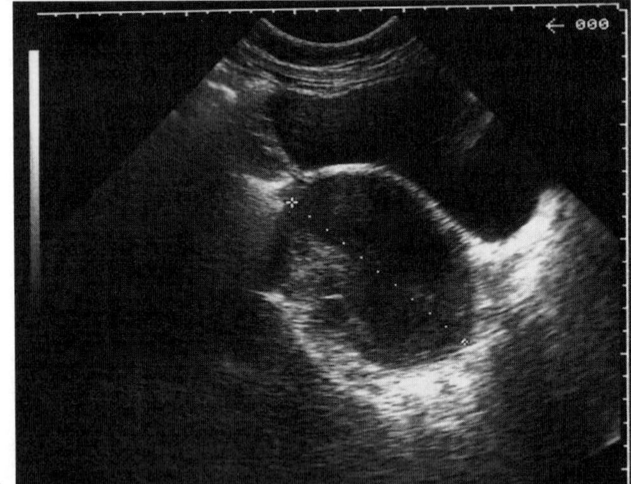
(b)

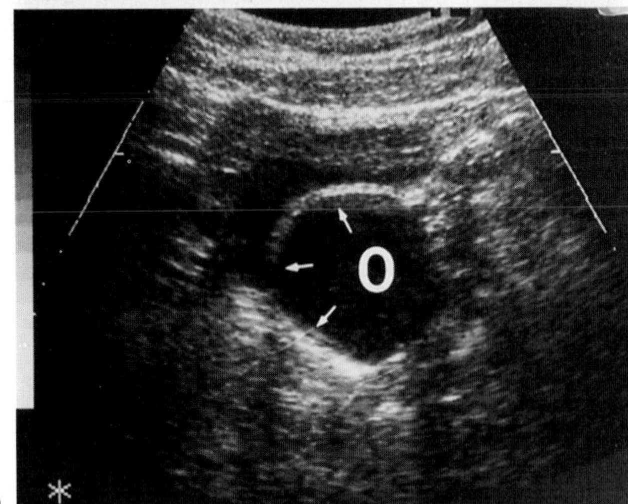

(c)

Fig. 33.22 (a) Transabdominal image of a unilateral solid ovarian mass containing dense irregular echogenic areas within it. (b) A solid ovarian mass with cystic areas present in a patient known to have endometriosis. (c) A thin rim of ovarian tissue (O) present in an ovarian mass. It was confirmed to be an endometrioma at surgery.

tumour as possible. Using an aggressive approach such cytoreductive surgery can clear the abdomen of macroscopic disease in 90% of cases. Like other gynaecological malignancy FIGO recommends an international staging scheme (Table 33.3). Chemotherapy is indicated in the management of all stages of ovarian cancer except stage Ia and Ib. Currently platinum-based treatments are most effective; cisplatin is well established though renal toxicity is problematic. Carboplatin is much less nephrotoxic and is being used increasingly. Taxol, a novel chemotherapeutic agent is now being used in ovarian disease and appears promising, particularly for previously platinum-resistant tumours. The overall 5-year survival rate in non-specialist units is 33%. For stages I and II the relevant figure is 63% but for stage III and IV the comparable figure is only 8%.

Screening for ovarian malignancy

In view of the improved survival associated with the early detection of ovarian malignancy, there has been increasing pressure to develop a screening programme. The tumour markers CA125 and carcinoembryonic antigen (CAE) were initially used but have a poor specificity and sensitivity. Campbell *et al.* [25] described transabdominal ultrasound as a possible tool for ovarian cancer screening. When used in a large-scale screening programme, however, the positive predictive value was poor—1.5% [26]. With the introduction of TVS, scoring systems based on tumour characteristics, such as the presence of septae/papillae, were devised. This improved the specificity of the technique to a degree [27]. Further work recognized that malignancy was associated with the development of new vessels. These vessels had a lower vascular impedance, demonstrated by Doppler ultrasound, when compared to the blood vessels normally present within the ovary [28,29]. Using one of these more sophisticated scoring systems [27], most malignant tumours will be correctly detected. However, many benign lesions still demonstrate these malignant features so that the positive predictive value remains poor.

New information on the role of genes in ovarian cancer is emerging but until the value of multi-parametric screening systems using TVS, tumour markers and genetics is more closely evaluated ovarian cancer screening should be restricted to well-conducted research studies such as the National Cancer Institute study on the early detection of ovarian disease [30].

The fallopian tube

Despite the advances of TVS for gynaecological ultrasound scanning, imaging the normal fallopian tube remains a diagnostic challenge, as the tube is normally small and has no fluid interface. The introduction of con-

Table 33.3 The FIGO staging classification for primary ovarian cancer

Stage	Features
I	Growth limited to ovaries
Ia	Growth limited to one ovary; no ascites; no tumour on external surface; capsule intact
Ib	Limited to both ovaries; no ascites; no tumour on external surfaces; capsule intact
Ic	Tumour stage Ia or Ib but tumour on surface of one or both ovaries; or with capsule ruptured; or with ascites present containing malignant cells; or with positive peritoneal washings
II	Growth involving one or both ovaries with pelvic extension
IIa	Extension and/or metastases to the uterus or tubes
IIb	Extension to other pelvic tissues
IIc	Tumour stage IIa or IIb and tumour on surface of one or both ovaries; or capsule ruptured; or ascites present containing malignant cells; or positive peritoneal washings
III	Growth involving one or both ovaries with extrapelvic peritoneal implants or positive retroperitoneal/inguinal nodes. Superficial liver metastasis equals stage III
IIIa	Tumour grossly limited to the true pelvis with negative nodes but with histologically confirmed microscopic seeding of abdominal peritoneal surfaces
IIIb	Tumour with histologically confirmed implants on abdominal peritoneal surfaces, none exceeding 2 cm in diameter; nodes are negative
IIIc	Abdominal implants greater than 2 cm in diameter or positive retroperitoneal inguinal nodes
IV	Growth involving one or both ovaries with distant metastases. If pleural effusion is present there must be positive cytology to allot a case to stage IV. Parenchymal liver metastasis equals stage IV

trast TVS, will enable visualization of the normal fallopian tube. In the meantime, however, the fallopian tubes are only visualized when there is fluid in the pelvis, such as blood or fluid from a ruptured corpus luteum/ovarian cysts or when gross pathology is present.

Ectopic pregnancy

Ectopic pregnancy is the implantation of the conceptus in a site other than the decidua of the uterine cavity. The vast majority, over 95% are sited in the fallopian tubes, but other sites include the ovaries, peritoneal cavity and cervix. Although only 1 in 300 pregnancies will be ectopic in site, ectopic pregnancies still accounted for almost 5% of maternal deaths in Britain during 1991–93 [31]. There is evidence that the number of ectopic pregnancies is climbing. Factors which adversely affect tubal motility and function such as the increased incidence of pelvic inflammatory disease (PID) and tubal surgery no doubt contribute to this rise. In addition, it is recognized that assisted conception techniques such as gamete intra-fallopian transfer (GIFT) and *in vitro* fertilization may predispose to this complication [32].

The ready availability of rapid urine pregnancy tests and quantitative serum estimations for β-HCG have revolutionized the diagnosis and management of early pregnancy and its complications. β-HCG is produced by the trophoblast and within days of implantation will be present in measurable quantities in serum. In normal pregnancy, serum levels of β-HCG double within 72 h.

ULTRASOUND FEATURES

Having confirmed a positive serum β-HCG, the location of the pregnancy must be established. Concomitant intra- and extrauterine pregnancies have been reported [33] but they are so rare that in practice if an intrauterine pregnancy is clearly demonstrated, and there are no adnexal masses, the diagnosis of an ectopic pregnancy may virtually be excluded. The presence of a gestation sac and embryo/fetal heart can be seen 1 week earlier with TVS than with conventional transabdominal ultrasound [34]. TVS has therefore become an integral part of the ultrasound work-up of a suspected ectopic pregnancy. The following descriptions refer to TVS. With this approach the chorionic sac can usually be identified in intrauterine pregnancies when the β-HCG is 500 mIU ml^{-1} or more [35,36].

A true gestation sac demonstrates a double echogenic ring representing the proliferative inner layer of cytotrophoblast cells and the outer syncytiotrophoblast layer. It is usually sited asymmetrically at the fundus. In contrast a pseudosac is often seen in the uterine cavity in the presence of an ectopically sited pregnancy. It is normally located in the centre of the uterine cavity and is characterized by a single echogenic ring which reflects the decidual response of the endometrium to a pregnancy. Intraluminal fluid or blood produces the echolucent portion of the pseudosac (Fig. 33.23).

An ectopic pregnancy will continue to grow until the tubal epithelium can no longer 'support' a pregnancy. As

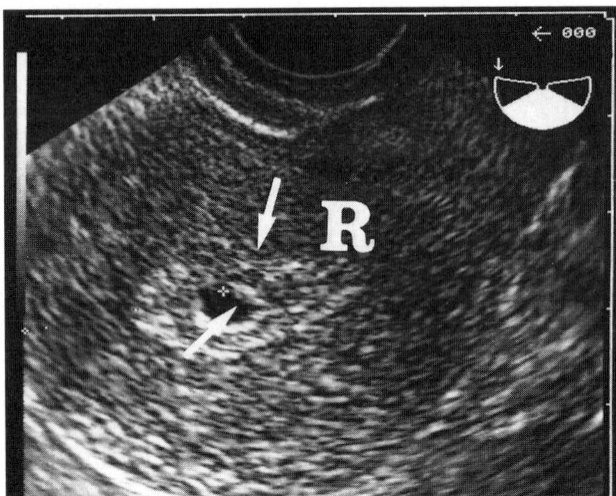

Fig. 33.23 A normal intrauterine gestation sac which is well defined and characterized by the presence of a double echogenic ring (R). In contrast the pseudosac seen in Fig. 33.22 is less well defined and has a single echogenic layer present.

with an intrauterine gestation, a sac will initially develop in the fallopian tube. Thereafter, with advancing gestation, a yolk sac, embryo and fetal heart may be detected. The presence of a definite fetal pole or yolk sac in an adnexal mass is diagnostic of an ectopic pregnancy. Frequently, however, these diagnostic features are not seen. Other ultrasound 'signs' suggestive of an ectopic pregnancy have been recognized of which the 'halo sign' or 'tubal ring sign' is the most well known [37]. This has been defined as a cystic area in the adnexa with an echogenic ring surrounded by a 2–4 mm sonolucent rim [38]. The halo is thought to be the tubal musculature and the echogenic rim, the chorion [39]. Care should be taken to exclude a corpus luteum which will normally be located on the peripheral edge of ovarian tissue (Fig. 33.24).

With continued stretching of the fallopian tube, erosion of the tubal musculature and bleeding into/around the sac will occur. Thereafter, the pregnancy may (a) reabsorb; (b) abort into the tubal lumen and from thence be extruded through the fimbrial end of the tube; and (c) rupture through the tubal wall. The latter two outcomes are associated with bleeding into the peritoneal cavity. The pouch of Douglas should therefore be specifically examined for free peritoneal fluid and blood clot (irregular echogenic material, often mobile). The absence of free fluid in the pouch of Douglas excludes any active intraperitoneal bleeding. If rupture has occurred, the fallopian tube will appear distended with irregular mixed echoes, reflecting blood clot with/around the tube.

The management of tubal pregnancy has advanced considerably in recent years with improved conservative

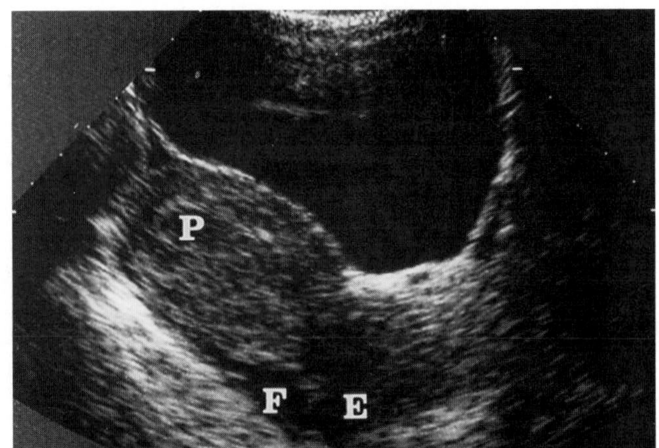

(a)

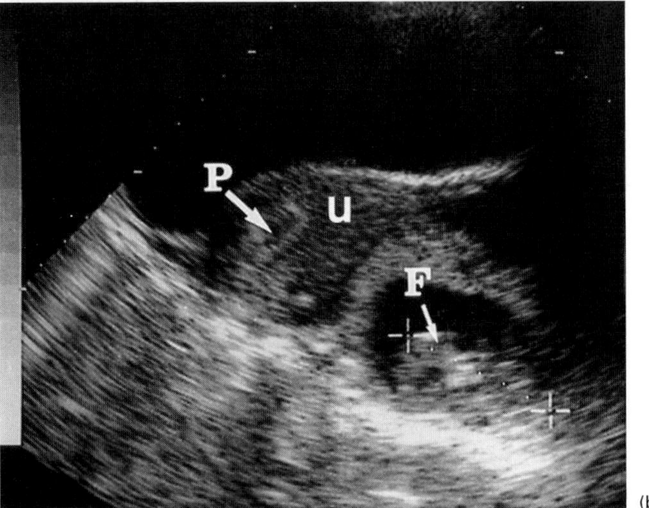

(b)

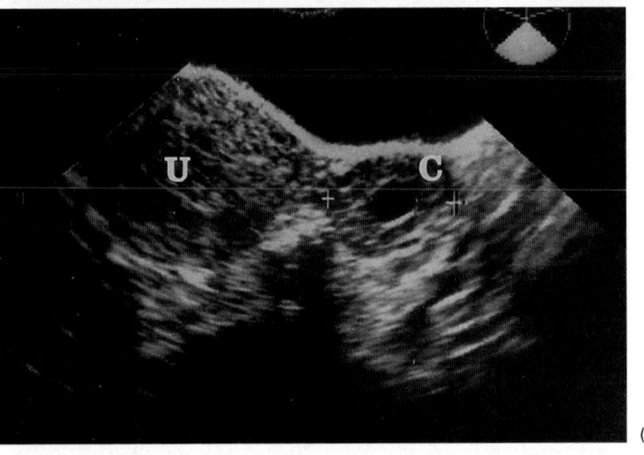

(c)

Fig. 33.24 Transabdominal image of the uterus containing a pseudosac (P) with a single echogenic ring. Fluid is present behind the uterus (F) and irregular echos (E) seen in the pouch of Douglas representing blood clot. (b) Transabdominal image of a fetal pole (F) located outside the uterus (U). The uterus contains a pseudosac (P). (c) Transabdominal image of a 'booking scan' at 7 weeks gestation. A cystic structure (C) is identified in the adnexa. It has no follicles and is therefore not an ovary, though the ovary was seen in close apposition. The uterus (U) was empty.

tubal surgery, which may be done laparoscopically, and increasing use of medical measures to prevent trophoblast invasion of the tube, based upon cytotoxic agents either injected through the laparoscope or given systemically. These improved management techniques depend, however, on the early diagnosis of ectopic pregnancy using serum β-HCG and TVS.

Tubal distension—PID

By definition, if the lumen of the fallopian tube is visualized it must be distended with fluid. The tubal contents may be sonolucent, reflecting serous fluid (hydrosalpinx) or partially echogenic when mucous or pus (pyosalpinx) are present. The most common cause of fluid within the fallopian tube is pelvic infection (PID). PID is an imprecise term which describes an acute inflammatory response in the uterus, fallopian tubes, ovaries and pelvic peritoneum as a result of ascending bacterial disease. The incidence is no less than 1% in women in the reproductive years and significantly higher in women aged between 15 and 24 years. The pathogenesis of primary PID is uncertain although much evidence appears to link sexually transmitted organisms such as *Trichomonas*, *Gonococcus*, *Chlamydia trachomatis*, *Bacteroides*, *Streptococcus* and *Mycoplasma*. Intrauterine devices should be removed in women suspected of PID and sent for bacteriological culture. Since ectopic pregnancy can mimic PID a pregnancy test and ultrasound examination should be performed.

In the presence of inflammation or pelvic infection, fluid may in addition be present in the pouch of Douglas, offering contrast which will outline the tube. In a small study Cacciatore *et al.* [40] identified 13 women who met stringent criteria for the diagnosis of endometritis. In 11 of these women thickened fluid-filled fallopian tubes were identified. Free pelvic fluid was also associated with PID but other workers have failed to identify purulent fluid in the pouch of Douglas in women confirmed at laparoscopy [41]. Antibiotic treatment aims to eliminate infection with minimal tubal damage.

In more severe pelvic infections a tubo-ovarian abscess may form. These will often result in tubal damage and usually occlusion. This can be recognized by the presence of multiple fluid filled, thick-walled cystic lesions in the adnexa. The ovarian portion can sometimes be distinguished by the presence of small follicles within it. The distended fallopian tube is usually wrapped around the ovary thus making definition difficult. At times the ovary and tube cannot be distinguished separately. Women with pelvic abscesses which do not respond to antibiotics require surgical drainage and this might either be achieved vaginally or abdominally.

Adequate treatment should minimize later problems and it is essential that sexual partners be treated. Failure to do so results in reinfection and this is particularly dangerous since a second infection results in infertility in 20% of cases. A third episode causes tubal occlusion in over 50% of cases. Women with a previous history of PID should undergo early ultrasound assessment in subsequent pregnancies since the risk of ectopic pregnancy is increased 10-fold.

Tubal patency

In women who appear to be ovulating, some form of assessment of tubal patency is required. In many centres laparoscopic hydrotubation is performed. During this procedure a dye is injected through the cervix and the laparoscopist can identify if there is free flow of this dye or evidence of tubal damage. While laparoscopy provides very full information on the pelvic organs, it carries the risks of general anaesthesia as well as those of the procedure itself which include damage to the bowel or bladder and large vessels.

Conventional X-ray hysterosalpingography has become established as a less invasive method of determining tubal patency. Further efforts to reduce the hazards in determining tubal patency have led to the use of ultrasound hydrotubation and ultrasound contrast hysterosalpingography. Mitri *et al.* [42] investigated the role of sonographic hydrotubation in an unselected population being investigated for infertility using between 10 and 20 ml of saline which was injected through the cervix. Saline is echolucent and while it delineates intrauterine pathology clearly, flow within the fallopian tubes is difficult to visualize beyond the proximal portion of the tubes. Reliable and reproducible information on tubal patency is therefore difficult to obtain. The introduction of an echogenic contrast agent Echovist in 1986 opened the way for more detailed and reliable assessment of fallopian tube patency. Since this is an echogenic medium, the presence of flow through each portion of the fallopian tube can be determined. The procedure requires a degree of technical expertise in order to obtain and interpret the views obtained but is well tolerated by most patients. In experienced hands, the detection rate for blocked fallopian tubes using hysterocontrast salpingography (HyCoSy) is around 100% and the concordance value between HyCoSy and other standard techniques such as hysterosalpingogram is around 90% [43,44]. False positive (blocked tubes which are actually patent) and false negative (tubes which appear patent but are not) results do occur but it should be remembered that false positive and false negative results will also occur with standard techniques such as laparoscopy and dye insufflation. HyCoSy is unlikely to ever completely replace hysterosalpingogram and laparoscopy but its introduction raises the possibility of an initial, rapid, outpatient assessment of both tubal and uterine pathology in an infertility clinic setting. Furthermore, well-controlled studies are required before such methods are introduced into routine clinical practice.

Lower genital tract

Vulval carcinoma comprises 4% of all gynaecological malignancies. It is usually a disease of postmenopausal women and with current population trends will be expected to increase in frequency. Pathologically the tumour is usually a squamous carcinoma and like cervical cancer a viral aetiology has been postulated. The diagnosis is based on histological features and the treatment is surgical. Radical or simple vulvectomy is indicated in all but the very unfit.

Vaginal carcinoma is rare and of uncertain aetiology. Intrauterine exposure to diethylstilboestrol, widely used in the 1950s in North America to reduce spontaneous abortion, increased the incidence of vaginal cancer in female offspring. Treatment is generally based on radiotherapy.

Conclusion

Ultrasound is no longer used simply to distinguish a cystic and solid mass within the abdomen and pelvis. With improved image resolution and software, subtle differences in tissue texture can be demarcated and pelvic organs clearly identified. Thus, it has become a significant tool in the diagnosis and management of many gynaecological problems. For the future, we look to the developments of three-dimensional imaging to improve further the definition and relationship of pelvic structures, and power Doppler to investigate the patterns of neovascularization associated with malignancy. In less than 30 years ultrasound has proved its worth and established itself firmly as a vital tool for the gynaecologist in the 21st century.

References

1 Donald, I., MacVicar, J., Brown, T.G. (1958) Investigation of abdominal masses by pulsed ultrasound. *Lancet* **i**, 1188–1195.

2 Fried, A., Oliff, M., Wilson, E. (1978) Uterine anomalies associated with renal agenesis: role of gray scale sonography. *American Journal of Radiology* **131**, 973.

3 Tulppala, M., Palosuo, T., Ramsay, T., Miettinen, A., Salonen, R., Ylikorkala, O. (1993) A prospective study of 63 couples with a history of recurrent spontaneous abortion: Contributing factors and outcome of subsequent pregnancies. *Human Reproduction* **8**, 764–770.

4 Nasri, M.N., Coast, G.J. (1989) Correlation of ultrasound findings and endometrial histopathology in postmenopausal women. *British Journal of Obstetrics and Gynaecology* **96**, 1333–1336.

5 Nasri, M.N., Shephard, J.H., Setchell, M.E., Lowe, D.G., Chard, T. (1991) Sonographic depiction of postmenopausal endometrium with transabdominal and transvaginal scanning. *Ultrasound in Obstetrics and Gynaecology* **1**, 279–283.

6 Karlsson, B., Granberg, S., Wikland, M., *et al.* (1995) Transvaginal ultrasonography of the endometrium in women with post-menopausal bleeding—a Nordic multicenter study. *American Journal of Obstetrics and Gynaecology* **172**, 1488–1494.

7 Dorum, A., Kristensen, B., Langebrekke, A., Sornes, T., Skaar, O. (1993) Evaluation of endometrial thickness measured by endovaginal ultrasound in women with post-menopausal bleeding. *Acta Obstetrica et Gynaecologica Scandinavica* **72**, 116–119.

8 Fischer, B., Costantino, J.P., Fisher, E.R., Wickerham, D.L., Cronin, W.M. (1994) Endometrial cancer in tamoxifen treated breast cancer patients: findings from the national surgical adjuvant breast and bowel project. *Journal of the National Cancer Institute* **86**, 527–537.

9 Kedar, R.P., Bourne, T.H., Powles, T.J., *et al.* (1994) Effects of tamoxifen on the uterus and ovaries of post-menopausal women in a randomised breast cancer prevention trial. *Lancet* **343**, 1318–1321.

10 Achiron, R., Lipitz, S., Sivan, M., *et al.* (1995) Changes mimicking endometrial neoplasia in postmenopausal, tamoxifen treated women with breast cancer: a transvaginal Doppler study. *Ultrasound in Obstetrics and Gynaecology* **6**, 116–120.

11 West, C.P. (1992) Uterine fibroids. In: Shaw, R., Soutter, P., Stanton, S. (eds) *Gynaecology*. Churchill Livingstone, London, pp. 397–412.

12 Bischof, P., Galfetti, M.A., Seydoux, J., Von Hospenthal, J.U., Campana, A. (1992) Peripheral CA 125 levels in patients with uterine fibroids. *Human Reproduction* **7**, 35–38.

13 FIGO (1990) Changes in gynecologic cancer staging by the International Federation of Gynecology and Obstetrics. *American Journal of Obstetrics and Gynecology* **162**, 610–611.

14 Kurjak, A., Shalan, H., Sosic, A., *et al.* (1993) Endometrial carcinoma in post-menopausal women: evaluation by transvaginal colour Doppler ultrasonography. *American Journal of Obstetrics and Gynaecology* **169**, 1597–1603.

15 Merce, L.T., Garcia, L., De La Fuente, F. (1991) Doppler ultrasound assessment of endometrial pathology. *American Journal of Obstetrics and Gynaecology* **70**, 525–530.

16 Hata, K., Hata, T., Manabe, A., Makihara, K., Kitao, M. (1992) Transvaginal Doppler ultrasound assessment of intratumoral haemodynamic change before and during hypertensive intra-arterial chemotherapy for uterine cancer. *Obstetrics and Gynaecology* **80**, 801–804.

17 Fox, R., Hull, M. (1993) Ultrasound diagnosis of polycystic ovaries. *Annals of the New York Academy of Science* **687**, 217–223.

18 Clayton, R.N., Ogden, V., Hodgkinson, J., *et al.* (1992) How common are polycystic ovaries in normal women and what is their significance for the fertility of the population? *Clinical Endocrinology* **37**, 127–134.

19 Polson, D.W., Adams, J., Wadsworth, J., Franks, S. (1988) Polycystic ovaries—a common finding in normal women. *Lancet* **i**, 870–872.

20 Whittemore, A.S., Harris, R., Intyre, J. (1992) Characteristics relating to ovarian cancer risk collaborative analysis of 12 US

case–control studies. II. Invasive epithelial ovarian cancers in white women. *American Journal of Epidemiology* **136**, 1184–1203.

21 Levine, D., Gosnik, B.B., Wolf, S.I., Feldesman, M.R., Pretorius, D.H. (1992) Simple adnexal cyst: the natural history in post-menopausal women. *Radiology* **184**, 653–659.

22 Caspi, B., Zalel, Y., Lurie, S., Elchlal, U., Katz, Z. (1993) Ultrasound-guided aspiration for relief of pain generated by simple ovarian cysts. *Gynaecology and Obstetrics Investigations* **35**, 121–122.

23 Konje, J.C., Speck, E.H., Chorlton, I. (1992) False negative ultrasound and aspiration cytology in a case of primary papillary serous cystadenocarcinoma of the ovary complicating pregnancy. *Journal of Obstetrics and Gynaecology* **12**, 245–246.

24 Wojcik, E.M., Selvaggi, S.M. (1994) Fine needle aspiration cytology of cystic ovarian lesions. *Diagnostic Cytopathology* **11**, 9–14.

25 Campbell, S., Goessens, L., Goswamy, R., Whitehead, M.I. (1982) Real time ultrasonography for the determination of ovarian morphology and volume. A possible early screening test for ovarian cancer. *Lancet* **i**, 425–426.

26 Campbell, S., Bham, V., Royston, P., Whitehead, M., Collins, W.P. (1989) Transabdominal screening for early ovarian cancer. *British Medical Journal* **299**, 1363–1367.

27 Lerner, J.P., Timor-Tritsch, I.E., Federman, A., Abramovich, G. (1994) Transvaginal ultrasonographic characteristics of ovarian masses with an improved weighted scoring system. *American Journal of Obstetrics and Gynaecology* **170**, 81–85.

28 Fleischer, A.C., Rodgers, W.H., Kepple, D.M., Williams, L.L., Jones, H.W. (1993) Color Doppler sonography of ovarian masses: a multiparameter analysis. *Journal of Ultrasound in Medicine* **12**, 41–48.

29 Kurjak, A., Schulman, H., Socisc, A., Zalud, I., Shalan, H. (1992) Transvaginal ultrasound, color flow and Doppler waveform of the post-menopausal adnexal mass. *Obstetrics and Gynaecology* **80**, 917–921.

30 Kramer, B.S., Gohagan, J., Prorok, P.C., Smart, C. (1993) A National Cancer Institute sponsored screening trial for prostatic, lung, colorectal, and ovarian cancers. *Cancer* **71**, 589–593.

31 (1996) *Report on Confidential Enquiries into Maternal Deaths in the United Kingdom 1991–1993*. HMSO, London, pp. 68–73.

32 Cohen, J. (1989) Outcome of IVF pregnancies in Europe. XIII World Congress on Fertility and Sterility, Marrakesh.

33 Funderburk, A.G. (1976) Bilateral ectopic pregnancy with simultaneous intra-uterine pregnancy. *American Journal of Obstetrics and Gynaecology* **119**, 274–275.

34 Pennell, R.G., Baltarowich, O.H., Kurtz, A.B., *et al.* (1987) Complicated first trimester pregnancies: evaluation with endovaginal US versus transabdominal technique. *Radiology* **165**, 79–83.

35 Bree, R.L., Edwards, M., Bohm-Velez, M., Beyler, S., Roberts, J., Mendelson, E.B. (1989) Transvaginal sonography in the evaluation of normal early pregnancy: correlation with HCG level. *American Journal of Roentgenology* **153**, 75–79.

36 Bernaschek, G., Rudelstorfer, R., Csaicsich, P. (1988) Vaginal sonography versus serum human chorionic gonadotrophin in early detection of pregnancy. *American Journal of Obstetrics and Gynaecology* **158**, 608–612.

37 Timor-Tritsch, I.E., Yeh, M.N., Peisner, D.B., Lesser, K.B., Slavik, T.A. (1989) The use of transvaginal ultrasonography in the diagnosis of ectopic pregnancy. *American Journal of Obstetrics and Gynaecology* **161**, 157–161.

38 Burry, K.A., Thurmond, A.S., Suby-Long, T.D., *et al.* (1993) Transvaginal ultrasonographic findings in surgically verified ectopic pregnancy. *American Journal of Obstetrics and Gynaecology* **168**, 1796–1802.

39 Timor-Tritsch, I. (1994) Transvaginal ultrasonographic findings in surgically verified ectopic pregnancy. *American Journal of Obstetrics and Gynaecology* **170**, 1205–1206 (letter).

40 Cacciatore, B., Leminen, A., Ingman Friberg, S., Ylostalo, P., Paavonen, J. (1992) Transvaginal sonographic findings in ambulatory patients with suspected pelvic inflammatory disease. *Obstetrics and Gynaecology* **80**, 912–916.

41 Patten, R.M., Vincent, L.M., WolnerHanssen, P., Thorpe Jr., E. (1990) Pelvic inflammatory disease: endovaginal sonography with laparoscopic correlation. *Journal of Ultrasound in Medicine* **9**, 681–689.

42 Mitri, F.F., Andronikou, A.D., Perpinyal, S., Hofmyer, G.J., Sonnendecker, E.W.W. (1991) A clinical comparison of sonographic hydrotubation and hysterosalpingography. *British Journal of Obstetrics and Gynaecology* **98**, 1031–1036.

43 Schlief, R., Deichert U. (1991) Hysterosalpingo-contrast sonography of the uterus and fallopian tubes: results of a clinical trial of a new contrast medium in 120 patients. *Radiology* **178**, 213–215.

44 Campbell, S., Bourne, T.H., Lan, S.L., Collins, W.P. (1994) Hysterosalpingo- contrast sonography (HyCoSy) and its future role within the investigation of infertility in Europe. *Ultrasound in Obstetrics and Gynaecology* **4**, 245–263.

Part 7
Obstetrics

Chapter 34: Introduction

J.R. MacKenzie

Historical background

The initial pioneering work in obstetric ultrasound was carried out by the late Professor Ian Donald and colleagues at the Glasgow Royal Maternity Hospital in the late 1950s and early 1960s. He continued with this work when he moved to the Queen Mother's Hospital in 1964. Initially many people were sceptical about the value and potential of ultrasound but time has proved them to be wrong.

There have been several major technological developments in ultrasound since the 1960s. A-scanning was initially used to measure fetal biparietal diameters and the subsequent development of B-scanning enabled the study of fetal growth to be undertaken. Its value in early pregnancy and in placental localization was realized and its ability to detect the fetal heart was appreciated. The initial pictures were entirely black and white and much valuable information was lost (Fig. 34.1). With the development of grey-scale ultrasound in the late 1970s it proved possible to identify intracranial and intra-abdominal anatomy. Real-time scanning was developed in the early 1980s and enabled fetal movement to be demonstrated. It also allowed scanning to be carried out more rapidly and more easily. In recent years the development of more sophisticated transducers has resulted in better resolution. Further improvements have been achieved with the development of pre- and postprocessing computer programs. Several companies are investigating the possibility of three-dimensional scanning. The more recent developments of duplex Doppler and colour flow Doppler systems have enabled fetal, placental and umbilical cord blood flows to be determined.

Recent years have also seen the publication of several large detailed texts on obstetric ultrasound and ultrasound of fetal abnormalities. This section aims to give a short overview of current obstetric ultrasound practice and hopefully to encourage the would be obstetric ultrasonographer to read or at least to dip into these larger texts (see further reading).

Ultrasound safety

For many years diagnostic ultrasound has been thought to be completely safe. However, many of the more sophisticated systems now use ultrasound power of increasing intensity and these levels are veering towards the output used in therapeutic ultrasound. There have been some reports of possible hazards in the literature in 1993, namely, an increased incidence of left-handedness together with a higher incidence of fetal growth retardation. Although these reports need to be verified they cannot be completely ignored and it is sensible only to use obstetric ultrasound for good clinical indications and to ensure that the power output utilized is the minimum required to produce acceptable diagnostic images.

Current controversies

For many years there has been an ongoing battle over who should carry out obstetric scans—obstetricians, radiologists, midwives or radiographers.

In reality it should not matter who carries out the scan provided the operators have received thorough training and are conversant with the ranges of normality and abnormality. If the scans are being carried out by non-medical personnel then adequate supervision by competent interested obstetricians or radiologists is essential.

People present during scanning

In recent years there has been a move towards allowing partners, relatives or friends to be present during obstetric scans. This can be distracting to the ultrasonographer and difficulties can arise if an abnormality is detected. In some instances it may be preferable to carry out the scan, determine that everything is satisfactory and then invite the partner to see the scan together with the 'patient'. The decision about whether other people are in the room during a scan must rest with the ultrasonographer.

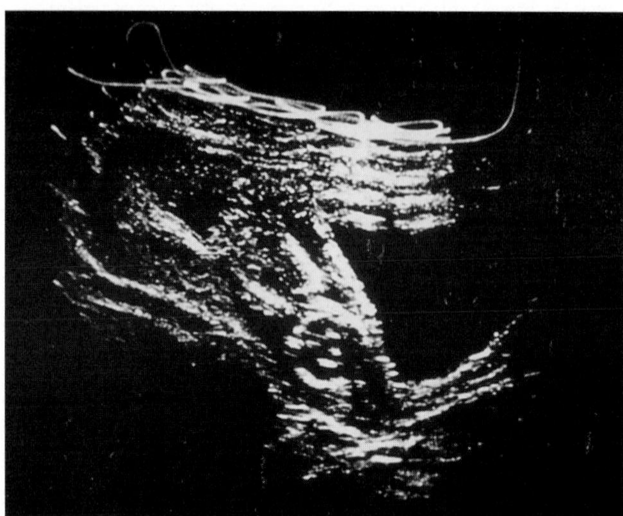

Fig. 34.1 B-scan of a 16–17-week fetus prior to the development of grey-scale ultrasound. The fetal head lies just above the cervix and the placenta is posterior.

The patient

Most pregnant women in the UK will have at least one ultrasound examination some time during their pregnancy. The exact timing and the reason for the scan will vary from place to place. A strong case can be made for carrying out a gestation assessment scan at the time of initial booking, a fetal anomaly scan at 18–20 weeks and a scan to assess fetal growth about 28–32 weeks. In many centres this is impossible, however, due to inadequate facilities and in these centres a protocol must be drawn up in consultation with the obstetricians listing the indications for obstetric scanning. In some hospitals the number of patients with no idea of their own dates will be found to be extremely high, and a gestational scan may well be routinely performed with other scanning only being carried out in high risk groups. In other hospitals the majority of patients may well know what their dates are and in this situation a detailed fetal anomaly scan, which also confirms dates, may be the only scan performed. It must always be borne in mind that some patients will refuse to have an obstetric scan or, whilst accepting a gestational assessment scan, may be unwilling to have a fetal anomaly scan on religious or ethical grounds.

Patient preparation

The decision as to whether the patient changes into a gown or is scanned in her own clothes should depend on the preference of the ultrasonographer and the patient. In first trimester scanning it is relatively easy to protect the patient's clothing from the acoustic gel but later on, with increasing abdominal girth, it may be considerably more pleasant for the patient to wear only her underwear and a hospital gown. Her pants can then be protected by a sheet which also covers her legs. The patient must remove her pants if she is having a vaginal scan.

If the patient is having an abdominal scan during the first or second trimester, or is being examined later for a possible placenta previa, she must have a full bladder at the commencement of the scan. Ideally she should be asked to drink about 2 pints of fluid, 30 min to 1 h before the scan. She should feel the need to micturate at the time the scan is performed but should not be absolutely desperate. An overfull bladder leads to a restless patient and may compress the uterus in very early pregnancy resulting in a misdiagnosis. In such circumstances the woman should be asked to partially empty her bladder and this can be achieved by pulling up the perineal muscles when a small amount of urine has been passed. If her bladder is inadequately full it may be impossible to identify the uterine fundus in first trimester scanning or to see the lower part of the spine if the baby is breech at the time of a detailed scan. If the patient is having a transvaginal scan she should be asked to empty her bladder completely prior to the commencement of the scan.

During an abdominal scan the patient should lie on a couch with her head slightly elevated. The ultrasonographer should face the patient. The technique used by some people where the ultrasonographer faces the patient's feet can cause confusion as to cranial and caudal, right and left and vaginal scanning becomes impossible. The argument that scanning in such a manner allows the patient to see the screen is unacceptable as most modern machines have monitors which can rotate as required. Some people prefer to scan without the patient or partner seeing the monitor until the ultrasonographer is happy that everything is satisfactory. At this point the monitor can be rotated and the patient and her partner can be shown the baby.

In the last trimester care must be taken to ensure that the patient does not become hypotensive in the supine position. The patient should be watched for any sign of restlessness or pallor and if this occurs or if she complains of feeling faint or sick she should be asked to roll over onto her left side when the feeling will rapidly disappear. It may be possible to conclude the examination with the patient in this position.

Ideally a vaginal scan should be carried out on a gynaecological couch where the patient's legs can be supported by stirrups. If such a facility is not available then the patient should lie with her bottom at the edge of the table resting her feet on two chairs placed at the end of the table. It is important to remember that this examination may cause embarrassment to the patient and steps should be taken to ensure that no one enters the room during the procedure.

It is helpful to explain to the patient precisely what one is going to do and to let them know that they will have an opportunity of seeing the baby themselves. It is beneficial to give the patient a picture of the baby to take away. However, care must be taken in explaining exactly what the picture shows.

Scanning technique

Abdominal or vaginal scanning

Vaginal scanning is of greater value than abdominal scanning in the first few weeks of pregnancy. The tip of the probe is in closer proximity to the uterus than with abdominal scanning, and detail is accordingly improved. This is particularly helpful if the uterus is retroverted or the patient is obese. However, the patient may be unwilling to have such a scan.

Selection of probe

A sector transducer with a small head is ideal in early pregnancy but a linear array transducer or curvilinear

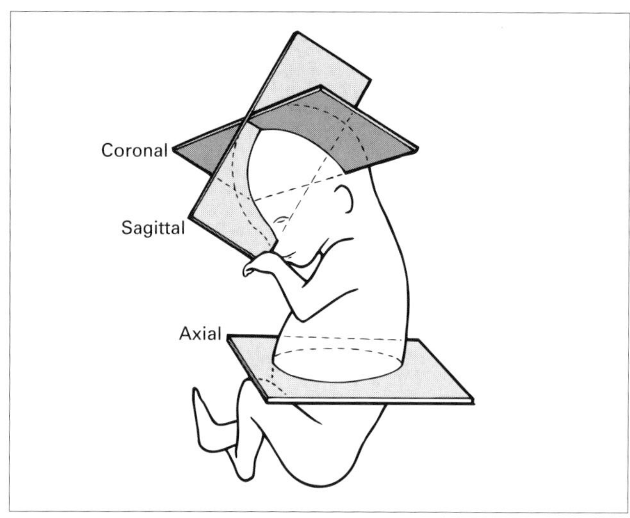

Fig. 34.3 The three scanning planes: coronal, sagittal and axial.

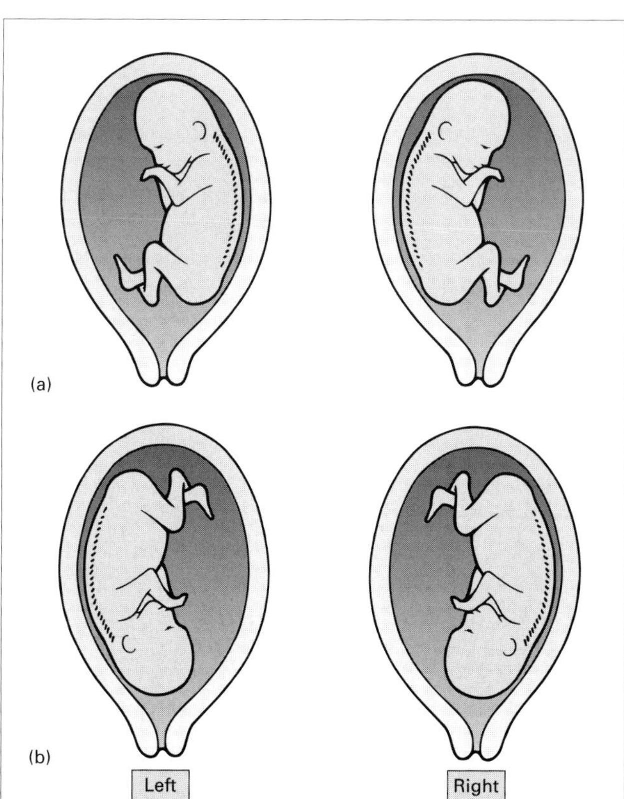

Fig. 34.2 Fetal lie: (a) breech and (b) cephalic showing right and left sides.

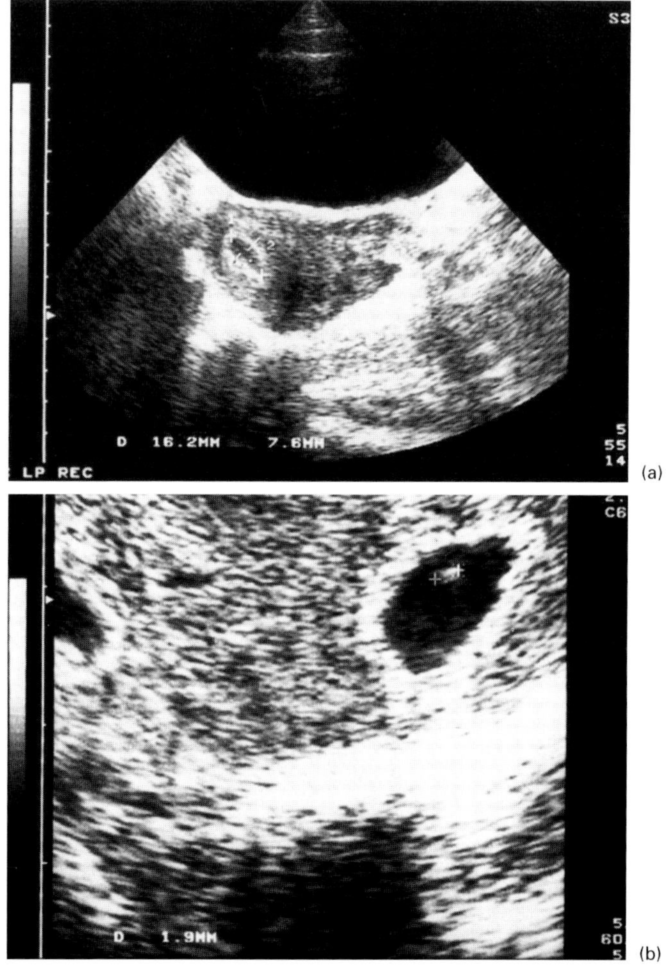

Fig. 34.4 (a) An abdominal scan at 5–6 weeks gestation showing the gestation sac (diameter marked with numbers 1 and 2) but no fetal pole. (b) A vaginal scan immediately afterwards demonstrating the fetal pole (1.9 mm).

transducer is preferable in the third trimester. Many people use a sector scanner for fetal anomaly work. A 7.5 or 5 MHz vaginal probe is preferable in the first trimester, a 5 MHz probe is commonly used for anomaly scanning but in the third trimester or in the obese patient, a 3.5 MHz probe is needed to ensure adequate penetration and detail.

Abdominal scanning

A rapid mid line longitudinal scan is performed initially and the probe is then moved to each side performing a parasagittal scan. The probe is rotated through 90° and three or four rapid transverse scans are performed. During this period the position of the fetal head, body and

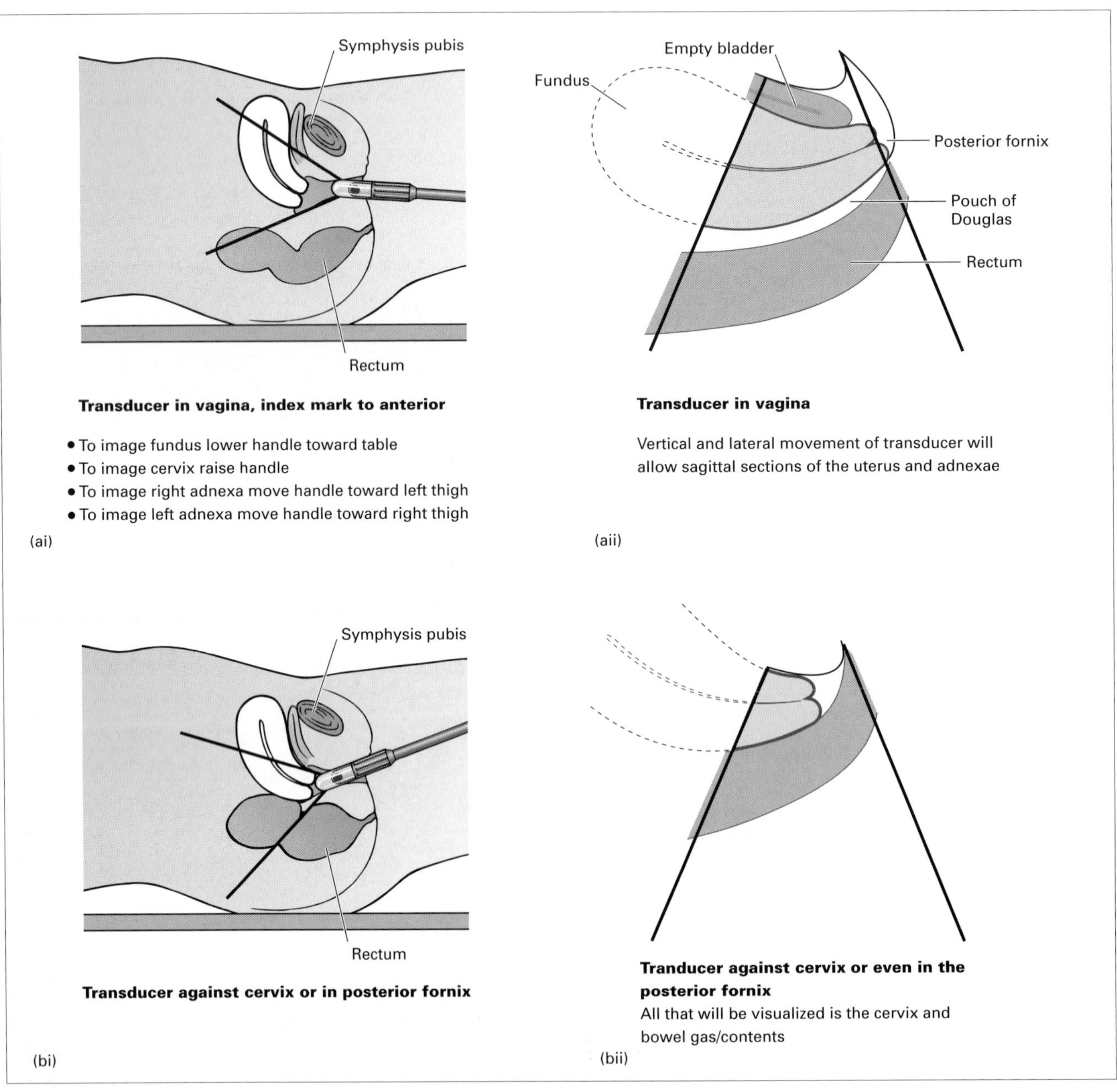

Fig. 34.5 Transvaginal ultrasound. (a) Normal anteverted uterus: (i) scan plane; (ii) sagittal image. (b) Transducer inserted too far: (i) scan plane; (ii) sagittal image. (c) Retroverted uterus: (i) scan plane; (ii) sagittal image. (d) Transverse plane: (i) scan plane; (ii) transverse image. (Courtesy of J. Macaulay, Glasgow Royal Maternity Hospital.)

limbs is assessed and the probe is then rotated so that a scan is performed through the long axis of the fetus. The appropriate measurements and, if indicated, the fetal anatomy can then be assessed. It is important that the parasagittal scans should extend out as far as the side walls of the pelvis and maternal abdomen so that adnexal masses can be excluded. The transverse scans should extend up to the uterine fundus and down to the bladder, again excluding adnexal pathology.

The lie of the fetus should be determined, i.e. cephalic, breech, transverse, oblique and the right and left sides of the fetus should be identified (Fig. 34.2). Further examination of the fetus can then be performed by scanning in the sagittal, coronal and axial planes (Fig. 34.3). The inexperienced ultrasonographer may find it helpful to use the pelvic bones of a skeleton and a doll to build up a three-dimensional image of the position of a fetus in the uterus.

Vaginal scanning

This technique is being used more frequently during the

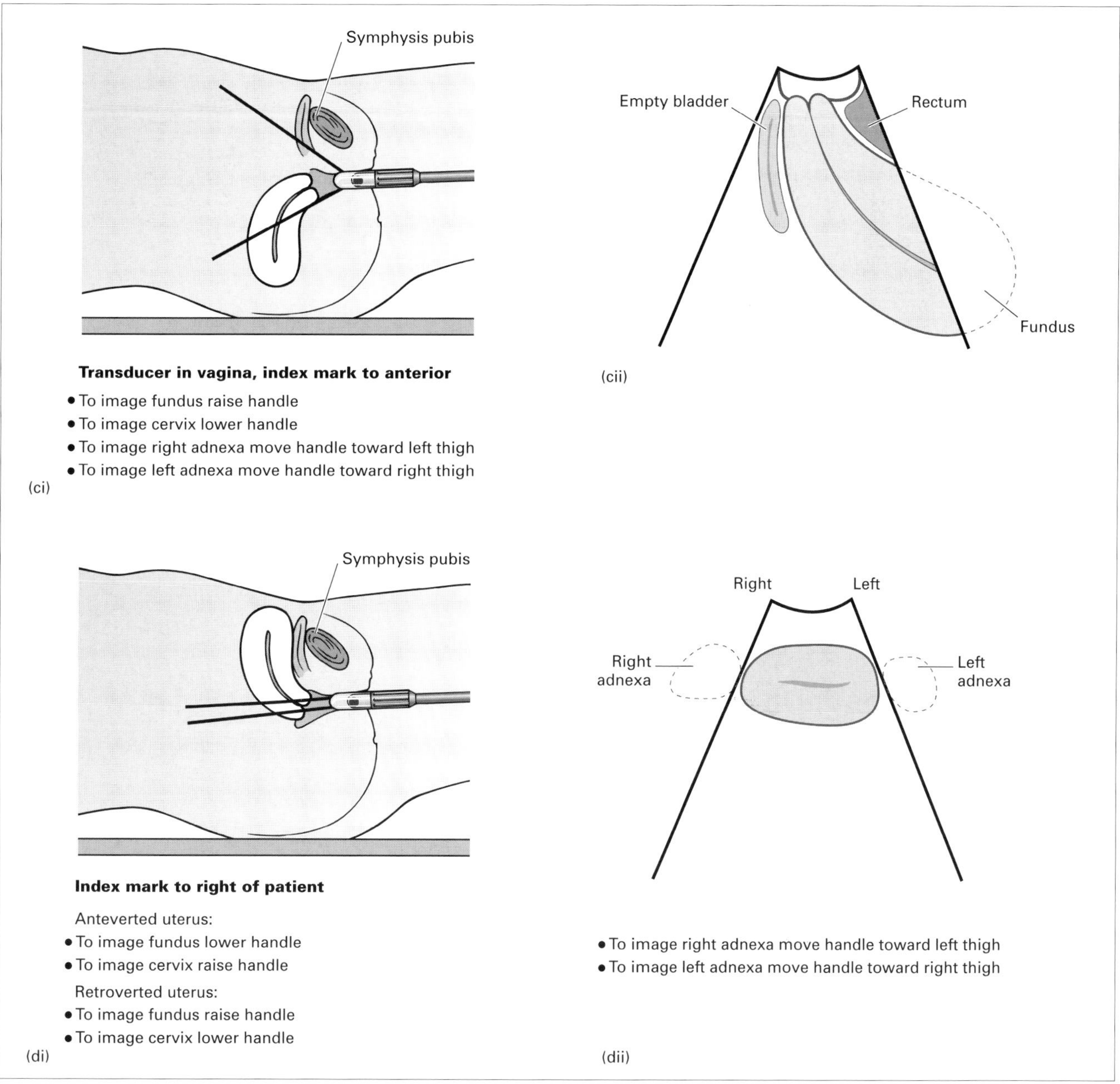
Symphysis pubis
Transducer in vagina, index mark to anterior
• To image fundus raise handle
• To image cervix lower handle
• To image right adnexa move handle toward left thigh
• To image left adnexa move handle toward right thigh
(ci)
Empty bladder
Rectum
Fundus
(cii)
Symphysis pubis
Index mark to right of patient
Anteverted uterus:
• To image fundus lower handle
• To image cervix raise handle
Retroverted uterus:
• To image fundus raise handle
• To image cervix lower handle
(di)
Right
Left
Right adnexa
Left adnexa
• To image right adnexa move handle toward left thigh
• To image left adnexa move handle toward right thigh
(dii)

Fig. 34.5 *Continued.*

first trimester. The ultrasound probe is situated closer to the developing embryo and enables a superior image to be obtained much earlier than on an abdominal scan (Fig. 34.4).

Most manufacturers provide details regarding cleaning and sterilization of vaginal probes and these instructions must be followed. Prior to scanning coupling gel is applied to the functional end of the probe and it is then covered by a condom. The application of gel to the covered transducer is not normally necessary. The patient's labia should be gently separated and the probe introduced into the vagina in such a position that a true sagittal section is obtained. Care must be taken not to insert the probe too far into the vaginal vault as this will significantly reduce the field of view. Orientation may be extremely difficult during the learning phase of the technique but with practice satisfactory images of the uterus and adnexal regions can be obtained by sliding the probe up and down the vagina, rotating the probe through 90° and angling the probe in a vertical or horizontal manner (Fig. 34.5). The uterus, ovaries, pouch of Douglas and internal iliac vessels can be identified early in the pregnancy.

Further reading

Chervenak, F.A., Isaacson, G.C., Campbell, S. (1993) *Ultrasound in Obstetrics and Gynaecology*. Little, Brown, Boston.

Chudleigh, P., Pearce, J.M. (1992) *Obstetric Ultrasound*. Churchill Livingstone, Edinburgh.

Dewbury, K., Meire, H., Cosgrove, D. (1993) *Ultrasound in Obstetrics and Gynaecology*. Churchill Livingstone, Edinburgh.

Harrington, K., Campbell, S. (1995) *A Colour Atlas of Doppler Ultrasonography in Obstetrics*. Edward Arnold, London.

Neilson, J.P., Chambers, S.E. (1993) *Obstetric Ultrasound*. Oxford Medical Publications, Oxford.

Nyberg, D.A., Mahony, B.S., Pretorius, D.H. (1990) *Diagnostic Ultrasound of Fetal Anomalies; Test and Atlas*. Year Book Medical Publishers, Chicago.

Whittle, M.J., Connor, J.M. (1989) *Prenatal Diagnosis in Obstetric Practice*. Blackwell Scientific Publications, Oxford.

Chapter 35: Fetal biometry

J.R. MacKenzie

Fetal measurements are usually carried out to assess gestation and fetal growth. Satisfactory assessment of the latter is dependent on the accurate knowledge of the former.

Gestational age assessment

The expected date of delivery (EDD) is calculated from the first day of the last menstrual period (LMP). This will be unreliable if the mother has 'got her dates wrong' or has no idea of her LMP. It is also dependent on a regular menstrual cycle of 28 days duration and may be affected by the recent cessation of the oral contraceptive pill. A short atypical period may also cause confusion.

In some centres a scan is carried out between 16 and 18 weeks to confirm the fetal gestation and to look for fetal abnormalities. However, in other maternity hospitals the incidence of wrong dates may be so high that it is sensible to carry out a gestation scan at the patient's booking visit. Several measurements can be carried out to assess gestation, some being more useful than others.

1 Gestation sac volume.
2 Crown—rump length (CRL).
3 Biparietal diameter (BPD).
4 Head circumference (HC).
5 Femoral length (FL).
6 Abdominal circumference (AC).
7 Thoracic circumference.

Gestation sac volume

The gestational sac can normally be identified at 3–4 menstrual weeks on transvaginal scanning and at 5 menstrual weeks on abdominal scanning. Tables are available which relate gestation sac volume to gestational age. In practical terms the measurement is of little value other than to demonstrate the presence of an intrauterine pregnancy. A fetal pole should always be visible in a sac that measures more than 2.5 cm^3 and if one is not seen a diagnosis of an anembryonic pregnancy is made (Fig. 35.1).

CRL

A fetal pole can be seen as early as 5 weeks transvaginally and from 6 to 7 weeks transabdominally. The CRL measurement is made from the tip of the crown to the tip of the rump (Fig. 35.2). Care should be taken not to include the lower limbs or a yolk sac in the measurement. With increasing age the fetus tends to flex and the assessment of CRL on a flexed fetus will be slightly inaccurate.

Longitudinal and transverse scans are obtained and the lie of the fetus is determined. A longitudinal view of a stretched fetus can then be obtained. The measurement is accurate to within ± 5–7 days. The accuracy falls off around 11 and 12 weeks due to increasing flexion of the fetus and after this gestation the BPD should preferably be obtained (Fig. 35.3).

A rough estimate of the gestation can be made by adding 6.5 to the CRL in cm, e.g. CRL 2.0 cm ≡ 8.5 weeks gestation, CRL 5.0 cm ≡ 11.5 weeks gestation.

BPD

This measurement is performed on a transverse or axial section of the head at the level of the thalami. Conventionally the measurement is made from the outer table of the near parietal bone to the inner table of the far parietal bone. The correct axial section is obtained by determining the fetal lie and obtaining a longitudinal section of the head and spine. The probe is then rotated through 90° to produce an axial section and is slid cranially and caudally until a section containing an anterior mid line echo, a mid line cavum septum pellucidum, a triangular area of reduced echoes pointing posteriorly due to the thalami and an area of increased echoes, posterior to this, due to the subarachnoid basal cisterns, is obtained (Fig. 35.4). If the axial view is too high there will be a continuous mid line echo from the anterior to the posterior part of the vault (Fig. 35.5). If the plane is too low a view of the orbits and nose will be obtained (Fig. 35.6).

In some instances the position of the fetus may make it impossible to obtain a true BPD. This can occur if the fetal

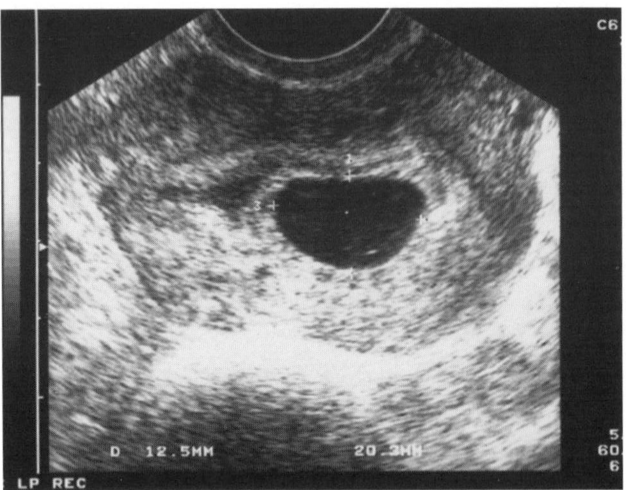

Fig. 35.1 Anembryonic pregnancy. There is a large gestation sac measuring 12.5 by 20.3 mm with no evidence of a fetal pole. The low echogenic area on the right represents a haemorrhage.

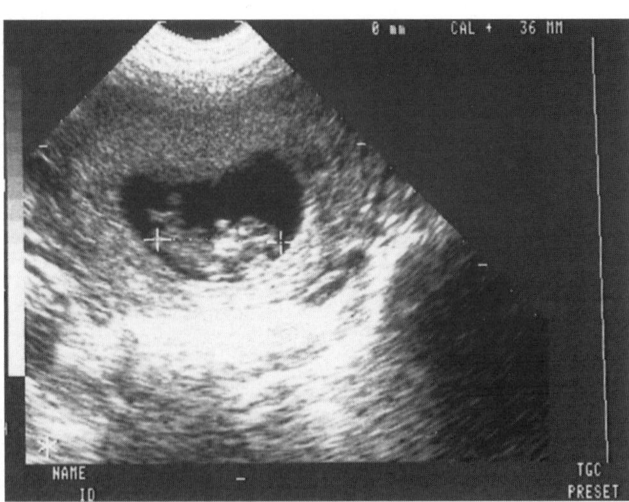

Fig. 35.3 Estimation of CRL in a 'flexed' fetus.

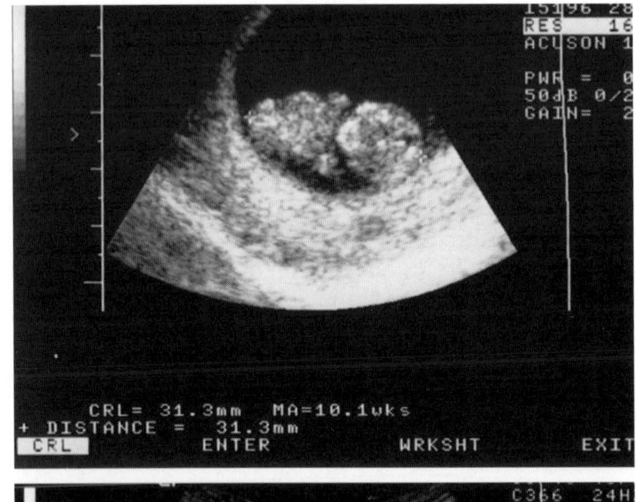

(a)

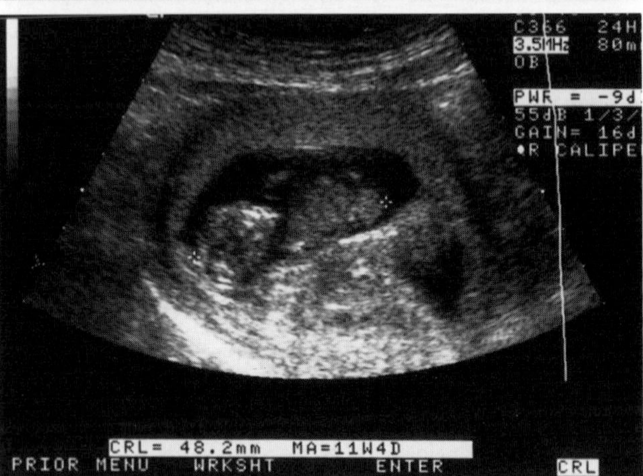

(b)

Fig. 35.2 (a) CRL using a vaginal probe. (b) CRL using an abdominal probe.

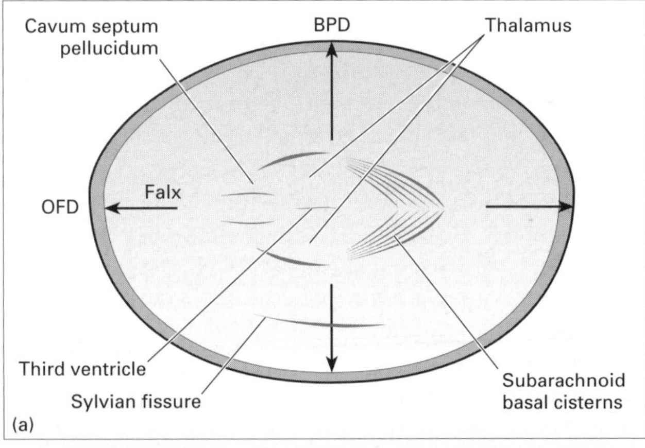

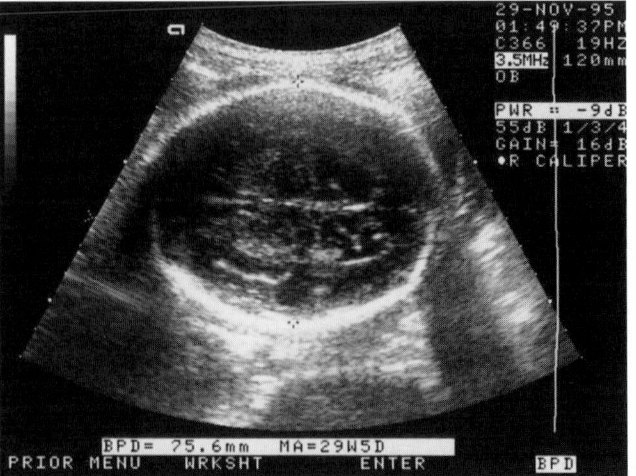

(b)

Fig. 35.4 Plane for measuring BPD: (a) diagram of intracranial anatomy, and (b) scan. BPD, biparietal diameter; OFD, occipitofrontal diameter.

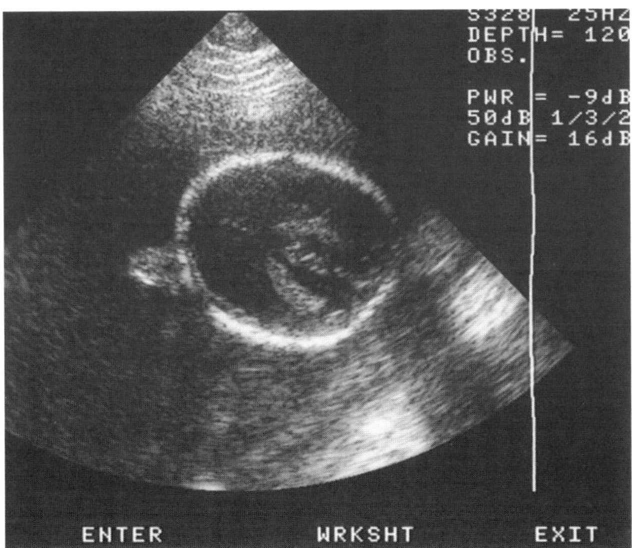

Fig. 35.5 Axial scan showing continuous mid line echo and prominent echogenic choroid plexuses. The plane is too high for BPD estimation.

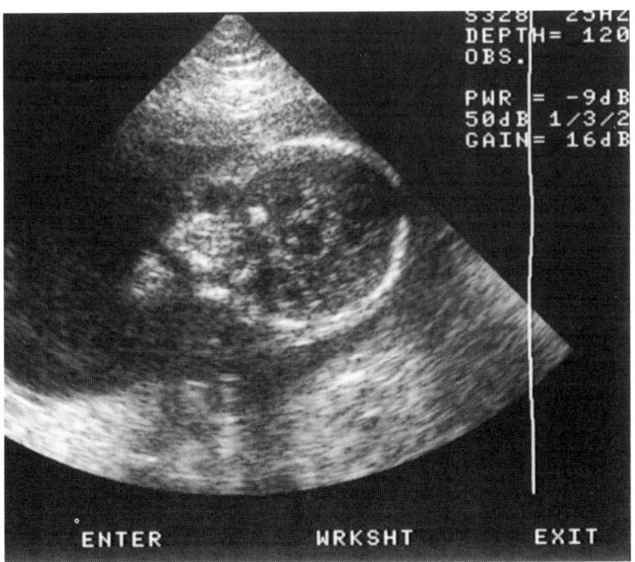

Fig. 35.6 Axial scan showing orbits and nose on right. The plane is too low for BPD estimation.

head is lying deep in the pelvis. It may be helped by filling the patient's bladder further or by tilting the woman head-down. It is also impossible to obtain the correct measurement in a fetus that is lying occipitoanterior or occipitoposterior. Again filling the bladder may be helpful but in some situations it may be simpler to rescan in a week's time.

The accuracy of the BPD varies with gestation and with the shape of the vault. The gestation will be underestimated if the head is doliocephalic or overestimated if it is brachiocephalic (Fig. 35.7). The cephalic index which is a measurement of the BPD divided by the occipitofrontal diameter ×100 should always be assessed. The index should lie between 75 and 85. An index below 75 indicates doliocephaly and above 85 brachiocephaly. In such cases the gestation will be more accurately assessed by the measurement of the HC using the same axial plane as the BPD estimation.

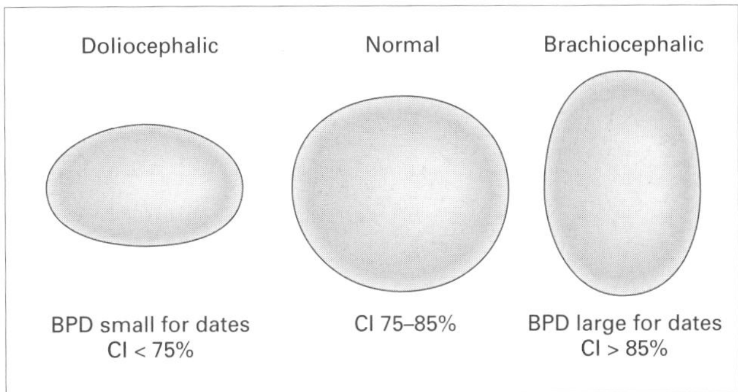

Fig. 35.7 Head shape and effect on biparietal diameter (BPD) and cephalic index (CI).

Up to 24 weeks gestation the BPD is accurate to within ± 5–7 days of positively known dates. Thereafter its accuracy becomes much less and by the third trimester can vary by up to ±3 weeks.

It is unhelpful, or even misleading, to attempt to assess gestation later in the pregnancy. In early pregnancy the fetus grows extremely rapidly and there is a significant difference in the measurements obtained week by week. However, during the last trimester growth slows significantly and the measurements only vary minimally from week to week leading to significant errors if an assessment of gestation is attempted.

HC

This measurement is assessed on the same axial section of the head as the BPD. The circumference can be measured using an ellipse (Fig. 35.8). Cursors are placed on the outer tables of the vault in the parietal areas and the ellipse is gradually increased in size until it encompasses the whole of the section through the vault. Alternatively, a series of dots can be drawn around the outer table of the vault using a joystick, a roller ball or a light pen.

If neither of these facilities is available the HC can be calculated from the BPD and the occipitofrontal diameter, HC = 1.62 (BPD + OFD).

The HC is more accurate than the BPD in assessing gestation if the fetal head is doliocephalic or brachiocephalic. The measurement is also of value in the assessment of fetal

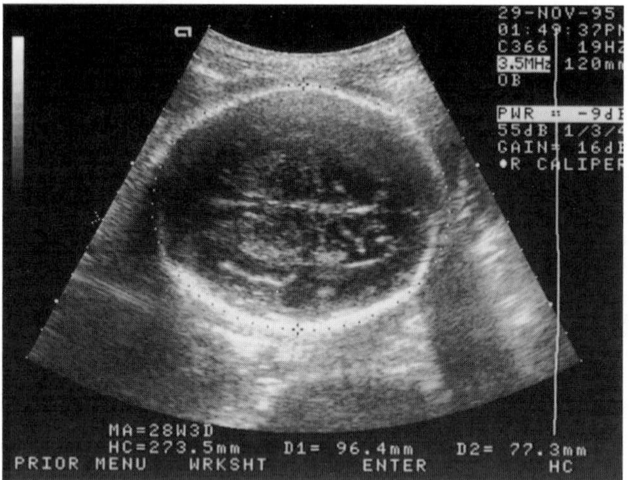

Fig. 35.8 Head circumference = 273.5 mm. Menstrual age, 28 weeks 3 days.

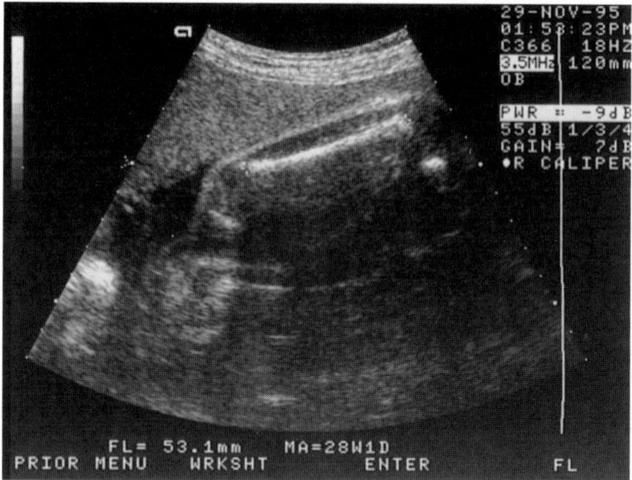

Fig. 35.9 Femoral length = 53.1 mm. Menstrual age, 28 weeks 1 day.

growth and can be used in assessing the presence of microcephaly or hydrocephaly. It is inaccurate in determining gestation in late pregnancy.

FL

This measurement is obtained by measuring the length of the ossified shaft of the femur. It should not include the measurement of the epiphyseal cartilages. It is of value in assessing the gestational age and is as accurate as the BPD. It can also be used in the subsequent assessment of fetal growth. It is particularly useful in the fetus where measurement of the BPD has proved impossible.

The best technique for obtaining this measurement is to scan the fetus transversely, sliding the probe caudally until a section of the femur is obtained. The probe can then be rotated until the maximum length of the femoral shaft is visible (Fig. 35.9). Care must be taken to ensure that the bone is not foreshortened or that a specular echo from the edge of the bone is not included.

AC

Although this measurement can be helpful in assessing gestational age its principal value is in growth assessment. The AC is measured through the liver at the level where the umbilical vein lies a third of the way along a line joining the anterior wall of the abdomen to the spine and is equidistant from the sides of the abdomen. The section is at right angles to the spine and frequently contains the stomach (Fig. 35.10). The circumference may be assessed using an ellipse or by drawing around the outer margin of the abdomen with a joystick, roller ball or light pen. If this facility is not available the circumference can be obtained

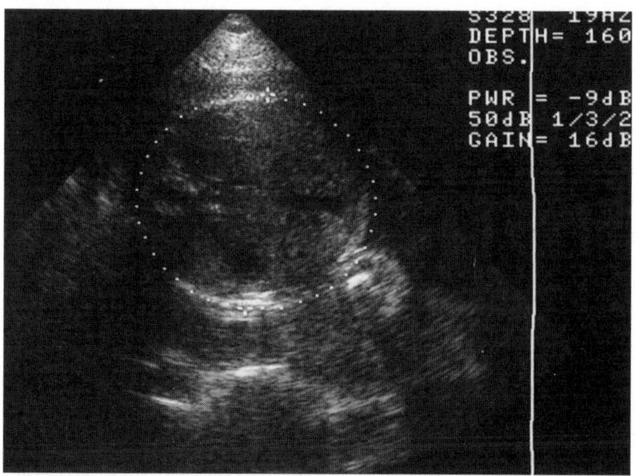

Fig. 35.10 Abdominal circumference = 235.6 mm. Menstrual age, 27 weeks 5 days.

from the transverse diameter (TAD) and anteroposterior diameter (APAD), AC = 3.14 (TAD/2 + APAD/2).

The correct section is obtained by scanning the fetus longitudinally and then rotating the probe through 90° at about the level of the heart. A four-chamber view of the heart is obtained and the probe is slid slowly in a caudal direction from this point. Ideally the outline of the abdomen should be circular. If it proves impossible to image the left portal vein then a section containing the fetal stomach is satisfactory. If the umbilical vein is seen throughout its length the section is oblique and the probe should be angled slightly until a true cross-sectional view is obtained particularly of the spine. The measurement becomes more difficult in the last trimester as the section may no longer be circular and may not fit entirely within the ultrasound screen.

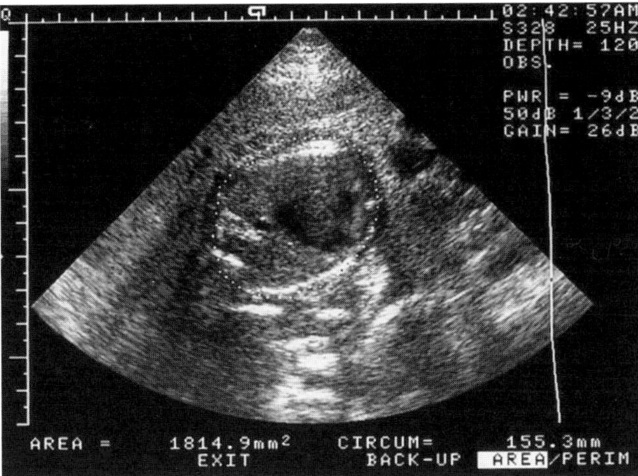

Fig. 35.11 Thoracic circumference in a fetus with pulmonary hypoplasia secondary to renal agenesis.

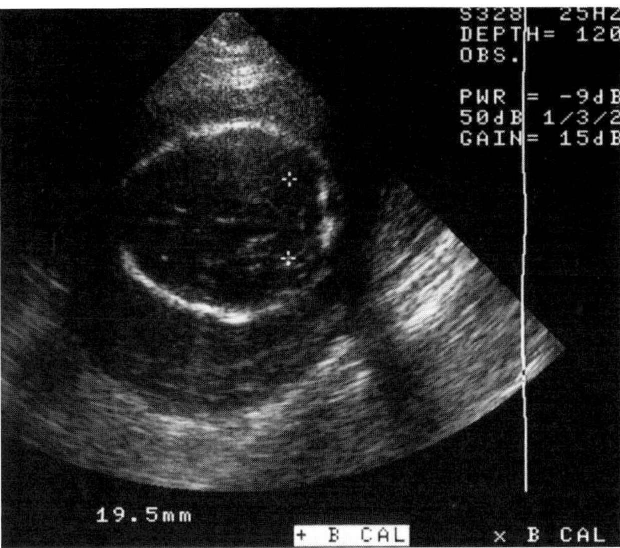

Fig. 35.12 Measurement of cerebellum. Distance = 19.5 mm which is equivalent to a gestation of 19.5 weeks.

Thoracic circumference

This circumference is measured at the same level as a four-chamber view of the heart and at right angles to the fetal spine. It is of particular value in cases where pulmonary hypoplasia may occur, e.g. severe fetal renal disease, premature rupture of membranes or severe intrauterine growth retardation (Fig. 35.11).

Other measurements

Tables are available relating the length of the humerus, radius, ulna and tibia to gestational age. These tables are not used routinely but are of value in suspected dwarfism. The cerebellar diameter in millimetres corresponds to the gestational age up to 25 weeks. The cerebellum is usually visualized by obtaining a BPD and then angling the posterior part of the probe slightly inferiorly (Fig. 35.12).

Tables are also available for measuring the orbital diameters, the binocular distance (distance from the outer wall of one orbit to the outer wall of the other orbit) and the interocular distance (distance between the inner walls of the orbit). These are of value in assessing possible abnormalities of the fetal face (Fig. 35.13).

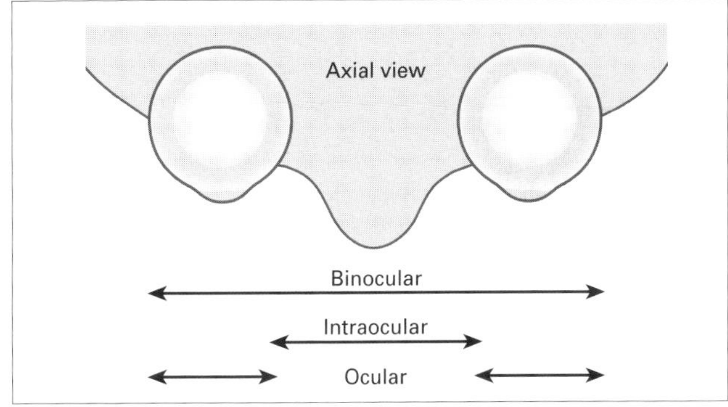

Fig. 35.13 Orbital measurements.

Ultrasound assessment of gestational age

Prior to commencing scanning the patient must be asked the date of her LMP, if the period was a normal one and if she has been on the oral contraceptive pill recently. It is also helpful to know if there has been any bleeding since she became pregnant. Using an obstetric dial calculator the patient's likely gestational age can then be determined.

Up to 14 weeks gestation the CRL of the fetus should be assessed and if this gives a gestational age within 5 days of the estimated age, the patient's own dates should be accepted as correct. Similarly if the patient is between 14 and 25 weeks the BPD, FL and AC should be assessed and the patient's own dates accepted as correct if these measurements are within 7 days of that date.

If the patient is uncertain of her dates, has been taking the contraceptive pill recently or has had some bleeding, then her own dates cannot be accepted as reliable and her gestational age must be determined from the measurement of CRL up to 14 weeks and BPD, FL and AC up to about 25 weeks. In some centres a second scan may be performed to confirm these dates but if the initial scans have been of good quality this should not be necessary.

Determination of gestational age after 25 weeks is known to be inaccurate and unless the patient is fairly definite about her own dates it can be impossible to actually determine the true gestational age. In these circumstances it is advisable to monitor fetal growth regularly and provided this continues at an acceptable rate, there should be no cause for anxiety.

Fetal growth

Normal fetal growth is determined by both genetic and environmental factors. The average Caucasian fetus in Britain weighs 1 kg at 28 weeks gestation, 2 kg at 32 weeks gestation and 3 kg at 36 weeks gestation. Most fetuses will grow steadily up to 38 weeks gestation when growth will decline slightly. Tables relating fetal weight to gestation are available for different populations and obviously the correct chart should be used.

Fetal growth can be assessed by the regular, usually monthly, assessment of BPD, HC, AC and FL. These measurements can then be plotted on appropriate charts and the growth pattern over a period of time assessed. For this it is essential to have an accurate knowledge of gestation obtained from positively known dates or preferably an early gestation scan. The ratio of HC to AC should be worked out and similarly plotted. Provided the curve for the measurements remains between the 90th and 10th centile and runs parallel to the centiles then the growth pattern can be accepted as normal (Fig. 35.14). Curves which rise above the 90th centile indicate fetuses which are large for gestational age (Fig. 35.15). Curves which fall below the 10th centile indicate that the fetus is small for gestational age (Fig. 35.16).

The fetal weight can be estimated from tables using the AC [1]; BPD and AC [2]; and the FL and AC [3]. Of the three tables the first is the least accurate as the AC can vary depending on whether the fetus is extended with consequent reduction in the AC or flexed up with consequent increase in the AC. The introduction of a second measurement such as BPD or FL increases the accuracy of the assessment but even so the estimation of weight can be out by ±10%. In late pregnancy it may be difficult to obtain a

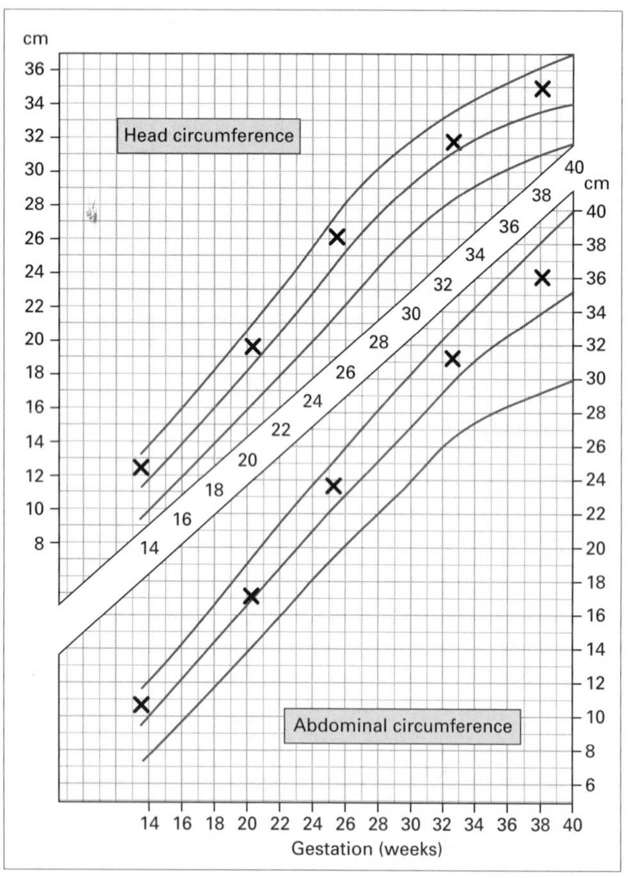

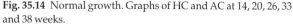

Fig. 35.14 Normal growth. Graphs of HC and AC at 14, 20, 26, 33 and 38 weeks.

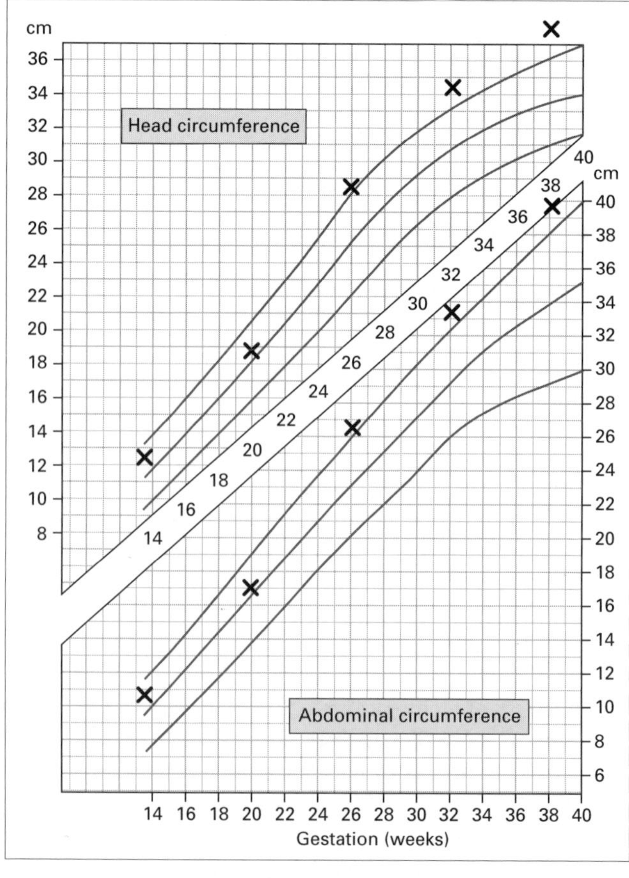

Fig. 35.15 Large for gestational age. Graphs of HC and AC.

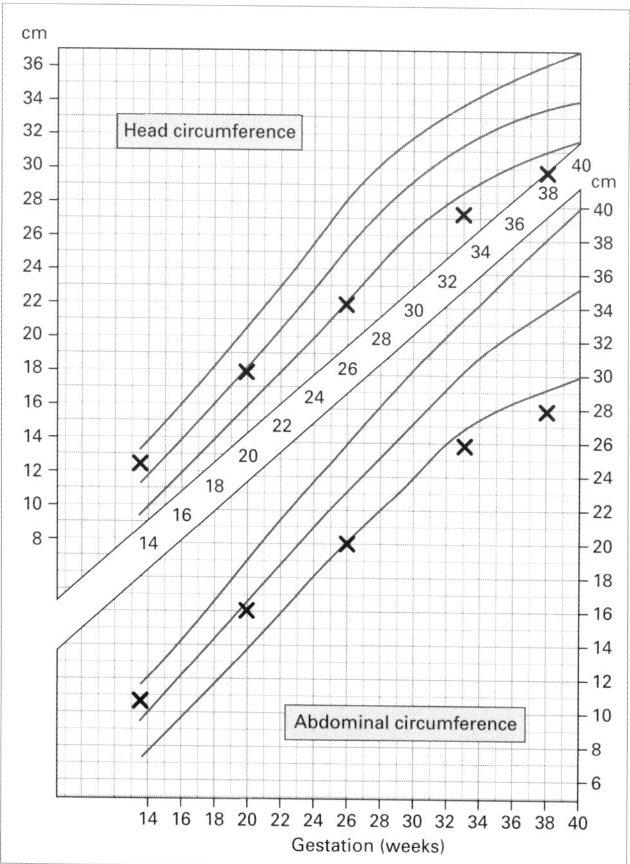

Fig. 35.16 Small for gestational age. Graphs of HC and AC.

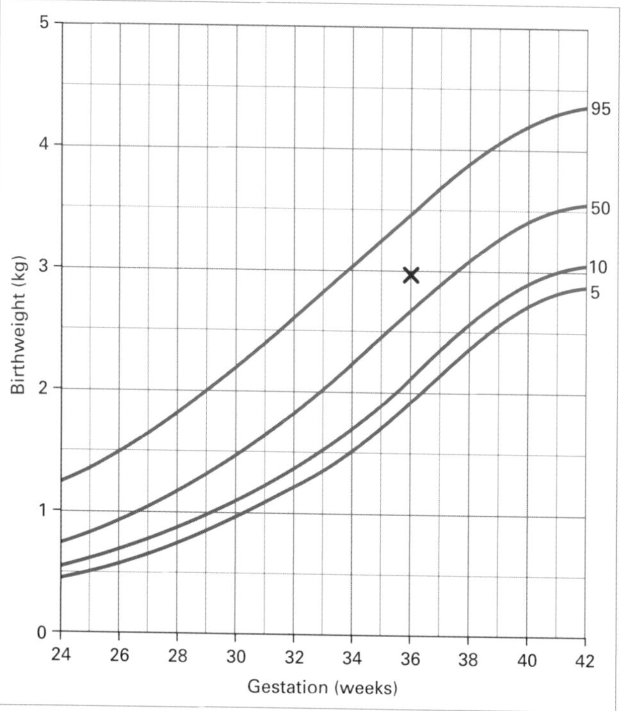

Fig. 35.17 Estimated fetal weight of a 36-week gestation fetus weighing 3 kg.

BPD and in this instance Hadlock's table relating FL and AC to weight is more useful.

Although an estimation of the weight may be useful in determining whether a fetus can be delivered early (Fig. 35.17), in practice it is more useful to follow the growth curves to determine whether the baby is large or small for gestational age.

Fetuses large for gestational age

The cause of most large fetuses is unknown but many will be genetic. A few are due to maternal diabetes mellitus and the mother should be screened to exclude this condition. The fetus may be noted to have scalp or trunk oedema secondary to the subcutaneous deposition of fat. The placenta is often increased in size in these fetuses. There is a higher incidence of fetal abnormality in the fetuses of diabetic mothers and a fetal anomaly scan should be carried out to exclude the 'VACTERL syndrome' (vertebral, anal, cardiovascular, tracheo-oesophageal, renal and limb abnormalities).

The main problem with the large fetus is the difficulty which may ensue at delivery due to cephalopelvic disproportion or shoulder dystocia. Fetal distress can develop resulting in birth asphyxia. The problem is particularly marked if there is a breech presentation and many obstetricians would automatically carry out a caesarean section for a large breech baby.

Fetuses small for gestational age

Confusion exists over the correct terms to apply to the 'small fetus'. A small for dates fetus is one whose weight is under the 10th centile for the gestational age at which it is delivered. Intrauterine growth retardation (IUGR) applies to a baby whose growth pattern has been less than expected. Using these definitions a fetus with IUGR may not necessarily be small for gestational age.

Fetal growth is best assessed by the regular measurement of several parameters which can then be plotted on charts. Two types of growth abnormality have been recognized and they can be picked up from the charts.

SYMMETRICAL GROWTH RETARDATION

This is a small but normally proportioned fetus and in most instances represents the lower end of the normal growth range. In these fetuses the growth curves for HC, AC, BPD and sometimes FL show a progressive falling off (see Fig. 35.16). Unfortunately, some of these small fetuses may be due to chromosomal abnormalities, infections or may be secondary to 'drugs'.

Causes

1 Idiopathic.
2 Congenital infections—toxoplasmosis, rubella, cytomegalovirus or syphilis.
3 Chromosome abnormality.
4 Fetal alcohol syndrome.
5 Heroin addiction.
6 Chronic maternal undernutrition.
7 Smoking.

When such a fetus is detected it is important to carry out a detailed fetal anomaly scan looking particularly carefully for any markers for chromosome abnormalities. Depending on the result of this examination, a decision over whether to karyotype the fetus should be made.

Thereafter the fetus should be carefully assessed with fortnightly growth measurements, biophysical profiles and Doppler assessment.

ASYMMETRICAL GROWTH RETARDATION

In this condition, which is usually the result of placental insufficiency, the fetal brain continues to grow at the expense of the fetal liver. The liver normally increases steadily in size throughout pregnancy due to accumulation of glycogen and similar substances. Liver growth falls off if there is a reduction in the supply of nutrients via the placenta. This in turn leads to a falling off in the growth of the AC. Despite the problem with the liver, the brain is still able to grow normally for some time and the BPD will continue to increase at a normal rate. However, in such fetuses the HC to AC ratio will become abnormal, the ratio showing gradual rise (Fig. 35.18).

This condition is particularly found in women who have had a previous baby who was small for dates and who have some form of materal vascular disease, e.g. hypertension, diabetes or collagen disorder.

The presence of asymmetric growth retardation may result in antenatal or perinatal asphyxia and there is a higher incidence of hypoglycaemia, hypothermia, necrotizing enterocolitis and pulmonary haemorrhage.

Fetuses with this problem should be monitored fortnightly for growth and should have a biophysical profile and Doppler assessment carried out. Weekly assessment of growth can be misleading as the error in such measurements may be greater than the actual amount which a fetus grows from week to week. The decision as to the

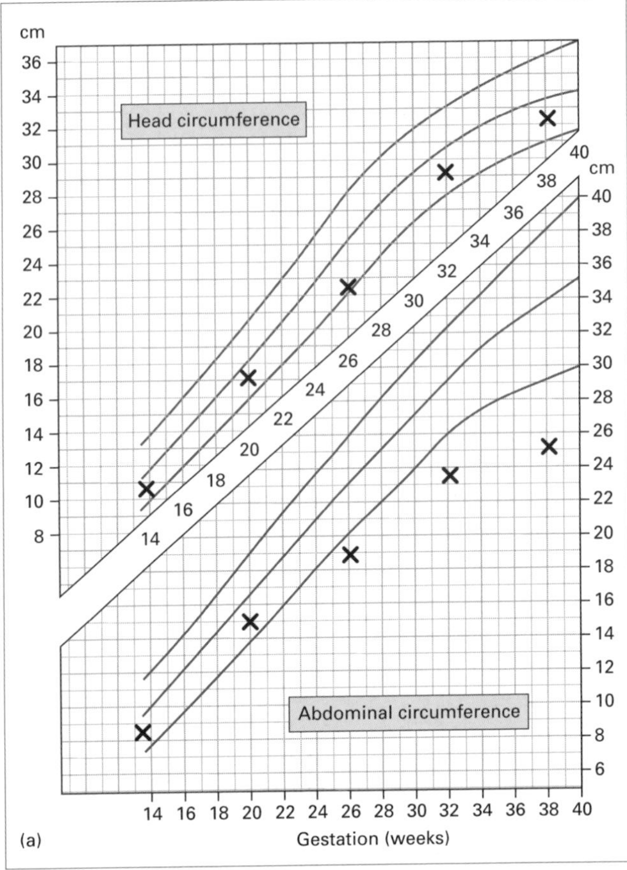

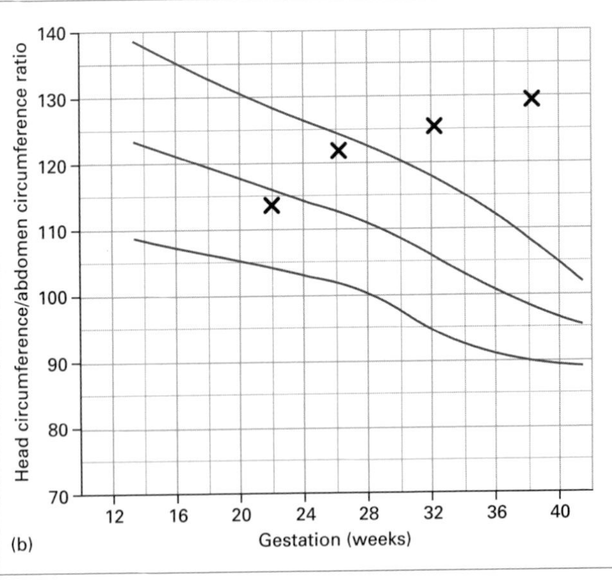

Fig. 35.18 Asymmetric growth retardation. (a) Graphs of HC and AC. (b) Graph of HC to AC ratio against gestational age.

correct timing of delivery will depend on the overall fetal well-being and this is discussed elsewhere.

Ideally all women should be offered fetal growth assessment but practically this is impossible in many centres and monitoring can only be offered to women perceived to be high risk:

1 Previous IUGR fetus.

2 Mothers with hypertension, diabetes mellitus or collagen disorders.

3 Mothers with recurrent antepartum haemorrhage.

4 Mothers with a raised serum α-fetoprotein but structurally normal fetus.

5 Heavy smokers, alcoholics or drug abusers.

Clinical assessment of fetal growth is poor, but measurements should be carried out if the size of the fetus appears small for dates. As many cases of IUGR are picked up by chance, growth assessment should be carried out routinely on any mother who is referred for ultrasound scanning in later pregnancy for any other reason, e.g. bleeding.

References

1 Campbell, S., Wilkin, D. (1975) Abdominal circumference in the estimation of fetal weight. *British Journal of Obstetrics and Gynaecology* **82**, 689–697.

2 Romero, R., Pilu, G., Jeanty, P., Ghidini, A., Hobbins, J.C. (1988) *Prenatal Diagnosis of Congenital Anomalies*. Appleton & Lange, Connecticut.

3 Hadlock, F.P., Harrist, R.B., Carpenter, P.J. (1984) Sonographic estimation of fetal weight. *Radiology* **150**, 534–540.

Chapter 36: The first trimester

J.R. MacKenzie

First trimester scanning

Scanning during the first 12 weeks of pregnancy is usually carried out to assess gestation or because the patient has presented with vaginal bleeding and/or pain. For many years scanning in early pregnancy was carried out abdominally and required the mother to have a full bladder. Underfilling or overfilling of the bladder could lead to an incorrect diagnosis. More recently there has been increased interest in the value of vaginal scanning during the first trimester. This disposes with the need for a full maternal bladder and in the hands of an expert the technique may frequently be of more value than abdominal scanning particularly in the obese patient or in the patient with a retroverted uterus.

Abdominal scanning can be carried out with a 5 MHz probe and vaginal scanning with a 7.5 or 5 MHz probe.

Before carrying out a scan in the first trimester it is helpful to know the exact date of the last menstrual period and whether the period was entirely normal. A history of previous pelvic infection or surgery should be obtained and it is useful to know if the patient has been using a contraceptive coil or has had *in vitro* fertilization (IVF) or gamete intrafallopian transfer (GIFT); the incidence of ectopic pregnancy is higher in these cases.

The gestation of a pregnancy is assessed from the start of the last normal menstrual period. Some 25 days after this an area of increased echoes develops within the uterus and is surrounded by thickened echo-poor endometrium. This may give rise to acoustic enhancement posteriorly and has been described as the intradecidual sign. A tiny gestation sac can be seen usually lying eccentrically in the uterus at 29 days. This can be detected by vaginal scanning at 4 weeks (Fig. 36.1) and becomes visible on abdominal scanning at 5 weeks (Fig. 36.2). The normal gestation sac is surrounded by a double concentric echogenic ring or crescent known as the double decidual sac sign (Fig. 36.3). The rings are believed to be due to the decidua capsularis and decidua parietalis. The double rings are useful in distinguishing a normal gestation sac from a pseudogestation sac and are present in about 70% of pregnancies.

The embryonic disc from which the fetus will develop forms during the fourth week of pregnancy. On one side of this disc is the amniotic cavity and on the other the yolk sac and developing extraembryonic coelom or chorionic cavity. A double bleb sign has been described on transvaginal scanning where the yolk sac and chorionic and amniotic cavities can be seen on either side of the embryonic plate (Fig. 36.4). This appearance is rarely seen on transabdominal scanning. The fetal heart can be detected at 5.5 weeks vaginally and at 6–7 weeks transabdominally. Fetal movement can be appreciated from 8 weeks and about this time the placental site can be determined.

An assessment of gestation can be made in the first trimester from measuring the diameter or volume of the gestation sac. In practice this is of little use. One of the most accurate means of assessing gestation is by measuring the crown–rump length and this is fully described in Chapter 35.

The presence of more than one gestational sac can be identified from 5 weeks onwards. However, before confirming the presence of a multiple pregnancy it is essential to identify a fetal pole within each sac and to demonstrate two or more fetal hearts. It is believed that up to 50% of twin pregnancies may result in the loss of one twin (Fig. 36.5).

The following features should be recorded during first trimester scanning.

1 Pregnancy site.
2 Number of sacs and gestational sac diameter.
3 Regularity of sac outline.
4 Presence and size of yolk sac.
5 Presence of embryo.
6 Crown–rump length measurement.
7 Presence or absence of cardiac activity.
8 Presence of intrauterine haematoma, placental bed abnormalities, extracoelomic fluid.
9 Presence of free peritoneal fluid.
10 Presence of adnexal masses.

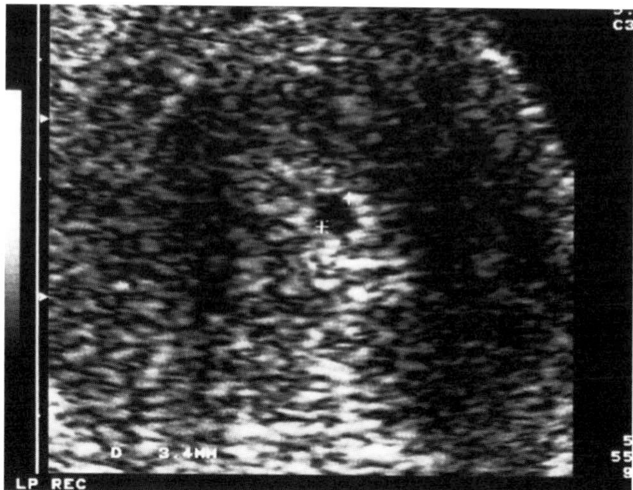

Fig. 36.1 Transvaginal scan showing a small gestation sac (4 weeks).

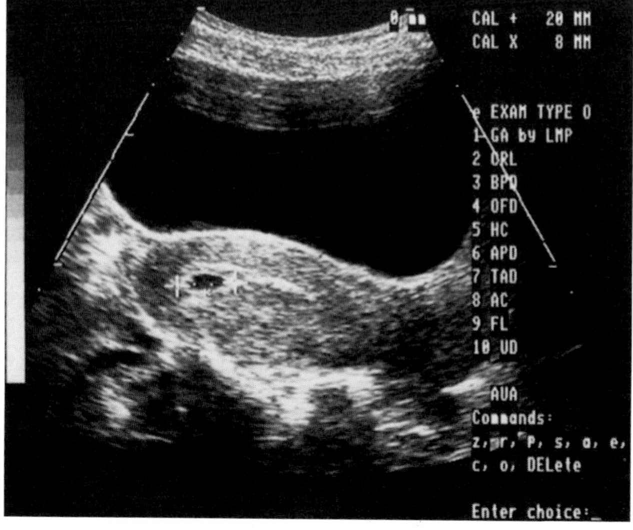

Fig. 36.2 Abdominal scan showing an eccentrically positioned small gestation sac (5 weeks).

First trimester problems

BLEEDING

An ultrasound examination is carried out in such cases to determine whether the pregnancy is continuing normally or not. It is essential to confirm the presence of fetal life and that the pregnancy is intrauterine. If the pregnancy is ongoing and the cervical canal is closed the patient is said to have a threatened abortion and follow-up scans will be indicated to assess subsequent development and to give maternal reassurance. In some instances the cervical canal will be open and in these cases it is inevitable that an abortion will occur (Fig. 36.6).

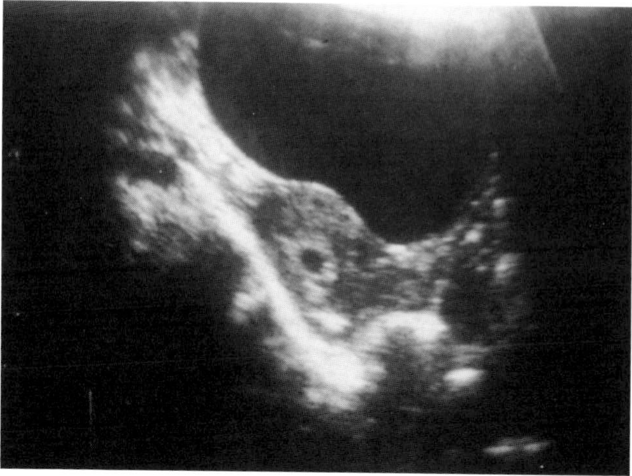

Fig. 36.3 Double decidual sign. Abdominal scan at 6 weeks gestation showing a double echogenic ring.

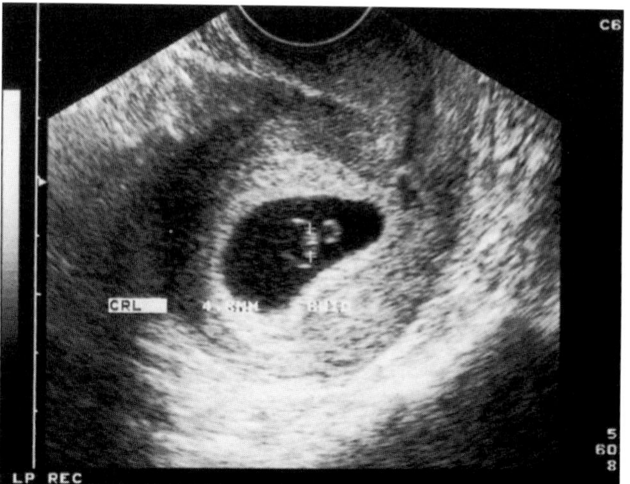

Fig. 36.4 Double bleb sign in a transvaginal scan at 6 weeks gestation.

In some cases a gestational sac will be identified and the fetal pole will be abnormally small for the size of the sac (missed abortion) (Fig. 36.7). Alternatively, there may be no evidence of a fetal pole (blighted ovum or anembryonic pregnancy). However, if the volume of the gestation sac is less than 2.5 cm^3 it must be remembered that a fetal pole can still develop normally. The outline of the gestation sac is frequently irregular or distorted in the presence of a missed abortion (Fig. 36.8).

When embryonic death is suspected two scans, 7 days apart should be performed and the diagnosis of missed abortion or anembryonic pregnancy (blighted ovum) should be confirmed by two experienced ultrasonographers. Bleeding may occasionally be due to a retroimplan-

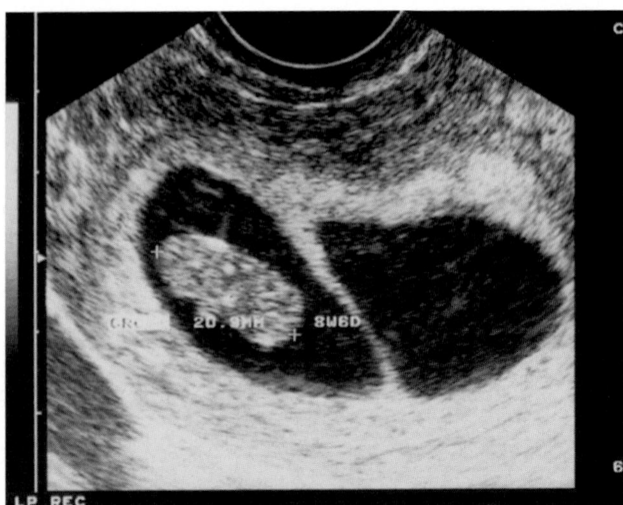

Fig. 36.5 'Twin pregnancy'. Transvaginal scan showing two gestational sacs, one of which contains an 8+ week pregnancy. The other sac is empty (anembryonic pregnancy or blighted ovum).

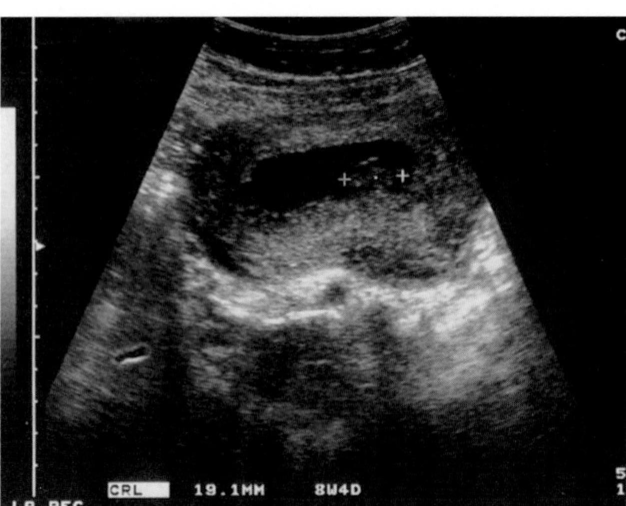

Fig. 36.7 Missed abortion. Large gestation sac containing a small fetal pole with no fetal heart beat.

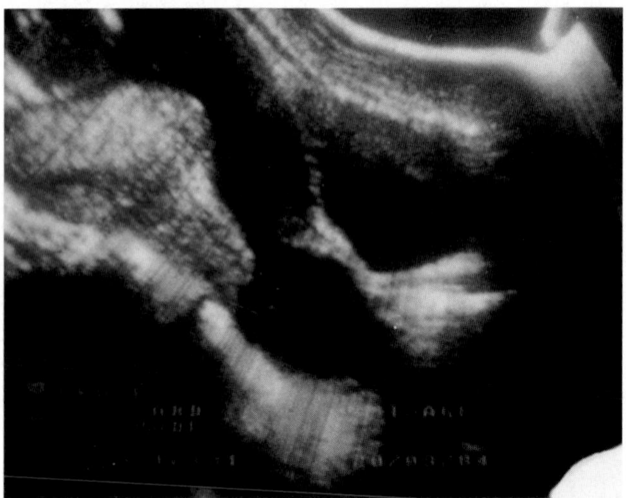

Fig. 36.6 Inevitable abortion. Abdominal scan at 15 weeks gestation in a patient with bleeding and pain demonstrating an open cervix.

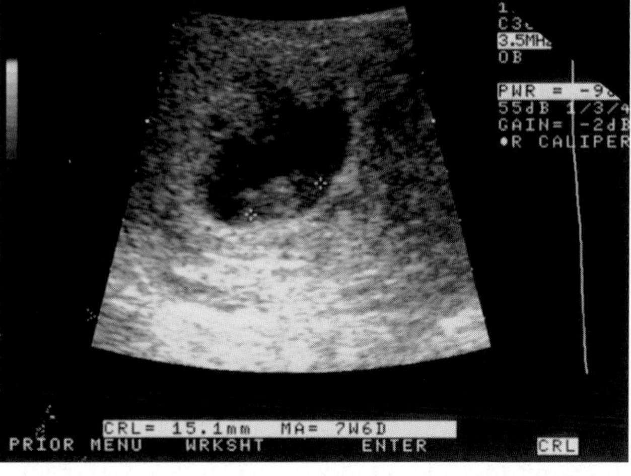

Fig. 36.8 Missed abortion 11.5 weeks. Crown–rump length is 15.1 mm which is equivalent to 7 weeks and 6 days. No FH. The wall of the sac is irregular.

tation bleed or subchorionic haemorrhage and an irregular transonic area may be identified near the gestation sac (see Fig. 35.1). These areas may be confused with an empty sac in a twin pregnancy.

A pseudogestation sac may occur with an ectopic pregnancy. The double decidual appearance will be absent and the walls may be irregular.

In the presence of an incomplete abortion the ultrasound picture of the uterus may be variable containing areas of both increased and decreased echoes due to retained blood clot and products of conception (Fig. 36.9).

HYDATIDIFORM MOLE

A mole is due to the proliferation of trophoblastic tissue rather than embryonic tissue. The incidence of a hydatidiform mole is around 1 in 3000 amongst Caucasians but this incidence rises to 1 in 300 amongst the Asian population. The patient usually presents with severe vomiting (hyperemesis gravidarum), painless vaginal bleeding and a uterus that is much larger than expected for her gestation. Ultrasound shows the presence of numerous cystic areas of varying sizes (Fig. 36.10). The appearance is

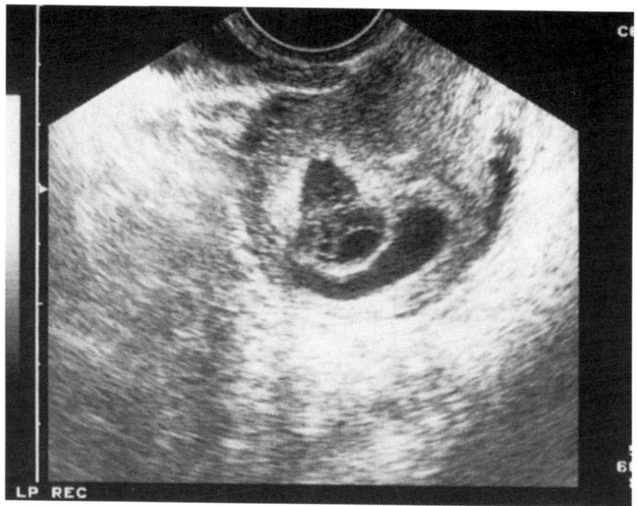

Fig. 36.9 Incomplete abortion. Vaginal scan showing cystic areas of varying size together with echogenic areas and a large transonic area. Appearances are due to retained products of conception and blood.

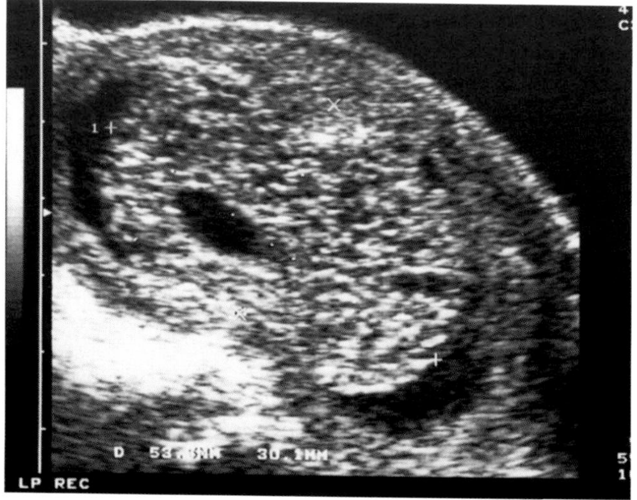

Fig. 36.10 Hydatidiform mole. Cystic areas of varying size showing an irregular gestation sac. The uterus is abnormally large for dates.

not dissimilar to that sometimes seen in an incomplete abortion. A molar pregnancy is sometimes associated with the presence of several large theca lutein cysts. Patients with a hydatidiform mole are at risk of developing a choriocarcinoma and they require serial estimations of β-human chorionic gonadotrophic. It has been suggested that Doppler flow studies may be helpful in the early diagnosis of a hydatidiform mole or in the detection of early recurrence. A partial mole has been described in cases of triploidy (an extra set of chromosomes).

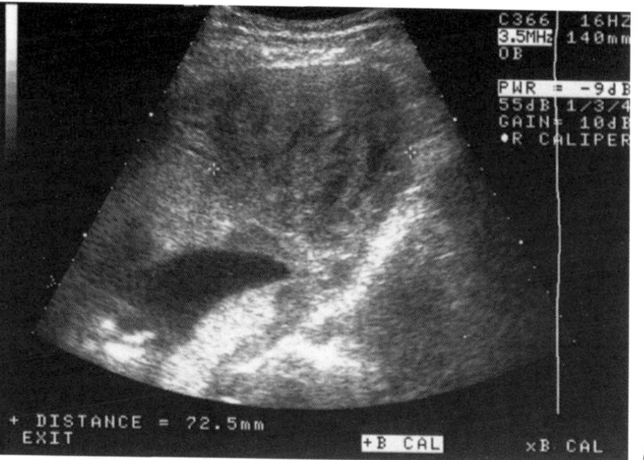

(a)

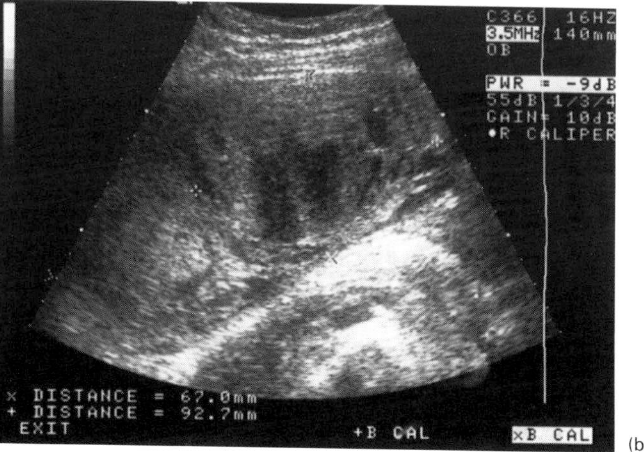

(b)

Fig. 36.11 Fibroid. A large fibroid measuring 7.2 × 6.5 × 9.3 cm complicating an IVF triplet pregnancy. (a) Longitudinal view; (b) transverse view.

ECTOPIC OR EXTRAUTERINE PREGNANCY

The possibility of this condition must be considered in any sexually active female of reproductive age who presents with bleeding and lower abdominal pain. This topic is fully covered in Chapter 33.

RELATED PROBLEMS

An ultrasound examination during the first trimester is helpful in diagnosing the presence of uterine fibroids and ovarian cysts. The incidence of fibroids increases with age. In many cases the fibroid presents no problem but if it is situated low in the uterus it could obstruct labour and necessitate a caesarean section. Central degeneration of a rapidly growing fibroid may take place and bleeding may occur into the centre of the fibroid. This results in severe localized pain and must be distinguished from a placental abruption (Fig. 36.11).

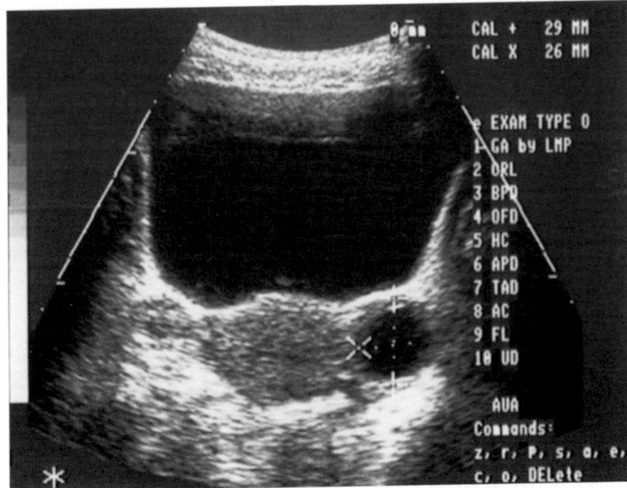

Fig. 36.12 Corpus luteum cyst. Left-sided corpus luteum cyst measuring 2.9 × 2.6 cm which had disappeared at a follow-up scan.

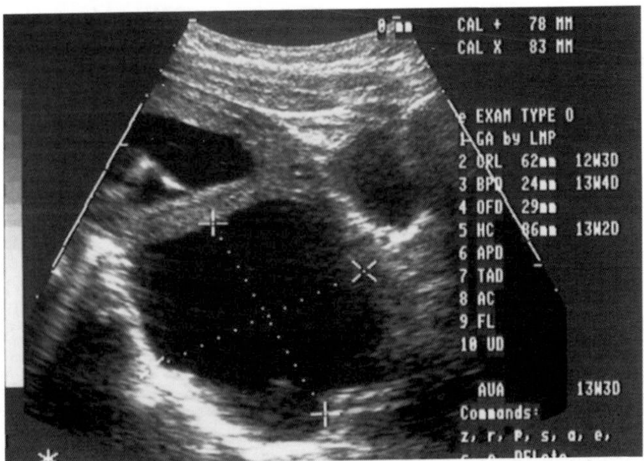

Fig. 36.13 Ovarian cyst. Large cyst in the pouch of Douglas (7.8 × 8.3 cm) which was eventually removed at 16 weeks gestation.

Ovarian cysts are commonly found in the early stages of pregnancy and are usually due to corpus luteum cysts. They result from human chorionic gonadotrophic stimulation. The cysts are usually small and disappear by 12 weeks gestation (Fig. 36.12). However, they can grow up to 10 cm and may become symptomatic due to torsion or bleeding. Many obstetricians favour the removal of large cysts which are still present at around 16 weeks gestation (Fig. 36.13).

A dermoid cyst may first come to light during pregnancy. These cysts can be of varying size and varying echogenicity. However, if they contain teeth, an area of high echogenicity with posterior acoustic shadowing will be demonstrated. Rarely a malignant ovarian tumour may be found during pregnancy.

Occasionally a pelvic kidney may be diagnosed for the first time as a mass posterior to the uterus.

Chapter 37: Fetal anomaly scanning

J.R. MacKenzie

Fetal anomaly scanning is usually carried out between 18 and 20 weeks gestation. Before attempting such scanning it is essential to have an excellent knowledge of normal fetal anatomy and to be familiar with the normal variations which can occur.

Normal fetal anatomy

Before looking at fetal anatomy in detail the uterus should be scanned rapidly to localize the placenta, to determine the number of fetuses that are present and to assess the position of the fetus (cephalic, breech, transverse or oblique). The position of the occiput is then determined and the fetal lie worked out, e.g. right occipitoanterior, occipitoposterior, and so on. The right- and left-hand sides of the fetus must then be ascertained. It must never be assumed that the fetal stomach is always on the left or that the cardiac apex points to the left. It is very disconcerting to discover at delivery that what was diagnosed as a right multi-cystic kidney turns out to a left one!

The fetus should be examined whenever possible in a logical manner and initially it is best to carry out the standard measurements of biparietal diameter, head circumference, abdominal circumference and femoral length. The fetal head should then be examined in detail. This is most successfully done by returning to the axial plane for the measurement of the biparietal diameter and checking the position of the cavum septum pellucidum and the thalami. The probe can then be slid slightly cranially when the lateral ventricles containing the hyperechoic choroid plexuses will be seen. Early in the second trimester the lateral ventricles and choroid plexuses take up most of the cranial vault (Fig. 37.1).

With the growth of the cerebral cortex the ventricles come to occupy a smaller area within the vault and the ventricular to hemispheric width ratio falls from around 75% at 15 weeks to 50% at 21 weeks and about 30% at term (Fig. 37.2). Some people routinely measure the anterior and posterior ventricular to hemispheric width ratios but providing the choroid plexus fills most of the atria and posterior parts of the ventricles this is unnecessary. The cerebral cortex may appear almost transonic in the latter part of the second trimester and this can lead to the false diagnosis of hydrocephalus (Fig. 37.3). This error should not occur if the position of the choroid plexus is carefully observed as it lies adjacent to the lateral wall of the ventricle.

The probe should now be angled down into the posterior fossa where the cerebellum and cisterna magna will be identified. The cerebellum consists of two circular hemispheres joined together by the vermis. The size of the cerebellum in millimetres is equal to the gestational age up to 26 weeks gestation. The cisterna magna appears as a transonic area between the cerebellum and the inner table of the vault. Its size increases with gestation but is usually about 5 mm. It should never be more than 10 mm (Fig. 37.4). The probe should now be moved back into the axial plane used for the biparietal diameter and then slid slightly caudally. The nose and orbits will be seen in cross-section. The interocular, binocular and orbital diameters are normally measured in this plane. By rotating the probe through 90° and sliding it anteriorly a view of the facial profile is obtained. The forehead, nasal bone, palate, lips, mouth and chin will be seen (Fig. 37.5). The probe can then be slid slightly to one side or the other and a coronal section of the face will be obtained. With practice it is possible to see the eyes, nose, nostrils, lips, mouth and chin (Fig. 37.6).

The probe should be rotated again to obtain an axial view through the lower cranial vault and should be moved slowly in a caudal manner so that sections through the fetal neck are obtained. The fetal spine will be noted in the posterior part of the neck and the neck should be closely examined for any abnormal cystic structures. The nuchal fat pad lies posterior to the cervical spine and this can be measured from the section used for assessing the cerebellum. The thickness of the soft tissues posterior to the occipital bone at this level should be less than 6 mm in the second trimester.

Moving caudally in an axial projection the fetal clavicles can be identified as symmetrical, curvilinear areas of increased echoes (Fig. 37.7). The thorax can now be exam-

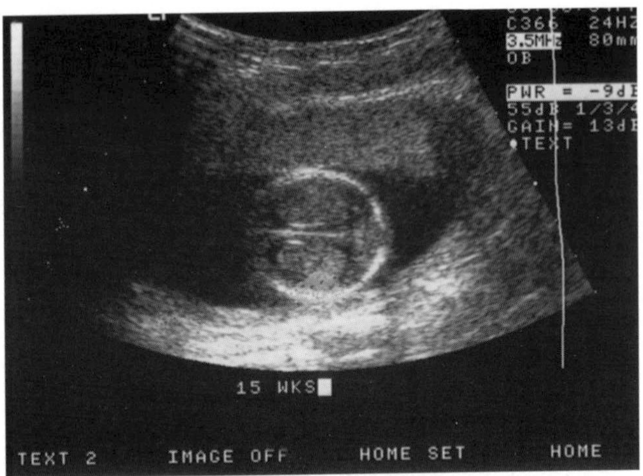

Fig. 37.1 Large echogenic choroid plexuses filling most of the vault at 15 weeks gestation.

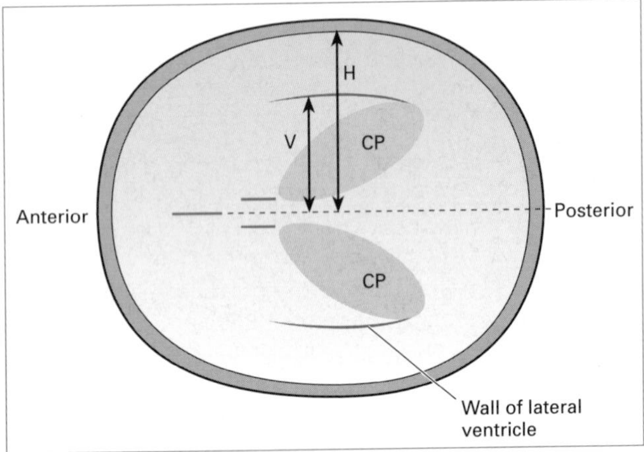

Fig. 37.2 Diagram showing measurements for ventricular to hemispheric ratio (V/H). CP, choroid plexus.

ined in detail. Echoes for the dorsal spine are situated posteriorly. The ribs are seen extending around the thorax from the spine. Most of the thorax is occupied by the lungs which have low level echoes. The fetal heart is situated in the anterior lower part of the thorax slightly to the left of the mid line. An axial view through the heart (four-chamber view) (Fig. 37.8) enables the ventricles, atria, patent foramen ovale, ventricular septum and the atrio-ventricular valves to be assessed. The ventricles should be of similar size and the atria of similar size. The left atrium is the chamber lying nearest the spine while the right ventricle is the most anterior chamber. Echoes within this ventricle are due to the presence of a moderator band. The atrioventricular valves, i.e. tricuspid and mitral, lie at the same level. The flap of the foramen ovale can be seen opening and closing. Rotating the transducer allows the

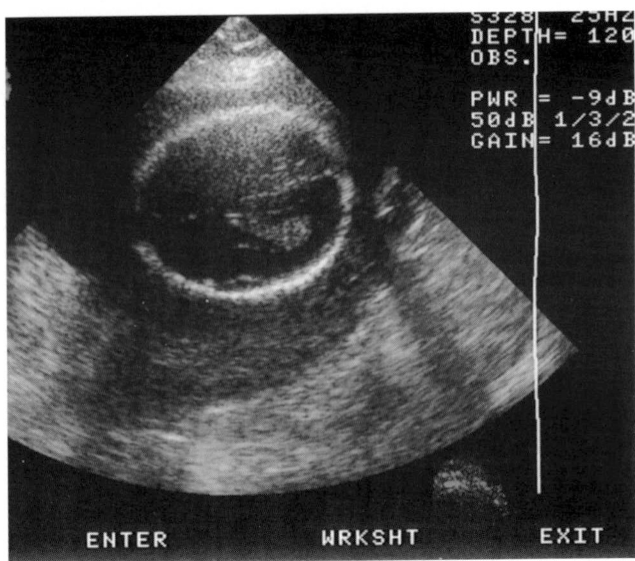

Fig. 37.3 Pseudohydrocephalus. The cerebral cortex appears transonic. The true position of the lateral ventricle is demonstrated by the position of the choroid plexus.

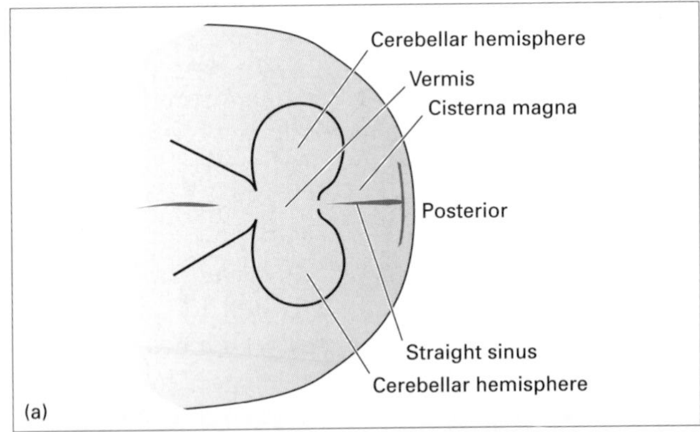

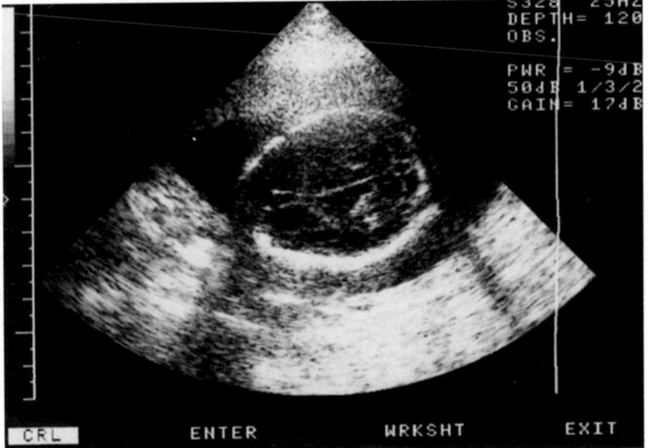

Fig. 37.4 Cerebellum and cisterna magna: (a) diagram and (b) scan.

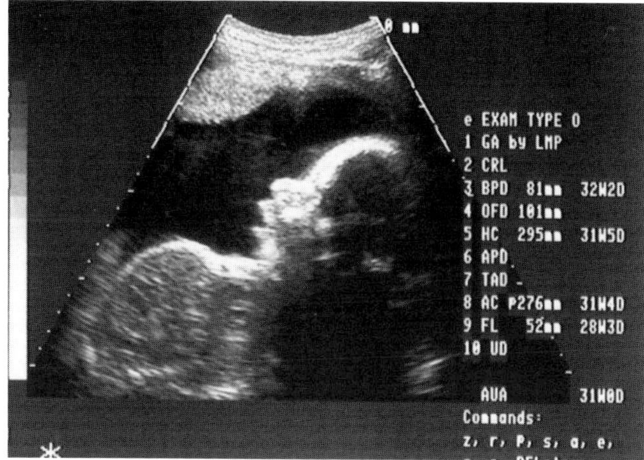

Fig. 37.5 Profile of a 32-week fetus with its mouth slightly open.

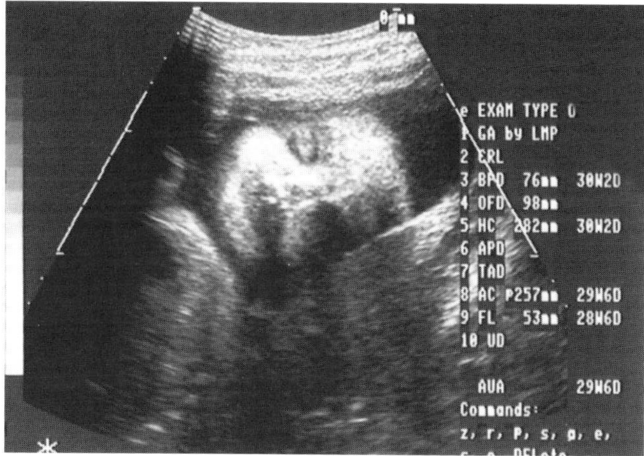

Fig. 37.6 View of the face showing eyes, nose and mouth.

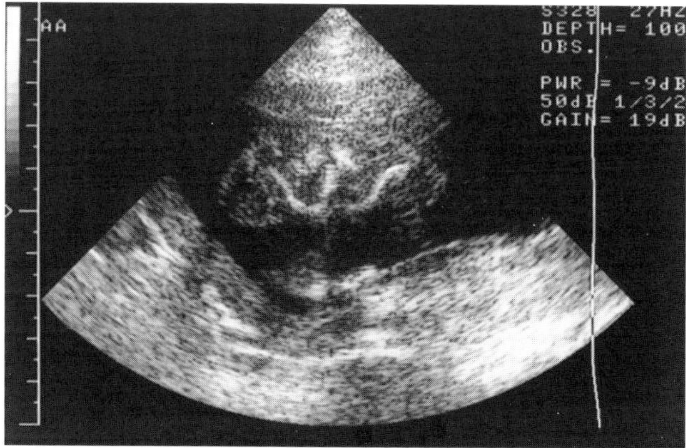

Fig. 37.7 Clavicles demonstrated on an axial scan.

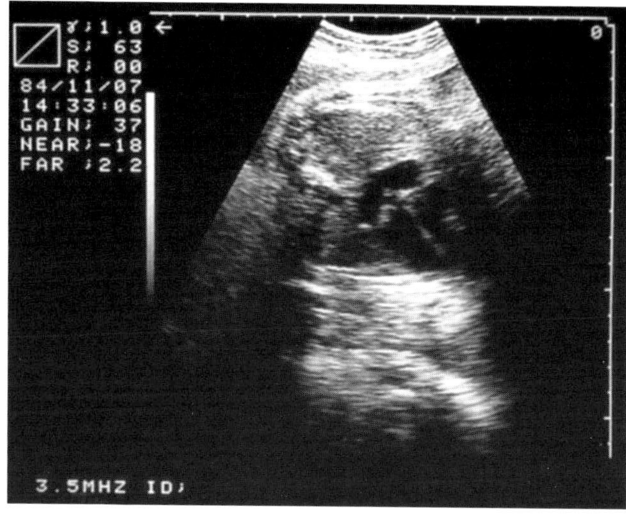

Fig. 37.8 Four-chamber view. An axial view of the atria, ventricles, patent foramen ovale and interventricular septum.

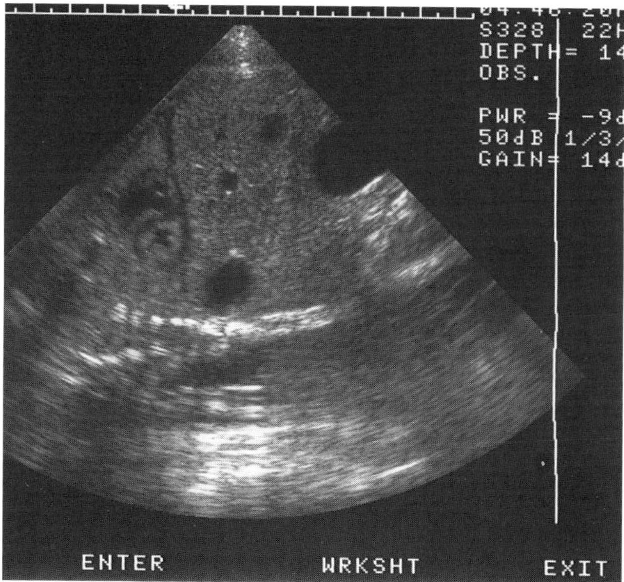

Fig. 37.9 Diaphragm. Transonic linear band separating the heart and lungs from the liver and stomach.

arch of the aorta to be seen in one direction and rotation in the other direction allows the pulmonary outflow tract to be assessed. The fetal heart rate varies from 120 to 160 beats min^{-1}. A rate below or above this should be regarded as abnormal. However, the rate may vary with fetal respiration and in the second trimester this may be quite marked. More detailed information on the fetal heart is given in Chapter 39.

The diaphragm can occasionally be positively identified as a linear area of decreased echoes between the fetal lungs and the fetal liver (Fig. 37.9). The fetal abdomen should be assessed in the axial, coronal and sagittal planes. It is often helpful to scan initially in the axial plane visualizing in turn the liver, stomach, kidneys, insertion of the umbilical cord and the bladder. The liver is normally situated in the right hypochondrium. There is frequently a small transonic area between the abdominal wall and the liver and this is a normal variant due to the abdominal wall musculature. The liver echoes are denser than those of the lungs. The umbilical vein enters the abdomen in the mid line and passes obliquely upwards and posteriorly through the liver (Fig. 37.10). At this point it divides and continues posteriorly and cranially as the ductus venosus which finally drains into the inferior vena cava (Fig. 37.11). The gallbladder may be seen as a small transonic organ lying to the right of the umbilical vein (Fig. 37.12). The stomach is a transonic structure which normally lies in the left hypochondrium. The spleen may be seen lying between the stomach and the lower rib cage in the upper abdomen. The size of the stomach varies considerably and if it is not visualized during the scanning period a follow-up scan should be arranged. Failure to visualize the stomach at any time, particularly if there is associated polyhydramnios must raise the possibility of an oesophageal atresia without a distal fistula.

The kidneys lie in the upper paravertebral regions on either side of the spine (Fig. 37.13) and can usually be identified in about 90% of cases after 17 weeks gestation. Some people find it easier to identify the kidneys initially in the axial plane (Fig. 37.14) whilst others find the parasagittal plane easier (Fig. 37.15). The echogenicity of the kidneys varies but they are usually surrounded by a rim of increased echogenicity due to perinephric fat. The renal pelvis may be visualized as a tiny central transonic area due to the presence of some urine. In the third trimester the renal pyramids are almost transonic in comparison with the renal cortex and this appearance has lead many people to assume that the kidneys are cystic (Fig. 37.16). Others have mistaken the pyramids for fetal

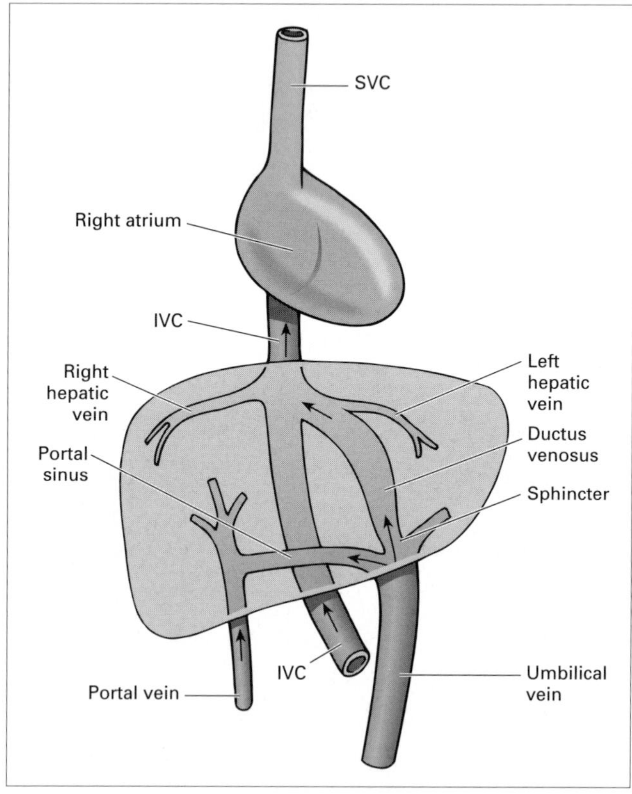

Fig. 37.11 Diagram of the pathway of the umbilical vein through the liver to the right atrium. IVC, inferior vena cava; SVC, superior vena cava.

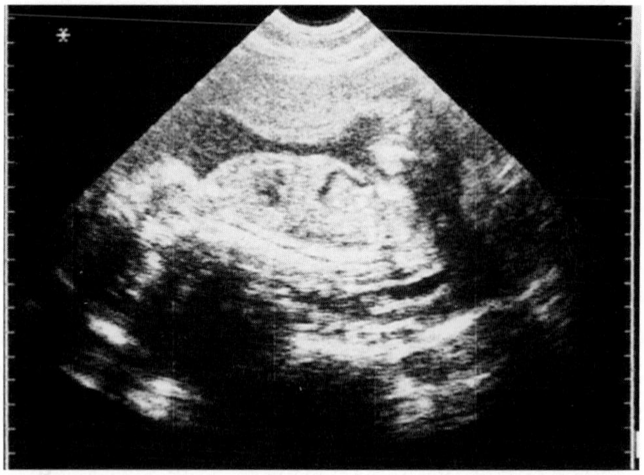

Fig. 37.10 Umbilical vein. Sagittal section showing the pathway of the umbilical vein from the abdominal wall obliquely and cranially through the liver towards the heart.

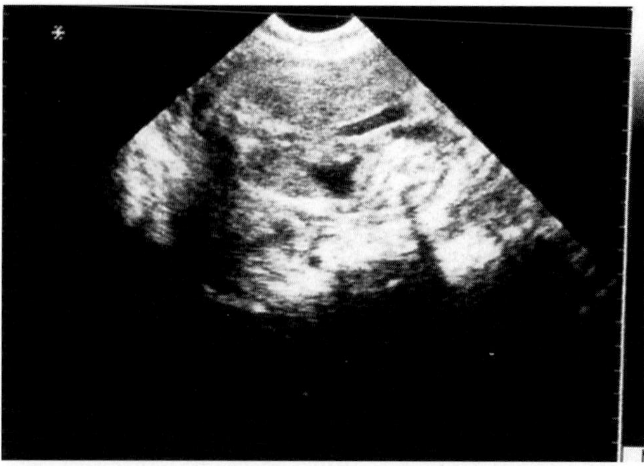

Fig. 37.12 Gallbladder. Axial scan of the upper abdomen demonstrating the gallbladder, umbilical vein and stomach.

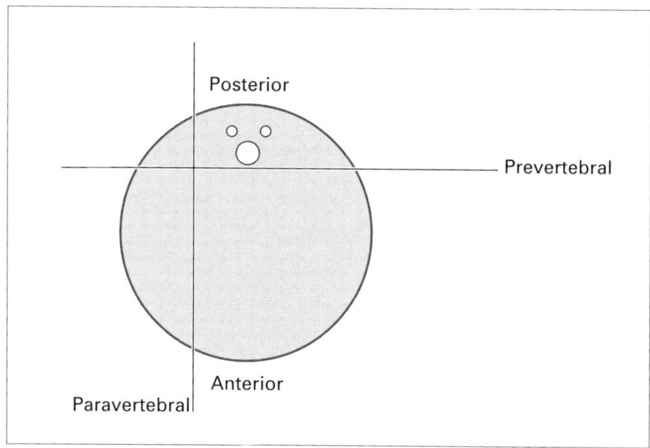

Fig. 37.13 Scanning planes in the upper abdomen.

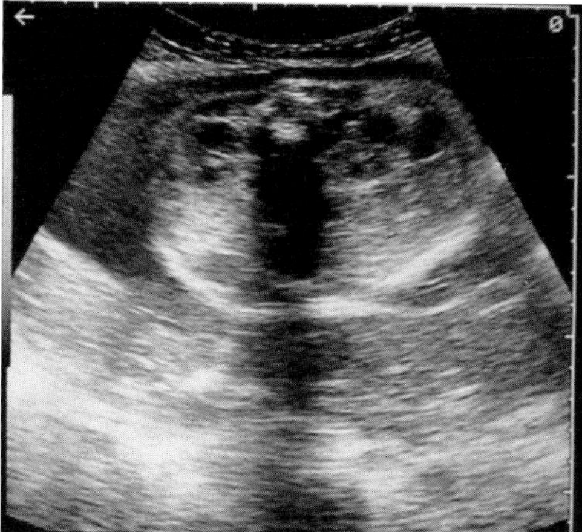

Fig. 37.14 Kidneys. Axial view showing the kidneys on either side of the spine.

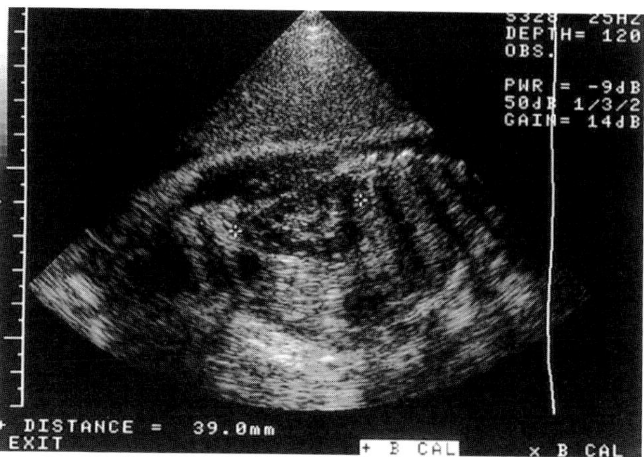

Fig. 37.15 Kidney. Parasagittal view of the kidney showing an echogenic pelvis and a slightly transonic cortex and medulla.

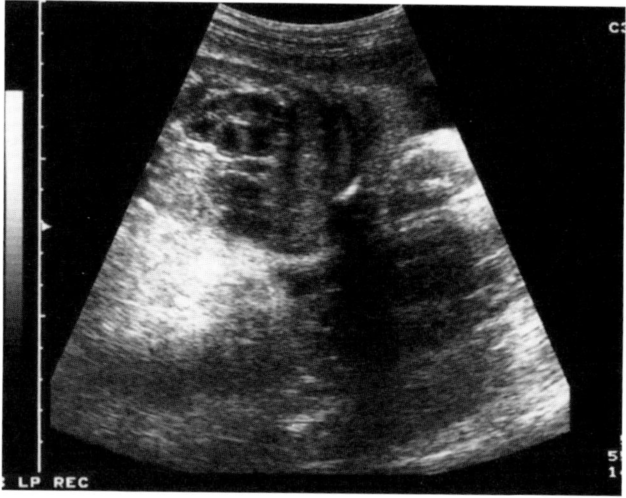

Fig. 37.16 Kidney. Scan in the last trimester demonstrating a slightly irregular echogenic outline of the kidney due to fetal lobulation. The transonic areas represent the renal pyramids.

lobulation. Fetal lobulation is described as a normal variant in the neonate and this may be identified antenatally. Tables are available for renal length and anteroposterior diameter. They are useful if the kidneys are suspected of being abnormally large or small. The ratio of renal circumference to abdominal circumference should lie between 0.27 and 0.30 throughout the second and third trimester. The significance to be attached to the size of the renal pelvis is one of the most controversial subjects in obstetric ultrasound at present. Dilatation of over 1 cm in the last trimester is abnormal and merits follow-up. Dilatation of less than 5 mm is probably of no clinical significance. The management of the fetus with dilatation of between 5 and 10 mm is uncertain and the best advice that can be given at present is for reassessment postdelivery.

The fetal bladder is identified as a transonic structure in the lower abdomen and can be seen to fill and empty in a cycle lasting from around 1 to 2.5 h (Fig. 37.17). If the bladder is not seen during the scanning period then reassessment at a later date is suggested. However, if the volume of amniotic fluid is normal it is unlikely that there is a significant bladder problem.

The fetal bowel is difficult to assess in the second trimester but transonic areas may be identified around the periphery of the abdomen in the third trimester due to the presence of fluid in the haustra of the colon. The aorta can be identified as a transonic pulsating linear structure in the posterior part of the abdomen lying anterior to the spine. The walls of the aorta are fairly echogenic. The division of the aorta into the right and left iliac arteries can frequently be identified (Fig. 37.18).

The fetal spine should be visualized in the axial, sagittal

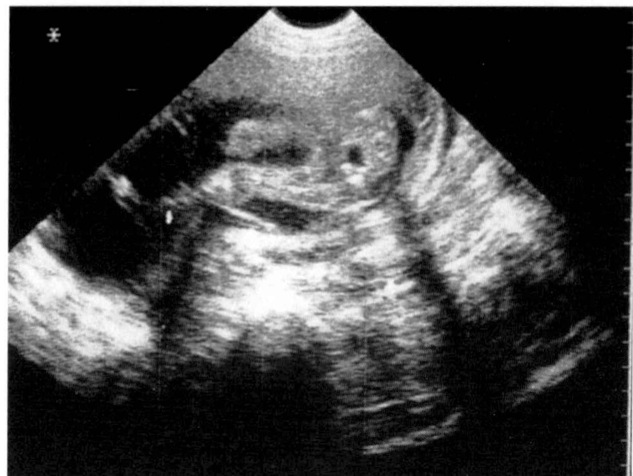

Fig. 37.17 Bladder. A scan of a small transonic bladder on the left with amniotic fluid trapped between the legs on the right.

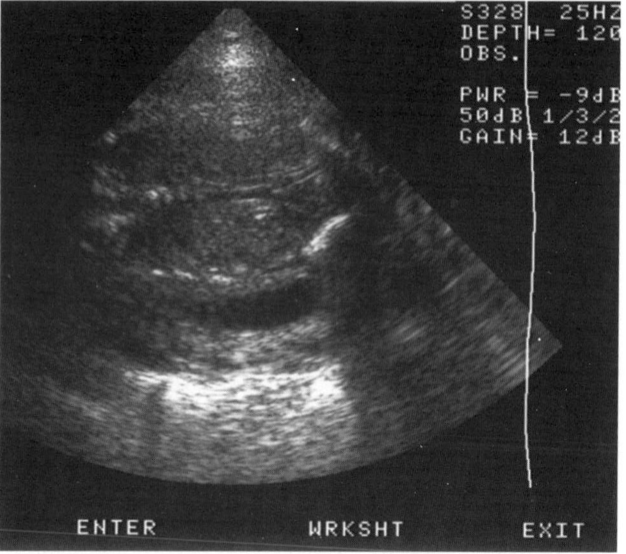

Fig. 37.18 Aorta dividing into right and left iliac arteries.

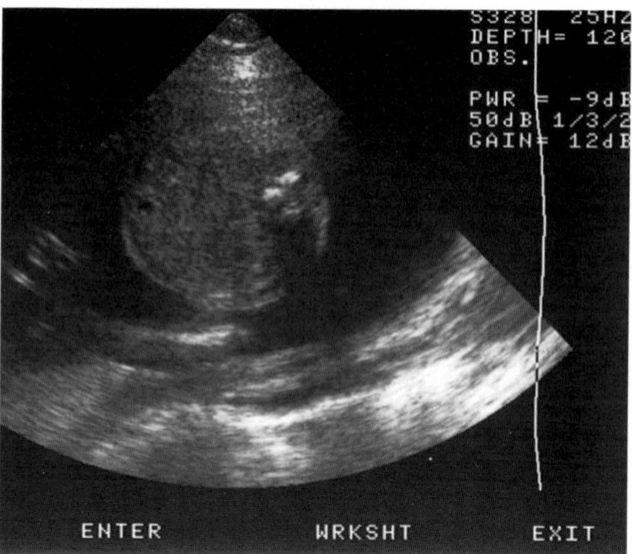

Fig. 37.19 Axial view of the spine showing echoes from the vertebral body and laminae, which is U shaped.

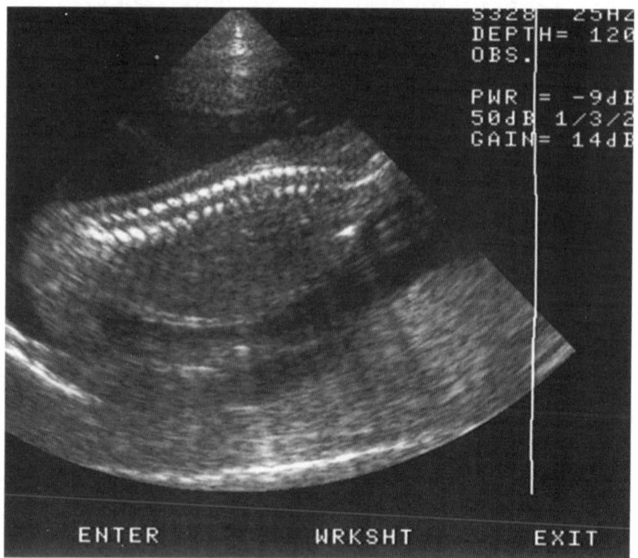

Fig. 37.20 Sagittal view of the lumbosacral spine and the overlying skin.

and coronal projections. The vertebrae have three ossification centres in fetal life, one for the vertebral body and one each for the laminae of the neural arches. These can be identified in transverse section and should have a U-shaped appearance (Fig. 37.19). The skin overlying the vertebrae should be visible throughout and the ossification centres should be assessed at each level from the cervical region down to the sacrum. Care should be taken to follow the normal spinal curvature. This curvature is best appreciated in the sagittal plane where the convex thoracic curvature and the concave cervical and lumbosacral curvatures are apparent (Fig. 37.20). The echoes for the sacrum should come to a point at the lower end of the sacrum. In the coronal projection the slight expansion of the interpedicular distance in the cervical and lumbar regions can be identified (Fig. 37.21). The examination of the spine should be performed after 18 weeks gestation as ossification of the sacral spine is not complete before this time.

The fetal sex can be determined from 14 weeks onwards provided a good view can be obtained between the fetal legs (Fig. 37.22). Care must be taken not to confuse male genitalia with the umbilical cord. It can be more difficult to

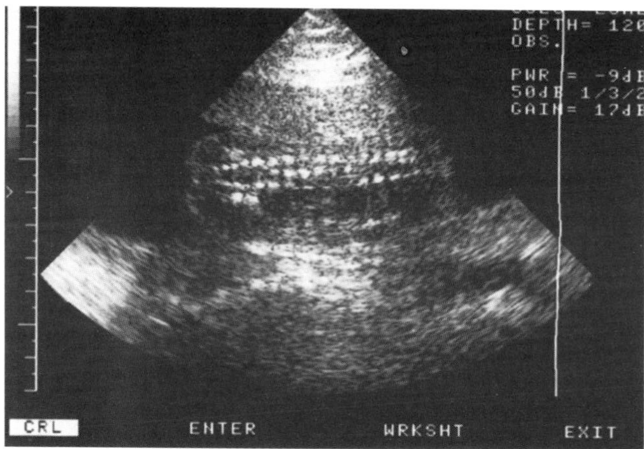

Fig. 37.21 Coronal view of the lumbosacral spine showing a slight, normal widening of the interpedicular distance in the lumbar area.

(a)

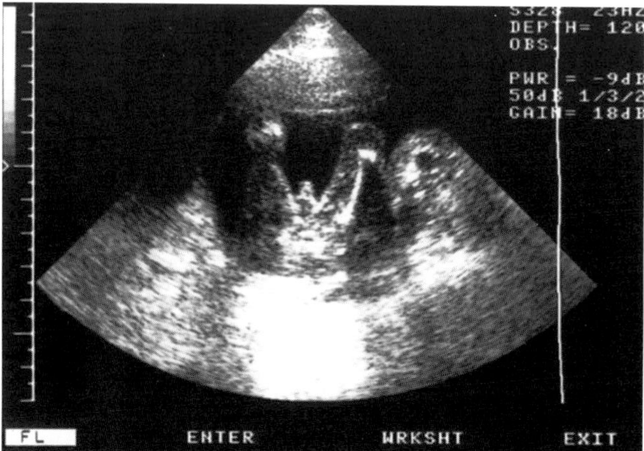

(b)

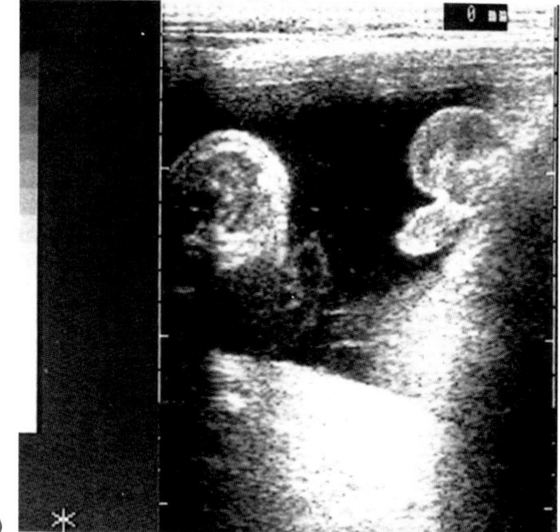

Fig. 37.22 Male fetus. (a) Scrotum and penis between the legs at 16 weeks gestation. (b) Scrotum and penis at 35 weeks gestation.

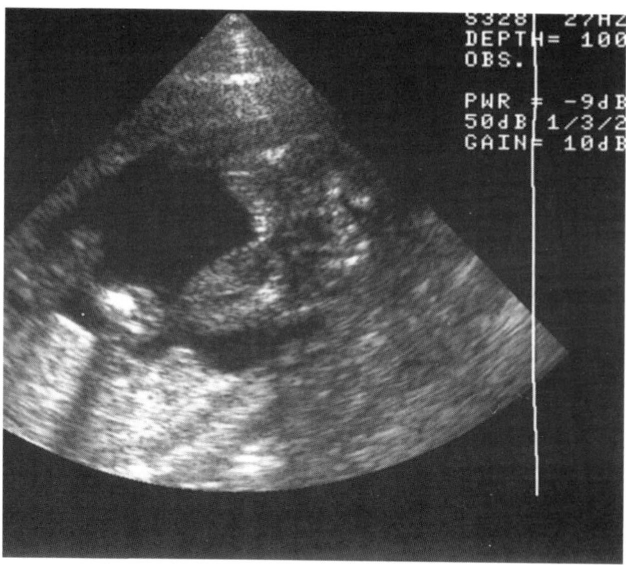

Fig. 37.23 Female infant.

determine the sex of the female infant (Fig. 37.23) as swollen labia can sometimes look very like a scrotum. Many parents are extremely eager to know the sex of the fetus and provided a good view of the perineum has been obtained it is reasonable to let them know the probable sex. They must, however, be informed of the pitfalls of such a diagnosis.

The fetal cord should always be assessed and should contain three vessels, a large non-pulsating vein and two smaller thick-walled pulsating arteries (Fig. 37.24).

Finally, the upper and lower limbs of the fetus should be looked at to check that all the bones are present and are of approximately the correct length. If possible the hands and feet should be examined and the presence of the correct number of fingers and toes determined. The ability to obtain good views of these is very much dependent on the fetal position, fetal activity and the amount of liquor.

Fetal anomaly scanning

The decision as to whether every woman is offered a detailed scan at around 18 weeks is totally dependent on the resources of each unit. In many centres there is inadequate staffing and there are inadequate high quality machines to offer such a routine service. However, as most fetal anomalies are picked up by chance rather than because there is a high risk, a strong argument can be made for attempting to scan everyone at 18 weeks. As the rate of picking up anomalies on such a programme will be low one must wonder whether it is cost-effective. In some centres fetal anomaly scanning is only carried out in so-called high risk groups.

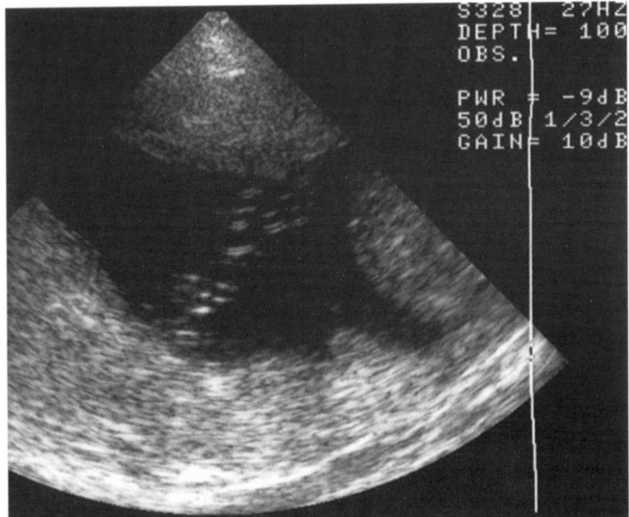

(a)

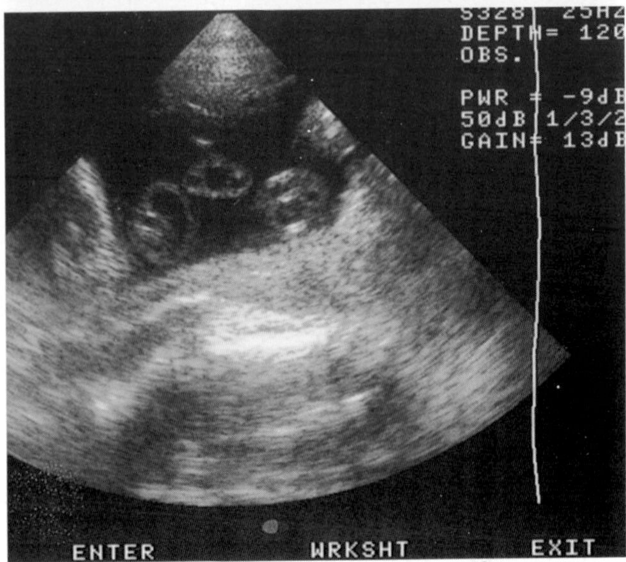

(b)

Fig. 37.24 Umbilical cord. (a) Longitudinal view; (b) transverse view.

The incidence of a major congenital abnormality in the UK is currently 2% with around a further 2% having a minor abnormality. The identification of a major abnormality will give the parents the option of having the pregnancy terminated if they so wish. If they decide to continue with the pregnancy the mode and place of delivery which is in the best interests of the fetus can then be determined. When such an abnormality is detected its presence should be confirmed by a second ultrasonographer and the parents should then receive appropriate counselling. It is often helpful to involve the paediatricians and paediatric surgeons at this stage so that a clear picture of the likely outcome and the problems which such a fetus would encounter can be fully discussed.

Fetal anomaly scanning should be offered in the following situations.

1 A family history of fetal abnormality.
2 Raised maternal serum α-fetoprotein.
3 Low maternal serum α-fetoprotein.
4 All patients having amniocentesis or chorionic villus sampling (CVS).
5 Patients taking certain drugs.
6 Patients with diabetes mellitus.
7 Patients with a multiple pregnancy.
8 Presence of polyhydramnios.
9 Presence of oligohydramnios.
10 Patients with a symmetrical growth retarded fetus.
11 Patients with a breech presentation who are going to be delivered by caesarean section.
12 Parental consanguinity.

Family history of fetal abnormality

Most congenital abnormalities are very unlikely to recur but a normal fetal anomaly scan at 18 weeks is extremely reassuring for the mother who has previously had a fetus with an abnormality, e.g. diaphragmatic hernia. Other abnormalities have a slightly increased risk of recurring (e.g. neural tube defect, congenital heart abnormality) and in these instances a normal scan is again reassuring. Yet other abnormalities recur frequently (e.g. the autosomal recessive condition of infantile polycystic kidneys, the sex-linked form of hydrocephalus) and in these cases it is important to make the diagnosis of a recurrence as soon as possible so that appropriate action can be taken if desired.

Raised maternal serum α-fetoprotein

Alpha-fetoprotein is a glycoprotein which is initially produced from the yolk sac in early pregnancy. Subsequently the major production is by the fetal liver but trace amounts are also produced by the stomach and small bowel. α-fetoprotein in the fetal serum is filtered through the glomeruli and reabsorbed by the tubules. However, a small amount passes down the ureters and into the bladder entering the amniotic fluid during micturition. α-fetoprotein can also leak into the amniotic fluid through skin defects, fetal autolysis, and so on. Its precise mechanism of entry into the maternal serum is uncertain but high levels can be encountered in the presence of placental abnormalities, and so on. Although the concentration of α-fetoprotein in the fetal serum peaks at around 13 weeks the maternal serum α-fetoprotein level peaks at 28–32 weeks.

In 1972 Brock and Sutcliffe [1] reported the findings of increased levels of amniotic α-fetoprotein in patients with anencephaly or spina bifida. In a collaborative study in the

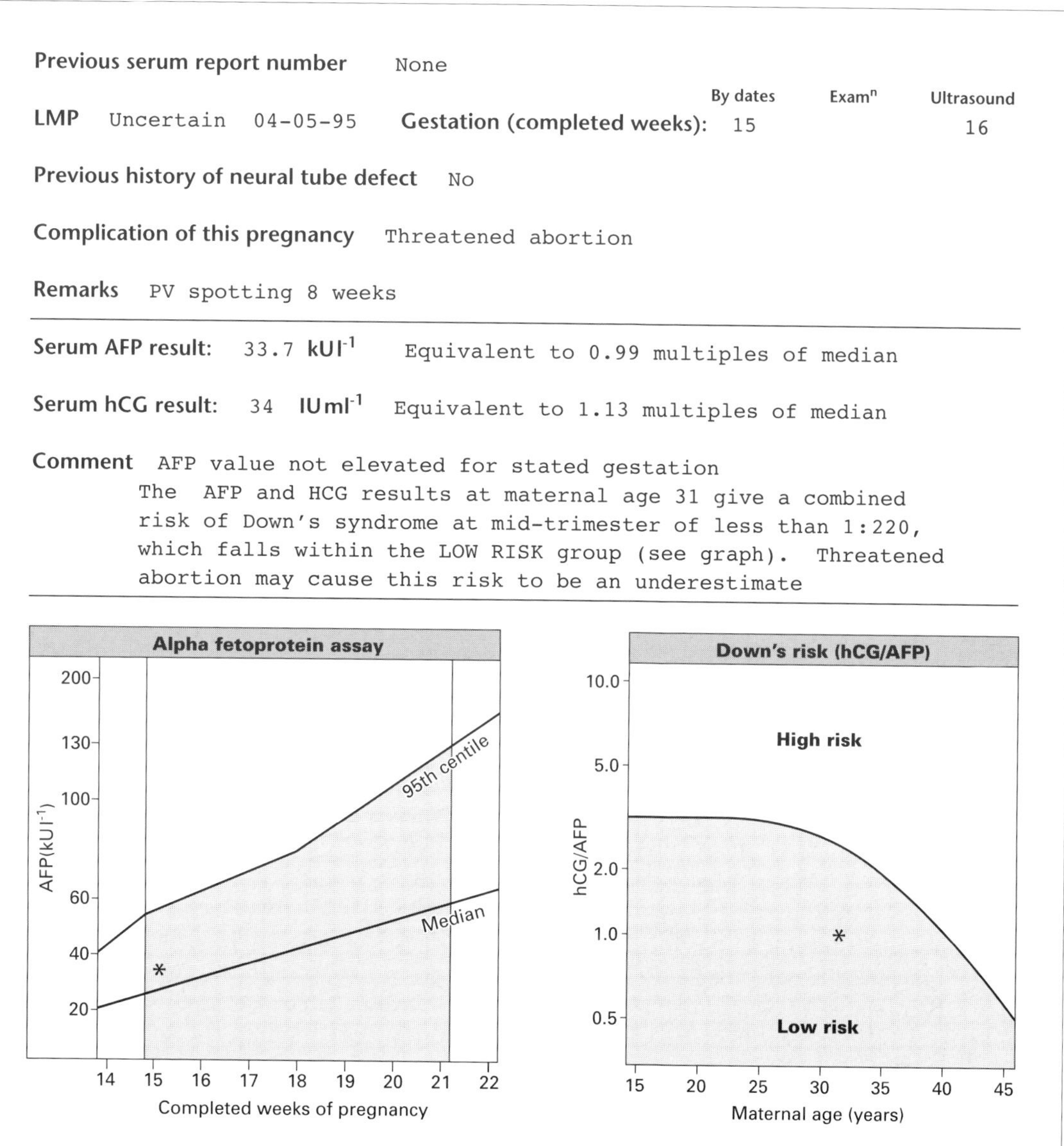

Previous serum report number None

			By dates	Exam^n	Ultrasound
LMP Uncertain 04-05-95	**Gestation (completed weeks):**		15		16

Previous history of neural tube defect No

Complication of this pregnancy Threatened abortion

Remarks PV spotting 8 weeks

Serum AFP result: 33.7 **kU l^{-1}** Equivalent to 0.99 multiples of median

Serum hCG result: 34 **IU ml^{-1}** Equivalent to 1.13 multiples of median

Comment AFP value not elevated for stated gestation
The AFP and HCG results at maternal age 31 give a combined risk of Down's syndrome at mid-trimester of less than 1:220, which falls within the LOW RISK group (see graph). Threatened abortion may cause this risk to be an underestimate

Fig. 37.25 A prenatal screening assay report as used in the West of Scotland Screening Programme.

UK it was subsequently found that 98% of anencephalics and 98% of open spina bifidas could be detected by the presence of elevated amniotic α-fetoprotein. The presence of acetylcholinesterase in the amniotic fluid increased the pick-up rate of neural tube defects to 99.5%. It was obviously impractical to offer amniocentesis to all patients and there was a slight risk associated with the procedure. Fortunately it was quickly realized that the level of α-fetoprotein in the maternal serum could be assessed and patients with abnormally high levels could then be offered amniocentesis. More recently it has become apparent that amniocentesis can be replaced by fetal anomaly scanning in the majority of instances.

Many centres now offer an α-fetoprotein screening programme. Unfortunately, there is a slight overlapping in the α-fetoprotein results from normal pregnancies and pregnancies with neural tube defects and this can result in a significant number of false positive and false negative readings. Most laboratories now determine their own cut-off point and this is usually 2 or 2.5 multiple of the median (MOM) (Fig. 37.25). The practice in most centres is to offer a fetal anomaly scan to anyone with readings above the cut-off point. Although the test was initially developed to identify patients with neural tube defects many causes for an elevated maternal serum α-fetoprotein have now been found.

Elevated serum α-fetoprotein

Incorrect dates. This is the commonest cause of an elevated α-fetoprotein and is due to the gestational age being underestimated at the time of carrying out the blood test. An early gestational age assessment should prevent this problem from arising.

Multiple gestation. Ten per cent of elevated maternal serum α-fetoprotein estimations are due to the presence of more than one fetus. Again this can be prevented by an early gestation scan. However, it must be remembered that there is a higher incidence of neural tube defects in twins than in singleton pregnancies and a detailed anomaly scan should be carried out if the α-fetoprotein estimation is above 3–3.5 MOM.

Intrauterine death. The α-fetoprotein level in these cases is extremely high and is felt to be due to the autolysis of fetal tissue.

Threatened abortion. The α-fetoprotein is frequently slightly elevated in patients who give a history of vaginal bleeding in the few days prior to the α-fetoprotein estimation.

Neural tube defects. There are three main tube defects, anencephaly, encephalocele and spina bifida. α-fetoprotein is felt to leak from the exposed neural tissue into the amniotic fluid and from there into the maternal serum. The levels in anencephaly are very high but may well be less marked in spina bifida. The level will be normal in patients with a closed spina bifida as no leakage of α-fetoprotein can take place. These abnormalities will be described in detail later.

Abdominal wall defects. Two principal defects give rise to an elevated serum α-fetoprotein, exomphalos and gastroschisis. The levels in gastroschisis are usually extremely high as loops of bowel are floating freely in the amniotic fluid and diffusion of fetal serum α-fetoprotein can readily take place into the fluid. The level may also be elevated in bladder extrophy and in a limb body wall abnormality.

Other abnormalities. An elevated maternal serum α-fetoprotein can also occur in some cases of gastrointestinal obstruction, such as oesophageal and duodenal atresia. It has been reported in several renal abnormalities, such as agenesis, obstruction and in particular congenital nephrosis; with sacrococcygeal teratomas, cystic hygromas, cyst adenomatous malformations and in several chromosome abnormalities.

Placental problems. The maternal serum α-fetoprotein is elevated in the presence of tumours of the placenta, such as chorioangioma and of the cord, such as haemangioma. An increased number of transonic areas are frequently observed in the placenta of patients with elevated α-fetoprotein and it has been suggested that episodes of fetomaternal transfusion have taken place in early pregnancy.

Unexplained. In the majority of patients undergoing ultrasound examination because of elevated maternal serum α-fetoprotein no abnormality of the fetus, placenta or liquor can be detected. However, many studies have indicated that such pregnancies are at increased risk of prematurity, low birth weight, intrauterine growth retardation and fetal mortality. Such patients should be regarded as at 'high risk' and should be very carefully followed up.

Low maternal serum α-fetoprotein

The association between a low maternal serum α-fetoprotein and chromosome abnormalities, such as trisomy 21, 18 and 13, was first reported by Merkatz *et al.* in 1984 [2]. The association between advancing maternal age and chromosome abnormalities had been well known for many years and many centres had been routinely offering chorionic villus sampling or amniocentesis to mothers over the age of 35 years. The identification of women with a maternal serum α-fetoprotein below 0.5 MOM should enable a further 25% of fetuses with trisomy 21 to be identified. In 1988 Wald *et al.* [3] reported that unconjugated oestriol levels were reduced in trisomy 21 and human chorionic gonadotrophin levels were increased. By using a combination of maternal age, α-fetoprotein, maternal serum unconjugated oestriol levels and the human chorionic gonadotrophin level, it has been possible to detect over 60% of fetuses with trisomy 21.

A fetal anomaly scan is not particularly helpful in patients with a low maternal serum α-fetoprotein as a normal scan will not exclude the presence of a chromosome abnormality. Some stigmata of a chromosomal lesion may be detected but ideally these patients should all have amniocentesis or chorionic villus sampling.

It is important to check that a patient with a low maternal serum α-fetoprotein has in fact been correctly dated. The presence of a long-standing intrauterine death or a hydatidform mole must also be excluded.

Patients having amniocentesis or CVS

The techniques and timing of these invasive procedures is discussed elsewhere. However, if they are performed before 18 weeks gestation the patient should be offered a detailed fetal anomaly scan to exclude a major fetal abnormality. It would be unhelpful to a patient to know that the fetus has a normal karyotype and to discover at delivery that it has a major abnormality, such as a diaphragmatic hernia, severe cardiac lesion, and so on.

Patients taking certain drugs

Because of the much publicized tragedy of thalidomide most patients are aware of the risks of taking drugs during pregnancy and keep it to a minumum. However, certain groups of patients may well be on long-term therapy for medical conditions or may take a short course of a drug without realizing that they are pregnant. Many drugs can be safely taken during pregnancy but others are known to be teratogenic. The effect that a drug may have depends on the stage of pregnancy during which it is taken.

In the pre-embryonic period which extends from conception to 17 days, a teratogenic drug will result in the destruction and absorption of the 'pregnancy'. The embryonic phase lasts from 18 to 55 days and during this time the organs are developing. Exposure to a teratogen at this time will result in the formation of abnormalities. If these abnormalities can be detected by ultrasound, it may be possible to diagnose them antenatally and give the parents the option of a termination. After 55 days the organs should be formed although they can be secondarily affected by some drugs, e.g. the development of a fetal goitre with carbimazole.

Certain groups of drugs are known to be teratogenic and should be avoided if at all possible during pregnancy, e.g. all forms of chemotherapy, some anticonvulsants, the vitamin A derivatives, lithium salts, stilboestrol and the coumarin anticoagulants.

In recent years the effects of alcohol on the fetus have been recognized and infants with the fetal alcohol syndrome may show evidence of microcephaly, facial hypoplasia and growth retardation.

The teratogenic effects of large doses of radiation have been recognized since the dropping of the atom bombs at Hiroshima and Nagasaki, and the nuclear testing in the Pacific Islands. The effects of small doses of radiation are more difficult to assess. The inadvertent use of diagnostic radiology in early pregnancy is unlikely to pose a problem. The exact timing of the exposure should be identified and if necessary a radiation physicist can be asked to assess the exact level of exposure. Maternal reassurance and a detailed anomaly scan at 18 weeks may well be all that is required. Exposure to radiation should be avoided throughout pregnancy if at all possible because of the minimal risk of carcinogenesis or genetic mutation. In each instance the possible risk to the developing fetus must be assessed against the need of the mother for the particular investigation.

Patients with diabetes mellitus

The incidence of fetal abnormality in insulin-dependent diabetics is about 10 times greater than that of the normal population. It is a particular problem in patients whose diabetes is poorly controlled. The anomalies encountered include congenital heart disease, renal, gastrointestinal and skeletal abnormalities, particularly the 'VACTERL' (vertebral, anal, cardiac, tracheo-oesophageal, renal and limb defects) and caudal regression syndromes. Babies of diabetic mothers frequently demonstrate macrosomia and there is an increased risk of pregnancy loss.

Patients with multiple pregnancy

The incidence of congenital abnormalities in twins is said to be 6–10% higher than in singleton pregnancies. It is now believed that this increased incidence is only related to monozygotic twins. Some of the abnormalities which have been described are believed to be due to thromboembolic insults, e.g. hydrocephaly, limb amputation, intestinal atresia or cardiac malformation. The possibility that the twins are conjoined must always be excluded.

Presence of polyhydramnios

Polyhydramnios is usually taken to refer to an amniotic fluid index (see Fig. 39.2) of greater than 2 litres. It is said to occur in around 1% of pregnancies. The majority of cases of polyhydramnios are idiopathic but the condition is also found in patients with diabetes mellitus and multiple pregnancy. Congenital abnormalities account for about one-fifth of cases and are usually abnormalities resulting in impaired fetal swallowing, e.g. anencephaly, or an upper gastrointestinal tract atresia resulting in impaired absorption of amniotic fluid by the bowel, e.g. oesophageal atresia or duodenal atresia.

Polyhydramnios may also occur in the presence of some genitourinary, lung or skeletal abnormalities.

An underlying cause for the condition is most likely to be found in cases where the polyhydramnios is severe.

Presence of oligohydramnios

There is no agreed volume of amniotic fluid which comprises oligohydramnios. Some workers define oligohydramnios as an amniotic fluid index of less than 5. Others measure the largest single pocket of amniotic fluid and if it is less than 3 cm or 1 cm, diagnose oligohydramnios. With practice a significant decrease in amniotic fluid volume can be assessed subjectively.

Oligohydramnios is due to intrauterine growth retardation, premature rupture of membranes, post-term pregnancies or fetal abnormalities involving the urinary tract. These abnormalities may be due to renal agenesis, bilateral renal obstruction or severe bilateral parenchymal disease. This topic is described in greater detail elsewhere.

Patients with a symmetrical growth retarded fetus

There is an increased incidence of chromosome abnormalities in such fetuses and a careful search for stigmata of such lesions should be made and karyotyping offered if they are found.

Patients with a breech presentation who are going to be delivered by caesarean section

Very occasionally a breech presentation may be due to some fetal abnormality resulting in inability of the head to descend into the pelvis, e.g. cystic hygroma of the neck. It is undesirable to perform a caesarean section if the fetus has a severe life-threatening abnormality and although it is technically difficult to perform a fetal anomaly scan at term, gross lesions such as hydrocephalus, can be excluded.

Parental consanguinity

There is an increased incidence of autosomal recessive disorders in children of parents who are blood relatives and the incidence of major congenital malformations rises to about 4%. Fetal anomaly scanning should be offered particularly if the couple have had a previously abnormal child.

References

1 Brock, D.J.M., Sutcliffe, R. (1972) Alpha-fetoprotein in the antenatal diagnosis of anencephaly and spina bifida. *Lancet* **ii**, 197–199.

2 Merkatz, I.R., Nitowsky, H.M., Macri, J.N., Johnson, W.E. (1984) An association between low maternal serum alpha-fetoprotein and fetal chromosomal abnormalities. *American Journal of Obstetrics and Gynaecology* **148**, 886–894.

3 Wald, N.J., Cuckle, H.S., Densem, J.W., *et al.* (1988) Maternal serum screening for Down's syndrome in early pregnancy. *British Medical Journal* **297**, 883–887.

Chapter 38: Fetal malformations

J.R. MacKenzie

Cerebral and spinal

This group of deformities is responsible for about 50% of the abnormalities which can be detected on antenatal ultrasound. The abnormalities are often major and may prove lethal or may result in severe chronic problems in later life.

Neural tube defects

This group of abnormalities comprises anencephaly, encephalocele and spina bifida. The incidence of neural tube defects varies throughout the world and for many years the west of Scotland, Fife, Wales and Northern Ireland had a particularly high incidence. Fortunately in recent years the true incidence of the condition has fallen and it is now found in 3.5 pregnancies per 1000 in the west of Scotland. The incidence of anencephaly and spina bifida is approximately equal. The cause of neural tube defects is unknown but is currently thought to be due to a deficiency of folic acid in the mother. There is a significant recurrence risk which rises to 3–5% after one neural tube defect and to 10% after two pregnancies involving a neural tube defect. Families where there is a close relative with spina bifida should be offered fetal anomaly scanning.

Mothers of fetuses with anencephaly and encephalocele will have a very high maternal serum α-fetoprotein (AFP). The AFP result is also elevated in fetuses with an open spina bifida but is normal if the spina bifida is closed.

Anencephaly

This condition is due to absence of the cerebral hemispheres and the cranial vault. There is normal development of the base of the skull and the brainstem and mid brain are present.

Although the condition is present as early as the embryonic stage of development it is usually only recognized in the early part of the second trimester. The advent of vaginal scanning has enabled it to be diagnosed a little earlier in some instances. The condition may be suspected in the first trimester if the crown–rump length is abnormally small for definitely known dates.

In the second trimester the absence of the vault will be apparent and it will be impossible to obtain a biparietal diameter. The orbits are noted to be prominent (frog's eyes) (Fig. 38.1). There is frequently polyhydramnios and because of this the fetus is often extremely active. On occasions it may be impossible to distinguish anencephaly from extremely severe types of microcephaly. Associated abnormalities are common and spinal dysraphism is present in up to one-third of fetuses.

The condition is lethal, the fetuses usually dying within a few hours of birth. Because of this termination of the pregnancy is usually acceptable to most parents.

Encephalocele

This abnormality is due to a defect in the cranial vault which allows the herniation of a meningocele (meninges plus cerebrospinal fluid) or encephalocele (meninges plus brain). The herniation is usually posterior though anterior encephaloceles may occur.

Ultrasonically a mass is seen in the mid line posteriorly or anteriorly. The mass may consist of fluid, brain or a combination of the two. If the mass is large it is most readily identified on an axial view of the vault at the level of the thalami (Fig. 38.2). Smaller posterior encephaloceles are more readily identified if the scanning plane is angled through the posterior fossa. The larger lesions are usually associated with microcephaly. In some instances the defect in the cranial vault may be visible particularly in the occipital region.

There is an extremely high incidence of hydrocephalus associated with the abnormality and there may also be spinal dysraphism. The condition is found in a variety of multiple anomaly syndromes, the commonest being the Meckel–Gruber syndrome. This is an autosomal recessive condition in which the fetus has infantile polycystic kidneys, an occipital encephalocele and polydactyly. There is a 1 in 4 chance of recurrence of this condition.

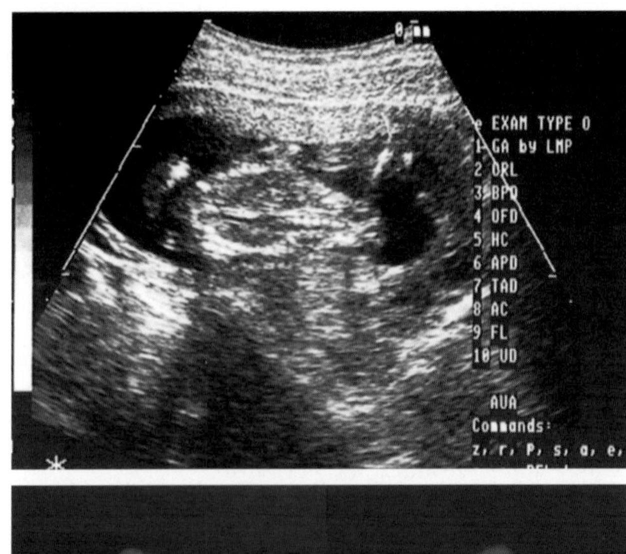

(a)

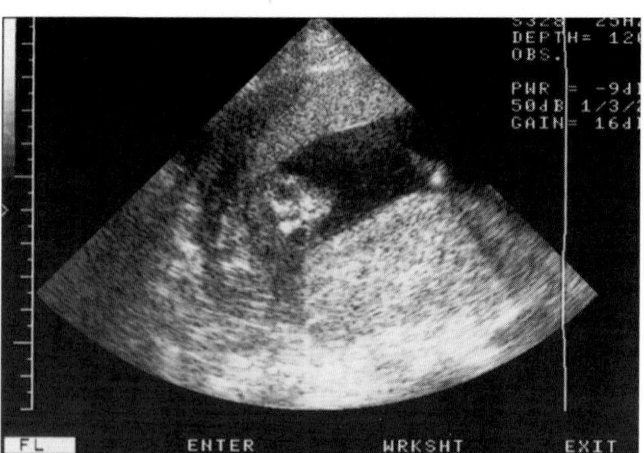

(b)

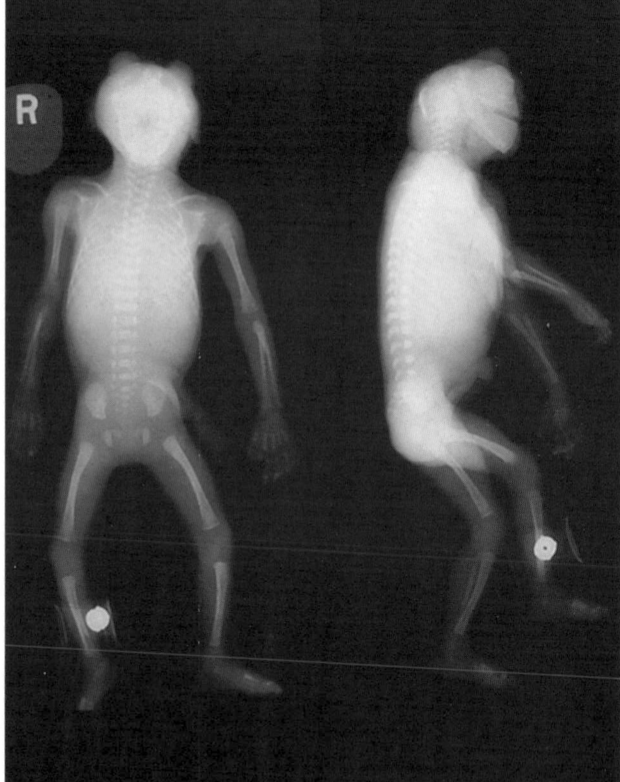

(c)

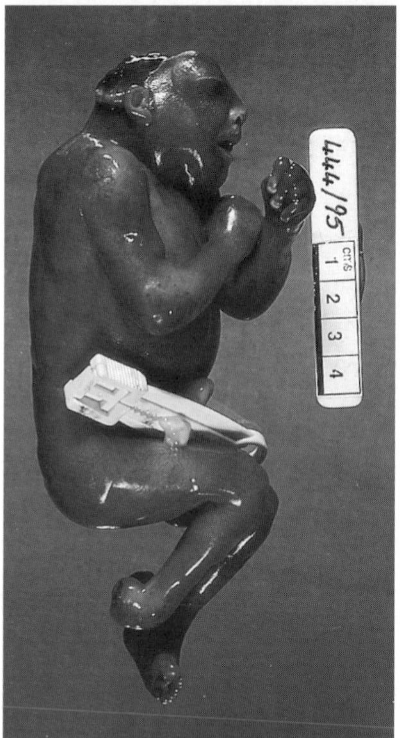

(d)

Fig. 38.1 Anencephaly. (a) Longitudinal scan of a fetus showing an absence of the cranial vault on the left of the scan. (b) Axial view of the hind part of the brain of the same fetus demonstrating the orbits and an absence of the vault. (c) X-ray of a fetus with anencephaly. (d) Pathological specimen. (Courtesy of Dr A. Howatson, Royal Hospital for Sick Children, Glasgow.)

The prognosis for encephaloceles depends on the size of the lesion and the amount of herniated brain within the lesion. A termination may well be a reasonable option for a fetus with a large lesion containing brain with associated microcephaly and hydrocephaly.

Spina bifida

Spina bifida is due to a defect involving the dorsal arch of the spine. In the two types which can be diagnosed antenatally there is protrusion of the meninges through the defect. In a meningocele the protrusion consists of meninges and cerebrospinal fluid. This form accounts for

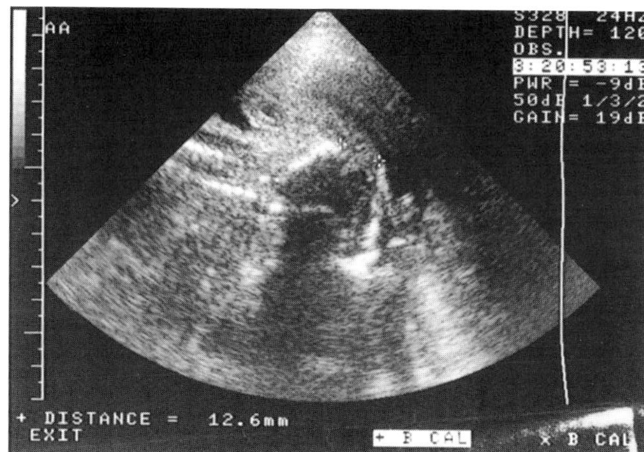

(a)

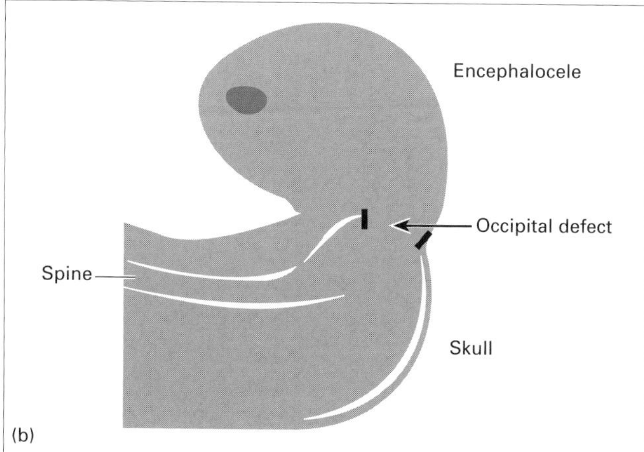

(b)

Fig. 38.2 Encephalocele. (a) A fetus with marked microcephaly and a large defect in the occipital bone through which the brain is herniating. (b) Diagram of the scan.

	Normal	Abnormal	
Sagittal			
Coronal			
Axial		Open lesion	Closed lesion

(a)

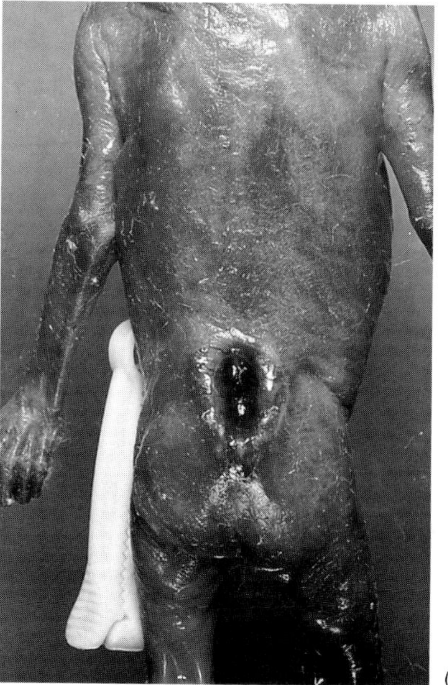

(b)

Fig. 38.3 Spina bifida. (a) Diagram of normal and abnormal spines in sagittal, coronal and axial planes. (b) Postmortem specimen of open lumbar spina bifida. (Courtesy of Dr A. Howatson, Royal Hospital for Sick Children, Glasgow.)

10% of those diagnosed antenatally. In a myelomeningocele as well as protrusion of meninges and cerebrospinal fluid, there is also involvement of neural tissue. This type accounts for 90% of prenatal spina bifida. A further division can be made into open and closed lesions. In a closed lesion the defect is covered with skin or with a thick membrane. In an open lesion the membrane is thin or may be absent allowing neural tissue to be exposed to the amniotic fluid. Leakage of fetal AFP occurs into the amniotic fluid in the presence of an open lesion and results in an elevated maternal serum AFP. About two-thirds of spina bifidas occur in the lumbosacral region.

In about 90% of cases of spina bifida the cerebellum is pulled down into the upper cervical region by tethering of the cord (Arnold–Chiari malformation type 2). This results in obliteration of the cisterna magna with the subsequent development of hydrocephalus.

The diagnosis of spina bifida depends on the identification of a defect in the posterior elements of the spine during an ultrasound examination. The spine should be assessed in three planes, the axial, sagittal and coronal (Fig. 38.3). In the axial plane the dorsal ossification centres will be found to diverge rather than converge. A related cystic mass may be apparent or the overlying skin may be deficient (Fig. 38.4). Care must be taken to carry out the examination perpendicular to each neural arch. A false positive diagnosis can occasionally occur if the spine is imaged obliquely and the body of one vertebrae is inadvertently linked with the ossification centres of another. In the coronal projection the echoes for the dorsal ossification centres will seem to diverge and the distance between the

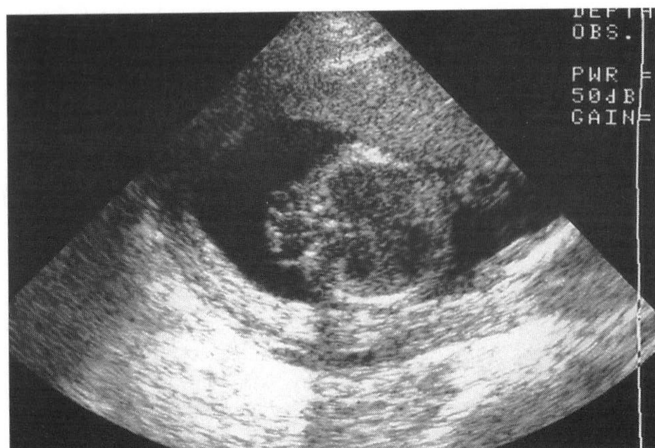

Fig. 38.4 Spina bifida. Axial view demonstrating a meningocele posterior to the spine at the level of the kidneys.

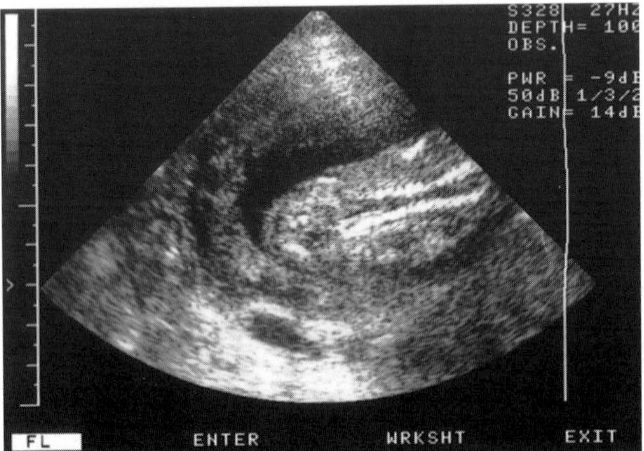

Fig. 38.5 Spina bifida. Coronal view showing a widening of the interpedicular distance in the lumbar region and disruption of the sacrum.

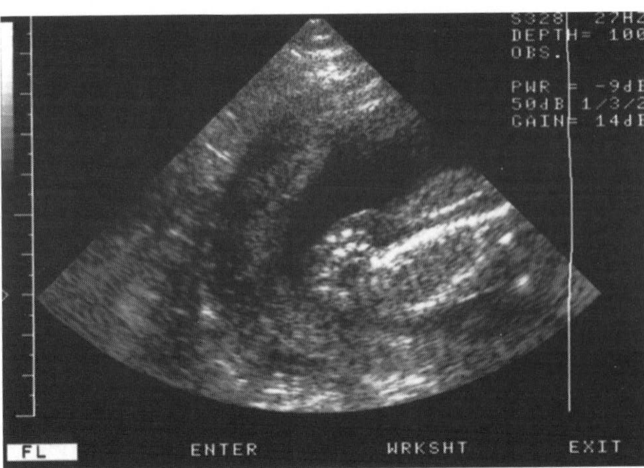

Fig. 38.6 Spina bifida. Sagittal view showing severe kyphosis with meningocele (same case as Fig. 38.5).

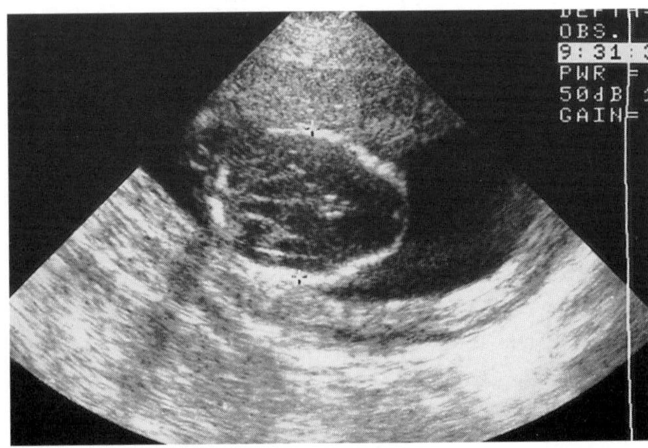

Fig. 38.7 Lemon sign. Axial scan of the vault with indentation of the frontal bones and mild hydrocephalus in a fetus with spina bifida.

centres will be increased (Fig. 38.5). The dorsal ossification centres will be absent or abnormally situated in the sagittal plane and again a cystic mass or absence of the overlying skin may be apparent (Fig. 38.6). A related scoliosis or kyphosis may be observed.

The diagnosis of a small spina bifida and in particular of a sacral spina bifida may be extremely difficult and the examination should always be carried out after 18 weeks gestation. In the majority of cases of spina bifida, there will be related intracranial abnormalities which are easier to detect.

1 Shape and size of vault. The biparietal diameter is frequently less than expected for a known gestation. The frontal bones at the level of the ventricles are indented up to about 24 weeks gestation (Fig. 38.7). This indentation was called the 'lemon' sign by Nicolaides *et al.* when they first described it in 1986 [1]. The sign is only rarely observed in normal fetuses. Care must be taken not to confuse the slight indentation normally seen immediately above the orbits for a lemon sign.

2 Hydrocephalus. Eighty per cent of fetuses with spina bifida will develop hydrocephalus antenatally. The severity varies from case to case. However, in many fetuses the biparietal diameter will still be within normal limits at term despite the ventricular dilatation. The hydrocephalus may be assessed by measuring the transverse atrial diameter which is normally less than 10 mm or by estimating the ventricular to hemispheric width ratio. The assessment of the position of the choroid plexus may be all that is necessary (Fig. 38.8).

3 Posterior fossa changes. As already indicated most of the fetuses have an Arnold–Chiari malformation. The

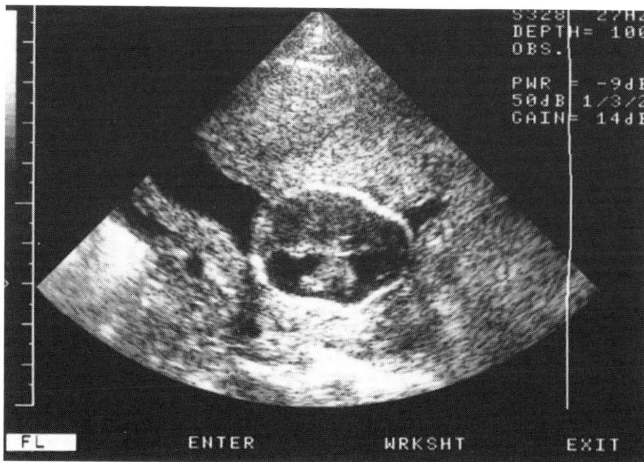

Fig. 38.8 Hydrocephalus—spina bifida. Severe hydrocephalus in a fetus with a large spina bifida (same case as Fig. 38.5). There is also a lemon sign.

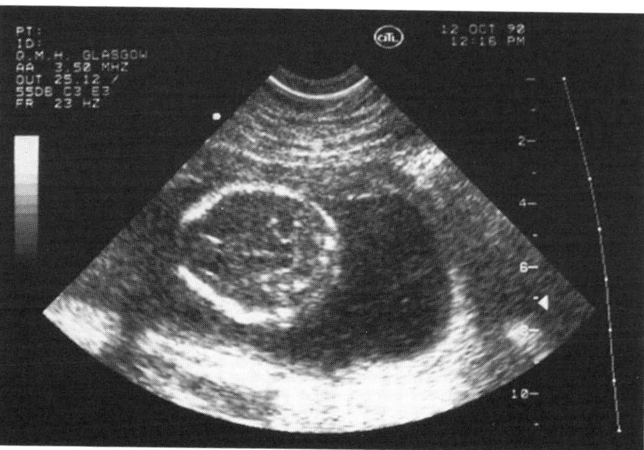

Fig. 38.9 Banana sign. The normal shape of the cerebellum is distorted and the cisterna magna is obliterated. (Courtesy of Dr M. McNay, Queen Mother's Hospital, Glasgow.)

configuration of the cerebellum is altered with loss of the cisterna magna. The shape of the cerebellum has been described as the 'banana' sign (Fig. 38.9). In some cases the cerebellum is so displaced into the upper cervical canal that it cannot be identified within the vault. This results in an 'empty posterior fossa' (Fig. 38.10).

The presence of any or all of these features is strongly suggestive of the diagnosis of spina bifida and an extremely careful search of the whole spine must be made to locate the position and size of the lesion. The prognosis for the condition depends on the size and position of the lesion and the severity of the related intracranial problems. A child with a small sacral lesion may have an excellent prognosis whereas the child with a larger thoracolumbar lesion will almost certainly require a ventricular shunt, will be confined to a wheelchair and will have bowel and bladder problems. Following the diagnosis of a fetus with spina bifida the parents should receive careful conselling and the assistance of a paediatrician or paediatric surgeon is invaluable.

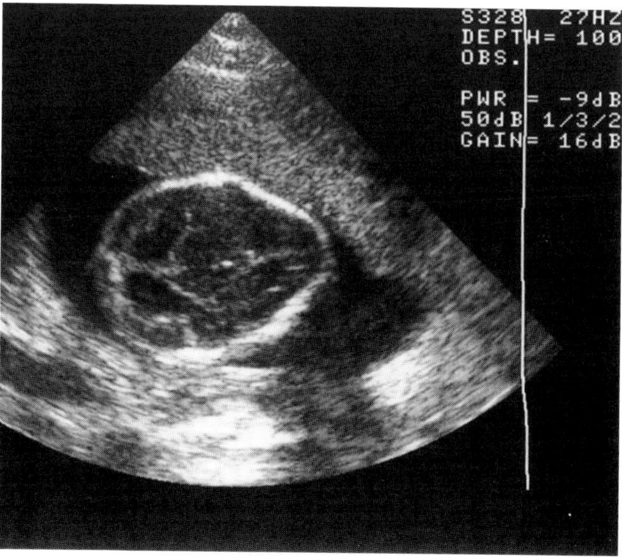

Fig. 38.10 Absent cerebellum. A fetus with severe spina bifida in whom the cerebellum cannot be identified. The posterior fossa is taken up by fluid.

Hydrocephalus

Hydrocephalus results from an abnormal amount of cerebrospinal fluid within the cranial cavities. Most cases are due to obstruction in the ventricular system (non-communicating hydrocephalus) or in the subarachnoid spaces (communicating hydrocephalus).

The commonest cause of hydrocephalus diagnosed antenatally is a neural tube defect (30%). Aqueduct stenosis accounts for about 20% of cases and the Dandy–Walker syndrome 5–10%. Hydrocephalus is frequently found in the multiple anomaly syndromes such as Meckel–Gruber and Apert's syndrome. It is also found in trisomy 18 and 13 and occasionally trisomy 21.

Hydrocephalus can be diagnosed simply by observing an increase in the amount of fluid in the ventricular system and noting the position of the choroid plexus relative to the walls of the ventricles. Normally the choroid plexus completely fills the lateral ventricles during the second trimester. With the accumulation of an increased amount of cerebrospinal fluid the choroid plexus moves away from the medial wall of the lateral ventricle and dangles down into the dilated ventricle (Fig. 38.11). The choroid plexus from the uppermost ventricle may herni-

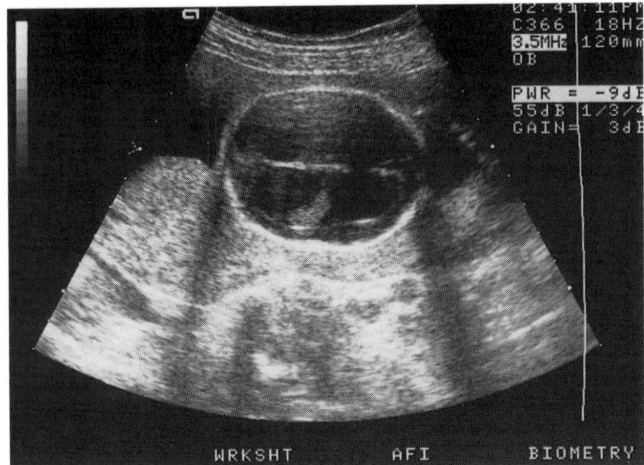

(a)

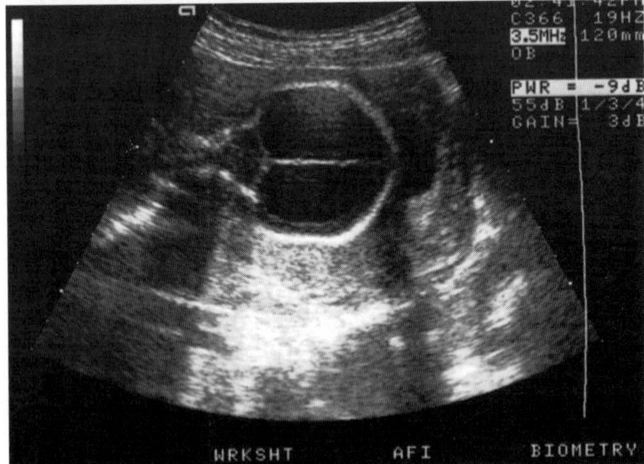

(b)

Fig. 38.11 Isolated hydrocephalus. (a) Axial view showing a 'dangling choroid plexus' and marked ventricular dilatation. (b) Coronal view of the same case.

ate into the lower ventricle. The ventricular to hemispheric width ratio has been used by some workers. A measurement is made from the mid line echo to the lateral wall of the lateral ventricle in the parietal region and from the same mid point to the inner table of the parietal bone. Tables are available relating the ratio to the fetal gestation.

Some workers have measured the ratios of the anterior horn to the hemisphere and the posterior horn to the hemisphere, whilst others find a measurement of the transverse atrial diameter to be of more value. This normally measures up to 10 mm and a measurement greater than this indicates a degree of ventricular dilatation.

Following the identification of hydrocephalus on ultrasound a careful search must be made for the primary cause of the condition, e.g. spina bifida, encephalocele. A search must also be made for any markers of a chromosome abnormality or any anomaly outwith the central nervous system.

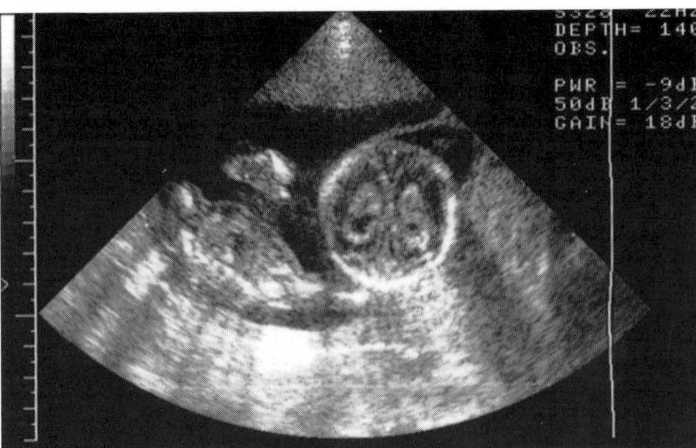

Fig. 38.12 Choroid plexus cysts. Bilateral cysts in a twin. There were no other abnormalities and the cysts resolved at 22 weeks. The twins were normal at birth.

The prognosis is dependent on the degree of hydrocephalus and the presence or absence of other abnormalities. If a decision is made to continue with the pregnancy it is helpful to monitor the size of the ventricles and of the cerebral cortex on a regular basis. The head size may increase markedly in the presence of a severe hydrocephalus and this will have implications for delivery. Intrauterine shunting of hydrocephalus has been attempted but the results have been discouraging.

Choroid plexus cysts

Choroid plexus cysts are thought to be due to the entrapment of cerebrospinal fluid in the villi of the choroid plexus. With increasing gestation the amount of stroma in the choroid plexus decreases and the fluid collections become smaller. Choroid plexus cysts occur at any age and are frequently found at autopsy in adults.

The cysts are identified as transonic areas within the echogenic choroid plexus. They are usually bilateral although a cyst in the near hemisphere may be obscured by reverberations. They vary in size from 3 mm to over 20 mm and they may be round or oval. The majority are single but multilocular cysts can occur (Fig. 38.12).

The exact incidence of choroid plexus cysts is unknown as many series are based on high risk pregnancies rather than the normal population. However, they probably occur in about 1% of pregnancies between 16 and 24 weeks. The majority of cysts become smaller between 20 and 24 weeks and have disappeared by 26 weeks.

The management of a fetus with a choroid plexus cyst is one of the most controversial topics in the current practice of fetal medicine. This is due to the association of the cysts with chromosome abnormalities particulary trisomy 18. Unfortunately, much of the data about the association has come from high risk pregnancies. This data suggests that the incidence of trisomy 18 in a pregnancy with a choroid plexus cyst is around 1%. This is greater than the risk of a 35-year-old woman having a fetus with trisomy 21 and here genetic testing would be routinely offered. Some perinatal specialists feel karotyping should be offered if a choroid plexus cyst is identified. Others believe that the true risk of the fetus having trisomy 18 is considerably less and that, provided the cysts disappear and there are no other abnormalities on a careful ultrasound examination, karotyping is not indicated. In our own series of 30 patients one was found to have trisomy 18 and in this fetus the cysts were large, multilocular and had not shown any decrease in size at 24 weeks.

Aqueduct stenosis

This condition accounts for just under 20% of the cases of hydrocephalus diagnosed antenatally. It is usually due to a congenital abnormality of the aqueduct resulting in atresia or stenosis. However, it can also result from intrauterine infection, haemorrhage or compression by an adjacent tumour. The possibility that it is due to an X-linked disorder must be considered in a male fetus.

The condition is characterized by dilatation of the lateral and third ventricles. The prognosis is dependent on the degree of dilatation.

Holoprosencephaly

Three types of this condition have been described, alobar, semi-lobar and lobar. The first two types can be diagnosed antenatally. The condition results from a failure of the forebrain to develop into the cerebral hemispheres and lateral ventricles. The condition is characterized by the presence of a single ventricle, the absence of the falx and the presence of fused mid line thalami.

There is a strong association between holoprosencephaly and trisomy 13, 18 and triploidy. Facial abnormalities are particularly common and should be carefully looked for. The majority of infants with this condition die shortly after birth, though the occasional child may live for up to 1 year.

Dandy–Walker syndrome

This condition is due to complete or partial absence of the cerebellum with cystic dilatation of the fourth ventricle and, in the majority of cases, hydrocephalus (Fig. 38.13). The condition is readily identifiable on ultrasound scanning. There is a high incidence of related abnormalities of the central nervous system, e.g. aqueduct stenosis or agenesis of the corpus callosum. Between a quarter and a half

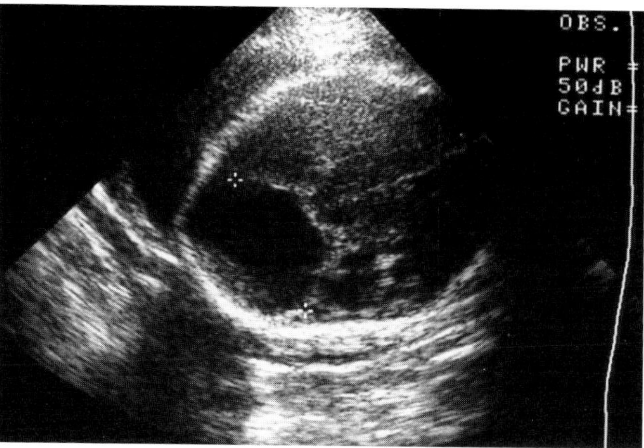

Fig. 38.13 Dandy–Walker syndrome. 'Cyst' occupying the posterior fossa and causing minimal hydrocephalus.

of the cases are found to have abnormalities outwith the central nervous system. The ultimate prognosis is very much dependent on the presence of these abnormalities.

Hydranencephaly

This rare abnormality is due to the absence of the cerebral hemispheres. It is thought to result from massive cerebral infarction secondary to the occlusion of the internal carotid arteries. Ultrasonically the falx can be identified within a fluid-filled head. The mid brain, basal ganglia and posterior fossa are normal. The condition may be confused with holoprosencephaly but in the latter condition there is no evidence of a falx.

Microcephaly

Microcephaly can be defined as a head size which is more than 3 standard deviations below the mean. The exact incidence is unknown, figures varying from 1 in 1000 to 1 in 50 000 births. It may occur as part of a syndrome and is then usually due to an autosomal recessive condition, e.g. Meckel–Gruber, Joubert's or Roberts' syndrome; an X-linked form has also been described. The condition may arise from exposure to infections such as rubella, cytomegalovirus or toxoplasmosis.

It may also occur as part of the fetal alcohol syndrome or may result from exposure to certain drugs (phenytoin, aminopterin). Exposure to radiation has also been implicated.

In severe cases the head size will appear too small for the remainder of the fetus. Less severe cases can be identified by plotting the growth in head size—either the biparietal diameter or preferably the head circumference—against gestation. The ratio of head circumference to

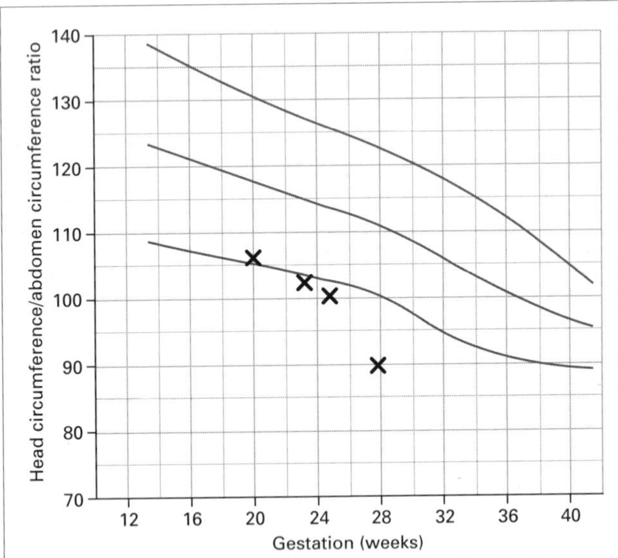

Fig. 38.14 Graph of head circumference to abdominal circumference ratio against gestational age in a fetus with microcephaly.

abdominal circumference is invaluable (Fig. 38.14). Unfortunately, in many instances the condition cannot be diagnosed until after 25 weeks. A view of the facial profile is sometimes helpful in demonstrating marked flattening of the frontal bone. A careful search should be made for other fetal abnormalities. Most of the fetuses with microcephaly will suffer from mental retardation.

Caudal regression syndrome

This condition is due to the complete or partial absence of the sacrum and/or lumbosacral spine. There may be a related abnormality of the lower limbs with fusion or absence. There is a strong association between this condition, the VACTERL syndrome (vertebral, anal, cardiac, tracheo-oesophageal, renal and limb defects) and poorly controlled diabetes mellitus. Sirenomelia (fusion of the lower limbs) is fatal. Prognosis for the other types of the abnormality is poor although children with sacral agenesis frequently survive with severe bladder problems.

Sacrococcygeal teratoma

This is a tumour which arises from the embryonic cells of the coccyx. It occurs in around 1 in 35000 births and female infants are more commonly affected. The tumour gives rise to elevated levels of maternal serum AFP. The tumour may be external, pelvic or intra-abdominal and the prognosis depends on whether the tumour can be complely excised. Residual tumour tissue may become malignant.

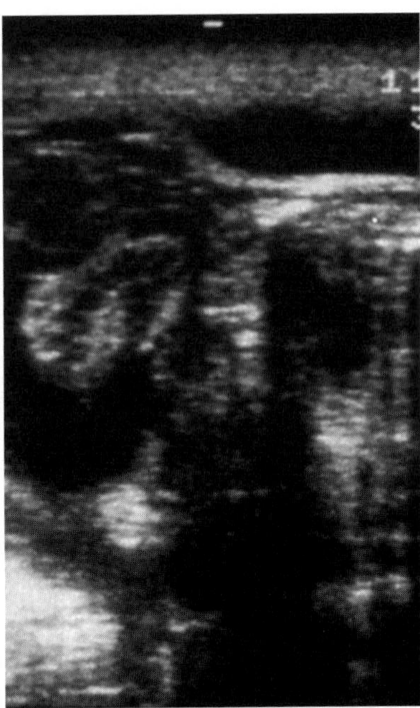

Fig. 38.15 Sacrococcygeal teratoma. A large mass at the lower end of the sacrum containing solid and cystic components in a 27-week fetus. The mass was successfully removed following delivery.

The tumour can be detected ultrasonically and may appear as a cystic, mixed solid and cystic, or entirely solid mass in relation to the sacrum with extension into the pelvic cavity or abdomen (Fig. 38.15). Polyhydramnios will be identified in three-quarters of the cases and in a quarter the fetus will be hydropic.

Other cerebral and spinal abnormalities

It is possible to diagnose several other intracranial abnormalities on ultrasound including agenesis of the corpus callosum, arachnoid cysts (Fig. 38.16), porencephaly and schizencephaly. Intracranial neoplasms have been detected. Intracranial haemorrhage has been recorded particularly in fetuses suffering from alloimmune thrombocytopenia.

Some skeletal abnormalities may be diagnosed from the antenatal appearance of the spine and cases of diastomatomyelia, hemivertebrae and scoliosis have been identified.

Face and neck

With the exception of cleft lip and palate, abnormalities of the face are rare. Whenever possible a careful examination of the eyes, nose, lips, palate and ears should be made. The interocular distance is increased in hypertelorism and this can occur in association with agenesis of the corpus callosum, an anterior encephalocele or as part of the median

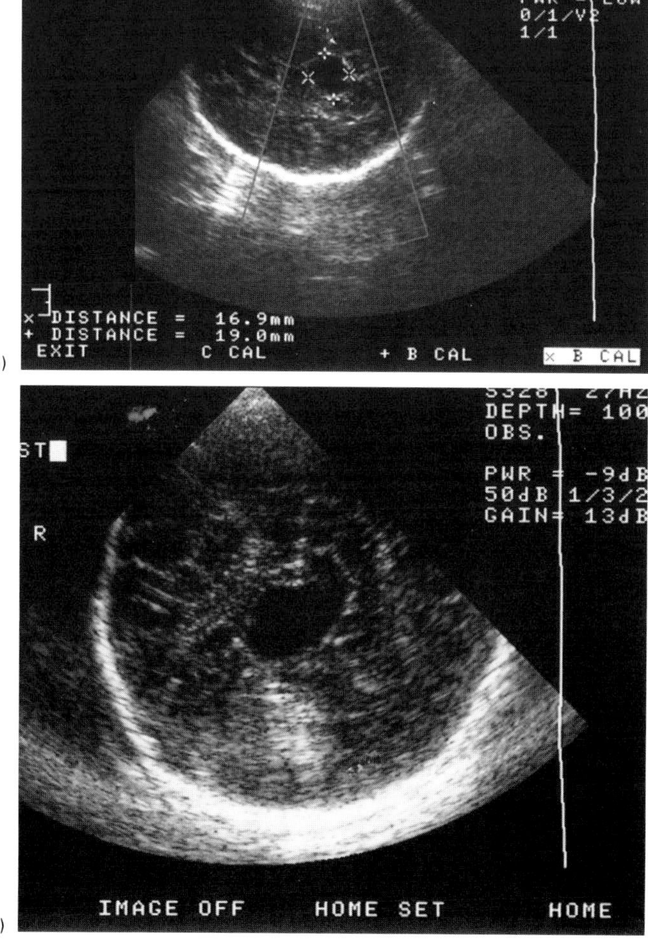

Fig. 38.16 Arachnoid cyst. Mid line cyst lying posterior to the third ventricle initially diagnosed at 25 weeks gestation. (a) Antenatal scan at 36 weeks. (b) Postnatal scan 4 weeks later. The neonate is well with no neurological problems.

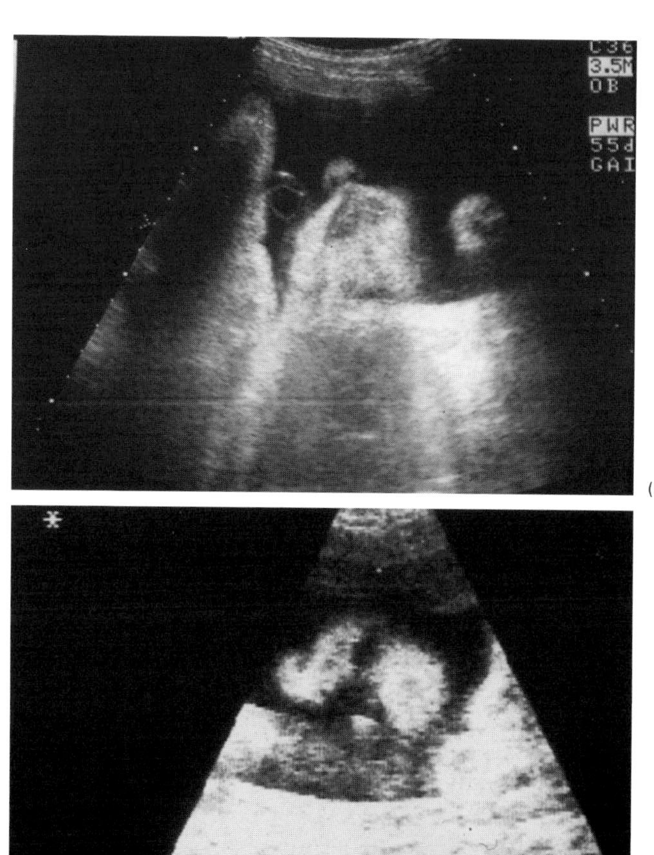

Fig. 38.17 (a) Normal view of the nostrils, lips and mouth. (b) Unilateral cleft in the right upper lip.

facial cleft syndrome. Hypotelorism is associated with holoprosencephaly. A proboscis is frequently found in association with this and there may be related orbital abnormalities such as cyclops. A large tongue (macroglossia) may be identified in the Beckwith–Wiedemann syndrome. The Pierre Robin syndrome is characterized by underdevelopment of the mandible (micrognathia) with a soft palate cleft.

Cleft lip and palate

This condition represents 10% of all congenital abnormalities and it may be complete or incomplete, unilateral or bilateral (Fig. 38.17). A cleft palate occurs in two-thirds of cases of fetuses with a cleft lip. The condition is frequently familial. One of the main benefits of identifying a cleft lip and/or palate antenatally is its known association with chromosome abnormalities particularly trisomy 13 and 18 and triplody. It is also associated with many malformations and syndromes such as holoprosencephaly, amniotic band syndrome and Meckel–Gruber syndrome.

Cardiothoracic and abdominal malformations

Cardiothoracic abnormalities

The heart is situated in the left side of the thorax. Part of the right and left atria normally lie outwith this quadrant. The apex of the heart is situated immediately behind the left chest wall. A four-chamber view of the heart can be obtained on a horizontal section just above the diaphragm. The atria are of the same size and the ventricles are of similar size up to 32 weeks gestation when the right ventricle may appear slightly larger than the left. The atrioventricular valves are situated at right angles to the ventriculoatrial septa. The foramen ovale is situated within the atrial septum with the flap opening towards the left atrium. About 95% of cardiac abnormalities which can be demonstrated on ultrasound will show some form of abnormality on the four-chamber view. Congenital heart disease occurs in 8 per 1000 live births and is an important cause of perinatal and neonatal death. Although the cause of most congenital heart lesions is unknown several risk factors have been identified.

1 Family history. Five per cent of cases are said to be due to some form of familial inherited disorder. A recurrence risk of 1 in 50 is given if there is a previous child with a congenital heart defect rising to 1 in 10 with two children affected. A similar risk is given if either parent had a congenital heart lesion.

2 Maternal diabetes. The incidence of congenital heart disease is five times greater in diabetics than in the normal population. Ventricular septal defects and transposition of the great arteries are the most likely abnormalities. The incidence can be minimized if control of the diabetes is adequate. Other maternal conditions such as collagen disorders and phenylketonuria are also associated with an increased risk of congenital heart disease.

3 Perinatal infections. There is an increased risk of pulmonary artery stenosis, patent ductus arteriosus and coarctation in infants whose mothers have contracted rubella in the first trimester. Cytomegalovirus infections have been associated with atrial septal defects and mitral stenosis.

4 Drugs. The risk of congenital heart disease is increased in mothers taking phenytoin, phenobarbitone, lithium and steroids including the oral contraceptive pill. Alcohol abuse has been linked with an increased incidence of atrial and ventricular septal defects.

5 Chromosome abnormality. There is an increased risk of congenital heart disease in fetuses with a chromosome abnormality particularly trisomy 21 and to a lesser extent trisomies 18 and 13.

Twenty-five per cent of infants with a congenital heart lesion have other abnormalities particularly in the central nervous system, the gastrointestinal system and the genitourinary system. A careful fetal anomaly scan is essential whenever a cardiac lesion is suspected antenatally. Twenty-five per cent of cases of fetal hydrops are due to an underlying congenital heart lesion and an expert assessment of the heart is essential in all such cases.

The lungs

The fetal lungs are clearly seen during the second trimester and their echogenicity can vary. The fetal thorax grows at a constant rate between 16 and 40 weeks and the ratio of chest circumference to abdominal circumference, head circumference, biparietal diameter and femoral length remains constant in normal pregnancies. The thoracic circumference is usually measured on an axial view at the same level as a four-chamber view, the skin and subcutaneous tissues being excluded. The ratio of thoracic circumference to abdominal circumference is of great value in the determination of pulmonary hypoplasia.

Normal fetal lung growth is dependent on the presence of adequate intrathoracic space and the presence of sufficient amniotic fluid. Four stages of normal development are described: the embryonic period, the pseudoglandular period, the canalicular phase and, finally, the alveolar phase. An abnormality may occur at any of these stages and may result in respiratory dysfunction following delivery.

It is important to determine the position of the heart in any assessment of the thorax. Mediastinal shift may result from the presence of a fluid collection in the thorax or a mass, or from an underlying congenital abnormality resulting in underdevelopment of a lung.

Pulmonary hypoplasia

Pulmonary hypoplasia occurs in about 1.5% of live births but is commoner in stillbirths and neonatal deaths. It is due to underdevelopment of the acini of the lung and the severity depends on the age of onset and the duration and severity of the precipitating factor.

Pulmonary hypoplasia usually occurs secondary to prolonged oligohydramnios and this in turn may be due to a severe renal abnormality, severe intrauterine growth retardation or premature rupture of the membranes. Pulmonary hypoplasia may also occur as a result of an intrathoracic mass lesion such as a diaphragmatic hernia, a cystadenomatous malformation or a large fluid collection. It may occur secondary to a skeletal dysplasia which affects the thoracic cage and has been described in some abnormalities of the cardiovascular and the central nervous systems, as well as in some chromosome abnormalities.

When pulmonary hypoplasia is suspected the thoracic circumference should be measured regularly and plotted against gestation (Fig. 38.18). A careful search should be made for a precipitating factor such as a renal abnormality. The presence of oligohydramnios may make the assessment of the fetus extremely difficult and this can be helped by the infusion of saline into the amniotic cavity.

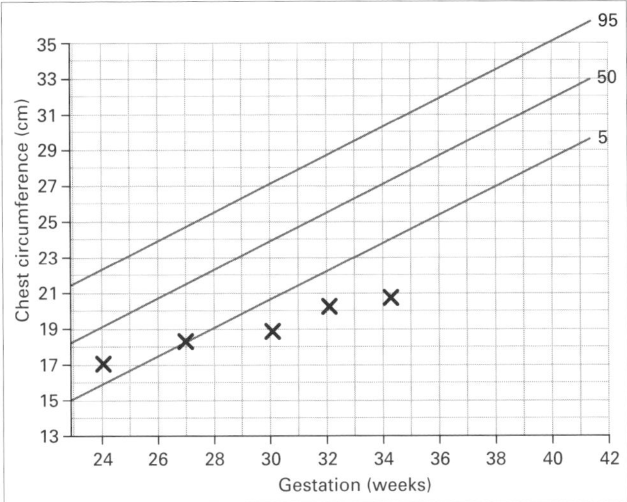

Fig. 38.18 A graph showing the thoracic circumference in a fetus with pulmonary hypoplasia due to posterior urethral valves.

This acts as a window allowing better visualization of fetal structures.

The prognosis of such fetuses is extremely poor, the neonate having severe respiratory distress with the development of pneumothoraxes shortly after delivery.

Congenital diaphragmatic hernia

Diaphragmatic hernias occur in 1 in 2000 births and in over 50% of cases there are other abnormalities. A recurrence risk of under 1% is given. Ninety per cent of diaphragmatic hernias occur posteriorly through a posterolateral defect in the pleuroperitoneal canal. This Bochdalek defect occurs on the left side in 75% of cases, but may occur on the right side or on both sides. Occasionally, the herniation may occur through the foramen of Morgagni just lateral to the retrosternal area.

Ultrasonically the condition can be recognized as early as 18 weeks and the initial clue is often the displacement of the heart due to herniation of bowel (Fig. 38.19) or liver (Fig. 38.20). It may be possible to identify the stomach or loops of bowel within the left hemithorax or less frequently the liver may be identified in the right hemithorax. The ipsilateral lung is compressed and the mediastinal shift results in compression of the contralateral lung. Hypoplasia of both lungs may develop and the outcome frequently depends on the degree of pulmonary hypoplasia.

A diaphragmatic hernia is frequently associated with other major abnormalities affecting the central nervous system, cardiovascular system, genitourinary system, muscular system and gastrointestinal tract. Chromosome

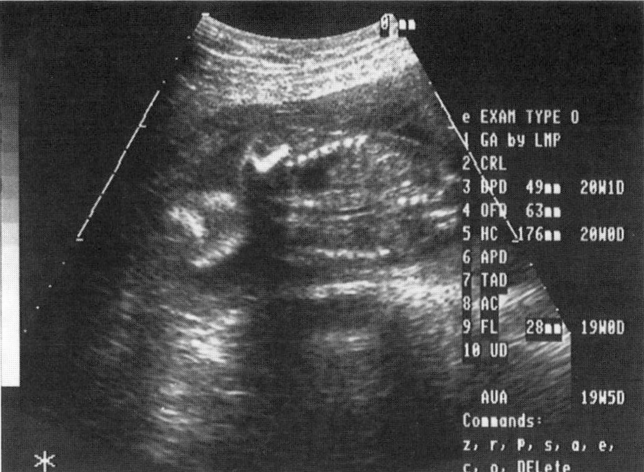

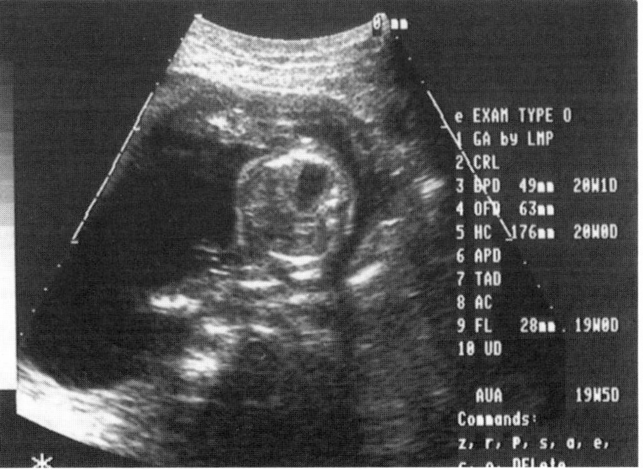

Fig. 38.19 Left sided diaphragmatic hernia. (a) Longitudinal and (b) axial scans showing a fluid-filled stomach in the left hemithorax at 20 weeks gestation. The baby survived for 10 days following delivery.

abnormalities are frequently found. Following the identification of a diaphragmatic hernia a careful search must be made for any other abnormality and karyotyping of the fetus should be carried out.

Despite early diagnosis and improvement in surgical management the mortality rate for an infant with a diaphragmatic hernia remains around 75%. Termination of the pregnancy may well be an option but if the pregnancy is continuing then delivery in a centre with immediate access to neonatal surgical care is recommended.

Thoracic masses

Several uncommon lung abnormalities may be mistaken for a diaphragmatic hernia. These abnormalities may be cystic, show increased echogenicity or show both features.

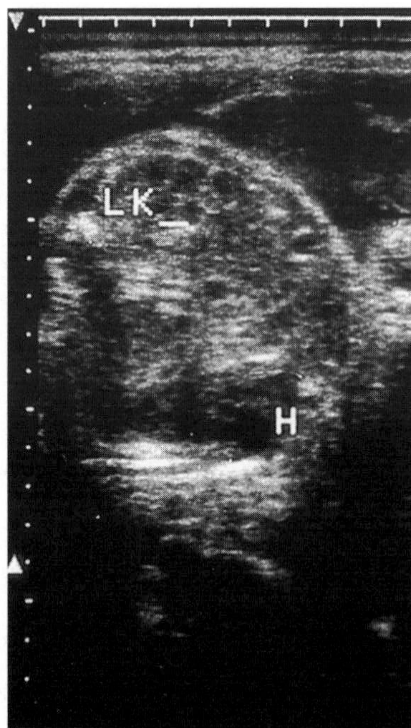

Fig. 38.20 Right-sided diaphragmatic hernia. Axial scan of the thorax with the heart (H) displaced to the right by a herniated liver and left kidney (LK). (Courtesy of Dr B. Muir, Simpson Memorial Maternity Pavilion, Edinburgh.)

CYSTADENOMATOUS MALFORMATION

This malformation is due to a hamartomatous lesion of the lung and usually presents with respiratory distress in the neonatal period. Three types are described.

Type 1 consists of several large cysts. There is usually mediastinal displacement away from the cysts. Pulmonary hypoplasia may develop but the prognosis is usually good.

Type 2 consists of numerous smaller cysts measuring under 1 cm in diameter. This type is usually associated with other severe abnormalities and the fetus rarely survives.

Type 3 presents as a solid echogenic mass, the prognosis being poor usually due to severe pulmonary hypoplasia.

All types may be associated with polyhydramnios and hydrops and the prognosis in these cases is poor.

BRONCHOPULMONARY SEQUESTRATION

This abnormality is due to a portion of the lung with an anomalous vascular supply usually from the descending aorta. The condition may be extralobar or intralobar. Ultrasonically, the sequestration usually appears as an echogenic mass related to the diaphragm.

THORACIC CYSTS

Thoracic cysts are usually due to bronchogenic, neurenteric or duplication cysts. The type of cyst may be suspected from its location and neurenteric cysts are usually associated with vertebral anomalies.

Abdominal abnormalities

These abnormalities can be divided into three main groups.

1 Abnormalities of the gastrointestinal tract.
2 Abdominal wall defects.
3 Abnormalities of the genitourinary tract.

Abnormalities of the gastrointestinal tract

Gastrointestinal abnormalities account for around 15% of abnormalities which can be detected antenatally. The abnormalities are usually characterized by polyhydramnios and bowel dilatation. Fetal swallowing commences at the beginning of the second trimester and small bowel peristalsis propels the amniotic fluid through to the large bowel where it is reabsorbed. Residual cells, lanugo hairs, vernix and mucoproteins collect in the large bowel as meconium. By term the colon is completely filled with meconium. The echogenicity of meconium varies depending on its water content.

The degree of polyhydramnios which occurs secondary to an obstruction is dependent on the level of obstruction, a proximal obstruction resulting in marked polyhydramnios and a distal obstruction in minimal polyhydramnios. There may in fact be a normal amniotic volume in the presence of a colonic obstruction.

It may be extremely difficult if not impossible to distinguish between large and small bowel dilatation ultrasonically. The large bowel is usually situated around the periphery of the abdomen with the small bowel being more centrally placed. Care must be taken not to confuse dilatation of the renal tract with a gastrointestinal abnormality. Likewise cystic abdominal masses may occur (ovarian cysts, hydrometrocolpos) which should be distinguished from dilatation of the bowel.

OESOPHAGEAL ATRESIA

This condition occurs in about 1 in 3000 deliveries and has a recurrence risk of less than 1%. There is, however, a threefold increase in neural tube defects in subsequent offspring. Five types of oesophageal malformations have been described but in about 90% of cases a tracheo-oesophageal fistula will be present and will enable amni-

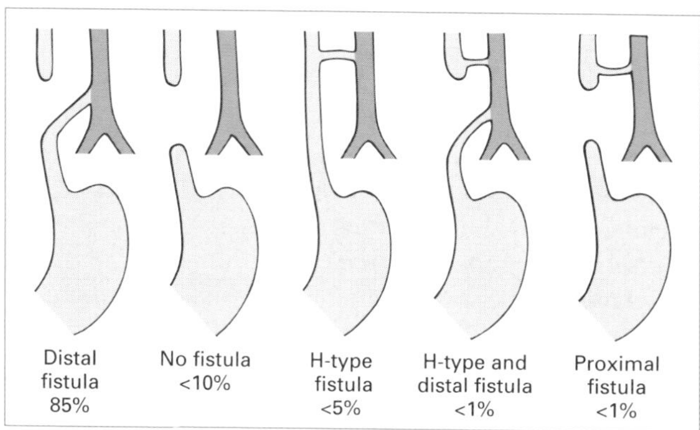

Fig. 38.21 Different types of oesophageal atresia and their rate of occurrence.

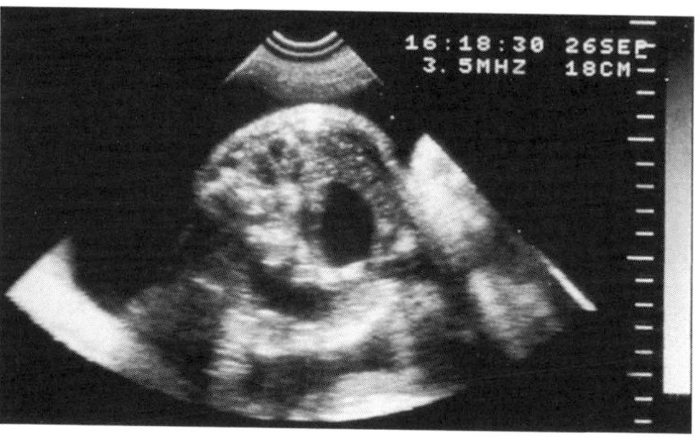

Fig. 38.22 Duodenal atresia. Axial scan of the upper abdomen showing fluid in the stomach and duodenum—'double bubble'. The fetus had trisomy 21.

otic fluid to pass down the trachea through the tracheo-oesophageal fistula and into the stomach (Fig. 38.21). The diagnosis of oesophageal atresia can never be confidently made antenatally but it must be strongly suspected in the presence of polyhydramnios and the inability to detect a fluid-filled stomach despite repeated ultrasound examinations. In over 50% of cases with oesophageal atresia, other abnormalities will be found and the ultimate prognosis is often dependent on these abnormalities. Oesophageal atresia is frequently associated with a well-defined group of abnormalities under the acronym of VACTERL. The condition is occasionally associated with chromosome abnormalities.

DUODENAL ATRESIA

Duodenal atresia occurs in 1 in 10000 births and 30% of cases are associated with trisomy 21. The obstruction occurs near the ampulla of Vater and is believed to be due to failure of recanalization of the duodenum in early development or to some form of vascular impairment of the duodenum. Distension of the stomach and duodenum occurs due to accumulation of swallowed amniotic fluid. This gives rise to a 'double bubble sign' (Fig. 38.22). The condition may be diagnosed as early as 18 weeks but frequently the diagnosis is delayed until polyhydramnios has developed. Dilatation of the duodenum may be confused with cystic masses in the right hypochondrium such as choledocal cysts but with careful scanning the duodenum will be found to be in continuity with the stomach.

Chromosomal abnormalities should be excluded by karyotyping and a careful search for other abnormalities particularly of the skeletal, gastrointestinal and cardiovascular systems should be made. The prognosis for fetuses with a normal karyotype and no concurrent abnormality is extremely favourable.

SMALL BOWEL OBSTRUCTION

This condition usually results from atresia or stenosis of the bowel and may occur anywhere within the small bowel but particularly in the distal ileum and proximal duodenum. The condition is believed to be due to vascular impairment during development.

Dilatation of the small bowel proximal to the site of obstruction will develop and with time polyhydramnios occurs. Other bowel abnormalities are frequently associated with small bowel atresia, e.g. malrotation, volvulus and duplication. However, it is uncommon for it to be associated with abnormalities outwith the gastrointestinal tract. The prognosis is dependent on the site and degree of bowel involvement and whether there is associated perforation with meconium peritonitis.

MECONIUM ILEUS

This condition is due to the presence of abnormally thick and sticky meconium in the distal ileum and is found in about 15% of fetuses who will subsequently prove to have cystic fibrosis. Ultrasonically, there is dilatation of bowel which is filled with echogenic meconium. Polyhydramnios may develop. The condition is frequently associated with volvulus, bowel atresia, perforation and the subsequent development of meconium peritonitis.

The presence of echogenic material in the bowel must always raise the possibility of a meconium ileus but a similar ultrasound appearance may be found if the blood supply is compromised or the fetus has trisomy 21, and it is frequently a normal variant.

MECONIUM PERITONITIS

This condition may occur following perforation secondary to meconium ileus with cystic fibrosis, as a result of bowel obstruction, secondary to an atresia or volvulus or it may be idiopathic. Linear areas of calcification will be noted in the inner aspect of the bowel wall, in relation to the liver edge or in the region of the mesentery. The condition is frequently associated with ascites. The prognosis depends on the underlying cause and surgery may well be indicated.

LARGE BOWEL ABNORMALITIES

Anorectal atresia has been recognized antenatally. The possibility of this abnormality must always be considered as part of the VACTERL syndrome.

Abdominal wall defects

This group of abnormalities occurs in 1 in 2000 live births. The condition is frequently detected antenatally as it is one of the causes of a high maternal serum AFP. Several types of abdominal wall defects are described.

1 Exomphalos or omphalocele.
2 Gastroschisis.
3 Ectopia cordis.
4 Body stalk anomaly or limb body wall complex.
5 Amniotic band syndrome.
6 Bladder or cloacal extrophy.

EXOMPHALOS

This condition is believed to occur in 1 in 5000 deliveries. It is characterized by a mid line defect in the abdominal musculature with herniation of intra-abdominal contents into the base of the umbilical cord. The herniated structures are surrounded by a membrane the outer wall consisting of amnion and the inner of peritoneum. Wharton's jelly is present between the walls (Fig. 38.23). Two types are recognized, those containing liver and those not containing liver. Up to 40% of cases are associated with a chromosome abnormality and the incidence is higher in cases which do not contain liver within the sac. There is also a very high incidence of other abnormalities, in particular cardiovascular abnormalities (30–50%) and abnormalities of the central nervous system, genitourinary system and gastrointestinal tract.

Exomphalos may be due to failure of the bowel to return to the intra-abdominal cavity about 12 weeks gestation. However, if liver is present within the sac then the condition may be due to failure of the body wall to close. Care must be taken not to diagnose the condition during the first trimester when the appearances may be entirely physiological. Ultrasound scanning will identify a mid line mass protruding from the abdomen with the umbilical cord entering the mass at its apex.

The membrane surrounding the sac may be difficult to identify but it does prevent the sac contents from floating freely in the amniotic cavity. The liver, stomach or loops of bowel may be noted within the sac. A careful examination of the heart, spine and renal tract is essential whenever the abnormality is identified and karyotyping should be offered.

The preferred mode of delivery is controversial, some believing that a caesarean section should be performed to prevent damage to the sac. However, if there are related abnormalities the prognosis for the fetus is poor and a vaginal delivery is preferable. Because of the covering membrane the AFP is not as high as in the presence of a gastroschisis.

GASTROSCHISIS

The incidence of gastroschisis is comparable with that of exomphalos. It has a much better prognosis, however, as it is very infrequently associated with other abnormalities. The condition is due to a small defect involving the abdominal wall in the paraumbilical region. Ninety per cent of defects are situated on the right. Bowel is extruded through the defect and is seen floating in the amniotic fluid. The umbilical cord can be identified entering the abdomen in a normal position (Fig. 38.24).

Prolonged contact of the bowel wall with urine in the amniotic fluid may result in bowel wall thickening and the development of areas of obstruction, ischaemia or perforation. Once the condition has been identified regular scanning should be performed to assess the condition of the bowel. Early delivery may be an option if the appearances suggest that the bowel is becoming compromised.

The ideal mode of delivering a fetus with gastroschisis is controversial, some believing that an elective caesarean section is preferable to a vaginal delivery. With the recent developments in neonatal and surgical techniques the prognosis for these fetuses has improved considerably and over 90% of them will now survive. Late complications may result from the fact that the bowel is malrotated.

The maternal serum AFP is extremely high in cases of gastroschisis due to leakage of AFP through the fetal bowel wall into the amniotic cavity.

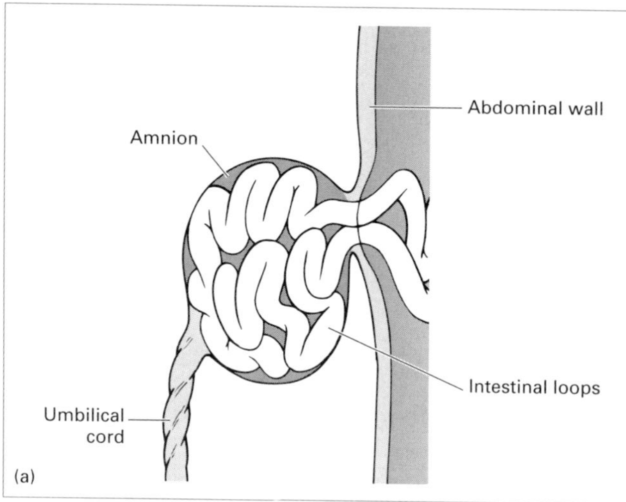

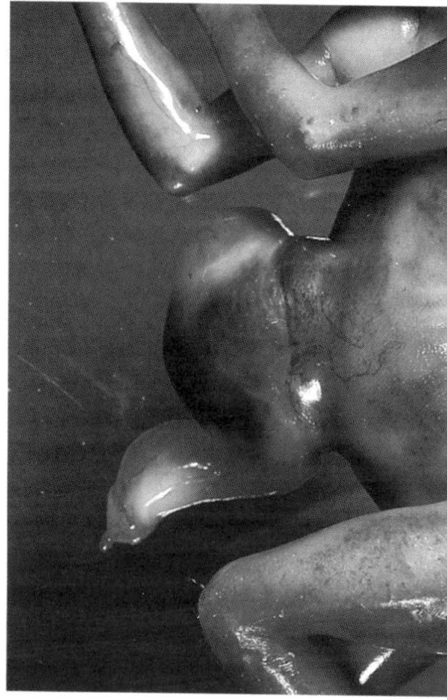

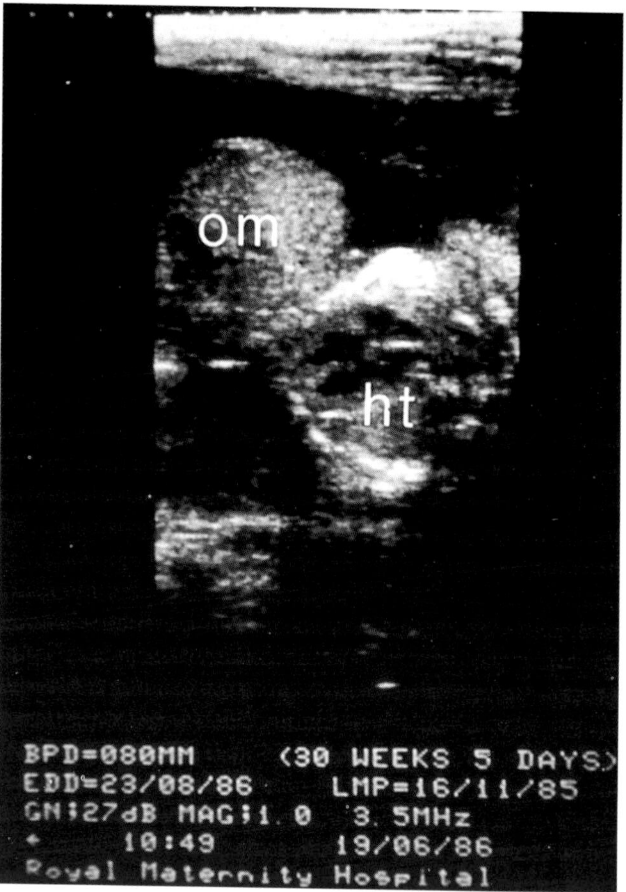

Fig. 38.23 Exomphalos. (a) Diagram. (b) Large exomphalos (om) containing liver and stomach. The mother presented initially at 30 weeks gestation; the fetus had trisomy 18. ht, heart. (c) Pathological specimen. (Courtesy of Dr A. Howatson, Royal Hospital for Sick Children, Glasgow.)

ECTOPIA CORDIS

This condition is rare but may be found in association with exomphalos. The heart will be noted to lie in an extrathoracic position. The prognosis for these fetuses is very poor.

BODY STALK ANOMALY

This lethal condition is characterized by defects in the thoracoabdominal area, the eviscerated organs forming a complex mass with the amniotic membrane. There are associated neurological abnormalities such as anencephaly, spina bifida and there is frequently a related scoliosis. Severe abnormalities of the limbs are common.

AMNIOTIC BAND SYNDROME

This is discussed under skeletal malformations (p. 575).

BLADDER AND CLOACAL EXTROPHY

These developmental abnormalities are rare and very few of them have been diagnosed antenatally.

Abnormalities of the genitourinary tract

Abnormalities of the renal tract are common. The exact incidence is unknown but some form of renal malformation is present in about 10% of live births. The prognosis of the abnormality varies from the insignificant slight pelvic dilatation to the lethal renal agenesis and is dependent on whether the condition is unilateral or bilateral.

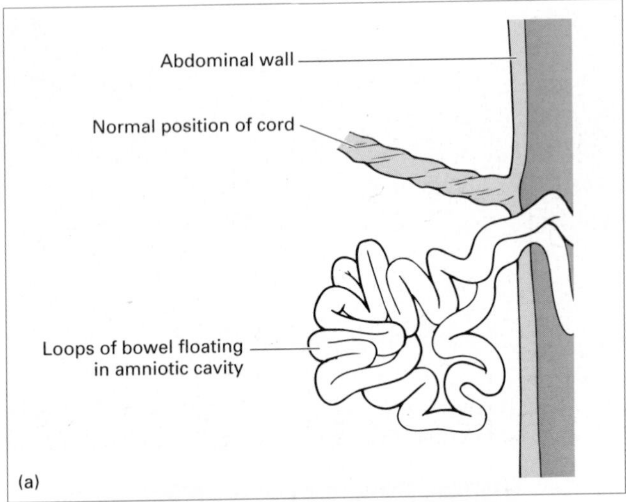

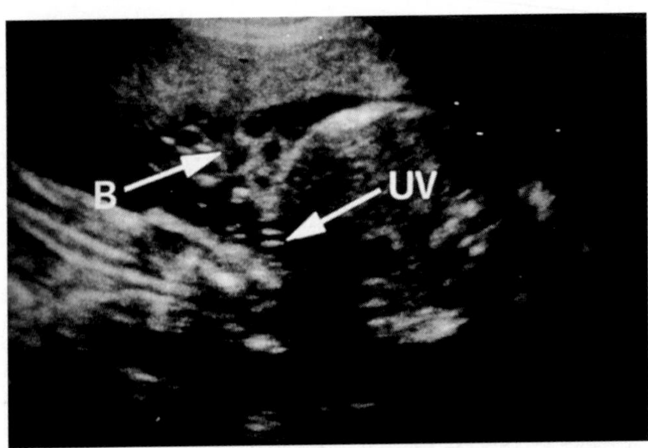

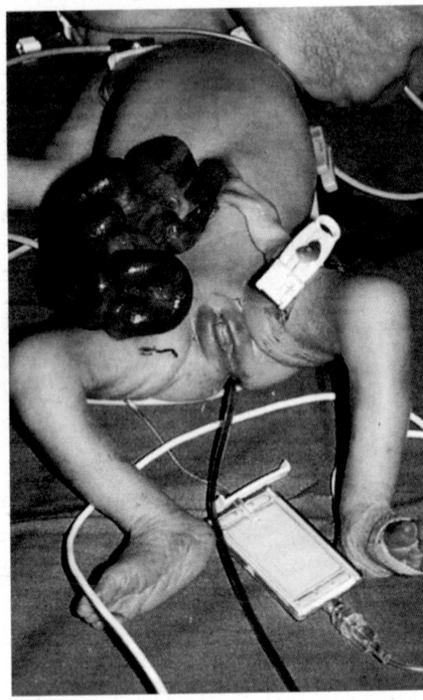

Fig. 38.24 Gastroschisis. (a) Diagram. (b) Loops of bowel (B) floating in amniotic fluid. There was a normal insertion of the cord (UV). (c) Neonate with gastroschisis; the baby did not survive. (Courtesy of Dr A. Howatson, Royal Hospital for Sick Children, Glasgow.)

An understanding of renal development and the production of amniotic fluid is helpful in the assessment of the renal tract. The first permanent nephrons appear at around 10 weeks gestation and at this time the kidneys begin to function. By 20 weeks one-third of the nephrons are present and the tubules have formed. Complete development of the kidneys is present by 35 weeks gestation. There is still some controversy about the exact mechanism of the production of amniotic fluid. However, most people believe that up to 10 weeks the amniotic fluid is an ultrafiltrate of maternal plasma. Between 10 and 20 weeks it is an ultrafiltrate of fetal plasma together with some fetal urine. The volume of fetal urine increases markedly between 20 and 30 weeks but fluid also comes from the gastrointestinal tract, respiratory tract and cord. From 30 weeks to term the volume of amniotic fluid is controlled by swallowing and urination. A reduced amniotic fluid volume may thus point to a renal problem.

Abnormalities of the renal tract can be divided into two principal types, those involving the renal parenchyma and those involving malformations of the drainage system.

PARENCHYMAL ABNORMALITIES

These can be subdivided into agenesis, cystic disease and dysplasia.

Renal agenesis

This condition may be unilateral or bilateral. The unilateral condition occurs in 1 in 1000 births and the bilateral in 1 in 3000 to 1 in 10000. A recurrence risk of 3.5–4.5% is given. Bilateral renal agenesis is characterized by severe oligohydramnios. It is impossible to identify the kidneys and bladder (Fig. 38.25). Two other conditions may give a similar ultrasound picture, severe intrauterine growth retardation and premature rupture of the membranes. Normally, the amniotic fluid acts as a window which allows good visualization of the fetus with the identification of the kidneys. Although it could be argued that the prognosis of a fetus with severe intrauterine growth retardation and premature rupture of the membranes early on is extremely poor, some of them do have a reasonable prognosis and it is important to differentiate the conditions. Some workers have used maternal intra-

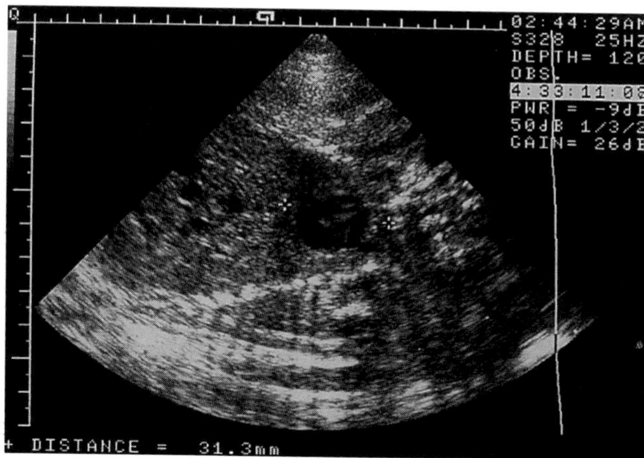

Fig. 38.25 Renal agenesis. Severe oligohydramnios with pulmonary hypoplasia in a fetus with renal agenesis.

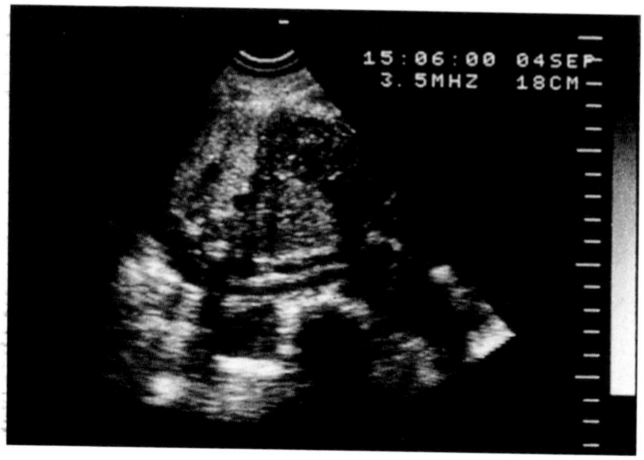

Fig. 38.26 Infantile polycystic kidneys. Axial scan showing large echogenic kidneys. The fetus died in the neonatal period.

venous frusemide in an attempt to encourage the baby to produce urine and fill the bladder whilst others have found this unsuccessful. In some centres saline is infused into the amniotic cavity and is used as a window to produce better images of the fetus. This procedure is not without risk, however, and care must be taken to avoid confusing the adrenal glands, which are often prominent in fetuses with renal agenesis, for the fetal kidneys.

Bilateral renal agenesis is associated with typical facial and limb abnormalities and with marked pulmonary hypoplasia, the appearance being known as Potter's syndrome. The bilateral condition is invariably lethal and termination may be offered if the condition is picked up early on and if there is no doubt about the diagnosis.

Renal cystic disease

There is disagreement amongst many experts as to the exact terminology which should be used in describing many of the types of renal cystic disease. The paediatric nephrologists use a simple classification: polycystic renal disease, multicystic dysplastic kidney disease and cortical dysplasia.

Polycystic renal disease. This can be divided into two types, infantile and adult.

1 Adult polycystic renal disease. This is an autosomal dominant with a recurrence risk of 50%. It is rarely diagnosed in the antenatal or perinatal period, cysts usually being detected on ultrasound in the late teens.

2 Infantile polycystic disease. This condition is an autosomal recessive with a recurrence risk of 25%. It occurs in 1 in 6000 to 1 in 16000 live births. Four types are described:

(a) the perinatal form is invariably lethal;

(b) the neonatal form usually results in death within 1 year;

(c) the infantile form;

(d) the juvenile form.

The infantile and juvenile forms are associated with hepatomegaly due to bile duct proliferation and portal fibrosis.

The fetal kidneys are large and echogenic (Fig. 38.26). This echogenicity is due to the presence of innumerable tiny cysts, echoes being reflected back from the walls of the cysts thus creating the impression of a solid mass. Occasionally, tiny transonic cystic areas may be identified. The condition can be diagnosed as early as 16 weeks but frequently the diagnosis cannot be made until 24 weeks. The prognosis is usually poor and is worse in cases with oligohydramnios and particularly large kidneys. Termination may well be an option particularly if there has been a previously affected child who has died from the condition.

The kidneys in a fetus with Meckel–Gruber syndrome have a similar appearance to infantile polycystic disease. In this condition there is an associated encephalocele which is usually situated posteriorly and the fetus may well have polydactly. A careful examination of the remainder of the fetus is imperative when infantile polycystic disease is suspected.

Multicystic dysplastic kidneys. The incidence of this condition is said to be 1 in 10000 births but the current incidence in the west of Scotland is around 6 per 10000 births. The bilateral condition is lethal. There is a 10–40% incidence of abnormality in the other kidney in the unilateral condition and careful postnatal follow-up is essential to assess the contralateral kidney adequately. A multicystic kidney consists of transonic areas of varying sizes and frequently the diagnosis is extremely easy (Fig. 38.27). However, the condition can be confused with hydronephrosis even in expert hands. The condition is invariably associated with an atretic ureter and the kidney will be non-functioning in around 90% of cases.

A ^{99m}Tc dimercaptosuccinic acid (DMSA) nuclear medicine scan may be helpful in confirming the absence of function when the infant is 1 month old (Fig. 38.28).

Previously, kidneys with multicystic disease have been removed because of the possibility of hypertension or malignancy. The current feeling is that this is unnecessary and regular ultrasound scanning postnatally confirms that the cysts become smaller and eventually completely disappear. As the ureter is atretic the kidney is at no risk of developing infection.

Cortical cystic dysplasia. This condition occurs secondary to renal obstruction resulting in abnormal development of the nephron system. The later the obstruction develops the less severe are the dysplastic changes. The cortex consists of tiny cysts and increased echogenicity is detected (Fig. 38.29).

MALFORMATIONS OF THE DRAINAGE SYSTEM

These abnormalities are mainly due to obstruction. Three levels of obstruction must be considered.

1 High—obstruction to the outflow of the renal pelvis.

2 Mid level—an obstruction occurring at the vesicoureteric junction.

3 Low—an obstruction affecting the bladder outlet, usually urethral valves or atresia.

High level obstruction

This normally results in a pelviureteric junction obstruction and may be unilateral or bilateral. The condition can be diagnosed from 16 weeks and careful follow-up should take place initially every 6 weeks and in the last trimester every 3 weeks. The degree of dilatation should be assessed by measuring the anteroposterior diameter of the renal pelvis at its mid point (Fig. 38.30). The thickness of the

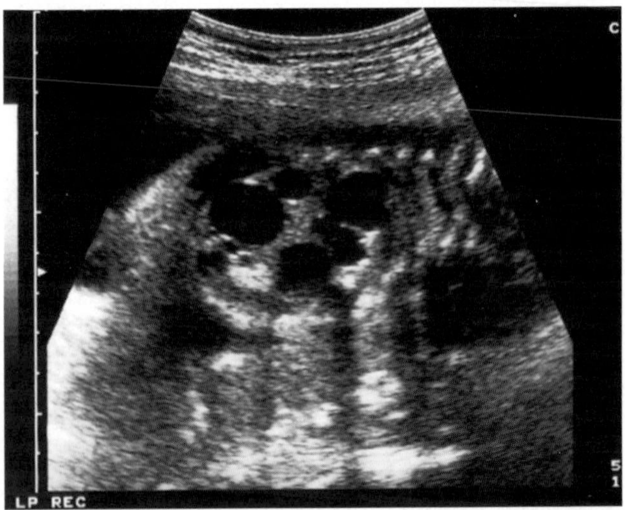

Fig. 38.27 Multicystic dysplasic kidney. This kidney consists of cysts of varying size; the contralateral kidney was normal.

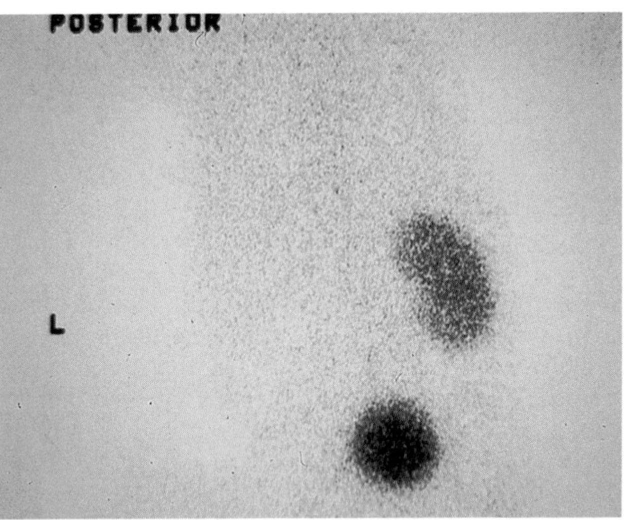

Fig. 38.28 ^{99m}Tc DMSA scan showing absence of function in a left multicystic kidney.

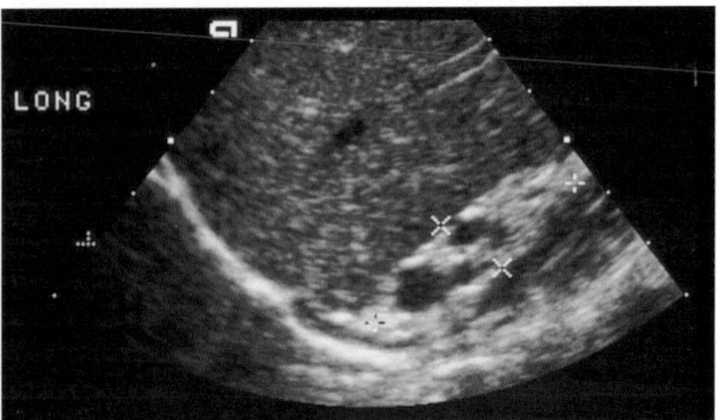

Fig. 38.29 Cortical cystic dysplasia. Antenatally, the right kidney was hydronephrotic. The postnatal scan shows the kidney to be small, with increased echogenicity and some cysts.

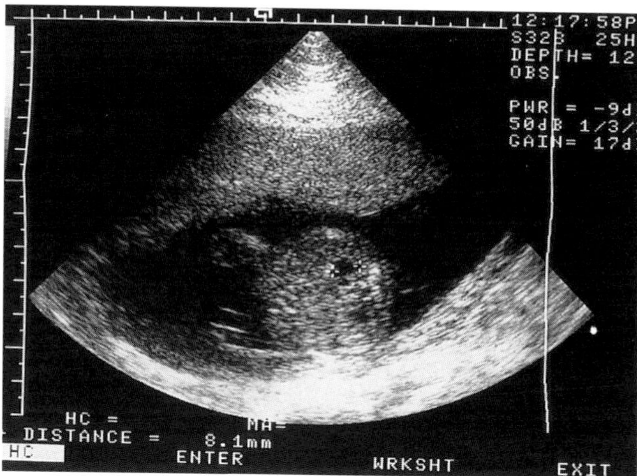

Fig. 38.30 Pelvic dilatation. Anteroposterior diameter of the renal pelvis is 8.1 mm.

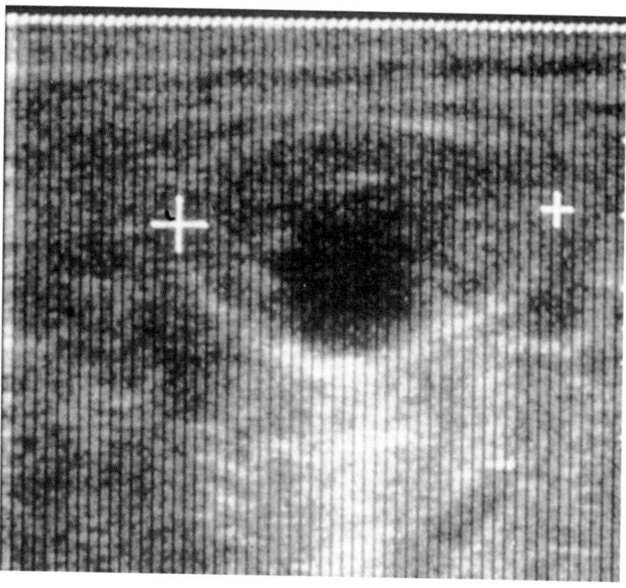

Fig. 38.31 Suspected pelviureteric junction obstruction. Minimal dilatation of the renal pelvis was found to be due to a prominent extrarenal pelvis postnatally.

renal cortex should also be measured. A fetus with unilateral hydronephrosis should be allowed to deliver at term and a follow-up ultrasound should be carried out 48–72 h following delivery. In the first 48 h following delivery a baby is frequently slightly dehydrated and a minimal hydronephrosis may be masked if the baby if scanned at that time. Nuclear medicine scans are valuable in assessing function and drainage and are usually performed at 1 month.

The prognosis with bilateral pelviureteric junction obstruction depends on the severity of the obstruction. In mild cases the dilatation will be minimal and the amniotic liquor volume will be normal. As the dilatation becomes more marked oligohydramnios will develop. If the condition is severe there will be marked oligohydramnios and pulmonary hypoplasia may also be present. The renal cortex may become echogenic due to cystic dysplasia. If this occurs in early pregnancy, termination may be an option. Early delivery may be considered but the neonate would be at great risk of developing severe pulmonary problems due to a combination of prematurity and pulmonary hypoplasia. The neonate may succumb from the respiratory problems rather than from the renal problems. *In utero* drainage has been attempted but there is a significant morbidity and mortality. It may be helpful to assess renal function by tapping each kidney and estimating the urinary sodium level. The prognosis is poor if the level is greater than 100 mmol l^{-1}.

In minimal hydronephrosis there will be dilatation of the renal pelvis (Fig. 38.31). As the hydronephrosis becomes more severe the pelvic dilatation will increase and the renal calyces will start to dilate up. The calyces may appear as cystic structures but they will be situated around the renal pelvis and will communicate with the pelvis (Fig. 38.32). It should thus be possible to distinguish this condition from a multicystic kidney. However, this is not always the case and a diagnostic problem can still persist postnatally. A DMSA scan may be useful in detecting whether the kidney is functioning or not. If there is no function then it is likely that the kidney is multicystic. If there is minimal function (i.e. <5%) then the kidney may be grossly hydronephrotic or multicystic. If there is reasonable function the kidney is hydronephrotic.

Mid level obstruction

This obstruction is less common than high level obstruction and is usually unilateral. There is dilatation of the pelvicalyceal system and ureter due to the vesicoureteric junction obstruction (Fig. 38.33). Occasionally mid level obstruction may be caused by a ureterocele blocking the lower end of the ureter draining the upper moiety of a duplex kidney. The ureterocele is identified as a transonic mass within the bladder and the upper moiety of the kidney will show increasing dilatation (Fig. 38.34). When the mid level obstruction is unilateral the fetus can be delivered at term and investigated postnatally. When the condition is bilateral oligohydramnios and pulmonary hypoplasia may develop.

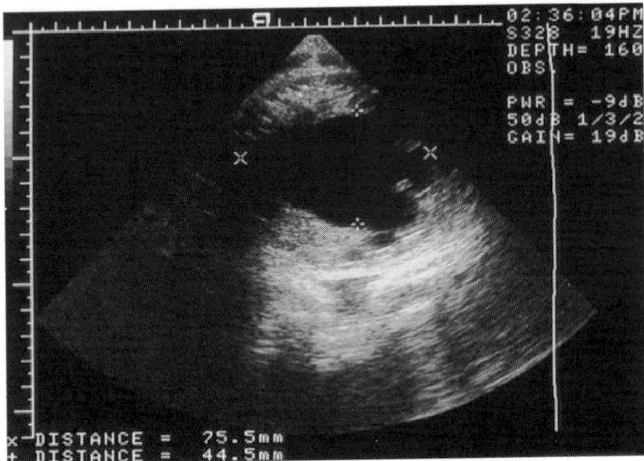

Fig. 38.32 Severe pelviureteric junction obstruction. Marked dilatation of the calyces and pelvis requiring postnatal surgery.

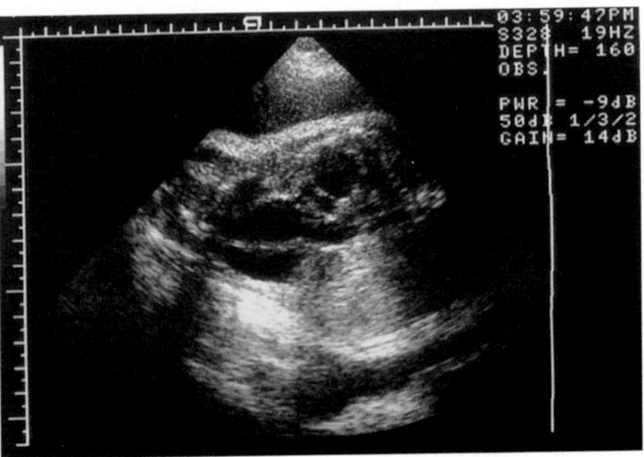

Fig. 38.33 Vesicoureteric obstruction. Dilatation of the renal pelvis and ureter down to bladder level.

Low level obstruction

This type of obstruction is usually due to some form of bladder outlet obstruction such as posterior urethral valves or urethral atresia. The bladder is usually extremely dilated and there is bilateral hydronephrosis and hydroureters. Depending on the severity of the obstruction cystic dysplasia, oligohydramnios and pulmonary hypoplasia may well develop. It is important to determine the gender of the fetus and, if the baby is male, the appearances will most probably be due to urethral valves. On occasions a dilated posterior urethra may be identified proximal to the valves (Fig. 38.35). The management of the pregnancy depends on the severity of the obstruction and the options of early delivery or termination must be considered. Renal function can be assessed

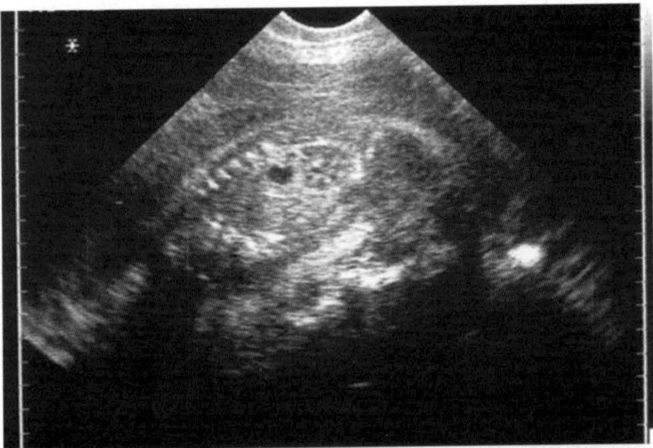

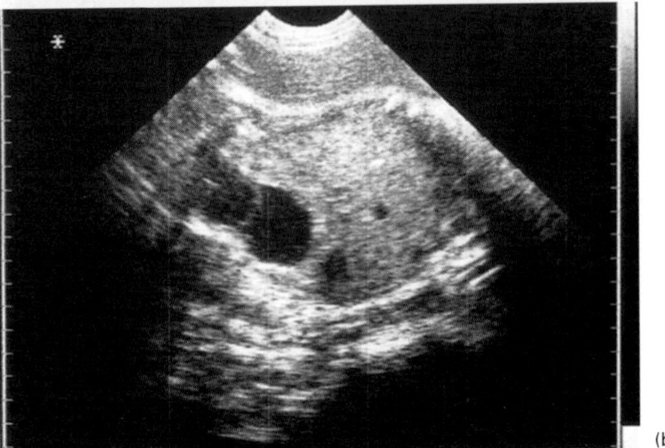

Fig. 38.34 Duplex kidney with ureterocele. (a) Dilated upper moiety with normal lower moiety; the upper moeity was non-functioning and removed at 3 months. (b) Ureterocele at the bladder base was removed following delivery.

by tapping the bladder and measuring the urinary sodium level. Some centres have shunted the bladder into the amniotic fluid but the results of this procedure have been disappointing.

Megacystis/megaureter situation

Dilatation of the kidneys and ureters is present in fetuses with this condition. The bladder may also be large. The exact cause of the condition is uncertain. Initially, in a male fetus a provisional diagnosis of posterior urethral valves may well be made. However, following delivery the urethra will be found to be normal.

Prune belly syndrome

This condition consists of an abnormality of the abdominal wall musculature together with a large hypotonic bladder, dilated ureters and cryptorchidism. Severe cases can be picked up early in pregnancy, the abdomen being distended and filled with fluid (Fig. 38.36). The thorax is small and many of the fetuses die *in utero*.

Vesicoureteric reflux

Minimal dilatation of the collecting system may be due to reflux and if the condition is marked and prolonged the kidneys will become dysplastic. Dilatation of the collecting systems may increase as the fetus empties its bladder (Fig. 38.37).

Minimal dilatation of the renal pelvis

Many fetuses are now being detected antenatally with minimal dilatation of the pelvis (Fig. 38.38). The management of such fetuses is uncertain and controversial. If the anteroposterior diameter of the pelvis is less than 5 mm at term then the condition can be regarded as insignificant and a variant of normal. If it is over 1 cm at term then the baby requires follow-up ultrasound postnatally and if the dilatation persists then more invasive tests may have to be considered such as a micturating cystogram to exclude reflux and nuclear medicine studies to assess function.

The significance of dilatation measuring between 5 and 10 mm is still unknown but from the local experience it is probably also insignificant, provided the kidneys are of normal size and configuration.

Minimal dilatation was originally thought to be a marker for trisomy 21 but it is now accepted that this risk is very low in the absence of other markers.

With the increased use of ultrasound antenatally more and more fetuses will be identified with a renal problem. Although such a diagnosis is upsetting for the parents it does mean that the baby can be adequately investigated and hopefully treated following delivery. It may prevent the baby from subsequently developing more serious renal problems, such as acute pyelonephritis, septicaemia or renal failure. The parents must always receive careful counselling whenever a renal abnormality is detected and it is invaluable to involve both the medical and surgical paediatricians.

FETAL GENDER

With careful scanning it is frequently possible to determine the sex of the fetus particularly if the fetus is male. However, it is possible to confuse the umbilical cord or swollen labia with the scrotum and great care must be taken with the information which is given to the parents. Small hydroceles are fairly frequently seen in term male infants (Fig. 38.39).

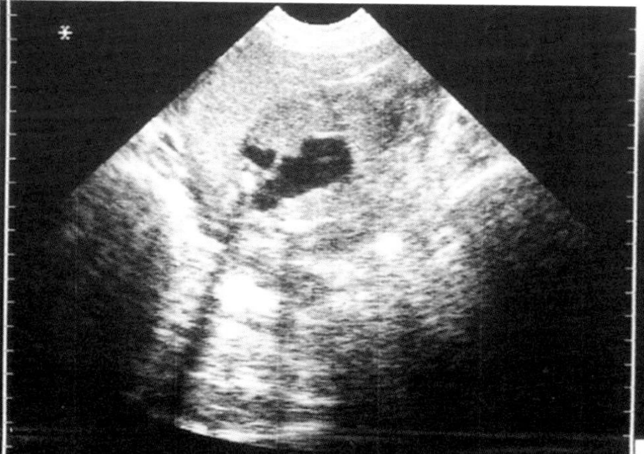

Fig. 38.35 Posterior urethral valves. Dilated bladder and posterior urethra in a 19-week fetus who also had severely dysplastic kidneys and gross oligohydramnios. The pregnancy was terminated.

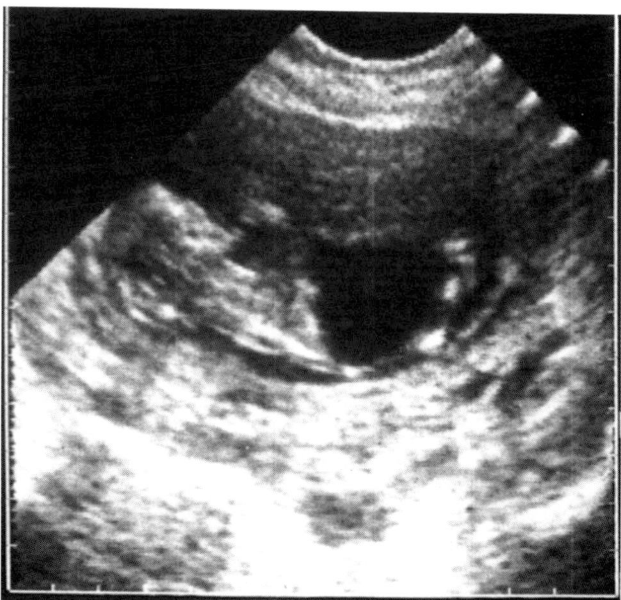

Fig. 38.36 Prune belly syndrome. Fetus at 14-weeks with a fluid-filled distended abdomen; there was subsequent intrauterine death.

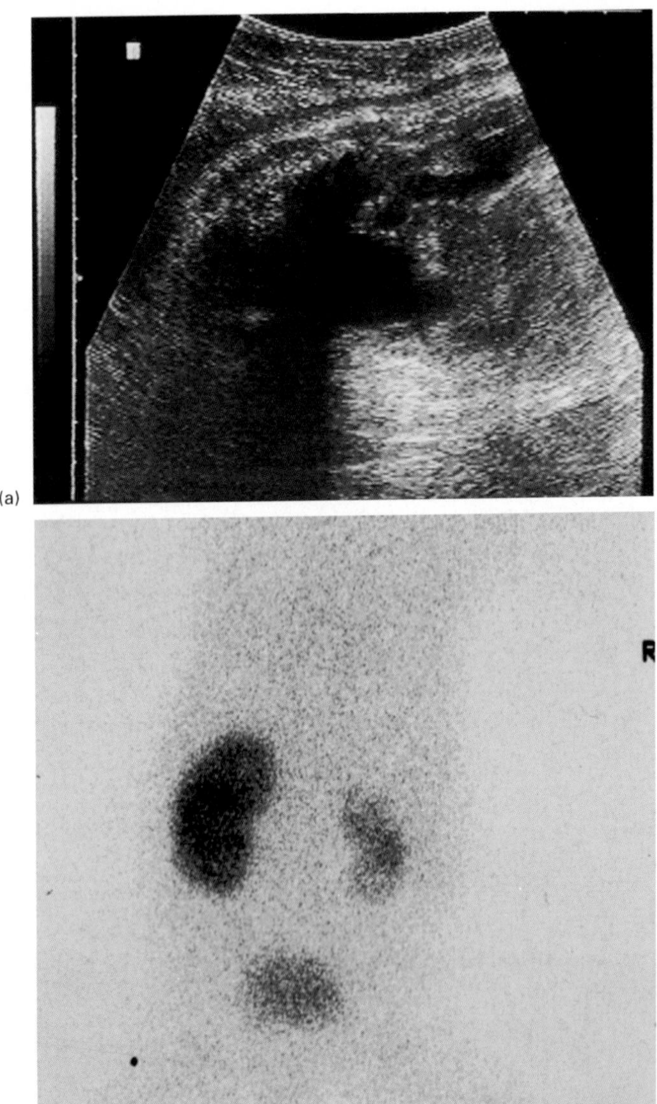

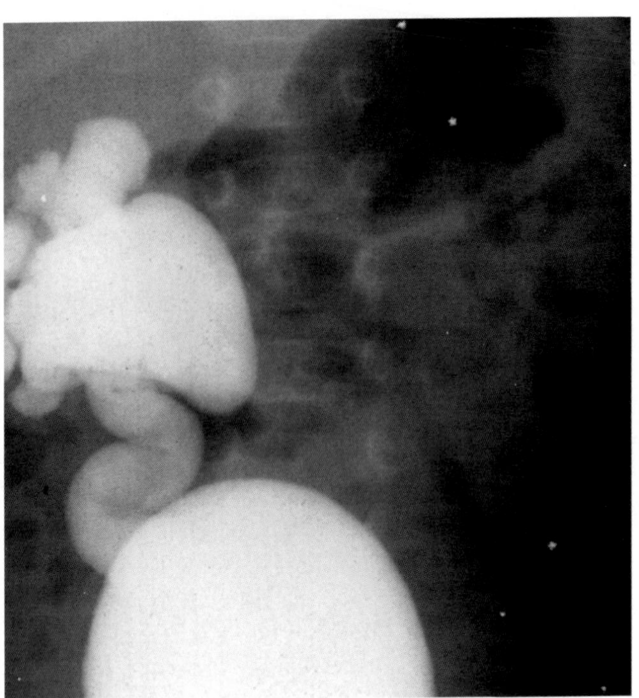

Fig. 38.37 Vesicoureteric reflux. (a) Dilatation of the right ureter during bladder emptying at 37 weeks gestation. The right kidney was smaller than the left kidney with a pelvis measuring 7 mm. (b) Marked right-sided reflux on micturating cystogram at 1 week following delivery. (c) ^{99m}Tc DMSA scan showing a small poorly functioning right kidney at 1 month.

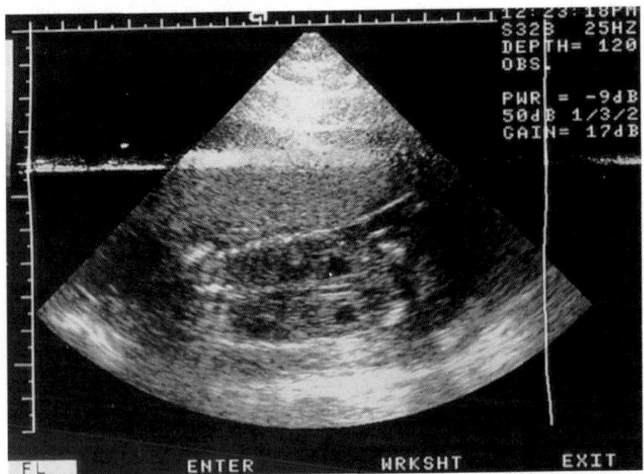

Fig. 38.38 'Dilated kidneys'. Minimal dilatation of both renal pelvises at 18 weeks gestation. The kidneys were normal following delivery.

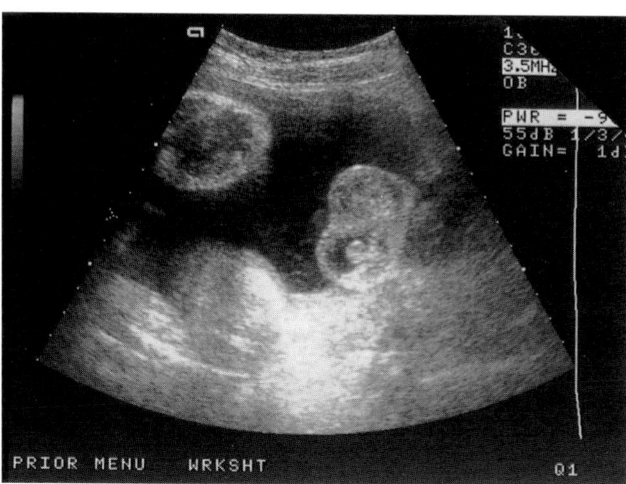

Fig. 38.39 Hydrocele. Fluid surrounding the left testis at 39 weeks gestation.

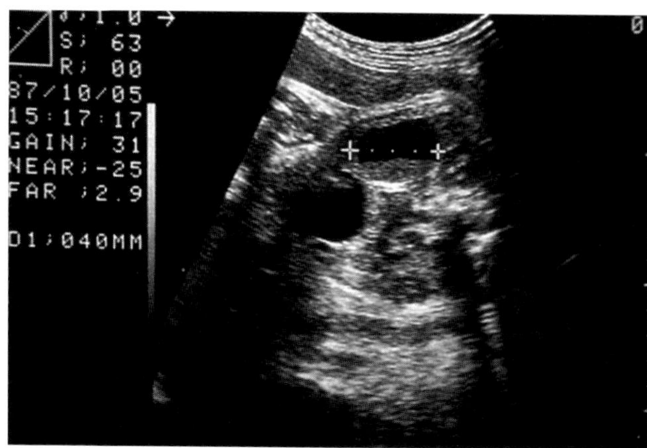

Fig. 38.40 Ovarian cyst. Fluid-filled structure lying in the right iliac fossa adjacent to the bladder containing debris due to haemorrhage. (Courtesy of Dr B. Muir, Simpson Memorial Maternity Pavilion, Edinburgh.)

OVARIAN CYSTS

Ovarian cysts can be identified as transonic masses on either side of the fetal bladder in female infants. Occasionally the cyst may contain debris secondary to haemorrhage (Fig. 38.40). Postnatal scanning should be carried out to confirm the diagnosis.

The condition must be distinguished from other cystic masses in the abdomen such as duplication cysts, mesenteric cysts, choledochal cysts or the less common cysts of the liver, spleen or urachus.

Other fetal abnormalities

Skeletal abnormalities

Skeletal abnormalities can be divided into malformations and dysplasias. An incidence of around 1 in 500 is recorded for major limb malformations and 1 in 5000 for dysplasias. The majority of abnormalities are detected by chance. However, if there is a family history of some form of dysplasia then a careful assessment of the whole of the skeleton is essential.

During a fetal anomaly scan the femoral length is routinely measured. The remaining long bones should be positively identified and the hands and feet seen. Measurements of the other long bones are not normally carried out unless there is a suspected abnormality.

Skeletal malformations

These usually take the form of absence or abnormality of part or of all of a limb. They may occur as a result of drug ingestion, as part of a syndrome or chromosome abnormality, or because of an amniotic band.

AMNIOTIC BAND SYNDROME

This condition occurs in 1 in 1200 births and is believed to be caused by rupture of the amnion resulting in the formation of fibrous bands which may then entrap part of the fetus resulting in amputations, constriction rings or lymphoedema. Facial clefts, abnormally situated encephaloceles and abnormalities of the chest and abdominal wall have also been recorded. The limb–body wall complex is believed to be a more severe lethal form of this abnormality with the addition of scoliosis and defects of the internal organs.

Amniotic bands are seen fairly often during routine scanning and it is important to check that they are not causing entanglement of the fetus. They are said to be extremely common in spontaneous abortion (Fig. 38.41).

RADIAL RAY DEFECTS

Absence of the radius is associated with several abnormalities such as the Holt–Oram syndrome (limb and cardiac abnormalities), TAR babies (thrombocytopenia and absent radius) and the VACTERL association. Radial ray defects are characterized by absence or abnormalities of the radius and lateral deviation of the hand. A careful search for abnormalities of the remainder of the fetus is essential.

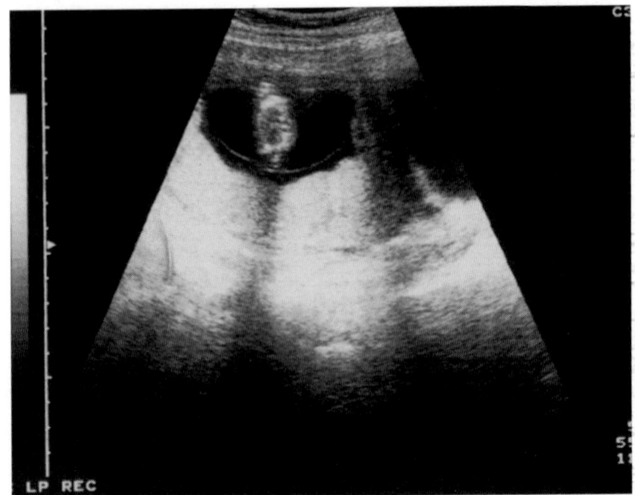

(a)

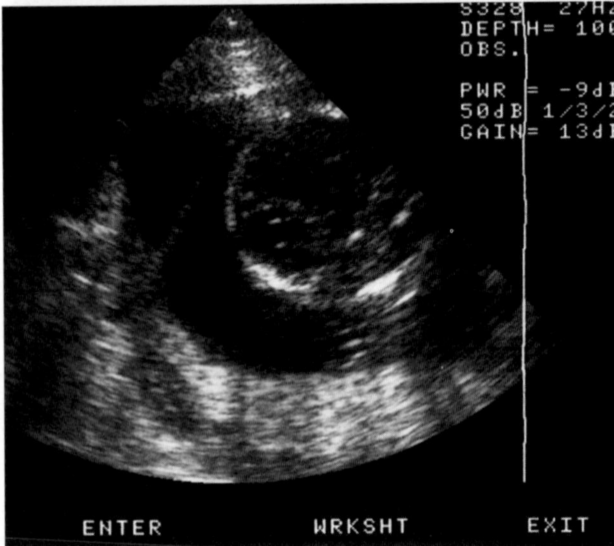

(b)

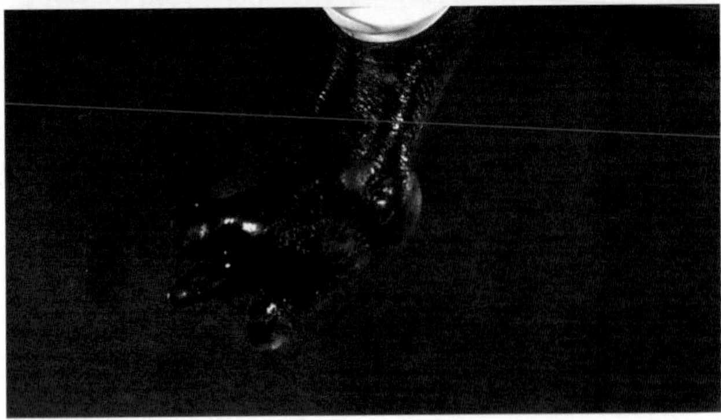

(c)

Fig. 38.41 Amniotic band. (a) 14 weeks gestation. (b) 25 weeks gestation. (c) Postmortem specimen of a hand where the fingers have been amputated. The fetus also had a severe facial cleft. (Courtesy of Dr A. Howatson, Royal Hospital for Sick Children, Glasgow.)

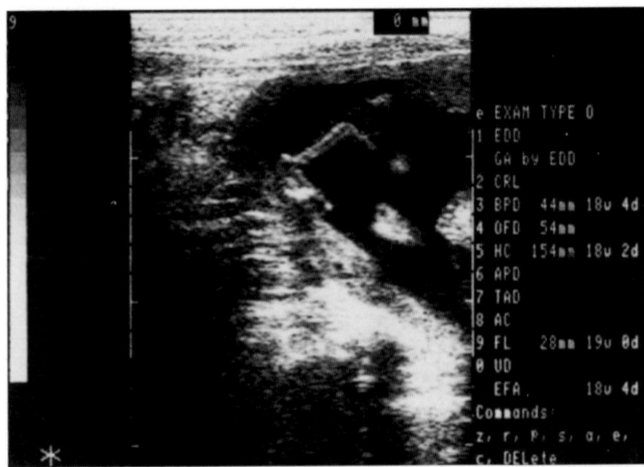

Fig. 38.42 Talipes. Severe inturning of the foot relative to the tibia and fibula.

TALIPES

Talipes occurs fairly commonly and the foot is usually plantar flexed and inverted. Whilst the finding may be isolated it is found in association with many other congenital abnormalities. Bilateral talipes usually accompanies severe oligohydramnios (Fig. 38.42).

HAND ABNORMALITIES

It is extremely time-consuming to diagnose abnormalities of the hand and detailed examination is usually carried out only if other abnormalities have already been identified. Clinodactyly (curving of any finger but usually of the little finger) may be seen in association with trisomy 21. Polydactyly (extra digit) may be an isolated abnormality but is found in trisomy 13 or the Meckel syndrome. Syndactyly (fusion of the digits) or ectrodactyly (split hands) may be found in several syndromes. Overlapping of the digits is typically associated with trisomy 18 and a 'hitchhiker thumb' is found in several types of dwarfism.

POSTURAL OR CONTRACTURAL ABNORMALITIES

These abnormalities are uncommon and usually develop as a result of severe oligohydramnios, extrinsic compression or the inability of the fetus to move. Four types of contractural abnormalities are described, arthrogryposis multiplex congenita and Pena–Shokeir phenotype being the most common.

Skeletal dysplasias

Skeletal dysplasias are uncommon and are usually inherited. Although over 100 separate dysplasias have been described the majority of those detected antenatally are cases of thanatophoric dwarfism, osteogenesis imperfecta, achondrogenesis and achondroplasia.

Initially most dysplasias are suspected because of the identification of shortening of the limb bones. This shortening may be identified in the second trimester but in some conditions may not be apparent until later.

It is important to have a logical approach to the diagnosis of skeletal dysplasia and this can be done by identifying the type of shortening.

1 *Micromelia*—shortening of all limb bones.
2 *Rhizomelia*—shortening of the proximal bones.
3 *Phocomelia*—absence of the middle part of an extremity.
4 *Mezomelia*—shortening of the distal long bones.

Following the identification of limb shortening it is important to determine whether the limb bones are straight or bowed. The bone density of the spine, skull and long bones should be determined. The head shape and the appearance of the soft tissues and hands should be assessed. The ratio of chest circumference to abdominal circumference should be measured.

Many skeletal dysplasias are lethal resulting in intrauterine death or death shortly after delivery. An accurate diagnosis of the type of dysplasia is important so that appropriate genetic counselling can be given. A postmortem examination and an X-ray of the fetus is essential in such cases.

OSTEOGENESIS IMPERFECTA

This abnormality is due to defective collagen and results in repeated fractures. Four types are described, I and IV are usually mild, and II and III are severe or lethal. The majority of cases identified antenatally are type II. The limbs are extremely short with bowing or angulation, the appearances being secondary to numerous fractures with callus formation. There is diminished bone density throughout. Poor ossification of the cranial vault allows extremely good visualization of the ventricular system and cortex. A pseudohydrocephalic picture may be produced.

Congenital hypophosphotasia may give similar ultrasound appearances to type II osteogenesis imperfecta. However, in this condition the bones are thin or even absent.

ACHONDROPLASIA

This condition is relatively common and in 80% of cases is due to a spontaneous mutation. The remaining cases are due to inheritance of an autosomal dominant condition. Initially the fetus appears normal but the femoral lengths become progressively short for gestational age (Fig. 38.43), and the cranial vault appears large with evidence of frontal bossing.

THANATOPHORIC DWARFISM

This is a lethal form of dwarfism and is characterized by marked shortening of the limbs with bowing of the femora (telephone receiver femora). The skull has a clover leaf configuration and the chest is small and hypoplastic (champagne cork appearance). The vertebral bodies are flattened (Fig. 38.44).

ACHONDROGENESIS

This is the second most common lethal form of short limbed dwarfism. It is inherited as an autosomal recessive trait. There is marked reduction in limb length with delayed or absent ossification of the vertebral bodies.

Fetal hydrops

Fetal hydrops is due to excess of fetal body water and may manifest itself as ascites (Fig. 38.45), pleural or pericardial effusions, oedema of the skin, polyhydramnios and increased thickness and echogenicity of the placenta. Two types are described, immune and non-immune.

IMMUNE HYDROPS

This condition is usually due to Rh (rhesus) isoimmunization and its incidence has fallen markedly during the last 20 years due to the use of prophylactic Rh immunoglobulin.

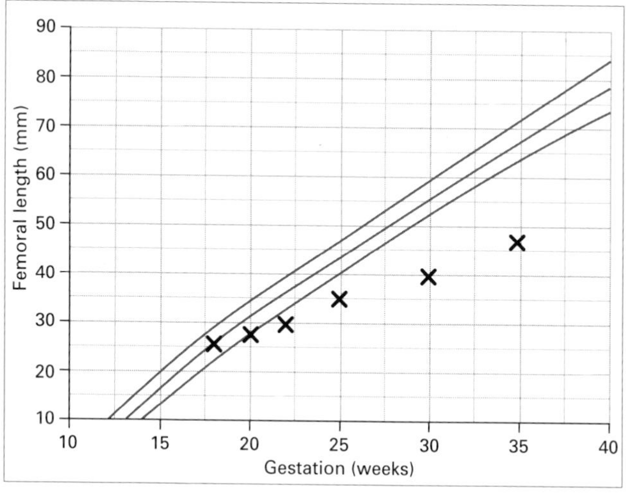

Fig. 38.43 Achondroplasia. A graph of the growth of the femur in a fetus with achondroplasia. (Redrawn from Warda *et al.*, 1985.)

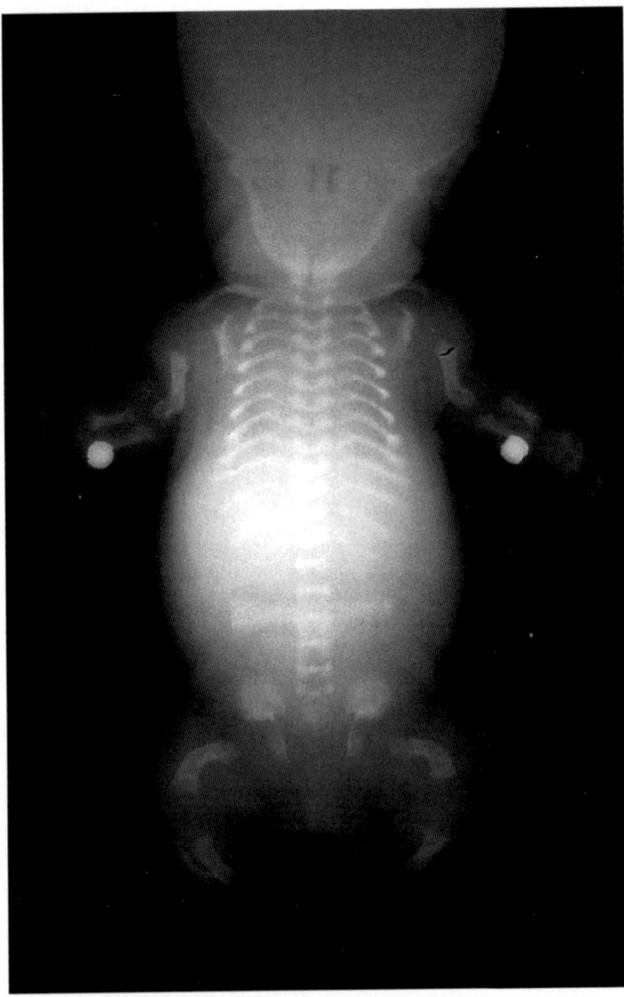

Fig. 38.44 Thanatophoric dwarf. An X-ray of an undiagnosed dwarf. The baby died shortly after delivery by caesarean section for fetal distress.

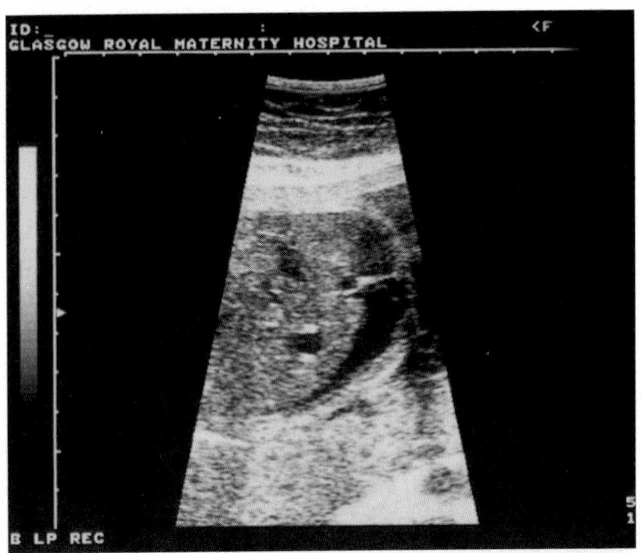

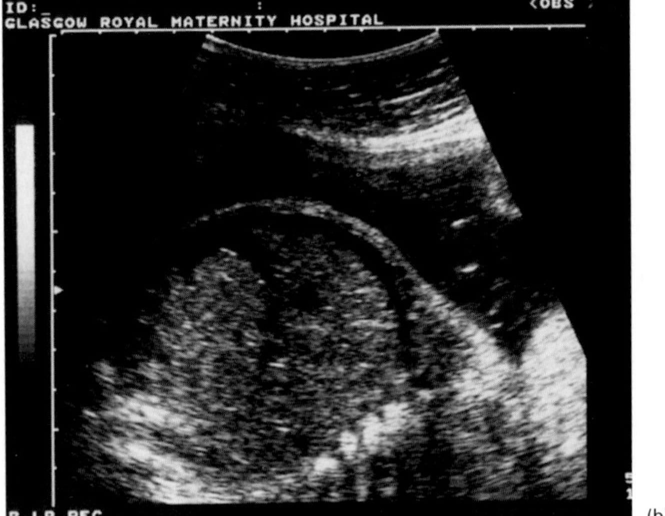

Fig. 38.45 Non-immune hydrops. (a) Axial and (b) parasagittal scans of the abdomen in a fetus with heart block showing extensive ascites.

Maternal antibodies develop when the mother is exposed to red cells which differ from her own. Fetal red cells do not normally cross the placenta. However, at the time of delivery or following fetomaternal haemorrhage, amniocentesis or CVS, fetal cells may enter the maternal circulation. Maternal antibodies are formed and these can cross the placental barrier freely. Binding of these antibodies to fetal antigens on the surface of fetal red cells leads to haemolysis with the development of fetal anaemia. Extramedullary erythropoiesis occurs with enlargement of the liver and the subsequent development of venous hypertension. Fetal ascites and placental oedema may then occur. Decreased protein synthesis results in hypoproteinaemia with further development of ascites. Fetal anaemia may result in cardiac failure.

The clinical management of such a pregnancy is outwith the scope of this text but regular scanning looking for the development of hydrops, amniocentesis and cordocentesis may be required. Intravascular transfusion has replaced intraperitoneal transfusion as the treatment of choice for affected fetuses.

The accumulation of ascitic fluid may be the first sign of fetal hydrops. Care must be taken not to confuse the rim of decreased echogenicity around the liver due to abdominal wall musculature with minimal ascites. With time thickening of the skin and subcutaneous tissues may develop in association with placental oedema and polyhydramnios. Enlargement of the liver and spleen may be identified and the ductus venosus may become dilated secondary to portal hypertension.

Isoimmunization may occur with other blood group antigens such as the Rh system (E and C), the Kell system and the Duffy system.

NON-IMMUNE HYDROPS

Non-immune hydrops now accounts for 90% of cases of fetal hydrops. With careful pre- and postnatal investigation the aetiology may be found in over 80% of cases. The overall prognosis for non-immune hydrops is poor with a mortality rate of up to 90%. Non-immune hydrops may result from heart failure, obstructed venous return, decreased plasma pressure, increased capillary permeability and lymphatic obstruction. Over 100 conditions have been described in association with non-immune hydrops and these can be summarized under the headings of infection; diseases of the heart, lungs or gastrointestinal tract; chromosome abnormalities; skeletal abnormalities; haematological abnormalities; neoplasms; and placental tumours (Table 38.1).

Following the identification of hydrops careful evaluation of both the mother and the fetus is necessary. Maternal blood should be obtained for antibody screening, assessment of carrier status for thalassaemia and for screening for congenital intrauterine infections (TORCH screen which includes *Toxoplasma*, other viruses, rubella, cytomegalovirus and herpes virus). Amniocentesis or cordocentesis may be helpful in the assessment of fetal karyotype, the presence of infection, and so on. The management of the fetus will depend on the underlying causes of the condition and its likely prognosis. Termination or preterm delivery may be options.

Table 38.1 Causes of non-immune hydrops

Infection	Cytomegalovirus
	Coxsackie virus
	Parvovirus
	Toxoplasmosis
	Syphilis
Heart disease	Cardiac arrhythmias
	Atrioventricular canal
	Hypoplastic left heart
Lung disease	Cystadenomatous malformation
Gastrointestinal disease	Diaphragmatic hernia
	Meconium peritonitis
Skeletal abnormalities	Sacrococcygeal teratoma
	Osteogenesis imperfecta
	Asphyxiating thoracic dystrophy
Chromosome abnormalities	Triploidy
	Trisomy 21
Haematological abnormalities	Twin-to-twin transfusion
	Thalassaemia
Neoplasm	Neuroblastoma
Placental tumours	Angioma

FETAL ASCITES

This may be seen in association with hydrops but may occur on its own due to abnormality of the gastrointestinal tract (e.g. meconium peritonitis) or urinary tract (e.g. following leakage of urine into the peritoneal cavity in association with severe renal tract obstruction).

Chromosome abnormalities

Chromosome abnormalities are common, the vast majority ending in early spontaneous abortion. Triploidy and trisomy 16 are particularly common in early abortions. 1 in 160 live births will be found to have a major chromosome abnormality. It has been recognized for some time that the risk of having a child with a chromosome abnormality increases with maternal age. For many years screening has been offered to mothers over the age of 35 years. More recently biochemical tests have become available which can highlight an at risk pregnancy in the younger maternal age groups. These tests are discussed in more detail in the sections on fetal abnormality and invasive procedures (pp. 550 and 593).

The possibility that a fetus has a chromosome abnormality may be raised at the time of a fetal anomaly scan. The identification of a marker for a specific defect will alert the ultrasonographer to carry out a careful search for any other associated abnormalities. Chromosome abnormalities are not usually associated with a solitary defect and their incidence increases markedly if more than one defect is found. The identification of such markers should result in appropriate counselling and karyotyping if the parents wish.

Recently Nicolaides *et al.* [2] has suggested that the most effective method of screening for chromosome disorders, particularly trisomy 21, is by measuring the nuchal translucency at 10–14 weeks (Fig. 38.46). Others have found it to be less helpful.

TRISOMY 21

This is one of the commonest chromosome abnormalities. Its incidence increases with maternal age, with a family history of Down's syndrome, and with low maternal serum AFP levels. Markers are as follows.

1 Cystic hygroma (Fig. 38.47).
2 Thickened nuchal fat pad (greater than 6 mm).
3 Cardiac abnormality (atrioventricular canal defect).
4 Duodenal atresia.
5 Clinodactyly.

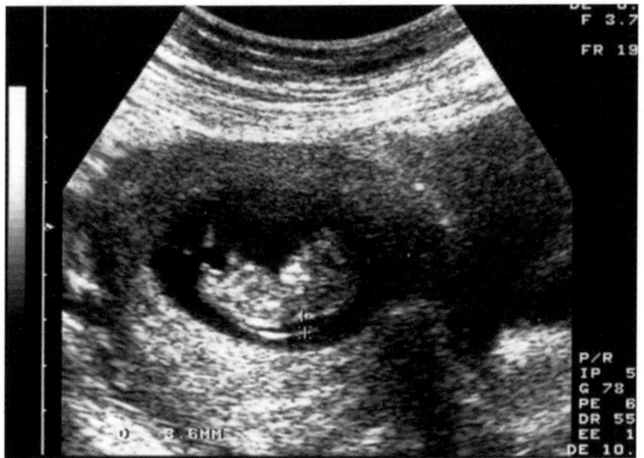

Fig. 38.46 Nuchal translucency. A fetus (10 + 5 weeks) with 3.6 mm nuchal lucency, which was not seen at follow-up at 12 weeks. There was a normal female karyotype at amniocentesis.

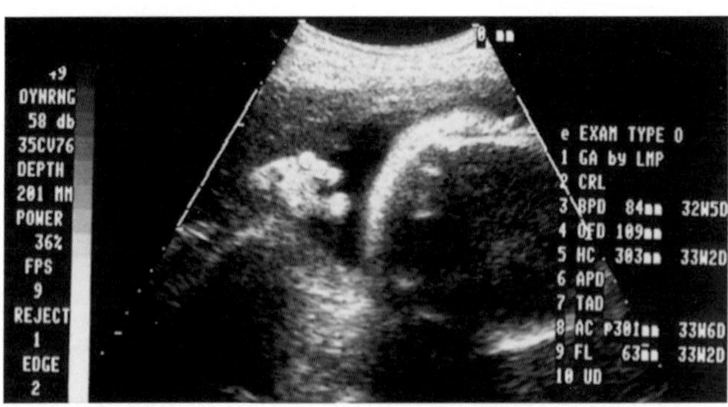

Fig. 38.48 Sandal gap. The space between the first and second toes in 33-week fetus which did not have trisomy 21.

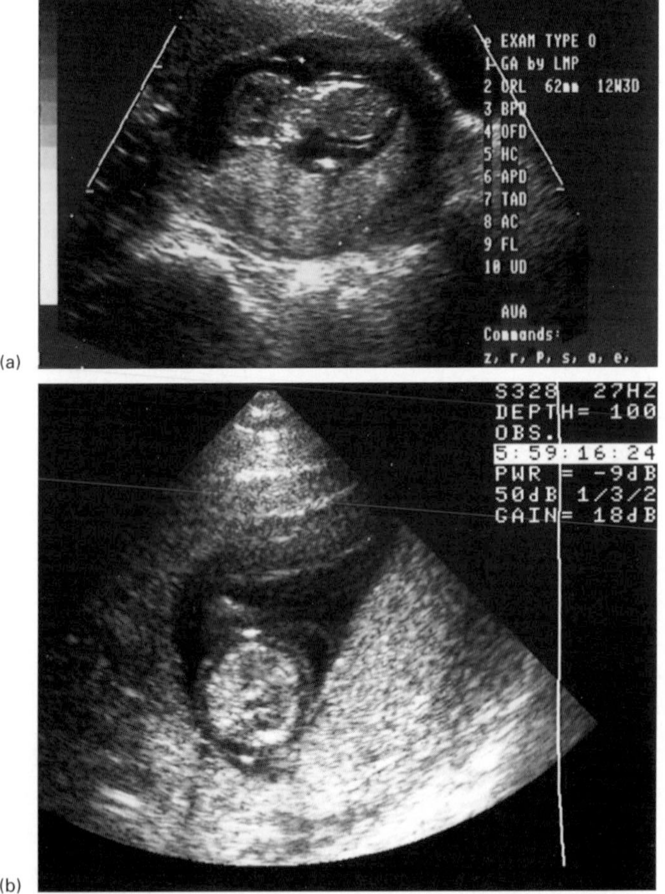

Fig. 38.47 Cystic hygroma. (a) Longitudinal and (b) axial scans of a fetus with trisomy 21 and an extensive hygroma posterior to the neck and around the trunk.

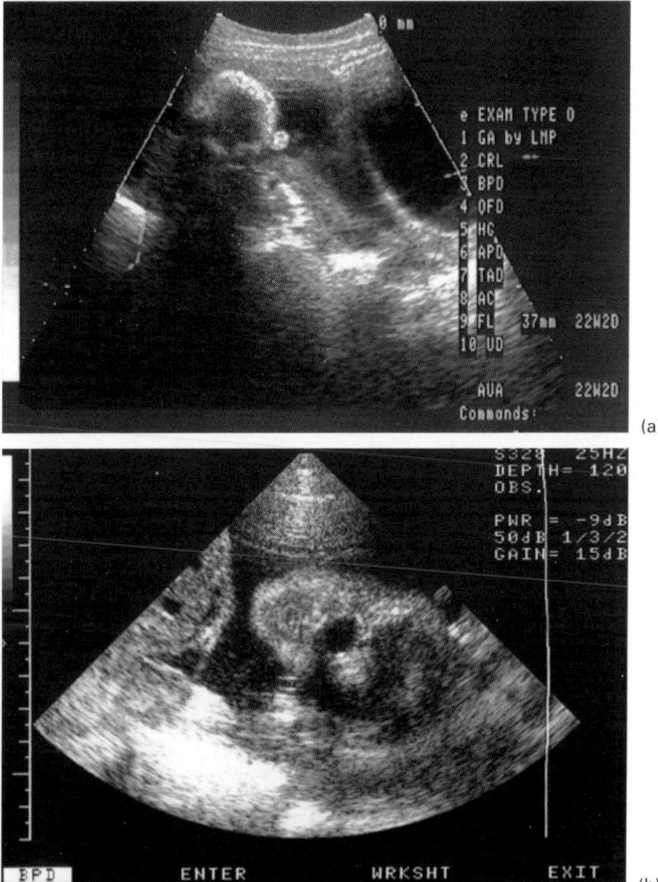

Fig. 38.49 Trisomy 18. A fetus with holoprosencephaly, cyclops and a proboscis. (a) Proboscis lying anterior to the frontal bone. (b) Single orbit in the middle of the face.

6 Sandal gap (increased space between first and second toes) (Fig. 38.48).

TRISOMY 18

This abnormality is not as common as trisomy 21 and frequently results in intrauterine death, stillbirth or death shortly after delivery (Fig. 38.49). Markers are as follows.

1 Choroid plexus cysts.
2 Holoprosencephaly.
3 Lateral facial cleft.
4 Diaphragmatic hernia.
5 Obstructive uropathy.
6 Exomphalos.
7 Rocker bottom feet.
8 Overlapping fingers.

TRISOMY 13 (PATAU'S SYNDROME)

An incidence of 1 in 6000 birth is recorded and this condition is said to account for 1% of spontaneous first trimester abortions. Markers are as follows.

1 Facial clefts.
2 Holoprosencephaly.
3 Agenesis of the corpus callosum.
4 Cardiac abnormalities.
5 Renal cystic dysplasia.
6 Rocker bottom feet.
7 Clindactyly or polydactyly.

TRIPLOIDY

This abnormality is common in early abortions. If the pregnancy continues there will be severe growth retardation and hydatidiform mole changes may be found in the placenta.

TURNER'S SYNDROME (45XO)

It is believed that the majority of such pregnancies end in early abortion. In the second trimester the fetus may present with a cystic hygroma. A congenital heart defect may also be present.

References

1 Nicolaides, K.H., Campbell, S., Gabbe, S.G., Guidetti, R. (1986) Ultrasound screening for spina bifida: cranial and cerebellar signs. *Lancet* **ii**, 72–74.

2 Nicolaides, K.H., Snijders, R.J.M., Gosden, C.M. (1992) Ultrasound markers of chromosomal abnormalities in 2086 fetuses. *Lancet* **340**, 704–707.

Chapter 39: Antenatal assessment of fetal health

A.M. Mathers

The purpose of antenatal fetal assessment is to predict, detect and therefore prevent fetal morbidity and mortality. Over the past decade the increasing range of ultrasound-based techniques, in tandem with the rapid expansion in laboratory technologies, has permitted unparalleled access to the fetus and its environment. This has lead to a greater understanding of the pathophysiology of many fetal disorders and the development not only of disease-specific testing regimes but also, in some cases, of life-saving fetal therapy. In the enthusiasm to embrace new techniques a widening gulf has appeared between what is possible and what is practical, with the obstetric sonographer straddling the gap. Antenatal fetal assessment is potentially time-consuming and, if poorly targeted, may result in inappropriate obstetric intervention which results in iatrogenic compromise. It is outwith the scope of this chapter to cover the wide range of clinical problems which prompt the obstetrician to ask for antenatal fetal assessment. Neither is its purpose to rationalize the different management strategies that may result from identical ultrasound findings being given to different obstetricians (or even the same obstetrician at a different time). The only way that fetal assessment can be used rationally and appropriately is by ensuring that the sonographer is an integral part of the perinatal team. This chapter describes the philosophy and pathophysiology underpinning non-invasive methods of fetal assessment and puts these into context with their use in clinical practice.

Development of biophysical monitoring

Since ancient times the association between maternal perception of fetal movements and fetal health has been recognized. In 1884, Playfair recommended the induction of labour 'on the mother feeling that the movements of her child are becoming less strong'. In 1903, Williams noted in his textbook that excess amniotic fluid (2 litres in his definition) was associated with fetal structural anomalies and 'weakness', while oligohydramnios was associated with fetal urinary tract abnormalities. He also noted that 'dry birth' was associated with slower progress in labour, meconium staining and fetal distress. The fetal heart was first heard in 1918 by F.I. Mayor of Geneva. This landmark in medical history was even more remarkable as he made the observation using only his ears, and through a corset! As his original purpose was to listen for sounds of the fetus splashing in amniotic fluid he was unwittingly embracing the concept of biophysical fetal monitoring, that is building a composite picture of fetal health by adding together multiple observations. In the early 20th century the main thrust of obstetric practice was aimed at successfully reducing the dreadful maternal mortality rates. The modern era of antenatal care which focuses on the 'fetus as a patient' as much as the mother's health was heralded by the birth of medical ultrasound in Glasgow in the late 1950s by Professor Ian Donald and co-workers and by the development of fetal heart rate monitoring in the 1960s by Hon. As paediatricians were increasingly able to offer more care to vulnerable neonates and at increasingly earlier gestational ages, the development and proliferation of real-time ultrasound equipment in the 1970s has allowed the establishment of an exciting interface between obstetric and paediatric services, perinatal medicine.

The fetus is susceptible to damage in many ways. As knowledge increased in the areas of genetic, infective, structural and isoimmunization disorders the contribution of hypoxic damage to perinatal mortality and morbidity has become increasingly important. It has been estimated that approximately 60% of perinatal morbidity and mortality is attributable to hypoxia.

Before the widespread use of antepartum fetal heart rate monitoring (AFHRM), it was assumed that the fetus was healthy if its mother remained well and the fetal heart was detectable. If maternal risk factors were identified an indirect assessment of placental function was attempted by measurement of oestriol and human placental lactogen in the maternal urine or serum. AFHRM looked at alterations in the fetal heart rate in relation to fetal activity and uterine activity and established itself as the gold standard predictor of fetal hypoxia. While this remains the case, it has become apparent that AFHRM has little value as a screening test and has a high false positive rate. A refinement of the test was introduced in which uterine contractions were stimulated by oxytocin either by intravenous infusion or by nipple stimulation. This 'contraction stress test' (CST), popular in the USA, still has an unacceptably high false positive rate between 50% and over 75%. There was considerable interest in ultrasound assessment of different types of fetal activity, and in 1980 Manning and Platt reported the first use of a composite 'biophysical profile score' (BPS), in which five variables were used in an effort to predict perinatal outcome (Table 39.1).

This system scored each variable as either 0 or 2 (maximum score 10). A modified BPS by Vintzileos added another variable, placental grading, and wider options with regard to scoring each variable. The advent of Doppler ultrasound and invasive fetal assessment via percutaneous umbilical vein sampling (PUBS, or cordocentesis), has broadened our knowledge of fetal pathophysiology. These developments have improved our understanding of the relative importance of each biophysical variable in determining fetal condition; however, there remain many controversial areas. There is increasing debate as to the potential for use and abuse of the BPS. As yet, Doppler information tends to be used as an additional test of the fetoplacental unit, rather than as an integral part of the BPS.

Sonographic assessment of fetal health

When the paediatrician approaches the newborn infant, the evaluation of health will be made from the history of the pregnancy and delivery, the morphology and nutritional appearance of the baby and by assessing the nature of basic reflexes. Metabolic, infective or genetic disorders, if suspected, may require blood analysis. A similar approach to assessment of fetal health is now possible which is flexible enough to avoid unnecessary study of normals and sensitive enough to determine fetal disease. A comprehensive description of obstetric risk factors necessitating the ultrasound evaluation of the fetus is outwith the scope of this book and other chapters deal with fetal growth, structural anomalies and invasive procedures (Chapters 35, 37, 38 and 40). The effective use of ultrasound-based fetal assessment is dependent on the interpretation of the results in the context of the individual case, e.g. concerns that a fetus is hypoxic become irrelevent if a lethal fetal anomaly is detected.

Concept of gradual hypoxia

Catastrophic obstetric events, e.g. massive placental abruption, which lead to acute fetal hypoxia cannot be predicted by the BPS: in such cases neonatal outcome is critically dependent on the rapid management of the underlying cause. Far more insidious and damaging is the development of metabolic acidosis secondary to chronic hypoxia. The effects on the fetus depend on the nature and duration of the hypoxic insult and the strength, frequency and duration of uterine activity. Labour may therefore be an intolerable insult in such fetuses and there is increasing evidence that the majority of infants who suffer from neurological damage, do so as a result of prelabour hypoxic insult.

Hypoxic stress induces two main fetal adaptations, alteration of central nervous system (CNS) mediated reflexes and redistribution of cardiac output. The consequence of these changes is that markers can be identified which differentiate 'acute' responses from chronic adaptations (Fig. 39.1).

Acute markers

Acute CNS-mediated markers are the ultrasound detectable signs of fetal tone (FT), fetal movements (FM),

Table 39.1 Modified biophysical profile (after Manning and Platt)

	Stage of development (weeks)	Criteria needed to score 2 points
FT subcortical area of cortex	7–8	1 Flexion/extension/flexion movement
FM cortex nuclei	9	3 gross movements in 30 min
FBM ventral fourth ventricle	20–21	30 s sustained activity in 30 min
AFHRM hypothalamus/medulla	28	Accelerative trace ('reactive')
qAFV alters with gestational age		1 × 2 cm deep, 1 cm wide cord-free pool

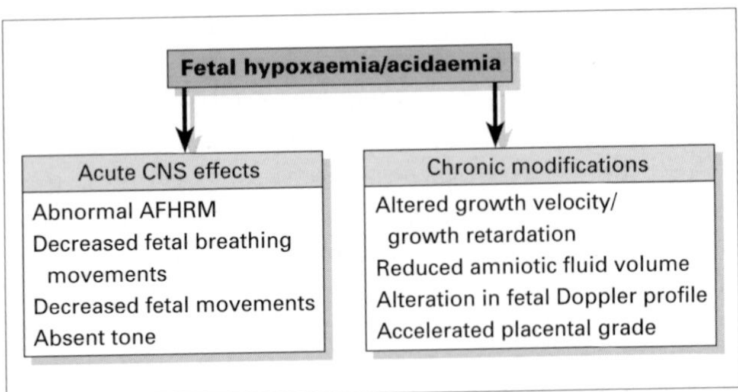

Fig. 39.1 Fetal adaptation to uteroplacental insufficiency. AFHRM, antepartum fetal heart rate monitoring.

fetal breathing movements (FBM) and fetal heart rate reactivity (demonstrated by AFHRM). Each of these variables are sequentially expressed, in the order as stated, as gestational age advances, and appear to be controlled by different areas of the fetal brain. The effect of hypoxic stress results in suppression of the most recently acquired reflex (e.g. fetal heart rate reactivity in the term fetus) and then serial suppression, in order, of the other variables. A higher oxygen concentration is required for newly developed centres controlling biophysical variables. Hypoxaemia results in acidaemia with a resultant sequential 'switching off' of each variable. Fetal pH data supports this concept. As pH falls below 7.2, fetal heart rate reactivity and then FBM are inhibited. When the pH is lower than 7.1, FM and, finally, FT cease. It can therefore be seen that the absence of FT is a grave prognostic sign whereas the presence of normal AFHRM excludes acidaemia. Unfortunately, the absence of a variable does not necessarily mean the fetus is acidaemic as each activity is subject to normal periodicity and can be influenced by changes in maternal metabolism particularly as a result of pharmacological agents. Individual characteristics of each component will be discussed with regard to periodicity, how the variable is assessed and how it is interpreted in the context of the BPS. Each variable will be described in the order that it develops during fetal life.

FT

Tone is the first variable to develop, appearing during the seventh and eighth weeks. It is thought that the controlling centre lies in the subcortical area of the cortex. Assessment of FT is arguably the most subjective part of the BPS. Tone is assessed by identifying at least one flexion/extension/return to flexion limb movement during the scanning period. The presence of normal FM implies normal tone is present and therefore would score 2 in the BPS. Absence of FM is counted as absent tone. A particularly ominous sign is persistent semi- or full limb extension and open hands. Patterns of periodicity have not been recognized.

FM

The FM control centre functions from 9 weeks and is located in the cortex nuclei. FM is scored when three or more gross body movements are observed within 30 min, simultaneous limb and trunk movements being counted as one. Less than three FM are awarded 0. There is a periodic pattern and a diurnal rhythm. With advancing maturity FMs initially increase in incidence reaching a maximum at 24–28 weeks gestation. During the last 10 weeks of pregnancy FM are present approximately 10% of the time and maximum activity occurs between 2100 and 0100 hours. The longest recorded episode of absent FM in the healthy human fetus is 75 min (from 24-h observations after 30 weeks gestation). In practice only 1% of fetuses will spend more than 45 min between episodes of FM. With advancing gestational age the quality and variety of movements alter and this is utilized for the study of fetal behavioural states. The study of fetal behavioural states is a research tool which correlates changes in AFHRM with fetal eye, breathing and body movements. These are outwith the remit of this chapter and will not be discussed further.

Maternal appreciation of FMs is extremely variable and the experienced ultrasonographer will often show vigorous FM to an unimpressed mother. There is no apparent effect on ultrasound-detected gross FM by social amounts of alcohol, smoking, maternal hyperglycaemia, hypercapnia, hyperoxia or by vigorous shaking of the maternal abdomen. The latent phase of labour has no effect on the incidence of FM; however, there is a significant decrease during the active phase.

FBM

The centre controlling this activity is located on the ventral surface of the fourth ventricle and begins to function around 20–21 weeks gestation. A score of 2 is awarded when at least 30 s of sustained FBM are seen in a 30-min period. Any less than this scores 0. FBM have been observed as early as 10 weeks gestation and increase in frequency until they are present for approximately 30% of the time during the last 10 weeks of pregnancy. FBM are episodic and a diurnal rhythm, which may be related to endogenous maternal cortisol levels, has been demonstrated in the last 10 weeks of pregancy. FBM episodes last between 20 and 60 min and alternate with periods of apnoea, the longest recorded period of apnoea in a healthy human fetus being 120 min.

FBM activity is markedly influenced by maternal glucose levels, and is significantly increased after meals. This has major implications when performing a BPS on a diabetic patient and it is therefore essential that normoglycaemia is confirmed at the time of the test. Smoking and chewing nicotine-containing gum results in a decrease in the incidence of FBM. Alcohol ingestion virtually abolishes FBM and this is not reversed by maternal glucose administration. Other CNS depressants also inhibit FBM. Hypercapnia and hyperoxia can increase FBM; however, the latter only occurs in the growth retarded fetus. There is a reduction in FBM in the 72 h prior to the commencement of labour, the mechanism of which remains unclear. It has been suggested that this may be useful in the diagnosis of impending preterm labour but this is unproven.

AFHRM

This is the variable that develops 'last' and is therefore the most sensitive to hypoxia. The centre is located in the posterior hypothalamus/medulla and fetal heart rate reactivity develops by the early third trimester. Like FM and FBM, AFHRM exhibits periodicity and diurnal variation. It is readily influenced by CNS depressants. AFHRM involves the assessment of changes in the fetal heart rate in response to FM and uterine activity. Occasionally the response to external vibroacoustic stimulation may be used. One of the first descriptions involved the use of an electric toothbrush on the maternal abdomen! Commercially available devices are now available. As AFHRM is the most widely used method of fetal assessment it is usually as a result of abnormal or equivocal tests that formal biophysical monitoring is initiated. The appropriate use and interpretation of this variable is crucial if inappropriate referrals for BPS are to be avoided; however, the scoring of AFHRM lies solely with the obstetrician and therefore will not be discussed further. In some centres, if there is a BPS of 8/8 on the ultrasound variables (i.e. FT, FM, FBM, amniotic fluid volume (AFV)), then AFHRM is not considered to be mandatory. As with most aspects of fetal monitoring this approach remains controversial.

Chronic markers

Acute markers reflect the immediate effects of hypoxaemia in the fetus and, if the scoring criteria are satisfied, a score of 8/10 is given. As discussed above these markers can be affected in numerous ways and do not necessarily reflect the effects of chronic intrauterine stress. The fetus may be found to be small; however, it may not be unhealthy. The separation of the constitutionally small fetus from the truly malnourished is fraught with difficulties. Given the significant perinatal mortality and morbidity of the small for gestational age fetus there has been a concentration on screening and diagnostic tests in this group. It must be remembered that the large fetus may be sick too and, although growing above a particular centile, may be failing to reach its growth potential because of pathological processes. Many obstetric ultrasound examinations are requests for fetal growth assessment and these examinations should include an assessment of the most important chronic marker of fetal condition, the AFV. This is such an important marker in the BPS, that extremely low AFV is given disproportionate weight when compared to the other variables. The use of other ultrasound markers of long-term fetal health, particularly fetal Doppler studies, and less importantly placental grading, merit discussion in this context although neither contribute to the BPS as described by Manning and Platt.

AFV

As described above, extremes in AFV have long been associated with fetal compromise. During the second half of pregnancy the main sources of amniotic fluid are the fetal kidneys and lungs. In animal models, reflex redistribution of blood away from the fetal kidneys and lungs results in oliguria. Oligohydramnios has been shown to be associated with a perinatal mortality rate of 89 in 1000 within 1 week of this finding and on this basis is considered to be the most important variable in BPS systems. Clinical assessments are notoriously unreliable and on the basis that 'seeing is believing', direct assessment using ultrasound was instantly attractive. There has been considerable debate regarding the optimal method of measuring AFV. The most commonly employed techniques are either by subjective assessment of volume by an experienced observer or a semi-quantitative method in which single or multiple pools of amniotic fluid are measured. Attempts to measure total intrauterine volume (TIUV) have fallen out of favour as a result of technological advances and the poor reproducibility of this laborious process.

The experienced sonographer will be able to divide AFV into broad categories, e.g. polyhydramnios or increased, normal, decreased and oligohydramnios; however, this technique is prone to considerable variability between and within observers. Manning and Platt proposed a semi-quantitative technique in their BPS wherein the depth of the maximum 1 cm wide, vertical pool, free of fetal parts and cord, was measured: qualitative AFV assessment (qAFV). They identified a significant association between a qAFV of <1 cm, intrauterine growth retardation and fetal anomaly. These findings were confirmed by Chamberlain who revised the qAFV cut-off to <2 cm. This group defined polyhydramnios as a qAFV of >8 cm.

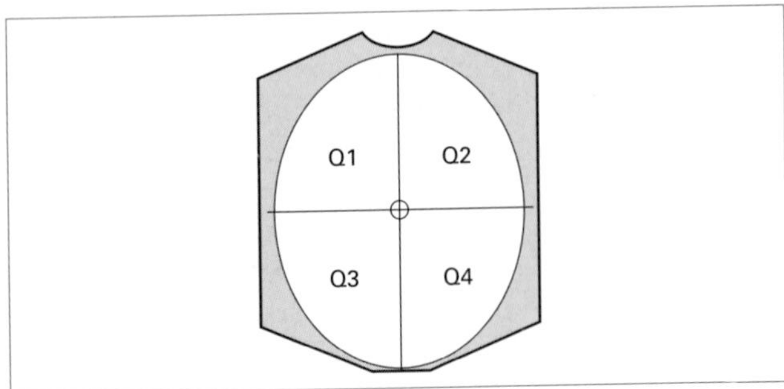

Fig. 39.2 Anatomical landmarks for determination of the four quadrant AFI.

Subsequent work indicated that qAFV varied considerably throughout pregnancy and suggested that qAFV had no advantage over subjective assessment. In an attempt to improve on these systems Phelan proposed the measurement of the amniotic fluid index (AFI), in which the maternal abdomen is divided into four quadrants (Fig. 39.2). The maximum vertical 1 cm pool in each is measured and the sum of the results represents the AFI. This appears to be both a reliable and reproducible technique and values during gestation have been defined from both cross-sectional and longitudinal datasets. The AFI rises from 20 weeks to plateau between 30 and 36 weeks thereafter declining to term. There is still debate as to the upper limits of the normal range; however, the AFI is currently the superior method for assessment of AFV and at present a score of <5 is considered to represent oligohydramnios. More work needs to be done to establish the efficiency of different levels of AFI in predicting complications.

Placental grading

Following the application of ultrasound in localization of the placenta, attempts were made to correlate an estimate of placental size (usually by a thickness measurement) with perinatal outcome, particularly in rhesus disease. As imaging improved, differences were recognized in the structural appearances of the placenta which lead to the system of placental grading proposed by Grannum. The grades were intended to reflect increasing placental maturity from 0 to 3; however, this correlation is not strong and the technique is not widely used in the UK. It is unusual to find a grade 3 placental maturity early in the third trimester and there is a correlation with placental abruption (14.8%) and abnormal fetal heart rate patterns in labour (44.4%). For this reason, Vintzileos included the placental grade in a modification of the Manning and Platt biophysical profile. It should be stressed that if reported, a clear distinction must be made between the placental grading and the placental site. As a numerical system is also used to describe the type of placenta praevia, confusion may occur with potentially disastrous consequences: in the author's unit, such a misinterpretation almost resulted in a caesarean section for an asymptomatic major placenta praevia which was actually a Grannum grade 3 placental maturity.

Doppler evaluation

The introduction of Doppler ultrasound in perinatal medicine lead to an initial flurry of excitement, which was subsequently tempered by extremely close scrutiny. Too often in the past new technologies have been introduced without rigorous evaluation with unfortunate results. Extensive research has demonstrated that Doppler evaluation of the uteroplacental circulation is a useful tool in the assessment of the high risk pregnancy. There are still controversial aspects of this technology relating not only to its eventual place as a diagnostic and monitoring tool but also regarding its safety, particularly with pulsed Doppler equipment. As there are still some uncertainties concerning the eventual role of Doppler evaluation of the fetal circulation, only a broad view will be taken highlighting the dilemmas faced in the clinical setting.

The principle of Doppler ultrasound velocimetry is that the frequency of sound reflected from moving objects is related to their velocity and direction. The frequency shift can be correlated with the velocity of blood; however, accurate quantification of flow is not yet reliable: this is critically dependent on the angle of insonation, the cross-sectional area of the vessel and possibly the blood viscosity. In the fetal circulation, estimates of volume flow would be related to the fetal weight and as this cannot be precisely defined it becomes clear why semi-quantitative assessments of flow characteristics are used in clinical practice.

Three waveform indices are commonly used, the systolic to diastolic (S/D or A/B) ratio, the resistance index (RI) and the pulsatility index (PI). These are relatively crude assessments of the waveform; however, more detailed analysis of the information contained in the waveform is not yet available. Individual centres often favour one index over the others and there has been considerable interest in the reproducibility and reliability of these measurements whether the results have been calculated automatically or manually.

Obstetric units usually have access to two types of Doppler equipment. Continuous wave Doppler (CWD) machines are available as relatively cheap, stand alone units. This is a simple, easy to learn technique, which is suitable for assessment of the fetal umbilical artery. The limiting factor is that it is indiscriminate. All moving objects within the beam are interrogated and therefore it is only possible to distinguish a particular vessel if it has a singular characteristic (e.g. the rate of the fetal heart). Pulsed wave Doppler (PWD) integrated with real-time imaging overcomes this problem. The structure of interest is visualized and a 'gate' placed over it. Only signals from within the target area are assessed. With the development of colour flow mapping (CFM) various regions of the fetal circulation are now accessible to study (Fig. 39.3). Ultrasound systems with pulsed Doppler facilities are relatively expensive but increasingly affordable. The main concern about widespread use of this technique remains over safety. Increased power outputs are required and a narrow area is exposed.

Until this concern is resolved by appropriately designed randomized controlled studies of sufficient power, PWD should be restricted to ethically approved research projects and high risk pregnancies where any perceived disadvantages are outweighed by potential advantages.

As a result of the technical restrictions described, research has focused on the use of CWD as a screening and simple diagnostic tool, and PWD as a means by which regional flow adaptations can be studied (e.g. fetal aorta, cerebral, carotid and renal arteries, inferior vena cava, intracardiac flows). PWD is useful for the non-invasive study of physiological and pathological adaptions to disease processes and in assessing the effects of pharmacological agents. In the compromised human fetus, regional changes in flow, as demonstrated by changes in waveform indices, are of considerable interest as they correspond to the changes seen in animal models.

Potential uses of Doppler in clinical practice

Abnormal flow velocity waveforms in the umbilical artery define a placental lesion which increases downstream resistance. Alterations in the flow characteristics of other fetal vessels are a response to this.

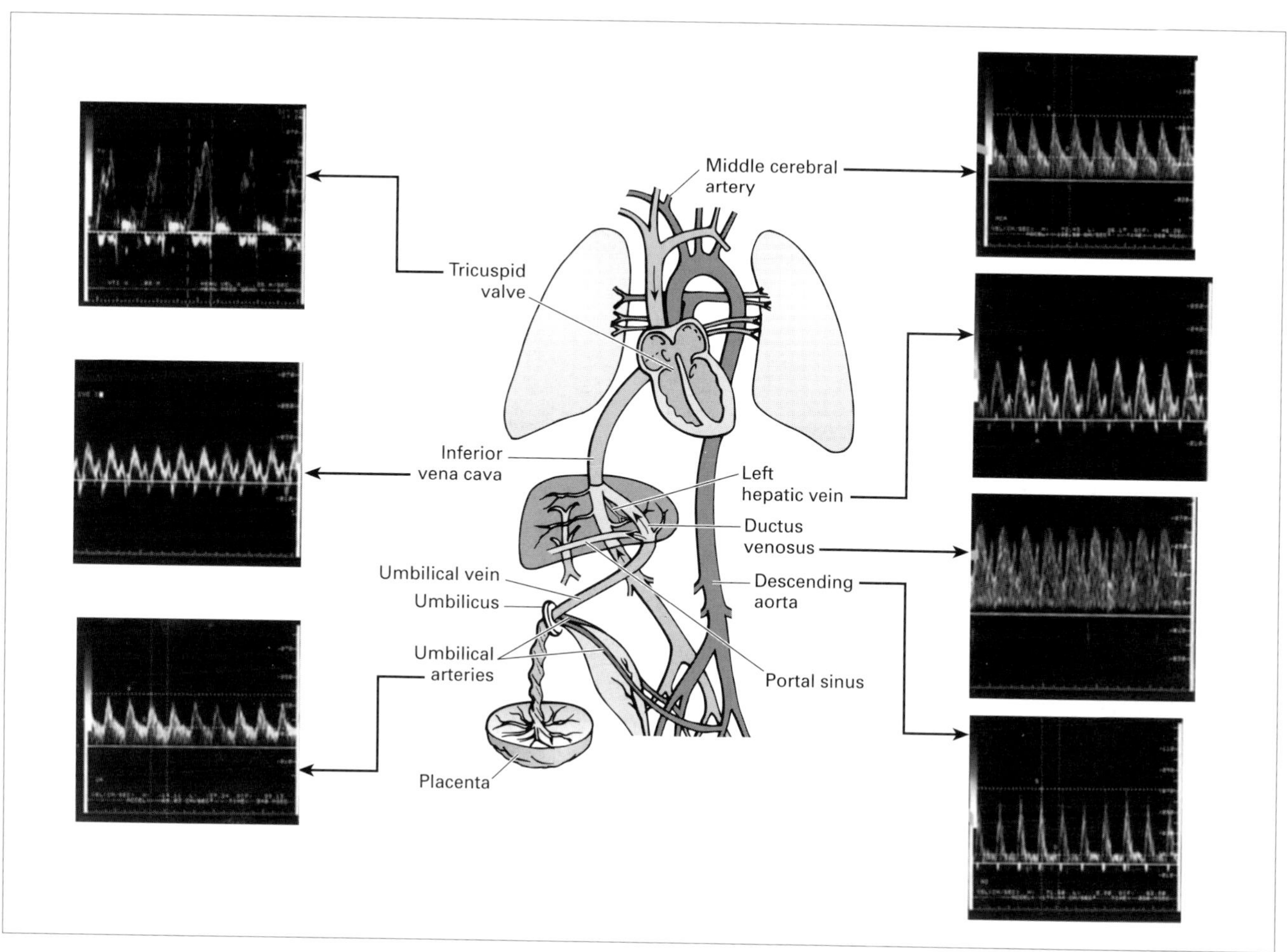

Fig. 39.3 Doppler assessment of different areas of the fetoplacental circulation.

Hypertensive disorders in pregnancy and many cases of pathological fetal growth retardation are associated with changes in the uteroplacental vasculature. Incomplete invasion of the spiral arteries results in the persistence of a high resistance system. In some cases the placental flow disturbances are focal rather than global. There was initial interest in the utilization of CWD as a screening tool which would identify high resistance in the maternal portion of the uteroplacental circulation; however, concern emerged regarding reproducibility and sensitivity. More recently a two-stage screening regime of sampling the uterine arteries using CFM and PWD and looking for a prediastolic notch as well as a high RI has attracted interest. The fetal umbilical artery is the only fetal vessel which can be assessed by CWD. In normal pregnancies, placental resistance falls with advancing gestational age, with a resultant increase in end-diastolic flow (EDF). While it is apparent that loss of EDF is an indicator of increased risk there is no evidence as yet from a randomized controlled trial that widespread introduction of screening the low risk population by this means would be efficient.

There is more convincing evidence to support the use of Doppler in high risk pregnancies. In the small for gestational age fetus with normal structure and liquor volume, the demonstration of normal umbilical indices is reassuring and uteroplacental insufficiency is less likely to be present (Fig. 39.4). If EDF is absent the fetus is at high risk of perinatal compromise and requires increased surveillence. Absent EDF may be present for weeks before other fetal assessments become abnormal. This is therefore a chronic marker of the fetal environment (cf. AFV). Eventually reverse flow in the umbilical artery may be seen (Fig. 39.5).

When PWD was introduced much attention was paid to the fetal aortic waveform. This is relatively easy to obtain but is angle dependent. Absent EDF here was initially thought to be a sign of imminent danger; however, it has become evident that, like the umbilical artery, changes can be present for several weeks. CFM has facilitated the study of other fetal vessels and much attention has been focused on the cerebral circulation. This is a high resistance system in the normal state. Hypoxia causes vasodilation and as a consequence the EDF component increases (Fig. 39.6). This is part of the brain-sparing protective mechanism and it has been suggested that intervention at this point may be more beneficial than waiting for the development of abnormalities in the acute CNS-mediated biophysical markers.

Attention has now been turned on adaptations to stress of the fetal venous systems. Flow in the umbilical vein is usually continuous. Pulsations in this system are seen in the first trimester probably due to ventricular wall stiffness at this stage. In the growth retarded fetus, pulsation in the umbilical vein indicates severe cardiac compromise and is associated with increased perinatal mortality (Fig. 39.7). There is still much to learn about the pathophysiological processes that lead to alterations in the various regional waveforms and indices. Doppler studies of multiple fetal vessels and fetal cardiac studies are providing fascinating insights into these mechanisms (Table 39.2).

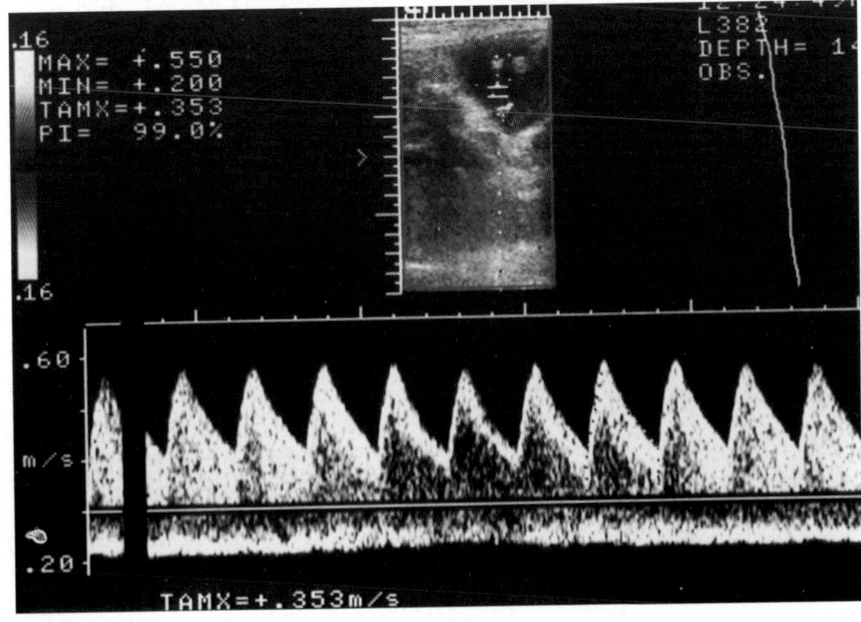

Fig. 39.4 Normal umbilical artery waveform. Note continuous even flow in umbilical vein (below line).

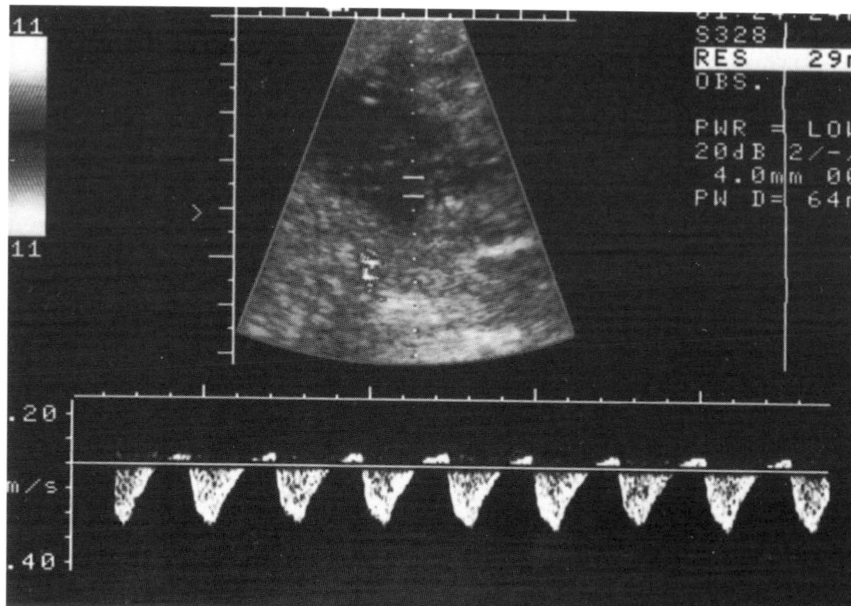

Fig. 39.5 Reverse EDF.

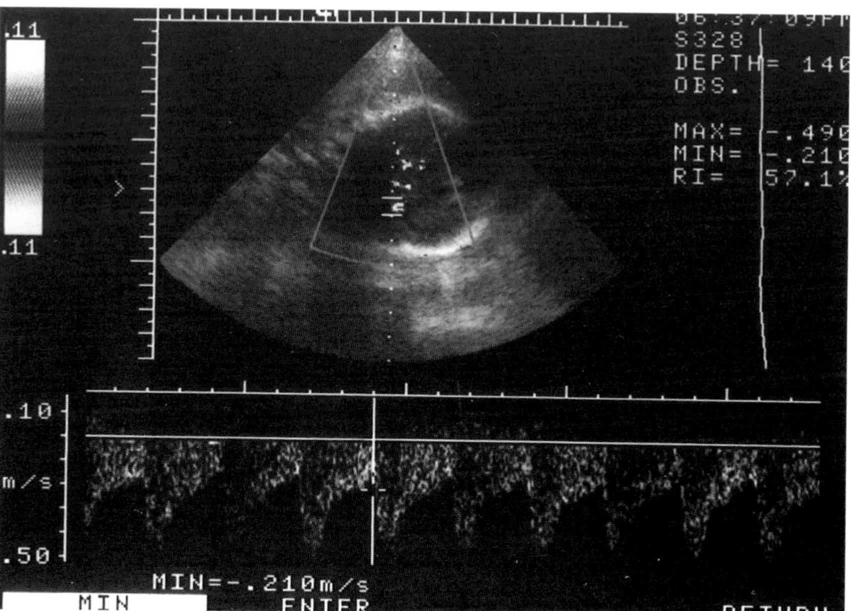

Fig. 39.6 Middle cerebral artery—vasodilatation.

Table 39.2 Guide to sequential changes in fetal circulation with uteroplacental lesion

Umbilical artery	Middle cerebral artery	Umbilical vein
Reduced EDF		
Absent EDF	Increased EDF	
Reverse EDF	Reduced EDF	Pulsations

As previously stated, new technologies have frequently been introduced into clinical practice without rigorous evaluation. The low perinatal mortality rates (PNMR) enjoyed today mean that increasing effort is required to identify the very small number of fetuses truly at risk without unnecessary study and intervention in the false positive population. The problems related to electronic fetal monitoring, practical and medicolegal, have tempered the initial enthusiasm that Doppler provides all the answers. Fetal Doppler assessment is undoubtedly destined to be an important investigative tool in the future

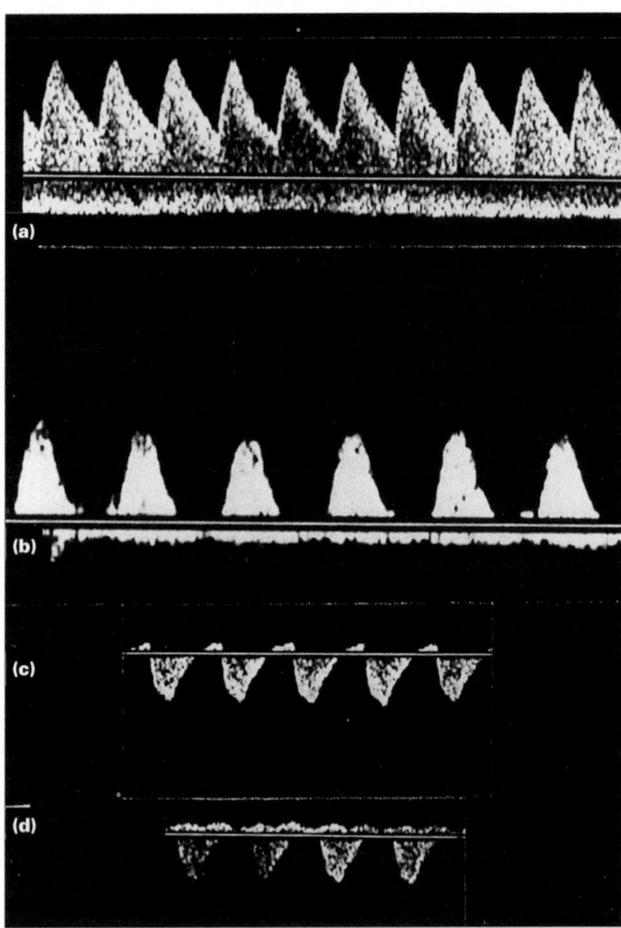

Fig. 39.7 Progressive deterioration in umbilical Doppler assessment. Case of severe pre-eclampsia with intrauterine growth retardation. Changes occurred between 23 and 26 weeks. (a) Normal waveform: note EDF and steady venous flow. (b) Absent EDF. (c) Reverse EDF. (d) Venous pulsations present above line. Reverse arterial flow continued. The picture is taken to emphasize the venous modifications.

but it is not yet clear as to what this role will be. It does help the clinician to identify a subgroup of fetuses compromised by a placental lesion. It remains to be proven that by closer study of the interrelationship of changes within the fetal arterial and venous systems fetal compromise will be detected at an earlier stage than at present with a subsequent improvement in the clinical outcome.

Antepartum fetal assessment in practice

Long before an ultrasound transducer is applied to the pregnant abdomen, the clinician should have clearly defined what is required from the investigation. The examination can then be performed by the appropriate level of practitioner, on a patient fully informed as to the nature and purpose of the test. There are of course circumstances in which a hitherto unsuspected problem is identified. Sonographers performing fetal assessments must be aware of when to refer cases for more detailed assessment. There is a disproportionate increase in the perinatal mortality rate in patients with recognizable high risk factors. Of these cases 10–20% will be attributable to a major fetal anomaly. It can therefore be argued that any patient requiring a full BPS should have their first assessment made by a sonographer competent in fetal anomaly scanning. If the pregnancy is truly high risk then there is a high likelihood of intervention and possibly preterm delivery. The detection of a major anomaly may completely alter subsequent obstetric management. Once a major structural anomaly is excluded, subsequent BPS can be performed by a less advanced sonographer.

Method of BPS

Initially the sonographer should obtain basic information regarding fetal heart activity, fetal number, lie and position. The placental site and morphology should be determined and some authors advocate that the position of the cord should be checked to exclude cord presentation. Fetal biometry should be performed, including biparietal diameter, head and abdominal circumference, and femoral length. A systematic fetal anomaly scan should then be conducted if required. It should be remembered that a previously negative anomaly scan at 18–20 weeks may not demonstrate some of the problems which manifest themselves in the third trimester (e.g. gastrointestinal atresias). The AFI or the maximum vertical pool should be measured and some practitioners may wish to record a subjective measure of AFV as described above. If there is a cord and fetal part free liquor pool greater than 2 cm deep and 1 cm wide a score of 2 is awarded.

A longitudinal view of the fetus is then obtained in order that the fetal face, forelimbs (particularly the hands) and fetal thorax can be visualized. The examination start time should be noted and observations continued until the following criteria are satisfied or 30 min have elapsed.

FBM

Discrete movements of the thorax causing descent and return to the original position of the diaphragm and abdominal contents. Fetal 'hiccups' are interpreted as a variant of normal fetal breathing activity. Different rates and patterns of FBM can be recognized; however, at present these are not given any clinical weighting. When 30 s of continuous fetal breathing has been observed, a score of 2 is awarded.

FM

These are defined as single or clusters of activity, involving the limbs and/or the fetal body. Three discrete movement episodes occurring within 30 min scores 2. While easily seen, movements of the lips, tongue and eyes are not included in the scoring system.

FT

This has always been the most criticized of the BPS variables and is the most sensitive to observer bias. The definition has been modified since the original description of the BPS and the assessment is now determined by fetal hand activity. At least one episode wherein the hand opens (with finger and thumb extension) and then returns to a close fist formation scores 2.

In the absence of such a movement, a score of 2 is awarded if the hand remains in fist formation throughout the entire scan period. In the presence of normal movements, tone is automatically awarded 2 points, unless the hand is persistently open (finger and thumbs extended).

The ultrasonographer can therefore award a score of 0 or 2 for each of the four variables (FBM, FM, FT, AFV). Scores of 0, 2, 4, 6 or 8 out of a possible 8 are therefore produced. The AFHRT result can then be scored, to complete the score out of 10.

If requested, Doppler investigations may then be performed but these results do not influence the formal BPS score awarded. In some North American centres AFHRM is only performed when at least one of the ultrasound variables is abnormal. Using this system less than 5% of patients require AFHRM and it is claimed that there is no change in the negative predictive accuracy; however, this remains controversial.

Which test, when and for how long?

The sonographer must work in liaison with clinicians in order to minimize the very real dangers of inappropriate testing and inefficient use of the sonographer's time. While North American centres have embraced the BPS as the gold standard method of fetal assessment, this is not the case in the UK. The main criticism of the BPS is not related to the logic of the test but rather to the lack of clear advantages over existing tests as demonstrated by randomized control trials. Another concern is the criteria used in considering the patient 'high risk'. Audits of large numbers of patients prospectively studied and managed by the formal BPS of Manning and Platt reveal impressive results regarding the PNMR (corrected and uncorrected for fetal abnormality) but need to be interpreted with caution. A large number of BPS examinations are performed for 'postdate' pregnancies. A satisfactory score (8/10 with normal fluid, 10/10), is associated with a PNMR <1/1000 within the following week. This reassures the clinician to postpone induction of labour when the cervix is unfavourable. Given the extremely low risk of fetal death occurring in this group any test of fetal well-being is likely to have a low false negative rate. This skews the outcome results to favour the positive predictive value of a normal BPS with regards to predicting continued fetal health. What is clear from the reported series is that there is a correlation between significant fetal compromise and low BPS scores and that the degree of acidosis correlates with the sequential loss of the CNS-mediated markers.

As with any test, abnormal results must be considered in the context of the existing clinical situation. Formal BPS should only be performed when abnormal results will prompt action. They are therefore inappropriate in the extremely premature infant or when the pregnancy cannot be prolonged in the interests of maternal safety. There is little need for full BPS in the patient with normal AFHRM and AFV or when the fetus is mature and the cervix is favourable. The place of BPS in the evaluation of multiple pregnancy is complicated by the usual clinical dilemma in such cases: is it justifiable to risk a seemingly healthy preterm infant for the benefit of a potentially compromised one? Other obstetric issues, particularly gestational age and parental wishes are often critical factors in such cases.

Some other common problems experienced with the BPS are worthy of consideration. If oligohydramnios is present, rupture of the membranes and renal tract anomalies must be excluded. Daily BPS appears to be useful in the conservative management of patients with preterm premature rupture of the membranes. If the oligohydramnios is 'unexplained', delivery is advocated because of the high associated PNMR (89 in 1000).

The gradual hypoxia concept suggests that in the presence of normal AFHRM and AFV, continuation of the BPS is unnecessary. Similarly, if for some reason AFHRM was not performed or the test was non-reactive (a common indication for BPS), the presence of fetal breathing with normal fluid would be reassuring and the test could be stopped. If fetal breathing was absent, the test should be continued. If FM and FT are present then the score would be 6/10 and therefore equivocal. Prolongation of the test beyond 30 min is indicated in order to differentiate hypoxia from a sleep state. Some centres have advocated the use of external vibroacoustic stimulation (VAS) in an effort to 'wake' the fetus from physiological sleep and thus decrease the examination time and possibly identify hypoxic fetuses more quickly. Such an intervention would alter the nature of the BPS from a test of adaptation to an assessment of response to stress. The normal sleep cycle of the human fetus increases in length with gestational age (up to 40–60 min). Prolonging the test up to this time is therefore advised. If the test remains equivocal, then the clinician has to consider retesting within 24 h (75% of retests are normal) or delivery. With scores of, or below, 4/10, delivery is indicated as there is a 60% PNMR and considerable morbidity associated with this group.

Conclusion

The development of ultrasound-based technologies allows the obstetric sonographer to perform antenatal assessments which mirror that of the neonatologist examining the newborn. Consequently, size and structure can be assessed, reflexes observed and invasive tests performed, if required, to check for biochemical, haematological, chromosomal or infective problems. In addition, the intrauterine environment can be assessed by looking at the AFV and placental grade, and regional blood flow can be studied using the Doppler principle.

There is still much to learn; however, it is possible to define fetal health and illness with increasing accuracy. This allows the development of monitoring regimes for the fetus which will complement the individualized care its mother should receive. As with all ultrasound-based technologies, the usefulness of antenatal fetal assessment is critically dependent on properly trained sonographers performing appropriate tests for the right indications as part of a multidisciplinary team.

Futher reading

Arduini, D., Rizzo, G. (1993) Doppler studies of deteriorating growth retarded fetuses. In: *Current Opinion in Obstetrics and Gynaecology*. Current Science, Philadelphia,pp. 195–203.

Chalmers, I., Enkin, M., Keirse, M. (eds) (1990) *Effective Care in Pregnancy and Childbirth*, vol. 1. Oxford University Press, Oxford.

Chervenak, F.A., Kurjak, A. (eds) (1996) *Current Perspectives on the Fetus as a Patient*. Parthenon Publishing, Lancs, UK.

Devoe, L.D. (ed.) (1994) *Clinics in Perinatology: Antenatal Fetal Assessment*. WB Saunders, Philadelphia.

Ingemarsson, I., Ingemarsson, E., Spencer, J.A.D. (1993) Antenatal cardiotocography. In: Ingemarsson, I., Ingemarsson, E., Spencer, J.A.D. (eds) *Fetal Heart Rate Monitoring*. Oxford University Press, Oxford, pp. 223–254.

Manning, F.A. (ed.) (1989) *Clinics in Perinatology: Fetal Monitoring*. WB Saunders, Philadelphia.

Manning, F.A., Platt, L.D., Sipos, L. (1980) Antepartum fetal evaluation: development of a fetal biophysical profile. *American Journal of Obstetrics and Gynaecology* **136**, 787–795.

Whittle, M.J. (ed.) (1987) *Fetal monitoring. Baillière's Clinical Obstetrics and Gynaecology*. Baillière Tindall, Eastbourne.

Chapter 40: Invasive prenatal diagnostic techniques

A.M. Mathers

The development of diagnostic amniocentesis in the 1960s ended the isolation of the fetus from laboratory-based science. Initially specimens were obtained by 'blind' needling, fetal transfusion was performed under image intensification and the fetus with hydrops fetalis was invariably doomed. Advances in allied sciences, particularly genetics, lead to new diagnostic and therapeutic possibilities. Fetal pathology was defined with increased accuracy. The development of fetoscopy in the 1970s allowed direct visualization of the fetal surface anatomy, access to the fetal vasculature, and biopsy of the fetal liver and skin. Thus it became possible to detect rare inherited disorders. However, fetoscopy carried a high fetal loss rate and was never widely available. As ultrasound imaging improved, the need for fetoscopy was largely replaced by the development of ultrasound facilitated biopsy of the fetus and its environment. As new techniques are developed and existing tests are refined, the sonographer must be familiar with all of the diagnostic and, increasingly, therapeutic options available. There is no place for practitioners to perform an 'occasional' invasive test and the highly specialized techniques (e.g. fetal transfusion, bladder shunting) should only be performed in regional referral centres with appropriate experience in the management of complex cases. The processes of counselling, screening for and diagnosis of fetal disorders are fraught with, at the very least, ethical, moral, legal and practical difficulties. This chapter focuses on the practical elements of invasive testing; however, it is essential that practitioners are conversant with the wider issues involved and the bearing these have on the service they provide, their patients and society in general (see further reading).

General considerations

The birth of a baby with a serious pathology may be regarded as a continuum from a blessing to a disaster. The single most important consideration relating to invasive tests is the comparative danger of iatrogenic compromise to the fetus in relation to the potential usefulness of the information obtained to its parents and the clinical team. Some patients will never consider prenatal testing as termination of an affected fetus would not be acceptable to them. Many are less certain.

It is vital that carefully structured comprehensive pretest counselling is available. Individual clinicians and patients may have very different perceptions with respect to the utility of a particular intervention. The process of investigation should be a stepwise continuum from the initial consultation through to the consequences of the result, whether this is positive, negative or, as is sometimes the case, equivocal (Table 40.1). Patients should be aware of what options are available to them once the results are available. These will include fetal therapy, birth with an anticipated disorder or termination of the pregnancy (Fig. 40.1). Patients should know if termination of the pregnancy will be an option and how this might be achieved. The practice of only offering a test if the patient would consider termination is to be deprecated. Prenatal diagnostic tests offer choice through knowledge. While some patients will elect to terminate the pregnancy, others will use the 'diagnosis to delivery' interval to make further choices as to the mode of delivery and to prepare for the birth of their baby. Every prenatal diagnostic service should have appropriately motivated and trained staff who can access relevent clinical and non-clinical support agencies and therefore facilitate parents in whatever course of action they embark upon. These services are of equal importance after the pregnancy ends.

Laboratory considerations

Prenatal diagnostic units must have excellent liaisons with relevent laboratory and clinical services. Staff need to be well trained and scrupulous in the correct labelling of specimens, accurate filling in of forms, administration of anti-D prophylaxis when required and transport arrangements. The establishment of designated 'sessions' for invasive procedures is a considerable advantage. This facilitates administration at the clinical and laboratory level and the training of medical and nursing staff.

Table 40.1 Options for prenatal screening/diagnosis

Preimplantation	
First trimester	CVS, amniocentesis, ultrasound
Second trimester	biochemical screening, ultrasound, invasive tests
Third trimester	ultrasound, invasive tests

Table 40.2 Patient groups presenting for invasive prenatal diagnosis

Pre-existing condition, e.g. parental translocation
Antenatal screen positive or abnormal scan finding
Late pregnancy complication, e.g. intrauterine growth restriction, polyhydramnios

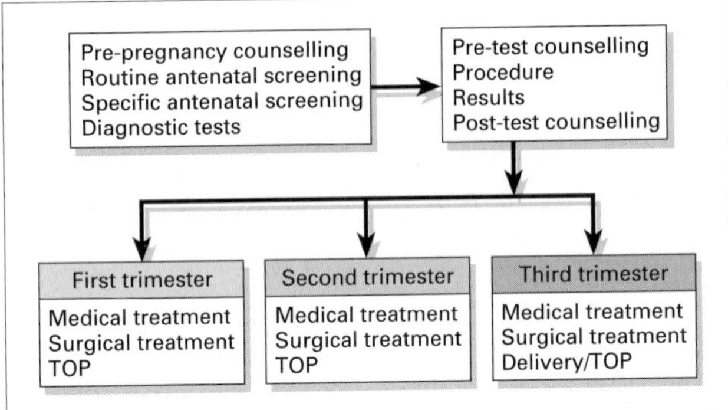

Fig. 40.1 Considerations for making a diagnosis in antenatal screening. TOP, termination of pregnancy.

The spectrum of tests available will depend on the nature of the unit and its technical and financial resources. Prearrangement of certain sophisticated investigations (e.g. DNA probes) is essential as the analysis may not be performed locally and will therefore have logistic and financial implications. The reference laboratory may need to be contacted about the availability and reliability of the investigation. A quality control may be requested, e.g. cord blood, and appropriate arrangements should be made.

Which test and when?

Invasive testing may be required in three broad instances (Table 40.2). Firstly, the patient may have a pre-existing condition which increases the risk of having an affected infant, e.g. advanced maternal age, balanced translocation, rhesus isoimmunization or previous fetal anomaly. Ideally, such patients will have been counselled prior to the pregnancy and clearly understand the utility of the tests offered. Secondly, the largest number of patients will be referred as a result of the biochemical screening programme designed to identify fetuses at risk of neural tube defects (NTD) and trisomies (the triple test) or, when a structural abnormality is detected during ultrasound examinations in the mid trimester. Since its introduction in the 1970s, biochemical screening using maternal serum α-fetoprotein (MSAFP) has had a major impact in the detection of NTDs. The realization that MSAFP could be used in association with other biochemical markers (human chorionic gonadotrophin (HCG), oestriol) to identify women with an increased risk of fetal autosomal trisomy, in particular trisomy 21 (low MSAFP, elevated HCG), when correlated with the maternal age risk, has resulted in a significantly increased detection rate of trisomic fetuses. Prior to the introduction of biochemical screening, the prenatal detection rate of trisomy 21 was approximately 15%, as most live births occurred in women under the age of 35 years. All pregnant women are 'at risk' of fetal aneuploidy. Biochemical screening is therefore an option for the entire pregnant population and is significantly more sensitive than simply asking the patient her age, the previous screening method employed. Widening the screening net is, of course, not without its problems. Patients often find it difficult to appreciate the differences between a screening and a diagnostic test and there are very real clinical difficulties encountered when giving numerical risk values to screen positives. The essential elements of a successful biochemical screening programme for NTD and trisomy 21 are the accurate assessment of gestational age and the provision of comprehensive pre- and post-test counselling, support and information. The practice of only informing screen positives of their results should be abandoned. Patients can experience considerable residual anxiety after such tests.

The third set of cases arise from the detection of an unexpected maternal or fetal complication (e.g. severe intrauterine growth restriction, non-immune hydrops, fetal anomaly, extremes of liquor volume), in which detailed knowledge of the fetal condition may be useful in determining management. Increasingly management options include the option of fetal therapy. While numerically the smallest group, such cases are often the most time-consuming and fraught with practical and philosophical difficulties. A multidisciplinary approach is essential and tertiary referral or consultation is often advantageous.

The decision to offer a particular test has to be governed by a balance of the relative risk of the procedure against its diagnostic accuracy and the time interval before the result is available (Table 40.3). A 3–4 week wait for an amniocentesis culture which might be acceptable to a 35-year-old

Table 40.3 Available prenatal invasive tests. Rapid exclusion of common trisomies possible using FISH analysis. Adequate anti-D must be given to non-immunized rhesus negative women

Amniocentesis	CVS	PUBS
Widely available	Limited availability	Limited availability
Gold standard	Transabdominal	Karyotype <4 days
Limited uses	Transcervical	Full serology possible
Culture 2–3 weeks	Karyotype <24 h	

PUBS, percutaneous umbilical blood sampling.

woman with no other risk factors for autosomal trisomy, would, however, be an inappropriate interval in a case of hydrops fetalis discovered at 32 weeks gestation. Patients quite rightly wish their anxieties to be resolved quickly and it should be remembered that one of the main attractions of chorionic villous biopsy was the utility of chromosomal analysis within 24 h, enabling the option of first trimester termination and therefore avoiding the difficulties of mid trimester abortion. Perhaps the most difficult dilemmas arise when the fetus is at a gestational age which is considered to be viable and therefore delivery is an option. Reconsider the case of the hydropic fetus discovered at 32 weeks gestation. A fetal blood sample will enable rapid determination of haematological indices; however, a fetal karyotype may not be available for 2–5 days. Even with the advent of the fluorescent *in situ* hybridization (FISH) technique there is a time window between test and result. The parents and clinicians have to determine a management plan should there be a deterioration in the fetal condition before the results are available. There are no easy answers for such clinical dilemmas, the important point is that there must be a clear understanding between the clinical team and the parents as to their options.

General technique and risks of invasive procedures

While there are individual logistic and laboratory considerations relating to the various techniques of invasive prenatal diagnosis, certain basic principles and risks are common to them all. The practice of performing an 'occasional' procedure should be discouraged and ideally each unit should have a designated team expert in these techniques. Trainees should start with amniocentesis and proceed through transabdominal chorionic villus sampling (CVS) before embarking on fetal blood sampling and similar fetal procedures. A standard approach to each technique is preferable. Most of the procedures are performed using spinal needles; however, different gauges and lengths are necessary depending on the intended procedure and patient characteristics.

Opinions differ as to the use of prophylactic antibiotics, maternal sedation or local anaesthetic for the more complicated techniques but these are preferable for a relatively prolonged procedure (e.g. fetal transfusion).

High resolution ultrasound equipment is vital. Two operators are preferable, one to insert the needle and one to aspirate the sample, although 'one handed' amniocentesis and CVS is possible. It is useful for there to be an assistant whose immediate job is to label and transfer specimens as required and give moral support to the patient if she is unaccompanied. The patient is placed in a comfortable supine position and a preliminary scan performed to confirm viability, further assess the fetus and establish the placental site and optimal needle tract. Some practitioners prefer to use a needle guide for insertions, others opt for a free hand technique. While needle guides help to build confidence early in the learning curve for the various procedures they are not infallible and, particularly for cord sampling, it is often necessary to release the needle and continue free hand, albeit in a narrower target area. Competence with both techniques is therefore necessary. After ensuring that all pieces of necessary equipment are readily available, the abdomen is cleaned with an antiseptic solution and the ultrasound transducer is placed in a sterile plastic bag containing coupling gel. Sterile gel is placed on the patient's abdomen. Holding the transducer in one hand the practitioner inserts the needle under continuous observation using a no-touch technique. It is sometimes useful for the assistant to stretch the skin with a gauze swab to prevent skin drag at the time of needle insertion. Once the specimen is obtained, the needle is withdrawn and the fetal heart rate is checked. As a transient bradycardia is not uncommon it is preferable to wait for about 30 s before demonstrating the fetal heart to the patient.

The specimen should be clearly labelled and sent to the laboratory as soon as possible. It is prudent to warn the laboratory in advance of the number and nature of specimens. Early recognition of 'lost' specimens is essential as they are usually retrievable and still suitable for analysis.

An appropriate dose of anti-D immunoglobulin should be given to all non-sensitized rhesus negative women (usually 250 IU if under 20 weeks, 500 IU thereafter). Maternal blood should be taken for a Kleihaur test which quantifies any fetomaternal haemorrhage which may have occurred and an appropriate further dose of anti-D immunoglobulin can therefore be given.

The patient should be warned that she may experience some abdominal cramp and be given suitable advice with regard to analgesia and a contact number if she is worried. Clear arrangements should be made regarding the receiving of results and follow-up.

All invasive procedures involve risk to the fetus. The main risk is of fetal death either as a direct result of the procedure (e.g. cord haematoma, exsanguination) or from an interval complication (e.g. chorioamnionitis, preterm labour). Fetal morbidity may occur as a result of premature prelabour rupture of the membranes resulting in pulmonary and postural problems or as a specific effect of the procedure (e.g. the association of limb reduction deformities with early CVS prior to 9 weeks). It cannot be overemphasized that failure to administer Anti-D immunoglobulin to rhesus negative mothers is a potent source of morbidity and litigation. Failure to culture cells successfully or the finding of karyotypic oddities may occur with any technique and these possibilities should be addressed during pretest discussions. Finally, it is prudent to offer a detailed anomaly scan to all patients who undergo invasive diagnosis in early pregnancy if this is not routinely performed.

Amniocentesis

Amniocentesis is the oldest invasive diagnostic test, remains the most widely available and is the technique that can be regarded as the gold standard for the diagnosis of chromosomal abnormalities. Initially used as a therapy for polyhydramnios, biochemical tests were developed to monitor rhesus disease and determine the likelihood of fetal lung maturity. Before the advent of high resolution ultrasound, amniotic fluid analysis of α-fetoprotein (AFP) and acetylcholinesterase activity was essential in the diagnosis of NTD. In the 1990s the commonest indication for amniocentesis is to detect chromosomal abnormalities. This is usually performed between 15 and 18 weeks gestation and there is usually a 2–4-week wait for culture results. The use of FISH analysis enables next day exclusion of the most common trisomies and determination of fetal sex but is not widely available. Culture failure may occur necessitating a further procedure, and further delay in obtaining a result. The development of CVS as a means for early diagnosis of chromosomal defects was greeted with tremendous enthusiasm which has been tempered by the subsequently discovered limitations of CVS and the advent of maternal serum screening for trisomy 21. The spotlight has returned to amniocentesis and in particular, early amniocentesis (EA) which can be performed as early as 7 weeks gestation. For various technical and practical reasons it is likely that if EA is of proven benefit it will be performed after 10 weeks; however, rigorous assessment by randomized control trial relating to risk–benefits is required before it becomes a common practice. While the loss rate from EA appears to be comparable to CVS, there remains concern about orthopaedic deformities (perhaps due to fluid leaks). The utility of measuring biochemical markers of NTDs from EA specimens remains unresolved.

Technique

For a diagnostic amniocentesis a 22-gauge spinal needle is sufficient. After insertion, 1–2 ml of fluid, which may be blood-stained, is removed and discarded; this is of particular importance when the procedure is being done for the assessment of rhesus disease. Thereafter, 15–20 ml of fluid is aspirated and the needle withdrawn. When the amniocentesis is performed for therapeutic reasons a 20 g needle is suitable (see below). As the needle is in the immediate vicinity of the fetus, it is sometimes necessary to nudge the inquisitive fetus gently out of the way of the needle. Occasionally a 'dry' amniocentesis tap occurs despite an apparently correct needle placement. This may be due to tenting of the amnion which has not been punctured. Advancement of the needle resolves this problem. If the needle is through the amnion and the tap remains dry, gentle pressure applied laterally to the uterus usually results in a successful aspiration. Replacing the stylet may help unblock a needle, it is extremely rare for a second puncture to be necessary. In cases where serial amniocentesis is required, it is reasonable to administer prophylactic antibiotics and send a portion of the specimen for bacteriological examination.

Early amniocentesis is performed from 10 weeks using the standard technique and 22-gauge needle. It is essential that the amnion, which has not yet fused with the chorion, is punctured, to avoid analysis of the extra-amniotic fluid. As previously stated this technique should be evaluated thoroughly prior to its widespread use.

Finally, there are unique problems when performing invasive tests in multiple pregnancies. Correct ascertainment of which sac has been sampled is crucial particularly in the absence of discordant anomalies or fetal sex. Some favour a double needle insertion, while others sample one and then advance the needle into the next sac. The practice of inserting methylene blue dye into one sac is no longer used as it is associated with an increased risk of fetal bowel atresia.

Indications for diagnostic amniocentesis

Apart from the detection of chromosomal anomalies, amniocentesis still has a role in several other obstetric pathologies, in particular the management of rhesus isoimmunization, where an indirect assessment of fetal haemolysis can be made from the optical spectrometry of bilirubin in the amniotic fluid. Occasionally, amniocentesis helps in the management of patients with suspected chorioamnionitis following preterm rupture of the membranes. Although such cases may have oligohydramnios, it is usually possible to locate a small cord free pool and the instillation, and later aspiration, of some sterile saline facilitates bacteriological assessment. In cases of severe oligohydramnios, the instillation of a large volume of Ringer lactate (e.g. 500 ml), at body temperature, enables a more comprehensive study of fetal anatomy, renal function and, of course, integrity of the amniotic sac. This technique is called amnioinfusion.

Indications for therapeutic amniocentesis

In certain cases reduction of the amniotic volume can be of benefit. The most common indication is in twin pregnancies complicated by twin-to-twin transfusion syndrome. This condition has a high perinatal mortality and morbidity and the only proven treatment to date is amnioreduction. Serial procedures are usually required, although occasionally a single procedure will suffice. The fluid should be withdrawn slowly and it would appear that large volume amnioreduction (i.e. several litres) can be safely achieved.

There is a limited role for amnioreduction to relieve maternal symptoms caused by severe polyhydramnios. Several litres of fluid may need to be removed. The use of a mechanical suction pump for large volume amnioreduction is recommended. This procedure can take up to an hour and it is important to ensure that the patient is in a comfortable well-supported position. A case can be made for the use of local anaesthetic, prophylactic antibiotics and tocolytic drugs in such cases. If serial amnioreduction is required then it is advisable to send subsequent samples for bacteriological examination.

Associated risks

Several studies have reported an increased pregnancy loss rate of between 0.5 and 1% above the background rate of mid trimester loss. These rates include pregnancies which were subsequently terminated for fetal anomaly. There is a higher loss rate when the MSAFP is elevated; however, high definition ultrasound examination has largely removed the need for amniocentesis as a means of diagnosing NTD. If the procedure is performed under optimal conditions for the detection of autosomal trisomies, it is reasonable to quote a 1 in 200 chance of miscarrying a genetically normal fetus as a consequence of the test. Individual departments are advised to audit their own performance and use this data for counselling their patients.

Future developments

One of the main concerns about EA is that the volume of fluid removed may represent up to 30% of the total amniotic fluid. A technique of amniofiltration is currently being evaluated whereby a closed filtration system allows the collection of a larger number of cells with the removal of only 1 ml of amniotic fluid.

CVS

The procedure of CVS, first introduced in Scandinavia in 1968, gained widespread acceptance during the 1980s. The principle of the test is that the fetal portion of the placenta, the chorion frondosum, has the same embryological origins as the fetus, and therefore this material can be used both to determine the fetal karyotype and for biochemical studies. The initial enthusiasm for CVS was understandable. Here was a technique applicable to the first trimester, from as early as 6 weeks, that allowed cytogenetic analysis within a few days. CVS was compatible with the new genetic technologies and patients could defer the announcement of a pregnancy until appropriate investigations were completed. If the fetus was affected, the option of first trimester suction termination was available, a technique which is safer and physically easier for the patient. The initial promise of CVS has been tempered somewhat by controversies regarding safety and accuracy. The development of maternal serum screening for trisomy 21, and the evolution of EA in tandem with faster cytogenetic analytical techniques have further diminished the need for first trimester CVS. Large collaborative studies of sufficient power have been performed which have helped to determine the utility of CVS compared to mid trimester amniocentesis. CVS will remain the technique of choice in first trimester diagnosis until alternative techniques have been similarly rigorously assessed.

As CVS is possible throughout pregnancy it remains an option for rapid karyotyping in later pregnancy. Patients electing to have biochemical screening may not find out they are screen positive until they are 17–18 weeks and may not receive an amniocentesis culture result for 3–4 weeks. Mid trimester CVS is an alternative to amniocentesis which appears to be at least as safe and will yield faster results.

Technique

CVS can be performed using a transabdominal (TA) or transcervical (TC) approach. The two techniques appear to be similar in safety and effectiveness; however, there is an obvious attraction to the TA technique as it is a technical analogue to amniocentesis. The TC technique is less 'patient friendly' for obvious reasons and is associated with more vaginal bleeding. It should be noted that the TA approach was developed in response to difficulties sampling some patients transcervically. The eventual technique employed will largely depend on the practitioner's preferences.

TRANSABDOMINAL CVS

An 18–20-gauge spinal needle is inserted into the placenta under direct ultrasound guidance (Fig. 40.2). Once in place, the sample is aspirated using a 10–20 ml syringe or a mechanical suction system. Alternatively, small biopsy forceps can be used, which is a particularly useful technique when a large sample is required for metabolic studies. Some practitioners place a small quantity of culture medium in the syringe. The needle tip is moved up and down within the placenta under direct vision, in order that an adequate sample is obtained. Repeat needle insertions are rarely required and diminish with operator experience. Occasionally, it is difficult to gain access to posterior placentae. Asking the patient to partially empty her bladder may help. If access remains difficult, deferring the procedure for a week usually converts a potentially difficult procedure into an easy one, as there is a tendency for the uterus to antevert as pregnancy advances and there is a larger placental bulk. When the uterus is retroverted an assistant may perform a vaginal examination and gently move the uterus and chorionic plate until access is possible.

TRANSCERVICAL CVS

This is performed with the patient in a modified lithotomy position, with a full bladder and for practical reasons is limited to the first trimester. A Cusco's speculum is inserted and the vagina and cervix swabbed with an antiseptic solution. The sampling instrument is then inserted into the placenta under ultrasound control, taking care to avoid the gestation sac. A suction cannula or biopsy forceps may be used. Vaginal bleeding is common and the patient should be aware of this.

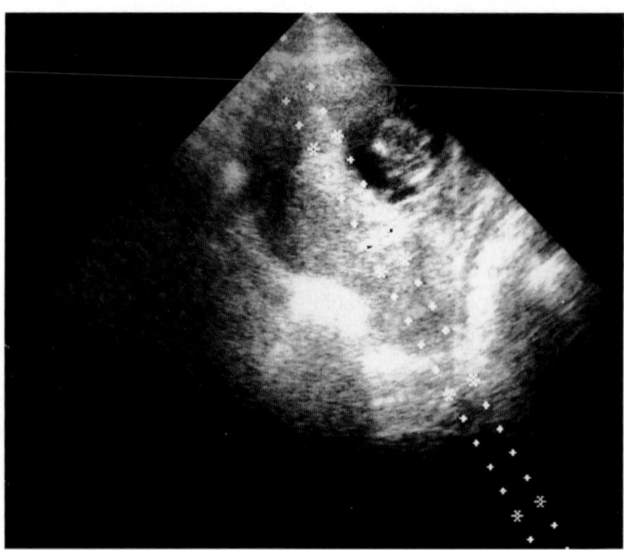

Fig. 40.2 Picture of needle tract for transabdominal CVS.

Indications for CVS

Karyotyping and metabolic analysis (e.g. gene probes) are indications for CVS. With regard to multiple pregnancy, whilst CVS has been employed here (both TC and TA) the problems are greater than with amniocentesis. Apart from the difficulties in identification of separate placentae, the problem of cell contamination of 4.6% is twice that found in singleton pregnancies. If the placentae are inseparable, and concordant results are found, normal or otherwise, a sampling error cannot be excluded and further testing by amniocentesis is necessary. This obviously limits the application of CVS in multiple pregnancies.

Associated risks and cytogenetic problems

The risk of iatrogenic loss after CVS depends more on the gestational age when it is performed and the experience of the practitioner rather than the number of needle insertions required to obtain an adequate sample.

In the first trimester there is an increased risk of miscarriage of 2–3% irrespective of whether a TA or TC technique is used. In the mid trimester the risk appears to be no greater than amniocentesis.

It should be established with the reference laboratory whether the results will be based on direct cytogenetic results (rapid analysis, but labour intensive), culture results (slower) or a combination of both, as this will influence both the patient's and clinician's choice of procedure.

There are two additional problems with CVS that have made the procedure controversial. The problem of placental mosaicism and the possibility that CVS can induce fetal limb deformities when used in the first trimester. When mutations occur in the first or second postzygotic divisions, chromosomal mosaicism affecting all the fetal tissues is the result. Confined placental mosaicism (CPM), is when a dichotomy exists between the chromosomal constitution of the fetal and placental tissues. This occurs with mutations which arise in the progenitor cells of trophoblast or extraembryonic mesoderm. Mosaicism can be a problem with any tissue sent for prenatal diagnosis, but difficulties arise much more commonly with CVS, with an overall incidence of 1–2%. The biological effect of mosaicism depends on the chromosomes involved, none the less the only method of establishing CPM from true mosaicism is to perform additional testing of fetal tissue. Patients undergoing CVS should as part of their pretest counselling be aware of a small risk that further tests, e.g.

amniocentesis, fetal blood sampling and detailed ultrasonography, may be necessary.

While large collaborative studies have demonstrated first trimester CVS to be a safe and reliable technique, with regards to miscarriage rates and accuracy, a possible causal relationship between the procedure and limb defects has been raised. The World Health Organization (WHO) CVS registry reviewed the incidence in 80051 births and found no increase over the accepted background rates of limb deformities in the general population. This issue has attracted considerable media attention and has diminished enthusiasm for the procedure. Elegant theories have been proposed regarding the genesis of such defects and risks assessed with regard to subsets of limb defects. At present there is data which supports a 0.3% (approximately 1 in 300) risk of CVS inducing transverse limb defects when it is performed between 8 and 12 weeks. Three factors appear to increase the risk: inexperience, rigid sampling devices (e.g. larger diameter Cook's catheter) and if the procedure is performed prior to 9 weeks. It should be remembered that patients undergoing first trimester CVS usually have a risk of abnormality in excess of 1 in 300 and in the case of recessive conditions a 1 in 4 risk. They should also have been quoted a 2–3% risk of miscarriage. The risk of limb defects must be placed in this context.

Percutaneous fetal blood sampling

The technique of percutaneous umbilical vein fetal blood sampling (PUBS) was initially described by Daffos in 1993. PUBS heralded a revolution in the understanding of fetal physiology and pathological processes and enabled the development of novel fetal therapies. Gestational age dependent normal ranges have been established for practically all conceivable blood parameters. The likelihood of a successful PUBS increases with advancing gestational age and in experienced hands and is usually successful after 18 weeks. PUBS is an exciting advance in fetal medicine, but it should be emphasized that outwith tertiary referral centres there will be relatively few cases identified per year in an average sized obstetric unit that will merit this investigation.

The procedure is mostly performed from the placental end of the umbilical cord (cordocentesis) PUBS is also possible in other sites of the cord, the intrahepatic portion of the umbilical vein and by direct puncture of the fetal heart (cardiocentesis). The common indications for PUBS are rapid karyotyping, investigation and management of rhesus disease and non-immune hydrops, suspected fetal infection, prenatal diagnosis of haemoglobinopathies and investigation of karyotypic dilemmas arising from other investigations (e.g. mosaics, failed cultures).

Technique

After completing a comprehensive fetal evaluation, the placental cord insertion site is identified if possible. Colour flow mapping can be extremely useful in difficult cases. Cord stability is an essential factor in successful PUBS. Attempting to puncture free loops is not only more difficult, but increases the risk of fetal movement dislodging the needle. A 20–22-gauge spinal needle is inserted under continuous ultrasound guidance along the chosen route. In some instances a tract through the placenta straight into the cord can be used and thus the amniotic cavity is not entered. If this is not possible the cord puncture is made transamniotically some 2–3 cm from the placental cord insertion. The aim is to insert the needle into the umbilical vein which is a large vessel and is less likely to constrict than the umbilical artery. The needle tip should be visible in the vessel. The vein is the vessel of choice for fetal transfusions and when a feticidal agent is being used in order that direct delivery occurs without placental passage. Access to a posterior cord root can be very difficult as can PUBS in cases of polyhydramnios.

Once the cord has been punctured, the assistant aspirates 2 ml of blood, which is preferably analysed immediately to check that it is indeed a pure fetal sample. Fetal and adult blood cell indices are markedly different, but additional confirmatory steps are usually advisable. These include the injection of a small amount of saline which will be visible as it induces turbulence in the vessel lumen. If no blood is obtained, gentle rotation of the needle may bring success without the need to advance the needle. After removing the specimen the needle is withdrawn and the fetal heart checked. Occasionally a stream of blood can be seen leaving the puncture site. This usually stops quickly.

Associated risks

This test is usually only performed in extremely high risk situations and therefore this has to be considered when discussing risks. The loss rate is higher when the fetus is significantly compromised and fetal death may occur as a sequela of its underlying condition, rather than as a direct result of the procedure. The overall risk is approximately 1%. This may be increased if the procedure is difficult and whether it is done for sampling blood or to perform a transfusion; overall risk also depends on the state of the fetus and the experience of the operator.

Immediate complications include cord trauma (laceration, haematoma), fetal bradycardia, vasospasm (particularly umbilical artery), thrombosis, embolism (air or clot) placental abruption, fetomaternal haemorrhage, bleeding after needle withdrawal, preterm labour and premature rupture of the membranes. Chorioamnionitis may be a factor in the latter two complications and may take some time to develop. The risks are increased with serial investigations and prolonged fetal insertion, e.g. transfusions.

Controversial aspects

The use of PUBS has revolutionized the approach to fetal disease. Certain aspects remain controversial such as the determination of fetal acidosis and the most appropriate place for fetal transfusion. There has been considerable interest in utilizing PUBS for the assessment of fetal acid–base status. This has resulted in a greater understanding of the relationship between abnormal biophysical variables, including Doppler, to particular degrees of fetal acidaemia. In turn this improved understanding of biophysical parameters has resulted in a review of how necessary PUBS is in confirmation of acidaemia in the absence of another indication to perform the investigation. Research continues for other markers which will help in the decision regarding delivery or surveillance.

In rhesus disease the original fetal therapy of intraperitoneal deposition of blood has been reintroduced in some centres at the same time as direct cordocentesis transfusion, as it lengthens the time interval between transfusions. Some centres now transfuse directly into the intrahepatic vein avoiding some of the problems associated with cordocentesis.

Additional invasive procedures

As a result of the wide range of pathologies which may present, it is occasionally necessary to perform other types of invasive procedures. The following procedures vary in their complexity. Diagnostic options and therapies are constantly being revised, modified and sometimes abandoned therefore liaison with a tertiary referral centre is advised.

It is likely that in many cases fetal karyotyping will be indicated. Each case must be considered on its own merits as to the most appropriate technique in order to minimize the number of needle insertions and in determining the optimal needle size.

Fetal aspiration

The most common indication for this technique is in the investigation of fetal obstructive uropathies which result in enlarged bladders. The urinary electrolyte concentrations have a use in determining which cases may be suitable for vesicoamniotic shunting. The procedure is relatively straightforward in experienced hands. It is possible to obtain a karyotype from the fetal urine and this is obviously of use if there is severe oligohydramnios and CVS or PUBS is not available.

There are very few indications for aspiration of other fetal cysts and this should only be considered if there is clear evidence that the mass is having an adverse effect on other organs. It is important to ensure such cysts are not vascular in origin and colour flow mapping is clearly of use for this purpose.

Investigation of anhydramnios/oligohydramnios

The technique of amnioinfusion is described above. After instillation of the fluid, the enhanced image facilitates a detailed structural survey of the fetus. The fetus will swallow the fluid if it is able, and the fetal stomach and bladder should subsequently fill. The use of colour flow mapping identifies the renal arteries if present. In equivocal cases, instillation of Ringer lactate into the peritoneal cavity allows demonstration of empty renal fossae; however, one must be aware of the possibility of aberrant renal location. The dynamic functional aspect of amnioinfusion is therefore important. Some workers recommend the administration of frusemide to the mother to stimulate fetal diuresis. Lastly, amnioinfusion is also a test of amniotic sac integrity and this should be assessed.

Feticide, fetal reduction and termination of pregnancy

Each unit should have a clearly understood philosophy regarding these complex areas and practitioners must be fully conversant with the relevant abortion legislation. Those who are involved in the counselling of patients in which termination of pregnancy is an option must be fully aware of the method likely to be used. In cases in which there is a possibility of the fetus being born with signs of life the option of feticide should be considered. This is achieved by insertion of a 20-gauge spinal needle into the fetal cardiac ventricle, and injection of a 15% solution of potassium chloride, in increments of 1 ml until asystole is confirmed. It is prudent to continue scanning for 30–60 s to confirm fetal death.

Patients with super multiple pregnancies may elect to have fetal reduction performed. It is best to perform this early and particularly before 16 weeks as there is a significant increase in miscarriage after this probably as a result of the increased volume of necrotic tissue. Fetal reduction is usually performed by the TA route but some practitioners utilize a TC approach. If feticide is considered when there is a discordant fetal anomaly in a multiple pregnancy it is important that chorionicity is established as there may be a shared circulation. In such cases the 'normal' twin may be compromised as a result of the feticide procedure. Novel techniques of non-pharmacological feticide have been used in such cases including mechanical occlusion of the umbilical cord.

It is better to avoid the sac immediately above the cervical os as there is a risk that necrotic tissue in this area may increase the risk of miscarriage. A 20–22-gauge needle of sufficient length is inserted into the fetal thorax and potassium chloride injected in 0.5 ml boluses. Serial follow-up scans are indicated. Reduction may be performed sequentially.

Future developments

The continuing increase in our understanding of genetics allied with technological advances in imaging and equipment, in tandem with the tendency for subspecialization and development of tertiary referral centres, has resulted in the conversion into science fact that which was previously in the realm of science fiction. In contrast there is considerable public debate concerning the 'new genetics' and the introduction of new medical technologies. The realities of resource availability and financial pressures exert a brake on the application of many available technologies.

Given the perceived success of mid trimester serum screening for NTD and more recently autosomal trisomies, it is likely that this will be able to be applied in the first trimester with reference to detection of chromosome disorders. This will result in the need for earlier confirmatory tests hence the continued interest in both EA and CVS. Accurate ultrasound dating is essential and there may be a place for the inclusion of morphological data in the assessment of risk. The association of increased nuchal translucency in fetuses affected with chromosomal anomalies may improve the accuracy of screening and help patients in their decision making. Increasingly transvaginal ultrasound is being used to identify structural abnormalities in the first trimester and the science of sonoembryology is evolving.

The application of more rapid analysis techniques will shorten the procedure to diagnosis interval. As previously mentioned FISH offers the rapid detection of certain chromosomal anomalies (e.g. trisomy 21) within 24 h, by applying a fluorescent tag onto a chromosome marker. This technique is of particular use in conjunction with second trimester screening as there is much parental anxiety during the wait for a culture result.

The option of fetal surgical interventions has led to the re-evaluation of fetoscopy and the development of embryoscopy. Minimal access surgical techniques (including laser) are being evaluated for fetal application.

While this is an exciting time in the evolution of fetal medicine and surgery there rightly remains public uncertainty about the application of these new techniques. A particular concern is the degree to which the fetus is aware and able to experience pain. This has yet to be clarified but some form of analgesia may be indicated particularly during complicated fetal interventions.

Finally, there is the possibility that one day 'non-invasive' prenatal diagnosis will be possible whereby fetal cells will be extracted and analysed from the maternal serum or from cervical specimens.

Further reading

Campbell, S., Harrington, K. (1993) Prenatal diagnosis. In: *Current Opinion in Obstetrics and Gynaecology*, vol. 5, no. 2. Current Science, Philadelphia, pp. 167–224.

Chevernak, F. (ed.) (1994) Prenatal diagnosis. In: *Current Opinion in Obstetrics and Gynaecology*, vol. 6, no. 5. Current Science, Philadelphia, pp. 435–478.

Chervenak, F.A., Kurjak, A. (eds) (1996) *Current Perspectives on the Fetus as a Patient*. Parthenon Publishing Group, Lancs, UK.

Lilford, R. (ed.) (1990) *Prenatal Diagnosis and Prognosis*. Butterworths.

McCullough, L.B., Chevernak, F.A. (1994) *Ethics in Obstetrics and Gynaecology*. Oxford University Press, Oxford.

Chapter 41: Sonographic examination of the placenta

A.M. Mathers

Antepartum haemorrhage and premature delivery are significant causes of perinatal and maternal morbidity and mortality. While there is a considerable body of literature concerning the fetus and the intrauterine environment, its place of residence (the uterus), and its means of escape, (the cervix) have received considerably less attention. Ultrasound placentography was first described by Gottsfield in 1966 and is established as the evaluation of choice in the diagnosis of placenta praevia (PP). An understanding of the relationship of the placental site to the lower pole of the uterus and cervix is essential if certain diagnostic pitfalls are to be avoided.

During pregnancy, the uterus undergoes dramatic anatomical changes, albeit gradually. Its length changes from 7.5 cm (non-pregnant) to over 20 cm, its weight from 40 to 1000 g. The upper portion is muscular, the cervix mostly connective tissue. Interposed between these is the isthmus which is about 1 cm long in the non-pregnant and by term will have elongated to create the lower uterine segment (LUS), which is 7–10 cm long. The LUS has relatively few muscle fibres and is much thinner than the upper segment of the uterus. It plays a relatively passive role in labour; however, a placenta which is even partially situated in the LUS will have embedded in tissue with poor contractility. This difference is clinically important: the upper segment after placental separation behaves as a 'living ligature', promoting rapid haemostasis. One legacy of PP is postpartum haemorrhage due to the relative inability of the LUS to perform this function.

The cervix will, of course, undergo considerable dilatation during the labour process; however, its length remains relatively static at approximately 3 cm until late pregnancy when it shortens. The sonographer has to take these changes into account when assessing placental site and cervical length if diagnostic errors are to be avoided.

Placental localization

Placental localization is a routine part of the basic obstetric ultrasound examination. Ideally the patient needs to have a relatively full bladder, but overdistension may result in the thin anterior and posterior walls of the LUS being opposed, creating a false impression of an extremely long cervix with or without a low lying placenta. A similar artefact may be produced by overzealous compression of the abdomen with the ultrasound probe. It is essential that such artefacts are recognized as the determination of placental position is defined by the relationship of the leading edge of the placenta to the internal os of the cervix. The LUS has no unique ultrasound features and the upper margin is usually assumed to be level with the upper edge of the full maternal bladder. As the LUS is rarely formed before 28 weeks, it is customary to describe a placenta encroaching on the cervix prior to 28 completed weeks as low lying. After 28 weeks, following traditional obstetric classification, a diagnosis of PP is made and a numerical type given to this (Fig. 41.1). The LUS continues to develop throughout the third trimester and therefore the degree of PP may change. Vaginal delivery may occur with 'minor' degrees of PP (types 1 and 2). 'Major' PP (types 3 and 4) invariably require delivery by caesarean section.

There are practical advantages in defining the degree of PP; however, it should be noted that all are associated with potential life-threatening haemorrhage. In addition to reporting the clinical type of PP, the distance, from the leading edge of the placenta to the internal os should be measured in centimetres as this allows the obstetric team the option of converting the sonographic findings into a clinical type of PP. This helps clinical management. A minor degree of PP in an asymptomatic patient may allow outpatient management; major degrees may require long-term inpatient care. A placental edge which is more than 5 cm from the internal os is unlikely to preclude an attempt at vaginal delivery.

The main pitfalls for the unwary are in defining the internal os and cervical length, mistaking Braxton Hicks uterine contractions for placental tissue, the effect of gestational age, posterior and lateral placental sites and some rarities.

The problem of defining the internal os is discussed above. It is occasionally possible to see the cervix when the

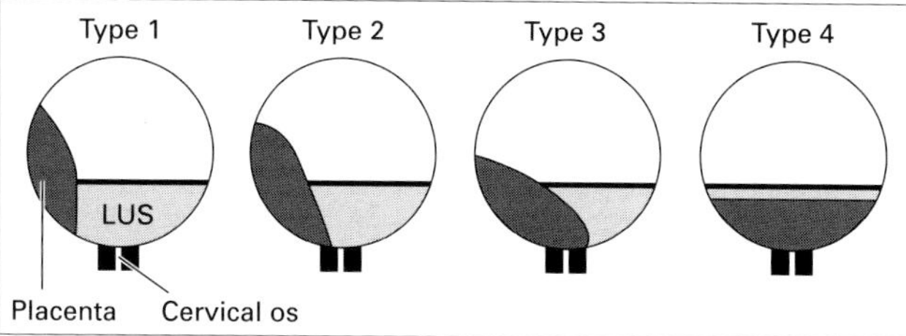

Fig. 41.1 Types of placenta praevia. The placental site (shaded) is related to the cervical os. The LUS lies under the thick black line.

patient's bladder is empty, using the amniotic fluid as an acoustic window. An alternative but rarely required strategy is to perform a careful transvaginal ultrasound examination. In general, using transabdominal sonography, one should be suspicious that extrinsic compression has occurred when the cervix is greater than 4.5 cm long. Occasionally uterine contractions will cause a bunching of the uterine wall which can be mistaken for placental tissues or a fibroid. Resolution of this problem is simple. Firstly, the chorionic plate should be identified as a bright linear line between the amniotic fluid and the placental bulk. Secondly, the placenta may be located elsewhere; and, thirdly, contractions are transient.

The relationship of gestational age to the development of the LUS is mentioned above. Between 16 and 20 weeks, 5% of placentas will appear to be low lying. The incidence of PP in the last trimester is 0.5%: it follows that once the LUS develops the vast majority of low lying placentas will in fact be localized in the upper segment. Opinions differ regarding the utility of telling an asymptomatic patient that the placenta is low early in pregnancy. There is a danger of inducing anxiety which will later be found to have been unnecessary in most cases. It is prudent to rescan the placenta which clearly covers the cervical os because this may persist as a major PP.

A further area of difficulty occurs when the placenta is posterior or laterally placed. Lateral placental sites are relatively uncommon but the sonographer should carefully assess the LUS contents from both anteroposterior and oblique angles. Posterior placentas are problematical when the presenting part of the fetus is low and interferes with image acquisition. This problem may be resolved by further bladder filling, scanning in an oblique lateral plane or by displacing the fetal part either by placing the patient in a slight head down position or by manually lifting the presenting part upwards. If it is still not possible to define the leading edge, then the option of transvaginal scanning should be considered. The alternative for the obstetrician, is to examine the suitably prepared patient in an operating theatre ready for immediate caesarean section if PP is diagnosed. This is rarely necessary except in dire emergency cases without ready access to a reliable ultrasound opinion.

A few rarities may cause problems. Extra satellite succenturate lobes of the placenta may be situated in the LUS despite fundal placement of the rest of the placental bulk. Alternatively, if the patient has been bleeding, an echogenic clot may be mistaken for placental tissue, or conversely, if the blood is transonic, as amniotic fluid. Finally, some placentas are very large either by chance or as a result of certain pathologies (e.g. maternal diabetes). The position of the leading edge should always be established. Identification that the placenta is in the fundus does not mean that it cannot also be in the LUS.

Other aspects of placentography

After PP has been excluded, the next most likely cause of antepartum haemorrhage is that of placental abruption, in which there is premature separation of a normally sited placenta. This condition is as frequent as PP. Major placental abruption is a clinical diagnosis which requires immediate action to save the baby and the mother. Ultrasound has an extremely limited role to play in such cases, but will help to identify fetal heart activity and exclude PP. When a large echogenic retroplacental clot is visible the baby is often dead. Many patients present to obstetric units with abdominal pain with or without vaginal bleeding and the possibility of a minor placental abruption is considered. Occasionally a small retroplacental clot is noted between the placenta and the myometrium although this often takes days to develop after the initial symptoms. A negative ultrasound examination neither confirms nor refutes this clinical diagnosis.

There is an association between unexplained antepartum haemorrhage and intrauterine growth restriction, and serial assessment of fetal growth and liquor volume should be considered in such cases.

The issue of placental grading, as described by Grannum, is covered in Chapter 39.

Other placental anomalies include placental lakes and placental cysts which appear to have no clinical significance. Placenta circumvallatum is extremely rare but is associated with fetal growth impairment, therefore serial growth assessment is indicated. Occasionally, dense, heterogeneous placental infarcts are visible, particularly in severe early onset pre-eclampsia.

Placental chorioangiomas are rare vascular tumours which are variable in appearance and may be associated with high output hydrops fetalis and growth impairment. Colour flow mapping is helpful due to the increased vascularity.

The cervix

If the cervix opens too early, miscarriage, preterm premature rupture of the membranes and preterm labour may occur. These conditions are a very significant cause of perinatal mortality and morbidity and their cause remains an area of intense research activity. Occasionally, the sonographer will identify that the cervix appears to be shortened or dilated, and sometimes there may be visible protrusion of the amniotic sac through the cervix into the vagina (Fig. 41.2). It is essential that this finding is confirmed on clinical examination as, occasionally, uterine contractions can induce a 'beaking' of the LUS above the internal os which mimics dilatation. If the cervix has indeed dilated and even if the membranes have prolapsed, it is still possible to salvage the pregnancy by reducing the sac and inserting cervical sutures as an emergency procedure.

In patients at high risk of preterm labour there is as yet no evidence to support serial measurement of cervical length. Because of the problem a full bladder can cause, current studies are evaluating the utility of transvaginal scanning for this purpose.

It is possible to identify suture material as a dense echo in the cervical tissue following surgery for cervical incompetence; however, this is of uncertain clinical value (Fig. 41.3).

The umbilical cord

The umbilical cord normally contains three vessels, a vein which carries oxygenated blood from the placenta, and two arteries that take deoxygenated blood back to the placenta. The vessels are supported by Wharton's jelly, which becomes sonographically detectable as pregnancy advances. In 1% of deliveries, only one artery is present and this is easily detectable as it produces a signet ring appearance, the vein being typically the larger vessel (Fig. 41.4). A single artery is associated with a higher incidence of congenital anomalies, intrauterine growth restriction, prematurity and perinatal mortality. A detailed anomaly scan and serial growth assessments are recommended;

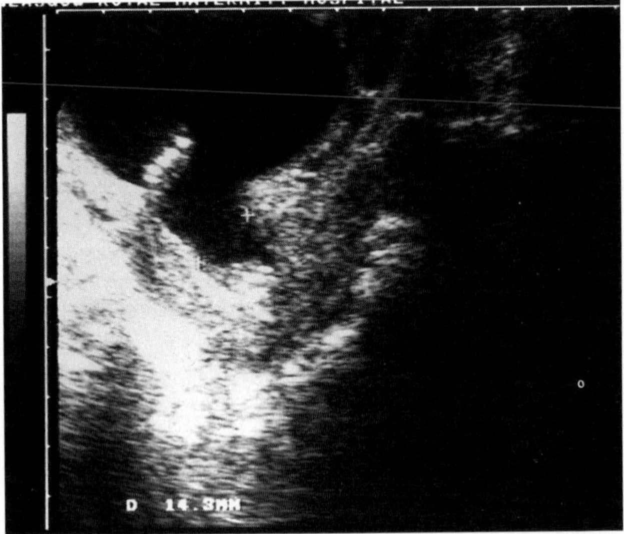

Fig. 41.2 Sagittal section of cervix. Amniotic sac protruding through dilated internal os into cervical canal.

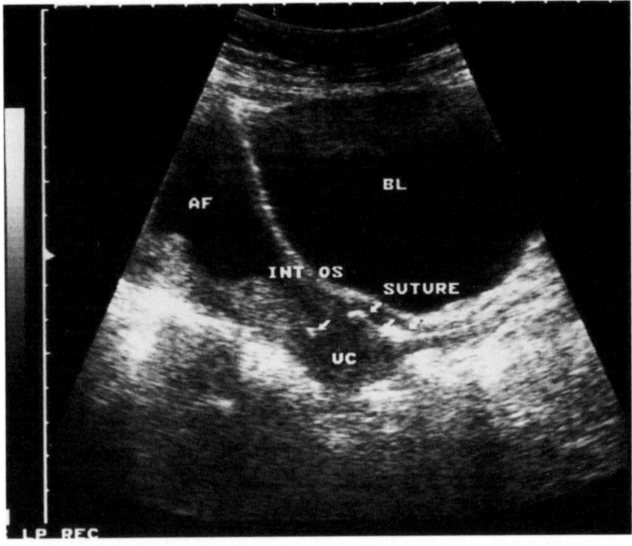

Fig. 41.3 Sagittal section after insertion of cervical suture (arrows) in same patient as in Fig. 41.2. Dense suture material is visible. AF, amniotic fluid; BL, bladder; INT OS, internal os; UC, uterine cervix.

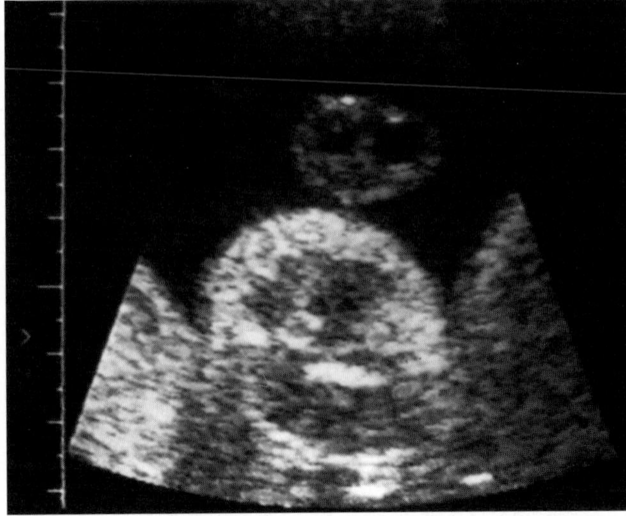

Fig. 41.4 Single umbilical artery with visible Wharton's jelly.

however, invasive prenatal diagnosis is not indicated if no structural markers are identified. Occasionally, there may be more than three cord vessels in rarities such as the twin reversed arterial perfusion sequence.

The integrity of the cord vasculature is vital for fetal life. The development of Doppler investigations has enabled the identification of rare anomalies of the cord. The use of colour flow mapping will help to differentiate vascular lesions (e.g. haemangiomas) from cystic anomalies (e.g. allantoid and omphalomesenteric cysts). High resolution ultrasound with or without the use of colour flow mapping will occasionally detect nuchal cord, cord presentations and may detect true knots. Nuchal cord occurs in at least 30% of deliveries and this finding should not affect obstetric management. Cord presentations require an urgent obstetric opinion but will often resolve spontaneously. Cord insertions distant from the placental mass (velamentous insertion), are sonographically detectable and are of greatest significance if located in the lower uterine segment: vasa praevia. If these vessels tear when the fetal membranes rupture rapid, usually fatal, fetal exsanguination occurs. Vasa praevia is associated with PP and succenturate placental lobes.

As the condition of the fetus is critically dependent on the integrity of the cord, it is recommended that serial assessments of fetal growth and health are performed and the obstetric team alerted when a cord anomaly is recognized.

Further reading

Chamberlain, G., Dewhurst, J., Harvey, D. (eds) (1991) Complications of pregnancy. In: *Illustrated Textbook of Obstetrics*, 2nd edn. Gower Medical, New York, pp. 86–89.

Chudleigh, P., Pearce, J.M. (1992) *Obstetric Ultrasound*. Churchill Livingstone, Edinburgh.

Fleischer, A.C., Romero, R., Manning, F.A., *et al.* (1991) *The Principles and Practice of Ultrasonography in Obstetrics and Gynaecology*, 4th edn. Prentice Hall, New Jersey.

Romero, R., Pilu, G., Jeanty, P., Ghidini, A., Hobbins, J.C. (1988) *Prenatal Diagnosis of Congenital Anomalies*. Appleton & Lange, California.

Chapter 42: Multiple pregnancies

J.R. MacKenzie

Twin pregnancies occur in 1 in 80 to 1 in 100 pregnancies. Twins may be either dizygotic (fraternal twins) arising from two fertilized ova or monozygotic (identical twins) arising from one fertilized ovum. Dizygotic twins account for about 70% of twins each ovum having its own placenta and amnion. The incidence of dizygotic twins increases with maternal age and family history, and it is commoner in certain ethnic groups. The incidence of monozygotic twins is about 30% and is the same throughout the world (Fig. 42.1).

The incidence of triplets (1 in 6000 pregnancies), quads (Fig. 42.2) or quins is very much less than that of twins but following the techniques of ovulation induction and *in vitro* fertilization the overall incidence of multiple pregnancies has risen.

Multiple pregnancies must be regarded as high risk pregnancies with increased perinatal complications and mortality. These problems are much commoner in monozygotic twins. There is also a significant increase in maternal problems such as hypertension, eclampsia, abruption and postpartum haemorrhage.

The majority of twin pregnancies can be identified by an early scan for gestational assessment (Fig. 42.3). It is important to determine whether they are monozygotic or dizygotic. Dizygotic twins are diamniotic and dichorionic with two amniotic cavities and two placentae. The placentae may be separate or fused. No vascular anastomosis exists between the placentae. The gender of the twins may be different. Monozygotic twins may have separate amniotic cavities and placentae (diamniotic, dichorionic), separate amniotic cavities but one fused placenta (diamniotic, monochorionic) or one amnionic cavity and one fused placenta (monoamniotic, monochorionic). Monochorionic pregnancies usually have vascular anastomosis in the placenta and this can give rise to problems such as twin-to-twin transfusion.

Following the diagnosis of a twin pregnancy the amnionicity and chorionicity should be assessed.

Dividing membrane

The presence of a membrane indicates that the pregnancy is diamniotic. If the membrane is thick (due to two layers of amnion and two of chorion), then the pregnancy is diamniotic dichorionic (Fig. 42.4). If the membrane is thin (two amnions) then the pregnancy is diamniotic monochorionic (Fig. 42.5).

Placenta

The presence of two separate placentae indicates that the pregnancy is dichorionic, diamniotic. Twin-to-twin transfusion will not occur. However, it must be remembered that the placentae may fuse and only a single large placenta will be identified.

Fetal gender

If the twins are of a different sex then they are dizygotic and must be dichorionic and diamniotic. However, twins can be of the same sex and can still be dizygotic or monozygotic.

Complications of twin pregnancy

Prematurity

Between a quarter and a half of twin pregnancies are delivered prior to term. This results in an increased mortality rate for twins when compared with singleton pregnancies. Early delivery is probably due to a combination of factors such as polyhydramnios, eclampsia, fetal distress and uterine distension.

Malpresentation

In around half of twin pregnancies one or both of the fetuses presents by the breech. The majority of twin pregnancies are now delivered by caesarean section in order to minimize birth trauma.

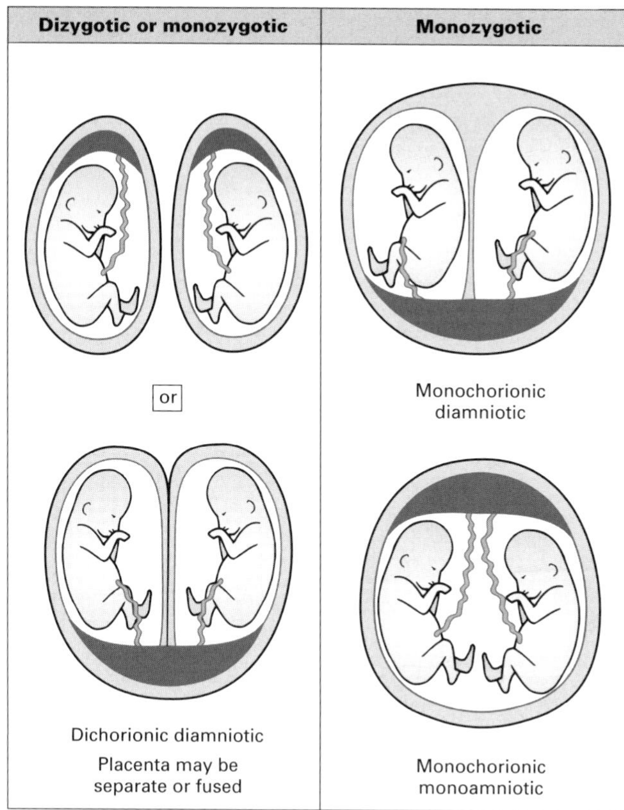

Fig. 42.1 Diagram showing different types of twins.

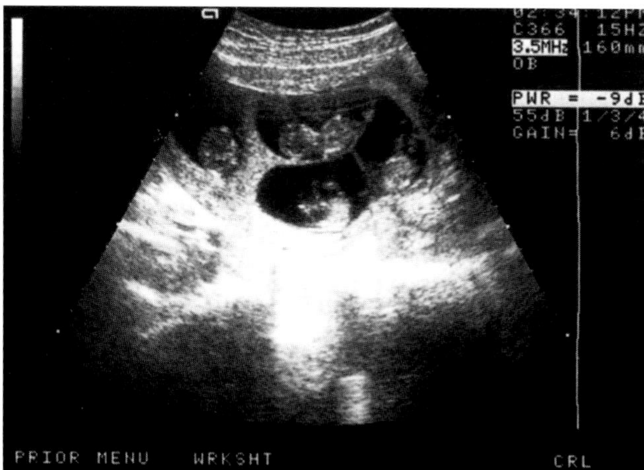

Fig. 42.2 Quads.

Intrauterine growth retardation

This is believed to affect 15–30% of twin pregnancies. Regular growth assessment is suggested and should include measurement of biparietal diameter, head circumference, abdominal circumference and femoral length. The fetal weight should be estimated and the head circumference to abdominal circumference ratio assessed. It is also important to measure the amniotic fluid volume in each sac. Growth impairment may well be identified after 28 weeks gestation and is usually of the asymmetric form. There is frequently a discrepancy in the growth of the twins but usually this does not cause a significant problem.

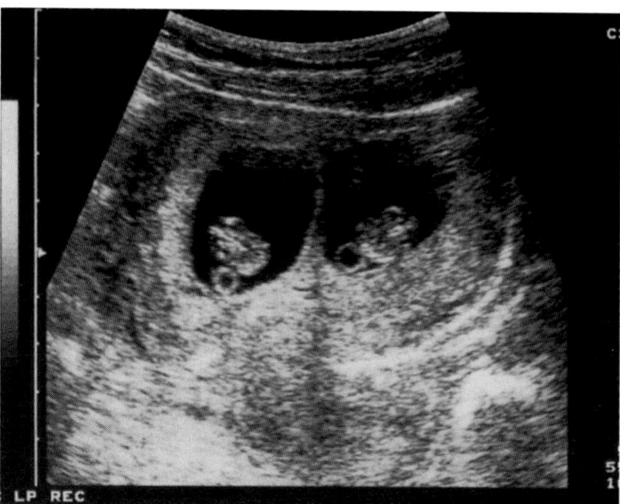

Fig. 42.3 Twins at 9 weeks gestation with separate sacs and prominent yolk sacs.

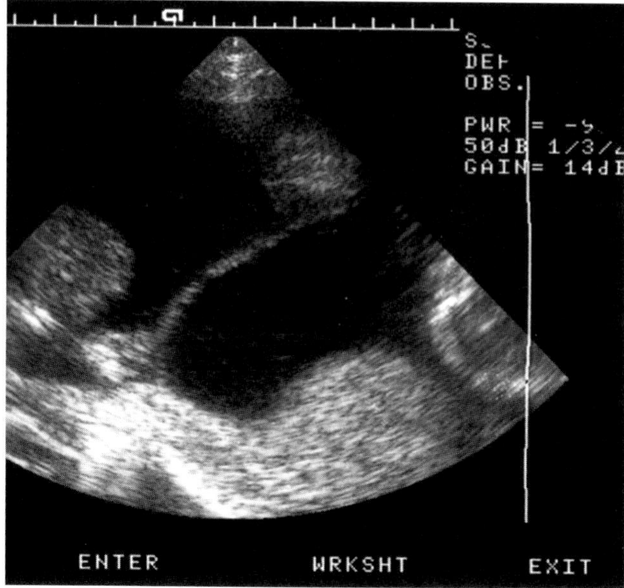

Fig. 42.4 Thick dividing membrane.

Polyhydramnios/oligohydramnios

Polyhydramnios is commoner in twin pregnancies than in single pregnancies. It may well lead to preterm delivery

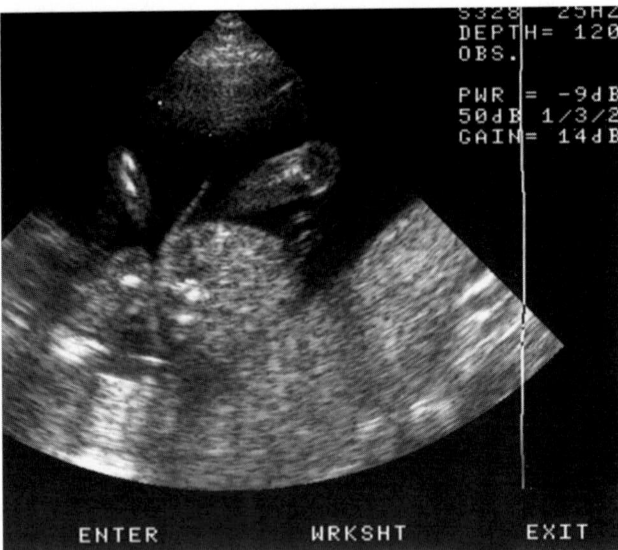

Fig. 42.5 Thin dividing membrane.

and is frequently associated with fetal abnormality. Careful examination of the twins to exclude neural tube defects, gastrointestinal abnormalities or hydrops is important. Marked polyhydramnios may occur in one sac with oligohydramnios in the other sac. There is a high incidence of perinatal mortality in such instances. The twin in the oligohydramniotic sac may become 'stuck'. The twin appears fixed to the uterine wall, even when the mother changes position. It is only with difficulty that a dividing membrane will be identified. If this problem is diagnosed before 26 weeks gestation the prognosis for both twins is extremely poor. After 26 weeks gestation the prognosis for the twin in the polyhydramniotic sac is reasonable although the 'stuck' twin usually succumbs.

Twin-to-twin transfusion

This problem only occurs in monochorionic twin pregnancies. It is believed to be due to the presence of vascular anastomosis in the placenta resulting in blood shunting from one fetus to the other. One twin becomes anaemic and the other has a fluid overload. The overloaded twin develops oedema and polyhydramnios. The donor twin is small with intrauterine growth regardation and there may be related oligohydramnios. The prognosis depends on the severity of the transfusion.

Intrauterine death

During the first trimester up to 20% of twin pregnancies positively identified on ultrasound will subsequently be found to be singleton pregnancies. The 'vanishing' twin is presumably resorbed. In later pregnancy death of one twin may result in the formation of a fetus papyraceous. This fetus undergoes necrosis and atrophy and may mummify. Death of a twin in later pregnancy may result in an abnormality in the remaining twin due to the passage of thrombotic material across the placenta to the live twin. This may cause embolization or thrombosis with the development of brain damage.

Conjoined twins or acardiac twins

The incidence of conjoined twins is extremely low and is estimated at 1 in 50000 births. The twins are monoamniotic and monochorionic. In any twin pregnancy where a dividing membrane cannot be identified it is important to scan the fetuses carefully to exclude any type of fusion disorder.

An acardiac twin pregnancy is one in which the abnormal twin has no vascular connection with the placenta and receives its blood supply from the normal twin. The abnormal twin is able to move but shows no cardiac motion. The mortality for the normal twin is high due to heart failure and prematurity.

Chapter 43: Maternal problems during and following pregnancy

J.R. MacKenzie

Ultrasound carried out during pregnancy usually concentrates on the contents of the uterus, in particular the fetus. The intercurrent problems or pregnancy related problems which the mother may have tend to be ignored. Maternal problems are usually related to the renal tract or to the gastrointestinal tract. Postpartum problems may be due to retained products of conception, problems secondary to caesarean section or bladder problems.

Renal tract problems

During pregnancy the renal tract undergoes changes, mainly those of dilatation. This dilatation affects the calyces, pelvises and upper two-thirds of the ureters. The ureters elongate and undergo kinking. There is no change in the lower third of the ureters or in the bladder. The dilatation is more marked on the right side than on the left side. It is believed to be secondary to the presence of an abdominal mass, to be hormonal and, on the right side, to be anatomical due to the position of the ureter as it crosses the pelvic brim in close relationship to the iliac artery and vein. There is also an 80% increase in renal blood flow in the first trimester, the right kidney being more affected than the left. The flow continues to increase symmetrically in the second trimester and decreases in the third trimester.

There is an increased incidence of pyelonephritis during pregnancy. This may be related to the dilatation previously described. Ultrasound is frequently used in the assessment of these women to exclude renal calculi, to check the thickness of the renal cortex and to look at the degree of dilatation of the kidneys. It may in fact prove difficult to differentiate physiological dilatation of a kidney from pathological dilatation. Localized tenderness frequently accompanies acute pyelonephritis and the mother will complain of pain during the renal scan (Fig. 43.1). Physiological dilatation decreases rapidly following delivery but may linger for up to 12 weeks postdelivery. Postnatal assessment should be delayed until then if practical.

In early pregnancy acute retention may develop if the uterus is retroverted and catheterization of the bladder may be needed to relieve the problem. Retention may occur postnatally due to diminished bladder tone and perineal trauma. It is occasionally helpful to scan the postnatal bladder before and following micturition.

The possibility that a pelvic mass is an ectopic kidney must be considered.

Gastrointestinal abnormalities

It is important to remember that abdominal pain in pregnancy may be incidental and due to problems such as appendicitis, cholecystitis, pancreatitis, intestinal obstruction or perforation. Obviously pregnancy related problems such as abruption, uterine rupture, fibroid degeneration and ectopic pregnancy must also be excluded. Gallstones may be identified incidentally whilst carrying out a renal or liver scan (Fig. 43.2).

Postpartum problems

Bleeding may be a problem immediately following delivery and in this situation ultrasound is likely to be unhelpful and should not be performed. Later in the puerperium ultrasound may be useful in the patient with an abnormally large uterus or who is continuing to pass clots. The uterine cavity may be filled with transonic material due to blood or there may be echogenic material due to clots, retained placental tissue or membranes (Fig. 43.3). Bright echoes within the endometrium may indicate the presence of infection. Extension of the infection to the myometrium results in areas of decreased echogenicity. These abnormalities are commoner following caesarean section.

Intrauterine contraceptive device

Postnatal scans are sometimes requested in patients who had an intrauterine contraceptive device at the time they became pregnant. This device may appear as a linear area of increased echoes during pregnancy or may be identified in relation to the uterine wall following preg-

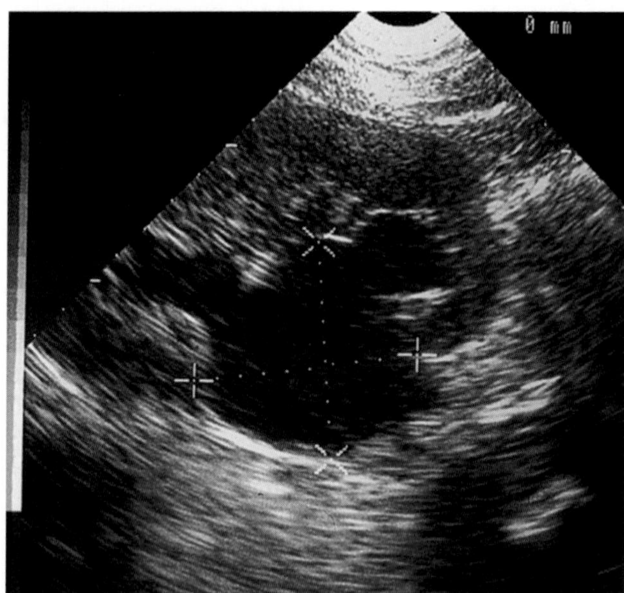

Fig. 43.1 Abnormal dilatation of the right kidney at 22 weeks in a patient with acute pyelonephritis.

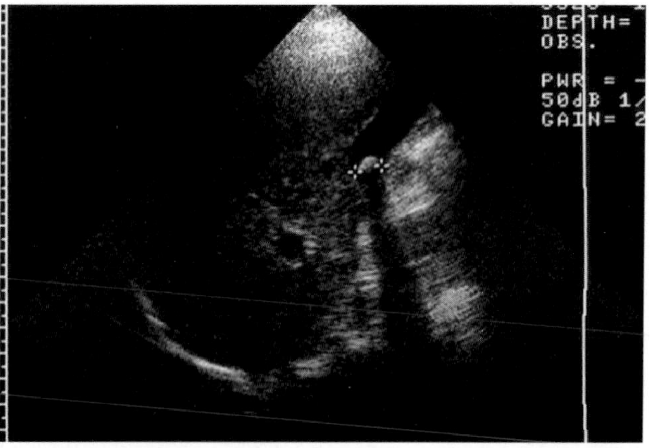

Fig. 43.2 Gallstone in patient with right hypochondrial pain in mid trimester.

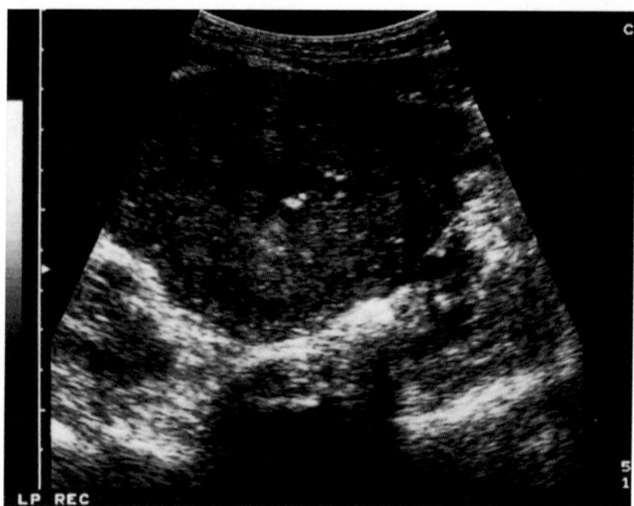

Fig. 43.3 Retained products of conception. Bulky postpartum uterus containing blood and retained products.

nancy. Failure to detect the coil within the uterus may mean that the coil has been extruded without the patient knowing or has perforated through the uterine wall and into the abdominal cavity. An X-ray of the abdomen is required to exclude this possibility.

Deep vein thrombosis

There is an increased risk of deep vein thrombosis during pregnancy and in the puerperium particularly following caesarean section. The technique for detecting deep vein thrombosis ultrasonically is discussed elsewhere.

Part 8
Paediatrics

Chapter 44: The brain

A.S. Hollman

Technique of cranial ultrasound

Ultrasound of the infant brain can be performed using the acoustic windows of the anterior and posterior fontanelles. The anterior fontanelle is usually much larger and allows access to most of the infant's brain. Valuable information about posterior structures can be obtained using the posterior fontanelle. Sonographic access can also be achieved through wide cranial sutures and (with transcranial ultrasound) through the thin squamous temporal bone. This method is particularly useful if the fontanelles have closed prematurely or imaging of suspected temporoparietal subdural fluid collections is required.

A wide range of transducer frequencies is essential. A 3 MHz probe is required for the infant with a very large head, 5 MHz is used for most babies and 7 MHz is employed for the premature infant. A linear 7 or 10 MHz probe is necessary to assess the subdural/subarachnoid space below the anterior fontanelle.

No special preparation is necessary for cranial ultrasound. In a well baby, the examination is best carried out in a radiology department. However, in critically ill and premature infants, the brain can be scanned with the infant relatively undisturbed in an incubator, thus avoiding heat loss or disturbances of mechanical ventilation and electrical monitoring. An oxygen head box will need to be removed and supplemental oxygen given by mask. The examination time should be kept to a minimum in a very sick premature infant, as the infant's condition often deteriorates with handling, resulting in bradycardia and hypoxia.

Coronal images are recorded initially with the 5 MHz sector transducer held parallel to the coronal suture. Anterior coronal images are made with the probe angled anteriorly to demonstrate both frontal lobes above the orbits. The probe is then progressively angled posteriorly until both occipital lobes are clearly demonstrated.

Similarly images are recorded by placing the transducer parallel to the sagittal suture. The probe is then angled from the centre to the left to demonstrate the temporal lobe and temporal fossa; the right side is then similarly imaged. The subdural and subarachnoid spaces below the anterior fontanelle should then be examined using a 7 MHz linear transducer.

The standard views obtained with a sector transducer include five coronal images and five sagittal images with additional views of any abnormality detected. The coronal sections from anterior to posterior pass through the following areas.

1 The frontal lobes (Fig. 44.1a).
2 The frontal horns of the lateral ventricles.
3 The mid line, through the third ventricle and foramen magnum (Fig. 44.1b).
4 The posterior lateral ventricles to show the tentorium and cerebellum (Fig. 44.1c).
5 The occipital lobes.

The sagittal scans are as follows.

1 Mid line sagittal section through the third and fourth ventricles, cerebellum and corpus callosum (Fig. 44.1d).
2, 3 Right and left parasagittal sections through the 'C' shape of both lateral ventricles to show the thalami and caudate nuclei (Fig. 44.1e).
4, 5 Right and left extreme parasagittal sections to show the sylvian fissures and temporal lobes (Fig. 44.1f).

Normal anatomy

The normal ultrasound appearance of the neonatal brain is shown in Fig. 44.1. Figures 44.1a–c show a standard series of coronal images obtained from a 1-month-old infant and Figs 44.1d–f show the sagittal images from the same child.

The complete ventricular system of the brain, the two lateral ventricles, third and fourth ventricle, can be well demonstrated by sonography [1]. The ventricles contain cerebrospinal fluid and the choroid plexus. The lateral ventricles are C shaped. The frontal horns are smaller than the occipital horns, and a minor degree of asymmetry in size between the two lateral ventricles is normal. The left lateral ventricle tends to be slightly larger than the right.

Ventricular size varies according to the gestation of the

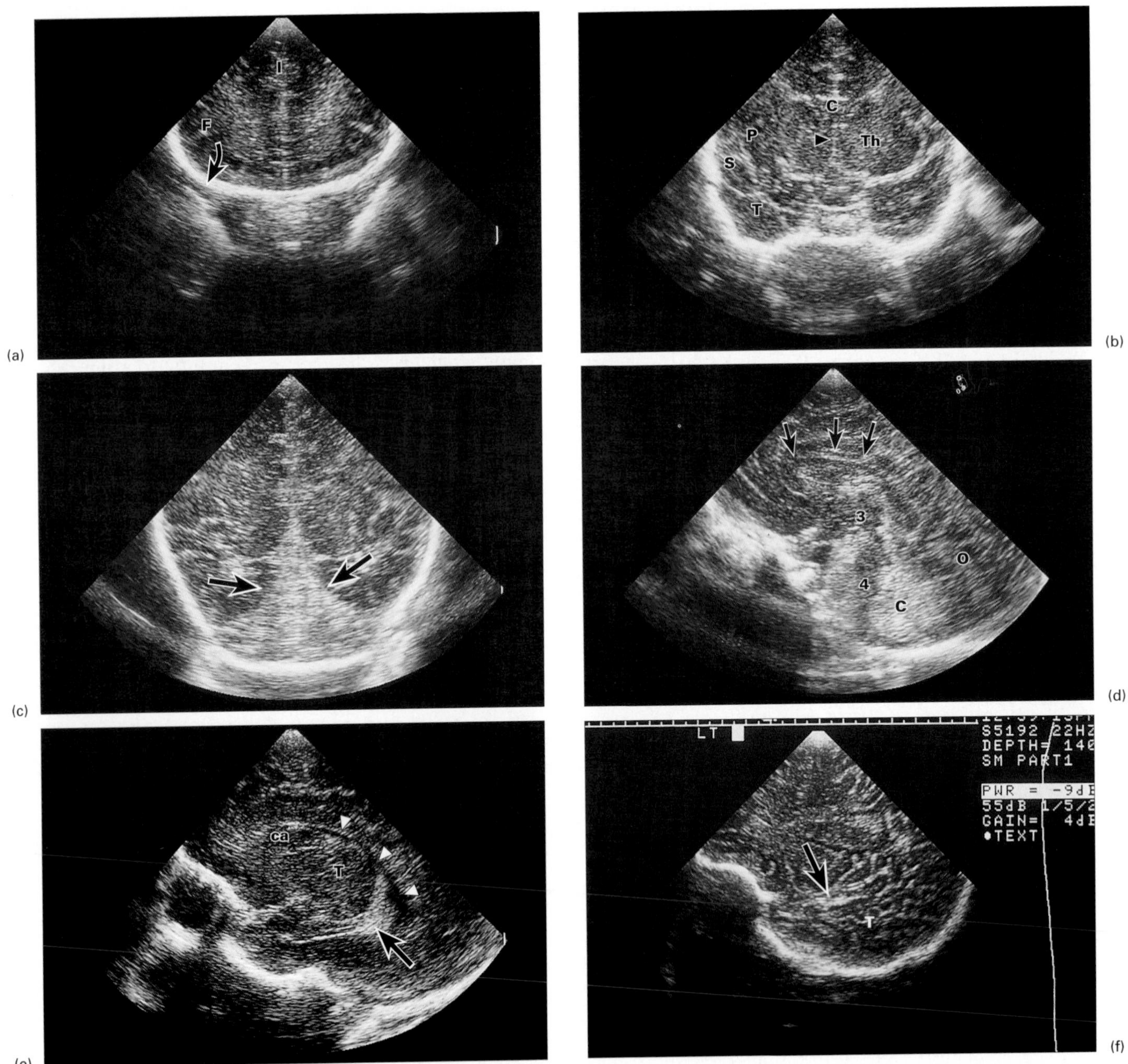

Fig. 44.1 Normal cranial ultrasound of a term infant aged 2 weeks. (a) Coronal scan through anterior cranial fossa showing orbital roofs (arrow). F, frontal lobe; I, interhemispheric fissure. (b) Coronal scan through middle cranial fossa. Arrowhead, third ventricle; C, corpus callosum; P, parietal lobe; S, sylvian fissure; T, temporal lobe; Th, thalamus. (c) Coronal scan through posterior cranial fossa demonstrating tentorium cerebelli (arrows). (d) Mid line sagittal scan through third (3) and fourth (4) ventricles. Arrows, corpus callosum; C, cerebellum; O, occipital lobe. (e) Parasagittal scan of normal C-shaped lateral ventricle (arrowheads). Arrow, choroid plexus; ca, caudate nucleus; T, thalamus. (f) Steep parasagittal scan showing the sylvian fissure (arrow) and temporal lobe (T).

infant [2,3]. In the premature infant, the walls of the lateral ventricles are well separated, but the walls are often opposed in term infants. The best method of recognizing ventricular dilatation is to measure the width of the lateral ventricles on a coronal scan at the level of the foramen of Munro. The upper limit of normal at term is 13 mm. The lateral ventricular ratio (LVR) is a reproducible method of expressing the degree of ventricular dilatation, especially when serial studies are to be performed. The LVR is the ratio of the width of the body of the lateral ventricle divided by half the internal parietal diameter (Fig. 44.1b). In fetal life, the ratio is as high as 0.5, but by term the normal range is 0.24–0.36 [4].

The choroid plexus in the lateral ventricle extends from the roof of the temporal horn posteriorly into the occipital horn and anterosuperiorly into the body of the ventricle as far as the foramen of Munro. There is no choroid in the frontal horn itself [5].

The choroid is relatively thin in the body and temporal horn, but is larger in the occipital horn and largest still around the trigone, where it forms the glomus.

The septum pellucidum is a mid line vertical septum beneath the corpus callosum, and this septum separates the anterior horns of the lateral ventricles from each other. Similarly, the septum vergae lies between the bodies of the lateral ventricles. In fetal life, these septae are fluid filled and known as the cavum septum pellucidum and cavum septum vergae. The potential space of the cavum septum vergae is usually obliterated by birth, and the cavum septum pellucidum is closed in 85% by 2 months of age. In premature infants, both these structures may be prominent.

Adjacent and lateral to the lateral and third ventricles are the paired thalami and caudate nuclei. Both are hypoechoic and have a similar echogenicity to the cerebral hemispheres. The pons and medulla are of medium echogenicity, and are best seen on a mid line sagittal scan. The cerebellum is more echogenic than the brainstem lying above the cisterna magna. The corpus callosum is hypoechoic and well demonstrated in a mid line sagittal scan and on coronal images forming the roof of the lateral ventricles.

The cerebral hemispheres are relatively echo-poor structures with increased echogenicity noticeable around the posterior aspects of the occipital lobes. This periarticular 'flare' is a common finding in premature infants, and a less common and less prominent finding in term infants. Provided the echogenicity of the flare is less than that of the choroid plexus it should not be confused with periventricular ischaemia.

The cisterna magna is an echo-free structure lying superior to the occipital bone and immediately below the inferior cerebeller vermis. Standardized measurements of the normal cisterna magna have been devised [6].

Intraventricular haemorrhage and ischaemia

The germinal matrix is largest in size from 24 to 32 weeks of gestation and lies just below the ependyma on the inferolateral aspects of the lateral ventricles. In premature infants, it is a highly vascular structure and following a hypoxic injury subependymal haemorrhage occurs, which can rupture through the ependyma into the ventricle (intraventricular haemorrhage) or into the brain substance itself (intracerebral haemorrhage).

The incidence of subependymal/intraventricular haemorrhage is 40% in infants under 32 weeks gestation or weight under 1500 g at birth. Two-thirds of these haemorrhages occur in the first 48 h and 90% occur during the first 6 days. About 80% of these haemorrhages are 'silent' with no obvious clinical manifestations, hence routine cranial ultrasound should be performed on such infants on days 1, 3 and 7, and at discharge. If an anomaly is demonstrated, then more frequent examinations may be necessary, particularly if the baby remains unstable.

The purpose of performing regular routine ultrasound is to demonstrate and grade the intraventricular haemorrhage as shown in Table 44.1 as this relates to the infant's prognosis and outcome [7].

A grade I haemorrhage comprises an isolated germinal matrix or a subependymal haemorrhage (Fig. 44.2a). The haemorrhage may be unilateral or bilateral, and appears as an echogenic lesion just anterior to the caudothalamic groove near the head of the caudate nucleus, in a non-dilated lateral ventricle [8]. A prominent choroid plexus may have a similar appearance but the choroid plexus does not extend anterior to the foramen of Munro. The haemorrhage usually resolves in a few days and in some cases becomes cystic in its centre (Fig. 44.2d).

A grade II haemorrhage is an intraventricular haemor-

Table 44.1 Grading and prognosis of infants with intraventricular haemorrhage

Grade	Type	Mortality (%)	Long-term neurological sequelae (%)	Hydrocephalus (%)
I	Subependymal haemorrhage	15	15	5
II	Intraventricular haemorrhage; no ventricular dilatation	20	30	25
III	Intraventricular haemorrhage; ventricular dilatation	40	40	55
IV	Intraventricular haemorrhage; intracerebral extension	60	90	80

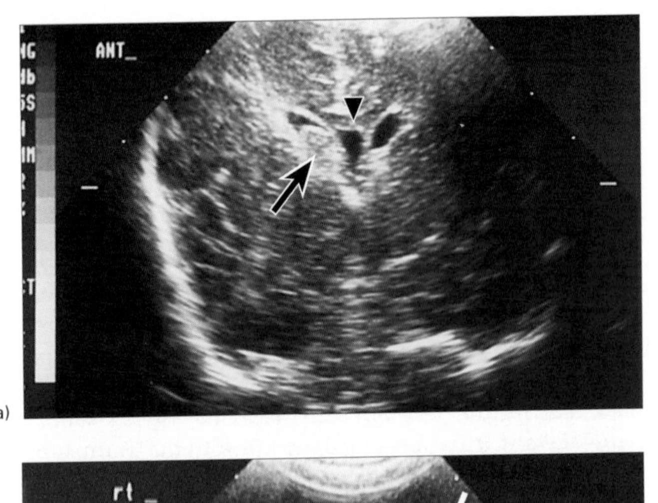

(a)

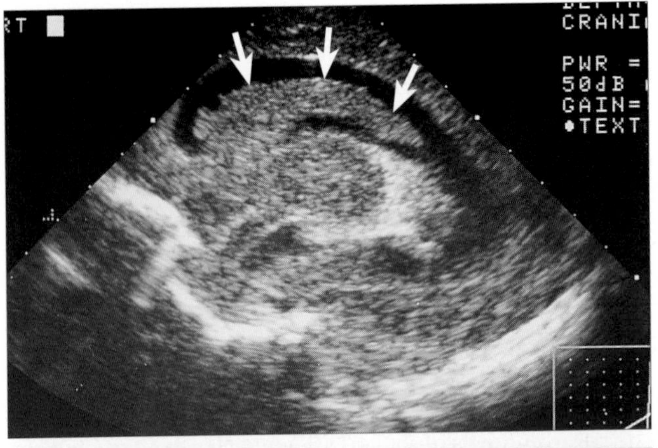

(b)

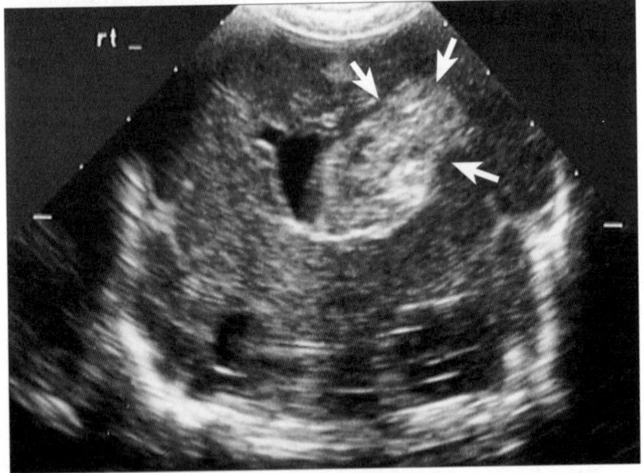

(c)

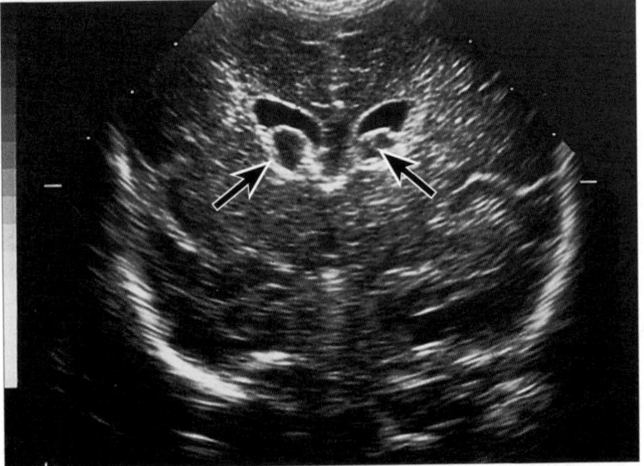
(d)

Fig. 44.2 Periventricular haemorrhage in preterm infant. (a) Grade I subependymal haemorrhage in left lateral ventricle and grade II intraventricular haemorrhage (arrow) in right lateral ventricle in 28-week preterm infant. Note: cavum septum pellucidum (arrowhead). (b) Grade III intraventricular haemorrhage in lateral ventricle in a parasagittal scan in 27-week preterm infant. The haemorrhage is seen as a discrete echogenic lesion within the dilated lateral ventricle (arrows). (c) Grade IV intraventricular haemorrhage in left lateral ventricle on mid coronal scan (arrows). Note: the haemorrhage extends into the parenchyma of the left parietal lobe. This gave rise to porencephalic cyst formation. (d) Resolving bilateral intraventricular haemorrhages. This preterm infant developed grade II intraventricular haemorrhages (arrows) and this scan was taken 2 weeks later. There was a reduction in echogenicity in the centre of the previously uniform echogenic lesion on a mid coronal scan.

rhage in part or all of a normal-sized lateral ventricle (Fig. 44.2a). A grade III haemorrhage is similar but the ventricle is mildly or moderately dilated (Fig. 44.2b), and the haemorrhage may form a C-shaped cast within it. These haemorrhages resolve over several weeks. A grade IV or intraparenchymal haemorrhage extends from the ventricle into the brain substance and appears as an echogenic lesion (Fig. 44.2c). They may be very small, or quite large affecting much of one cerebral hemisphere. Most commonly the frontal and parietal lobes are affected. When these haemorrhages resolve, the affected brain substance may undergo cystic change to form a porencephalic cyst, an area of cerebromalacia communicating with the lateral ventricle.

Grade III and IV haemorrhages may be complicated by the development of hydrocephalus with ventricular dilatation [9]. In the majority of cases, the hydrocephalus resolves or becomes arrested, and relatively few infants require ventricular shunting.

Periventricular leukomalacia

Ischaemia of the deep white matter adjacent to the lateral ventricles results in cystic necrosis called periventricular leukomalacia. This is particularly common in premature infants with birth weights under 1500 g, for whom the incidence is between 8 and 17%. Infarction occurs at the vulnerable watershed boundaries between the anterior and middle cerebral arteries, and the middle and posterior cerebral circulation.

The clinical outcome is often poor. The least severely affected infants develop mild cerebral palsy but many have severe neurological handicap such as spastic quadriplegia and a small proportion die [10–13].

Ultrasound is the most sensitive imaging modality to screen for and to diagnose periventricular leukomalacia in the initial stages. The earliest feature, seen in the first 2 weeks, is increased periventricular echogenicity (Fig. 44.3a). The sites most commonly affected are the white matter adjacent to the frontal horns of the lateral ventricles and the trigones of the lateral ventricles. The lesions can be small and difficult to differentiate from the normal peritrigonal flare, or they can be large and extend deep into the white matter. Ultrasound cannot differentiate between haemorrhagic and non-haemorrhagic infarction.

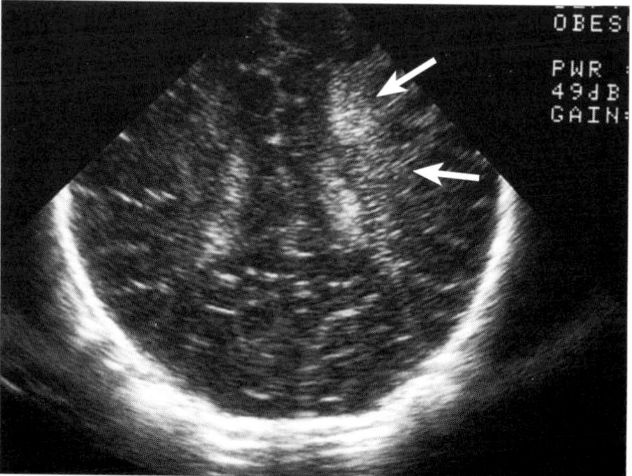

(a)

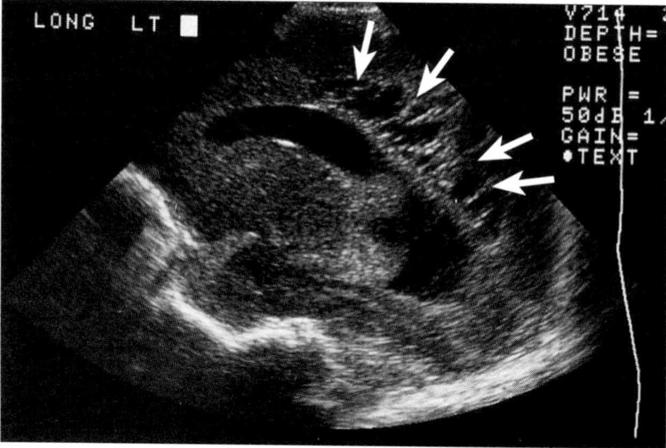

(b)

Fig. 44.3 Periventricular leukomalacia. (a) Coronal scan of a 27-week premature infant showing left-sided periventricular echogenicity in the periventricular white matter posteriorly (arrows). (b) Cystic periventricular leukomalacia on a parasagittal scan of a 26-week-old preterm infant who is now 3 weeks old. There are multiple small cysts in the parenchyma (arrows) adjacent to the mildly dilated left lateral ventricle.

Within 2–3 weeks the infarction may become cystic and multiple cysts are seen in the periventricular white matter (cystic encephalomalacia) [14]. The cysts may be small and only several millimetres in diameter, or they may be up to 1 cm in size, for which the prognosis is worst. The cysts do not usually communicate with the lateral ventricles themselves (Fig. 44.3b).

Eventually diffuse cerebral atrophy may ensue with dilated lateral ventricles and increased extra-axial cerebrospinal fluid (CSF) spaces around the brain. Magnetic resonance imaging (MRI) provides the best means of follow-up for periventricular-leukomalacia to assess myelination and the brain parenchyma as the loss of white matter is not well demonstrated by ultrasound [15,16].

Subdural haemorrhage

Subdural haemorrhages in neonates may arise following birth trauma, particularly as a result of rapid delivery or difficult breech delivery. In infancy, such haemorrhages occur following accidental or non-accidental injury, and as a result of rapid decompression of dilated ventricles in infants with hydrocephalus treated with ventricular shunts. The haemorrhages arise as a result of rupture of superficial cerebral bridging veins that traverse the subdural space, or by tearing of the dura, tentorium or falx. Common sites for subdural collections include a parafalcine location adjacent to the interhemispheric fissure. Collections also occur adjacent and lateral to the parietal, frontal and temporal lobes.

Detection of subdural haemorrhages may be difficult particularly if the anterior fontanelle is small (Fig. 44.4a). High resolution linear 7 or 10 MHz probes are required to detect fluid in the interhemispheric fissure and immediately under the fontanelle (Fig. 44.4b). Axial transtemporal scans may detect laterally placed parietal or temporal subdural haematomas.

Recent haemorrhages appear as echogenic extracerebral collections, whilst older haemorrhages become echo-free. Large parietal or temporal collections cause displacement of the adjacent brain, compression of the ipsilateral ventricle and shift of mid line structures. Parafalcine subdurals widen the interhemispheric fissure.

Ultrasound is not a reliable method of confirming or excluding this diagnosis, nor is it effective for estimating the size of the haemorrhages. Small subdural haemorrhages are easily missed, and accurate dating of the haemorrhages cannot be made. This may be important if the injury is non-accidental. Subarachnoid haemorrhages or communicating hydrocephalus may be difficult to differentiate from subdurals on ultrasound. Computed tomography (CT) or MRI should be performed as the imaging modalities of choice.

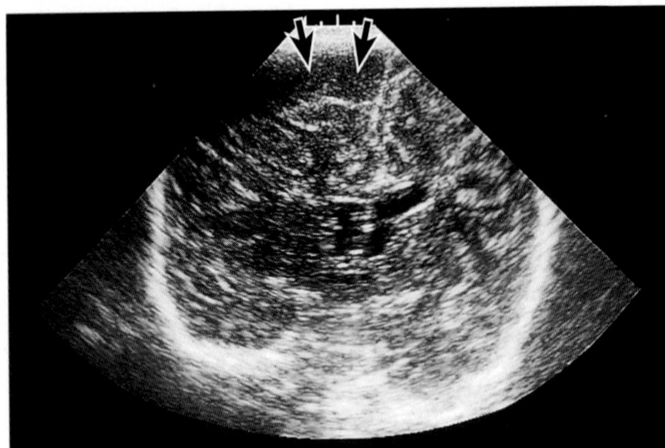
(a)

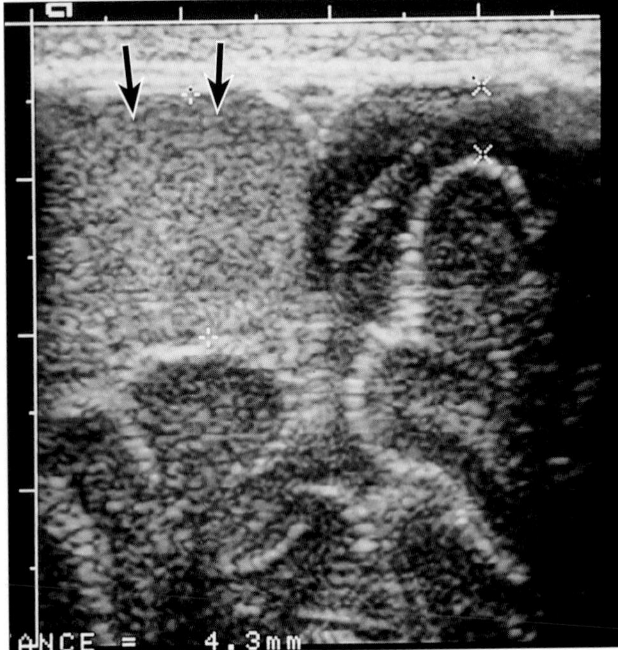

(b)

Fig. 44.4 Subdural haemorrhage. (a) Mid coronal sector scan of a 7-month-old infant presenting with seizures and a bulging fontanelle showing right subdural (arrows). (b) Linear high frequency coronal scan through the fontanelle better demonstrates the large right subdural haemorrhage (arrows). Non-accidental injury was suspected but not proven.

Subarachnoid haemorrhage

Subarachnoid haemorrhage results from bleeding of small vessels in the subarachnoid space, due to trauma (accidental and non-accidental), or from hypoxia when intracerebral lesions commonly accompany the haemorrhage. Ultrasound is unreliable to detect subarachnoid haemorrhage. The interhemispheric fissure and the sylvian fissure may be widened and the subarachnoid space may be increased in width with increased echoes within the fluid. This is best shown using a high frequency linear probe. There may be difficulty differentiating subdural from subarachnoid fluid. Occasionally, the dura is well visualized. CT rather than MRI should be performed if this diagnosis is suspected.

Intracerebral haemorrhage

Most intracerebral haemorrhages result from extension of intraventricular haemorrhages in preterm infants. Spontaneous intraparenchymal haemorrhages do occur, but are less common and most are supratentorial. Coagulation defects, bleeding diatheses, trauma, haemorrhage into an arteriovenous infarct or an underlying arteriovenous malformation may all produce these haemorrhages (Fig. 44.5).

On cranial ultrasound an area of abnormally increased echogenicity in the cerebral cortex or basal ganglia is demonstrated. Haemorrhages may be multiple and vary in size. If solitary, they may be difficult to differentiate from an infarct or a tumour.

Cerebral infarction

Cerebral infarction in infancy is uncommon. Predisposing factors include meningitis, trauma [17], birth asphyxia, prematurity and congenital heart disease. Clinical features are non-specific and include seizures, lethargy and hypotonia. The prognosis varies according to the severity and extent of the infarction.

In the acute situation, the infarct is recognized on ultrasound as a focal area of increased echogenicity with loss of gyral definition and absence of arterial pulsations (Fig. 44.6). At follow-up, there is return of vascular pulsations and the infant becomes cystic [18]. The territorial distribution of the infarct makes the diagnosis likely.

Neonatal asphyxia in term infants

Perinatal asphyxia has been defined by the American Academy of Paediatrics in 1986 as an Apgar score of 0–3 at 10 min, early neonatal seizures and prolonged hypotonia. The incidence ranges from 3.7 to 9 per 1000 live births, and may result in a severe hypoxic ischaemic encephalopathy leading to death or severe mental handicap.

In a premature infant asphyxia results in injury of the periventricular white matter producing periventricular haemorrhage and periventricular leukomalacia as there is a predominance of blood vessels directed centrally until 32 weeks. In the term infant a different pattern of injury is recognized, mainly affecting the cerebral cortex, white matter, basal ganglia, cerebellum and brainstem. Four patterns of injury are recognized.

1 Cortical necrosis affecting the cortex of cerebrum and cerebellar cortex.

(a)

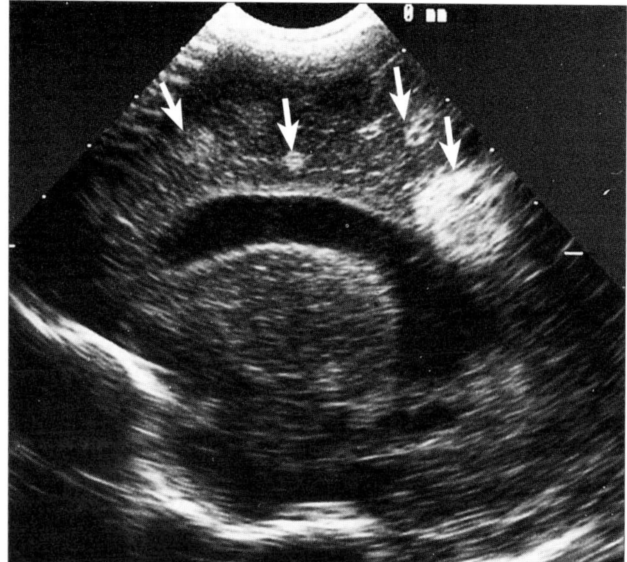

(b)

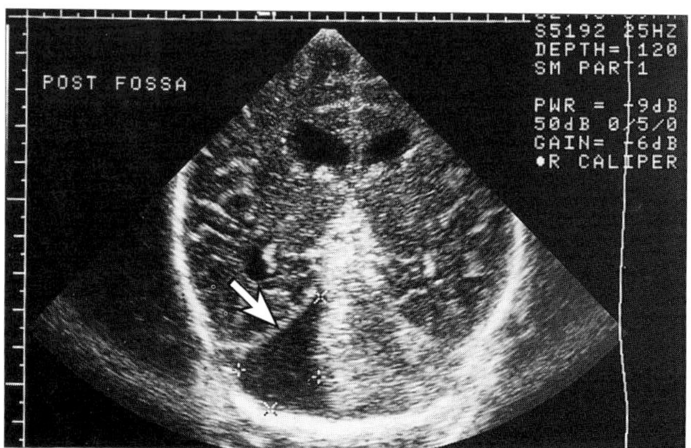

Fig. 44.5 (a) Multiple intracerebral haemorrhages from vitamin K deficiency on a parasagittal scan of a 6-week-old exclusively breast-fed term infant (arrows). The haemorrhages are seen as multiple different-sized echogenic lesions in frontal and parietal lobes and thalamus. (b) Right posterior fossa haemorrhage shown on a posterior coronal scan of a 1-week-old term infant. The haemorrhage is shown as an echo-free triangular lesion (arrow) and was a complication of anticoagulation whilst the infant was on ECMO.

2 Basal ganglia ischaemic injury.
3 Watershed infarcts in the boundary zones between the major cerebral arteries.
4 Infarction of periventricular white matter resulting in periventricular leukomalacia.

Mild asphyxia may result in cerebral oedema, which can resolve completely. If the hypoxic ischaemic injury is more severe, cerebral infarction occurs, and leads to necrosis and cavitation. The end result will be an ischaemic encephalomalacia. The clinical effects depend on the gestational age of the infant, the timing of the event and the severity of the infarction.

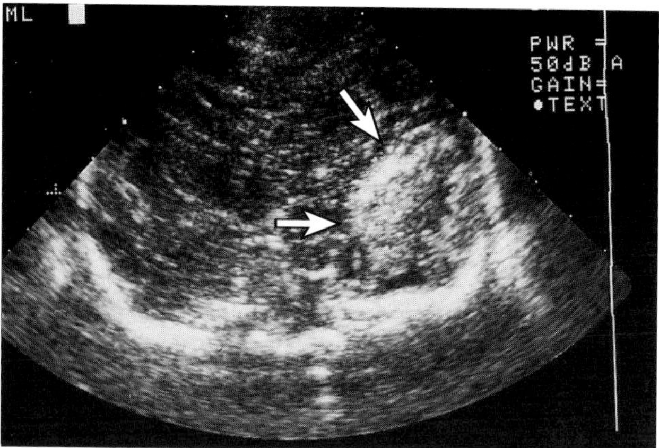

Fig. 44.6 Cerebral infarction. This 10-day-old infant presented with seizures. Mid coronal scan demonstrates a well-defined echogenic lesion in the left temporal lobe (arrows). CT scan confirmed an infarct. The cause of the infarct is unknown.

Ultrasound plays a limited role in the diagnosis and demonstration of the extent of the hypoxic ischaemic injury. It is an insensitive technique, and the changes are poorly demonstrated by this modality.

In the first few days of life, sonography may show focal or diffuse poorly defined areas of increased echogenicity in the cerebral hemispheres, and if the cerebral oedema is diffuse, the ventricles will be small due to compression. There may be poor definition of the normal cerebral gyri and there may be absence or diminution of vascular pulsation within the affected cerebral vessels. Pulse Doppler examination of the cerebral arteries may show reduced or absent flow. In the basal ganglia and thalami there may be focal echogenic lesions known to be associated with a poor clinical outcome [19]. Like the premature infant, changes of periventricular haemorrhage and periventricular leukomalacia may also be observed. The ultrasonic examination may be entirely normal.

At follow-up several days later, areas of infarction may appear as focal increased echoes. Several weeks later, if encephalomalacia has developed, cerebral atrophy develops with dilated ventricles and increased fluid in the extra-axial spaces, with or without calcification in the parenchyma and cystic changes in the white matter.

Alternative imaging techniques have proved useful. CT better demonstrates the early changes, particularly the cerebral oedema best seen on day 3 following the insult. MRI is of value for follow-up examinations, as it does not show the acute ischaemic changes as well as CT does in the neonate. The sensitivity of SPECT to detect hypoxic ischaemia changes seems similar to ultrasound [20].

Ultrasound has been shown to be useful in predicting prognosis of these asphyxiated infants. If the ultrasound examination shows the parenchyma to be abnormal, then

90% of these infants will die or will have neurological sequelae, while 10% with a normal ultrasound will have an abnormal neurological outcome [21].

Hydrocephalus

Dilatation of the cerebral ventricles is common, and is due to an imbalance between production of CSF and its resorption, resulting in ventricular dilatation, thinning of the brain substance and a rise in intracranial pressure. Hydrocephalus can be divided into two types: obstructive, from mechanical obstruction in the ventricular system, or communicating, in which there is failure of resorption or excessive CSF production.

The commonest causes in infancy are neural tube defects, posthaemorrhagic hydrocephalus particularly in premature infants and following meningitis. Less common causes include craniostenosis, other cerebral malformations such as Dandy–Walker malformation, cerebral tumours and migration disorders.

In hydrocephalus, ultrasound is used to confirm or refute the clinical diagnosis, to indicate whether the hydrocephalus is obstructive or communicating, and if possible to identify a cause. The lateral ventricles are dilated, and measure over 10 mm in depth or width, which is thought to be the upper limit of normal. As the hydrocephalus progresses, frequently the occipital and superolateral aspects of the lateral ventricles become most dilated. The thinning of the cerebral cortex is readily demonstrated. The third ventricle may also be dilated, and above its upper limit of normal of 5 mm (Fig. 44.7a). The fourth ventricle should also be assessed for dilatation as well as the subarachnoid spaces. Increase in depth of the extra-axial CSF spaces suggests communicating hydrocephalus.

Follow-up cranial ultrasound is possible as often as the clinical situation demands. Meticulous attention must be placed to ensure the serial scan cuts are performed in identical fashion using the same field of view to allow direct comparison to be made.

The LVR or ventricular to hemispheric index is used to indicate the severity of hydrocephalus [22]. This is a ratio of the distance between the outer aspects between the lateral ventricles divided by the distance from inner table across the brain to the other. Rapidly increasing or progressive increase in ventricular size usually means that ventricular shunting is required.

After ventricular shunting, ultrasound is used to iden-

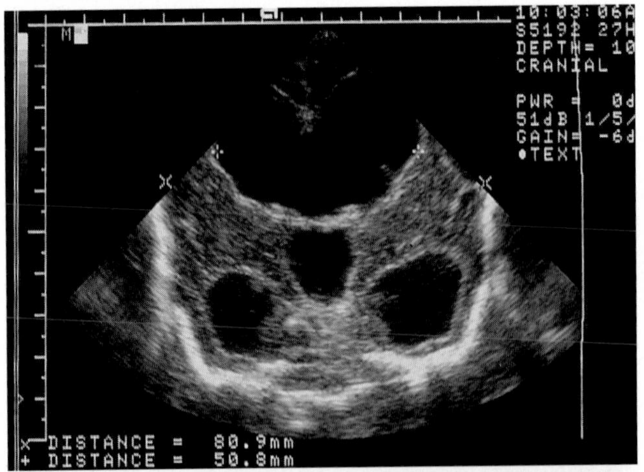

(a)

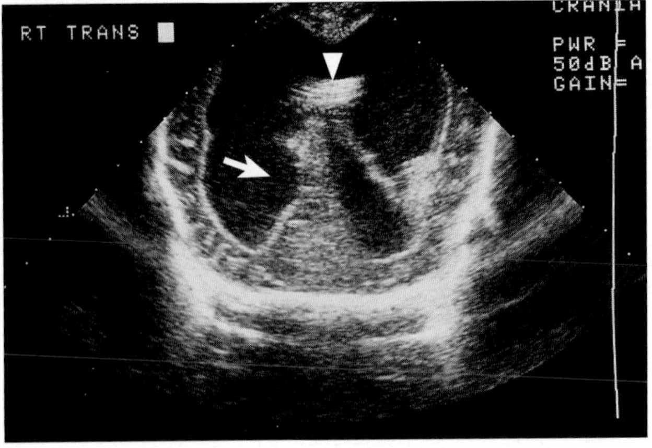

(b)

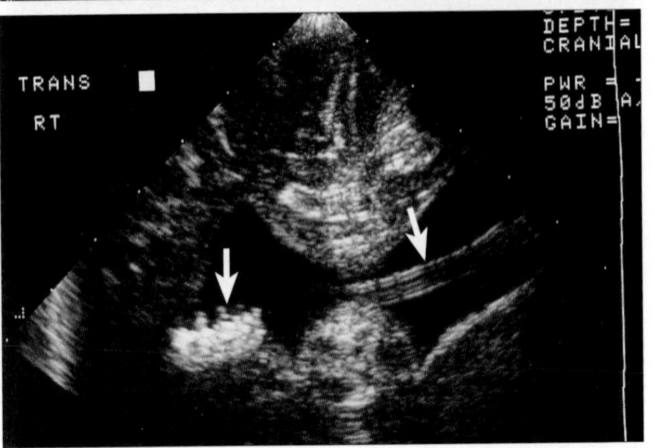

(c)

Fig. 44.7 Hydrocephalus. This infant was born at 28 weeks gestation and developed posthaemorrhagic hydrocephalus 3 weeks following intraventricular haemorrhage in the early neonatal period. (a) Coronal scan demonstrates moderately dilated lateral and third ventricles. (b) This premature infant with posthaemorrhagic hydrocephalus underwent a ventricular peritoneal shunt for worsening hydrocephalus. The shunt became infected and the coronal scan demonstrates the ventricular shunt *in situ* (arrowhead) with increased echogenicity of the CSF within the dilated ventricles (arrow). Ventricular tap confirmed infected CSF. (c) Ventricular shunt placement can be monitored using ultrasound. This coronal scan demonstrates a left-sided shunt crossing the mid line and the tip lies in the right lateral ventricle (arrows).

tify the position of the proximal shunt within the ventricle, to monitor changes in ventricular size and to look for complications of shunting which include the development of subdural collections, infection, haemorrhage and an encysted fourth ventricle (Figs 44.7b,c).

Further imaging is required such as MRI or CT, when ultrasound fails to demonstrate the cause of the hydrocephalus to further delineate complex malformations, to differentiate severe hydrocephalus from hydranencephaly and after the anterior fontanelle closes.

Infection

Infection may occur antenatally or may be acquired after birth. Any site in the central nervous system may be affected.

Intrauterine infection

The TORCH group of congenital or intrauterine infections (toxoplasmosis, other (syphilis), rubella, cytomegalovirus, herpes simplex) produce chronic inflammatory and destructive lesions within the brain, which may be detected *in utero* or *ex utero* by ultrasound.

Congenital toxoplasmosis infection results in focal areas of cerebral calcification within the basal ganglia, the cerebral cortex and in a periventricular distribution. There is often associated hydrocephalus. Hydranencephaly has been reported.

Congenital cytomegalovirus infection typically is associated with extensive periventricular calcification, although other cerebral lesions involving the cortex, cerebellum and brainstem are reported. Increased ventricular size is common. Radiating linear echogenic lines in the basal ganglia (Fig. 44.8a) are due to a mineralizing vasculopathy, and are seen in cytomegalovirus and in some other congenital infections [23]. Affected infants often are microcephalic with chorioretinitis.

In congenital rubella, infants have microcephaly, hydrocephalus with subependymal pseudocysts and basal ganglia calcification.

Meningitis

Infection of the meninges is commonest in the first month of life, in which *Escherichia coli* and group B streptococci are the commonest infecting organisms. The diagnosis is made by lumbar puncture or by transfontanelle tap of CSF. Ultrasound imaging is required if complications develop such as a rapidly increasing head size, a tense anterior fontanelle, deterioration in conscious level, a focal neurological deficit or seizures.

Apart from the routine cranial ultrasound, detailed ultrasound of the extra-axial CSF spaces is necessary to

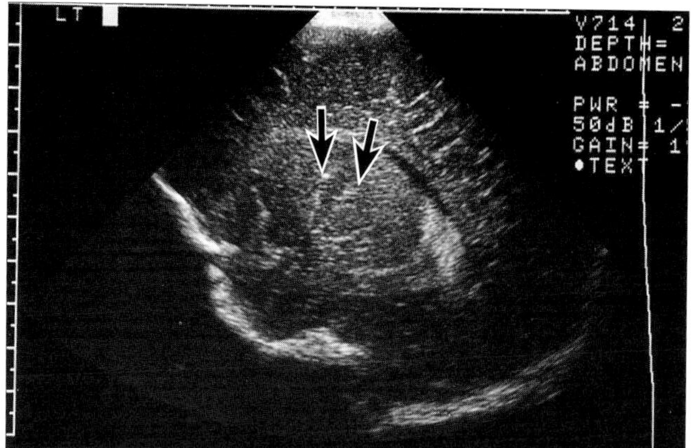

(a)

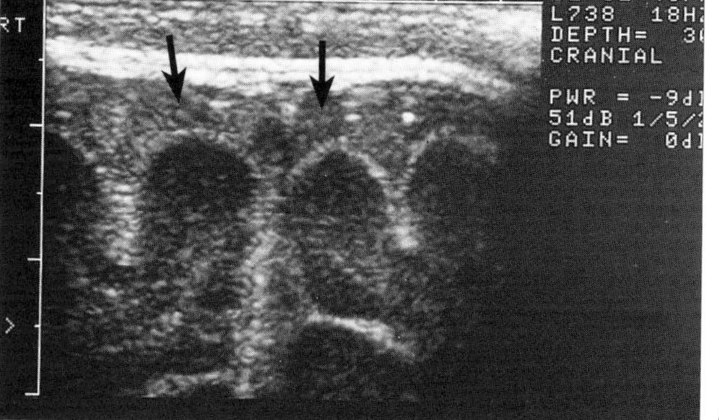

(b)

Fig. 44.8 Infection. (a) Parasagittal scan of left thalamus in an 8-week-old infant with failure to thrive. There are radiating echogenic lines in the thalamus which were shown to be secondary to congenital cytomegalovirus infection (arrows). (b) Coronal scan using a 7 MHz linear probe demonstrates echogenic material in the extra-axial spaces (arrows). Transfontanellar CSF tap confirmed bacterial meningitis with group B streptococci.

document the size of subdural effusions, to look for loculated fluid collections and to assess the cerebral sulci. Features seen in meningitis include increased echoes in CSF, in the extra-axial spaces (Fig. 44.8b) and within the ventricles, or even a fluid/pus level. The walls of the lateral ventricles may be bright indicating ventriculitis and the sulci over the brain surface may be thickened. Hydrocephalus may develop, and a discrete cerebral abscess or infarct can occur [24]. If the infection is severe, diffuse parenchymal infection/infarction can occur, which is better demonstrated on CT. The ventricles can be tapped under ultrasound guidance [25].

Colour Doppler imaging of CSF flow in the aqueduct may be useful in infants with meningitis. The detection of CSF flow may indicate the existence of ventriculitis [26].

Congenital malformations

Congenital malformations of the brain refer to those anomalies that are present before or at birth [27]. A variety of these malformations can be diagnosed by sonography [28].

Agenesis of the corpus callosum

The corpus callosum is a mid line interhemispheric commissure which allows axons from the two cerebral hemispheres to cross the mid line to share information. Agenesis of the corpus callosum may be due to congenital absence in which it fails to develop between the 10th to the 20th weeks of gestation, secondary to intrauterine infarction of the anterior cerebral artery resulting in its loss.

In isolated agenesis of the corpus callosum, there are no other associated cerebral abnormalities and the child is often asymptomatic. Complex agenesis is associated with many anomalies including Arnold–Chiari type II malformation, mid line interhemispheric cyst and lipoma, cerebral heterotopias, Dandy–Walker cyst, encephalocele and holoprosencephaly. The clinical features of seizures and mental retardation often related to the associated condition.

Corpus callosum agenesis may be partial, in which only the posterior aspect of the splenium, is usually absent, or complete, in which the whole structure is absent. In complete agenesis, ultrasound demonstrates the normal corpus callosum to be absent. The frontal horns of the lateral ventricles are widely separated, the medial borders appear concave, and the lateral borders are sharply angulated (Fig. 44.9a). There is often colpocephaly with dilatation of the occipital horns. The third ventricle is displaced upwards and may be interposed between the bodies of the lateral ventricles [29]. The pericallosal and cingulate sulci are absent.

On a mid line sagittal scan, the sulci and gyri have a radial pattern extending down to the third ventricle, the so-called 'sun-burst' pattern [30] instead of their normal pattern of paralleling the corpus callosum and cingulate sulcus. The associated anomalies may be clearly demonstrated on ultrasound such as interhemispheric cyst, Dandy–Walker cyst and hydrocephalus, whereas others such as heterotopias often require other imaging modalities such as MRI for adequate demonstration.

In partial agenesis, the ultrasonic features are more subtle. The anterior aspect of the corpus callosum is often present and the radial pattern of the gyri and sulci are only seen radiating into the roof of the third ventricle posteriorly.

Septo-optic dysplasia

Optic nerve hypoplasia, absence of the septum pellucidum and pituitary hypothalamic insufficiency comprise the condition known as septo-optic dysplasia. A wide range of neurological and endocrine disorders are associated with this condition, including structural malformations of the brain and various hormone deficiencies. Cranial ultrasound may demonstrate absence of the septum pellucidum in about half of the cases (Fig. 44.10). Flattening of the roofs of the frontal horns and pointing of the floors of the lateral ventricles with absence of the septum pellucidum can be shown. Hypoplasia of the

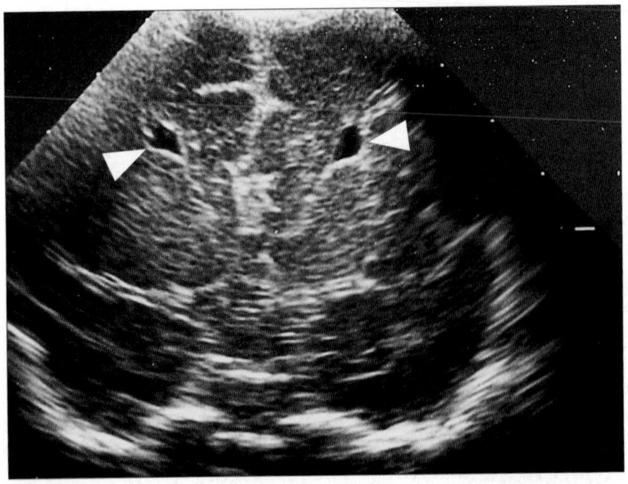

Fig. 44.9 This 10-week-old infant has complete agenesis of the corpus callosum. This coronal scan demonstrates the frontal horns of the lateral ventricles are widely separated with a sharply angulated lateral border (arrowheads). The corpus callosum is absent from the roof of the lateral ventricles.

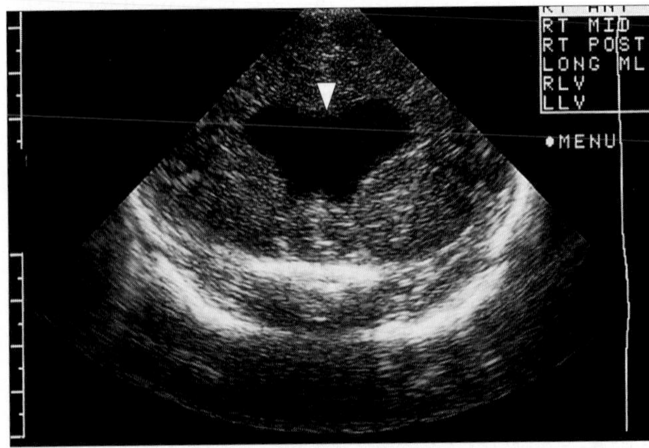

Fig. 44.10 Agenesis of septum pellucidum. This 8-week-old infant presented in the neonatal period with hypoglycaemia. He was shown to have pituitary insufficiency and bilateral optic nerve hypoplasia. Coronal ultrasound scan demonstrates absence of the septum pellucidum (arrowhead) and mildly dilated lateral ventricles. A diagnosis of septo-optic dysplasia was confirmed.

septum pellucidum is difficult to appreciate on ultrasound, but is well demonstrated on MRI.

Other anomalies frequently demonstrated include hydrocephalus (38%), porencephaly (24%), absence (partial or complete) of the corpus callosum (14%) and schizencephaly [31]. Typically there is bilateral optic hypoplasia and dilatation of the suprasellar and chiasmatic cisterns in this syndrome, but CT or MRI would be necessary to demonstrate this.

Hydranencephaly

Hydranencephaly is a severe brain defect in which the cerebral hemispheres are replaced by thin-walled membranous cyst. The basal ganglia and cerebellum are usually normal. The cause is not clear. The lesion may arise as the result of *in utero* occlusion of both carotid arteries causing cerebral infarction or as the result of intra-uterine infection. The affected neonates are markedly retarded, often microcephalic, with a skull which transilluminates and on electroencephalography (EEG) there is absence of cerebral electrical activity.

Ultrasound shows absence of the cerebral hemispheres with a large fluid-filled supratentorial component (Fig. 44.11) divided by a recognizable mid line falx. The occipital lobes are frequently present as are the inferior aspects of the temporal lobes. The basal ganglia and cerebellum appear normal. There may be difficulty distinguishing this condition from severe hydrocephalus, in which a thin rim of cerebral cortex persists around the dilated lateral ventricles, and from alobar holoprosencephaly in which the falx cerebri is absent. CT or MRI may be needed to make this distinction possible.

Spinal dysraphism—neural tube disorders

Dysraphism of the spine or neural tube defect constitute one of the commonest congenital malformations occurring with an incidence of approximately 1–2 per 1000 births. The prognosis depends on the extent and site of the lesion. Anencephaly is the most severe malformation and is incompatible with life, and there is absence of all cerebral structures above the level of the brainstem, and hence failure of either cerebral hemispheres to develop.

Encephalocele is the herniation of cerebral tissue through a mid line defect in the skull, usually in the occipital region. Ultrasound of encephalocele itself will confirm the presence and volume of brain tissue within the sac. Cranial ultrasound will indicate if hydrocephalus coexists and if there are other associated malformations.

Myelomeningocele and meningocele of the spinal cord are associated with the Arnold–Chiari type II malformation of the brain in 90% of these cases. In all infants with these spinal defects, cranial ultrasound as a baseline should be performed before surgery is carried out. The features of an Arnold–Chiari type II malformation include a low lying ovoid cerebellum which extends down to or through the foramen magnum. The cisterna magna is obliterated. The fourth ventricle may be more difficult to visualize as it is elongated and displaced downwards (Fig. 44.12). The third ventricle is larger than usual with a prominent intermediate mass. The posterior horns of the lateral ventricles are often more dilated than the frontal horns (colpocephaly), and there may be hydrocephalus. The frontal horns have a typical shape of bat-wing appearance [32] with anterior and inferior pointings.

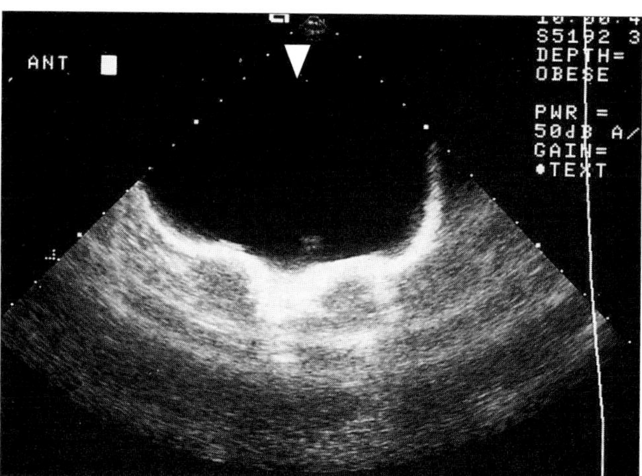

Fig. 44.11 Hydranencephaly. Anterior coronal scan shows absence of the cerebral hemisphere with a large fluid-filled supratentorial components (arrowhead). The baby died after several days.

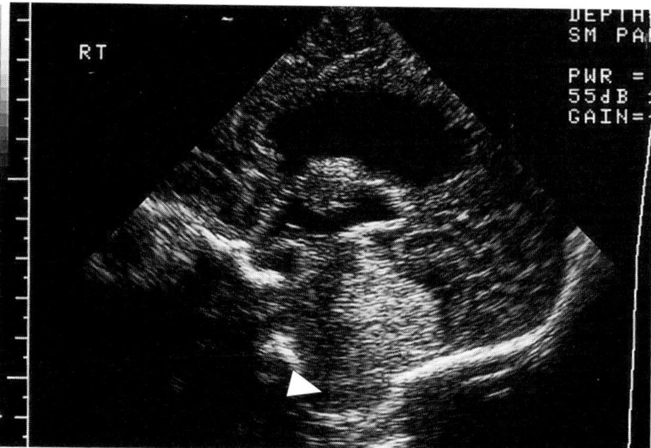

Fig. 44.12 Arnold–Chiari type II malformation of posterior fossa. Mid line sagittal scan of a 3-month-old infant with thoracolumbar myelomeningocele demonstrates downward displacement of the fourth ventricle and inferior aspect of the cerebellum (arrowhead).

Following closure of the spine defect, repeat cranial ultrasound is frequently necessary if the head size shows a rapid increase indicating worsening of the hydrocephalus.

Dandy–Walker syndrome

Dandy–Walker syndrome comprises the following triad: cystic dilatation of the fourth ventricle, aplasia or hypoplasia of the cerebellar vermis and hydrocephalus. The aetiology is unknown. One theory suggests the lesion arises around the sixth to eighth week of fetal life due to atresia or the foramen of Magendie and Luschka. This syndrome is associated with various central nervous system anomalies and others including polycystic kidneys, cardiac anomalies and polydactyly/syndactyly.

Many cases are now diagnosed antenatally [33], whilst others present in infancy with hydrocephalus and developmental delay. In later childhood, posterior fossa symptoms of ataxia, headache and vomiting would be typical.

Cranial ultrasound demonstrates cystic and disproportionate dilatation of the fourth ventricle, causing upward displacement of the tentorium. The cerebellar vermis is absent and there is anterolateral displacement of the cerebellar hemispheres and brainstem. There is hydrocephalus of the lateral and third ventricles. Various associated central nervous system anomalies may be demonstrated including holoprosencephaly, agenesis of the corpus callosum, encephaloceles and cerebral heterotopias.

The Dandy–Walker variant is a less severe anomaly with agenesis of the inferior aspect of the cerebellar vermis. The fourth ventricle is less dilated and communicates posteriorly with a posterior fossa cyst. This condition is also associated with similar anomalies of the central nervous system.

Vein of Galen malformation

Vein of Galen aneurysm is an arteriovenous malformation in which various cerebral arteries drain directly into the venous component which is a large vein of Galen. The arterial supply may include the anterior and posterior choroidal arteries, the superior cerebellar artery and the anterior cerebral arteries. Clinical presentation in the neonatal period is of congestive cardiac failure. A cardiac ultrasound will have been performed and no structural abnormality of the heart found, but often a large dilated superior vena cava is noted. A cranial bruit will often be present. In later infancy, babies present with hydrocephalus or seizures and in childhood with headaches or cerebral haemorrhage.

Ultrasound demonstrates the vein of Galen aneurysm as a large pulsatile cystic lesion behind the third ventricle draining into a huge straight sinus and lateral sinuses (Fig. 44.13a). On colour Doppler ultrasound, markedly increased venous flow in the dilated vein is easily shown and the diagnosis is rapidly confirmed [34] (Fig. 44.13b).

Associated hydrocephalus is common as the dilated vein compresses and obstructs the cerebral aqueduct. Ischaemia of the cerebral hemispheres is common and arises from stealing of the blood from the cortex through the arteriovenous shunt. This may be difficult to demonstrate on sonography, but a diffuse increase in echogenicity of the parenchyma may be evident and cerebral atrophy can result and will be seen later in infancy.

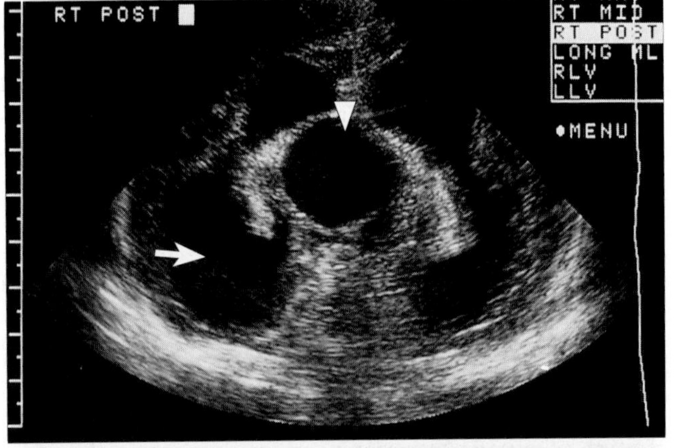

(a)

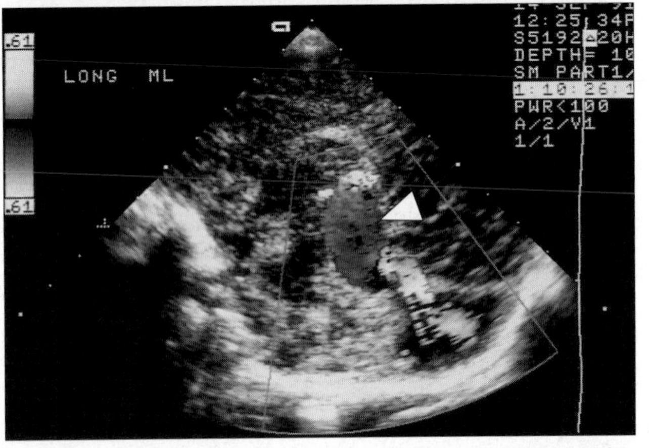

(b)

Fig. 44.13 (a) Vein of Galen malformation. A posterior coronal scan performed on the first day of life shows the mid line dilated vein of Galen (arrowhead) associated with hydrocephalus (arrow). This malformation had been diagnosed antenatally. (b) Colour Doppler ultrasound of a 2-day-old male infant presenting with intractable cardiac failure. The sagittal scan demonstrates a dilated vein of Galen (arrowhead) with an enlarged straight sinus and transverse sinus. For colour, see Plate 44.13 (between pp. 308 and 309).

Tuberous sclerosis

This syndrome is usually inherited as an autosomal dominant condition and is characterized by the clinical triad of epilepsy, mental retardation and adenoma sebaceum. Within the brain there are tubers (neuroglial nodules) in the cortex and subependymal lesion typically in the bodies and inferior horns of the lateral ventricle. The tubers can obstruct the ventricle, can often calcify and may become malignant. There may be cardiac (rhabdomyomas) and renal tumours (hamartoma/angiomyolipoma).

CT or MRI of the brain are the most sensitive imaging modalities to demonstrate the cerebral tubers. Ultrasound may demonstrate small echogenic nodules in the wall of the lateral ventricles with or without ventricular dilatation (Fig. 44.14).

Holoprosencephaly

Holoprosencephaly is a cerebral malformation due to a disturbance in the first trimester in the development of the prosencephalon or primitive forebrain. The prosencephalon fails to divide into the two cerebral hemispheres resulting in a fused single ventricle. This condition is subdivided into three groups according to severity. The most severe type with the worst prognosis is alobar holoprosencephaly, semi-lobar has an intermediate prognosis and lobar holoprosencephaly the least severe malformation.

Typically there are facial anomalies, usually associated with the alobar type including cyclopia, microphthalmia, hypotelorism and cleft lip and palate. Microcephaly is common, but hydrocephalus may be present. Cardiac, endocrine and renal anomalies are associated as is polydactyly and syndactyly.

In alobar holoprosencephaly, there is a single inverted U-shaped ventricle overlying the fused thalami, with absence of the third ventricle. This is best shown on coronal scans (Fig. 44.15). The interhemispheric fissure and corpus callosum are absent.

Lobar holoprosencephaly is the least severe form and may be difficult to diagnose on ultrasound. There is agenesis of the septum pellucidum and the frontal horns of the lateral ventricles have a 'squared off' appearance. MRI can elegantly demonstrate that there is fusion of grey/white matter of the inferior aspect of the cerebral hemisphere across the mid line. The ventricles, thalami and falx appear normal.

In semi-lobar type, the posterior horns of the lateral ventricles are separate, but there is fusion of the anterior horns. The interhemispheric fissure is present posteriorly. The thalami may be fused and the third ventricle is incorporated into the monoventricle.

Neuronal migration disorders: lissencephaly, schizencephaly and grey matter heterotopia

LISSENCEPHALY

This is a malformation resulting from arrest in normal neuronal migration. The brain is smooth without gyri formation (agyria) or has a few broad shallow gyri (pachygyria). Affected infants often have microcephaly, seizures and severe developmental delay. Lissencephaly is not well demonstrated on sonography. The lateral ventricles

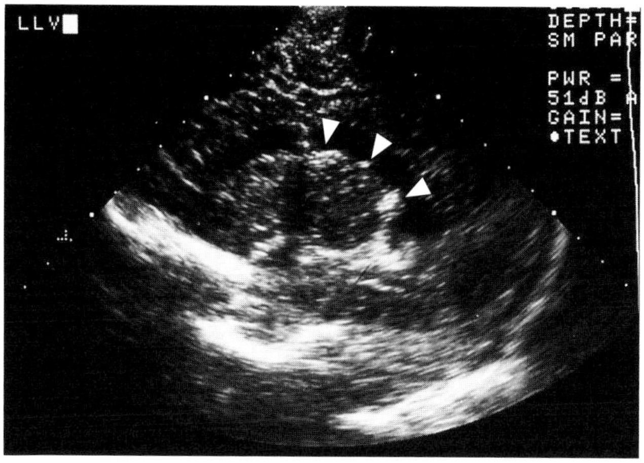

Fig. 44.14 Tuberous sclerosis. Nine-month-old infant with seizures. Parasagittal scan of both lateral ventricles demonstrates multiple discrete echogenic foci lying in a periventricular distribution (arrowheads). CT scan confirmed calcified tubers of tuberous sclerosis.

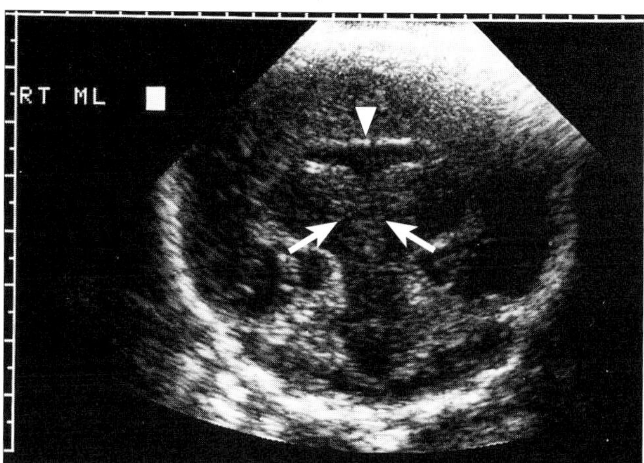

Fig. 44.15 Holoprosencephaly. One-week-old infant with microcephaly and mid line facial defects. Mid line coronal ultrasound shows a single inverted U-shaped ventricle (arrowhead) with fused thalami (arrows).

are often dilated, particularly the posterior horns (colpocephaly). The sylvian fissures are wide, and the smooth brain surface is much better shown by MRI or CT [35] (Fig. 44.16b,c).

SCHIZENCEPHALY

This is a migration disorder with a cleft-like defect in the cerebral hemispheres. The cleft extends from the subarachnoid space to communicate with the ventricle and is lined with cortical grey matter. This condition is associated with absence of septum pellucidum, absence of corpus callosum and grey matter heterotopia. Affected patients present with mental retardation, seizures and failure to thrive.

Type I or closed lip schizencephaly may be difficult to visualize on sonography. These clefts are usually bilateral and best demonstrated on T_1-weighted MRI. Ultrasound of type II or open lip schizencephaly shows a large fluid-filled CSF space between the clefts, often associated with dilated ventricles and absence of septum pellucidum. The clefts are usually bilateral, can be asymmetrical and occur anywhere in the cerebral hemisphere.

GREY MATTER OR CORTICAL HETEROTOPIAS

These are focal ectopic areas of grey matter found within the white matter or subependymal region. They arise from an arrest of normal axial neuronal migration. They usually occur in association with other disorders of neuronal

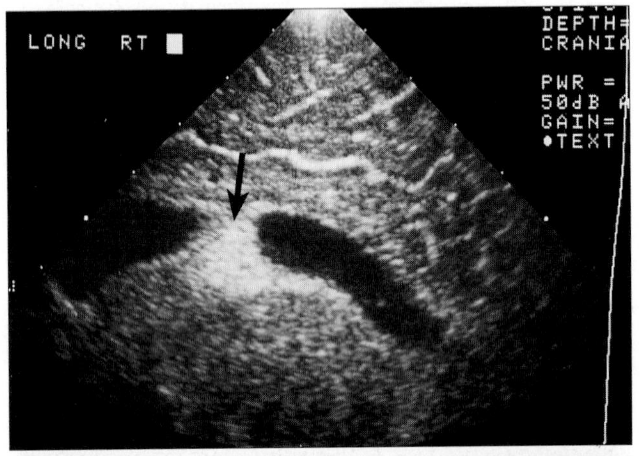

(a)

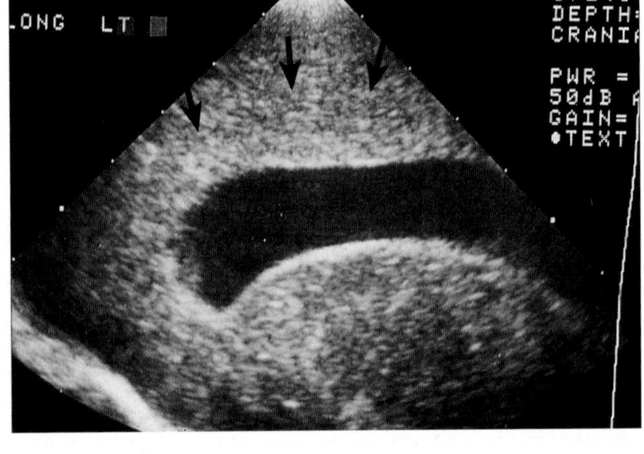

(b)

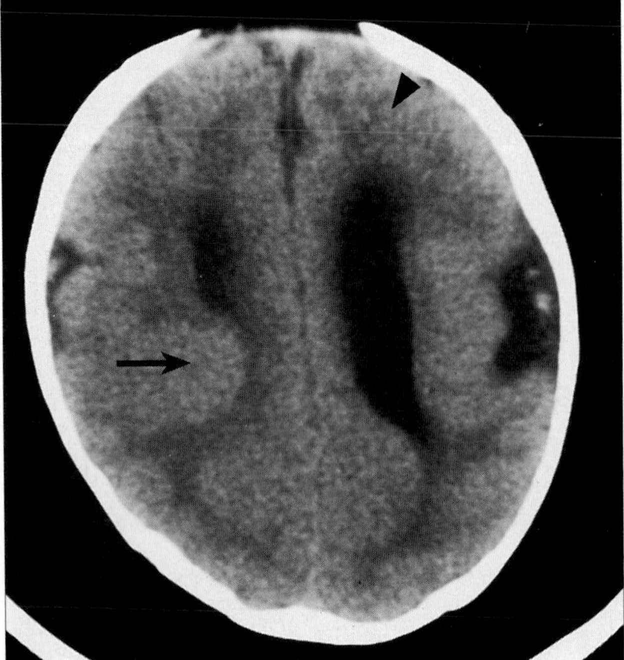
(c)

Fig. 44.16 Cerebral heterotopia is uncommonly demonstrated on ultrasound. (a) Parasagittal scan of right lateral ventricle demonstrates heterotopic grey matter protruding into right lateral ventricle (arrow) in an 8-week-old infant with seizures. (b) Lissencephaly. Parasagittal scan of left lateral ventricle of same term infant demonstrates absence of normal gyral pattern (arrows). (c) CT scan of this infant with neuronal migration disorder shows cerebral heterotopia (arrow) and lissencephaly with smooth shallow gyral pattern (arrowhead).

migration such as schizencephaly and lissencephaly, but occasionally occur in isolation, when children present with refractory epileptic seizures.

They are difficult to recognize on ultrasound, as the echogenicity of the ectopic grey matter is not usually sufficiently different to the surrounding white matter. They can cause distortion and indentation of the wall of the lateral ventricle if they occur in a subependymal location (Fig. 44.16a,c). MRI is the only reliable imaging method to demonstrate such a lesion.

Space-occupying cerebral lesions

Arachnoid cysts

Arachnoid cysts are the most common benign intracranial cysts. The cysts lie in an extracerebral location between the dura and the brain; the wall is lined by arachnoid and the cyst is filled with CSF. They are most commonly located in the suprasellar region, the cerebellopontine angle, behind the cerebellum or in the sylvian fissures. They occur less commonly in the interhemispheric fissure or at the cerebral convexities.

If the cysts are large, they can obstruct the ventricular system and then they may be diagnosed in infancy with an enlarging head size or focal bulging of the skull. Later in childhood, the child may develop headaches or seizures. They are often diagnosed as an incidental finding when imaging is carried out for other reasons such as a head injury.

On cranial ultrasound, the cyst appears as a well-defined fluid-filled lesion displacing the adjacent brain. The cyst wall is too thin to be demonstrated. There may be associated hydrocephalus, if the cyst obstructs the ventricular system. Unlike the porencephalic cyst, the cyst does not communicate with the ventricles. Arachnoid cyst may occur in association with other cerebral malformations, such as alobar holoprosencephaly and agenesis of the corpus callosum. CT may be necessary to confirm the diagnosis, and to differentiate it from other similar lesions such as a cystic tumour.

Porencephalic cyst

A porencephalic cyst is defined as a fluid-filled cavity within the cerebral hemisphere that communicates with the ventricle and/or the subarachnoid space. Most porencephalic cysts are acquired arising from destruction of brain tissue as a result of periventricular/intracerebral haemorrhage, birth trauma, cerebral infection or following hydrocephalus. Less commonly these cysts may be congenital in origin and possibly occur following intrauterine cerebrovascular accident. Infants may have hemiparesis, mental retardation and seizures.

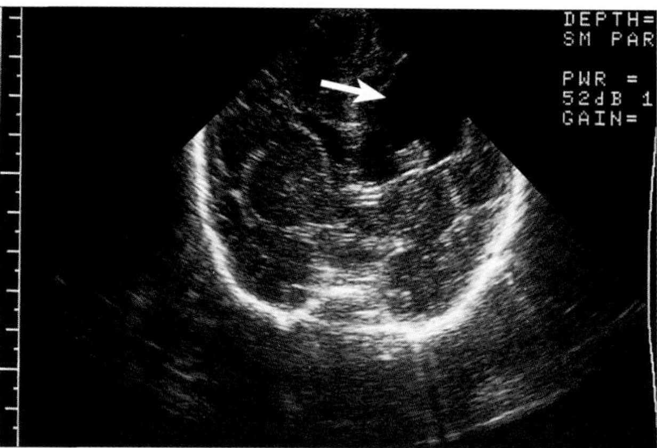

Fig. 44.17 Mid line coronal scan of a 3-month-old infant with left porencephalic cyst (arrow). Born at 29 weeks gestation, he developed left intraventricular haemorrhage which ruptured into the left parietal lobe. The grade IV haemorrhage resolved to leave this area of encephalomalacia communicating with the lateral ventricle.

A fluid-filled cavity is demonstrated by ultrasound with the brain substance itself, and communicating with the ventricle. The cyst size is variable. The ventricle is usually slight to moderately dilated (Fig. 44.17).

Cerebral tumours

Brain tumours in infancy are rare; only 3% of all cerebral tumours in childhood present before the age of 12 months. The commonest types of tumour are neuroectodermal tumours and gliomas [36]. Other tumours include choroid plexus papilloma, arachnoid cysts and teratomas. Infants usually present with features of raised intracranial pressure with an increasing head size but some infants are diagnosed antenatally.

On cranial ultrasound, most tumours appear as large echogenic lesions, some are mixed solid and cystic (Fig. 44.18), and few are entirely cystic. The lesions are often poorly defined and most infants have associated hydrocephalus due to the large size of the lesion. Neuroectodermal tumours tend to be supratentorial solid tumours with calcification and cystic spaces. Gliomas may be located above or below the tentorium and are usually echogenic tumours. Ultrasound cannot predict the histological type and a pathological diagnosis is necessary. MRI and CT are also necessary to demonstrate accurately the limits of the tumour which ultrasound cannot.

Pulsed Doppler and colour flow imaging

The intracranial vasculature of the infant can be elegantly demonstrated using pulsed Doppler and colour flow

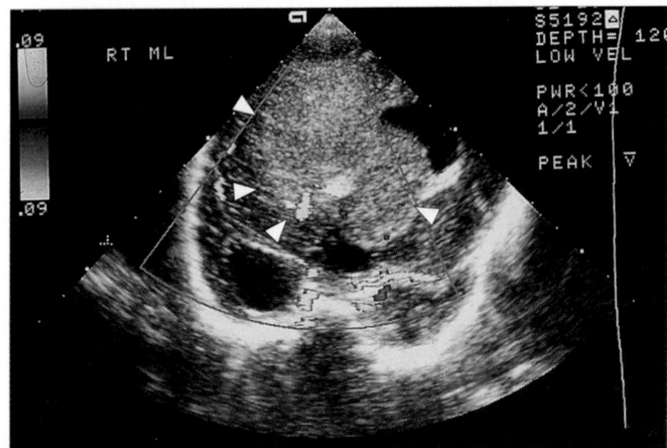

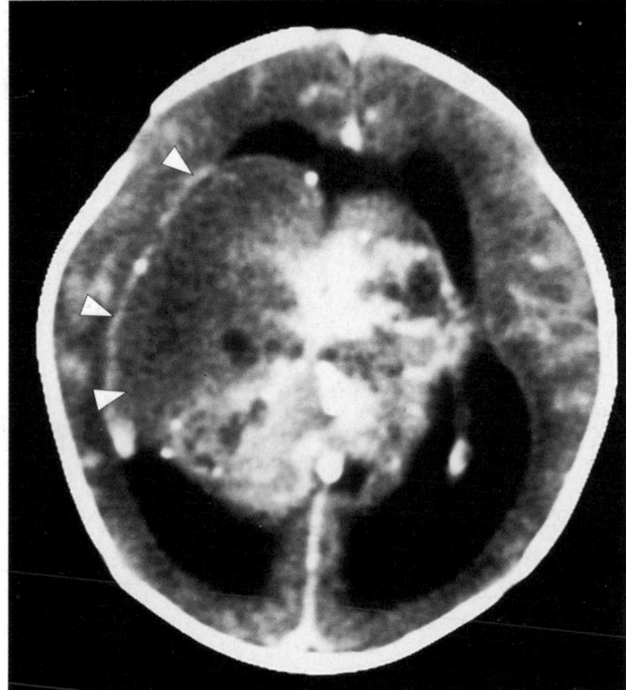

Fig. 44.18 (a) Mid line coronal scan of a 1-day-old infant with a congenital pineal tumour (arrowheads). Antenatal ultrasound in the third trimester had shown this large mid line solid cerebral tumour. (b) CT scan of the brain confirms centrally placed cerebral tumour (arrowheads). Biopsy was performed but the pineal tumour was considered inoperable. For colour, see Plate 44.18 (between pp. 308 and 309).

imaging [37–40]. There has been some concern about the safety of pulsed Doppler to examine the vasculature of the neonatal brain, although as yet there is no evidence to suggest any biological injury. The examination should be kept as short as possible. Colour flow imaging uses lower power levels and therefore theoretically should be safer.

Using the anterior fontanelle as an acoustic window, the anterior cerebral artery, pericallosal artery, the basilar and internal carotid arteries are best evaluated. The middle and posterior cerebral arteries are best sampled using an axial scan with a transtemporal approach [41]. These two latter vessels can be imaged successfully through the anterior fontanelle but, if velocity measurements are necessary, the θ angle would be too high to make accurate measurements possible.

With increasing age, both the absolute systolic and diastolic velocity within the intracranial vessels increase [42]. The resistive index (RI) in normal full-term infants is 0.75 or 75%. The RI decreases with increasing age due to reduced vascular resistance in the brain.

Intracranial pathology associated with an increase in RI includes germinal matrix haemorrhage, periventricular leukomalacia, intracerebral haemorrhage, hydrocephalus (Fig. 44.19), cerebral oedema and subdural fluid collections [43]. However, extracranial disease also may account for a rise in intracranial RI such as a patent ductus arteriosus, hypotension and cardiac failure.

A lowered RI is seen in neonatal asphyxia (vasodilatation from carbon dioxide accumulation) and in infants with intrauterine growth retardation.

Measuring the RI after surgical intervention has been shown to be of some value as the RI will fall if the hydrocephalus has been successfully shunted or if the subdural haemorrhage is successfully evacuated.

Colour flow imaging is of considerable benefit to assess arteriovenous malformations in the brain such as the vein Galen aneurysm, as the diagnosis can be rapidly confirmed. It has also been of value to assess changes in cerebral blood flow in the right cerebral hemisphere when an infant requires extracorporeal membrane oxygenation (ECMO) therapy in which the right carotid artery is ligated. The blood flow in the right internal carotid artery can be demonstrated, and the adequacy of collateral flow in the brain can be assessed [44–46].

Disproportionate head size

Infants with a large head can be rapidly and safely assessed by cranial ultrasound. The clinician will be concerned that the infant has hydrocephalus or a structural abnormality, in which clinical symptoms and signs are often surprisingly absent.

The ultrasound technique employed will be to confirm or exclude dilated ventricles, assess the brain parenchyma itself, exclude a structural malformation or space-occupying lesion and ensure the extra-axial CSF spaces are not abnormally increased in width, as would be seen in recent or old subdural haemorrhages or communicating hydrocephalus.

Most infants with a large head who are examined will have parents who have large heads and the cause will be

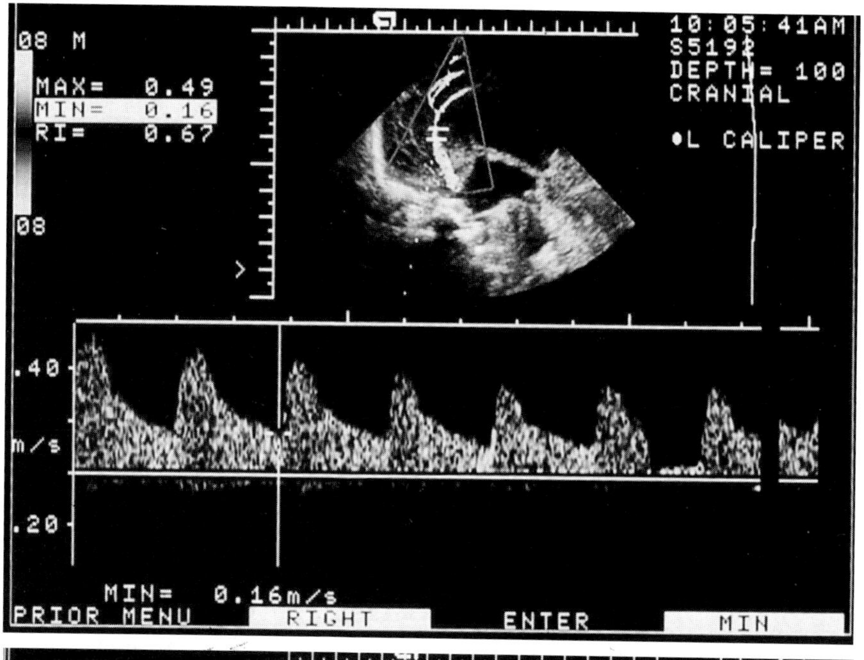

(a)

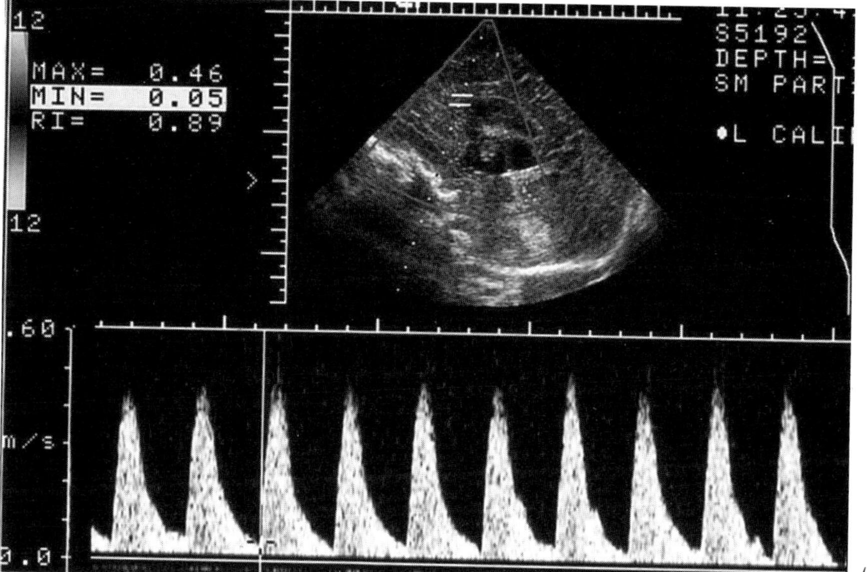

(b)

Fig. 44.19 (a) Normal pulsed Doppler of anterior cerebral artery in an infant with mild hydrocephalus. There is good diastolic flow and the RI is normal at 0.67. (b) One-week-old infant with acute hydrocephalus following closure of myelomeningocele. The RI is elevated at 0.89, the maximum systolic velocity has increased and the diastolic flow has decreased. At surgery for ventricular shunt the intracerebral pressure was considerably elevated at 35 mmHg.

genetic and of no clinical importance. These infants are well, have no neurological signs and the head grows along the same centile. Ultrasound in benign macrocrania will often demonstrate slightly larger lateral ventricles than usual, and subarachnoid spaces often slightly wider than usual. The brain substance itself will be entirely omcreasomg normal. Unless the increasing head size continues to accelerate, no further imaging or alternative technique is necessary.

Similarly, premature infants who sometimes show rapid increase in occipitofrontal circumference due to catch-up growth can be examined to exclude hydrocephalus.

References

1 Appareti, K.E., Johnson, M.L., Rumnack, C. (1983) Ultrasound evaluation of the neonatal brain In: Hagen-Ansert, S.L. (ed.) *Textbook of Diagnostic Ultrasonography*. Mosby, St Louis, pp. 270–284.

2 Pasto, M.E. (1990) Ultrasound measurement of the central nervous system. In: Goldberg, B.B., Kurtz, A.B. (eds) *Atlas of Ultrasound Measurements*. Year Book Medical, Chicago, pp. 20–30.

3 Soni, J.P., Singhania, R.U., Sharma, A. (1992) Measurement of ventricular size in term and preterm infants. *Indian Pediatrics* **29**, 55–59.

4 Garrett, W.J. (1983) The brain and cerebral ventricles. Cross-sectional echography of the brain. In: Morley, P., Donald, G., Sanders, R. (eds) *Ultrasonic Sectional Anatomy*, 1st edn. Churchill Livingstone, Edinburgh, pp. 1–11.

5 Fiske, C.E., Filly, R.A., Callen, P.W. (1981) The normal choroid plexus: ultrasonographic appearance of the neonatal head. *Radiology* **141**, 467–471.

6 Goodwin, L., Quisling, R.G. (1983) The neonatal cisterna magna: ultrasonic evaluation. *Radiology* **149**, 691–695.

7 Bowerman, R.A., Donn, S.M., Silver, T.M., Jaffe, M.H. (1984) Natural history of neonatal periventricular/intraventricular hemorrhage and its complications. Sonographic observations. *American Journal of Roentgenology* **143**, 1041–1052.

8 Bowie, J.D., Kirks, D.R., Rosenberg, E.R., Clair, M.R. (1983) Caudothalamic groove: value in identification of germinal matrix haemorrhage by sonography in preterm neonates. *American Journal of Roentgenology* **141**, 1317–1320.

9 Pellicer, A., Cabanas, F., Garcia-Alix, A. *et al.* (1993) Natural history of ventricular dilatation in preterm infants: prognostic significance. *Pediatric Neurology* **9**, 108–114.

10 Jongmans, M., Henderson, S., de Vries, L., Dubowitz, L. (1993) Duration of periventricular densities in preterm infants and neurological outcome at 6 years of age. *Archives of Disease in Childhood* **69**, 9–13.

11 Trounce, J.Q., Rutter, N., Levene, M. (1986) Periventricular leucomalacia and intraventricular haemorrhage in the preterm neonate. *Archives of Disease in Childhood* **61**, 1196–1202.

12 Ringelberg, J., van de Bor, M. (1993) Outcome of transient periventricular echodensities in preterm infants. *Neuropediatrics* **24**, 269–273.

13 van de Bor, M., den Ouden, L., Guit, L.G. (1992) Value of cranial ultrasound and magnetic resonance imaging in predicting neurodevelopmental outcome in preterm infants. *Pediatrics* **90**, 196–199.

14 de Vries, L.S., Eken, P., Dubowitz, L.M.S. (1992) The spectrum of leukomalacia using cranial ultrasound. *Behavioural Brain Research* **49**, 1–6.

15 de Vries, L.S., Eken, P., Groenendaal, F., *et al.* (1993) Correlation between the degree of periventricular leukomalacia diagnosed using cranial ultrasound and MRI later in infancy in children with cerebral palsy. *Neuropediatrics* **24**, 263–268.

16 Flodmark, O., Lupton, B., Li, D., *et al.* (1989) MR imaging of periventricular leukomalacia in childhood. *American Journal of Roentgenology* **152**, 583–590.

17 Zepp, F., Bruhl, K., Zimmer, B., Schumacher, R. (1992) Battered child syndrome: cerebral ultrasound and CT findings after vigorous shaking. *Neuropediatrics* **23**, 188–191.

18 Hernanz-Schulman, M., Cohen, W., Genieser, N.B. (1988) Sonography of cerebral infarction in infancy. *American Journal of Roentgenology* **150**, 897–902.

19 Cabanas, F., Pellicer, A., Perez-Higueras, A., Garcia-Alix, A., Roche, C., Quero, J. (1991) Ultrasonographic findings in thalamus and basal ganglia in term asphyxiated infants. *Pediatric Neurology* **7**, 211–215.

20 Shankaran, S., Kottamasu, S.R., Kuhns, L. (1993) Brain sonography, computed tomography and single-photon emission computed tomography in term neonates with perinatal asphyxia. *Clinics in Perinatology* **20**, 379–395.

21 Siegel, M.J., Shackelford, A.S., Perlman, J.M., Fulling, K.H. (1984) Hypoxic-ischemic encephalopathy in term infants: diagnosis and prognosis evaluated by ultrasound. *Radiology* **152**, 395–399.

22 Warren, P.S., Garrett, W.J., Kossoff, G. (1983) The infant brain. In: Goldberg, B.B., Wells, P.N.T. (eds) *Ultrasonics in Clinical Diagnosis*, 3rd edn. Churchill Livingstone, Edinburgh, pp. 158–166.

23 Teele, R.L., Hernanz-Schulman, M., Sotrel, A. (1988) Echogenic vasculature in the basal ganglia of neonates: a sonographic sign of vasculopathy. *Radiology* **169**, 423–427.

24 Fisher, R.M., Lipinski, J.K., Cremin, B.J. (1984) Ultrasonic assessment of infectious meningitis *Clinical Radiology* **35**, 267–273.

25 Han, B.K., Babcock, D.S., McAdams, L. (1985) Bacterial meningitis in infants: sonographic findings. *Radiology* **154**, 645–650.

26 Tatsuno, M., Hasegawa, M., Okuyama, K. (1993) Ventriculitis in infants: diagnosis by colour Doppler flow imaging. *Pediatric Neurology* **9**, 127–130.

27 Castillo, M., Dominguez, R. (1992) Imaging of common congenital anomalies of the brain and spine. *Clinical Imaging* **16**, 73–88.

28 Babcock, D.S. (1986) Sonography of congenital malformations of the brain. *Neuroradiology* **28**, 428–439.

29 Warren, M.E., Cook, J.V. (1993) Case report: agenesis of the corpus callosum. *British Journal of Radiology* **66**, 81–85.

30 Atlas, S.W., Shkelnik, A., Naidich, T.P. (1985) Sonographic recognition of agenesis of the corpus callosum. *American Journal of Roentgenology* **145**, 167–173.

31 Zeki, S.M., Hollman, A.S., Dutton, G.N. (1992) Neuroradiological features of patients with optic nerve hypoplasia. *Journal of Ophthalmology and Strabismus* **29**, 107–112.

32 Babcock, D.S., Han, B.K. (1981) Cranial sonographic findings in meningomyelocele. *American Journal of Roentgenology* **136**, 563–569.

33 Fileni, A., Colosimo, C., Mirk, P., *et al.* (1983) Dandy–Walker syndrome: diagnosis *in utero* by means of ultrasound and CT correlations. *Neuroradiology* **24**, 233–235.

34 Tessler, F.N., Dion, J., Vinuela, F., *et al.* (1989) Cranial arteriovenous malformations in neonates: color Doppler imaging with angiographic correlation. *American Journal of Roentgenology* **153**, 1027–1030.

35 Barkovich, A.J., Chuang, S.H., Norman, D. (1988) MR of neuronal migration anomalies. *American Journal of Roentgenology* **150**, 179–187.

36 Wong, H.-F., Ng, S.-H., Wai, Y.-Y., Wan, Y.-L., Kong, M.-S. (1995) Congenital extracranial meningioma. *Pediatric Neurology* **25**, 173–174.

37 Taylor, G.A., Phillips, M.D., Ichord, R.N., *et al.* (1994) Intracranial compliance in infants: evaluation with Doppler US. *Radiology* **191**, 787–791.

38 Raju, T.N.K. (1991) Cerebral Doppler studies in the fetus and newborn infant. *Journal of Pediatrics* **119**, 165–174.

39 Horgan, J.G., Rumack, C.M., Hay, T., *et al.* (1989) Absolute intracranial blood flow velocities evaluated by duplex Doppler sonography in asymptomatic preterm and term neonates. *American Journal of Roentgenology* **152**, 1059–1064.

40 Mitchell, D.G., Merton, D., Desai, H., *et al.* (1988) Neonatal brain: color Doppler imaging. II. Altered flow patterns from extracorporeal membrane oxygenation. *Radiology* **167**, 307–310.

41 Grant, E.G., White, E.M., Schellinger, D., *et al.* (1987) Cranial duplex sonography of the infant. *Pediatric Radiology* **163**, 177–185.

42 Yoshida, H., Yasuhara, A., Kobayashi, Y. (1991) Transcranial Doppler sonographic studies of cerebral blood flow velocity in neonates. *Pediatric Radiology* **7**, 105–110.

43 Quinn, M.W., Levene, M.I. (1994) Changes in cerebral artery blood flow velocity after intermittent cerebrospinal fluid drainage. *Archives of Disease in Childhood* **70**, F158.
44 Mitchell, D.G., Merton, D., Needleman, L., *et al*. (1988) Neonatal brain: color Doppler imaging. I. Technique and vascular anatomy. *Radiology* **167**, 303–306.
45 von Allmen, D., Babcock, D., Matsumoto, J., *et al*. (1992) The predictive value of head ultrasound in the ECMO candidate. *Journal of Pediatric Surgery* **27**, 36–39.
46 Canady, A.I., Fessler, R.D., Klein, M.D. (1993) Ultrasound abnormalities in term infants on ECMO. *Paediatric Neurosurgery* **19**, 202–205.

Further reading

Anthony, M.Y., Levene, M.I. (1993) Doppler of the neonatal brain. In: Cosgrove, D., Meire, H., Dewbury, K. (eds) *Abdominal and General Ultrasound*, vol. 2. Churchill Livingstone, Edinburgh, pp. 945–956.

Barkovich, A.J. (1995) *Pediatric Neuroimaging*, 2nd edn. Raven Press, New York.

Levene, M.I., Williams, J.L., Fawer, C.L. (1985) *Ultrasound of the Infant Brain*. Spastic International Medical Publications, London.

MacDonald, L.M. (1993) The neonatal brain. In: Cosgrove, D., Meire, H., Dewbury, K. (eds) *Abdominal and General Ultrasound*, vol. 2. Churchill Livingstone, Edinburgh, pp. 917–944.

Ryan, S. (1994) Cranial ultrasound in the newborn. In: Carty, H., Shaw, D., Brunelle, F., Kendall, B. (eds) *Imaging Children*. Churchill Livingstone, Edinburgh, pp. 1426–1439.

Siegel, M.J. (1991) Brain. In: Siegel, M.J. (ed.) *Pediatric Sonography*. Raven Press, New York, pp. 9–62.

Teele, R.L., Share, J.C. (1991) Cranial ultrasonography. In: Teele, R.L., Share, J.C. (eds) *Ultrasonography of Infants and Children*. WB Saunders, Philadelphia, pp. 1–56.

Chapter 45: The abdomen

P.R. John

Ultrasound is used extensively in the assessment of infants and children with abdominal abnormalities. The real-time nature of the examination, its multiplanar capabilities and absence of ionizing radiation make it ideal for paediatric practice. There is a large variation in body size of infants and children attending for ultrasound examinations and having a variety of transducers available to deal with this is an advantage. Using small amounts of gel applied to the transducer is helpful as children can be frightened when gel is liberally squirted over the abdomen. For diagnostic scanning (including complex Doppler cases) sedation is not routinely required. When fasting is required in infants (i.e. less than 12 months of age) 3h is usually adequate (e.g. leaving out one feed is often sufficient in breast/bottle-fed infants). Fasting in older children is for 4–6h. If a full urinary bladder is required scanning at the end of a feed in babies and shortly after drinking if children are in nappies can be helpful. Table 45.1 briefly outlines the preparation that is needed for abdominal scanning and also describes scan techniques that can help to demonstrate the area of interest. A successful examination not only requires skill in dealing with children and their carers but also flexibility in scanning techniques. Scan techniques will need to be modified in the presence of certain congenital disorders, e.g. children with situs inversus and scoliosis.

Hypertrophic pyloric stenosis

This is a common paediatric disorder where the circular muscle of the pylorus is hypertrophied. Its aetiology, however, remains obscure. Non-bilious, sometimes projectile vomiting in a 2–6-week-old male infant is the classical presentation. The definitive treatment is surgical relief of the obstruction by pyloromyotomy; however, surgery is not an emergency procedure. The diagnosis may be confirmed by the experienced paediatrician carrying out a 'test feed' and palpating the hypertrophied pylorus. Imaging is reserved when the clinical findings are unclear or equivocal [1].

Although the diagnosis of hypertrophic pyloric stenosis (HPS) can be made with an upper gastrointestinal contrast examination, ultrasound is now the preferred method of imaging as the thickened pyloric muscle can be visualized [2]. If the presentation is atypical and the ultrasound findings are difficult to interpret then a repeat ultrasound examination 24h later should be undertaken. For the examination the infant is placed in the supine position and turned with its left side raised. This promotes antral distension with fluid. If there is no fluid in the antrum then a small sterilized water feed of 20ml is given (either orally or via a nasogastric tube). Ultrasound is carried out with a 5–10MHz linear transducer, scanning initially longitudinally over the epigastrium to locate the pylorus and then rotating the transducer transversely aligning it with the long axis of the channel (Fig. 45.1a,b). Overdistending the stomach with fluid displaces the pylorus posteriorly, making assessment difficult. Also the pylorus may erroneously appear thickened if the transducer is tangential rather than aligned along the true long axis of the pylorus. The ultrasound criteria for the diagnosis of HPS include a muscle thickness of 3.5mm or greater, a channel length of 17mm or greater, no or minimal passage of gastric contents through the channel and gastric peristalsis ending at the pylorus [3–7] (Fig. 45.1c). Equivocal muscle thickness measurements are more likely to occur in preterm than term infants [8]. Measuring the volume of the pylorus relative to the infant's weight can also confirm the diagnosis of HPS [9]. With an experienced examiner, if the pylorus is difficult to visualize and provided the stomach is not overdistended, then it is likely that there is no HPS. Gastro-oesophageal reflux may be seen during the examination if the gastro-oesophageal junction is examined in infants with HPS. It has been suggested that there is an increased incidence of renal anomalies in infants with HPS, e.g. pelviureteric junction obstruction, duplex and horseshoe kidneys [10]. Scanning the kidneys and urinary tract at the time of the pyloric examination is recommended. Following surgery the pyloric muscle returns to normal within 2–12 weeks [11,12].

Table 45.1 Patient preparation and scanning techniques

Area to be examined	Patient preparation	Scan technique
Liver	No preparation	Patient supine; subcostal/intercostal approach; longitudinal and transverse scans
Biliary tract	Fast	Patient supine/right side raised/ erect; suspended respiration (if possible); longitudinal and transverse scans
Spleen	No preparation	Patient supine/left side raised; longitudinal and transverse scans in coronal plane
Pancreas	Fast (usually)/ scan after water	Patient supine/erect; scan through left liver/spleen; transverse scans (coronal through spleen)
Adrenal glands (identified more easily during infancy)	No preparation	Patient supine/side raised; scan through liver/ spleen; longitudinal and transverse scans
Kidneys and bladder	No preparation	Patient supine (kidneys and bladder), side raised/decubitus and prone (kidneys); longitudinal and transverse scans (kidneys and bladder)
Gastrointestinal tract	No preparation/scan after sterile water solution	Patient supine/side raised; longitudinal and transverse scans of whole abdomen; compression scan in right iliac fossa
Pelvis	Full bladder	Patient supine; longitudinal and transverse scans

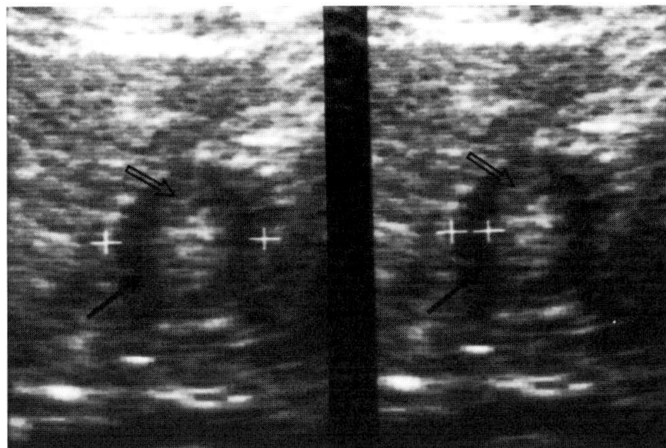
(a)

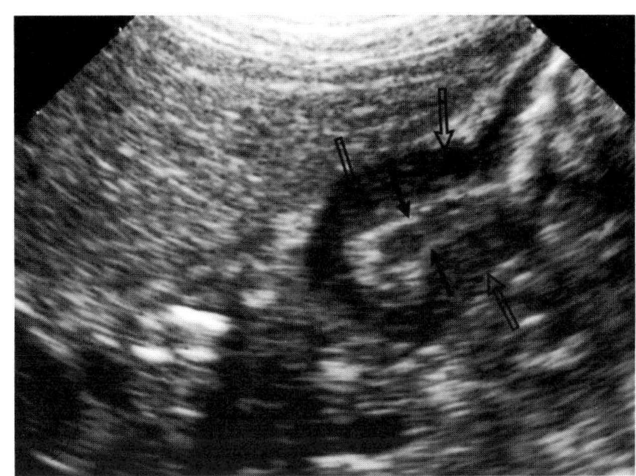
(b)

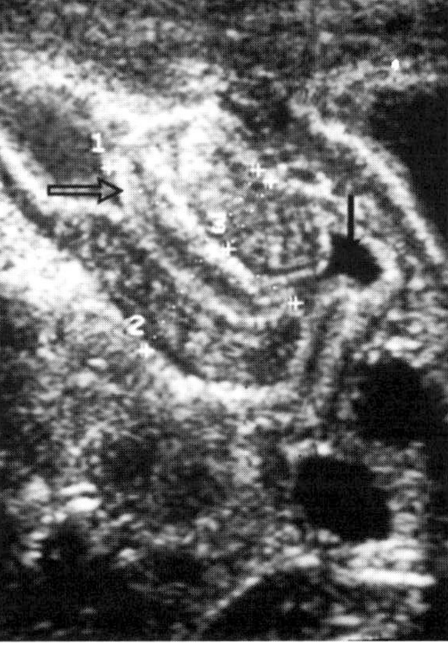

(c)

Fig. 45.1 Hypertrophic pyloric stenosis. (a) Transverse scan of the pylorus showing a thickened outer hyporeflective muscle layer (black arrows) and central hyper-reflective mucosa. Note the normal muscle artefact at the 6 o'clock position with increased reflectivity due to anisotropy (this is also seen at the 12 o'clock position, open arrows). (b) Longitudinal scan. The hyporeflective muscle (open arrows) surrounds the echogenic mucosa of the pyloric channel (black arrows). A small amount of fluid can be seen in the channel in HPS, though antral fluid does not pass through the channel in significant amounts. (c) Longitudinal scan showing an elongated pyloric canal (1), a widened pyloric transverse diameter (2) and thickened pyloric muscle (3). Normal folded mucosa (open arrow) can be seen within the pyloric channel. There is a small amount of fluid present in the first part of the duodenum (black arrow).

Intestinal obstruction

Small bowel obstruction in the neonatal period is most commonly due to meconium ileus, bowel atresias and malrotation whilst in older children intussusception (see below), malrotation and incarcerated hernias are the main causes (Fig. 45.2). Appendicitis (see below) and adhesions can also cause small bowel obstruction. Large bowel obstruction in the neonatal period is most commonly due to Hirschsprung's disease and anorectal malformations. Sonography is not usually required in the assessment of the majority of children with intestinal obstruction; however, it can show for example an intussusception (see below), ascites and dilated fluid-filled bowel loops.

Appendicitis

Most children presenting with acute appendicitis have typical clinical features and can undergo surgery. However, nearly one-third of children present atypically and are a clinical diagnostic challenge. It is this group that can benefit from ultrasonography with the graded compression technique [13]. Although it is difficult in children with significant pain and marked ascites, ultrasound can be helpful in establishing the diagnosis with a sensitivity and specificity between 80–94% and 90–95%, respectively [14–17]. The inflamed appendix is non-compressible, has an outer wall diameter of greater than 6 mm and shows a hypervascular wall on Doppler (Fig. 45.3a,b). This is in comparison to the normal appendix which is partially compressible, has an outer wall diameter of less than 6 mm and shows only a few Doppler vascular signals in its wall. Perforation occurs in up to one-third of children with appendicitis and abscess formation is the major complication (Fig. 45.3c). With perforation pericaecal fluid, loss of the echogenic submucosa and prominent pericaecal fat can be seen on ultrasound. Abscess formation generally occurs in the right lower quadrant and may extend into the pelvis or upper abdomen. An appendix abscess appears as a hyporeflective or complex mass. Increased central flow around the appendix stump or peripherally around the abscess can be seen in perforation [18]. A careful ultrasound examination should be performed of the entire abdomen and pelvis in children with acute abdominal pain suspected of having appendicitis as only 25% of children will have appendicitis. Ultrasound may be helpful in identifying other causes in such situations [19].

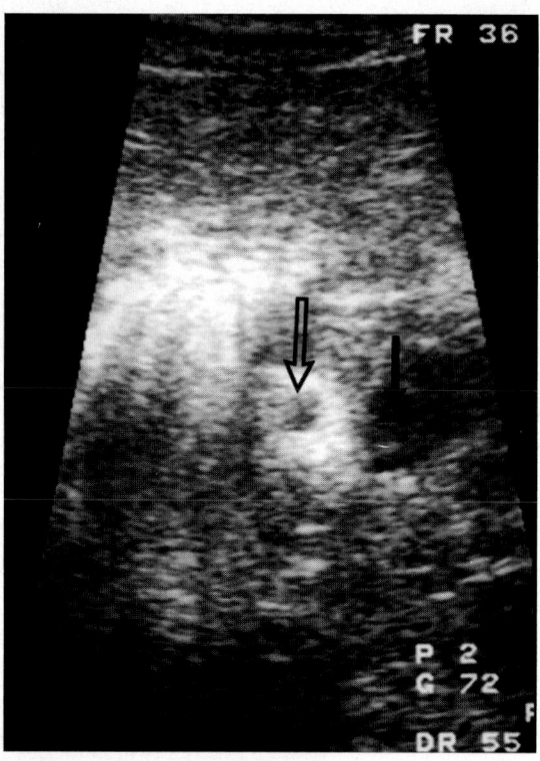

Fig. 45.2 Midgut malrotation. Transverse scan through the upper abdomen showing the reversal of the normal relationship of the superior mesenteric vessels with the superior mesenteric vein (black arrow) present on the left aspect of the superior mesenteric artery (open arrow). Infrequently this can be seen without midgut malrotation. An upper gastrointestinal contrast study is still the 'gold standard' test for midgut malrotation.

Intussusception

In this condition bowel (the intussusceptum) prolapses into caudad bowel (the intussuscipiens) which can result in intestinal obstruction. Most intussusceptions (approximately 90%) are ileocolic, i.e. the ileum prolapses into colon, though ileoileocolic, colocolic and ileoileal can occur. Idiopathic intussusception occurs predominantly in children aged between 3 months and 3 years of age, classically presenting with vomiting, abdominal pain, a palpable abdominal mass and red current jelly stools. Most (approximately 90%) are believed to be due to enlarged lymphoid follicles (Peyer's patches) in the terminal ileum. In children over the age of 5 years there are probably pathological lead points, e.g. Meckel's diverticula, polyps and duplications. Ultrasound can confirm the diagnosis and is generally undertaken for unusual cases and not used as a routine screening tool. If there is enough clinical suspicion of the diagnosis then the infant should have the benefit of an enema (using air or water-soluble contrast) even if the ultrasound is normal. Plain films of the abdomen may suggest an intussusception and if there is enough clinical suspicion of the diagnosis the infant should proceed to enema. When using ultrasound the

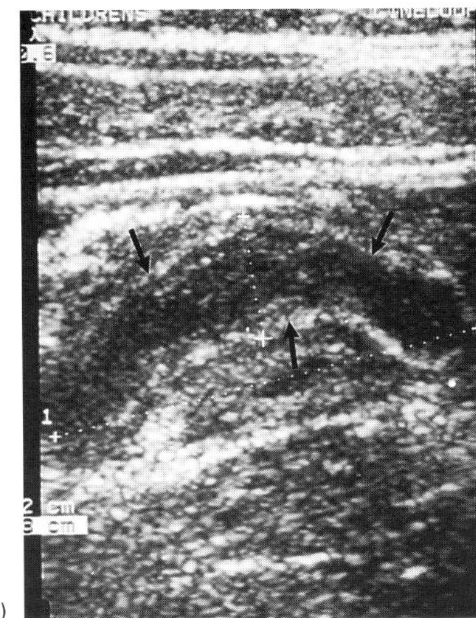
(a)

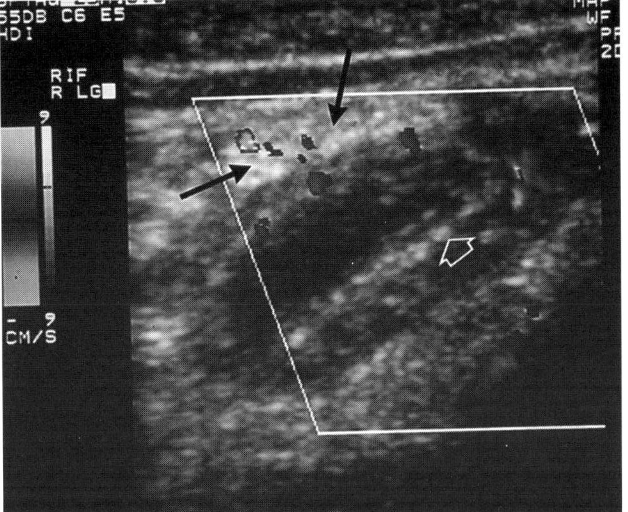

(b)

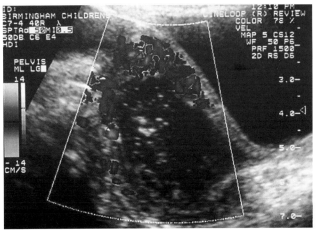

(c)

Fig. 45.3 Acute appendicitis. (a) Longitudinal scan with compression with a linear 5–10 MHz probe in the right lower quadrant. A non-compressible, blind-ending, distended and fluid-filled appendix is shown with its echogenic mucosa (arrows). (b) Longitudinal scan. There is some increased vascularity in the inflamed appendix (the normal appendix has no demonstrable colour flow on Doppler imaging). Note the prominent echogenic pericaecal fat due to inflammation (black arrows) and echogenic appendiceal mucosa (open arrow). (c) Appendiceal abscess. Longitudinal scan showing a pelvic abscess from a perforated appendix with peripheral hypervascularity around the collection. Appendiceal abscesses can be limited to the right lower quadrant or extend into the pelvis or upper abdomen. For colour, see Plate 45.3 (between pp. 308 and 309).

whole abdomen and pelvis should be scanned carefully paying particular attention to scanning the colon in longitudinal and transverse, moving the transducer clockwise around the abdomen with the infant supine and commencing in the right lower quadrant. The intussusception in transverse can have a 'target' appearance with several hyporeflective concentric rings surrounding and echogenic centre, a thick-walled 'doughnut' appearance with an echogenic centre and a thick hyporeflective outer rim or a complex echogenic appearance [20–22] (Fig. 45.4a). On longitudinal scans the intussusception appears reniform in shape (Fig. 45.4b). Other findings seen in intussusception include lead masses, obstructed small bowel which is dilated and fluid-filled and free peritoneal fluid [20,23–25]. Absent blood flow in the intussusception on colour Doppler suggests gangrenous bowel [26,27]. Once intussusception has been diagnosed then a radiological enema reduction (pneumatic or hydrostatic) should be carried out provided there is no evidence of peritonism. Hydrostatic reductions can be monitored with ultrasound. Enema reductions can be safely performed by experienced radiologists working closely with a paediatric surgical team.

Abdominal masses (Table 45.2)

Ultrasound easily differentiates non-malignant conditions, e.g. hydronephroses from solid abdominal tumours which may be malignant. Every child who presents with an abdominal mass should initially have the benefit of an ultrasound examination. It can direct further imaging and other necessary investigations. Renal masses are the commonest cause of an abdominal mass. In neonates hydronephrosis, and older infants and young children Wilms' tumour, account for the majority of renal masses.

Hydronephrosis

Obstructive uropathies and vesicoureteric reflux can

Table 45.2 Causes of neonatal abdominal masses

Site of origin	Cause	Ultrasound findings
Kidney	Hydronephrosis	See text
	Multicystic dysplastic kidney [32,33] (Fig. 45.5)	Renal cysts of variable size and shape, no communication between cysts, absent renal pelvis, absent/dysplastic renal parenchyma, contralateral renal anomalies, e.g. pelviureteric junction obstruction/reflux (in 10–20%)
	Autosomal recessive polycystic kidney disease [32,34]	Bilateral enlarged and diffusely echogenic kidneys (numerous 1–2 mm cysts), pyramids echogenic, echolucent rim in peripheral renal parenchyma, unilateral renal enlargement (rare), macrocysts sometimes in medulla
	Mesoblastic nephroma [35]	Large well-defined low reflective tumour; hyporeflective centre, hypo-/hyper-reflective rings surrounding tumour
	Renal vein thrombosis [36,37] (Fig. 45.6)	Kidney initially hyper-reflective and enlarged, after 1–2 weeks reflectivity decreases and then becomes echogenic, thrombus in renal vein and IVC
	Renal ectopia	Ectopic position of kidney (may be fused to normal opposite kidney), kidney may have abnormal shape, unusual calyces and tilted axes
	Wilms' tumour	See text
Genital tract	Hydrometrocolpos [38]	Tubular fluid-filled dilated vagina and uterus (vagina larger than uterus), fallopian tube may be fluid filled, hydronephrosis (from obstruction)
	Ovarian cyst	May be large extending into the abdomen, haemorrhage causes fluid/debris level in cyst, with torsion small multiple peripheral cysts in enlarged ovary
Gastrointestinal tract	Bowel duplication cyst [39]	Most common at ileocaecal valve/terminal ileum, less than 6 cm diameter, wall 2–3 mm thick
	Mesenteric cyst	Uni- or multilocular cyst, larger than duplication cysts, debris in cyst (due to infection/haemorrhage)
Retroperitoneum	Adrenal haemorrhage [40,41] (Fig. 45.7)	Unilateral (usually right)/bilateral; mixed reflective mass becomes hyporeflective, then disappears often leaving calcified focus
	Neuroblastoma	See text
	Germ cell tumour (most common is teratoma) [42]	Presacral location, benign tumours predominantly cystic and malignant tumours predominantly solid
Liver and spleen	Hepatoblastoma	See text
	Hepatic cyst [43]	Solitary cyst in right liver (and incidental finding)
	Choledochal cyst [44,45] (Fig. 45.8)	Well-defined cyst at porta hepatis, intrahepatic bile duct dilatation
	Splenic haematoma [46]	Parenchymal fluid collection

cause hydronephrosis. In the neonate pelviureteric junction obstruction, posterior urethral valve, duplex systems, vesicoureteric junction obstruction, vesicoureteric reflux and prune belly syndrome can cause hydronephrosis [28–30] (Fig. 45.9). Separation of the central echoes of the collecting system in the kidney is the main finding on ultrasound in hydronephrosis. It is well recognized that a false negative ultrasound examination can occur in the first few days after birth secondary to the relative dehydration that exists in the neonate [31] and therefore you may need to repeat the examination after the first few days of life.

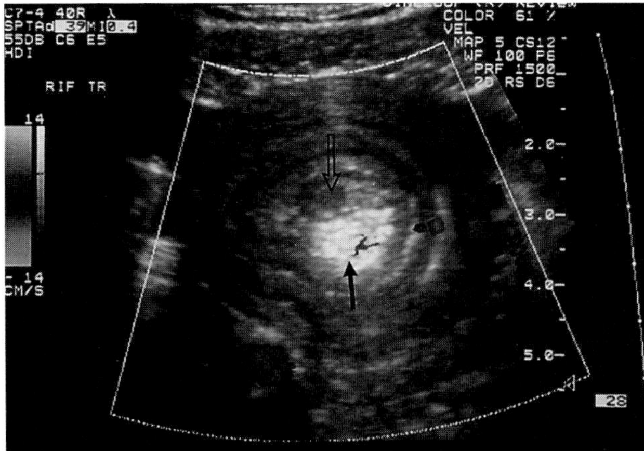

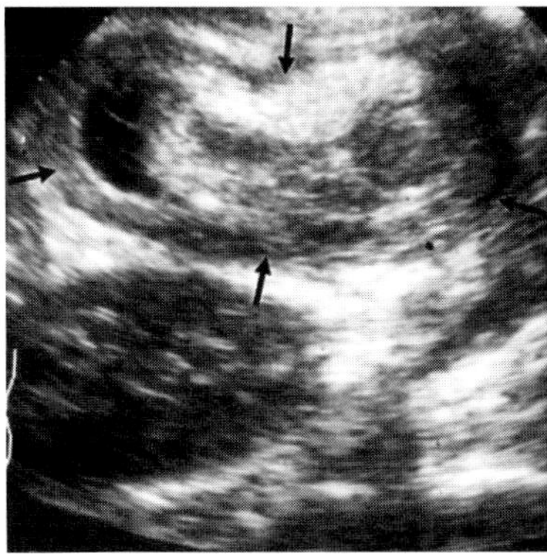

Fig. 45.4 Intussusception. (a) Transverse colour Doppler scan with typical target sign of multiple layers and concentric rings due to the invagination of the bowel wall. The reflectivity and number of concentric rings depends on the degree of oedema and impaction of mucosal and serosal layers. An invaginated echogenic mesentery is shown (black arrow). Fluid trapped in the mesentery (open arrow) can look like a cyst. Blood flow in the intussusception is in keeping with a viable bowel. (b) Longitudinal scan showing a reniform or 'pseudo-kidney' shape to the intussusception (arrows). For colour, see Plate 45.4 (between pp. 308 and 309).

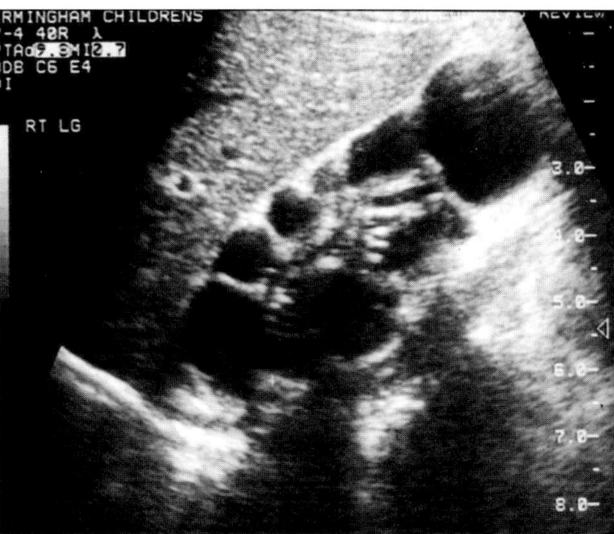

Fig. 45.5 Multicystic dysplastic kidney. Longitudinal scan showing kidney replaced with cysts of varying size, no identifiable renal pelvis and absent renal parenchyma. There is no communication between the cysts.

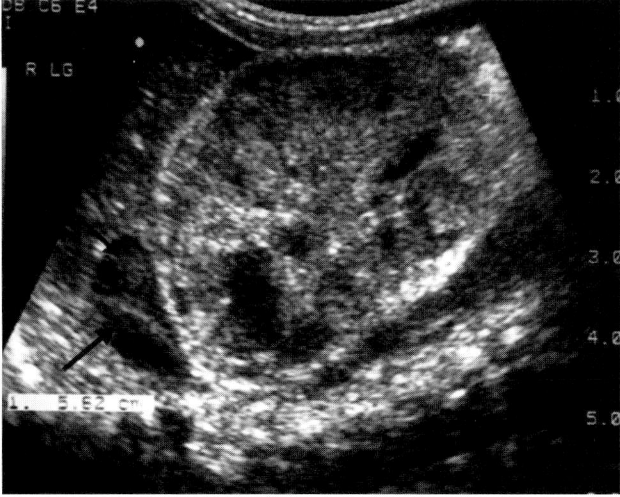

Fig. 45.6 Acute neonatal renal vein thrombosis. Longitudinal scan showing an enlarged kidney with increased parenchymal reflectivity and loss of the normal corticomedullary differentiation. There is associated adrenal haemorrhage (arrows).

Solid abdominal tumours

The three commonest malignant abdominal tumours seen in infants and young children are Wilms' tumour (or nephroblastoma), neuroblastoma and hepatoblastoma. The correct staging of solid abdominal tumours is vital so that children can receive appropriate treatment. Ultrasound alone cannot accurately assess these tumours and computed tomography (CT), magnetic resonance imaging (MRI), nuclear medicine and occasionally angiography are needed. Ultrasound can, however, be very helpful in the initial assessment and the points to try and identify are as follows.

1 The anatomical location of the lesion, e.g. whether it is retroperitoneal, and its size and organ of origin (e.g. if it arises from the liver/kidney/adrenal).

2 The nature of its margins (i.e. well or ill defined) and its consistency, i.e. solid/cystic/mixed solid and cystic elements.

3 The relationship to adjacent structures and other viscera (e.g. whether it displaces or encases the abdominal aorta and inferior vena cava (IVC)).

4 The presence of local spread out of the tumour (e.g. either direct spread or to local lymph nodes; involvement is difficult to detect on ultrasound).

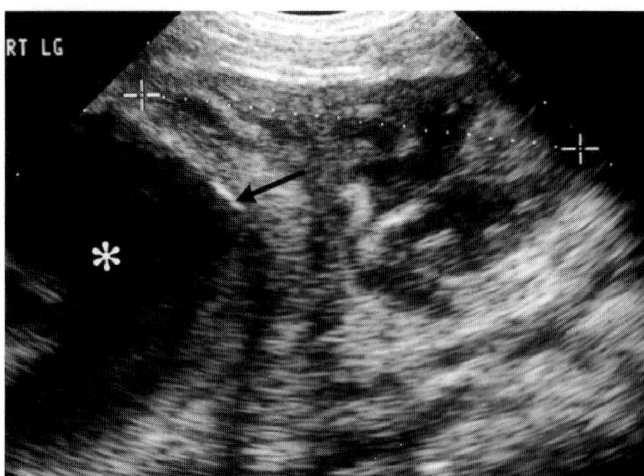

Fig. 45.7 Adrenal haemorrhage. Longitudinal scan showing a large hypoechoic haemorrhage (*) indenting the upper pole of the kidney (arrow). Temporal changes occur in haemorrhage reflectivity (initially the haemorrhage is of mixed reflectivity, which becomes hyporeflective after several days and then becomes echogenic due to calcification).

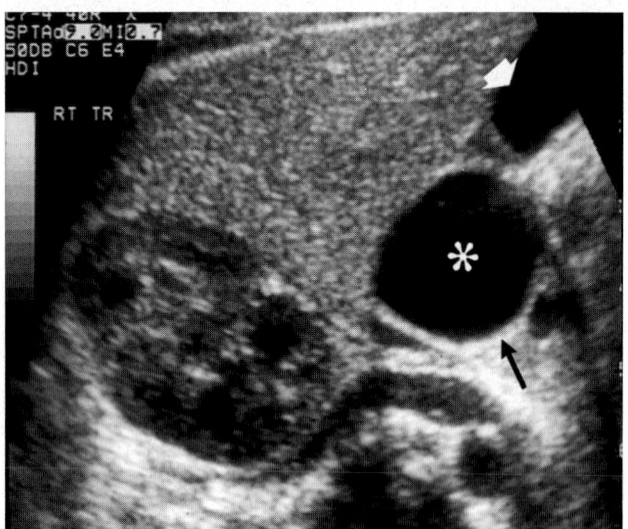

Fig. 45.8 Choledochal cyst. Transverse scan showing a well-defined cyst at the porta hepatis (*). The gall bladder (white arrow) is adjacent and separate from the cyst. The cyst wall has a single layer (black arrow), unlike duplication cysts which can have several layers. The diagnosis preoperatively can be confirmed by nuclear medicine.

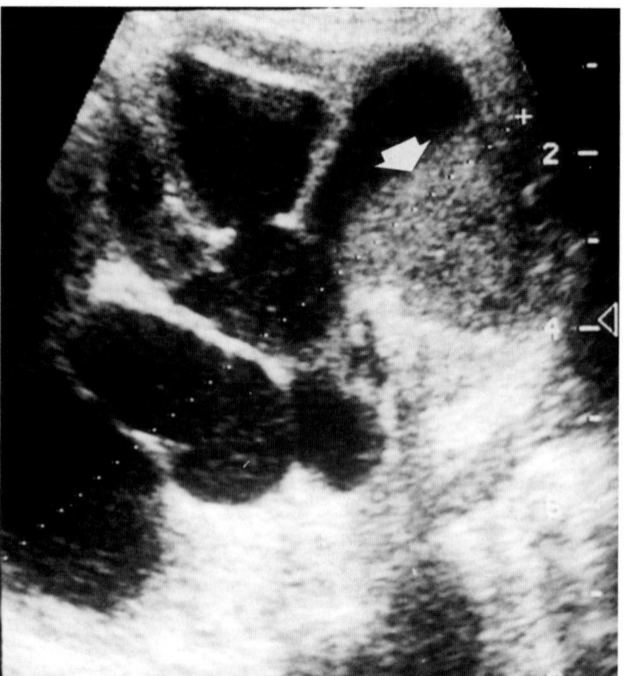

(a)

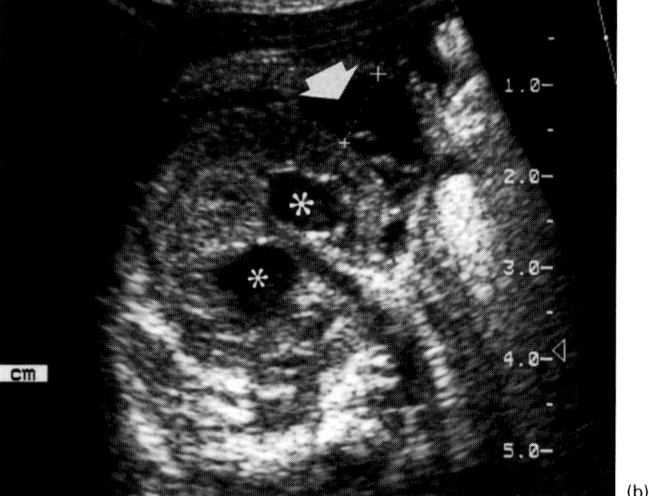

(b)

Fig. 45.9 Hydronephrosis. (a) Longitudinal scan showing dilated calyces containing echogenic debris in the lower pole due to pus, i.e. there is a pyonephrosis (arrow). The collecting system was obstructed secondary to a posterior urethral valve. (b) Transverse scan with hydronephrosis from an upper tract obstruction secondary to a posterior urethral valve. A perforation resulting in a urinoma (arrow) has occurred. The calyces (*) in the hydronephrotic kidney are less dilated following perforation. A posterior urethral valve is the commonest cause of urinomas and ascites in term male infants.

5 The presence of distant spread, e.g. liver mestastases.
6 The local effects, e.g. venous involvement and hydronephrosis.

Wilms' tumour

This is both the commonest renal neoplasm and malignant abdominal tumour in childhood. The mean age of presentation is 3 years. Children present with a palpable mass, abdominal pain, haematuria or fever. Hypertension is commonly present.

The tumour is usually large (e.g. can be 12 cm in diameter) on presentation with well-defined margins replacing most of the involved kidney. Compressed normal renal tissue may be seen. The tumour is commonly a little more echogenic than liver and homogeneous, frequently containing echo-poor and echogenic areas due to haemorrhage, necrosis and rarely calcification [47–51] (Fig. 45.10a). Calyceal dilatation may be seen due to tumour obstruction of the collecting system. Vascular invasion involving the renal vein, IVC, right atrium and other IVC tributaries such as the hepatic veins can occur and can be

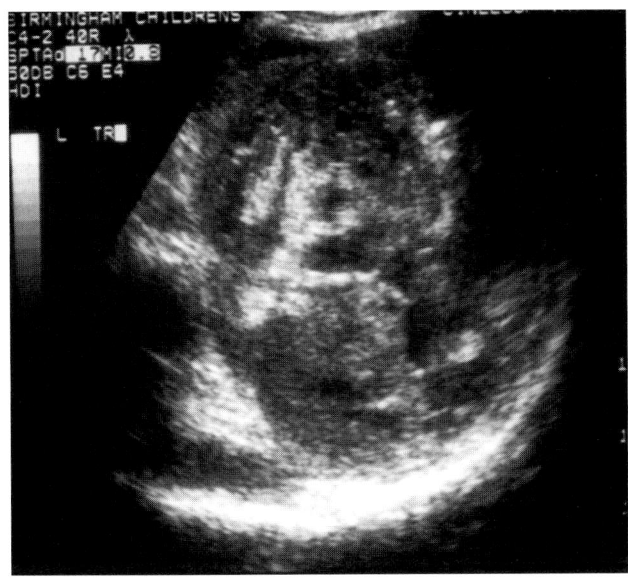

(a)

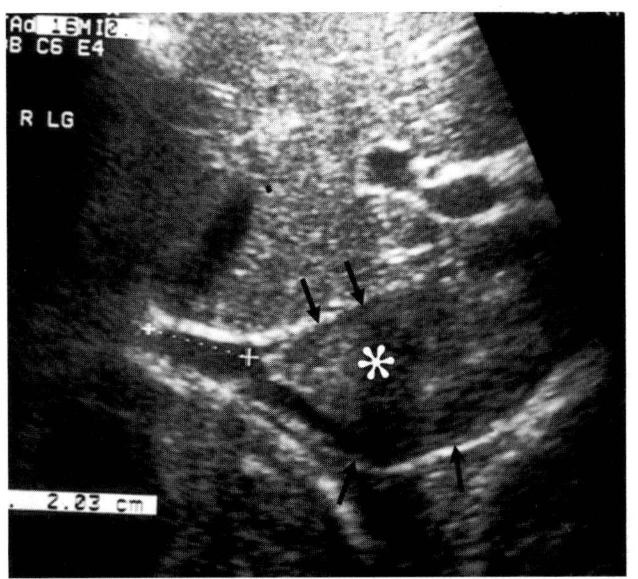

(b)

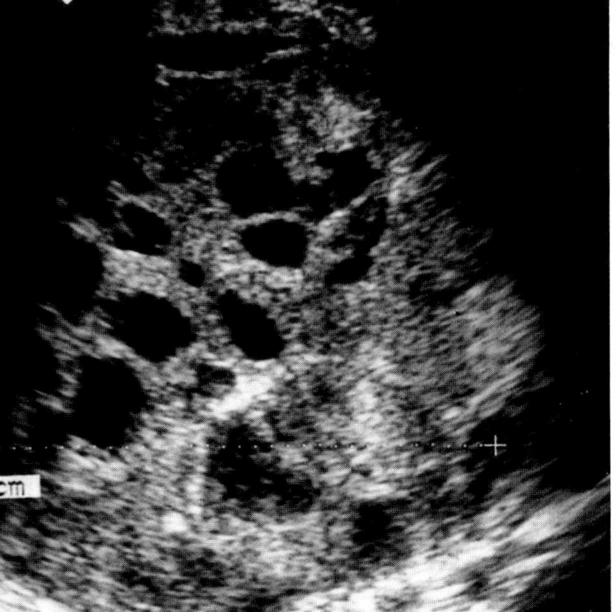

(c)

Fig. 45.10 Wilms' tumour. (a) Transverse scan of a kidney which is replaced by a large heterogeneous, highly reflective Wilms' tumour with well-defined margins. It is difficult in this case to identify normal renal tissue. The heterogeneity of the tumour is due to haemorrhage and necrosis. Some tumours, although echogenic, are more homogeneous. (b) Wilms' tumour with venous extension. Longitudinal scan showing IVC expansion (arrows) by an intraluminal echogenic tumour thrombus (*). There is no extension of tumour into the right atrium. (c) Following chemotherapy multiple cystic areas in the tumour due to necrosis can be seen.

well seen on ultrasound (Fig. 45.10b). With large tumours and extensive local spread there is displacement rather than encasement of major retroperitoneal vessels such as the aorta and IVC. Of tumours 5–10% will be bilateral at presentation and 12% of Wilms' tumours will have metastasized by presentation, e.g. to the lungs and sometimes to the liver.

The treatment of Wilms' tumour involves surgery (with nephrectomy) and chemotherapy. If children receive chemotherapy before surgery, tumours may shrink in response to the chemotherapy and cystic necrosis can be seen within the tumour (Fig. 45.10c). The survival of children with Wilms' tumour is generally good and depends on staging (determined by imaging and surgical findings) with a 5-year survival of 90% in those with a 'favourable' tumour histology.

Neuroblastoma

This is the commonest malignant tumour in infancy and may be present at birth. The mean age at presentation is approximately 2 years with the majority under 5, commonly presenting with a palpable mass. Systemic symptoms of fever, weight loss, anaemia, hypertension and irritability are sometimes seen. These tumours arise from neural crest tissue and consequently arise anywhere along the sympathetic chain or in adrenal medulla. Tumour occurs in the adrenal gland in 40% of cases. Ultrasound confirms the retroperitoneal site of the tumour and often its origin. The tumour is usually solid with a heterogeneous echo texture, has ill-defined margins and within the tumour there is often punctate calcification identified as echogenic foci with acoustic shadowing and cystic haemorrhage and necrosis seen as areas of low echogenicity (Fig. 45.11). Typically, it spreads directly along the retroperitoneum across the mid line encasing vessels (whereas Wilms' tumours displace vessels) [52,53]. Dumb-bell tumours occur in 15% of cases as tumour spreads into the spinal canal through the intervertebral foramina. A cystic variant of these tumours usually occurs in babies of less than 3 months of age or as an antenatal finding [54]. Metastases are present in 70% at presentation. At less than 1 year of age liver, marrow, skin and lymph nodes are most likely to be involved. Children of more than 1 year of age are most likely to have metastasis in the bony cortex, lymph nodes, liver and marrow. Skull metastases may have large soft tissue components and dural lesions may widen skull sutures.

The prognosis is generally poor with a cure rate of approximately 35%. Staging depends on a combination of imaging, surgery and histopathology results. The prognosis is better in young children. Spontaneous resolution of

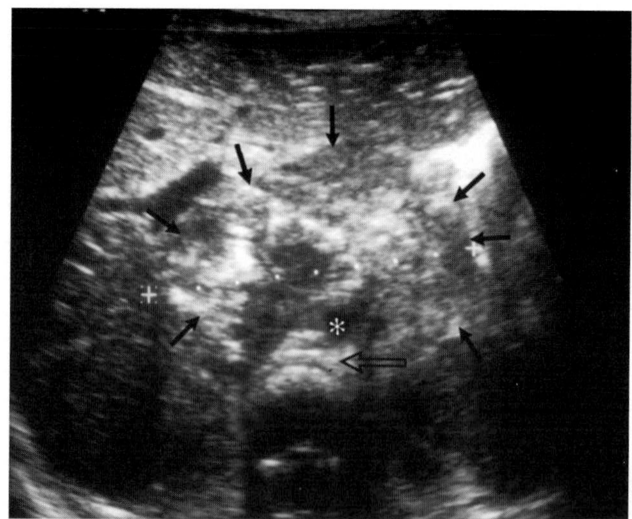
(a)

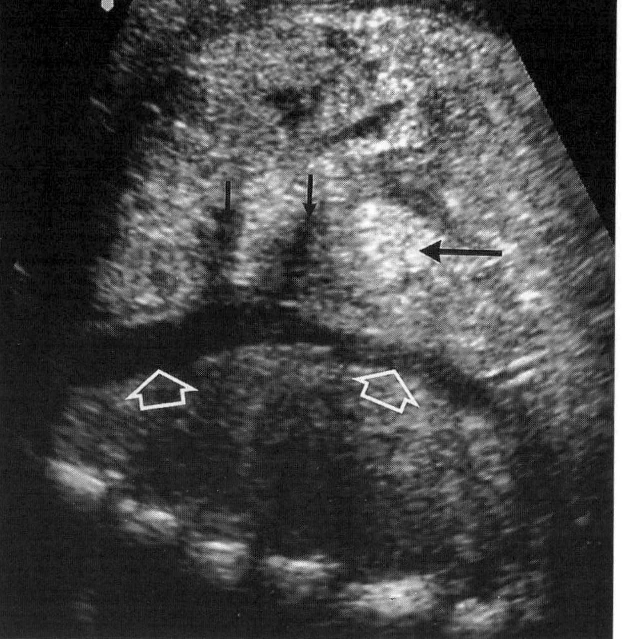
(b)

Fig. 45.11 Neuroblastoma. (a) Left adrenal neuroblastoma. Transverse scan across the upper abdomen showing a solid heterogeneous retroperitoneal tumour with ill-defined margins (black arrows) spreading across the midline. The abdominal aorta (*) is uplifted from the spine (open arrow) and encased by tumour. (b) Longitudinal scan showing typical appearance with a large retroperitoneal solid tumour. The heterogeneous appearance (long arrow) is due to haemorrhage, necrosis, cystic change and calcification. Punctate calcification in the neuroblastoma does not always produce acoustic shadowing. The aorta (open arrows) is uplifted off the spine by tumour infiltration. The coeliac trunk and superior mesenteric artery (short arrows) are encased by tumour.

the malignant tumour by maturation to a benign ganglioneuroblastoma may occur.

Hepatoblastoma

These tumours are the third most frequent neoplasm in children after Wilms' tumour and neuroblastoma. They are usually large at presentation and most present with a right upper quadrant mass. Serum measurement of α-fetoprotein is useful in diagnosis and monitoring. Associations with hepatoblastoma include familial polyposis coli and the Beckwith–Wiedemann syndrome. The tumour on ultrasound appears commonly as a poorly marginated heterogeneous hyperechogenic mass (containing calcification) with echo-poor areas of haemorrhage and necrosis (Fig. 45.12). Tumour margins are difficult to accurately assess on ultrasound. Vascular invasion, highly suspicious of malignancy, can sometimes be seen [55–57]. It is usually confined to one lobe, but may be multicentric, and rarely diffusely infiltrative which will give a heterogeneous echo pattern and vascular distortion. Hypertrophy or atrophy of normal liver can occur secondary to vascular or biliary compromise. Tumour biopsy to establish histology is not always undertaken. These patients are treated initially with chemotherapy and provided disease is confined to the liver cures can be achieved at surgery with tumour resection [58]. If tumour is unresectable and confined to the liver then liver transplantation may be considered. Metastatic disease is most commonly seen in the lungs, being present in 10% of patients at diagnosis. The number of liver segments involved, spread to hepatic vessels and IVC, local spread outside the liver and the presence of distant metastasis are all important in assessing resectability and therefore as many imaging modalities should be used as is necessary to provide a full evaluation. Survival is very unlikely unless the tumour is completely excised.

(a)

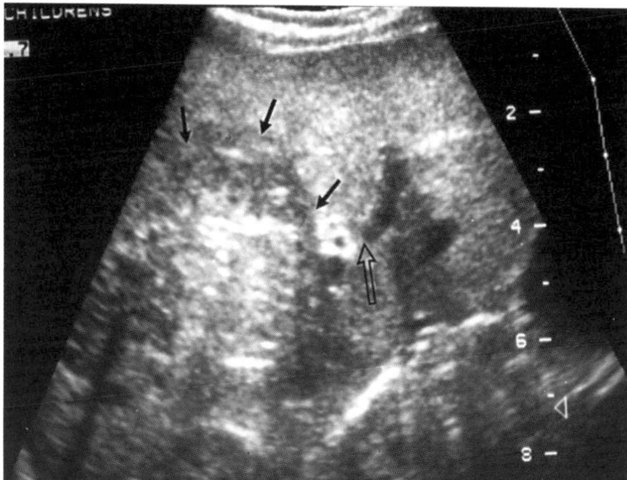

(b)

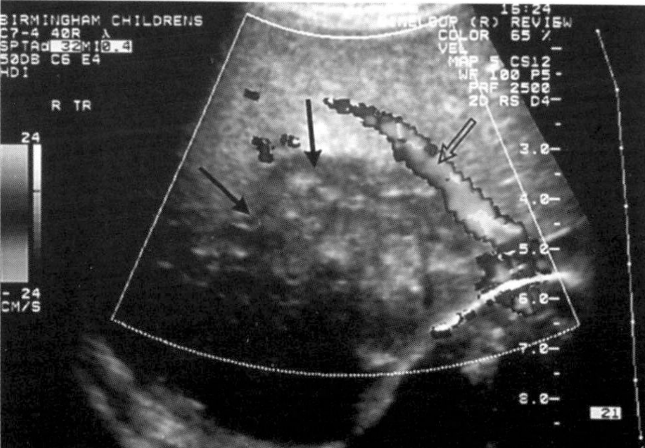

Fig. 45.12 Hepatoblastoma. (a) Transverse scan showing an echogenic tumour in the right liver with partially ill-defined margins (black arrows). The left portal vein is truncated and involved by tumour (open arrow). (b) Large right hepatic tumour (black arrows). There is no tumour on the left side of the middle hepatic vein (open arrow). No right hepatic vein is seen—it is likely that tumour is compressing rather than invading it. For colour, see Plate 45.12 (between pp. 308 and 309).

Ascites

There are numerous causes of ascites. Tables 45.3 and 45.4 briefly outline the causes seen in the neonatal period and older infants and children. Ascites can appear anechoic or with internal echoes and can be free flowing or loculated. The reflectivity of the fluid may suggest the nature of the

Table 45.3 Neonatal ascites

Urinary tract	Posterior urethral valve; congenital nephrosis
Gastrointestinal	Meconium peritonitis
Liver and biliary	Biliary atresia; congenital infection; bile duct perforation
Cardiovascular	Congenital heart disease; vascular malformation
Chyle	Lymphatic obstruction; thoracic duct trauma
Infection	Congenital (syphilis, toxoplasmosis, cytomegalovirus)
Tumours	Hepatoblastoma
Intraperitoneal haemorrhage	Coagulopathy; ischaemic bowel

Table 45.4 Ascites in older infants and children

Cardiovascular	Heart failure (from any cause); severe anaemia
Liver and biliary	Cirrhosis from any cause (e.g. biliary atresia); extrahepatic portal hypertension; Budd–Chiari syndrome
Renal	Acute and chronic renal failure (e.g. reflux, glomerulonephritis, nephrotic syndrome)
Gastrointestinal	Perforated viscus, ischaemic/infarcted bowel; inflammatory bowel disease; protein-losing enteropathy
Peritoneal	Bleeding, chyle, inflammation, pancreatitis
Neoplasia	Ovarian; lymphoma
Other causes	Cerebrospinal fluid shunt; malnutrition and collagen vascular disease

fluid, e.g. transudates (in cardiac failure and liver disease), chyle, urine, cerebrospinal fluid and bile are generally echo-free. Complex ascitic fluid (which is of variable echogenicity) is due to exudates with protein or blood causing the echogenic appearance. Haemorrhagia, inflammation, neoplasia and sometimes chyle cause complex ascites.

References

1 Breaux, C.W. Jr, Georgeson, K.E., Royal, S.A., Curnow, A.J. (1988) Changing patterns in the diagnosis of hypertrophic pyloric stenosis. *Pediatrics* **81**, 213–217.

2 Teele, R.L., Smith, E.H. (1977) Ultrasound in the diagnosis of idiopathic hypertrophic pyloric stenosis. *New England Journal of Medicine* **296**, 1149–1150.

3 Graif, M., Itzchak, Y., Avigad, I., Strauss, S., Ben-Ami, T. (1984) The pylorus in infancy: overall sonographic assessment. *Pediatric Radiology* **14**, 14–17.

4 Haller, J.O., Cohen, H.L. (1986) Hypertrophic pyloric stenosis: diagnosis using US. *Radiology* **161**, 335–339.

5 Hayden, C.K. Jr, Swischuk, L.E., Lobe, T.E., Schwartz, M.Z., Boulden, T. (1984) Ultrasound: the definitive imaging modality in pyloric stenosis. *Radiographics* **4**, 517–530.

6 Keller, H., Waldmann, D., Greiner, P. (1987) Comparison of preoperative sonography with intraoperative findings in congenital hypertrophic pyloric stenosis. *Journal of Pediatric Surgery* **22**, 950–952.

7 Stunden, R.J., LeQuesne, G.W., Little, K.E.T. (1986) The improved ultrasound diagnosis of hypertrophic pyloric stenosis. *Pediatric Radiology* **16**, 200–205.

8 Bisset, R.A.L., Gupta, S.C. (1988) Hypertrophic pyloric stenosis, ultrasonic appearances in a small baby. *Pediatric Radiology* **18**, 405.

9 Carver, R.A., Okorie, M., Steiner, G.M., *et al.* (1987) Infantile hypertrophic pyloric stenosis—diagnosis from the pyloric muscle index. *Clinical Radiology* **38**, 625–627.

10 Atwell, J.D., Levick, P. (1981) Congenital hypertrophic pyloric stenosis and associated anomalies in the genitourinary tract. *Journal of Pediatric Surgery* **16**, 1029–1035.

11 Okorie, N.M., Dickson J.A.S., Carver, R.A., Steiner, G.M. (1988) What happens to the pylorus after pyloromyotomy? *Archives of Disease in Childhood* **63**, 1339–1340.

12 Sauerbrei, E.E., Paloschi, G.G.B. (1983) The ultrasonic features of hypertrophic pyloric stenosis, with emphasis on the post-operative appearance. *Radiology* **147**, 503–506.

13 Pulyaert, J.B.C.M. (1986) Acute appendicitis: US evaluation using graded compression. *Radiology* **158**, 355–360.

14 Rubin, S.Z., Martin, D.J. (1990) Ultrasonography in the management of possible appendicitis in childhood. *Journal of Pediatric Surgery* **25**, 737–740.

15 Sivit, C.J. (1993) Diagnosis of acute appendicitis in children: spectrum of sonographic findings. *American Journal of Roentgenology* **161**, 147–152.

16 Siegal, M.J., Carel, C., Surratt, S. (1991) Ultrasonography of acute abdominal pain in children. *Journal of the American Medical Association* **266**, 1987–1989.

17 Vignault, F., Filiatrault, D., Brandt, M.L., Garel, L., Grignon, A., Ouimet, A. (1990) Acute appendicitis in children: evaluation with US. *Radiology* **176**, 741–744.

18 Quillan, S.P., Siegal, M.J. (1994) Appendicitis: efficacy of colour Doppler sonography. *Radiology* **191**, 557–560.

19 Siegel, M.J. (1992) Acute appendicitis in children: the role of US. *Radiology* **185**, 341–342.

20 Alzen, G., Funke, G., Truong, S. (1989) Pitfalls in the diagnosis of intussusception. *Journal of Clinical Ultrasound* **17**, 481–488.

21 Bowerman, R.A., Silver, T.M., Jaffe, M.H. (1982) Real-time ultrasound diagnosis of intussusception in children. *Radiology* **143**, 527–529.

22 Swischuk, L.E., Hayden, C.K., Boulden, T. (1985) Intussusception: indications for ultrasonography and an explanation of the doughnut and pseudokidney signs. *Pediatric Radiology* **15**, 388–391.

23 Itagaki, A., Uchida, M., Ueki, K., Kajii, T. (1991) Double target sign in ultrasonic diagnosis of intussuscepted Meckel diverticulum. *Pediatric Radiology* **21**, 148–149.

24 Patenaude, Y., Jequier, S., Russo, P. (1993) Pediatric case of the day. *Radiographics* **13**, 218–220.

25 Swischuk, L.E., Stansberry, S.D. (1991) Ultrasonic detection of free peritoneal fluid in uncomplicated intussusception. *Pediatric Radiology* **21**, 350–351.

26 Quillin, S.P., Siegel, M.J. (1993) Colour Doppler US of children with acute lower abdominal pain. *Radiographics* **13**, 1281–1293.

27 Lam, A.H., Firman, K. (1992) Value of sonography including colour Doppler in the diagnosis and management of long standing intussusception. *Pediatric Radiology* **22**, 112–114.

28 Brown, T., Mandell, J., Lebowitz, R.L. (1987) Neonatal hydronephrosis in the era of sonography. *American Journal of Roentgenology* **148**, 959–963.

29 Kasper, T.E., Osborne, R.W. Jr, Semerdjan, H.S., Miller, H.C. (1976) Urologic abdominal masses in infants and children. *Journal of Urology* **116**, 629–633.

30 Paltiel, H.J., Lebowitz, R.L. (1989) Neonatal hydronephrosis due to primary vesicoureteral reflux: trends in diagnosis and treatment. *Radiology* **170**, 787–789.

31 Laing, F.C., Burke, V.D., Wing, V.W., Jeffrey, R.B. Jr, Hashimoto, B. (1984) Postpartum evaluation of fetal hydronephrosis: optimal timing for follow-up sonography. *Radiology* **152**, 423–424.

32 Hayden, C.K. Jr, Swischuk, L.E. (1991) Renal cystic disease. *Seminars in Ultrasound CT and MR* **12**, 361–373.

33 Sanders, R.C., Hartman D.S. (1984) The sonographic distinction between neonatal multicystic kidney and hydronephrosis. *Radiology* **151**, 621–625.

34 Hayden, C.K. Jr, Swischuk, L.E., Smith, T.H., Armstrong, E.A. (1986) Renal cystic disease in childhood. *Radiographics* **6**, 97–116.

35 Grider, R.D., Wolverson, M.K., Jagannadharao, B., Graviss, E.R., O'Connor, D.M. (1981) Congenital mesoblastic nephroma with cystic component. *Journal of Clinical Ultrasound* **9**, 43–45.

36 Hricak, H., Sandler, M.A., Madrazo, B.L., Eyler, W.R., Sy, G.S. (1981) Sonographic manifestations of acute renal vein thrombosis; an experimental study. *Investigative Radiology* **16**, 30–35.

37 Paling, M.R., Wakefield, J.A., Watson, L.R. (1985) Sonography of experimental acute renal vein occlusion. *Journal of Clinical Ultrasound* **13**, 647–653.

38 Sailer, J.F. (1979) Hematometra and hematocolpos: ultrasound findings. *American Journal of Roentgenology* **132**, 1010–1011.

39 Teele, R.L., Henschke, C.I., Tapper, D. (1980) The radiographic and ultrasonographic evaluation of enteric duplication cysts. *Pediatric Radiology* **10**, 9–14.

40 Mittelstaedt, C.A., Volberg, F.M., Merton, D.F., Brill, P.W. (1979) The sonographic diagnosis of neonatal adrenal haemorrhage. *Radiology* **131**, 453–457.

41 Pery, M., Kaftori, J.K., Bar-Maor, J.A. (1981) Sonography for diagnosis and follow-up of neonatal adrenal haemorrhage. *Journal of Clinical Ultrasound* **9**, 397–401.

42 Hogge, W.A., Thiagarajah, S., Barber, V.G., Rodgers, B.M., Newman, B.M. (1987) Cystic sacrococcygeal teratoma: ultrasound diagnosis and perinatal management. *Journal of Ultrasound Medicine* **6**, 707–710.

43 Quillin, S.P., McAlister, W.M. (1992) Congenital solitary nonparasitic cyst of the liver in a newborn. *Pediatric Radiology* **22**, 543–544.

44 Kangarloo, H., Sarti, D.A., Sampl, W.F., Amundson, G. (1980) Ultrasonographic spectrum of choledochal cysts in children. *Pediatric Radiology* **9**, 15–18.

45 Torissi, J.M., Haller, J.O., Velcek, F.T. (1990) Choledochal cyst and biliary atresia in the neonate: imaging findings in five cases. *American Journal of Roentgenology* **155**, 1273–1276.

46 Lupien, C., Sauerbrei, E.E. (1984) Healing in the traumatised spleen: sonographic investigation. *Radiology* **151**, 181–185.

47 De Campo, J.F. (1986) Ultrasound of Wilms' tumour. *Pediatric Radiology* **16**, 21–24.

48 Cremin, B.J. (1987) Wilms' tumour: Ultrasound and changing concepts. *Clinical Radiology* **38**, 465–474.

49 Hartman, D.S., Sanders, R.C. (1982) Wilms' tumour versus neuroblastoma: usefulness of ultrasound in differentiation. *Journal of Ultrasound Medicine* **1**, 117–122.

50 Jaffe, M.H., White, S.J., Silver, T.M., Heidelberger, K.P. (1981) Wilms' tumour: ultrasonic features, pathological correlation and diagnostic pitfalls. *Radiology* **140**, 147–152.

51 Reiman, T.H., Siegel, M.J., Shakelford, G.D. (1986) Wilms' tumour in children: abdominal CT and US evaluation. *Radiology* **2**, 25–28.

52 Bousvaros, A., Kirks, D.R., Grossman, H. (1986) Imaging of neuroblastoma: an overview. *Pediatric Radiology* **16**, 89–106.

53 Daneman, A. (1988) Adrenal neoplasms in children. *Seminars in Roentgenology* **23**, 205–215.

54 Atkinson, G.O. Jr, Zaatari, G.S., Lorenzo, R.L., Gay, B.B. Jr, Garvin, A.J. (1986) Cystic neuroblastoma in infants: radiographic and pathologic features. *American Journal of Roentgenology* **146**, 113–117.

55 Boechat, M.I., Kangarloo, H., Gilsanz, V. (1998) Hepatic masses in children. *Seminars in Roentgenology* **23**, 185–193.

56 Brunelle, F., Chaumont, P. (1984) Hepatic tumours in children: ultrasonic differentiation of malignant from benign lesions. *Radiology* **150**, 695–699.

57 De Campo, M., De Campo, J.F. (1988) Ultrasound of primary hepatic tumours in childhood. *Pediatric Radiology* **19**, 19–24.

58 Stringer, M.D., Hennayake, S., Howard, E.R., *et al.* (1995) Improved outcome for children with hepatoblastoma. *British Journal of Surgery* **82**, 386–391.

Part 9
Musculoskeletal System

Chapter 46: The musculoskeletal system

E.G. McNally

Muscle, tendon and ligament injury

Muscle injury

Normal muscle comprises echo-poor fascicles, surrounded by reflective fibroadipose septa. The septa are arranged in a regular herringbone fashion which is disrupted following injury. Trauma can result in a tear, haematoma, compartment syndrome or myositis ossificans. On occasions the differential diagnosis between a tear and haematoma may be difficult. Definitive diagnosis of a muscle tear can be made when there is discontinuity of the fibroadipose septa (Fig. 46.1), or when the disrupted ends of the tear can be identified. This latter sign has been referred to as the 'bell clapper' sign [1] (Fig. 46.2) and implies severe injury. More subtle tears are seen as areas of decreased reflectivity without septal disruption (Fig. 46.3). The majority of haematomas are well-defined lesions, their ultrasound pattern depending on their age. Fresh blood is reflective [2] and remains so for 2–3 days, gradually decreasing in reflectivity over time. Tears also result in echo-poor lesions, but are less sharply defined than haematomas. Dynamic scanning can also assist in distinguishing haematomas from tears which appear to increase in size during contraction whereas haematomas do not [3]. Haemorrhage can occur into a pre-existing tumour. Though this is uncommon, it is prudent to continue to observe a haematoma until it resolves fully or reduces to a constant small size. In time, reflective foci of calcification and eventually ossification may develop. In post-traumatic myositis ossificans, sonographic evidence of calcification precedes plain film changes and may appear as early as 2–3 weeks after injury [4]. A plane of separation from underlying bone differentiates from parosteal osteogenic sarcoma. Myositis ossificans can demonstrate variable appearances on ultrasound, including increased vascularity at the periphery.

Tendon injury

Normal tendons appear as fine parallel lines of increased reflectivity interspersed with echo-poor tendon fibrils (Fig. 46.4). With high resolution equipment, the tendon sheath is seen as a thin highly reflective structure surrounding the tendon [5]. Tendons must be examined with a perpendicular ultrasound beam, as they appear echo-poor (mimicking tendinitis) when examined obliquely [6] (Fig. 46.5). This is termed anisotropy and can be a particular problem at the tendon insertion, where fibres follow an oblique course close to bone and appear hyporeflective. Care must be taken to avoid misdiagnosis of tendinitis at these sites.

Acute trauma can result in a tear, which can be partial or complete. Complete tears appear as a disruption of the normal linear reflective structure of the tendon with separation of the tendon ends. During healing, the tendon ends may be joined by a reflective fibrous scar [7] (Fig. 46.6) and differentiation of the normal tendon ends can be difficult . Acoustic shadows from the true tendon ends can help to assess the size of the tendon gap. Dynamic scanning is also helpful.

Partial tears appear as small hypoechoic areas within the tendon that do not traverse it. An intratendinous haematoma has a similar appearance but is less common. Recurrent subthreshold trauma may also result in intratendinous hypoechoic areas, similar to a partial tear, but within an enlarged tendon [7] (Fig. 46.7). This is termed tendinitis; in chronic lesions calcification may develop. The normal tendon sheath is difficult to visualize. Using high frequency probes it can be identified and is usually less than 1 mm thick [8]. Hypoechoic fluid filling the surrounding tendon sheath can occur with either bacterial or viral tenosynovitis (Fig. 46.8), but bacterial infection is more likely to cause an increase in tendon diameter [9]. Reflective debris may be present and also suggests bacterial infection. Adhesions between the tendon and tendon sheath can occur following trauma, surgery or pyogenic infection. The range of movement of a tendon can be tested on dynamic scanning. Restricted movement of the tendon will occur if there are adhesions between the tendon and its sheath [10]. This can occur following surgery or pyogenic tenosynovitis.

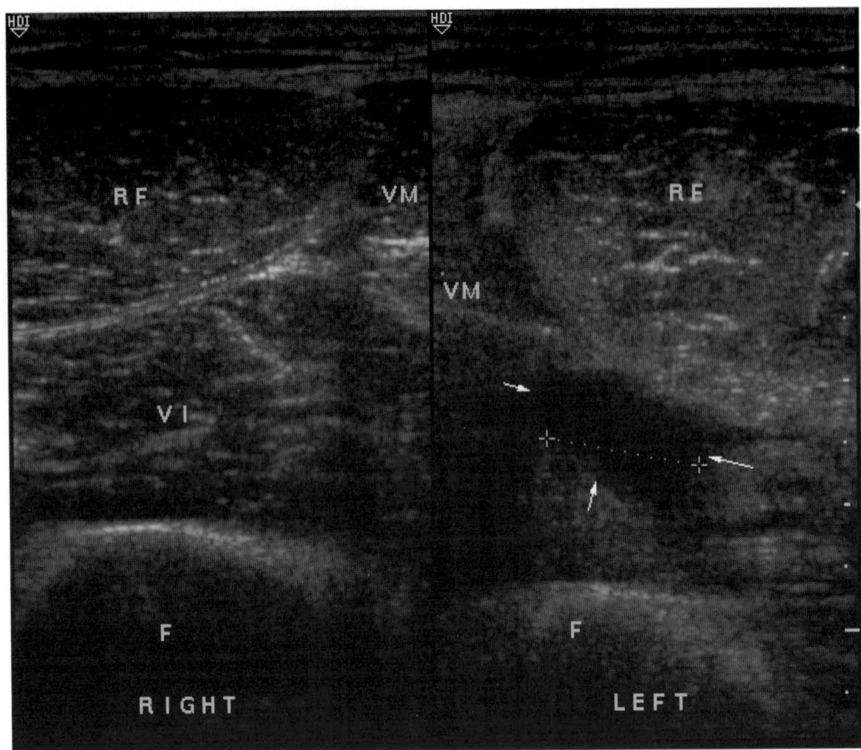

Fig. 46.1 A muscle tear: note the disrupted muscle fibres (small arrows) on the vastus intermedius (VI) on the left compared with the normal right side. F, femur; RF, rectus femoris; VM, vastus medialis.

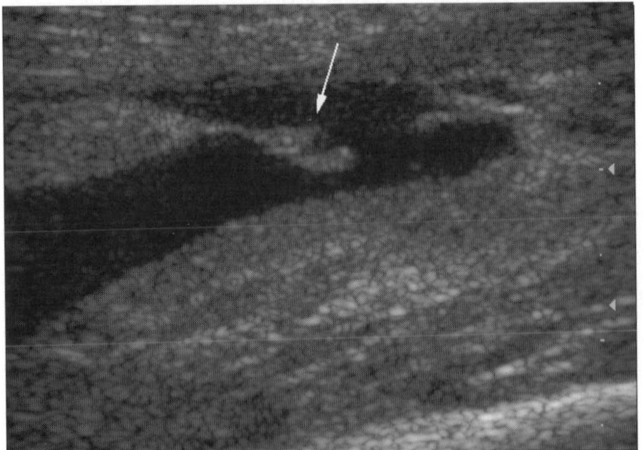

Fig. 46.2 Bell clapper sign (arrow) of severe muscle injury.

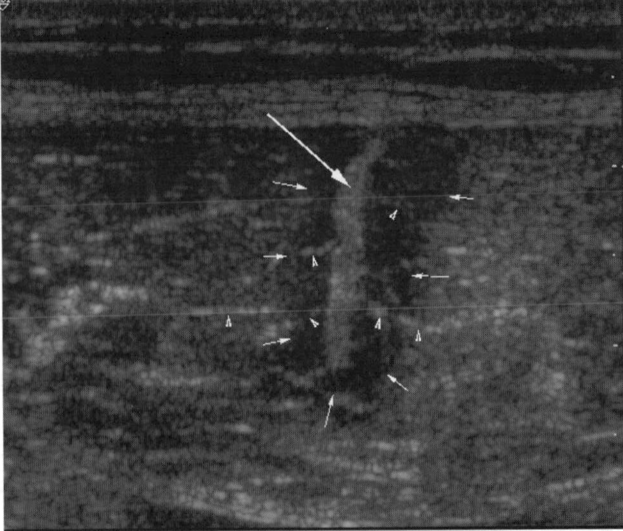

Fig. 46.3 A more subtle muscle tear with oedema (small arrows) surrounding the large central septum (large arrow) of the rectus femoris muscle. Note the integrity of the secondary septae (arrowheads).

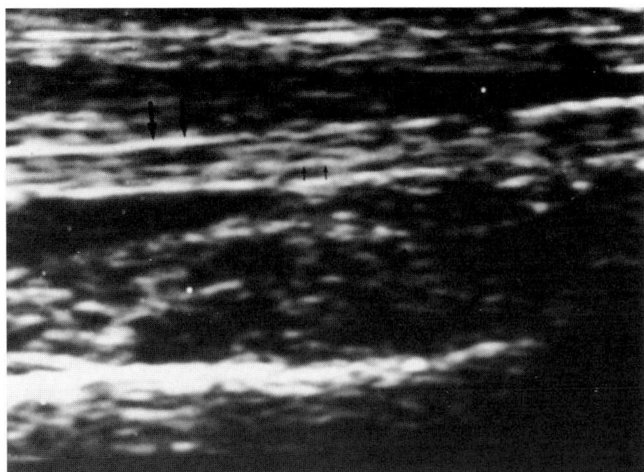

Fig. 46.4 Normal flexor digitorum profundus tendon. The reflective tendon sheath (large arrows) surrounds the echo-poor tendon fibrils, with interspaced connective tissue strands (small arrows).

(a)

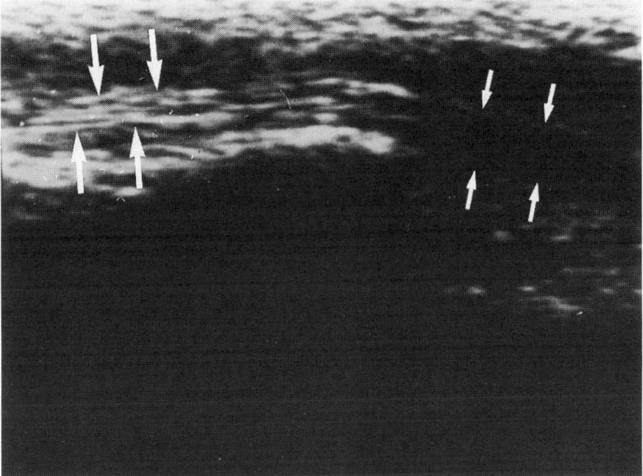

(b)

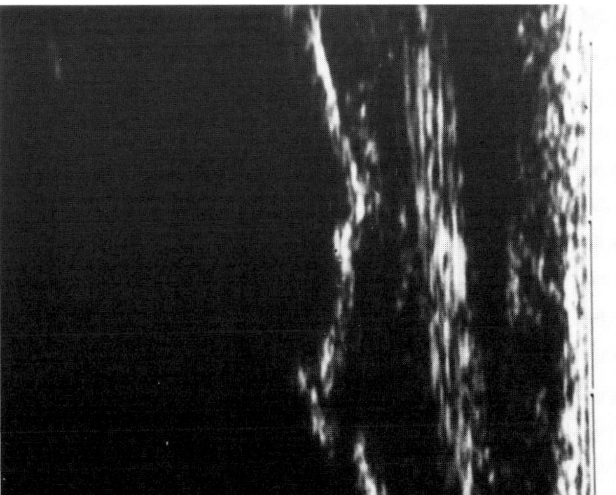

Fig. 46.5 (a) Normal posterior tibialis tendon (large arrows). The distal tendon appears echo-poor as it rounds the medial malleolus (small arrows). (b) Moving the probe inferiorly brings the tendon perpendicular to the beam and normal reflectivity is restored.

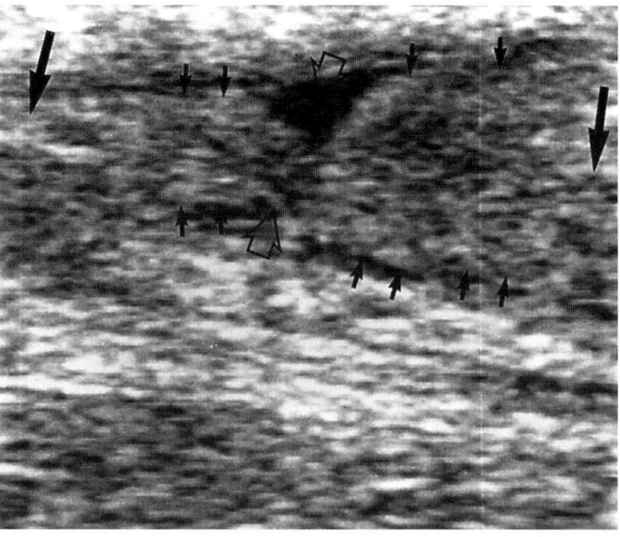

Fig. 46.6 Complete Achilles tendon tear. A fluid-filled gap can be seen traversing the tendon (large open arrows). The ruptured tendon ends (large black arrows) are separated from each other by heterogeneous granulation tissue (small black arrows).

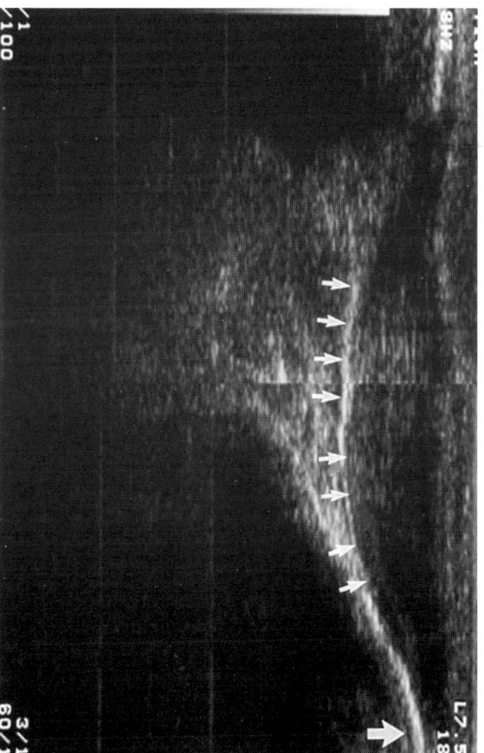

Fig. 46.7 Chronic Achilles tendinitis (composite image). The tendon thickened and fusiform shaped from origin to insertion into the calcaneum (large arrow). The small arrows outline the anterior border of the enlarged heterogeneous tendon.

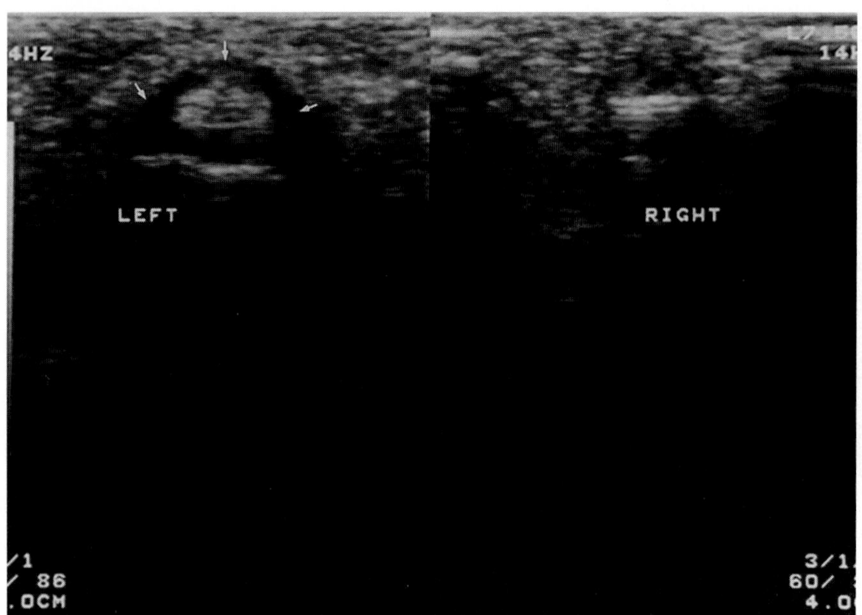

Fig. 46.8 Tenosynovitis. An echo-poor cuff of fluid surrounds the left flexor indicis tendon on this transverse section (arrows). Compare with the normal right side.

Ligament injuries

Ligament injuries can be divided into acute and chronic. Acute lesions can be further divided into ligament sprain, partial tear and complete tear. Sprains are diagnosed when an intact ligament is surrounded by fluid. Partial tears are seen as focal thinning of the ligament with surrounding fluid but with some intact fibres. With complete tears, there is separation of the ligament ends with fluid communicating across the tear. Chronic tears are seen as ligamentous thickening which can either be focal or involve the entire ligament. Calcification can occur with chronicity.

Miscellaneous post-traumatic findings

Ultrasound is useful in the search for non-radio-opaque foreign bodies. In many cases, a history of penetrating injury is not obtained and patients present with an abscess. A careful search should be made in these patients for the culprit, which is often a small splinter of wood or a thorn. Foreign bodies of less than 1 mm are difficult to locate. Metal is most easily seen and fragments as small as 0.5 mm may be identified. Wood has to measure 0.7 mm, glass greater than 2 mm and plastic greater than 4 mm to be seen [11]. With very large foreign bodies, only the reflective leading edge will be seen with the remainder of it obscured in the acoustic shadow or reverberation artefact. The exact size may therefore be underestimated. Correlation with plain films is recommended when a foreign body is located to avoid misdiagnosing sesamoid bones or areas of soft tissue calcification as foreign bodies [12]. Inclusion cysts are usually hypoechoic although the presence of keratin can result in small foci of increased reflectivity. Other post-traumatic abnormalities that are readily detectable include post-traumatic bursitis and pseudoaneurysms. The faint periosteal reaction that occurs with stress factors can be identified and is often associated with soft tissue hypoechoic oedema.

Soft tissue masses

Ultrasound is useful for confirming the presence of a soft tissue mass, determining whether it is cystic or solid and demonstrating its relationship to surrounding structures and assessing its vascularity. A negative ultrasound examination excludes tumour or abscess. In cases where a mass is palpable but ultrasound is negative a fascial herniation of muscle or lipoma should be considered. Occasionally, the former can be confirmed by contracting the involved muscle.

Once identified, the mass lesion can be further characterized by magnetic resonance imaging (MRI) or biopsied under ultrasound control (Fig. 46.9). Less often a specific diagnosis can be made prior to biopsy. Increased reflectivity within a mass suggests fat, acute haemorrhage [13] or fibrosis [14]. One-third of lipomas are hypoechoic and 20% show a mixed pattern [13]. Liposarcoma is also most commonly reflective and may contain echo-poor strands (Fig. 46.10). The more aggressive liposarcomas may contain little evidence of fat on any imaging technique.

Fluid-filled cystic lesions can be readily identified as echo-poor structures. Lymphoma and neuromas are also of quite low reflectivity [15] and need to be differentiated. In the case of tumours of neural origin, the adjacent nerve can often be identified as a structure similar in appearance

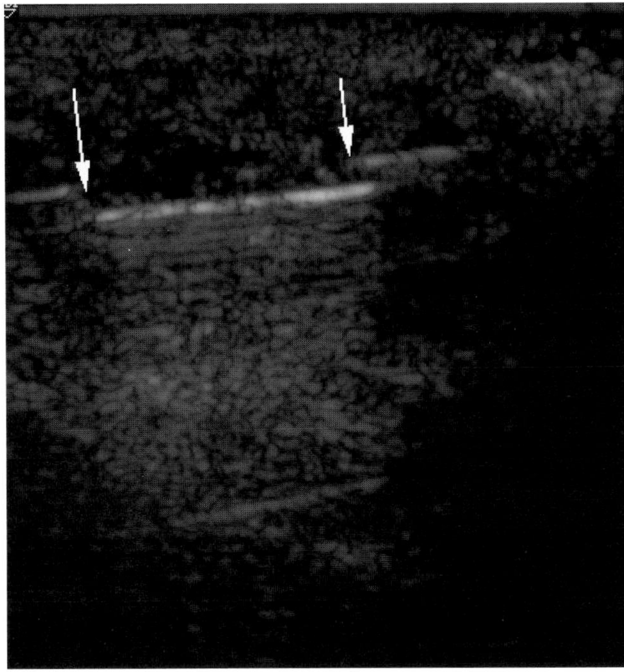

Fig. 46.9 Ultrasound is an excellent means of biopsying soft tissue lesions. The needle can be tracked with great accuracy. Here the open port of a tru-cut needle is clearly demonstrated (between arrows).

to a tendon but which does not move when adjacent muscles contract. To differentiate cystic lesion from homogeneous echo-poor solid masses, it is useful to compare the lesion with a known fluid-filled structure, increasing the gain until artefactual echoes begin to appear in the fluid. When the gain is then reduced slightly, true cystic lesions should still appear anechoic. A colour flow facility is also useful to assess solid lesions and, in particular, vascular lesions prior to biopsy.

Soft tissue abscesses are relatively hypoechoic, but can be either well defined or poorly marginated. Reflective foci may be identified in surrounding musculature indicating a secondary inflammatory reaction [16]. Compression with the probe can help to confirm the thick fluid content and colour flow may reveal high vascularity within the capsule. Percutaneous drainage can also be performed under ultrasound guidance, the most common organism isolated being *Staphylococcus aureus*.

The thickness of the echo-poor cartilage cap of an osteochondroma can be reliably measured. A thickness of greater than 15 mm is suspicious for chondrosarcomatous change [17]. Ultrasound is generally poor at distinguishing benign from malignant lesions as often benign lesions have less well-defined margins [13] and vice versa. If malignancy is confirmed full local and systemic staging is indicated and ultrasound has no role to play in this regard. Choi *et al.* [18] compared the use of ultrasound with MRI for the detection of sarcoma recurrence following surgery, and found it as good as MRI. Ultrasound was poor in the

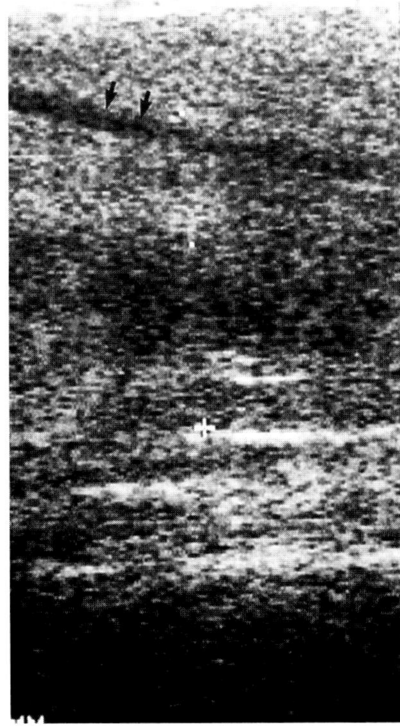

(a)

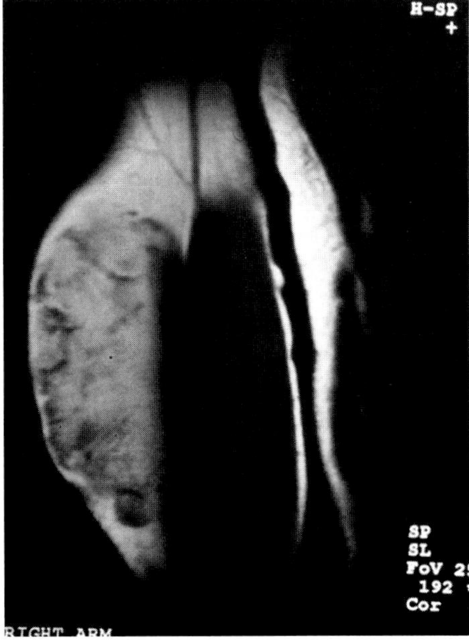

(b)

Fig. 46.10 (a) Ill-defined reflective mass with echo-poor strands (arrows). (b) MRI confirms diagnosis of liposarcoma.

immediate postoperative period as granulation tissue, haemorrhage, oedema or abscess cannot be reliably distinguished from recurrence or residual tumour, though the use of enhancing agents has yet to be assessed. Any echo-poor mass arising later than 6 months after surgery should be biopsied.

The upper limb

The shoulder

BICEPS TENDON

Injuries to the biceps tendon are best detected with the patient seated. The operator can stand either in front of or behind the patient. The patient places the dorsum of the hand on the ipsilateral knee and axial and longitudinal sections (Fig. 46.11) are obtained. Slight pressure with the distal end of the probe can improve visualization of the tendon in longitudinal section. The tendon of the long head of biceps, which normally measures 4 mm in diameter, is easily identified within the bicipital groove (Fig. 46.12). Tears, tendinitis, tenosynovitis and subluxation (Fig. 46.13) can be appreciated. Tendon subluxation is characterized by pain and an audible click. Dynamic scanning with internal and external rotation will demonstrate the tendon subluxing, usually medially, over the lesser tuberosity.

THE ROTATOR CUFF

Rotator cuff tears often present with pain, reduced range of motion and weakness, though many are asymptomatic. Clinical examination may reveal tenderness over the insertion of the supraspinatus tendon and diminished range of abduction with weakness and atrophy of the supraspinatus muscle. On occasion, an actual defect may be palpated.

The cuff is best seen with the arm adducted and internally rotated [19]. Images should be obtained in the transverse and longitudinal planes, beginning anteriorly. On the transverse anterior image, the reflective leading edges of the coracoid and the humeral head should be identified. The round reflective structure lateral to the coracoid is the

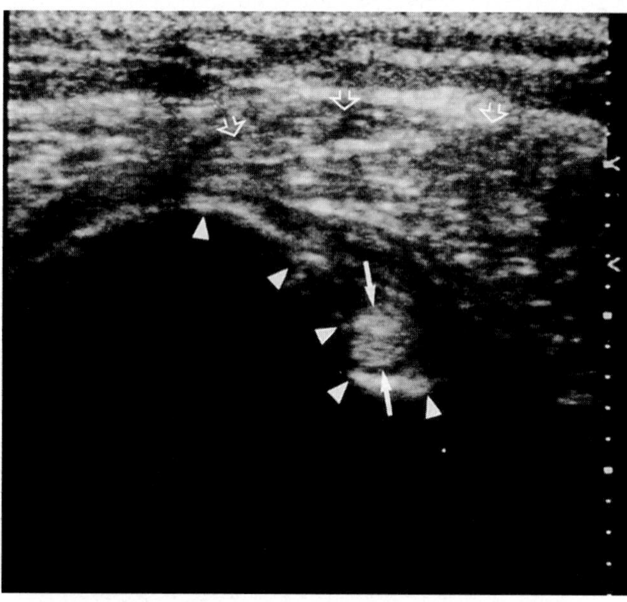

Fig. 46.12 Transverse section of biceps tendon in groove (white arrows). Humeral head (arrowheads) and deltoid (open arrows) overlie.

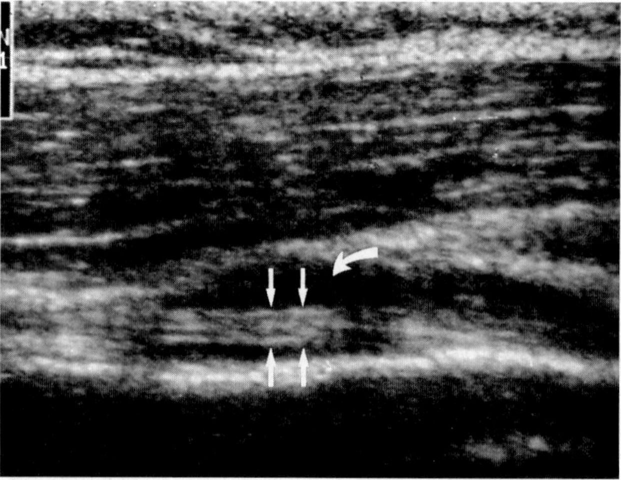

Fig. 46.11 Longitudinal section of biceps tendon (straight arrows). A little fluid surrounds the tendon in the sheath (curved arrow).

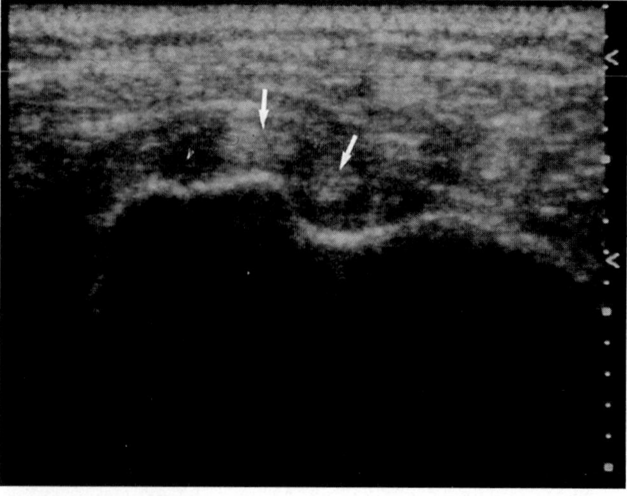

Fig. 46.13 Split biceps tendon (arrows) with subluxation of medial slip over lesser tuberosity.

biceps tendon, which in turn lies medial to the anterior edge of the supraspinatus tendon. This is an important anatomical landmark, as many tears begin in this area.

The normal tendon is a wide structure measuring 4–6 cm from front to back; it is wedge shaped in sagittal section and is normally thinner posteriorly [20]. Thinning in this context must not be misdiagnosed as a tear. Comparison with the contralateral shoulder is useful.

A large number of signs have been described in patients with tears. These include: focal discontinuity (Fig. 46.14), non-visualization of the tendon (Fig. 46.15), focal thinning (Fig. 46.16), increased reflectivity of the cartilage surface [21], hypoechoic foci, reflective foci or linear reflective bands [20,22–26]. Of these, the first four appear to be the most reliable. Crass *et al.* [23] have had success in using hyperechoic foci, suggesting that they represent granulation tissue within a tear; however, hyperechoic foci can be due to pathology other than tears. for example calcification, various artefacts [25] or even as a normal variant. Care is therefore needed with this sign.

Additional support for the diagnosis of a tear can be obtained by detecting fluid in the subacromial bursa and in the biceps tendon sheath [27]. Neither of these signs is specific to a rotator cuff tear, but their presence should alert the operator to a careful search for one. Considerable fluid in one compartment, with no fluid in the other is evidence against a full thickness tear as it implies there is no communication between the two spaces. Identification of the inferior epimysium of the deltoid muscle can also be helpful. Normally this is a reflective line, convex superiorly, separating the supraspinatus from the deltoid. In the presence of a tear, the deltoid drops into the space created by the tear. The hyperechoic line becomes flattened or concave superiorly [25]. Hypoechoic areas can also occur with partial tears, but they do not completely traverse the tendon.

With increasing age the reflectivity of supraspinatus decreases and approaches that of the deltoid. This may give a false impression of non-visualization of the tendon with the 'deltoid' in direct contact with the humerus mimicking a complete rotator tear. Comparison with the contralateral shoulder should again avoid this pitfall [28]. Other potential pitfalls include: (a) slight heterogeneity encountered in normal patients; (b) a normal area of discontinuity identified in the sagittal plane representing the intra-articular biceps tendon within the anterior part of the supraspinatus (anterior interval); (c) an hyperechoic area representing the biceps tendon itself; and (d) shadows cast on the tendon from the normal intermuscular septa of the deltoid. Finally subacromial tears may be missed unless an axial scan plane is used. This pattern is fortunately uncommon.

The size of rotator cuff tears as determined by ultrasound correlates well with defects identified at arthrogra-

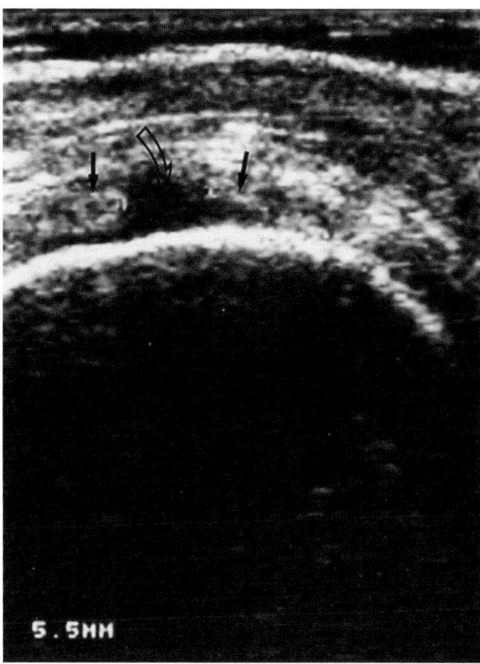

Fig. 46.14 Focal discontinuity in supraspinatus tendon indicating a tear. The separated tendon ends (black arrows) outline the fluid-filled tear (open curved arrow).

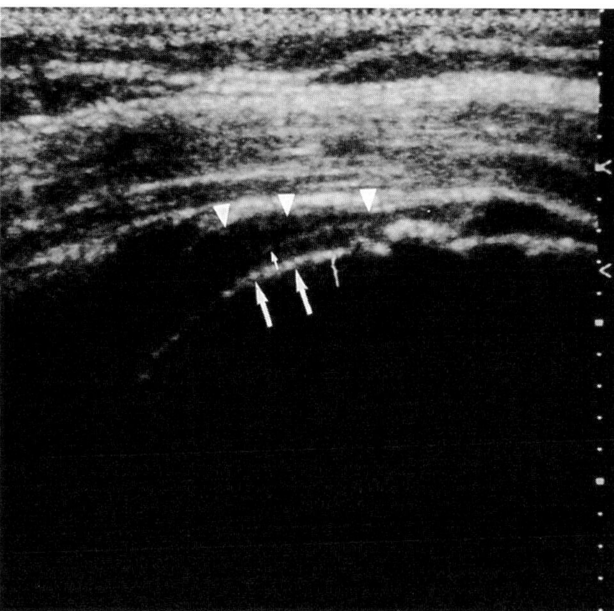

Fig. 46.15 Non-visualization of cuff. Deltoid muscle (arrowheads) rests directly on the articular surface of the humeral head (small arrow). Subcartilage cortex of humeral head (large arrows).

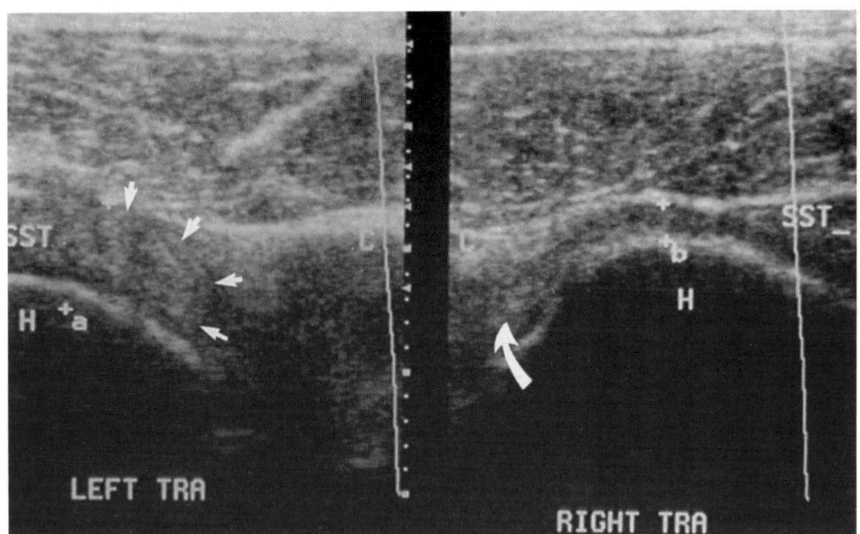

Fig. 46.16 Focal discontinuity of anterior portion of right supraspinatus tendon (SST)—compare with the normal left side. C, coracoid process; H, humeral head; arrowheads, anterior edge of normal left SST; curved arrow, right intra-articular biceps tendon.

phy [29]. Tears can be divided into partial thickness (either joint or bursal surface), full thickness (both surfaces involved) or complete (involving a large portion of the tendon which usually retracts). There is debate as to the surgical management of partial thickness tears. The author's view is that the overall size of the lesion is the important determinant—a large lesion with a few intact fibres, and therefore a partial tear, is likely to be more significant than a tiny full thickness tear measuring less than 5 mm. With this approach, ultrasound is effective in differentiating tears that are likely to require surgical repair from those that can be treated either conservatively or with subacromial decompression. Several studies have compared the accuracy of ultrasound against arthrography and MRI [26,29,30] with varying outcomes. Improvements in technology and the use of the more reliable signs have had a profound effect on the accuracy of this technique, with good results only possible with the highest resolution equipment. A recent study carried out by the author demonstrated a 91% sensitivity, 94% specificity, 81% negative predictive and 97% positive predictive value, with an overall 92% accuracy in the detection of full thickness tears when compared with surgery. A 5–12 MHz variable frequency linear array (ATL) probe was used.

Evaluation of the postoperative rotator cuff is difficult as the tendon is normally reflective at the site of repair. The only reliable sign of a retear is a defect or gap [31]. Clear demonstration of fluid bridging a gap in the re-attached tendon (Fig. 46.17) and loss of normal transmitted movement on dynamic assessment are suggestive of a re-tear, but studies with surgical correction are lacking.

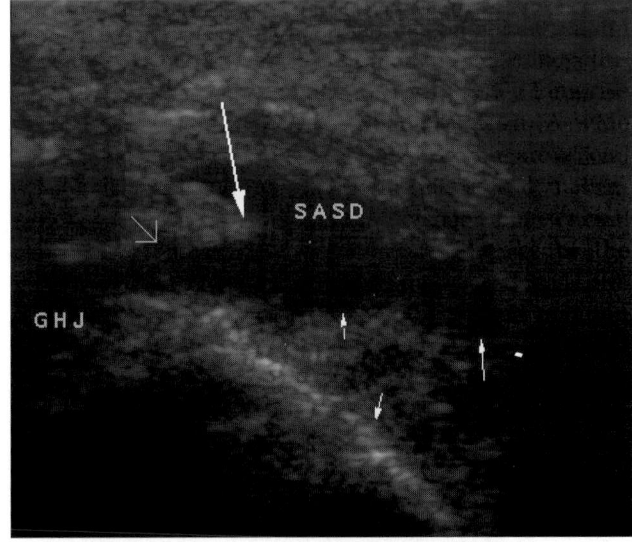

Fig. 46.17 Postoperative cuff repair. Fluid traverses (thin arrow) between the bursa (SASD) and the glenohumeral joint (GHJ). The supraspinatus tendon end lies apparently free within the fluid (long arrow) and separate from an inflammatory mass at the normal site of re-insertion (smallest arrows).

The elbow

The elbow is best examined with the patient seated and arms resting on the examination table. The operator sits opposite. Three positions are adopted in turn. The first has both hands and wrists fully supinated and resting on the table side by side. The elbow is extended. This position is used to examine the medial structures, anterior joint space and biceps tendon. The wrists are then pronated to 90° and can be clasped into the praying position (Fig. 46.18).

The lateral structures including the common extensor origin can be compared. From this position, one wrist is fully pronated, and turned through 180° so that the finger tips point towards the patient rather than the operator. This will also necessitate flexion at the elbow to 90° whilst raising the arm above the table (Fig. 46.19). The dorsum of

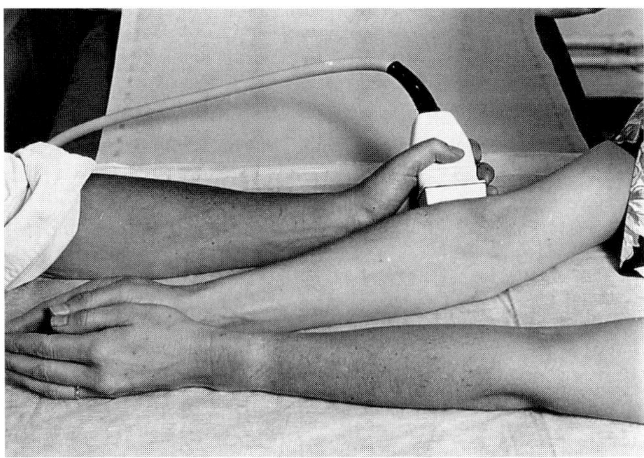

Fig. 46.18 Praying position for examining the lateral epicondyle and common flexor origin.

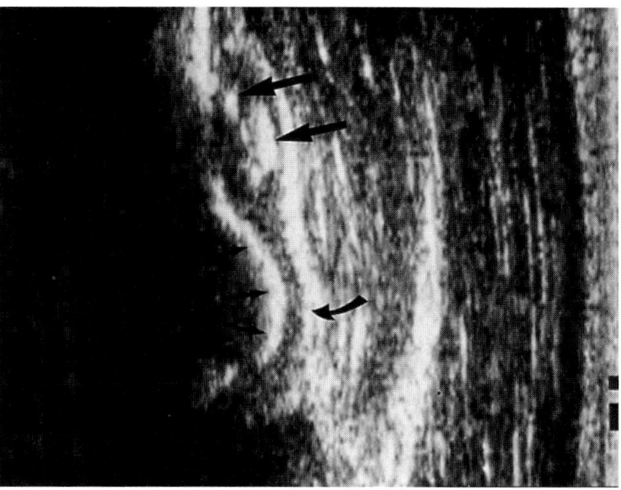

Fig. 46.20 Loose bodies in the olecranon fossa (large arrows), posterior humerus (small arrows) and capsule (curved arrow).

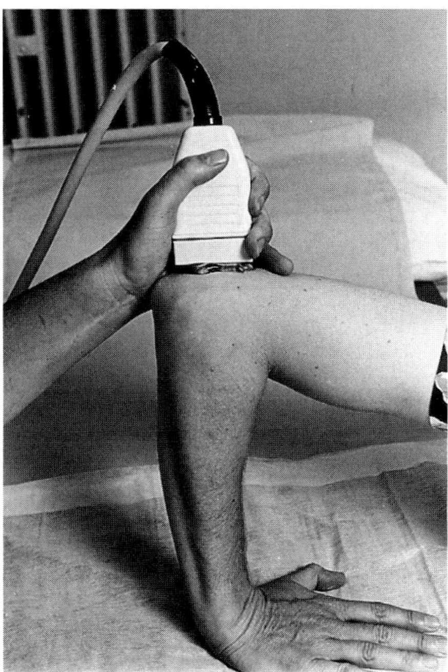

Fig. 46.19 Position for examining triceps tendon and posterior fat pads. If required, a large volume of gel can be used and the probe 'floated' on the surface creating good stand-off.

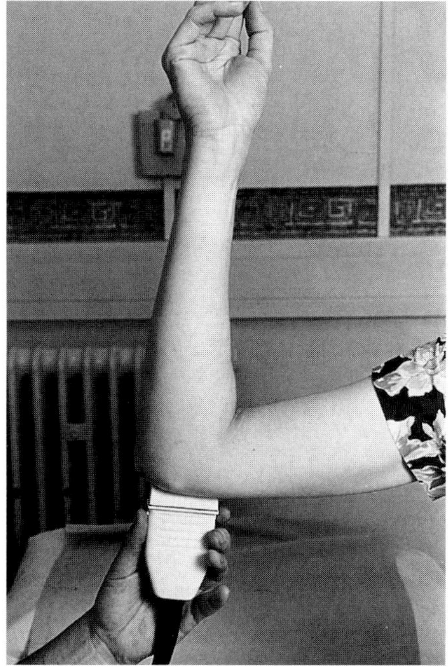

Fig. 46.21 Position for examining for elbow effusion and loose bodies.

the arm is now parallel to the table top which allows the triceps and the posterior joint space to be examined for loose bodies (Fig. 46.20) and displaced fat pads. The probe can be rested on the dorsal aspect of the arm to visualize these structures. One disadvantage of this position with respect to the examination of the posterior joint space is that joint fluid, if present, will gravitate to the anterior compartment away from the probe. To overcome this, the arm can be externally rotated through 180° so that the forearm is now directed towards the ceiling (Fig. 46.21). The posterior joint space can be examined from the underneath and should now be maximally distended. This is a particularly good position to examine for loose bodies.

Ultrasound findings in epicondylitis include enthesopathy, tendinitis or bursitis. The common flexor origin as it arises in the medial epicondyle can be identified as a triangular-shaped structure arising deep to the pronator teres muscle. The medial collateral ligament, injured in throwing sports, can be seen deep to this. The common extensor has a similar bright triangular appearance (Fig. 46.22). Chronic tendinitis, bursitis and tears of the biceps tendon insertion can occur. The obliquity of the tendon as it approaches its insertion makes assessment difficult. Axial views can be helpful. The brachial vessels are a useful marker to assist in locating the biceps tendon. The triceps tendon is less commonly injured. Other potential applications in the elbow include assessment of osteochondral lesions of the capitellum and differentiating stable from unstable fractures of the lateral mass. The precise role in these areas has yet to be defined.

The wrist and hand

Ultrasound of the wrist is indicated for the detection of ganglia and other masses, assessment of tendon disease and nerve entrapment (carpal tunnel and Guyon canal). With modern equipment, stand-off is no longer necessary; stand-off gel blocks and saline bags are difficult to control, but if required, large volumes of coupling gel with the probe 'floating' on the surface improves visualization of superficial structures. Another useful technique is to place the patient's hand in shallow water and 'float' the probe on the surface (Fig. 46.23). It is mandatory to check with the manufacturer before attempting this manoeuvre, but it is possible with the majority or probes.

The median nerve is best found by beginning in the mid forearm with the transducer in the axial plane. The nerve is easily seen between the superficial and deep muscle compartments, where it can be traced to the carpal tunnel (Fig. 46.24). Ultrasound findings in carpal tunnel syndrome include alterations in the calibre of the median nerve (thickened proximal to and flattening within the tunnel) and bowing of the flexor retinaculum [32]. The nerve measures approximately 8 mm within the flexor retinaculum, and is oval in cross-section, normally three times wider than it is thick. Changes occur as a result of the increased pressure within the flexor retinaculum and are therefore present regardless of the underlying cause of the carpal tunnel syndrome [33]. Local causes such as flexor tenosynovitis or a ganglion cyst may be identified.

Ganglia present a variable appearance depending on

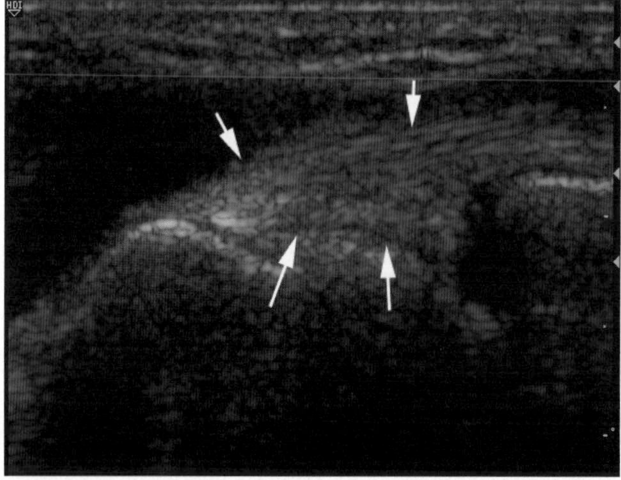

Fig. 46.22 Common extensor origin (lateral) (between arrows).

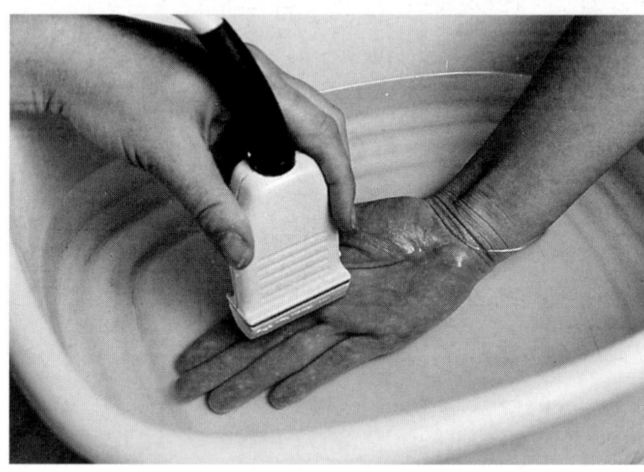

Fig. 46.23 Water bath technique for examining very superficial structures in the hand and wrist.

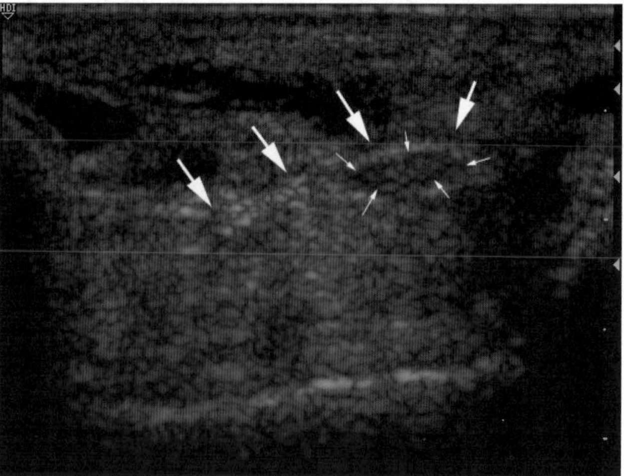

Fig. 46.24 Axial section through the carpal tunnel. Note the median nerve (between small arrows) which is of lower reflectivity than the adjacent tendons and lies deep to the flexor retinaculum (long arrows). The median nerve can also be differentiated from the tendons by asking the patient to move their fingers. The nerve will remain static while the tendons move. Using colour flow will augment this phenomenon.

their age. Newer lesions are thin walled anechoic structures. Older cysts show irregular internal echoes and thicker walls [34]. An origin from an adjacent ligament, most commonly the scapholunate ligament, may be demonstrated (Fig. 46.25). Ganglia are most frequently found on the dorsum of the wrist. Cystic tenosynovitis has a similar appearance but has a more longitudinal appearance, lying along the tendon sheath [34] without a communication to the underlying joint. Occasionally, ganglia need to be differentiated from normal joint recesses. Compression ultrasound will compress a recess while a ganglion remains tense (Fig. 46.26).

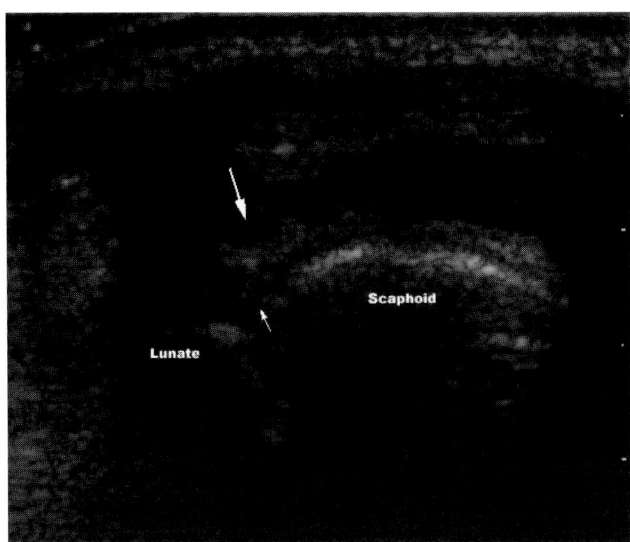

Fig. 46.25 Axial section over the dorsum of the wrist demonstrating a poorly reflective ganglion with a neck (large arrow) extending towards the scapholunate ligament (small arrow).

More distally the flexor tendons can be traced to their insertions. The flexor digitorum superficialis lies anterior to flexor digitorum, encircling it to insert onto the middle phalanx. Tendinitis, tenosynovitis and rupture have the same appearances as elsewhere, As the flexor tendons are contained in a synovial sheath and lie along the concavity of the phalanges, they may appear relatively echo-poor due to the obliquity of the interrogating beam. Occasionally, the sheath that contains the flexor tendon can be disrupted and bow-stringing occurs where there is increased distance between the tendon and the underlying phalanx compared with adjacent uninvolved fingers.

Thickening of the extensor pollicis brevis and the abductor pollicis longus tendons have been described in de Quervain's tenosynovitis [35]. The ultrasound findings in patients with rheumatoid arthritis include hypoechoic thickening of tendon sheaths [8], tenosynovitis, joint effusions, bursitis, erosions and rheumatoid nodules.

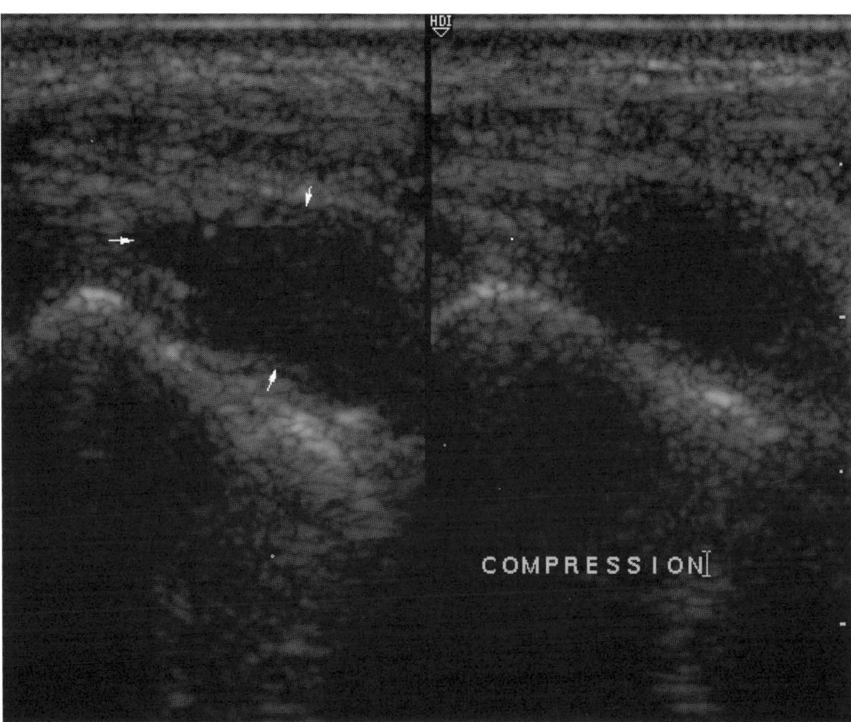

Fig. 46.26 Compression ultrasound of a ganglion (between arrows). The lesion does not alter with compression.

Rheumatoid nodules are generally not associated with posterior acoustic shadowing whereas gouty tophii are [36]. Within the affected tendon sheath, the flexor tendons are generally well defined. Any irregularity of their surface suggests direct tendon involvement by the disease process. Ultrasound can also be used to monitor the effects of treatment [37] and in the postoperative patient when function has not been restored following repair [38].

The lower limb

The hip

DEVELOPMENTAL DYSPLASIA OF THE HIP

Hip instability is common, occurring in approximately 15 in 1000 infants. True dislocation is uncommon, seen in only 1–2 in 1000. A further 1–2 in 1000 will demonstrate acetabular dysplasia. Risk factors for developmental dysplasia of the hip (DDH) include breech presentation, female infants and first born, a family history and some congenital spine, foot and neck anomalies [39]. The prevalence is higher in several American Indian tribes, in regions of Japan and Scandinavia, and much lower in Africa. The left hip is more commonly affected than the right.

Anatomy

The normal cartilagenous femoral head measures 1.2–2.1 cm in diameter in the neonate to 6-month age group [39]. It sits in the acetabulum which comprises a superficial layer of articular cartilage, resting on a band of hyaline cartilage and the bony acetabulum. The acetabulum is deepened by the cartilagenous labrum, which is acoustically reflective [40]. Inferiorly the labrum is completed by the transverse acetabular ligament, which gives rise to the ligamentum teres. This intra-articular structure is not usually identified when the femoral head is ossified, but is readily seen in neonates and infants when it appears as a broad reflective band within the joint [40], inserting into the fovea centralis of the femoral head. The triradiate cartilage is identified as a defect between the ilium and ischium medially. The entire joint is contained within the capsular–ligamentous complex which is reflective. The intracapsular fat pad, called the pulvinar, is also reflective.

In the neonate, the femoral head is composed of cartilage. The ossification centre normally appears between the second and eighth month, earlier in girls. The earliest changes occur as a result of a confluence of epiphyseal vessels, seen as an area of increased reflectivity within the femoral head. Calcification and ossification ultimately limit visualization of the acetabulum by ultrasound. The appearance and development of the ossification centre is often delayed in DDH, although some asymmetry in size may simply reflect normal variation [41].

Ultrasound assessment

Ultrasound affords a considerably better delineation of the relationship between the femoral head, acetabulum and labrum than plain films. Complete assessment involves a static examination of joint morphology, followed by a dynamic assessment of the relationship between the femoral head and acetabulum during posterior and lateral stress.

Static examination

Transducer position. The femoral head has been likened to a ball resting on the spoon of the acetabulum, with the handle of the spoon represented by the reflective lateral border of the ilium. To obtain a coronal image, the transducer position should be adjusted so that the ilium forms a straight line when viewed horizontally and forms a sharp angle as it meets the bony acetabular roof at the promontory. The acetabulum should appear deep, the labrum and the triradiate cartilage clearly visible. Often a small hyper-reflective focus is seen at the junction of the bony roof and the triradiate cartilage on a good coronal section. Slight anterior and posterior movement of the probe will bring the bony pubis and ischium into view respectively. If the plane of scanning is too far anterior or posterior, acetabular depth may be underestimated. Rotating the probe through 90° yields the axial scan plane. On this view, approximately equal portions of the femoral head lie anterior and posterior to the triradiate cartilage; however, displacement of 2–3 mm in an otherwise normal hip [39] is acceptable.

Infant position. The infant can be placed supine or decubitus; the former is often used in conjunction with a sling, the latter with a foam restraint. If the child is particularly distressed, the examination can be carried out with the infant in the arms of a parent.

For screening a large number of infants, a single coronal view of the flexed hip in the lateral decubitus position is efficient. In this position the normal anatomical structures are easily identified, and the relationship of the femoral head to acetabulum reliably assessed (Fig. 46.27). Harcke and Grissom [42] evaluate the hip in a variety of additional positions, beginning with a transverse view with the hip in neutral, moving to transverse with hip flexed, in both abduction and adduction, and ending with a coronal view with the hip in flexion. Using multiple planes may give a better assessment of stability during movement, and allow abnormalities found in one position to be confirmed in another. However the examination is prolonged which is important if a screening programme is being considered. A prolonged examination may also result in the child becoming agitated, thus obscuring subluxation on the stress test due to increased muscle tension.

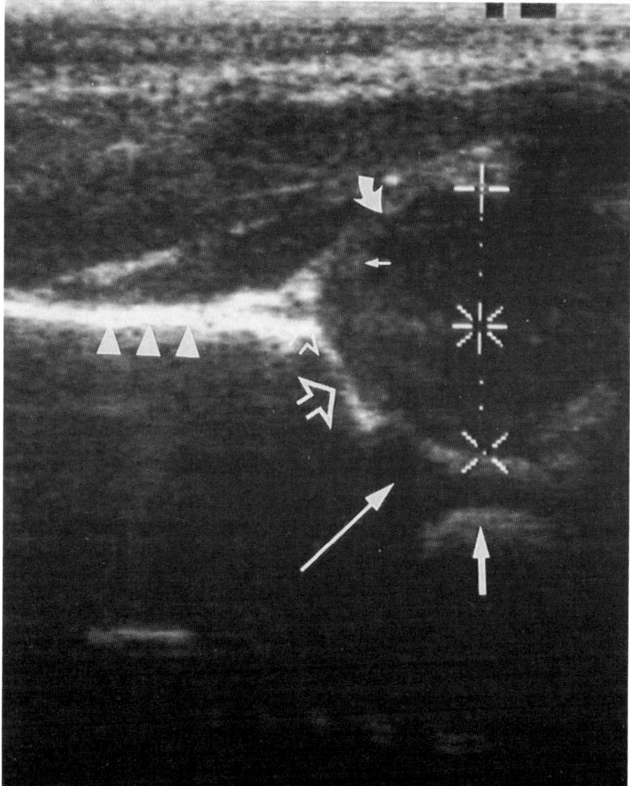

Fig. 46.27 Infant hip. Coronal section with cursors showing diameter of femoral head. Slightly less than 50% of the head is covered classifying it as borderline. The ischium (medium arrow), triradiate cartilage (long arrow), bony acetabular roof (large open arrow), promontory (small open arrow), reflective labrum (small arrow) and reflective capsular complex (curved arrow) are all easily seen. The baseline (arrowheads) is used to calculate the bony and cartilage roof angles. The α angle is formed between the baseline and the bony roof line and the β angle between the baseline and the tip of the labrum.

Schler *et al.* [43] found that the addition of transverse scanning advocated by Harcke did not add any additional diagnostic information.

The European approach, pioneered by Graf recommends a coronal scan plane. The acetabulum is divided into four morphological types (I–IV) based on the relationship of the bony roof line and cartilage roof line to a baseline. The baseline is represented by a line drawn along the horizontal lateral iliac margin (see Fig. 46.27). The bony roof line is from the promontory (small open arrow in Fig. 46.27) to the superolateral margin of the triradiate cartilage. The cartilage roof line is drawn from the promontory to the tip of the labrum. The angle between the baseline and the bony roof line is designated the α or bony angle (normal >60°); the angle between baseline and cartilage roof line is called the β or cartilage angle (normal <77°). Graf's classification is outlined in Table 46.1.

Other authors advocate a subjective assessment of femoral head coverage by the bony and cartilagenous acetabulum. The proportion of femoral head that lies above and below the baseline can be assessed from the static picture, often without the need for actual measurements. This assessment correlates well with the absolute measurements of the acetabular angle [44]. Morin *et al.* [44] determined that the radiographic acetabular angle was always normal in hips where femoral head coverage exceeded 58% and always abnormal when coverage was less than 33%. These measurements are based on plain film correlations and are probably overcautious. It is likely that the majority of hips with more than 40% coverage will develop normally. Certainly over 50% is a safe limit. The major difference between the two systems of classification is that femoral head coverage takes little account of the unossified roof cartilage. A large cartilage anlage may be associated with a normal femoral head coverage but is likely to have a more shallow bony roof angle. Whether this is clinically significant is not certain.

A dislocated femoral head is easily detected in any position. It is usually found lateral, posterior and superior to the acetabulum. The joint capsule may also be thickened and the acetabular cartilage may be displaced superiorly

Table 46.1 Graf classification of acetabular dysplasia

Type	Subtype	Bony angle	Cartilage angle	Notes
I	a	Normal (>60°)	Normal (<77°)	Sharp promontory
	b	Normal (>60°)	Normal (<77°)	Rounded promontory
II	a	Decreased (>50°)	Normal (<77°)	Age under 3 months
	b	Decreased (>50°)	Normal (<77°)	Age over 3 months
	c	Deficient (>43°)	Normal (<77°)	
	d	Deficient (>43°)	Increased (>77°)	
III	a	Poor (<43°)	Increased (>77°)	Normal roof cartilage
	b	Poor (<43°)	Increased (>77°)	Reflective roof cartilage
IV		Poor (<43°)	Increased (>77°)	Dislocated

and stretched with increased reflectivity. Gentle abduction in these infants usually reduces the hip, unless reduction is prevented by an inverted labrum, hypertrophy of the ligamentum teres, intra-articular fat pad, hour-glass deformity or transverse acetabular ligament. Reduction is usually necessary for complete assessment of the acetabulum, which is difficult to see with the head dislocated. Intrauterine dislocation or instability can lead to a notched acetabular promontery. When the hip reduces spontaneously, this may be the only residual sign.

Assessment of stability

Assessing acetabular depth is only part of the examination and is followed by an assessment of femoral head stability during stress. A simple method of stressing the joint is, for the left hip, to place the infant in the right lateral decubitus position. The tip of the probe is gripped between the thumb and index finger of the right hand with the palm and remaining fingers placed against the child's buttock and lower back to provide posterior support. The hip and knee are flexed, and the knee rests in the palm of the left hand with the middle finger extended along the inner left thigh. When a coronal image has been obtained, gentle posterior pressure with the left palm on the knee, followed by abduction pressure on the inside of the left thigh with the examiner's left middle finger, may reveal posterior and lateral motion of the femoral head. The pressure required is minimal and should not upset the infant; indeed a false negative examination may result if the child becomes distressed, as muscular contraction can stabilize an otherwise subluxable femoral head. It is also important to refrain from applying counterpressure with the probe as this too will prevent subluxation.

Smaller degrees of movement are more readily appreciated when successive pressure/relaxation cycles are applied. In many cases increased echogenicity will be noted within the joint during the stress manoeuvre; these are normal and represent the appearance of multiple microbubbles, the ultrasound equivalent of the vacuum phenomenon.

Subluxation in the early postpartum period is physiological and may persist up to 30 days of age. Keller *et al.* [45] measured the degree of subluxation in 40 normal neonates during the first 2 days of life and noted a mean subluxation of 3.2 mm (range 1–6 mm) with greater subluxation on the left. Subluxation beyond the neonatal period is uncommon but to what degree it is important is unclear, and an arbitrary measurement of 2 mm is the upper limit. Additional abnormalities that can be seen in hips with a tendency to sublux are a thickened stretched joint capsule, increased reflectivity of the cartilage anlage and flattening of the posterior bony acetabulum [46].

Ultrasound in the management of DDH

Diminished abduction, poor movement of the affected limb and asymmetric skin creases provide clues, but clinical examination (Ortolani's sign and Barlow's test) will only detect 50% of cases of DDH, an equal number will present as late 'missed' dislocation [47]. All clinically unstable hips are detected by competent ultrasound. Ultrasound also finds many more 'abnormalities', particularly acetabular dysplasia, in clinically normal babies; it has been assumed that, within this group, are the hips that, had they not been detected by ultrasound, would have progressed to late dislocation. A controlled trial comparing treatment with non-treatment in this group has yet to be performed. Ultrasound findings include abnormal morphology and occult instability. The question as to which of these, if either, is the more important remains unresolved, despite a vast literature.

The natural history of ultrasound-detected abnormalities in clinically stable hips has been assessed in a number of studies albeit with relatively small numbers. Gardiner and Dunn [48] found 15 morphologically abnormal hips (Graf grade IIc or worse) in 158 clinically normal high risk babies. None were treated and all were normal at 6 months. Rosendahl *et al.* [49] did not treat 50% of a group of babies with abnormal morphology and, again, all developed normally. However, Castelein *et al.* [50] evaluated a group of 101 babies who were clinically normal but had abnormal morphology on ultrasound. None were treated and four were described as having dysplasia at 6 months. The severity of dysplasia at birth did not correlate with outcome [50]. In Gardiner and Dunn's group, there were also three morphologically normal hips that demonstrated instability on ultrasound. On follow-up, one of these became morphologically abnormal and was treated.

It is important to understand the natural history of occult hip dysplasia and instability, and in particular the tendency for 'abnormalities' to resolve spontaneously, if a screening programme is to be considered. An ultrasound examination detects many more abnormalities than clinical examination and advocates of neonatal hip screening claim that if all babies are examined close to birth, late DDH is eradicated. Conversely, only a relatively small proportion of babies with detectable abnormalities will require treatment [48], generally some form of harness, for which there is a small but definite association with avascular necrosis. In some centres the percentage of screened babies who are treated is high, thus increasing the risk of iatrogenic avascular necrosis and potentially causing more long-term disability than the underlying problem of DDH. Conversely, ultrasound can reduce unnecessary treatment in other areas. Berman and Klenerman [51] showed that the demonstration of a normal acetabulum on ultrasound meant that 14 of 17 infants with clinical instability were not treated and developed normally.

The cost of screening all infants is high. In addition to preliminary examinations, even in experienced hands, repeat scan rates of up to 10–40% can place a considerable burden on health resources. Despite this, the cost may be less than the cost of treating missed DDH. One of the main difficulties is that controlled trials of treatment versus non-treatment are lacking, and until they are available controversy is likely to remain.

One approach that has been suggested is to recommend ultrasound on a subpopulation of babies with a known risk factor for DDH. Risk factors include a first-degree family history of DDH, breech presentation at birth, an abnormality (click or clunk) found on physical examination or an associated congenital anomaly (spinal, foot anomaly or torticollis). While this has been the policy adopted in many centres, it is likely that this more limited approach will not detect all cases of acetabular dysplasia, as not all infants with the disorder have one of the commonly recognized risk factors.

The higher prevalence of both abnormal morphology and ultrasound instability at birth suggests that if screening is to be performed, then it is best done when the infant is at least 4 weeks of age. After this age, physiological subluxation is uncommon and the number of ultrasonographically immature hips will be reduced. Abnormalities present at this stage are often treated as many orthopaedic surgeons feel that the earlier that treatment is instituted, the better the outcome. Better results may, however, simply reflect the inclusion of large numbers of babies who would have resolved spontaneously without any form of treatment.

Treatment

The hip that is dysplastic, and clinically and sonographically unstable, is generally treated. Morphologically 'abnormal' hips are more prevalent at birth, seen in about 10% of infants falling to about 5% over 2 weeks [48]. Several different types of splints are in use including Pavlik, Von Rosen, modified Denis Browne and the Frejka pillow. The last has been associated with a particularly high rate of avascular necrosis [52]. It is generally recommended that treatment with a harness has failed if the hip has not reduced within 3 weeks of treatment. A high risk of failure is present in hips that do not reduce at first assessment and bilateral dislocation in infants over 7 weeks of age at the onset of treatment [53]. This group often fail with other methods of closed reduction.

Ultrasound can be used to assess reduction and stability within the harness, and can be used to confirm normality at the end of the treatment period. Harnessing appears to be effective in the management of the subluxed, but not dislocated hip, which requires more effective splinting. Regular monitoring of stability using ultrasound is recommended, particularly in the older age groups and in those with higher grades of dislocation. The incidence of avascular necrosis depends on the degree of dislocation at diagnosis, ranging from 1% for minor, to nearer 15% for severe dislocation.

Ultrasound can also be used to assess reduction following open or closed reduction and spica casting. A window is cut medial or lateral to the affected hip. Windows are immediately repaired following the ultrasound examination. To allay concerns over cast stability caused by cutting a window, computed tomography (CT), or preferably MRI, are now used to assess reduction following casting.

PAINFUL HIP IN OLDER CHILDREN

Painful hip is one of the commonest causes of non-traumatic, acute paediatric presentations in orthopaedic practice and ultrasound plays a pivotal role in its assessment. In the majority of cases the underlying cause is benign, usually transient synovitis, a disorder that is still incompletely understood but with self-limiting and short-lived symptoms. The majority of children will settle within 5 days without specific treatment.

INVESTIGATION OF IRRITABLE HIP

Plain films are of no value in the assessment of effusion and ultrasound should be the primary investigation. Local anaesthetic cream is applied to the skin anterior to the affected hip as soon as the patient presents to hospital. The optimal time for examination depends on the anaesthetic preparation used, but is between 30 min and 1.5–2 h later. The hip is examined with the child supine using an anterior approach. A high frequency linear array transducer is optimal and the probe is aligned along the femoral neck by rotating it approximately 45° from sagittal. Easily identified landmarks include the femoral capital epiphysis, the physis itself and the femoral neck. More anteriorly echo-poor cartilage is identified overlying the femoral head. More superficially still, a reflective band representing the anterior capsule is identified and can be traced inferiorly to its insertion on the femoral neck. The capsule is displaced anteriorly in the effused hip (Fig. 46.28). The degree of displacement is measured by the maximum distance between the anterior capsule and femoral neck. The thickness of articular cartilage overlying the femoral head can also be measured at this time.

There is varied opinion as to what constitutes a normal anterior joint space [54]. Adam *et al.* [55] suggests 2 mm as

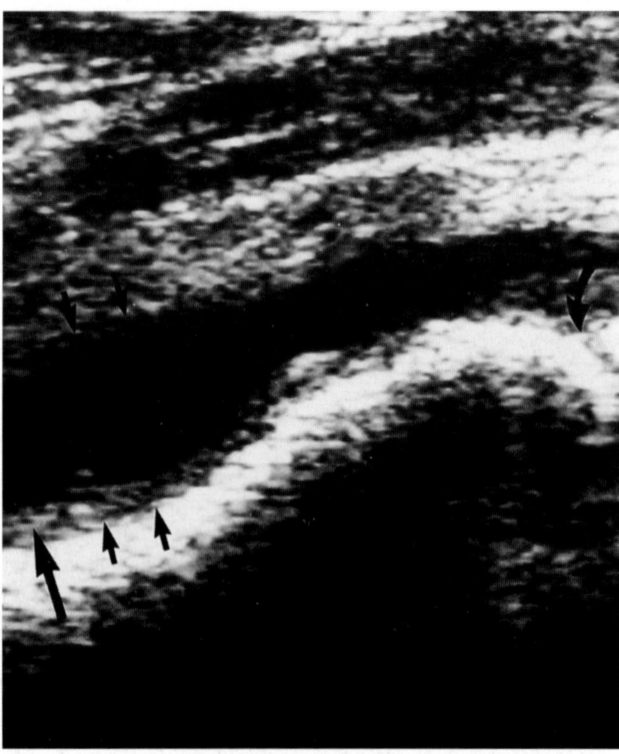

Fig. 46.28 Effused hip. The anterior joint space is increased (small arrows). Minimal synovial thickening is present (large arrow). The physis is a useful landmark (curved arrow).

the upper limit of normal. Alexander *et al.* [56] defines less than 2.3 mm as normal, but notes that greater distances may be normal if symmetrical. Asymmetry is the most useful sign and a greater than 2 mm difference between sides should be regarded as abnormal. The size of an effusion does not determine its nature, though the largest effusions are often seen in association with benign transient synovitis [56].

There are several pitfalls for the unwary. The iliopsoas muscle, which overlies the anterior capsule, is relatively echo-poor and can masquerade as an effusion particularly if examined obliquely, resulting in anisotropy. A true effusion has a convex upper border rather than flat as is the iliopsoas. The undistended capsule is concave. Compression of the anterior synovial space occurs with the hip in the external rotation, and the space may also decompress if the femoral head subluxes as a consequence of the effusion. The subluxed hip can be identified by an increased distance between the acetabular rim and the physis.

If an effusion is present, in the author's centre, aspiration using a 21-gauge needle is carried out. An anterior approach is recommended. The probe is placed vertically over the most distended part of the capsule. As the needle is to be inserted at right angles to the skin, the probe must be held vertically over the point of maximum distension. The mid points of the ends and sides of the probe are then marked on the skin, and the probe removed (Fig. 46.29). The skin is punctured at the centre of the four marked points and the needle advanced slowly in a single motion. Gentle traction is applied on the syringe plunger as soon

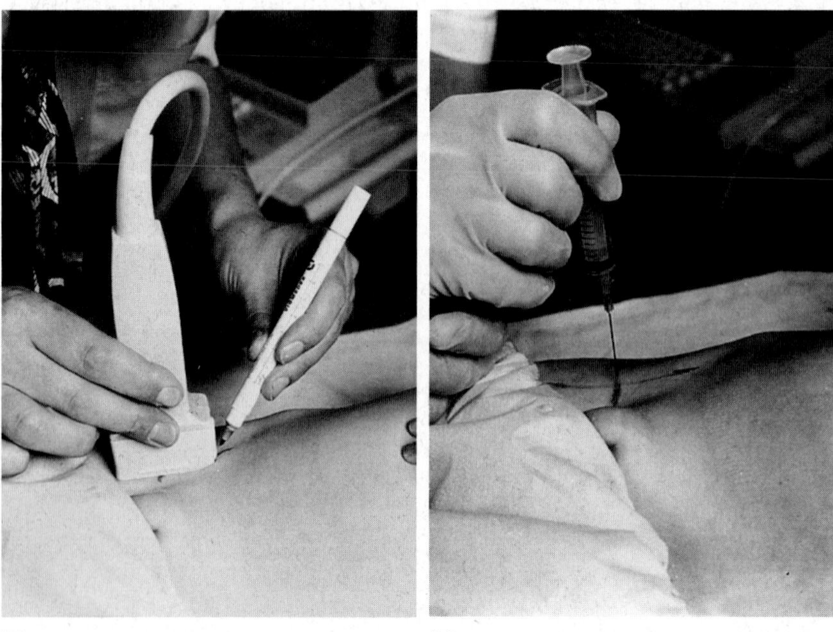

(a) (b)

Fig. 46.29 Hip aspiration technique. (a) The transducer is vertically over the point of maximal capsular distension and the mid points marked. (b) A vertical puncture without screening is used.

as the skin is breached. Scanning during needle insertion and advancement is not necessary. Aspiration should be as complete as possible, as this may result in more rapid resolution of symptoms and a shorter hospital stay [57]. There is good correlation between the size of the effusion [58], pain intensity, restriction of movement [59] and intra-articular pressure.

TRANSIENT SYNOVITIS

The diagnosis of transient synovitis is only suggested when other conditions are excluded and signs and symptoms subside without complications. Children present with a 1–7-day history of pain and limitation of movement. The incidence is approximately 0.2% and up to 25% will have recurrent episodes [56]. A seasonal variation has been reported, with more cases occurring when respiratory tract infection is common [56], though this has not been the experience at the author's unit. Approximately 75% have an effusion, and the condition is more common in boys, with a ratio to girls of 2.5 to 1. There is no site predisposition. Resolution occurs in 75% within 2 weeks [56]. Persisting effusion is suggestive of another cause, and Perthes' disease should then be considered.

SEPTIC ARTHRITIS

Because of the devastating consequence of bacterial infection within the joint, early diagnosis is mandatory. Typically the effusion is reflective [60] with synovial thickening. Thickening of the anterior capsule is seen in about 50% [61] but this sign also occurs in transient synovitis [62]. While the majority of effusions in septic arthritis are reflective [60], some are echo-free [63]. As there are no absolute differences between the clinical presentation or sonographic appearance of a septic effusion and transient synovitis, aspiration is recommended in all cases. Indeed if septic arthritis is strongly suspected clinically, aspiration should be performed if no effusion is demonstrated. Particulate matter in the absence of blood is usually associated with sepsis.

PERTHES' DISEASE

The ultrasound findings in Perthes' disease include effusion, thickening of femoral head articular cartilage, fragmentation of the epiphysis and increased femoral anteversion [64] (Fig. 46.30). A difference in thickness of greater than 3 mm in the articular cartilage between sides is significant. Cartilage overlying the femoral head only should be included, and it is therefore easier to measure cartilage anteriorly where the femoral head is not covered by acetabulum. The absence of cartilage asymmetry does not exclude the condition, as the disease may be bilateral. An effusion is more common in the early stages of the disease [65].

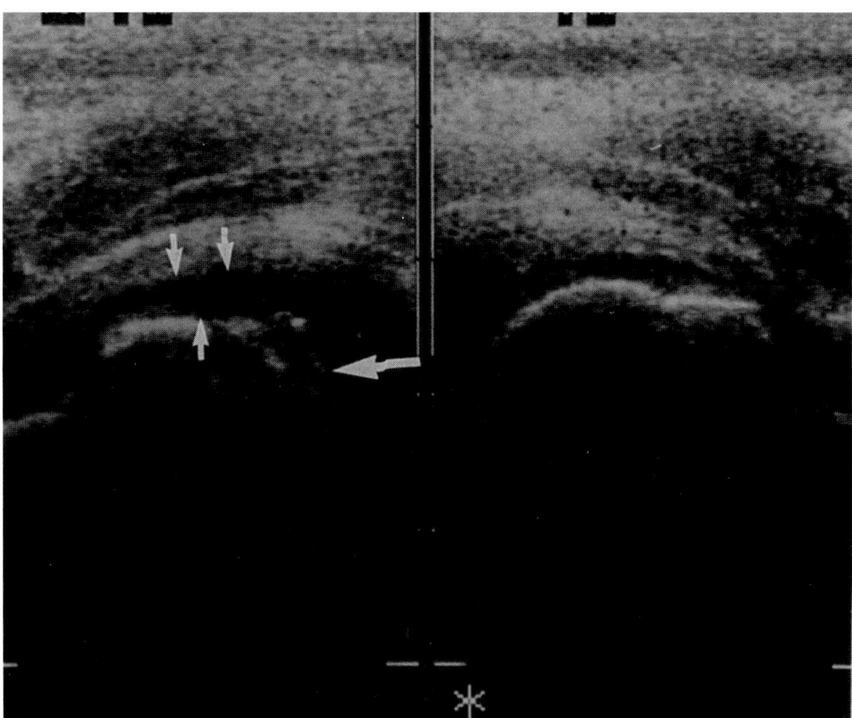

Fig. 46.30 Perthes' disease. Note the fragmented epiphysis (large arrow) and thickened cartilage (small arrows) compared to the contralateral normal side.

Meyer's dysplasia is a condition of unknown aetiology which is associated with irregularity of the femoral head. The process is benign, bilateral and symmetrical and the hip always develops normally. It is not associated with effusion.

SLIPPED CAPITAL FEMORAL EPIPHYSIS

Children with slipped capital femoral epiphysis (SCFE) are older than patients with transient synovitis or Perthes' disease; the mean age from several series is 11 years, whereas the mean age in transient synovitis and Perthes' disease is 6.7 years [58]. The ultrasound signs of SCFE include a step in the anterior physeal outline and diminished distance between the anterior acetabular rim and the femoral metaphysis [66]. An effusion is seen in about half of cases and is more likely when the onset is acute. The anteroposterior film fails to show displacement in 14% of cases [66], a frog-leg view is necessary to detect these. Ultrasound provides an accurate measurement of the physeal step and the degree of metaphyseal shortening in the acute slip, without the need for ionizing radiation [66]. In chronic SCFE measurements of the physeal step are unreliable due to metaphyseal remodelling [66].

The place of MRI in SCFE remains to be established. A T_1-weighted image orientated along the femoral neck provides an elegant view of the displacement and the quantity of new bone formation at the site of periosteal stripping. In clear-cut cases MRI probably does not add significantly to the diagnosis but where there is diagnostic difficulty it may have a role.

MISCELLANEOUS

Ultrasound can also be used to assess traumatic separation of the proximal, femoral and humeral epiphysis due to birth injury [67]. Sonography has also been used in the assessment of juvenile chronic arthritis [59], particularly in the assessment of the severity of the synovitis prior to synovectomy.

IMAGING PROTOCOL IN CHILDREN WITH IRRITABLE HIP

Plain films are poor at detecting effusions and in children under the age of 8 years there is general agreement that ultrasound should be used as the screening method. Over the age of 8 radiography should also be employed to detect SCFE. Some centres limit this to a frog-leg view only, which is also sufficient to detect the majority of significant pathologies including Perthes' disease.

If no effusion is demonstrated on ultrasound, consideration should be given to other potential causes of pain referred to the hip, such a discitis or other spinal disorders. Clinical hip irritability strongly suggests disease within the hip itself and if symptoms fail to resolve MRI is indicated.

There is disagreement as to the correct management of children with effusions, with some workers supporting a conservative, observational approach and others recommending aspiration in all cases. Transient synovitis and septic arthritis present similar clinical features and the ultrasound appearance of the effusion does not reliably distinguish between them. A pyrexia and leucocytosis is inconstant. Klein *et al.* [68] in a small series of 21 patients found the erythrocyte sedimentation rate (ESR) elevated to greater than 20 in 95%. Others have found the ESR less reliable. Septic arthritis is rare accounting for less than 5% of patients presenting with an irritable hip, but consequences of misdiagnosis of septic arthritis are devastating and irreversible damage can occur in a matter of days. Hip aspiration appears to be a benign procedure with no reported cases of iatrogenic sepsis and is regarded by many as little more invasive than obtaining a blood sample.

If symptoms settle, and do not recur, then no further imaging is necessary. Patients who fail to settle with symptoms persisting for more than 10 days should be more intensively investigated to exclude Perthes' disease [63] or the uncommon association of osteomyelitis with a sterile effusion.

ULTRASOUND OF THE ADULT HIP

Ultrasound can be helpful in the patient with a total hip replacement to detect complications. In the immediate postoperative period, disruption of the normal tissue planes can create diagnostic difficulties. Poorly reflective areas can represent haematomas or sepsis [69] which can be differentiated by ultrasound-guided biopsy. Biopsy/aspiration should be limited to patients in whom there is a strong clinical suspicion of sepsis as needling of haematomas is imprudent and may itself induce infection. In the late postoperative period, ultrasound can be used to detect effusions and guide biopsies of the pseudocapsule when infection is suspected. Not all effusions signify loosening or infection; some resolve with conservative treatment [69]. Ultrasound is also useful in demonstrating trochanteric and iliopsoas bursitis [70]. The latter can occasionally extend superiorly into the pelvis and retroperitoneum. In the absence of infection, a guided steroid injection may provide relief. Ultrasound to detect the associated effusion has been suggested as a screening test for intra-articular femoral neck fracture when radiographs are negative. Not all fractures are associated with effusion however.

The knee

Ultrasound is used to examine the extensor mechanism, collateral ligaments and periarticular cysts (popliteal and meniscal). It was previously used to evaluate the anterior cruciate and menisci, a task now performed by MRI.

LIGAMENTS AND TENDONS

The extensor mechanism, comprising the patella, patellar and quadriceps tendons, are particularly suitable to ultrasound examination. The origin of the patella tendon, from the base of the patella, shows some variation in shape. It is conical in active athletes and ribbon-like in sedentary individuals [71]. In transverse section, the patella tendon appears oval, measuring 3–6 mm in anteroposterior and 20 mm in lateral diameter.

A variety of pathological conditions can be demonstrated. Patellar tendinitis can be either diffuse, with an enlarged diffusely hypoechoic tendon [71], or focal. Focal tendinitis usually occurs near the upper insertion where it is known as 'jumper's knee', as it is particularly common in basketball, volleyball and soccer. The lesion, which is caused by repetitive microrupture, appears as a cone-shaped poorly reflective area, exceeding 0.5 cm in length, at the centre of the patella tendon [72]. Occasionally small sonolucent areas, of less than 3 mm in length in the centre of the tendon close to the apex of the patella, may be seen in normal knees. To be considered significant sonolucent lesions must measure more than 0.5 cm. Jumper's knee has to be distinguished from Sinding–Larsen–Johansson disease which is an osteochondrosis of the patella. In this entity the lower pole of the patella is fragmented. The equivalent, and more common, condition at the tibial insertion of the patellar tendon is Osgood–Schlatter disease which has similar ultrasound findings. These entities are diagnosed clinically but ultrasound can be useful in confirming atypical cases and by demonstrating associated infrapatellar bursitis. De Flaviis *et al.* [73] divides the appearances at the tibial tuberosity into four types depending on the appearances of both patellar tendon and ossification centre.

The cruciate ligaments can be demonstrated, but ultrasound has taken a subsidiary role to MRI. The posterior cruciate is more readily identified and can be seen via a posterior approach as a low reflective inserting at a point where the posterior tibial margin assumes a more sloped rather than flattened shape. The collateral ligaments are well seen (Fig. 46.31).

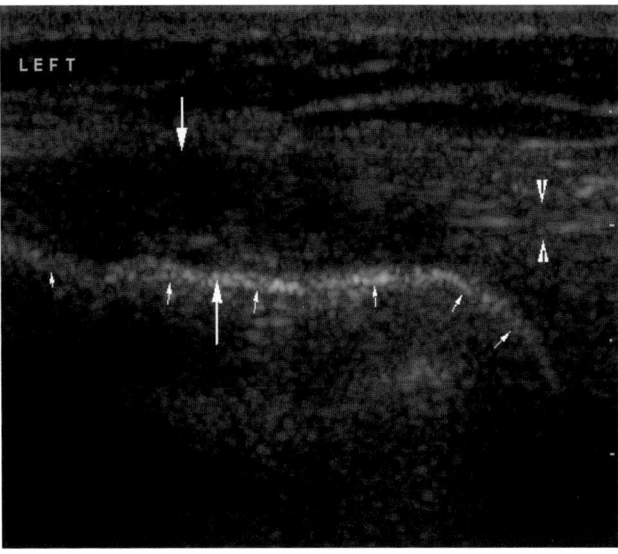

Fig. 46.31 Chronic tear to the medial collateral ligament. The ligament is swollen (large arrows) and has lost the normal reflectivity (arrowheads). Small arrows delineate the medial femoral condyle.

ARTICULAR CARTILAGE

The articular cartilage of the weight-bearing surface of the femoral condyle and intercondylar notch can be evaluated in the flexed knee. Unfortunately, patients with arthritis, in whom it is most desirable to examine articular cartilage, often find full flexion difficult and therefore portions of the weight-bearing surface may be obscured. When it is visualized, articular cartilage is seen as an echo-poor band with anterior and posterior reflective margins. The cartilage–bone interface appears more reflective than the superficial synovial space–cartilage interface. Normal weight-bearing cartilage is 1.2–1.9 mm thick, slightly less over the medial femoral condyle [74]. Clarity and sharpness of cartilage correlate better with clinical status than absolute thickness measurements due to the wide range of normal. The patellar articular surface cannot be evaluated.

Ultrasound can differentiate effusion from synovitis and guide biopsy. The suprapatellar pouch is particularly accessible in this regard and it is also possible to identify synovial plica in this area [75]. The response of thickened synovium to therapy can be followed [76].

POPLITEAL CYSTS

Synovial extensions, including popliteal cysts, can be differentiated from popliteal artery aneurysms and tumours of the popliteal fossa. A popliteal cyst typically communicates with the knee joint via a small neck between the medial head of gastrocnemius and the semi-membranosis tendon. When this neck is identified, a confident diagnosis can be made. Rupture of a popliteal cyst can mimic a deep venous thrombosis, and ultrasound can be useful in distinguishing these entities. Not all echo-poor structures posterior to the knee joint are popliteal cysts. It is usually easy to distinguish popliteal artery aneurysm; however, some poorly reflective tumours, in particular neurogenic tumours, can cause confusion.

THE MENISCII

The normal meniscus appears as an homogeneous reflective triangular structure. The posterior horn is more readily seen than the body or anterior horn. The lateral meniscus is particularly difficult to visualize [77]. In *in vitro* studies in cadaveric knees, Richardson *et al.* [78] was able to demonstrate tears as small as 2 mm if they were vertically oriented, and 4–5 mm if they were horizontal or radial. Improvement in equipment now means that even smaller lesions can be detected. Associated meniscal cysts have similar appearances to ganglia and can appear either of increased or decreased reflectivity. It is doubtful that ultrasound will replace MRI in the assessment of internal derangement due to the ability of MRI which can more reliably assess the cruciate ligaments and the inability of ultrasound to detect trabecular microfracture.

The ankle and foot

ACHILLES TENDON

The normal Achilles tendon measures 5 mm thick and 13 mm wide in adults and comprises six to eight hyperechoic bands representing the connective tissue between the tendon fascicles [79]. It has a well-defined reflective margin with fine parallel internal echoes. The diagnosis of acute complete rupture is usually made clinically. Complete tears are seen as discontinuity of this normal pattern, with intervening haematoma or, in the case of chronic healed tears, reflective fibrous scar tissue. Chronic tears may be overlooked clinically because intervening scar tissue may fill the normally palpable defect and collateral muscles may give a false negative Thompson's test [80] (a positive test occurs when the foot fails to plantar flex on squeezing the calf). Ultrasound is useful to assess the position of the tear and estimate the size of the gap. The majority of tears occur within the tendon itself between 4 and 6 cm above its insertion. The second commonest location is at the musculotendinous junction. Ultrasound is useful in identifying these tears which are not amenable to surgical repair. Partial tears may show as areas of localized thinning, contour abnormalities, irregular acoustic shadowing, peritendinous fluid and thickening of the severed ends of the tendon [79].

Tendinitis is seen as a focal hypoechoic enlargement of the tendon. Fluid, haematoma or oedema may be identified in the paratenon, in the pretendinous bursa or surrounding soft tissue. Chronic tendinitis is seen as a diffuse heterogeneous, but predominantly echo-poor swollen tendon, usually involving the medial portion of the tendon and occasionally with calcification. The proximal and middle thirds are more frequently involved than the distal third. A normal sonogram in a symptomatic patient with a short duration of history will reliably predict a successful response to conservative treatment [79].

LATERAL LIGAMENTS

The lateral ligament complex of the hindfoot comprises three ligaments. The weakest, and the first to tear during inversion injury, is the anterior talofibular ligament. Disruption of this ligament does not appear to render the ankle unstable. The most important ligament in this regard is the calcaneofibular ligament. With the hindfoot plantar flexed, this ligament runs in the horizontal plane and can be identified as a linear high signal structure deep to the peroneal tendons. The posterior talofibular ligament comprises multiple fascicles. It is much stronger than the other two components and rarely tears.

HINDFOOT TENDONS

The three medial tendons are the tibialis posterior, the flexor digitorum and the flexor hallucis tendons. Complete tears of the first of these are relatively common in middle-aged women and are a common cause of peroneal flat foot. Tibialis posterior is located by placing the probe on the medial malleolus and gently moving it posteriorly until the tendon is encountered. Care should be taken not to confuse it with flexor digitorum which lies on its posterior surface. The posterior tibial vessels lie posterior to the flexor digitorum tendon and provide a useful landmark. Reflectivity within all three tendons will change as they round the medial malleolus due to anisotropy. Reorientation of the probe into the horizontal plane will restore reflectivity in the normal tendon. At this point, a search can be made for ganglion cysts, anomalous muscles and vascular anomalies in the region of the tarsal tunnel, which can all present with posterior tibial nerve entrapment (tarsal tunnel syndrome). On the lateral side, peroneus brevis lies anterior to the peroneus longus tendon. Chronic trauma can result in splitting or rupture, more usually of the peroneus brevis, or anterior dislocation of the tendons around the lateral malleolus.

The plantar fascia is divided into two bundles and the more medial of these is more commonly involved with plantar fasciitis. When affected, the fascial bundle appears

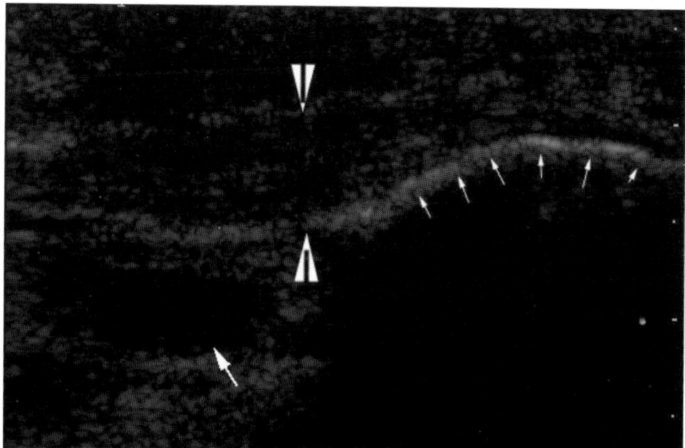

Fig. 46.32 Swollen plantar fascia (arrowheads) with surrounding fluid (large arrow). The small arrows outline the os calcis.

swollen, heterogeneous and of reduced reflectivity (Fig. 46.32). Largely a clinical diagnosis, ultrasound has a confirmatory role and can assist with guided injections.

THE MID AND FOREFOOT

Common mid and forefoot masses include plantar fibroma, hamartoma, lipoma, ganglia and Morton's neuroma. The former are to be distinguished from the rarer and more sinister infantile and juvenile fibromatosis which are more often associated with lesions on the palm of the hand. Hamartomas more commonly occur on the dorsum of the foot, though they have little regard for tissue planes. Morton's neuromas are perineural fibrosis of interdigital nerves and are often associated with bursitis in the adjacent intermetatarsal space. They are best examined from below with counterpressure from the examiner's finger pressing from above in the intermetatarsal space. They appear as poorly defined areas of low reflectivity. Pressure often elicits a typical sensation that is referred into the toes.

Ultrasound in limb lengthening

The technique of lengthening bone by distraction osteotomy, pioneered by Illizarov in Russia, is now used extensively worldwide. An external fixation device is placed above and below the site to be lengthened and the bone incised. After a postoperative period of 5–14 days the osteotomy is slowly distracted at a rate of approximately 1 mm per day. The distraction continues until the desired length is reached and the bone gap allowed to heal. If the rate of distraction is too rapid, bone cysts form within the distraction site (Fig. 46.33). These are mechanically weak and impair healing. If the distraction rate is too slow a callus bridge may form, preventing further distraction.

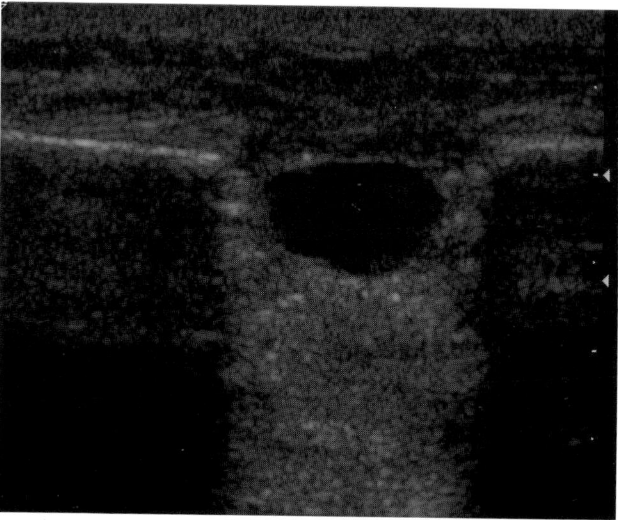

Fig. 46.33 Fluid-filled cyst within an osteotomy gap during limb lengthening.

The gap created by the distraction can be measured on both plain films and ultrasound. Plain radiography visualizes the bone ends (the bone gap). Healing of the fracture site results in the formation of mature callus at the separated bone ends which is not visible on plain radiography. Ultrasound visualizes the gap between the mature callus (ultrasound gap) (Fig. 46.34). These are not the same except in the early phase of treatment. The difference between the bone gap and ultrasound gap defines the amount of mature callus that has formed.

During the first 7–10 days, no identifiable callus forms, and the bone gap is equal to the ultrasound gap. This phase is called the lag period. A number of patients have a prolonged lag period lasting up to 25 days. After the lag period, the rate of callus formation shows one of three patterns.

1 Callus formation increases in proportion to the bone gap. This is the optimal situation with good rates of healing and fewer complications.

2 Rate of callus formation slower than rate of bony distraction. This implies an impaired rate of healing. If this is not recognized early, bone cysts and other complications, including fracture and angulation may occur.

3 The rate of callus formation is faster than the rate of distraction. Increased healing may bridge the bone gap, and prevent further distraction. Increasing the distraction rate is not always an option, as the rate is limited by the ability of surrounding soft tissues to be lengthened. These patients can be difficult to manage.

Ultrasound can also be used to assess the quality and quantity of callus formed in the gap. Ideally this should be a uniform parallel lamellar pattern without echo-poor areas. Young *et al.* [81] aspirated echo-poor areas within

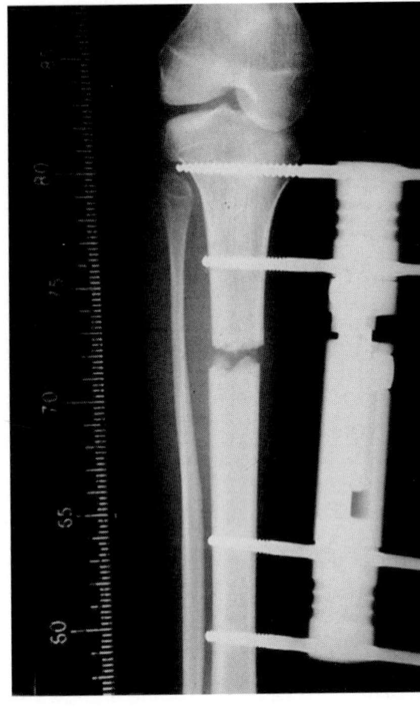

(a)

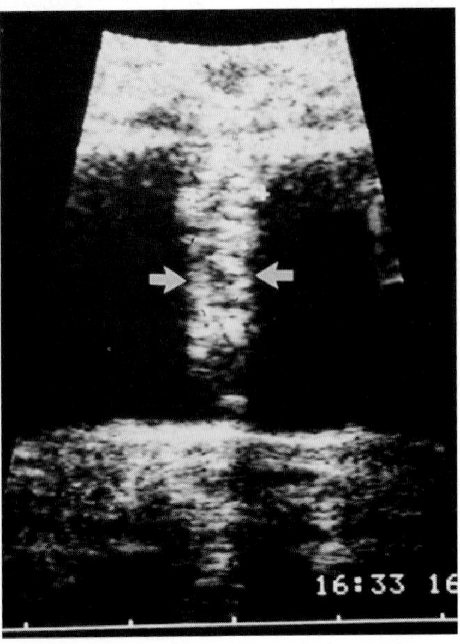

(b)

Fig. 46.34 (a) Osteotomy with distraction apparatus. The scale on the left is used to measure the bone gap. (b) The ultrasound gap is measured on a longitudinal image (arrows).

the bone gap and found them to be fluid-filled cysts. Cyst formation can be reversed by stopping or reversing distraction [82].

Ultrasound in orthopaedic measurement

Ultrasound has been used for a variety of orthopaedic measurements including femoral anteversion, femoral torsion and limb length discrepancies. A detailed description of the methodology is well described in the literature and is beyond the scope of this chapter [83].

References

1 Fornage, B.D., Touche, H., Raguetem, *et al.* (1982) Accidents musculares du sportif. Apport originale di l'ultrasonographie. *Nouvelle Presse Medicin* **11**, 571.

2 Corlho, J.C.U., Sigel, B., Ryva, J.C., *et al.* (1982) B-mode sonography of blood clots. *Journal of Clinical Ultrasound* **10**, 323–327.

3 Fornage, B.D., Touch, D.H., Segal, P., Rifkin, M.D. (1983) Ultrasonography in the evaluation of muscular trauma. *Journal of Ultrasound Medicine* **2**, 549–554.

4 Fornage, B.D., Eftekhari, F. (1989) Sonographic diagnosis of myositis ossificans. *Journal of Ultrasound Medicine* **8**, 463–466.

5 Dillehay, G.L., Deschler, T., Rogers, L.F., *et al.* (1984) The ultrasonographic characterization of tendons. *Investigative Radiology* **19**, 338–341.

6 Fornage, B.D. (1987) The hypoechoic normal tendon. *Journal of Ultrasound Medicine* **6**, 19–22.

7 Fornage, B.D., Rifkin, M.D. (1988) Ultrasound examination of tendons. *Radiology Clinics of North America* **26**, 87–107.

8 Fornage, B.D. (1989) Soft-tissue changes in the hand in rheumatoid arthritis: evaluation with ultrasound. *Radiology* **173**, 735–737.

9 Jeffrey, R.B., Laing, F.C., Schechter, W.P., Markison, R.E., Barton, R.M. (1987) Acute suppurative tenosynovitis of the hand: diagnosis with ultrasound. *Radiology* **162**, 741–742.

10 Kanavel, A.B. (1943) *Infections of the Hand*. Lea and Febiger, Philadelphia, pp. 241–242.

11 Little, C.M., Parker, M.G., Callowich, M.C., Sartori, J.C. (1986) The ultrasonic detection of soft tissue foreign bodies. *Investigative Radiology* **21**, 275–277.

12 Fornage, B.D., Sehernberg, F.L. (1986) Sonographic diagnosis of foreign bodies of the distal extremities. *American Journal of Roentgenology* **147**, 567–569.

13 Fornage, B.D., Tassin, G.B. (1991) Sonographic appearances of superficial soft tissue lipomas. *Journal of Clinical Ultrasound* **19**, 215–220.

14 Rubenstein, W.A., Gray, G., Auh, Y.H., *et al.* (1986) CT of fibrous tissues and tumors with sonographic correlation. *American Journal of Roentgenology* **147**, 1067–1074.

15 Hughes, D.G., Wilson, D.J. (1986) Ultrasound appearances of peripheal nerve tumours. *British Journal of Radiology* **59**, 1041–1043.

16 van Sonnenburg, E., Wittich, G.R., Casola, G., Cabrera, O.A., Gosink, B.B., Resnick, D.L. (1987) Sonography of thigh abscess: detection, diagnosis, and drainage. *American Journal of Roentgenology* **149**, 769–772.

17 Malghem, J., Vande Berg, B., Noel, H., Maldague, B. (1992) Benign osteochondromas and exostotic chondrosarcomas:

evaluation of cartilage cap thickness by ultrasound. *Skeletal Radiology* **21**, 33–37.

18 Choi, H., Varma, D.G.K., Fornage, B.D., Kim, E.E., Johnston, D.A. (1991) Soft-tissue sarcoma: MR imaging vs sonography for detection of local recurrence after surgery. *American Journal of Roentgenology* **157**, 353–358.

19 Crass, J.R., Craig, E.V., Feinberg, S.B. (1987) The hyperextended internal rotation view in rotator cuff sonography. *Journal of Clinical Ultrasound* **15**, 416–420.

20 Bretzke, C.A., Crass, J.R., Craig, E.V., Feinberg, S.B. (1985) Ultrasonography of the rotatory cuff. Normal and pathologic anatomy. *Investigative Radiology* **20**, 311–315.

21 Van Holsbeek, M.T., Kolowich, P.A., Eyler, W.R., *et al.* (1995) US depiction of partial-thickness tear of the rotator cuff. *Radiology* **197**, 443–446.

22 Nelson, M.C., Leather, G.P., Nirschl, R.P., Pettrone, F.A., Freedman, M.T. (1991) Evaluation of the painful shoulder. *Journal of Bone and Joint Surgery* **73A**, 707–715.

23 Crass, J.R., Craig, E.V., Feinberg, S.B., *et al.* (1984) Ultrasonography of the rotator cuff: surgical correlation. *Journal of Clinical Ultrasound* **12**, 487–492.

24 Drakeford, M.K., Quinn, M.J., Simpson, S.L., Pettine, K.A. (1990) A comparative study of ultrasonography and arthrography in evaluation of the rotator cuff. *Clinical Orthopaedics and Related Research* **253**, 118–122.

25 Middleton, W.D. (1992) Ultrasonography of the shoulder. *Radiology Clinics of North America* **30**, 927–940.

26 Mack, L.A., Matsen, F.A., Kilcoyne, R.F., Davies, P.K., Sickler, M.E. (1985) US evaluation of the rotator cuff. *Radiology* **158**, 205–209.

27 Middleton, W.D., Reinus, W.R., Totty, W.G. (1985) Ultrasonography of the biceps tendon apparatus. *Radiology* **157**, 211–215.

28 Middleton, W.D., Edestein, G., Rhinus, W.R., Totty, W.G., Murphy, W.A. (1986) Pitfalls in rotator cuff sonography. *American Journal of Roentgenology* **146**, 555–560.

29 Middleton, W.D., Edelstein, G., Reinus, W.R., Melson, G.L., Totty, W.G., Murphy, W.A. (1985) Sonographic detection in rotator cuff tears. *American Journal of Roentgenology* **144**, 349–353.

30 Brandt, T.D., Cardone, B.W., Grant, T.H., Post, M., Weiss, C.A. (1989) Rotator cuff sonography. A reassessment. *Radiology* **173**, 323–327.

31 Crass, J.R., Craig, E.B., Feinberg, S.B. (1986) Sonography of the post-operative rotator cuff. *American Journal of Roentgenology* **146**, 561–564.

32 Buchberger, W., Schon, G., Strasser, K., Jungwirth, W. (1991) High resolution ultrasonography of the carpal tunnel. *Journal of Ultrasound Medicine* **10**, 531–537.

33 Mesgarzadeh, M., Schneck, C.D., Bonakdarpour, A., Amitabha, M., Conway, D. (1989) Carpal tunnel: MR imaging. 11. Carpal tunnel syndrome. *Radiology* **171**, 749–754.

34 De Flaviis, L., Nessi, R., Del Bo, P., Calori, G., Balconi, G. (1987) High resolution ultrasonography of wrist ganglia. *Journal of Clinical Ultrasound* **15**, 17–22.

35 Fornage, B.D., Schernberg, F.Z., Rifkin, M.D. (1985) Ultrasound examination of the hand. *Radiology* **155**, 785–788.

36 Tiliakos, N., Morales, A.R., Wilson, C.H. Jr (1982) Use of ultrasound in identifying tophaceous versus rheumatoid nodules. *Arthritis and Rheumatology* **25**, 478–479.

37 Spiegel, T.M., King, W., Weiner, S.R., Paulus, H.E. (1987) Measuring disease activity: comparison of joint tenderness, swelling and ultrasonography in rheumatoid arthritis. *Arthritis and Rheumatology* **30**, 1283–1288.

38 McGeorge, D.D., McGeorge, S. (1990) Diagnostic medical ultrasound in the management of hand injuries. *Journal of Hand Surgery* **15B**, 256–261.

39 Novick, G.S. (1988) Sonography in paediatric hip disorders. *Radiology Clinics of North America* **26**, 29–53.

40 Yousefzadeh, D.K., Ramilo, J.L. (1987) Normal hip in children: correlation of US with anatomic and cryomicrotome sections. *Radiology* **165**, 647–655.

41 Harcke, H.T., Lee, M.S., Sinning, L., Clarke, N.M.P., Borns, P.F., MacEwen, G.D. (1986) Ossification centre of the infant hip: sonographic and radiographic correlation. *American Journal of Roentgenology* **147**, 317–321.

42 Harcke, H.T., Grissom, L.E. (1990) Performing dynamic sonography of the infant hip. *American Journal of Roentgenology* **155**, 837–844.

43 Schuler, P., Feltes, E. Kienapesel, H., Griss, P. (1989) Ultrasound examination for the early determination for dysplasia and congenital dislocation of neonatal hips. *Clinical Orthopaedics and Related Research* **258**, 18–26.

44 Morin, C., Harcke, H.T., MacEwen, G.D. (1985) The infant hip: real time ultrasound assessment of acetabular development. *Radiology* **157**, 673–677.

45 Keller, M.S., Weltin, G.G., Rattner, Z., Taylor, K.J.W., Rosenfield, N.S. (1988) Normal instability of the hip in the neonate: US standards. *Radiology* **169**, 733–736.

46 Boal, D.K.B., Schwenkter, E.P. (1985) The infant hip: assessment with real time ultrasound. *Radiology* **157**, 667–672.

47 Leck, I. (1986) An epidemiological assessment of neo-natal screening of dislocation of the hip. *Journal of the Royal College of Physicians* **20**, 56–62.

48 Gardiner, H.M., Dunn, P.M. (1990) Controlled trial of immediate splinting versus ultrasonographic surveillance in congenitally dislocatable hips. *Lancet* **336**, 1553–1556.

49 Rosendahl, K., Markestad, T., Lie, R.T. (1992) Ultrasound in the early diagnosis of congenital dislocation of the hip. Significance of hip stability versus acetabulum morphology. *Paediatric Radiology* **22**, 430–433.

50 Castelein, R.M., Sauter, A.J.M., De Vlieger, M., Van Linge, B. (1992) Natural history of ultrasound hip abnormalities in clinically normal newborns. *Journal of Paediatric Orthopaedics* **12**, 423–427.

51 Berman, L., Klenerman, L. (1986) Ultrasound screening for hip abnormalities: preliminary findings in 1001 neonates. *British Medical Journal* **293**, 719–722.

52 Heikkila, E. (1988) Comparison of the Frejka pillow and the Von Rosen splint in the treatment of congenital dislocation of the hip. *Journal of Paediatric Orthopaedics* **8**, 20.

53 Viere, R.G., Birch, J.G., Herring, J.A., Roach, J.W., Johnstone, C.E. (1990) Use of the Pavlik harness in congenital dislocation of the hip. *Journal of Bone and Joint Surgery* **72A**, 238.

54 Royle, S.G. (1992) Investigation of the irritable hip. *Journal of Paediatric Orthopaedics* **12**, 396–397.

55 Adam, R., Hendry, G.M.A., Moss, J., *et al.* (1988) Arthrosonography of the painful hip in childhood: a review of 1 year's experience. *British Journal of Radiology* **59**, 205–208.

56 Alexander, J.E., Seibert, J.J., Glasier, C.M., *et al.* (1989) High-

resolution hip ultrasound in the limping child. *Journal of Clinical Ultrasound* **17**, 19–24.
57 Wilson, D.J., Green, D.J., MacLarnon, J.C. (1984) Arthrosonography of the painful hip. *Clinical Radiology* **35**, 17–19.
58 Bickerstaff, D.R., Neal, L.M., Booth, A.J., Brennan, P.O., Bell, M.J. (1990) Ultrasound examination of the irritable hip. *Journal of Bone and Joint Surgery* **72B**, 549–553.
59 Rydhom, U., Wingstrand, H., Egund, N., Elborg, R., Forsberg, L., Lidgren, L. (1986) Sonography, athroscopy, and intracapsular pressure in juvenile chronic arthritis of the hip. *Acta Orthopaedica Scandinavica* **57**, 295–298.
60 Zieger, M.M., Dorr, U., Schulz, R.D. (1987) Ultrasonography of hip joint effusions. *Skeletal Radiology* **16**, 607–611.
61 Dorr, U., Zieger, M., Hauke, H. (1988) Ultrasonography of the painful hip. *Pediatric Radiology* **19**, 36–40.
62 Miralles, M., Gonzalez, G., Pulperio, J.R., *et al.* (1989) Sonography of the painful hip in children: 500 consecutive cases. *American Journal of Roentgenology* **152**, 579–582.
63 Shiv, V.K., Jain, A.K., Taneja, K. (1990) Sonography of hip joint in infective arthritis. *Journal of the Canadian Association of Radiology* **41**, 76–78.
64 Terjesen, T. (1993) Ultrasonography in the primary evaluation of patients with Perthes' disease. *Journal of Paediatric Orthopaedics* **13**, 437–443.
65 Wirth, T., LeQuesne, G.W., Paterson, D.C. (1992) Ultrasonography in Legg–Calve–Perthes disease. *Paediatric Radiology* **22**, 498–504.
66 Kallio, P.E., Lequesne, G.W., Paterson, D.C., Foster, B.K., Jones, J.R. (1991) Ultrasonography in slipped capital femoral epiphysis. *Journal of Bone and Joint Surgery* **73B**, 884–889.
67 Diaz, M.J., Hedlund, G.L. (1991) Sonographic diagnosis of traumatic separation of the proximal femoral epiphysis in the neonate. *Pediatric Radiology* **21**, 238–240.
68 Klein, D.M., Barbera, C., Gray, S.T., Spero, C.R., Perrier, G., Teicher, J.L. (1997) Sensitivity of objective parameters in the diagnosis of pediatric septic hips. *Journal of Clinical Orthopaedics* **338**, 153–159.
69 Foldes, K., Gaal, M., Balint, P., *et al.* (1992) Ultrasonography after hip arthroplasty. *Skeletal Radiology* **21**, 297–299.
70 Meaney, J.F., Cassar-Pullicino, V.N., Etherington, R., Ritchie, D.A., McCall, I.W., Whitehouse, G.H. (1992) Ilio-psoas bursa enlargement. *Clinical Radiology* **45**, 161–168.
71 Forage, B.D., Rifkin, M.D., Touche, D.H., Segal, P.M. (1984) Sonography of the patella tendon: preliminary observations. *American Journal of Roentgenology* **143**, 179–182.
72 Kalebo, P., Sward, L., Karlsson, J., Peterson, L. (1991) Ultrasonography in the detection of partial ligament ruptures (jumper's knee). *Skeletal Radiology* **20**, 285–289.
73 De Flaviis, L., Nessi, R., Scaglion, R., Blconi, G., Albisetti, W., Derchi, L.E. (1989) Ultrasonic diagnosis of Osgood–Schlatter and Sinding–Larsen–Johansson diseases of the knee. *Skeletal Radiology* **18**, 193–197.
74 Aiscen, A.M., McCune, W.J., MacGuire, A., *et al.* (1984) Sonographic evaluation in the cartilage of the knee. *Radiology* **153**, 781–784.
75 Derks, W.H., De Hoog, E.P., Van Ling, E.B. (1986) Ultrasonographic detection of the patella plica in the knee. *Journal of Clinical Ultrasound* **14**, 355–360.
76 Cooperberg, P.L., Tsang, I., Truelove, L., *et al.* (1978) Grade scale ultrasound in the evaluation of rheumatoid arthritis of the knee. *Radiology* **126**, 759–763.
77 Coral, A. (1993) Ultrasound in diagnosis of the knee. *British Medical Ultrasound Society* **1**, 12–16.
78 Richardson, M.L., Selby, B., Montana, M.A., Mack, A.L. (1988) Ultrasonography of the knee. *Radiology Clinics of North America* **26**, 63–75.
79 Kainberger, F.M., Enger, A., Barton, P., Huebsch, P., Neuhold, A., Salomonowitz, E. (1990) Injury of the Achilles tendon: diagnosis with sonography. *American Journal of Roentgenology* **155**, 1031–1036.
80 Inglis, A.E., Sott, W.N., Sculco, T.P., *et al.* (1976) Ruptures of tendo Achillis. An objective assessment of surgical and non surgical treatment. *Journal of Bone and Joint Surgery* **5BA**, 990–993.
81 Young, J.W.R., Kostrubiak, I.S., Resnik, C.S., Paley, D. (1990) Sonographic evaluation of bone production at the distraction site in Illizarov limb-lengthening procedures. *American Journal of Roentgenology* **154**, 125–128.
82 Derbyshire, N.D.J., Simpson, A.H.R.W. (1992) A role for ultrasound in limb lengthening. *British Journal of Radiology* **65**, 576–580.
83 Kumar, F., Joseph, B., Verghese, J., Ghosh, M.K. (1992) Measurement of femoral torsion with ultrasound: evaluation of a new technique using reference lines on the posterior surface of the femur. *Journal of Clinical Ultrasound* **20**, 111–114.

Index

Note: Page numbers in *italic* refer to figures and/or tables